Prevention and Control of Nosocomial Infections

Prevention and Control of Nosocomial Infections

Edited by

Richard P. Wenzel, M.D.

Professor of Medicine and Preventive Medicine
Director, Division of Clinical Epidemiology
Department of Internal Medicine
Director, Hospital Epidemiology Program
University of Iowa Hospitals and Clinics
Iowa City, Iowa

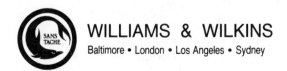

WILLIAMS & WILKINS
Baltimore • London • Los Angeles • Sydney

Editor: Timothy H. Grayson
Associate Editor: Carol L. Eckhart
Copy Editor: Deborah K. Tourtlotte
Design: Bert Smith
Illustration Planning: Wayne Hubbel
Production: Raymond E. Reter

Accurate indications, adverse reactions, and dosage schedules for drugs are provided in this book, but it is possible that they may change. The reader is urged to review the package information data of the manufacturers of the medications mentioned.

Printed in the United States of America

Library of Congress Cataloging-in-Publication Data

Main entry under title:

Prevention and control of nosocomial infections.

Includes bibliographies and index.
1. Nosocomial infections. 2. Hospitals—Sanitation. I. Wenzel, Richard P. (Richard Putnam), 1940–   [DNLM: 1. Cross Infection—prevention & control. WX 167 P944]
RA969.P74 1986   614.4′8   85-16932
ISBN 0-683-08923-4

Composed and printed at the
Waverly Press, Inc.

86 87 88 89 90 91
10 9 8 7 6 5 4 3 2 1

Preface

Although it is a relatively new field in a young science, hospital infection control has made important strides in the last 5 years. It can be stated with confidence that at least 5% of patients entering United States hospitals will develop a nosocomial infection, that the attributable mortality for the 120,000 or more institutionally acquired bloodstream infections is approximately 25%, and that by the most conservative estimates hospital-acquired infections represent a leading cause of death.

Data accumulated recently suggest that such infections add significantly to the expected length of stay for patients and, thus, comprise a direct economic burden of $5 billion to $10 billion. In the current era of reimbursement based on a limited number of diagnosis-related groups (DRGs), nosocomial infections have been recognized by administrators and government officials as an important economic priority. Furthermore, the risk of such infections has been the subject of enhanced scrutiny by legal and administrative factions and is increasingly recognized by patients as a serious consequence of hospitalization.

This book was written by practicing experts providing state-of-the-art information on the causes, prevention, and implications of nosocomial infections. The authors have endeavored to indicate, whenever possible, where information is lacking and which practices are carried out with no supportive evidence for their efficacy. The book, therefore, is intended for the advanced practitioner, the infection control director, and those wishing to go beyond the basics.

As editor, it has been a privilege working with such a distinguished group of contributors who gave up professional and family time in the preparation of this book. Only friends who are also dedicated colleagues would do so much. I wish to acknowledge the skill and energies of Patti Miller, M.S., Deborah Crickenberger, Stella King, and Kathryn Beall in preparing manuscripts, working with both authors and publisher, and managing day-to-day details.

RICHARD P. WENZEL, M.D.

Contributors

Robert C. Aber, M.D.
Vice Chairman, Department of Medicine
Chief, Infectious Diseases and Epidemiology
The Milton S. Hershey Medical Center
The Pennsylvania State University
College of Medicine
Hershey, Pennsylvania

Richard L. Barr, M.A.
Clinical Computing Laboratory
Department of Medicine
University of Virginia School of Medicine
Charlottesville, Virginia

James F. Childress, Ph.D.
Commonwealth Professor of Religious
    Studies
Professor of Medical Education
Department of Religious Studies
University of Virginia
Charlottesville, Virginia

Burke A. Cunha, M.D.
Infectious Disease Division
Winthrop-University Hospital
Mineola, New York

Richard E. Dixon, M.D., F.A.C.P.
Department of Medicine
Helen Fuld Medical Center
Trenton, New Jersey
Hahnemann University
Philadelphia, Pennsylvania

Gerald R. Donowitz, M.D.
Assistant Professor of Medicine
University of Virginia Medical Center
Charlottesville, Virginia

Leigh G. Donowitz, M.D.
Assistant Professor in Pediatrics and
    Anesthesiology
University of Virginia Medical Center
Charlottesville, Virginia

David S. Fedson, M.D.
Head, Division of General Medicine
Associate Professor of Medicine
Department of Internal Medicine
University of Virginia Medical Center
Charlottesville, Virginia

E. Lee Ford-Jones, M.D.
Assistant Professor of Pediatrics
Division of Infectious Diseases
The Hospital for Sick Children
University of Toronto
Toronto, Ontario, Canada

Richard A. Garibaldi, M.D.
Hospital Epidemiologist
Professor of Medicine
Department of Medicine Health Center
University of Connecticut School of
    Medicine
Farmington, Connecticut

Peter A. Gross, M.D.
Director, Department of Medicine
Chief, Infectious Disease Section
Hackensack Medical Center
Hackensack, New Jersey
Professor of Medicine
New Jersey Medical School
University of Medicine and Dentistry of
    New Jersey
Newark, New Jersey

Bruce H. Hamory, M.D.
Associate Professor of Medicine
Hospital Epidemiologist
University of Missouri-Columbia
Columbia, Missouri

A. Lex Hampton, M.D.
Assistant Professor
Division of Infectious Disease
University of Florida Medical Center
Gainesville, Florida

Walter J. Hierholzer, Jr., M.D.
Professor of Medicine
Hospital Epidemiologist
Yale University School of Medicine
New Haven, Connecticut

James M. Hughes, M.D.
Director, Hospital Infections Program
Center for Infectious Diseases
Centers for Disease Control
Public Health Service
U.S. Department of Health and Human
  Services
Atlanta, Georgia

William R. Jarvis, M.D.
Director, Hospital Infections Program
Center for Infectious Diseases
Centers for Disease Control
Public Health Service
U.S. Department of Health and Human
  Services
Atlanta, Georgia

Donald L. Kaiser, Dr.P.H.
Associate Professor of Medicine
Director, Clinical Computing Laboratory
Department of Medicine
University of Virginia Medical Center
Charlottesville, Virginia

Thomas F. Keys, M.D.
Department of Infectious Disease
Cleveland Clinic Foundation
Cleveland, Ohio

F. Marc LaForce, M.D.
Medical Service
Veterans Administration Medical Center
Division of Infectious Diseases
Department of Medicine
University of Colorado School of Medicine
Denver, Colorado

Elaine Larson, Ph.D., F.A.A.N.
M. Adelaide Nutting Chair in Clinical
  Nursing
The Johns Hopkins University
School of Nursing
Baltimore, Maryland

Jerome F. Levine, M.D.
Assistant Attending
Infectious Disease Section
Hackensack Medical Center
Hackensack, New Jersey
Clinical Assistant
Professor of Medicine
New Jersey Medical School
University of Medicine and Dentistry of
  New Jersey
Newark, New Jersey

C. Glen Mayhall, M.D.
Associate Professor of Medicine
Hospital Epidemiologist
Medical College of Virginia
Virginia Commonwealth University
Richmond, Virginia

**Harry C. Nottebart, Jr., J.D., M.D.,
    F.C.L.M., F.A.C.P.M., F.A.C.P., F.C.A.P.**
Clinical Associate Professor of Medicine
University of Virginia School of Medicine
Charlottesville, Virginia
Associate Clinical Professor of Pathology
Medical College of Virginia
Richmond, Virginia

William E. O'Brien, B.Sc., R.Ph.
Director, Materials Management
The Milton S. Hershey Medical Center
The Pennsylvania State University
  College of Medicine
Hershey, Pennsylvania

James E. Peacock, Jr., M.D.
Assistant Professor of Medicine
Division of Infectious Diseases
Bowman Gray School of Medicine
Wake Forest University
Winston-Salem, North Carolina

James E. Pennington, M.D.
Associate Professor of Medicine
Harvard Medical School
Associate Chief of Infectious Diseases
Brigham and Women's Hospital
Boston, Massachusetts

Richard A. Peterson, M.S.L.S.
Head Reference Librarian
Assistant Professor
Claude Moore Health Sciences Library
University of Virginia Medical Center
Charlottesville, Virginia

Samuel Ponce de Leon R., M.D.
Hospital Epidemiologist
Assistant Professor of Medicine
Infectious Diseases Department
Instituto Nacional de la Nutricion
Mexico, DF, Mexico

Patricia A. Ristuccia, M.S.
Director, Microbiology Research
Therapeutic Research Institute, Inc.
Sarasota, Florida

William A. Rutala, Ph.D., M.P.H.
Research Assistant Professor
Division of Infectious Diseases
The University of North Carolina at Chapel
  Hill
School of Medicine
Chapel Hill, North Carolina

Louis D. Saravolatz, M.D.
Clinical Associate Professor of Medicine
University of Michigan Medical School
Division Head
Infectious Diseases and Hospital
  Epidemiology
Henry Ford Hospital
Detroit, Michigan

William Schaffner, M.D.
Professor of Medicine
Departments of Medicine and Preventive
  Medicine
Vanderbilt University School of Medicine
Nashville, Tennessee

Robert J. Sherertz, M.D.
Assistant Professor
Division of Infectious Disease
University of Florida Medical Center
Gainesville, Florida

Robert L. Thompson, M.D.
Division of Infectious Diseases
Central Hospital
Group Health Cooperative of Puget Sound
Seattle, Washington

Timothy R. Townsend, M.D.
Associate Professor of Pediatrics
Division of Infectious Diseases
The Johns Hopkins University School of
  Medicine
Hospital Epidemiologist
The Johns Hopkins Hospital
Baltimore, Maryland

Richard P. Wenzel, M.D.
Professor of Medicine and Preventive Med-
  icine
Director, Division of Clinical Epidemiology
Department of Internal Medicine
Director, Hospital Epidemiology Program
University of Iowa Hospitals and Clinics
Iowa City, Iowa

Margaret Lynn Yonekura, M.D.
Assistant Professor of Obstetrics and
  Gynecology
Women's Hospital
Los Angeles, California

Contents

Chapter 1

The Control of Infections in Hospitals: 1750 to 1950

F. Marc LaForce, M.D.

INTRODUCTION

An inevitable consequence of agreeing to write a historical piece is the realization that one cannot do justice to the topic. This chapter will discuss the rise of hospitals, the statistical definition of hospital infections, and the means by which these infections were controlled. Surgical and puerperal infections will be stressed. Fortunately, a great deal of primary material is easily available in 20th-century journals and monographs, and whenever possible these sources were used. A specific effort was made at understanding the evolution of a statistical approach to hospital infections. For that reason more space will be given to the work of individuals who have studied nosocomial infections statistically. Important contributors, such as Holmes and Lister, are dealt with briefly, as neither counted cases. Conversely, data from Semmelweis, Farr, Nightingale, Simpson, and Meleney are reviewed as they provide an important statistical perspective. This presentation ends somewhat arbitrarily in the 1950s when hospital epidemiology as we know it today came into being.

THE RISE OF HOSPITALS

It is impossible to consider a history of nosocomial infections without discussing how hospitals came to be. Today's large hospital is a modern, complex institution offering a wide variety of diagnostic and therapeutic services. To many, Americans hospitals are synonymous with high quality, albeit expensive, health care. Such was not always the case. In earlier days only the poor went to hospitals while the upper classes were cared for at home.

Other than Roman military hospitals, there was little institutionalized medical care in Western Europe until the rise of the monastic orders in the Middle Ages. St. Benedict counseled: "Before all things and above all things, let care be taken of the sick" (1). Hence, infirmaries were almost always built as part of monasteries. The monastery plan of St. Gall devoted one-tenth of its site to health services and included an infirmary complex, a house for physicians with a pharmacy and a sick ward, a house for bleeding, two bath houses, and a medicinal herb garden (1). Monastic infirmaries were used for sick monks, travelers, and visitors and ranged in size from small houses with one or two beds to well planned hospitals in the larger abbeys.

In the later Middle Ages, as prosperity increased, guilds began caring for their sick. This trend led to increased secularization of health services. Monks and nuns still provided the bulk of the nursing care, but local authorities were in charge. By the end of the 15th century, Europe was well served by a network of hospitals. These hospitals were, of course, subject to external influences. The dissolution of the monasteries by Henry VIII, which followed the break of English monarchy from Rome, is one such example. Over a short period of time a major part of the English hospital system simply disappeared. This led to the development of English voluntary hospitals which were administered by towns or parishes. The Elizabethan Poor Law made parishes responsible for the care of their lame and poor. This system seemed to have met health care needs for the poor and infirm until the rapid urbanization of the 18th and 19th centuries.

The rise of absolutist monarchies on the continent led to the construction of hospitals for the poor. General hospitals were created in France during the rule of Louis XIII and Louis XIV. In addition, as cities grew, new hospitals were built. By 1840 there were 114 provincial hospitals in England (2). This expansion was paralleled in Europe. However, the conditions in some of the larger hospitals were somewhat primitive.

The Hotel Dieu in Paris was founded in the 7th century and grew bit by bit over the centuries.

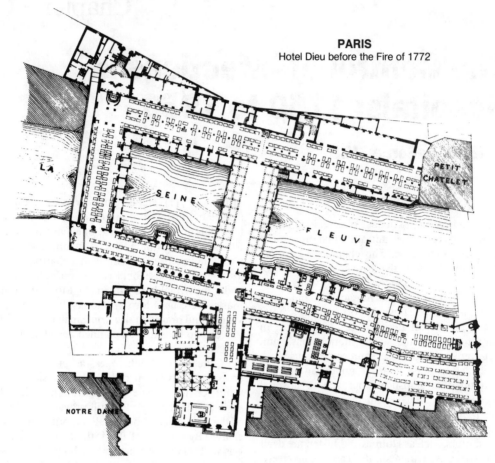

Figure 1.1. **Hotel Dieu in Paris prior to the 1772 fire. Note the large open wards and relation to the Seine River.**

It was the sole Parisian hospital prior to the Renaissance. The hospital spanned the Seine River and was severely damaged by a series of fires in the 18th century. In the latter part of the 18th century the hospital had about 1000 beds but never fewer than 2000 to 3000 patients (Fig. 1.1). During epidemics it was said that the census went above 7000 (3). As many as eight patients shared a single bed, and at times beds were used in shifts.

Patients were fed twice a day, and the quality of the food varied according to the hospital census and the level of almsgiving. Basic foods included bread and meat stews. Fresh fruits and vegetables were not emphasized. Wine was given daily, and it is said that the night attendants were given 3 pints of wine nightly (4, 5).

Wounds were washed daily with a sponge which went from patient to patient. All wounds became infected. Mortality after amputation was

about 60% (4, pp 48–50). Only the maternity and surgical wards were heated, and drinking water came directly from the Seine. The maternity ward was located in the basement, and frequently the Seine rose to empty its water and garbage onto the floor of the maternity ward (4). Puerperal fever was common, and one epidemic in 1746 killed 19 of 20 women.

As bad as this may seem, it was argued that the only other alternative, being out on the street, was worse. Diderot's *Encyclopedia* described the Hotel Dieu in 1765 as follows: "It is the largest, has the greatest number of patients, and is the richest and the most frightful of hospitals" (4).

On the whole, British hospitals seemed to fare better. For one thing they were cleaner (6, pp 97–122). The following orders were issued to all new patients admitted to the Manchester Infirmary in 1771: "(1) That every patient has clean sheets upon their admission, (2) that they have clean sheets at least once in three weeks, and (3) that two patients be not suffered to be in the same bed except that there is no spare bed in the house" (6, p 103).

Early physicians were aware that certain diseases like smallpox could spread to hospitalized patients, and the practice of segregating certain patients was accepted. Leprosariums were common during the Middle Ages. In the 15th century, Venetian authorities established lazarettos where plague victims were confined. The segregation of smallpox and fever cases was formalized in England in the early 19th century when fever hospitals were established (6, pp 61–74). The statistical evidence for the efficacy of isolation of infected patients was fragmentary. One attempt compared the nosocomial spread of typhus in the London Fever Hospital and general hospitals (7). The 1080 typhus cases admitted into the Fever Hospital resulted in 27 nosocomial cases, of whom 8 died. On the other hand, 272 cases admitted to six general hospitals led to 71 nosocomial cases, of whom 21 died. Thus, nosocomial spread of typhus occurred once for every 4 cases admitted to a general hospital, whereas 1 hospital-acquired case occurred for every 40 cases admitted to the Fever Hospital.

By 1850, the demand for hospital beds had increased dramatically in European cities. Resources were stretched and were often insufficient to provide acceptable hygienic practices. Hospital-related mortality, particularly on surgical and obstetric services, increased dramatically.

PUERPERAL FEVER

The delivery of babies in hospitals is a relatively recent phenomenon, and it was not until 1940 that 50% of U.S. births occurred in hospitals. The wealthy and middle classes had their children at home until hospitals were shown to be safe. The poor and unwed had no such options, and urban maternity hospitals were built in the 18th and 19th centuries to care for them and also to serve as clinical teaching facilities as men began assuming the control of midwifery. Mortality rates in these units were notoriously high; so much so that Thomas Lightfoot writing in the (1850) *London Medical Times* suggested that hospitals had become "the gates which lead (women) to death" (8).

Several astute clinicians in the late 19th and early 20th centuries had commented on the apparent contagiousness of puerperal fever. It was just such an observation that led Oliver Wendell Holmes to review the medical literature and to publish his 1843 essay on the contagious nature of puerperal fever (9). In an astonishingly precise paper, Holmes traced the evidence that puerperal fever was a contagious disease and outlined measures that had to be taken to minimize the spread of illness. The paper had little impact on the practice of midwifery and was later rediscovered as a classic example of keen insight into a clinical problem.

Little changed until the clinical studies of Semmelweis. Reading his monograph, *The Etiology, the Concept and the Prophylaxis of Childbed Fever*, requires time and patience (10). Despite the repetition, one can admire the completeness with which he analyzed his data and the integration of new observations into a basic hypothesis that puerperal fever was a contagious disease spread by physicians and midwives when their hands were contaminated with necrotic material.

Semmelweis's story is a familiar one but worth retelling. He graduated from the University of Vienna Medical School in 1844 at the age of 26. Three years later, he was appointed as an Assistant in the Maternity Department of the Allegemeines Krankenhaus in Vienna. The Vienna School was then at its zenith with outstanding pathologists and clinicians such as Rokitansky and Skoda. Students from all over Europe came to study in and enjoy Vienna. The Allegemeines Krankenhaus housed Europe's largest obstetric department. The poor and the unwed presented themselves for obstetric care. On admission they signed a form, whereby they were cared for at no cost in exchange for being used as "teaching material" for students and midwives.

The Vienna Lying-in Hospital was divided into two contiguous divisions. The First Division was a medical student teaching service, while the Second Division was staffed by midwife trainees. Admissions alternated between divisions every 24 hours. Semmelweis reviewed maternal deaths in the two divisions and noted that while almost 10% of women delivered by Division I physicians and students died, only 3% of women bedded in Division II, hence delivered by midwives, died. His first step was to search for more cases, and he learned that several sick women in Division I were transferred to a general hospital. If they died at the general hospital, their death did not appear in the Division I Lying-in figures.

He immediately rejected the hypothesis that a miasma was responsible for puerperal fever since this was inconsistent with the low and high rates on two contiguous wards. Rather he concluded that the high puerperal fever rates were the results of factor(s) within Division I. He studied and rejected seasonality and crowding as important factors and showed that there was no correlation between number of births and the death rate. If anything, Division II with the lower death rate was more crowded, since women knowing of the high mortality in Division I waited until they could be admitted to Division II.

He rejected socioeconomic class, food, water, laundry and ventilation as factors, since they were the same in both divisions. Division II favored a lateral position at delivery whereas Division I used the prone position. To insure that conditions were as comparable as possible, Semmelweis changed Division I to the lateral position for delivery, but no decrease in mortality rates occurred.

He noted some positive correlations: (a) any woman with prolonged labor was at increased risk of disease; (b) children born of mothers who developed puerperal fever were more likely to become ill; (c) women who had street births or premature labor were far less likely to develop puerperal fever; (d) most cases of childbed fever occurred sporadically, but frequently entire rows of women in Division I would become ill; and (e) when puerperal fever occurred in Division II, it never clustered or spread in rows.

It was at this time that Semmelweis made a key observation which led him to formulate his hypothesis. One of his close friends, a forensic pathologist, Professor Jacob Kolletschka died suddenly while Semmelweis was vacationing. While performing an autopsy, Kolletschka was stuck in the finger by a student's knife. He soon developed an acute infection and died. Semmelweis reviewed Kolletschka's autopsy and noted that the findings were similar to those seen in women dying from puerperal fever. He made the remarkable deduction: "Not the wound but the contamination of the wound by cadaveric material was the cause of death" (10).

Semmelweis analyzed his observations according to this hypothesis, and everything fit. Medical students did autopsies; hence, Division I had high mortality rates; midwife trainees did not do autopsies, a fact which explained the low Division II mortality rates; women in extended labor were examined more frequently than others which increased their risk, while women who delivered on the street were, of course, not examined prior to delivery and consequently had low rates of childbed fever.

He reasoned that if his hypothesis was correct, disinfection of hands could break the transmission of disease from cadaver to pregnant woman. On May 15, 1847 he posted an order that all students scrub their hands in chlorinated lime until the cadaver smell was gone from their hands. The results of this intervention were dramatic and are shown in Table 1.1. In 1848, the following year, 3556 deliveries were done in Division I with only 45 maternal deaths (1.3%). Division II mortality rates that year were 1.2%.

Semmelweis made other important observations. A patient with carcinoma of the uterus with a foul-smelling discharge was examined, and 11 of the next 12 women to deliver developed puerperal fever. Semmelweiss correctly concluded that puerperal fever could be spread from necrotic discharges from living patients, as well as autopsy material. He insisted that students now wash their hands between examinations. Sometime later he also correlated epidemics of puerperal fever with the reuse of soiled laundry. Lastly, he confirmed his observations in the laboratory where he showed that purulent material when introduced into the vagina and uterus of a rabbit a short time after delivery could cause a fatal disease characterized by extensive inflammation.

In writing that has a contemporary ring, he identified puerperal fever as a disease of medical progress. After reviewing maternal mortality data back to 1784, he noted that prior to the development of the Anatomic School in Vienna, puerperal fever rates were low. It was only with the development of scientific medicine with its emphasis on the autopsy, that puerperal fever rates at the Allegemeines Krankenhaus soared (Table 1.2).

Semmelweis's classic monograph was published in 1860, 13 years after his initial observations. Some have suggested that he did not receive

Table 1.1. Division I Births and Maternal Deaths, Allegemeines Krankenhaus (Vienna Lying-in), April to December 1847*

Month	Births	Deaths	Mortality Rate (%)
April	312	57	18.3
May†	294	36	12.2
June	268	6	2.4
July	250	3	1.2
August	264	5	1.9
September	262	12	5.2
October	278	11	3.9
November	246	11	5.0
December	273	8	2.9

* Data from Semmelweis (10).
† Indicates introduction of chlorine hand washes.

Table 1.2. Mortality Rates, Vienna Lying-in Hospital, 1784 to 1848*

Years	Medical Teaching	No. of Deliveries	Maternal Deaths	Mortality Rate (%)
1784–1822	Preanatomic	71,395	897	1.2
1823–1846	Postanatomic	28,429	1509	5.3

*Data from Semmelweis (10).

due recognition for his work because he failed to publish his observations quickly. This may be true but cannot detract in any way from the insight and careful analysis contained in his publication. The first 100 pages of his monograph provide a powerful argument that contact spread with cadaveric or necrotic material could account for virtually all cases of puerperal fever.

Semmelweis was keenly aware that he had been responsible for many cases of puerperal fever; he noted, "Because of my convictions, I must here confess that God only knows the number of patients that have gone prematurely to their graves by my fault. I have handled cadavers extensively, more than most accoucheurs. As painful and depressing, indeed, as such an acknowledgment is, still the remedy does not lie in concealment and this misfortune should not persist forever, for the truth must be made known to all concerned" (10).

The rest of Semmelweis's story is not a pretty one. In the midst of his clinical success his appointment as an Assistant in Obstetrics ended and was not renewed. Embittered, he fled to Budapest where he repeated his clinical studies and was elected Professor of Obstetrics in 1855. In 1860, he published his findings and was soon embroiled in acrimonious controversy with several continental obstetricians (11). By 1865, Semmelweis's performance had deteriorated. He was periodically psychotic and was committed to an asylum where he died that year. Over time virtually all of his observations were confirmed.

FLORENCE NIGHTINGALE AND WILLIAM FARR

Florence Nightingale's triumphs in Crimea have been well chronicled (12). Against a hostile, entrenched military bureaucracy she convincingly showed that safe food and water and a clean environment could result in a major decrease in death rates in a military hospital. Her interest in hospital hygiene never waned, and throughout her long career she proved to be a very able lobbyist.

In 1856 she met William Farr and soon became interested in his statistical interpretation of health data. At that time Farr, the Registrar-General, was the premier British health statistician. Farr and Nightingale quickly recognized each other's strengths, and their active collaboration spanned the next 20 years (13).

One of their first efforts was an analysis of the mortality data from Crimean military hospitals and mortality among soldiers in general (14). They chose to compare the health of soldiers against a civilian standard. The differences in death rates were impressive; males of military age in England and Wales from 1839 to 1853 had an annual mortality rate of 9.2/1000 compared to 35.0/1000 for servicemen. Farr also calculated the numbers of military lives that could be saved each year if civilian rates were in effect. Farr and Nightingale showed that most of the excess military mortality was due to contagious diseases and crowding. Their work led to improved hygienic practices and a standardized reporting system for army deaths.

Farr had long been interested in hospital mortality and had asked that standard forms be used to report hospital deaths. Nightingale shared Farr's interest in hospital mortality. In 1863, she published the third edition of *Notes on Hospitals*, a book which had a major impact on health care in England, and it is worth perusing even today (3). On page 3 she reproduced a table of mortality for the principal hospitals of England which had originally been prepared and published by Farr for the Reports of the Registrar-General (Table 1.3). She concluded "that the most unhealthy hospitals are those situated within the vast circuit of the metropolis" and made the striking statement that "in all probability a poor sufferer would have a much better chance of recovery if treated at home."

The response to her conclusions was rapid and vigorous (15–18). Two key points were challenged: (*a*) the method by which mortality rates were calculated and (*b*) the comparability of cases in large and small hospitals. Rather than using admissions or discharges as the denominator for the calculation of mortality rates, Farr chose the average number of beds occupied *in a single day* as his denominator (Table 1.3). This bed-specific

Table 1.3.   Mortality in the Principal Hospitals of England, 1861*

	No. Patients 8 April 1861†	Avg. No. Patients‡	No. of Deaths	Mortality (% of Patients)
106 Hospitals	12,709	120	7,227	56.9
24 London hospitals	4,214	176	3,828	90.8
12 Hospitals, large towns	1,870	156	1,555	83.2
25 County and provincial hospitals	2,248	90	886	39.4
30 Other hospitals	1,136	38	457	40.2
13 Naval and military hospitals	3,000	231	470	15.7
1 Royal infirmary (Margate)	133	133	17	12.8
1 Metro infirmary (Margate)	108	108	14	13.0

* Table prepared by William Farr and published in Nightingale's *Notes on Hospitals* (3).
† Column lists the number of patients in hospitals on April 8, 1861.
‡ Column lists average number of hospitalized patients on a single day per hospital (data not used to calculate rate but to give an idea as to the average size of the hospitals generating data; see the text for details).

attack rate was calculated as the number of deaths occurring during a year divided by the number of beds that were occupied on a single day (19). It is in this way that mortality rates of 91% for London hospitals were derived. Farr argued that the risk of death in the hospital was fundamentally related to the concept of bed-year exposure much the same way that army regimental mortality rates are based on person-years. Farr's technique was severely criticized because it did not take into account length of stay and generated such high mortality rates. To most physicians and hygienists it seemed more logical to express mortality rates on the basis of deaths and admissions or discharges. Farr's disclaimer that since each bed saw "on the average" 10 patients, that simply dividing his mortality column by 10 would correct for this problem. However, Farr never furnished corroborative data on length of stay.

Farr and Nightingale lost the argument. The British medical establishment chose to accept the results of another study on English hospitals commissioned by the Privy Council of the City of London prepared by Drs. Holmes and Bristow which concluded that large hospitals were as safe as small ones (20, 21).

Before leaving *Notes on Hospitals*, one needs to be aware of a few more points. With great clarity Nightingale suggested that there was a direct relationship between the sanitary conditions of a hospital and postoperative complications, such as gangrene, erysipelas, and pyemia. She proposed a comprehensive reporting system for deaths in hospitals suggesting that ward sisters could maintain these statistical records. This is

Table 1.4.   Mortality of Matrons, Sisters, And Nurses by Age in 15 London Hospitals Compared to the Female Population of London*

	Annual Mortality per 1000			
Ages	Matrons, Sisters, and Nurses (1848–1857)		Female Population of London	
	All Diseases	Zymotic Diseases†	All Diseases	Zymotic Diseases†
25–35	15.9	9.5	9.9	2.2
36–45	15.8	10.9	14.6	2.7
46–55	17.8	11.9	20.4	3.2
56–65	46.4	14.3	36.0	4.9

* Table prepared by William Farr and published in Nightingale's *Notes on Hospitals* (3).
† Zymotic diseases are defined as contagious diseases.

probably the first reference to surveillance of hospital-acquired infections by nurses.

The book also contains Farr's interesting analysis of mortality among hospital employees, which showed that mortality from contagious (zymotic) diseases was more common among hospital personnel and that being a matron, sister, or nurse was a significant health risk (Table 1.4).

SIMPSON AND THE AMPUTATION SURVEY

Surveys are used frequently by hospital epidemiologists to gather data. An early survey which played a major role in the history of hospital epidemiology was one made by Dr. James Simpson on mortality following amputations. Simpson, Professor of Midwifery at the University of

Table 1.5.   Mortality after Amputation: Simpson Survey, 1869*

Site of Amputation	Simpson Survey			Metropolitan Hospitals		
	No. of Procedures	Deaths	Fatality Rate (%)	No. of Procedures	Deaths	Fatality Rate (%)
Thigh	670	124	18.5	935	435	46.5
Leg	618	81	13.1	613	270	44.0
Arm	433	19	4.3	297	110	57.0
Forearm	377	2	0.5	244	40	16.4
Total	2098	226	10.8	2089	855	41.0

* Data from Simpson (22).

Edinburgh, was already famous for the introduction of chloroform as an anesthetic agent. He was also very much concerned with the mortality associated with operative procedures and was convinced that the building of large municipal hospitals was a major contributing factor to hospital mortality.

In 1860 Simpson began surveying country practitioners on the number and type of amputations that the physician had done, the socioeconomic class of the patient, the reason for amputation, and the results (22). He felt that amputations were valid for comparison because they did not require a great deal of surgical skill and were performed frequently enough to generate sufficient data. Simpson specifically avoided practitioners in towns and cities. He obtained data on 2098 amputations from 394 practitioners. He then compared his statistics to similar data from 11 large metropolitan hospitals (Table 1.5). On the basis of this data, he concluded that country amputations were 5 times as likely to be successful than those done in the city. Simpson then added the Farr touch by calculating the excess number of deaths associated with amputations done in the city.

Predictably there was a vigorous response to his papers. Holmes, an earlier outspoken critic of Nightingale and Farr, challenged each of Simpson's points (23). He suggested that Simpson collected data only from successful surgeons and proposed that there had to be differences between country and city patients. He simply did not believe the physicians in Simpson's series who stated that they had never seen pyemias, tetanus, or erysipelas in their practice. To document that some of these infections were, in fact, community-acquired, Holmes published a remarkable table which documented some community-acquired and nosocomial infections at St. George's Hospital in London from 1865 to 1868 (Table 1.6). About half of these infections were classified as nosocomial.

Table 1.6.   Infections at St. George's Hospital, 1865–1868*,†

Infection	Community Acquired (No.)	Hospital Acquired (No.)	Total
Erysipelas	80	43	123
Diffuse cellulitis	55	13	68
Sloughing and phagedema	55	60	115
Pyemia	9	81	90
Total	199	197	396

* Total admissions from 1865 to 1868 were 8392.
† Data from Holmes (23).

One of Simpson's main points was that the building of permanent large hospitals was an important factor in the high mortality associated with hospitals. Simpson favored hospitals that could be taken down and set up as sheds, a suggestion which seemed to upset Holmes more than anything else. Holmes felt that for the poor, the dust of hospitals was probably better than the dust of their homes, and he finished by conceding that although postamputation mortality in city hospitals was high, "much of the mortality I believe to be inevitable" (23).

Simpson wasted no time in answering, and within 2 weeks he rebutted Holmes's points and added data from 3000 amputations done in provincial hospitals (24). He published a dramatic table showing that death rates after amputations increased with the size of the hospital (Table 1.7).

Analysis of the causes of death after amputation provided Simpson with yet another powerful argument (Table 1.8). The leading cause of death after country amputations was shock, whereas pyemia accounted for 60% of deaths occurring in large hospitals. Simpson ended his paper with some clear statements: "Surgical patients in surgical wards seem sometimes to have pyemia or surgical fever induced by the accidental inoculation of the morbific secretions formed in the

Table 1.7.   Mortality after Limb Amputation by Size of Hospital and Degree of Isolation*

Size of Hospital	Death Rate
300–600 beds	1 in 2½ die
100–300 beds	1 in 4 die
25–100 beds	1 in 5½ die
Less than 25 beds	1 in 7 die
Isolated rooms (country practice)	1 in 9 die

* Data from Simpson (24).

Table 1.8.   Causes of Death after Amputation: Simpson Survey and St. George's Hospital*

Cause of Death	St. George's (London) (41 Cases)	Country Practice (173 Cases)
	%	%
Shock	5.0	36.4
Pyemia	58.5	4.6
Exhaustion (no hemorrhage)	17.0	16.2
Exhaustion (with hemorrhage)	9.7	5.2
Visceral diseases	9.7	12.7
Inflammation and gangrene	2.4	10.4
Tetanus		6.3
Other injuries	2.4	7.5

* Data from Simpson (24).

bodies of other patients affected" (24). The doctrine of contact spread of infectious particles is as clearly articulated as in Semmelweis's monograph. Secondly, he emphasized, somewhat incorrectly, that a concentration of sick people invariably led to pollution of air and spread of disease by contamination of air. As evidence he cited the example of how much the odor from a case of empyema permeated an entire hospital. Lastly, he came down strongly on the side of isolation and emphasized the general premise that the fewer patients per room, the less likely infection would spread to others.

As a body of information, Simpson's survey was a remarkable piece of work. He knew of the fearsome mortality after amputation in large hospitals, and he correctly reasoned that if crowding and concentration of sick were important, then he should be able to document low postamputation mortality if he canvassed physicians who performed amputations at home. His data were persuasive and his published rebuttals to Dr. Holmes were measured and precise, and included corroborative statistics from France, England, and Scotland.

LISTER AND ANTISEPSIS

The following rather depressing statement by a Norwich surgeon in 1874 accurately depicted what a surgeon operating in a large hospital could expect: "I have unwillingly, and almost tremblingly proceeded to operate in the hospital. . . . I come to the conclusion in my own mind that pyemia, if it does not find its birthplace, does find its natural home and resting place in hospitals; and although the hospital may not be the mother of pyemia it is its nurse" (25).

The savior of the municipal hospital was Lister. While Simpson documented the danger of a major surgical procedure in a large general hospital, Lister corrected it. He integrated new advances in microbiology into a comprehensive hypothesis on how wounds became infected; and having done so, he developed a technique to prevent infection.

Lister did his medical training in London. He went to Edinburgh in 1847 to study with Syme, who was then considered to be one of the finest surgeons in the British Isles. He married Syme's daughter, and his stay in Scotland lasted 25 years. In 1860 at the age of 33 Lister was chosen Professor of Surgery at the University of Glasgow. While in Glasgow Lister's attention was drawn to the studies of Pasteur, who had shown that the air was contaminated with living germs. Pasteur had also convincingly shown that fermentation and putrefactions resulted from the growth of germs. Lister reasoned that if the above principles were correct, microbes might be responsible for wound suppuration. Furthermore, infection could be prevented by killing organisms in a wound and by preventing contaminated air from coming into contact with these wounds.

Lister chose to test his idea in patients with compound fractures who were known to have a dismal prognosis. He packed the wounds of these patients with lint soaked in carbolic acid. Lister chose carbolic acid as an antiseptic largely because the neighboring town of Carlisle had used it to improve a sewage problem. Initially, he used a 10% solution but soon decreased the concentration to 2.5%. To facilitate wound care he made a putty impregnated with carbolic acid and used it as an external dressing. His clinical success was dramatic since heretofore invariably fatal wounds were now being healed (26).

Lister published his results in 1867. Surprisingly, his chief detractor was Simpson, who chided Lister for not being original or scholarly, since carbolic acid had been used by the French for years. Lister responded to these points by claiming no priority for the use of carbolic acid but insisting that his approach was a new one.

He continued to experiment with his techniques and was soon soaking his fingers and ligatures and cleansing operative sites with carbolic acid prior to surgery. He reasoned that if his infection rates had fallen because of exclusion of airborne bacteria, it might be safer to operate in an environment where airborne bacteria had been killed. Therefore, he introduced a carbolic acid spray to be used during surgery.

Lister clearly articulated the reasoning behind his antiseptic system, and his results were published primarily as a series of case reports. He used few statistical summaries and this review of his collected papers succeeded in identifying only one table which summarized his early results (27) (Table 1.9). Nonetheless, the types of cases that were responding to his method were so dramatic as to guarantee interest in the procedure.

Over the next 20 years his technique gradually spread. Buttressed by new and irrefutable microbiologic studies the concept became clear that bacteria caused wound infections and, just as importantly, that bacteria could be killed.

Lister succeeded primarily because he used cleaner instruments than his predecessors. During World War I, Wright and Fleming showed that leukocytes, not antiseptics, killed bacteria in wounds (28, 29). Lister's emphasis on airborne bacteria was only partially correct as most of the wound contamination he prevented had come from dirty hands, instruments, and dressings. It was only decades later that a true appreciation of the role of airborne bacteria in wound infections became clear.

1890 TO 1950

German surgeons in particular accepted Lister's methods (30). From antisepsis it was but a short intellectual jump to asepsis. Bacteria could be destroyed by heat; and by 1910 sterile instruments, gowns, masks, and gloves were standard in large university hospitals. It is impossible to overstate the impact that these developments had on the practice of surgery. Surgical procedures now could be truly elective and innovative.

Gloves were an important advance. In 1889 Halstead at the Johns Hopkins Hospital asked the Goodyear Rubber Company to make two pairs of rubber gloves because his operating room scrub nurse, whom he would later marry, was allergic to the corrosive sublimate hand rinse (31).

Table 1.9. Mortality after Amputation*

Year	Total	Deaths	Mortality Rate (%)
1864–1866 (before antiseptic method)	35	16	46
1867–1869 (after antiseptic method)	40	6	15

* Data from Lister (27).

Gradually the idea took hold that gloves should be worn to protect the patient, and by 1899 some surgeons at Johns Hopkins were using gloves in clean cases. Before long the morning coat was discarded and white aprons and gowns were donned. The switch to green was made later for eye comfort. Masks soon followed as microbiologists measured the microbial soilage which occurred during conversation. Several surgical clinics emphasized silence during surgery to limit bacterial contamination, and it was not unusual for Cushing to perform 4- and 5-hour operations in silence (4, p 490). Sterilizers completed the evolution to a truly aseptic approach—everything to come into contact with the patient had to be sterile.

The application of the aseptic technique brought surgical infections under control. New surgical procedures and approaches were developed, but few statistical data were published on wound infections. What data were available suggested that elective clean surgery could be done with wound infection rates between 2 and 5% (32). The issue of postoperative wound infection largely disappeared as an important issue, and few surgeons studied the problem.

Important exceptions included Devenish and Miles (33) in England and Meleney, a New York surgeon and bacteriologist (34). Meleney emphasized the need to keep records, and he developed an active surveillance system for wound infections. He investigated epidemics of wound infections and made important contributions on the importance of silk as a suture material and the need to search for carriers during staphylococcal and streptococcal epidemics. The changes that were instituted resulted in a decrease in wound infection rates at the Presbyterian Hospital in New York City from 14% in 1925 to 4.8% in 1933 (35).

Other hospital-acquired infections were largely ignored. One important exception is the 1929 study by Cuthbert Dukes on catheter-associated urinary tract infections. Dukes noted that urinary tract infection invariably occurred after rectal surgery because of the need for an indwelling bladder catheter. He clearly recognized the problem of asymptomatic bacteriuria and commented on the "unobtrusive character of these infections" (36). Dukes introduced a quantitative measure of infection in the urinary tract which utilized the number of leukocytes in urine. He published standards showing that less than 10 leukocytes/ml was normal and greater than 100 leukocytes/ml was consistent with infection as defined by positive cultures. He measured urine leukocytes on a daily basis in patients with indwelling catheters and defined the following course of events: Urine was sterile until the second or third day when staphylococci or coliforms were isolated; on the sixth to eighth day a marked increase in urine leukocytes to levels between 100 and 1000 cells/ml occurred. He stressed three points: (a) the certainty of infection, (b) the punctual onset of bacteriuria and the increase in urine leukocytes, and (c) the unpredictability of the course of the infection.

In men the indwelling catheter was usually plugged with a wooden peg which was periodically removed to drain the bladder. Dukes felt that the wooden peg became contaminated and, in turn, contaminated the urine. He experimented with other urinary drainage techniques. Open drainage to a sterile bottle was not successful. In 20 patients he used a drainage system with a Y-shaped junction which allowed for intermittent irrigation of the drainage tubing and bladder with an antiseptic solution (Fig. 1.2). Using this system in 20 patients, 8 remained free of infection, 4 developed urethritis, and 8 developed a urinary tract infection. Those patients who ultimately became infected did so much later than would have been normally expected without the rinsing procedure.

In a remarkable paper Dukes clearly described the hazards of indwelling catheterization, proposed a simple quantitative laboratory method to determine whether infection was present, and tested a urinary drainage system which prevented infection in two-thirds of patients in whom it was tested.

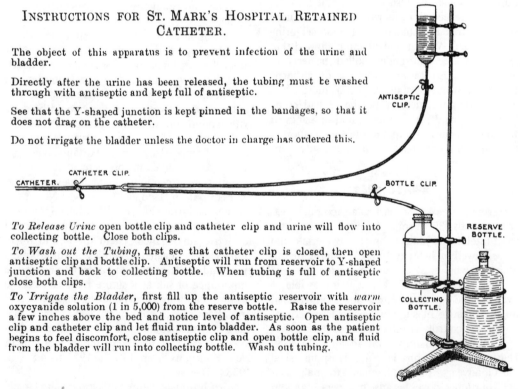

Figure 1.2.   Instructions for indwelling catheter care as prepared by Cuthbert Dukes (see the text for details).

Antibiotics were a major advance. In 1935, sulfonamides were introduced, and serious streptococcal and staphylococcal infections could now be cured. The introduction of penicillin after World War II was even more dramatic. Surgery entered what was then felt to be a golden era. Infections might occur but there now were potent, relatively nontoxic drugs which could prevent septicemia and cure infections. The concept of prophylactic use of antibiotics to prevent infections after surgical procedures was introduced. Unfortunately the experiemntal design for many of these studies was poor, and it was not until the 1960s that definitive studies were being published.

During the 1950s severe epidemics of nosocomial staphylococcal infections in surgical and pediatric units were being reported in Europe and America. This pandemic was the main impetus for the development of hospital epidemiology as a recognized discipline. If one had to define the beginning of the modern era, the Communicable Disease Center-sponsored meeting on staphylococcal infections in 1958, and the 1960 publication of *Hospital Infections* by R.E.O. Williams and his associates seem appropriate (37). Williams's book discussed a variety of nosocomial infections and emphasized the importance of an infection officer. Lastly, work by Moore and his colleagues firmly established the point that an "infection control sister" could serve a key role in hospital infection control activities (38).

The discipline of hospital epidemiology is now well established, but young enough so that many of us have seen and helped it evolve over the last 30 years. In reflecting on the enormous progress that has been made over the last 150 years, one inevitably concludes that those individuals who not only have had good ideas but the energy to test their concepts and to analyze their results have had the greatest role in this success.

Acknowledgment. The author gratefully acknowledges the secretarial assistance of Ms. Jo Ann Esposito.

References

1. Price L: *The Plan of St Gall in Brief.* Berkeley, University of California Press, 1982.
2. Buer MC: *Health, Wealth, and Population in the Early Days of the Industrial Revolution.* London, Routledge and Kegan Paul, 1968, pp 126–136, 164–179, 193–209, 268–273.
3. Nightingale F: *Notes on Hospitals*, ed 3. London, Longman, 1863.
4. Wangensteen OH, Wagensteen SD: *The Rise of Surgery.* Minneapolis, University of Minnesota Press, 1978.
5. Goldin G: A walk through a ward of the eighteenth century. *J Hist Med* 22:221–138, 1967.
6. Woodward J: *To do the Sick No Harm: A Study of the British Voluntary Hospital System to 1875.* London, Routledge and Kegan Paul, 1974.
7. Murchison C: On the isolation of infectious diseases. *Med Times Gaz* 1:210–211, 1864.
8. Lightfoot T: Some practical observations on the disease usually called puerperal fever. *Lond Med Times* 21:;463–465, 1850.
9. Holmes OW: The contagiousness of puerperal fever. *N Engl Q J Med Surg* 1:503–530, 1842–3.
10. Semmelweis IF: *The Etiology, the Concept and the Prophylaxis of Childbed Fever.* Pest, CA Hartleben's Verlag-Expedition, 1861 (translation by FP Murphy republished, Classics of Medicine Library, Birmingham, 1981).
11. Nuland SB: The enigma of Semmelweis—an interpretation. *J Hist Med* 34:255–272, 1979.
12. Cook E: *Life of Florence Nightingale.* London, Macmillan, 1913, vol 2.
13. Farr, Florence Nightingale, and medical services. In Eyler JM: *Victorian Social Medicine: The Ideas and Methods of William Farr.* Baltimore, Johns Hopkins University Press, 1979, pp 159–189.
14. Cohen IB: Florence Nightingale. *Sci Am* 250:128–137, 1984.
15. Editorial: Relative mortality in town and country hospitals. *Lancet* 1:248–250, 1864.
16. Book review: Notes on hospitals. *Med Times Gaz* 1:129–130, 1864.
17. Holmes T: Mortality in hospitals. *Lancet* 1:338–339, 365–366, 1864.
18. Bristowe JS: Mortality in hospitals. *Lancet* 1:451–452, 1864.
19. Farr W: Hospital mortality. *Med Times Gaz* 1:242–244, 1864.
20. *Sixth Report of the Medical Officer of the Privy Council, 1863.* London, 1864.
21. Bristowe JS, Holmes T: Hospital hygiene no. I and II. *Lancet* 2:498–500, 532–533, 700–702, 1864.
22. Simpson JY: Our existing system of hospitalism and its effects. *Edinb Med J* 14:816–830, 1084–1115; 15:523–532, 1869.
23. Holmes T: On hospitalism. *Lancet* 2:194–196, 229–230, 1869.
24. Simpson JY: Some propositions on hospitalism. *Lancet* 2:295–297, 332–335, 431–433, 475–478, 535–538, 698–700, 1869.
25. Ashhurst AP: The centenary of Lister (1827–1927). A tale of sepsis and antisepsis. *Ann Med Hist* 9:205–221, 1927.
26. Lister J: On a new method of treating compound fracture, abscess, etc. with observations on the conditions of suppuration. *Lancet* 1:326, 357, 387, 507; 2:95, 1867 (in vol 2, *Collected Papers*, Oxford, 1909; republished Classics of Medicine Library, Birmingham, 1979.
27. Lister J: On the effects of the antiseptic system of treatment upon the salubrity of a surgical hospital. *Lancet* 1:40, 400, 1870; In vol. 2 *Collected Papers*, Oxford, 1909; republished, Classics of Medicine Library, Birmingham, 1979).

28. Wright AE: Address on wound infections; and on some new methods for the study of the various factors which come into consideration in their treatment. *Proc. R Soc Med* 8:41–86, 1915.
29. Fleming A: The action of chemical and physiological antiseptics in a septic wound. *Br J Surg* 7:99–129, 1919.
30. Upmalis IH: The introduction of Lister's treatment in Germany. *Bull Hist Med* 42:221–240, 1968.
31. Fulton JF: *Harvey Cushing.* Springfield, Charles C Thomas, 1946, p 238.
32. Beckman EH: Complications following surgical operations. *Surg Gynecol Obstet* 18:551–555, 1914.
33. Devenish EA, Miles AA: Control of *Staphylococcus aureus* in an operating theatre. *Lancet* 1:1088–1094, 1939.
34. Meleney FL, Whipple AO: A statistical analysis of a study of the prevention of infection in soft part wounds, compound fractures, and burns with special reference to the sulfonamides. *Surg Gynecol Obstet* 80:263–296, 1945.
35. Meleney FL: Infection in clean operative wounds. *Surg Gynecol Obstet* 60:264–276, 1935.
36. Dukes C: Urinary infections after excision of the rectum; their cause and prevention. *Proc R Soc Med* 22:269, 1929.
37. Williams REO, Blowers R, Garrod LP, Shooter RA: *Hospital Infection.* London, Lloyd-Luke (Medical Books), 1960.
38. Gardner AMN, Stamp M, Bowgen JA, Moore B: The infection control sister. *Lancet* 2:710–711, 1962.

Chapter 2

The Global Impact of Hospital-Acquired Infections

William Schaffner, M.D.

Nosocomial infections are a global problem; in every hospital of the world some patients acquire infections after they are admitted to the institution. Recognition of the problem and defining its characteristics have varied considerably from country to country, however. Over the past 30 years hospital infection control has evolved in certain developed countries to the point that it is now a recognized professional discipline; many hospitals in these countries support infection control activities. Hospital epidemiologists in such institutions have established definitions of nosocomial infections, have employed a variety of surveillance methods for their detection, have analyzed the occurrence of nosocomial infections for predisposing patient risk factors, and have implemented numerous control measures designed to prevent their occurrence. As the contents of this volume indicate, these efforts continue at an intense pace, both to improve on past performance and to cope with the ever expanding developments in medical science and changes in the delivery of health care.

Although enormous progress has been made in the practice of hospital infection control, recognition of the problem has not proceeded equally, even among the developed countries. It is only within the past decade that health professionals in certain developed countries have begun to address infection control issues. Because they have access to an accumulated body of knowledge, it is anticipated that they will be able to progress comparatively rapidly as they adapt these prevention concepts to their own health care cultures and traditions.

Understandably, it is in the developing world that hospital infection control practices remain the most rudimentary. Nevertheless, many of these countries have invested in building large hospitals modeled on those in the developed world. This trend, for better or worse, is likely to continue. These new institutions include many of the high technology features with which the reader is familiar: renal dialysis and transplantation wards, intensive care units, and sophisticated support facilities. In addition to the well known infection hazards associated with this technology, hospitals in the developing nations must also cope with the risks presented by the classic communicable diseases which remain endemic in their societies. Thus, the problems which challenge hospital infection control in the developing world are even greater than those in developed nations.

METHODS FOR MEASURING THE OCCURRENCE OF NOSOCOMIAL INFECTIONS

Measurement of the magnitude of disease occurrence in populations serves a multiplicity of essential functions. Without that information, health policy remains uninformed. With that information, the relative burden of illness produced by various diseases can be compared; disease distribution by age, sex, race, socioeconomic status, occupation, geographic location, and the like can be assessed; the costs of disease and losses of productivity also can be calculated. Health policy planners use such data to establish goals for health improvement and to make those hard decisions which allocate support for primary care networks, hospital construction, nutritional supplementation, nursing education, immunization programs, and the host of other competing demands for the limited resources available. The explosion of medical technology and the escalating costs of delivering health services to a growing population recently have made even the highly developed countries aware that they must curtail the proportion of their national resources which is allocated to health. The developing nations, of course, have severely limited budgets; appropriate allocation of resources is consequently even more important to them.

Thus, a critical first step in the campaign to reduce nosocomial infections is an assessment of the magnitude of the problem. Although the hospital infection literature is enormous, this goal has not yet been achieved for most countries because the available data are so heterogeneous. Many investigators have provided prevalence and incidence data from their own hospitals, have surveyed selected patient populations thought to be at high risk (neonates and immunocompromised patients, for example), or have focused on the infection hazards of special care wards (burn units, intensive care units) or certain procedures (urinary catheterization, surgery). These investigations have provided the body of information which is elaborated in this volume and which is used by infection control teams to define and prevent nosocomial infections in their own hospitals. However, methodologic problems have made it difficult to compare these studies directly. Thus, one must view comparisons between countries and, indeed, between hospitals within the same country with caution.

Fortunately, the World Health Organization (WHO) recently has undertaken a major initiative in the area of hospital infection control (1). WHO Scientific Working Groups were convened to consider the interrelated problems of hospital-acquired infections (2) and the increasing trend toward antibiotic resistance among bacterial pathogens (3). Working independently, both groups of experts recommended that an international surveillance program be undertaken that would define the epidemiologic characteristics of nosocomial infections and would be coordinated with a survey of the antibiotic resistance patterns of nosocomial bacterial pathogens. A critical achievement was the elaboration of a set of common definitions and agreed upon methods of data collection and recording. These will go far toward resolving the methodologic roadblocks which have hampered previous investigators and will permit a more secure comparison of results from the participating countries.

As a result of these agreements established by the Working Groups in 1983, WHO initiated a voluntary worldwide program of collaborative prevalence surveys of nosocomial infections and antibiotic resistance among the member nations. The main objectives of the survey were:

"to identify determinants and mechanisms and quantify patterns of hospital infections and assure valid comparison;

to identify individuals and populations at greatest risk;

to evaluate the benefit of different methods used in the prevention, management, surveillance and control of nosocomial infections, including their cost effectiveness" (1).

These surveys are preceded by regional training sessions to enhance the comparability of the final results. Also, recognizing that the resources of the member nations vary considerably, the program permits a country to participate to a degree consistent with its own current involvement with hospital infection control and its available resources. At the time of this writing, the international prevalence survey process is under way. It is anticipated that the results will provide a major impetus in the campaign to prevent nosocomial infections and curtail the spread of antimicrobial resistance in both the developed and the developing nations of the world.

THE DEVELOPED COUNTRIES

Despite the methodologic difficulties alluded to in the preceding section, two developed countries, the United States and England, have undertaken national prevalence surveys of nosocomial infections. Each survey was performed using standardized internal definitions and methods. Although their approaches were similar, there were, once again, sufficient differences in the methods employed that the results cannot be directly compared.

In the mid-1970s Haley and colleagues at the Centers for Disease Control (CDC) conducted the rigorous and extensive Study on the Efficacy of Nosocomial Infection Control (SENIC Project) which produced a sample-based estimate of the magnitude of the nosocomial infection problem in acute care hospitals in the United States (4). They concluded that the national nosocomial infection rate in acute care institutions was approximately 5.7 infections/100 patients admitted, a figure which was consistent with estimates derived from previous studies performed at the CDC and by investigators at individual hospitals. They also pointed out that the risk of acquiring nosocomial infections was distinctly higher in larger hospitals, particularly those which would be designated tertiary care or referral medical centers. When ranked according to the site of infection, urinary tract infections were the most common (42% of all nosocomial infections), followed by surgical wound infections (24%), pneumonia (10%), bacteremia (primary and secondary combined, 5%), and all other types of nosocomial infection (19%). During the period encompassed by the SENIC Project it was estimated that 2.1 million nosocomial infections occurred in the United States each year. The diagnosis and therapy of these infections and the prolongation of hospital stay that they incurred resulted in calculated additional costs of approximately a billion dollars annually (5).

The other large prevalence survey was conducted in 1980 among 43 general hospitals in England and Wales (6). In this study, 9.2% of all patients surveyed had a hospital-acquired infection. The investigators used somewhat different definitions of nosocomial infections than did their counterparts in the United States, and they also included several specialty areas of the hospital (neonatal units, orthopaedic surgery, and the like) in their survey which had been excluded from the SENIC Project. It is thought that these variations account, at least in part, for the difference in overall nosocomial infection rates in the two studies. The ranking according to the site of nosocomial infection in the British study found that nosocomial urinary tract infections occurred most frequently (40% of the total), followed by surgical wound infections (25%), lower respiratory tract infections (20%), and skin infections (17%). Thus, these distributions of nosocomial infections by site in the two studies were remarkably similar.

THE DEVELOPING COUNTRIES

The available survey data on the occurrence of nosocomial infections in the hospitals of developing nations are meager and often inconsistent. However, the literature contains a considerable number of reports of outbreaks of nosocomial infections which have occurred in hospitals located in the developing world. Although biased, a review of such outbreaks is instructive, providing insights into the daunting circumstances encountered by those who take up the challenge of preventing hospital-associated infections with very modest resources.

It is obvious that the many developing nations are not alike; their highly dissimilar geographic locations, cultures, languages, and stages of economic development are apparent. Likewise, their health care resources, medical care delivery systems, ratios of physicians and nurses to population, and their culturally determined attitudes and practices regarding disease vary enormously. Even within countries, the hospital facilities in the capital city and major population centers usually are far more sophisticated than those available to rural populations. These considera-

tions vitiate attempts at generalization. Nevertheless, because many readers have not had the opportunity to work in the developing world, a few comments seem appropriate to provide an appreciation of the hospital environment in many nonindustrialized nations.

The classical community-acquired infectious diseases, largely eliminated or controlled in the developed nations, continue to occur commonly in many developing countries. These include tuberculosis, leprosy, salmonellosis (including typhoid fever), shigellosis, measles, and other vaccine-preventable diseases. Lolekha, a physician trained in hospital epidemiology in the United States, has analyzed the experience at a major teaching hospital in Bangkok, Thailand (7). He and his co-workers reported that approximately 75% of patients admitted to the medical and pediatric wards had community-acquired infections on admission; the comparable proportion on the surgical and gynecologic services was 35%. These are greatly in excess of the proportions one would experience in Europe or North America. Community-acquired infections, thus, regularly strain the ability of hospitals to isolate patients properly. Indeed, the census of some hospitals often exceeds their bed capacity, requiring that more than one patient occupy the same bed (8). The concept of interrupting transmission took on new meaning when a colleague visiting Thailand recently found a patient with typhoid fever sharing a bed with a patient with leukemia (KE Nelson, personal communication, 1985). Under such conditions periodic nosocomial outbreaks of infections caused by traditionally community-acquired pathogens are to be expected. Indeed, sporadic outbreaks of measles are a feature of many pediatric wards in the tropics.

Adding to the congestion in the open, crowded wards are the patients' families, who may take up temporary residence in the hospital to provide the patient food, care, and comfort (9). Sinks and toilets may be unavailable, the water supply not potable, and electric power uncertain. Critical supplies—such as syringes, needles, gloves, antimicrobials, laboratory reagents, and bacteriologic media—are often difficult to obtain on a regular basis. Because antibiotic disks are costly, a hospital laboratory in Guatemala is able to provide susceptibility data on bacterial isolates for only part of the year (CA Ramirez, personal communication 1985).

Hospitals may elect to produce their own supplies, such as intravenous fluid. When it cannot be packaged in individualized sterile bottles, hospitals in countries such as China have adopted the practice of using bottles with removable bottoms, thus permitting the addition of fluid while the infusion is running. Sterilization and disinfection are often rudimentary. Used intravenous needles may be removed, wiped with an alcohol-soaked pledget, and then used again in another patient (9). Last, housekeeping practices can vary from meticulous to quite casual.

Diarrheal Disease

In the developed world, nosocomial gastroenteritis accounts for a very small proportion of hospital-acquired infections. The situation in the tropics is quite different; nosocomial gastroenteritis is omnipresent and may achieve epidemic proportions regularly. The pathogens often remain unidentified. Western and colleagues have described such circumstances well (9):

"In one capitol city in the teaching hospital of the national medical school, three separate outbreaks of diarrheal disease occurred in the premature nursery during the past year. The average census of the nursery was 12 to 15 infants. In each instance, the attack rate was 100% (all the children became infected), and the mortality rate was 100% (all the children died). The pathological agent was never identified and no epidemiological investigation was undertaken to identify the probable sources of the outbreaks.

At the only pediatric hospital in one Central American country, the occurrence of diarrheal disease in children frequently exceeds 100% during hospitalization. In other words, if a child did not suffer from diarrhea on admission, it was virtually certain he would acquire an enteric infection before death or discharge. Multiple episodes are common, especially in high-risk, malnourished children."

Two bacterial pathogens, *Salmonella* and *Vibrio cholerae*, have been repeatedly reported to produce nosocomial outbreaks of diarrhea, especially in premature nurseries, nurseries for normal babies, and pediatric wards. These outbreaks tend to be prolonged, involve large numbers of patients, and are associated with a high mortality rate.

An unusually protracted outbreak of *Salmonella bareilly* gastroenteritis took place in a hospital in Sri Lanka (10). Lasting just over 2 years, it involved 516 infants, most premature, as well as adult patients and staff members. It was thought that the organism initially was introduced by an infected mother and was then spread by close contact. It soon became part of the environmental flora and was recovered from sinks, weighing scales, and prepared milk, as well as from pads of gauze that had been wrapped about the outlets of water faucets to act as filters for particles of rust. Eventually, it was discovered that faulty plumbing had permitted waste water to enter the hospital's fresh water lines; virtually the entire hospital's water system had become contaminated with *Salmonella*.

Demonstrating that nosocomial neonatal salmonellosis knows no geographical bounds, epidemics recently have been reported from Taiwan (11) and Guatemala (12). In Taiwan, 109 infants were involved; both prematurity and increased duration of hospitalization were found to be risk factors for acquiring the infection. The organism responsible for the outbreak in Guatemala was susceptible only to chloramphenicol and produced 23 cases of neonatal meningitis; all were fatal.

Like salmonellosis, hospital outbreaks of cholera usually affect neonatal units and pediatric wards and the epidemic strains are usually resistant to multiple antibiotics (8, 13). Crowding and lack of secure isolation facilities greatly contribute to spread of the infection. Repeated outbreaks of cholera have been reported, for example, from Dar es Salaam, Tanzania, where two or three babies were placed in each crib and children ate with their fingers from communal plates (8). A combination of control measures, including cohorting and the use of prophylactic tetracycline, helped to end the outbreaks.

Viral Infections

The lack of diagnostic facilities has hampered the assessment of viral disease in the developing countries. Most authorities, however, believe that viral infections account for a significant proportion of febrile illness and that nosocomial viral infections are common. Hepatitis B is probably the most important viral nosocomial infection in the developed world; its nosocomial role in the developing world remains undefined. Because needles are often not sterilized adequately and are commonly used in several patients, the opportunity for transmission of hepatitis B certainly exists.

Nosocomial varicella among hospital workers, especially young nurses, may be more common in certain developing countries than in the developed parts of the world (14). Young staff members apparently are more apt to be susceptible and are likely to acquire varicella when they are exposed to the disease in the course of their early ward activities. The susceptibility of young nurses in the tropics to varicella can have a direct bearing on infection control programs in the temperate zone. When such nurses are recruited to work in hospitals in the developed countries they can acquire varicella from their patients and become the source of a nosocomial outbreak (14).

Somewhat greater attention has been directed to understanding the epidemiology of "exotic" viral infections, such as those due to the Lassa, Ebola, and Marburg viruses and, more recently, the Crimean-Congo hemorrhagic fever virus (15). Capable of being spread by blood and possibly by body fluids, the greatest concern has been that these viruses could be imported into developing countries and produce a nosocomial outbreak. Based on the experience of the last decade, this risk seems reassuringly low (16).

Contaminated Environment

Bacterial contamination of the hospital environment still produces occasional outbreaks of infection in the developed world. Because standards of environmental hygiene, disinfection, and sterilization vary so widely in the hospitals of the developing countries, it is not surprising that similar episodes have occurred in these circumstances. Most of these episodes have not been published, but have been noted in correspondence with colleagues. In Thailand, a teaching hospital experienced over 100 infections caused by *Pseudomonas cepacia* which was traced to contaminated disinfectant used in the operating room. The organism also was recovered from unsterilized distilled water which was used throughout the hospital. Somewhat later, 43 cases of nosocomial septicemia due to *Serratia marcescens* were traced to injections of contaminated diluted atropine which also had been used in the operating room (S Lolekha, personal communication, 1984). Although many hospitals in the developing world now use closed systems for draining urinary catheters, limited economic circumstances compel some institutions to use open systems. Some have created homemade "semiclosed" systems, only to discover that they are constantly violated by nurses and physicians. A recent survey in a Guatemalan hospital recorded an infection rate of 65% when clean catch urine samples were obtained 48 hours after catheter removal (CA Ramirez, personal communication, 1985).

During the early 1960s several large outbreaks of bacteremia occurred in the United States and England which were caused by intrinsically contaminated intravenous fluid. The developing world has not been spared similar episodes. In 1983, pyrogenic reactions were associated with intravenous fluids from one manufacturer in Guatemala (CA Ramirez, personal communication, 1985), and in 1981, Greek hospitals experienced a national epidemic of sepsis caused by *Enterobacter cloacae* and *Enterobacter agglomerans* which resulted from contamination of fluids produced by the single local manufacturer (17). Goldmann has expressed his concern that similar episodes in countries without substantial microbiologic and epidemiologic resources might go unrecognized (18). Indeed, inadequate manufacturing practices are probably most likely to occur in those areas of the world least prepared to recognize intravenous fluid-associated septicemia.

CONCLUSIONS—AND FORWARD

The foregoing has been a brief overview of the importance of nosocomial infections around the globe. Even without comprehensive population-based surveillance data, widespread experience and anecdotal reports lead inevitably to the conclusion that hospital-associated infections are a large and costly problem everywhere. Because the problem already has attracted sustained attention in many developed countries, the emphasis of the discussion has been on the developing world. There the problem still lies dormant: unrecognized, undefined, and sometimes denied. Many countries are spending a significant proportion of their limited resources to provide improved diagnostic and therapeutic facilities for their populations. To have these efforts negated by the morbidity, mortality, and costs consequent to nosocomial infection is a tragedy.

Fortunately, we sense the nascent stirrings of recognition and action. Several national infection control programs have been established (19) and the leadership of WHO is expected to stimulate further activity. But we should make haste slowly. The methods employed in the developed nations cannot simply be transplanted into the hospitals of the developing world. The problems are more extensive, the available resources are more modest, and the cultural context is different. Solutions will evolve if we can work together and learn from each other. Reducing the risk of nosocomial infections in all of the hospitals of the world should be the next grand goal of all practitioners of infection control.

References

1. Velimirovic B: Hospital infections from the WHO perspective. *Infect Control* 4:364–366, 1983.
2. *Surveillance, Control and Prevention of Hospital-Acquired (Nosocomial) Infections 1981—Report of a Scientific Group.* Geneva, World Health Organization, 1981.
3. *Antimicrobial Resistance—Report of a Scientific Working Group.* Geneva, World Health Organization, 1981.
4. Haley RW, Culver DH, White JW, Morgan WM, Emori TG: The nationwide nosocomial infection rate. A new need for vital statistics. *Am J Epidemiol* 121:159–167, 1985.
5. Haley RW: Preliminary cost-benefit analysis of hospital infection control programs (the SENIC Project). In Daschner F (ed): *Proven and Unproven Methods in Hospital Infection Control. Proceedings of an International Workshop at Baiersbronn, Germany. September 24–25, 1977.* Stuttgart, Gustav Fischer Verlag, 1978, p 93.
6. Meers PD, Ayliffe GAJ, Emmerson AM, et al: Report on the National Survey of Infection in Hospitals, 1980. *J Hosp Infect* 2 (suppl):1–51, 1981.
7. Lolekha S, Ratanaubol B, Manu P: Nosocomial infection in a teaching hospital in Thailand. *Philippines Soc Microbiol Infect Dis J* 10:103–114, 1981.
8. Mhalu FS, Mtango FDE, Msengi AE: Hospital outbreaks of cholera transmitted through close person-to-person contact. *Lancet* 2:82–84, 1984.
9. Western KA, St John RK, Shearer LA: Hospital infection control—an international perspective. *Infect Control* 3:453–455, 1982.
10. Mendis NMP, De La Motte PU, Gunatillaka PDP, Nagaratnam W: Protracted infection with *Salmonella bareilly* in a maternity hospital. *J Trop Med Hyg* 79:142–150, 1976.
11. Nursery epidemic of *Salmonella cerro* in a Taipei hospital. *Epidemiol Bull Republ China* 1:9–11, 1985.
12. Cabrera-Meza G, Meneses LF, Rosales JM, Melgar R: Unusual cause of neonatal meningitis: *Salmonella enteritidis* serotype poona. Report of a nosocomial outbreak (abstract). *Pediatr Res* 15:520, 1981.
13. Field Epidemiology Training Programme. Annual Report 1982–1983 (Cholera in Samut Sakhon, Thailand). *WHO Weekly Epidemiol Rec* 58:345–352, 1983.
14. Venkitaraman AR, John TJ: The epidemiology of varicella in staff and students of a hospital in the tropics. *Int J Epidemiol* 13:502–505, 1984.
15. Crimean-Congo hemorrhagic fever—Republic of South Africa. *MMWR* 34:94–101, 1985.
16. Cooper CB, Gransden WR, Webster M, King M, O'Mahony M, Young S, Banatvala JE: A case of Lassa fever: experience at St. Thomas's hospital. *Br Med J* 285:1003–1005, 1982.
17. Matsaniotis NS, Syriopoulou VP, Theodoridou MC, Tzanetou KG, Mostrou GI: *Enterobacter* sepsis in infants and children due to contaminated intravenous fluid. *Infect Control* 5:471–477, 1984.
18. Goldmann DA: Intravenous fluid contamination, Aegean-style. *Infect Control* 5:469–470, 1984.
19. Ponce de Leon Rosales S: Nosocomial infection control in Latin America: we have to start now. *Infect Control* 5:511–512, 1984.

Chapter 3

Costs of Nosocomial Infections and Benefits of Infection Control Programs

Richard E. Dixon, M.D., F.A.C.P.

For many years, the economic costs of nosocomial infections were largely hidden from hospitals and individual practitioners and were seen as primarily important at a national, macroeconomic level. The majority of hospitals were able to pass along the excess costs associated with these infections to patients or their insurance or other third-party payers. Most hospitals were also able to defray many of the costs of infection prevention and control programs. Thus, the economic consequences of nosocomial infections were mainly the concerns of hospital epidemiologists, public policy analysts, and economists, not hospital administrators or practicing physicians.

Even without economic incentives to reduce the risk of nosocomial infections, a substantial proportion of United States hospitals voluntarily developed infection control programs in the early 1970s (1), and standards published by the Joint Commission on Accreditation of Hospitals in 1976 (2) hastened that development. But throughout this period when infection control programs were being developed, concerns were expressed about both the economic costs of nosocomial infections and the costs of programs designed to prevent them.

Fundamental changes in health care financing, which began in the mid-1970s and accelerated in the early 1980s, have changed the ways that hospitals and other providers evaluate the economic consequences of nosocomial infections. New reimbursement systems, exemplified by the Federal Medicare Prospective Payment System (PPS), shift the economic consequences of nosocomial infections back to hospitals. As a result, hospitals have a strong incentive to reduce economic losses attributable to nosocomial infections, but they must also be certain that infection control programs are economically efficient.

MEDICAL CARE REIMBURSEMENT SYSTEMS

Physicians and hospitals in the United States have traditionally charged patients retrospectively for each service provided or activity performed. These charges have not been standardized but have largely been determined by decisions of individual providers and influenced by local practices. Charges have not necessarily borne a predictable relationship to the costs of providing those services, however; costs of providing care to indigent patients have been spread among patients able to pay either directly or through insurance or other third-party payers (3), and some of the costs of expensive services were shifted to other, less expensive services (4).

This simple fee-for-service approach to health care financing has gradually eroded during the past several decades. As third-party payers became responsible for paying the majority of American hospital costs, they began to establish reimbursement rates for hospitals and physicians, to determine which services are reimbursable, and otherwise to influence hospital and practitioner charges and practices.

Changes in health care economics accelerated when medical costs began to rise rapidly in the mid-1970s. The medical component of the Consumer Price Index (CPI-M) rose only slightly faster than the overall CPI (CPI-W) from 1968 to 1974 (average of 0.27%/year) but rose 0.9%/year faster in the next 7-year period from 1975 to 1981. In the most recent 3-year period (1982 to 1984), it increased even faster, an average of 4.23%/year. As a result, the CPI-M was 20% higher than the CPI-W at the end of 1984 (5). Health care accounted for progressively larger fractions of the Gross National Product (GNP) during the same period. In 1965, the year before the Federal Medicare and Medicaid programs were introduced, health care accounted for 5.9% of the GNP (6); by 1977, it accounted for 8.8% (6); and it comprised 10.5 to 11% of the GNP in 1982 (7). Health care expenditures became increasingly large segments of federal and state budgets during these periods, and governments along with business, labor organizations, and other groups expressed increasing unwillingness to pay these rising costs, leading to increasing pressure for costs to be limited.

In response to these economic pressures, various experimental cost containment programs were begun by hospitals, medical societies, insurors, and governments. A New Jersey experimental program in prospective hospital rate setting formed the basis for a Medicare reimbursement system, the Federal Prospective Payment System, authorized by the Tax Equity and Fiscal Responsibility Act (TEFRA) of 1982 and the Social Security Ammendments the following year (8).

The Federal PPS established a formula to reimburse hospitals prospectively for care of Medicare beneficiaries and thereby canceled the traditional fee-for-service payment for these patients. The PPS formula is complex, but it basically reimburses hospitals a fixed fee that depends upon the patient's principal diagnosis. The formula allocates each of more than 60,000 potential standard diagnoses (9) to one of 467 diagnosis-related groups (DRGs) (10, 11). The PPS establishes a basic fee for each of these DRGs since each DRG is generally designed to combine similar conditions that, on the average, consume equivalent economic resources. At the present time (1985), DRG reimbursements are slightly modified by selected hospital characteristics, such as whether the hospital has major teaching responsibilities, and by hospital location. Reimbursements are not influenced by differences in care provided for

individual patients, however. Thus, for example, payment is the same for treating a patient with uncomplicated chronic obstructive pulmonary disease (COPD) as for treating a patient with COPD who requires management in an intensive care unit.

The DRG that determines reimbursement is based first on the patient's principal diagnosis, which is defined as the condition that, after study, is determined to be responsible for the patient's admission. Next, patients who have major surgical procedures related to that diagnosis are placed into one of 199 surgical DRGs, and remaining patients are placed into one of 268 nonsurgical DRGs (Table 3.1).

Principal diagnosis and the presence or absence of a surgical procedure are the sole factors that determine DRG placement for 198 diagnostic groups. However, as shown in Table 3.1, age or the occurrence of other secondary diagnoses determines DRG placement for other patients. For example, craniotomy procedures are paid at different rates for patients 18 years of age and older than for younger patients. DRG assignment may also be influenced by the occurrence of co-morbid conditions, which are defined as significant coincident illnesses or complications that occur during hospitalization. Over 2800 potential complications and co-morbid conditions are listed, selected because they would be expected to prolong length of stay by at least 1 day in more than 75% of instances (10). These secondary diagnoses are quite varied, however, and include such serious conditions as cerebrovascular accident, pulmonary embolism, and *Candida* endocarditis. They also include diagnoses that may represent nonspecific, transient, or even trivial conditions, such as hypovolemia, mild malnutrition, lumbar puncture reaction, and cachexia. Nosocomial infections are included in the list of complicating and co-morbid conditions as "infectious compli-

Table 3.1. Influences of Surgical Procedures, Age, Complications, and Co-morbidity on DRG Assignment

	Surgical Number (%)	Nonsurgical Number (%)	Total Number (%)
Unaffected DRGs	89 (19.1)	109 (23.3)	198 (42.4)
Age-dependent DRGs	24 (5.1)	37 (7.9)	61 (13.1)
Co-morbidity-dependent DRGs	8 (1.7)	6 (1.3)	14 (3.0)
Age, complication, and co-morbidity-dependent DRGs	78 (16.7)	116 (24.8)	194 (41.5)
Total	199 (42.6)	268 (57.4)	467 (100.0)

cation of medical care," postoperative infection, and the like.

For a large number of conditions, paired DRGs are available that are based on both age and the occurrence of a co-morbid condition or complication (Table 3.1). A patient who is less than 70 years of age and has no complication or co-morbid condition is paid at a lower rate than the patient who is 70 or older or who has one or more complications or co-morbid conditions. The occurrence of a nosocomial infection will shift patients who are less than 70 years of age and have no other significant secondary diagnoses, into higher paying DRGs, but it will not affect DRG placement of a patient 70 or older or one who already has a co-morbid condition or has already suffered a complication of hospitalization. Thus, a 65-year-old woman with a principal diagnosis of "simple pneumonia," which allows a higher DRG reimbursement if age is greater than 69 or if a complicating or co-morbid condition is present, would generate a higher reimbursement if she acquired nosocomial septicemia and had no other significant medical conditions. However, her care would not be reimbursed at a higher rate for the septicemia if she had diabetes mellitus as a co-morbid condition, since she would have already been eligible for reimbursement in the higher rate DRG.

The PPS system has numerous profound implications for hospitals and infection control programs. First, hospitals are generally unable to recoup costs of activities such as infection control programs other than through increased efficiency in patient care. Second, it is apparent that many nosocomial infections and other complications will not lead to higher reimbursement.

Prospective payment using a DRG-based approach may have even broader economic implications in the future. The Federal PPS does not apply to non-Medicare patients, nor is it used to reimburse physicians or other providers at the present time. Several states now use the system for all payers, however, making it difficult for hospitals to shift unrecovered expenses to other third-party payers or to other patients. In addition, other third-party payers are considering implementing similar programs. Since physicians are not paid by DRGs at present, PPS has no direct effect on physicians' incomes. However, physicians in all-payer DRG states have had lower rates of income growth than physicians in other states (12). DRG-based systems have been proposed for reimbursing physicians as well, however, and physicians and other providers will

likely face increased economic incentives to prevent avoidable complications if such a system is implemented.

COSTS OF NOSOCOMIAL INFECTIONS

Nosocomial infection costs may be considered from several viewpoints. They affect the national economy, and health economists can calculate their net costs and benefits at that level. At the other pole of the economic analysis, they affect the individual patient with infection. Although the costs to individuals have been evaluated for some diseases, their effects on individual patients with nosocomial infection have not been evaluated systematically. Rarely does any patient pay the exact cost of nosocomial infection, however, since third-party payers spread the economic costs of illnesses among their beneficiaries, and hospitals spread the costs of nosocomial infections and infection control programs among infected as well as uninfected patients. As a result, nosocomial infections also profoundly affect hospitals and third-party payers.

National Impact of Nosocomial Infections

Nosocomial infections have direct and indirect costs. Direct costs are defined as the specific costs incurred in treating an illness and include hospital per diem charges, costs of medications and other treatments, physician fees, and the like. Indirect costs include such items as losses of economic productivity and the costs of pain, suffering, and infirmity.

Direct Costs

Many investigators have studied the direct costs attributable to nosocomial infections and have reported a broad range of costs (13). Most of these studies have actually evaluated hospital charges rather than true costs, although these terms have often been used interchangeably. True cost estimates would be preferred, but they are difficult to determine.

Different techniques have been used to evaluate excess charges resulting from nosocomial infections (13, 14), and these differences account in large part for the variability in results reported. Most often, investigators have compared charges incurred by infected patients with charges of similar patients who did not acquire nosocomial infection. The accuracy of these estimates is obviously determined by the similarity of the infected and uninfected groups. Since severely ill patients have not only a higher risk for nosocomial infection (15) but also higher risks for other complications and tend to generate higher charges than less seriously ill patients, studies that use only few and simple variables, such as age, sex, or major diagnosis, as controlling factors tend to report higher charge differences than those that use more complex variables to compare infected and uninfected patients. On occasion in such studies, the investigator is unable to identify any uninfected patient who can be compared with a patient with nosocomial infection, further complicating analysis of these comparison studies.

In order to avoid the problems of comparison studies, other investigators have attempted to evaluate individual patients and define, for each, specific charges that were attributable to the nosocomial infection (13). It is often difficult to determine whether a test or procedure was performed solely because of a nosocomial infection, of course, and it is difficult to evaluate the effect of observer bias in these studies.

Despite these methodologic problems in defining direct charges, all studies indicate that nosocomial infections prolong hospital stay substantially and cause large expenditures of extra resources. A conservative estimate of excess charges is listed in Table 3.2.* Using national incidence estimates (18), the average direct charges for nosocomial infections appear to be greater than $2.5 billion/year in the United States (Table 3.2).

Indirect Costs

Indirect costs of nosocomial infections have not been adequately evaluated. They include losses in personal income or tax revenue due to illness and costs of retraining and replacing workers who are ill or who die. Reductions in productivity are major indirect costs. Changes in medical practice may lead to subtle indirect costs, as when broad spectrum and very expensive antimicrobial agents are used in preference to less expensive antibiotics because of the prevalence of multiple drug-resistant nosocomial pathogens. Less objective effects are even more difficult to measure. How can one measure the losses that occur when investments in education and training fail to bear fruit because of serious illness or premature death, for example? Attempts to assign monetary value for pain, suffering, and disability that result from illness have produced inconsistent results (19).

Indirect cost calculations are further complicated by the need to assign monetary value to

---

* All financial estimates are standardized to a 1984 base-year by using changes in the medical component of the Consumer Price Index (5) as an adjustment factor.

items that have political or ethical overtones. Some economists consider persons past the arbitrary retirement age of 65 to have no positive economic benefit to society so that all health care expenditures for such persons are a net economic loss. If one accepts this viewpoint, prevention of a nosocomial infection might actually be costly if it thereby allows a person to live longer, to collect economic benefits from society, and to acquire another more expensive illness at a later time. It is obvious, therefore, that indirect cost estimates often reflect the political and ethical views of the person making the projection. But despite the problems in calculating indirect costs, it is very likely that these costs are quite high.

Hospital Costs

So long as hospital costs of nosocomial infections could be passed directly along to third-party payers or shifted from one payer to another, hospitals had few direct economic incentives to prevent or control nosocomial infections. Nonetheless, U.S. hospitals invested heavily in developing infection control programs during the period before those programs were required by accrediting agencies and well before prospective payment systems were introduced (1). Now that such systems are being used to reimburse hospitals, it is essential for hospitals to evaluate their experiences to determine the economic gains or losses from their infection control programs.

Although national statistics may not be precisely accurate when applied to individual hospitals, they can be used to estimate individual hospitals' costs. Using conservative projections for prolongations of stay and excess charges attributable to nosocomial infections (see Table 3.2, for example), a hospital can use its own case mix and DRG data to determine the extent to which excess PPS reimbursements defray nosocomial infection costs. An example of such an approach is shown below. Few such studies have been reported in the literature thusfar, but those that have been reported indicate that only a relatively small fraction of nosocomial infections occur in individuals who have not already qualified for the highest allowable DRG reimbursement because of age or prior complications or co-morbid conditions (20).

COST-BENEFIT ASSESSMENTS OF NOSOCOMIAL INFECTION CONTROL PROGRAMS

The Study on the Efficacy of Nosocomial Infection Control (SENIC) project, conducted by the Centers for Disease Control, found that up to

Table 3.2. Estimated Excess Charges and Prolongation Lengths of Stay Attributable to Nosocomial Infections, U.S., 1984 Dollars

Infection Site	Excess Charge/Patient Day*	Excess Days of Stay*	Extra Physician Charges†	Average Charge/Patient	Annual U.S. Number Infections‡·§	Total Excess Direct Costs, U.S.§
Surgical wound	324	6.0	0	2656	510	1,354,560
Urinary tract	265	1.2	48	366	903	276,318
Respiratory	385	4.0	160	1700	227	385,900
Bacteremia	324	7.0	280	2548	103	262,440
Other sites	265	4.2	168	1281	405	518,805
All infections					2,148	2,798,023

* Adapted from Dixon (16) and adjusted to 1984 dollars by change in CPI-M (5).
† Estimated to be $40/day for follow-up visits (17); no added surgeons' fees are included for surgical wound infections.
‡ Estimated number in 1976 (18).
§ Thousands.

one-third of nosocomial infections can be prevented by effective infection control programs. Hospitals without effective programs actually had a temporal rise in infection rates from 1970 to 1976 of from 9 to 31% at various sites, but effective programs reduced infection rates during the same period from 7 to 48% (Table 3.3) (21).

It is not possible to establish a cost-benefit ratio for infection control programs that will be applicable to every hospital, since hospitals have different resources and infection control problems. Nonetheless, costs and benefits can be estimated for an average hospital. For purposes of illustration, consider a hypothetical hospital that is relatively typical of many United States hospitals; it has an average census of 250 patients (excluding newborn infants) and provides broadly based primary and some secondary level care. Such a hospital has 12,000 adult and pediatric admissions each year, of whom about 5,500 have surgical procedures.

Based on findings from the SENIC project (18, 21), this hypothetical hospital would have approximately 713 infections/year without an effective infection control program but only 487 infections with a uniformly effective program. The direct hospital charges for the excess services consumed by these infections would amount to approximately $800,000/year without an effective infection control program, and an effective program would save the hospital almost $250,000 annually (Table 3.4).

The projected $250,000 annual savings/250 occupied beds is a crude approximation at best. The actual savings to be derived from an infection control program might be far greater, at least in some hospitals. For example, the projection uses very conservative estimates of the excess costs

Table 3.3. Changes in Nosocomial Infection Rates: 1970 to 1976, Hospitals with and without Effective Programs*

Infection Site and Patient Risk Category	Hospitals with Very Effective Programs	Hospitals with Ineffective Programs
Surgical wound		
High risk	−48.0	+13.8
Low risk	−23.6	+21.3
Urinary tract		
High risk	−35.8	+18.5
Low risk	−41.6	+30.7
Pneumonia		
Surgical patients	−7.3	+9.3
Medical patients	—†	+10.0
Bloodstream		
All patients	−27.6	+25.5

* Modified from Haley et al (21).
† Programs rated as "moderately effective" had a reduction of 7.7% in the period (21).

resulting from nosocomial infections, and many investigators have projected far higher costs (13, 22–24). Use of these higher cost projections would substantially magnify both the costs of preventable infections and the savings from an effective program. Since it is an average, the projection also minimizes the savings that would occur in a hospital that treats large numbers of high risk patients or provides sophisticated care. Furthermore, although the projection adjusts costs to 1984 dollars, it uses estimates of infection rates and infection control program benefits that were derived from 1976 data. The SENIC project found that infection rates were actually increasing in hospitals without effective programs, although they were falling in hospitals with such programs (21). Thus, the benefits of a control program may

Table 3.4. Estimated Annual Nosocomial Infection Cost Savings by Introducing Effective Infection Control Program in Hypothetical 250-Bed Hospital

Infection Site	Infections without Any Program	Infections with Effective Program	Infections Prevented*	Average Cost/Infection†	Total Savings†
Surgical wound	186	120	66	1944	128,304
Urinary tract	283	195	88	318	29,574
Respiratory	74	58	16	1540	24,640
Bacteremia	34	22	12	2268	15,216
Other sites	136	92	44	1113	48,972
Total	713	487	226		246,706

* Difference between numbers of infections without program and with program.
† Direct hospital costs, not including physicians' fees, 1984 dollars.

be even greater in the 1980s than they were in the mid-1970s. On the other hand, the projection assumes that a hospital that introduces an infection control program will be able to achieve maximal benefits at every site of infection, and this seems unlikely, at least initially. Moreover, hospitals that treat low risk patients or provide only relatively unsophisticated services would benefit relatively less. Nonetheless, it seems quite likely that a 700-bed hospital that provides sophisticated tertiary level care might avoid $1 million or more in excess charges by instituting a highly effective infection control program.

Some of the excess costs of nosocomial infections can be recovered. Where hospital payment continues to be reimbursed on a retrospective basis for services rendered, patients or their third-party payers can be charged. For patients covered by DRG-based systems, however, excess costs can only be recovered if an infection shifts the patient into a DRG that pays more for complications (Table 3.1). Preliminary data suggest that relatively few of the excess costs of nosocomial infections will be recovered by this mechanism, however (20).

Although the introduction of an effective infection control program would be expected to save substantial amounts of unreimbursed costs, such programs are expensive, and their costs are not directly reimbursed under most prospective payment systems. In the SENIC project, four components of infection control programs were found to be generally necessary to assure program effectiveness: (a) having a physician interested and active in infection control efforts; (b) having one infection control practitioner for every 250 beds; (c) conducting active surveillance for nosocomial infections; and (d) providing feedback of infection rates to surgeons. Additional factors were identified for infections at individual sites, such

as having effective control programs to prevent intravenous device-associated bacteremias (21).

Personnel would account for substantial costs in our hypothetical hospital. The SENIC findings suggest that at least one infection control practitioner and a part time infection control physician would be required (21). Their activities often require clerical and computer support. Changes in patient care practices may also be costly, although effective infection control programs tend to reduce expensive and unnecessary activities, thereby providing additional cost savings (1, 25). No data are available to provide a firm basis for estimating the costs of a fully effective hospital infection control program for our hypothetical hospital, but a reasonable estimate is that approximately $60,000 might be required each year for a typical 250-bed hospital.

Larger or more complex institutions would require larger infection control budgets, although certain costs, such as those for data processing or clerical support, are unlikely to increase in proportion to hospital size. Smaller hospitals would require a smaller budget for infection control, although, here too, savings are unlikely to be proportional to bed capacity. For example, an infection control practitioner who works only part time does not seem to be as effective, in general, as one who works full time; and it is unlikely that a practitioner working 8 hours/week in a 50-bed hospital would be as effective as a full time practitioner in a 250-bed institution.

As illustrated in Table 3.5, the hypothetical hospital used in this example benefits substantially by introducing an effective infection control program. It is highly probable that actual hospitals will find equally large savings. But each hospital would need to determine the proportion of excess costs from nosocomial infections that could be recouped from patients or their third-

Table 3.5. Annual Costs and Benefits of Infection Control Program in Hypothetical 250-Bed Hospital

Estimated reduction of direct costs from infections prevented	$246,700
Estimated program expenses	60,000
Hospital savings	$186,700

party payers as well as the likely costs of an infection control program in order to determine the magnitude of the benefits that are likely to accrue from an active infection control program. It must be remembered that cost effectiveness is not the only determinant of the value of a program, though; hospitals have traditionally chosen to implement programs that improve patient care. Infection control programs are demonstrably successful in reducing patient morbidity (21). Fortunately, they appear to be financially beneficial to the hospital as well.

References

1. Haley RW, Shachtman RH: The emergence of infection surveillance and control programs in US hospitals: An assessment, 1976. *Am J Epidemiol* 111:574–591, 1980.
2. Joint Commission on Accreditation of Hospitals: *Accreditation Manual for Hospitals.* Chicago, JCAH, 1976.
3. Ginzburg PB, Sloan FA: Hospital cost shifting. *N Engl J Med* 310:893–898, 1984.
4. Finkler SA: The distinction between cost and charges. *Ann Intern Med* 96:102–109, 1982.
5. US Department of Labor, Bureau of Labor Statistics: *C.P.I. Detailed Report.* Sup. Doc. No. L2.38/3:984/6. Washington, DC, US Government Printing Office, July 1984.
6. Young DW, Saltman RB: Medical practice, case mix, and cost containment: a new role for the attending physician. *JAMA* 247:801–805, 1982.
7. Ginzberg E: The monetarization of medical care. *N Engl J Med* 310:1162–1165, 1984.
8. Inglehart JK: Medicare begins prospective payment of hospitals. *N Engl J Med* 368:1482–1432, 1982.
9. Health Care Financing Administration: *The International Classification of Diseases, 9th Revision, Clinical Modification.* Public Health Service, US Department of Health and Human Services (DHHS Publication No. (PHS) 80-1260), 1980.
10. St Anthony Hospital: *The Physician's DRG Working Guidebook.* Louisville, KY, St Anthony Hospital, 1984.
11. Fetter RB, Shin Y, Freeman JL, Averill RF, Thompson JD: Case mix definition by diagnosis-related groups. *Med Care* 18 (suppl):1–53, 1980.
12. Zukerman S, Becker ER, Adams EK, Musacchio RA, Sreckovich C: Physician practice patterns under hospital rate-setting programs. *JAMA* 252:2589–2592, 1984.
13. Haley RW, Schaberg DR, VonAllmen SD, McGowan JE: Estimating the extra charges and prolongation of hospitalization due to nosocomial infections: a comparison of methods. *J Infect Dis* 141:248–257, 1980.
14. Freeman J, McGowan JE: Methodologic issues in hospital epidemiology. III. Investigating the modifying effects of time and severity of underlying illness on estimates of cost of nosocomial infections. *Rev Infect Dis* 6:285–300, 1984.
15. Hooton TW, Haley RW, Culver DH, White JW, Morgan WM, Carroll RJ: The joint associations of multiple risk factors with the occurrence of nosocomial infection. *Am J Med* 70:960–970, 1981.
16. Dixon RE: Effect of infections on hospital care. *Ann Intern Med* 89 (part 2):749–753, 1978.
17. Dixon RE: Economic costs of respiratory infections in the United States. *Am J Med* 78:45–51, 1985.
18. Haley RW, Culver DH, White JW, Morgan WM, Emori TG: The nationwide nosocomial infection rate. A new need for vital statistics. *Am J Epidemiol* 121:159–167, 1985.
19. Avorn J: Benefit and cost analysis in geriatric care. Turning age discrimination into health policy. *N Engl J Med* 310:1294–1301, 1984.
20. Beyt BE, Troxler S, Caveness J: Prospective payment and infection control. *Infect Control* 4:161–164, 1985.
21. Haley RW, Culver DH, White JW, Morgan WM, Emori TG, Munn VP, Hooton TM: The efficacy of infection surveillance and control programs in preventing nosocomial infections in US hospitals. *Am J Epidemiol* 121:182–205, 1985.
22. Rose R, Hunting KJ, Townsend TR, Wenzel RP: Morbidity/mortality and economics of hospital-acquired blood stream infections: a controlled study. *South Med J* 70:1267–1269, 1977.
23. Green JW, Wenzel RP: Postoperative wound infection: a controlled study of the increased duration of hospital stay and direct cost of hospitalization. *Ann Surg* 185:264–268, 1977.
24. Spengler RF, Greenough WB: Hospital costs and mortality attributed to nosocomial bacteremias. *JAMA* 240:2455–2458, 1978.
25. Daschner FD: Practical aspects for cost reduction in hospital infection control. *Infect Control* 5:32–35, 1984.

Chapter 4

Current Legal Issues

Harry C. Nottebart, Jr., J.D., M.D., F.C.L.M., F.A.C.P.M., F.A.C.P., F.C.A.P.

INTRODUCTION

The legal principles which are applied to cases involving infection control, nosocomial infections, infections generally, and related topics are hundreds and sometimes thousands of years old. Even the Mosaic Code (see for example Deut. 23:12–13) contains provisions for practices that when implemented provided for good infection control whether that was the primary purpose or not.

There is not a great deal written specifically about this subject. See inter alia Nottebart (1), Nottebart (2), and related works cited therein. There have been discussions of individual important cases such as *Helman* (3) and *Kapuschinsky* (4) as well as nosocomial infections in hospital employees (5) including laboratory employees (6).

This chapter reviews the background of the legal system and infection control and then examines cases from 1978 to early 1985.*

LEGAL SYSTEM

The legal system in our country has developed over hundreds of years and is the descendant of the English common law system. (Louisiana is, of course, the exception. Its heritage is the French Code Napoleon originally.) It is an adversarial system. That means that two parties are opponents and each side attempts to present the facts and opinions in the best light for his side of the controversy. In civil, i.e., noncriminal, cases the party suing is the plaintiff and the party being sued is the defendant. (In criminal cases the plaintiff is the state, sometimes called prosecution, and the accused is still the defendant.) Because medical malpractice is a form of negligence, an unintentional tort, or civil wrong, criminal law will not be considered in the discussion that follows.

---

*From a strictly legal viewpoint one might see the Annotation in 96 A.L.R.2d 1205 (1963).

A law suit begins when a suit is filed with a court of appropriate jurisdiction. It includes a statement as to injuries sustained and damages incurred. Within a specified time period the person being sued (defendant) responds with a statement that answers or admits the various allegations in the complaint. There follows a period of pretrial pleadings and discovery. The purpose of these is to clarify the issues involved so that when there is a trial only those issues specifically in controversy are tried. That is, at the trial evidence is presented on both sides of the issue and then a trier of fact (jury or judge if no jury) determines the "facts" based on the evidence presented. This usually means determining which witnesses are believed and which testimony is accepted as true. In medical malpractice cases the testimony is often by expert witnesses so it is a matter of which expert or experts the trier of fact believes.

This pretrial process is designed to limit valuable and scarce court time to hearing testimony about issues in question. If the incident in question occurred on July 4 and both the plaintiff and defendant agree that whatever happened did happen on July 4, then there is no need to present a long line of witnesses or documents trying to prove that it occurred on July 4—it is accepted as "fact." Sometimes in medical cases one might not totally agree with some of the items that have been accepted as "fact." However, if accepted by both sides, these may be considered the "facts" for that case.

The whole process involving pretrial, trial, and appeal may be considered as a pyramid with many, many claims at the bottom, a fewer number of law suits filed above the claims, an even fewer number of cases which actually go to trial above the suits filed, and a very few cases which get to appellate courts at the top of the pyramid.

Settlements can occur anywhere along this process. Settlements or claims dismissed, dropped, or otherwise not pursued are *not* reported in the legal literature.

For the most part only opinions rendered at appellate level are reported in the legal literature. By the time a case gets to the appellate level, the facts have been stipulated or determined by the trier of fact (the jury) at the trial level. At the appellate level the issues are those of law, not fact. The facts of an individual case are generally pertinent only to that case, but the principles of law which apply to the facts have widespread application. These principles of law apply not only to the case at hand but to other plaintiffs and defendants in other suits. Because of this wider applicability, the appellate decisions are reported, i.e., published, for all to read and be guided thereby. Therefore, it is the legal principles that are important in these reported, appellate opinions. Only those facts which relate to the legal principles are included in the appellate opinions.

This explains why some of the facts that physicians might want to see in a reported case are not present; they are immaterial to the legal principles involved in the appeals. But, of course, these facts may have been very important from the medical diagnosis, treatment, or management aspects of the case. These all came out at the trial, or at least one hopes they did, and the trier of fact (the jury, if it is a jury trial) determined the facts which were at issue. These facts which have been determined are then taken as given by the appellate court in considering the issues of law.

It is sometimes difficult to accept or believe that these are now the "facts." It is sometimes incredible what has gotten admitted and was not challenged so that it is considered fact. This can occur with expert opinion as well. That is, if testimony is not challenged or if no evidence is entered to contradict the other testimony then that testimony is taken as a given.

If one reads very many cases involving infectious diseases and clinical microbiology one sees frequent examples of poor information or even misinformation which have been admitted as expert testimony; with no testimony to the contrary, this information becomes the "facts" in the case. This is due in part to the fact that infectious disease specialists and clinical microbiologists are reluctant to be expert witnesses (for either side). The result is poor expert testimony and even poor law as a result.

Some fault also lies with some of the attorneys who use this expert testimony. Some do not bother to understand the technical issues and sometimes do not even ask those questions which would elicit the appropriate information from the expert. This sometimes happens even when the expert has tried to indicate what is at issue medically. There are even a few attorneys who want expert witnesses but then do not pay any attention to what they say and almost ignore the medical issues. These are often then the same ones who blame the expert if the attorney loses the case. This experience is usually so distasteful that the conscientious expert is so appalled by the whole business that he will rarely, if ever, again be willing to be an expert witness. To those who have suffered through such an experience, or who may endure such in the future, remember that attorneys are just like physicians in this regard. There are those who are unprepared and inept and with whom it is painful and disappointing to work, but there are also those highly competent, extremely intelligent ones with whom it is a pleasure to work. It should be obvious then, that the number of reported (appellate) cases is only a very small fraction of all claims that were originally made, or suits filed, or even trials that preceded the appeals.

PROCEDURAL ISSUES

There are also cases which involve infectious disease or medical microbiology issues, but the decision or disposition of the case may be based on some other issue(s), even a procedural issue. In these cases those aspects in which one is most interested may not be discussed at all. In legal parlance they may not reach those substantive, as distinct from procedural, issues. One example of this is *Anderson v. Lutheran Deaconess Hospital* 257 N.W.2d 561 (1977), in which the plaintiff allegedly suffered an injury, *Haemophilus parainfluenzae* endocarditis. There could have been many interesting aspects of this case from a medical viewpoint. However, the case was decided on the issue of whether it had been filed soon enough. The defense raised the issue of statute of limitations. That is, the attorney for the defense made a motion that the case be dismissed because it was not filed soon enough. That is, it was filed after the statute of limitations for that kind of action had expired. The motion for dismissal was granted by the trial judge, and it was affirmed on appeal. That action disposed of the case before any evidence was presented, yet that was as final a disposition as if days of evidence had been presented and a decision made based on the medical aspects. Although it may seem strange to those in the field of medicine, it is reasonable and straightforward to those in law.

It is probably too obvious, but from the above

discussion one should realize that legal reports should not be used as a source of definitive medical facts. One should never confuse what has been "proved" in a law suit and what is accepted as true medically. There is a great difference even in what is meant by a proposition being proved in law versus medicine (7).

Suppose one had an interest in looking up law suits involving a certain organism or a certain kind of infection. In the medical literature these might well be terms indexed by *Index Medicus, Science Citation Index, Excerpta Medica, Biological Abstracts*, etc and it would be straightforward, if tedious, to search for articles published on any of these topics.

The legal literature is not indexed this way. Diseases and organisms are not indexed, and there is no way of finding the kinds of law suits as postulated above. One can review the legal indexes for Hospitals, Malpractice, Negligence, and similar terms and then find the kinds of cases in which one is interested by scanning all of those—a very time-consuming process. One can rely, in part, on various services that abstract various kinds of cases. Of those, one that is usually readily available to health professions is *The Citation*, a bimonthly publication of the American Medical Asociation that abstracts many cases involving hospitals, physicians, and nurses.

Once one finds one or several cases involving the topic one wants, the search becomes easier. Many prior cases are likely to be cited in the opinion, so one has those citations. Subsequent cases can be found by using *Shepherds*, which gives subsequent citations of the case one has already found. By following those citation trails and other cases to which those cases lead, one can often rapidly develop a comprehensive view of the legal literature on a particular topic.

Of course one reason that the legal literature is not indexed by organisms and diseases, as we might wish, is that for the purposes of the law specific organisms or diseases *may not* be pertinent. It is the legal principles which are important, and that is how cases are indexed. Malpractice or negligence principles applicable to one case are applicable to others even though the specific facts, organisms, diseases, etc are different in every case.

Another aspect to consider is the state to state variation. Statutory law and precedents in one state may well determine the outcome of litigation in that state so that decisions from other states or jurisdictions may not be applicable. This should be remembered in reading about cases from other jurisidictions. Cases from other jurisdictions should be considered as guides or possibly trends, but they are not absolutely determinative of any particular litigation.

Perhaps it is obvious to all, but legal citations are in a different format from medical citations. The legal citation contains a number (volume number), a series of letters (abbreviations of the specific reporter being cited), another number (the first page of the specific report being cited), and finally the year of the report in parentheses.

NEGLIGENCE

As mentioned above, medical malpractice is a form of negligence, and so the plaintiff in attempting to prove medical malpractice has to prove the same elements as negligence.

There are four elements to prove negligence:
1. A duty or standard of care;
2. A failure to perform the duty or to meet the standard of care;
3. An injury that resulted from the failure to perform the duty or to meet the standard of care;
4. Measurable damages resulting from the injury due to the failure to perform the duty or to meet the standard of care.

Although these may seem simple and even obvious, there have been many, many cases involving these elements.

Duties or standards of care can be established in many different ways. Hospital policies and procedures establish duties or standards of care. So do state licensure requirements and probably even Joint Commission on Accreditation of Hospitals (JCAH) standards of a JCAH-accredited hospital.

In actions involving physician care, duties or standards of care are established by expert witnesses. That is why some law suits against physicians fail; there is no expert testimony establishing the duty or standard of care. Because there has been difficulty at times in obtaining expert witnesses to testify as to the standard of care, plaintiffs have often tried to invoke the doctrine or principle of *res ipsa loquitor*. If *res ipsa loquitor* is applied, then expert testimony is not needed. There are three elements needed to invoke this doctrine:
1. The event that occurred does not occur unless there is negligence by someone.
2. The parties or equipment involved were all under the control of the defendant(s).

3. The plaintiff had no control over any of the parties or equipment and did nothing himself to cause the injury that occurred.

If these three elements are present, then the plaintiff does not have to present testimony as to the duty or standard of care and that the defendant was negligent.

Recently there have been cases involving an injury that occurred after an operation or other procedure and the plaintiff alleged negligence, as usual, but also alleged lack of informed consent. Often the plaintiff cannot show that the operation or procedure was done negligently, but there was a terrible result in spite of the fact that the operation or procedure was performed appropriately and competently. Plaintiffs are now arguing that even though there may not have been negligence in the performance of the operation or procedure, there was a terrible result and if they had known of the possibility of such a result they never would have consented to such a procedure. Therefore there was a lack of *informed* consent. This is certainly a trend that could have devastating applications. For one view of this see Nottebart (8).

PRECEDENTS

Perhaps one ought to know that in the legal literature sometimes older is better. Medically, of course, we all feel that newer is better. We sit around talking about the most recent issue of the *New England Journal*, *JAMA*, the *Annals*, etc. Often the newest information changes or modifies what was known before, so keeping up to date is important. Of course there are new changes in the law as well. New laws are passed, courts hand down decisions which interpret and modify previous rulings, and courts even hand down decisions which radically change what had previously been understood about a segment of the law. However, in spite of these changes there is an antiquarian tendency in the law to feel that older is better. That is, if one can cite precedents that are hundreds of years old that have been followed continuously, that is viewed as representing a sound and even fundamental principle. It has stood the test of time; it is not ephemeral or a fad. Some lawyers may even feel it reflects the depth and breadth of their research and preparation.

HISTORICAL BACKGROUND OF INFECTIONS AND THE LAW

Many of the early cases involve smallpox and some scarlet fever. They might even be consid-

ered the acquired immune deficiency syndrome (AIDS) of their time.

The earliest case I have found so far involves an attempt by some to get an injunction to prevent the building of an "Inoculation Hospital" where there would be people infected with smallpox. No injunction was granted (*Baines v. Baker* 1 Amb. 158, S.D. *Anon.* 3 ATK 750 (1752)). In *Rex v. Sutton* 4 Burr. 2116 (1767) Sutton was indicted for maintaining a nuisance in keeping a house for inoculating for smallpox. Neighbors were as concerned then as they are now about sick patients in their neighborhood.

In *Rex v. Vantandillo* 4 Maule & Selwyn 73 (1815) a mother carried her 1-year-old child who was infected with smallpox along a public highway exposing people passing by and near dwelling places. The court noted that there was a danger of infecting others with smallpox and it was an "evil example" to others. The mother was imprisoned for 3 months for this crime. In *Rex v. Burnett* 4 Maule & Selwyn 272 (1815) the defendant was an apothecary who had inoculated several children with smallpox. When ill with this contagious disease he carried them or caused them to be carried along the public highway, exposing many people to this contagious disease. The crime was not the inoculating for smallpox even, as one judge noted, after the introduction of vaccination, but the crime was exposing and endangering the public. The apothecary was sentenced to 6 months in prison. One can imagine how different infection control might be if these precedents were followed.

In a later case, *Board v. Bisshopp* 2 C.P.Div. 187 (1877) a doctor walking with a person with scarlet fever was held not to have exposed the public to the contagious disease. The doctor was held not to have been in charge of the person with scarlet fever.

In *Best v. Stapp*, cited in a footnote in *Board v. Bisshopp* 2 C.P.Div. 191 (1877), a lodging house keeper sued a lodger who knowingly introduced into the house children infected with scarlet fever. As a result the plaintiff (the lodging house keeper) lost four of his children. He was awarded £120 for the medical expenses and funerals of his four children.

In all of these cases the issue was whether someone with a contagious disease or in charge of someone with a contagious disease so acted to expose the public, or segments thereof, to that contagious disease.

Besides physically exposing someone to a contagious disease one might expose one by giving bad advice to someone who relied on that advice, or by not taking precautions necessary to prevent carriage of the contagious disease between patients.

In an early 20th-century case in the United States, *Skillings v. Allen* 143 Minn 323, 173 N.W. 663 (1919), a physician was sued because he advised a mother and father that they could safely visit their daughter whom he had hospitalized with scarlet fever. He also said that they could safely take their daughter home and that there was no danger of communicating the disease. As a result of relying on his advice both parents contracted scarlet fever. The defendant physician demurred, that is, he said that this was not a claim that was compensable by a legal action. This was overruled by the trial court and affirmed by the Minnesota Supreme Court.

In one of the cases cited in *Skillings v. Allen, Piper v. Menifee* 12 B.Mon.(Ky.) 465, 54 Am Dec. 547 (1851) a physician was said to be liable to a patient for communicating smallpox to the patient after the physician had attended other patients with smallpox. The physician had said that there was no danger to the patient because he would change clothes after seeing the smallpox patients.

In a lawsuit against a physician for transmitting smallpox to a patient and his children *Haas v. Tegtmeier* 128 Ill.App. 280 (1906), 225 Ill. 275, 80 N.E. 130 (1907) there was evidence that defendant physician took every reasonable care and precaution, and there was evidence that the patient and his children were exposed to smallpox through others besides the physician. The physician was not held liable for transmitting smallpox to this family.

There are several modern cases which involve further extensions of this kind of responsibility and possible liability.

In *Gill v. Hartford Accident Indemnity Co.* 337 So.2d 420 (1976) an appellate court said that a physician of one patient had a duty to warn other patients or their physicians of a contagious disease in his patient where there was a risk that this disease might be transmitted to others. (See previous summary (2).)

In *Derrick v. Ontario Community Hospital* 47 Cal.App.3d 145, 120 Cal.Rptr. 566 (1975) the physician and the hospital where a patient with an unnamed contagious disease was hospitalized failed to report this contagious disease to the local health officer as required by law. After the patient

was discharged from the hospital, apparently this contagious disease was communicated to the plaintiff, who sued physician, hospital, patient, and patient's mother. An appellate court held that there was a cause of action, that is, there was an injury for which there was a remedy at law, but there might be some difficulty in proving that the failure to report was the proximal cause of the plaintiff's injuries. (See previous summary (2) and previous discussion (9).)

Gammill v. U.S. 727 F.2d 950 (1984) seems to go the other way. A contract physician of the federal government did not report a case of hepatitis as required by state law. The patient with hepatitis had children who were in day care with a husband and wife. The husband contracted hepatitis and sued the physician and the federal government as emloyer. The trial court and appellate court held that he had no claim.

In *Lipari v. Sears, Roebuck & Co.* 497 F.Supp. 185 (1980) the court said that a " ... physician patient relationship gave rise to a duty to warn third persons of possible exposure to contagious diseases." This is not specifically the holding of this case but is dicta in the opinion.

ANTIBIOTICS

Antibiotics and other anti-infectives have been known to cause side effects virtually since they were first given to human beings. In recent years these side effects have been the reason behind more and more law suits. The obvious trend is toward liability for more and more of the side effects even when the side effects could not be anticipated or when the side effects were well known. There is an expectation that antibiotics will be 100% efficacious with 0% side effects or toxicity. Anything less than this unachievable goal is unacceptable by much of the public and therefore actionable.

Besides the increasing JCAH requirements (guidelines or standards) demanding more and more in the way of monitoring the use of all drugs in the hospital and the increasing emphasis on medical staff quality assurance with a specific thrust on evaluation and continuous ongoing monitoring of antibiotic usage by written objective criteria, there have also been more and more law suits involving the use of antibiotics. For a general discussion see Nottebart (10).

Brannan v. Lankenau Hospital 417 A.2d 196 (1980). During esophagoscopy for removal of a piece of roast beef, the forceps opened suddenly. There was no visible evidence of perforation but shortly thereafter the patient's temperature, pulse, and respiration increased. A clinical diagnosis of perforated esophagus was made and antibiotics were ordered. The first dose of antibiotics was not given for 4 hours. Subsequently the patient had a stroke and lost the use of his right arm and leg. The issue was whether antibiotics had been administered at the earliest opportunity and whether the delay caused any of the damages.

Crowe v. John W. Harton Memorial Hospital 579 S.W.2d 888 (1979). The patient was given the wrong drug by a hospital nurse. The hospital admitted liability but argued that limit of liability was $20,000 by statute. The trial court agreed, and it was affirmed on appeal.

Doss v. U.S. 659 F.2d 863 (1981). A patient had a swollen right foot. He went to a podiatrist, who recommended an operation that the patient could not afford. He went to a Veterans Administration (VA) hospital where he was noted to have an increased temperature, pulse, and blood pressure, and he was sent to an orthopaedic clinic on an emergency basis. The patient was sent home and told to return in 4 days. When he returned, a white blood cell count and sedimentation rate were ordered. The physician did not order a culture and sensitivity, aspirate fluid, or do an incision and drainage but did prescribe cephalexin. Four days later the patient's foot "burst" and drained. The patient was diagnosed as having gas gangrene and a below-the-knee amputation was done. The patient was awarded $291,500 plus $30,000 for attorneys' fees.

Drexel v. Union Prescription Centers, Inc. 582 F.2d 781 (1978). A patient had a prescription for Aldactone, and when he returned to the pharmacy for refill he was given coumadin. He developed massive injuries as a result and died. The issue was whether the patient's estate could sue the franchisor of the pharmacy involved.

French Drug Company, Inc. v. Jones 367 So.2d 431 (1978). A physician prescribed Ethatab, and the pharmacy dispensed Estratab (an estrogen). This error was not discovered for a year. The patient suffered breast enlargement and impotence. A jury award of $135,000 to the patient was affirmed.

Garza v. Keillor 623 S.W.2d 669 (1981). A patient with a compound fracture of the right forearm had been placed in a cast of the arm and antibiotics were prescribed. An infection developed, but no Gram stain or culture and sensitivity were done. The patient developed a clostridial infection, and after a series of operations his right

arm was amputated below the elbow. There were significant issues of facts so that a directed verdict was not appropriate and there needed to be a trial on the merits.

Kernall v. U.S. 558 F.Supp. 280 (1982). A patient had a needle stuck in the wrist and an infection developed. A VA hospital allegedly treated this infection inappropriately. The patient was awarded $28,209.65.

Killeen v. Reinhardt 419 N.Y.S.2d 175 (1979). A patient was pregnant and had asthma. She had difficulty in breathing and was admitted to the hospital. She died on the third day in hospital, and the immediate cause of death was determined to be bronchial pneumonia. The patient's estate sued the hospital and the physicians but settled with the physicians prior to trial for $265,000. The trial proceeded against the hospital. The hospital was allegedly negligent in administering cephalothin to someone who was allergic to penicillin. A jury found against the hospital; the apportioned award would have been $275,000, but this was reversed and remanded for a new trial for the jury to specify on which theory of negligence they based their verdict.

King v. Retz 454 N.Y.S.2d 594 (1982). This case did not involve an antibiotic, and it has been discussed before (10). The patient died of malignant hyperthermia, and his estate alleged that death was due to the hospital's not having dantrolene. Dantrolene was widely used to treat malignant hyperthermia, and the patient's estate alleged that it was negligent to operate a hospital without having the drug available.

Leary v. Rupp 280 N.W.2d 466 (1979). A patient with sore throat, fever, and headaches was treated with Polycillin because she was allergic to penicillin[!]. After her reaction to the Polycillin she was treated with prednisone and improved. More than 5 years later she was diagnosed as having aseptic necrosis of her legs that was probably caused by the drugs she had taken. The appellate court reversed the verdict for the physician based on the statute of limitations.

Lennon v. U.S. 579 F.2d 12 (1978). A patient had badly fractured a leg in an auto accident. At the trial the judge found that insufficient cultures were taken of the wound and that improper antibiotics were administered. Subsequently osteomyelitis developed in the leg and it was eventually amputated. An award of $600,000 to the patient was affirmed on appeal.

McLean v. U.S. 613 F.2d 603 (1980). A physician prescribed Pronestyl for his patient, but an

Air Force pharmacy filled the prescription with Prostaphlin. The patient sued the federal government, and a trial court found for the federal government. The appellate court reversed, saying that the patient was entitled to recover damages for pain, suffering, and mental anguish during the 26 days he continued to have palpitations while on the wrong medicine.

O'Connell v. Albany Medical Center Hospital 475 N.Y.S.2d 543 (1984). A patient was treated with penicillin and "Cefadyl, a broad base antibiotic." The patient's culture revealed that the bacteria were not sensitive to the penicillin. The organisms were sensitive to 10 different antibiotics, but none of those antibiotics were prescribed for another 24 days after the culture report was returned. The expert testifying for the plaintiff was of the opinion that had proper antibiotics been prescribed, the patient's infection would have been cleared, thus increasing the chances of a successful skin graft, shortening his hospital stay, and probably reducing his permanent disability. The patient was awarded $150,000 and his wife $50,000.

Pharmaceutical Manufacturers Association, v. Whalen 446 N.Y.S.2d 217 (1981). In a suit challenging the constitutionality of a law allowing generic substitution, the law was held to be constitutional.

Richardson v. Lutheran Hospital of Brooklyn 417 N.Y.S.2d 526 (1979). A patient with intestinal blockage was operated on and 6 days later died of general sepsis. His wife sued the hospital alleging, inter alia, that the hospital did not administer the required amount of antibiotics. She won $470,000 for his wrongful death. A trial court set aside this verdict as excessive. The appellate court agreed and remanded for new trial on damages only.

Ullman v. Grant 450 N.Y.S.2d 955 (1982). A patient had a prescription for Septra D.S., and a physician had authorized generic substitution. The pharmacist filled the prescription with Bactrim D.S. When the patient had a drug reaction, he sued the pharmacy. The court found the pharmacy not liable and said that a pharmacist would not be negligent in making a generic substitution unless he knowingly dispensed an inferior drug (10).

U.S. v. Evers 643 F.2d 1043 (1981). A physician was not found guilty under Food and Drug Administration (FDA) laws of misbranding when he prescribed a drug for a use not approved by the FDA.

Wade v. Thomasville Orthopedic Clinic, Inc. 306 S.E.2d 366 (1983). A patient was hospitalized for 54 days for a fractured leg. He had had a Foley catheter in during virtually the entire stay. A urinary tract infection was found 8 days prior to his discharge. It was alleged that the antibiotics prescribed were not effective against the organism in the urine. The defendant clinic defended on the ground that the statute of limitations had passed, and won.

Waits v. U.S. 611 F.2d 550 (1980). A patient with compound fractures of his right hip and leg was treated with pins placed in the leg, and traction was used. An infection developed in a pin track. Empiric treatment with cephalexin was started. However, culture and sensitivity ordered December 26, 1972 were not reported until after January 5, 1973. On January 5, 1973 he was transferred to another hospital where culture and sensitivity and other studies revealed osteomyelitis due to *Escherichia coli* and *Pseudomonas*. Both of these organisms were resistant to the cephalexin which had been prescribed. His right leg was amputated. In the lawsuit the plaintiff (patient) won $266,823.36.

Westphal v. Guarino 394 A.2d 377 (1978). A patient had chills, headaches, and nausea and was diagnosed as having influenza. He was admitted to one hospital on February 6, 1972, was transferred to a second hospital on March 23, and died March 29. A death certificate gave cerebral infarction due to brain abscess due to meningitis as the cause of death. An autopsy showed no evidence of meningitis. The patient's widow sued, claiming there was negligence in diagnosing subarachnoid hemorrhage rather than a bacterial infection. She also claimed that there was negligence in administering an antibiotic which masked the growth of the bacteria. A trial court verdict for the defendant physicians was reversed on appeal because the trial court had excluded testimony of two of the plaintiff's expert witnesses; the case was remanded for a new trial.

Wilson v. Stilwill 309 N.E.2d 898 (1981). A patient had infection in the right arm postoperatively. He was treated with antibiotics after a culture and sensitivity were performed. Subsequently, his arm was permanently paralyzed. The trial court directed a verdict in favor of the hospital and the orthopaedic surgeon. It was affirmed on appeal, and it was noted that infections can occur without negligence.

Zito v. Friedman 430 N.Y.S.2d 78 (1980). The defendant oral surgeon had been treating the plaintiff, who had severe trauma to the jaw, with antibiotics for more than a month. The defendant stopped antibiotics and asked the plaintiff to return in 1 week for re-evaluation. The plaintiff did not return for more than 3 weeks. Later, when the patient sued the oral surgeon, one of the allegations was that stopping the antibiotics was negligence. The judgment for the plaintiff was reversed, and the case was dismissed. With respect to stopping antibiotics the court said, "At its worst, it would have been an error in professional judgment, and not malpractice." One is not liable for "a mere error of judgment, provided he does what he thinks is best after careful examination."

There are, of course, many other law suits involving side effects of one sort or another. See Table 4.1 for a listing of some that have been decided recently.

Some earlier cases involving immunizations have been discussed previously (11, 12).

Table 4.1. Recent Law Suits Involving Adverse Effects of Antibiotics or Vaccines

Case and Citation	Drug and Alleged Injury	Case and Citation	Drug and Alleged Injury
Addision v. Health and Hospital Governing Commission of Cook County 371 N.E.2d 1060 (1977).	Cephalothin in penicillin allergy.	Ezagul v. Dow Chemical 598 F.2d 727 (1979).	Quadrigen. Encephalopathy.
Bass v. Barksdale 671 S.W.2d 476 (1984).	INH and Ethambutol. Vision loss.	Fraley v. American Cyanamid Co. 570 F.Supp. 497 (1983).	Polio vaccine.
Berwald v. Kasal 301 N.W.2d 499 (1980).	Gentamicin. Myocardial infarction.	Givens v. Lederle 556 F.2d 1341 (1977).	Oral polio vaccine. Paralysis in recipient's mother.
Bluestein v. Upjohn Co. 430 N.E.2d 580 (1981).	Clindamycin. Colitis.	Grant v. Parke, Davis & Co. 544 F.2d 521 (1976).	Quadrigen.
Bonney v. Upjohn Co. 342 N.W.2d 551 (1983).	Lincomycin. Psychologic and physical disorders.	Griffin v. U.S. 351 F.Supp. 10 (1972).	Oral polio vaccine. Paralysis in recipient.
Bristol-Myers Co. v. Gonzales 561 S.W.2d 801 (1978).	Kanamycin and neomycin. Deafness.	Grinnell v. Pfizer 79 Cal.Rptr. 369 (1969).	Oral polio vaccine. Paralysis in recipient.
Calabrese v. Trenton State College 413 A.2d 315 (1980).	Rabies vaccine. Neurologic problem.	Grodin v. Grodin 301 N.W.2d 869 (1980).	Tetracycline. Discolored teeth. (See discussion (13)).
Callan v. Nordland 448 N.E.2d 651 (1983).	Neomycin.	Hawkes v. Mt. Sinai Hospital 426 N.Y.S.2d 745 (1980).	Sulfa drug in patient allergic to sulfa.
Caron v. U.S. 548 F.2d 366 (1976).	DPT, oral polio vaccine, and typhoid vaccine. Seizures and mental retardation.	Hawkins v. Greenberg 304 S.E.2d 922 (1983).	Sulfa vaginal suppositories. Anaphylactic reaction.
Daniels v. Hadley Memorial Hospital 566 F.2d 749 (1977).	Penicillin. Anaphylactic reaction.	Hawkins v. Richardson Merrell 249 S.E.2d 286 (1978).	Sulfa vaginal suppositories. Anaphylactic reaction.
Davis v. U.S. 642 F.2d 328 (1981).	Oral polio vaccine. Paralysis in recipient.	Hitchcock v. U.S. 665 F.2d 354 (1981).	Rabies vaccine. Neurologic problems.
Dunn v. Lederle Laboratories 328 N.W.2d 576 (1982).	Oral polio vaccine. Paralysis in recipient's mother.	Jackson v. State of Louisiana 428 So.2d 1073 (1983).	INH. Hepatitis.
Edwards v. St. Mary's Hospital 327 N.W.2d 377 (1982).	Penicillin. Cardiovascular collapse, coma, and death.	Javitz v. Slatus 461 N.Y.S.2d 44 (1983).	Clindamycin.
Ewell Engineering & Contracting Co. v. Cato 361 So.2d 728 (1978).	Gentamicin. Loss of vestibular function.	Knox v. Eli Lilly 592 F.2d 317 (1979).	Killed polio vaccine. Paralysis.
		Kubrick v. U.S. 581 F.2d 1092 (1978). 100 Sup.Ct. 352 (1979).	Neomycin. Bilateral nerve deafness.

Kukowski v. Piskin 327 N.W.2d 832 (1982).	Ethambutol. Vision loss.
Lemar v. U.S. 580 F.Supp. 37 (1984).	DPT and oral polio vaccine. Infantile spasm syndrome.
Loge v. U.S. 662 F.2d 1268 (1981).	Oral polio vaccine. Paralysis in recipient's mother.
Lurus v. Bristol Laboratories 574 P.2d 391 (1978).	Kanamycin. Hearing loss.
Maher v. Worker's Compensation Board 190 Cal.Rptr. 904 (1983).	Antituberculosis medicine. Adverse reaction.
Mauldin v. Upjohn Co. 697 F.2d 644 (1983).	Clindamycin. Colitis.
McCarthy v. Bristol Laboratories 401 N.Y.S.2d 509 (1978). 449 N.Y.S.2d 280 (1982).	Kanamycin and Cephalothin. Injuries including blindness.
Mercurdo v. County of Milwaukee 264 N.W.2d 258 (1978).	Penicillin. Ischemic necrosis after skin infiltration.
Mielke v. Condell Memorial Hospital 463 N.E.2d 216 (1984).	Gentamicin. Vestibular dysfunction.
Mitchell v. Parker 315 S.E.2d 76 (1984).	Gentamicin. Renal damage.
Moncrief v. Fuqua 610 S.W.2d 720 (1979).	Cycloserine. Encephalitis.
Moodie v. Santoni 441 A.2d 323 (1982).	INH. Hepatitis and death.
Morris v. Parke, Davis & Co. 573 F.Supp. 1324 (1983).	DPT.
Muilenberg v. Upjohn Co. 320 N.W.2d 358 (1982).	Clindamycin. Colitis.
O'Brien v. Angley 407 N.E.2d 490 (1980).	Gentamicin. Partial hearing loss and vestibular dysfunction.
Oksenholt v. Lederle Laboratories 656 P.2d 293 (1982).	Ethambutol. Blindness.
Peltier v. Eldredge 345 N.W.2d 605 (1983).	Gentamicin, neomycin. Hearing loss.
Perkins v. Windsor Hospital 455 A.2d 810 (1982).	Metronidazole.
Phillips v. Mease Hospital and Clinic 445 So.2d 1058 (1984).	Antibiotics. Injuries.
Pratt v. Stein 444 A.2d 674 (1982).	Chloramphenicol and neomycin. Deafness.
Reis v. Pfizer 402 N.Y.S.2d 401 (1978).	Oral polio vaccine. Paralysis in recipient.
Richards v. Upjohn Co. 625 P.2d 1192 (1980).	Neomycin, polymycin, and bacitracin. Deafness.
Rodriquez v. Jackson 574 P.2d 481 (1977).	Streptomycin. Vestibular dysfunction.
Salter v. Upjohn Co. 593 F.2d 649 (1979).	Clindamycin. Death.
Sanderson v. Upjohn Co. 578 F.Supp. 338 (1984).	Clindamycin. Death.
Santoni v. Moodie 452 A.2d 1223 (1982).	INH. Hepatitis.
Scales v. U.S. 685 F.2d 970 (1982).	Rubella vaccine. Congenital rubella.
Schering Corp. v. Giesecke 589 S.W.2d 516 (1979).	Gentamicin and kanamycin. Deafness.
Schindler v. Lederle Laboratories 725 F.2d 1036 (1983).	Oral polio vaccine. Paralysis in recipient.
Sewell v. Wilson 641 P.2d 1070 (1982).	Gentamicin. Vestibular and auditory dysfunction.
Sheehan v. Pima County 660 P.2d 486 (1982).	Oral polio vaccine. Death in recipient's father.

Table 4.1.—Continued

Case and Citation	Drug and Alleged Injury	Case and Citation	Drug and Alleged Injury
Sheffield v. Eli Lilly & Co. 192 Cal.Rptr. 870 (1983).	Killed polio vaccine. Encephalitis.	Werner v. Upjohn Co. 628 F.2d 848 (1980).	Clindamycin. Colitis.
Sheridan v. U.S. 542 F.Supp. 1243 (1982).	Sulfa. Agranulocytosis and death.	Willoughby v. Wilkins 310 S.E.2d 90 (1983).	Gentamicin. Deafness.
Stanback vs. Parke, Davis & Co. 657 F.2d 642 (1981).	Influenza vaccine. Guillain-Barré syndrome.	Wolfgruber v. Upjohn Co. 436 N.Y.S.2d 614 (1980).	Clindamycin. Colitis.
Timm v. Upjohn Co. 624 F.2d 536 (1980).	Clindamycin. Colitis.	Wright v. U.S. 507 F.Supp. 147 (1980).	Penicillin. Anaphylactic reaction.
Walton v. Pfizer & Co. 590 P.2d 1190 (1978).	Vaccines. Paralysis in lower extremities.		

COMMITTEE RECORDS

The availability of medical records to plaintiffs in law suits has been a major issue in a large number of cases. This has been discussed previously (14, 15).

At this point only five cases seem to mention infection control committee minutes or records specifically.

In *City of Edmond v. Parr* 587 P.2d 56 (1978) the records of the hospital infection control committee and records of an investigation of a staphylococcal infection at the time of a plaintiff's infection were protected. That is, the plaintiff could not get them.

In *Farley v. County of Nassau* 459 N.Y.S.2d 470 (1983) infection committee minutes were not subject to disclosure to the plaintiff.

In *Sherman v. District Court in and for the City and County of Denver* 637 P.2d 378 (1981) the court took the very narrow view that the only records protected were those protected by statute. This statute protected records submitted as required by state or federal law as part of utilization review function. The appellate court sent the case back to the trial court for a determination of this issue.

In *Spears v. Mason* 303 So.2d 260 (1974) the plaintiff was allowed access to hospital infection committee reports as they related to the patient's case and the time he was hospitalized.

In *Young v. King* 344 A.2d 792 (1976) plaintiff was allowed access to hospital infection committee records as they related to the patient's infection and death.

Other than these few cases involving infection control committees specifically, there are many others involving peer review committees or even specific committees or records.

First, there will be a brief outline of cases in which discovery of records or some information was allowed. Then there is Table 4.2, which lists cases in which peer review or other committees' minutes or reports were protected from discovery.

Baxter County Newspapers, Inc. v. Medical Staff of Baxter General Hospital 622 S.W.2d 495 (1981). (Arkansas) A credentials committee hearing was required to be public. This was not specifically protected by statute.

Carroll v. St. Luke's Hospital of Newburgh 457 N.Y.S.2d 128 (1982). Peer review committee records were discoverable.

Gadd v. News-Press Publishing Co., Inc. 412 So.2d 894 (1982). (Florida) The personnel files of staff physicians and utilization review records of a public hospital could be inspected by a news-

Table 4.2. Cases in Which Peer Review or Other Committees' Minutes or Reports Were Protected from Discovery

Case and Citation	Court Ruling	Case and Citation	Court Ruling
Attorney General v. Bruce 335 N.W.2d 697 (1983).	Peer review records did not have to be disclosed to state attorney general.	Hollowell v. Jove 279 S.E.2d 430 (1981). 628 F.2d 513 (1980).	Confidentiality of medical records protected by statute but not retroactively.
Beth Israel Hospital and Geriatric Center v. District Court in and for the City and County of Denver 683 P.2d 343 (1984).	Hospital review committees' records were protected.	Holly v. Auld 450 So.2d 217 (1984).	Statute protecting records of medical review committees applies to other actions besides medical malpractice.
Brandwein v. Gustman 367 So.2d 725 (1978).	Report of a hospital committee that investigated staff members was protected.	Jenkins v. Wu 468 N.E.2d 1162 (1984).	Medical peer review records were protected.
City of Williston v. Roadlander 425 So.2d 1175 (1983).	Medical review committee records were protected.	Kappas v. Chestnut Lodge 709 F.2d 878 (1983).	Transcripts of medical review committees were protected.
Coburn v. Seda 677 P.2d 173 (1984).	Regularly constituted hospital committees whose duties were to review and evaluate quality of care were protected.	Long v. Pinto 179 Cal.Rptr. 182 (1981).	Committee member's letter to Board of Medical Quality Assurance was protected.
Daly v. Genovese 466 N.Y.S.2d 428 (1983).	Peer review committee records were not discoverable in a defamation action.	Matviuw v. Johnson 444 N.E.2d 606 (1982).	Statute protected hospital medical committees' reports but not retroactively.
Danklef v. Wilmington Medical Center 429 A.2d 509 (1981).	Credentials committee records could not be subpoenaed.	McClatchy Newspapers v. University of California at Davis Medical Center Docket #300115, January 20, 1982.	Medical staff minutes and audits of use of clindamycin and cephalosporins were protected.
Eubanks v. Ferrier 267 S.E.2d 230 (1980).	Medical review committee records were privileged and nondiscoverable.	Mennes v. South Chicago Community Hospital 427 N.E.2d 952 (1981).	Records concerning credentialing were not discoverable.
Franco v. District Court in and for the City and County of Denver 641 P.2d 922 (1982).	A suspended surgeon could not obtain records of peer review committees.	Morse v. Gerity 520 F.Supp. 470 (1981).	Peer review committee records were not discoverable.
Griffin v. Cortland Memorial Hospital 446 N.Y.S.2d 430 (1981).	Hospital staff have qualified privilege in what they say about patients in chart and to physicians and hospital personnel.	Murphy v. Wood 667 P.2d 859 (1983).	Records of tumor board meetings were not discoverable.
Hayden v. Foryt 407 So.2d 535 (1981).	There is a privilege for medical staff discussion about quality of work of physician.	Palmer v. City of Rome 466 N.Y.S.2d 238 (1983).	Pathology reports were not discoverable.
		Parkson v. Central DuPage Hospital 435 N.E.2d 140 (1982).	Hospital records did not have to be disclosed to other patients.
		Parkway General Hospital v. Allinson 453 So.2d 123 (1984).	Medical staff review committee minutes were protected.

Table 4.2.—*Continued*

Case and Citation	Court Ruling	Case and Citation	Court Ruling
Posey v. District Court in and for the Second Judicial District 586 P.2d 36 (1978).	Records of hospital review committee were protected.	Segal v. Roberts 380 So.2d 1048 (1979).	Hospital committee's records were protected.
Qasem v. Kozarek 716 F.2d 1172 (1983).	Individuals on credentials committee were protected by statute from civil liability as long as acting in good faith.	Sitva v. State of New York 441 N.Y.S.2d 43 (1981).	Records of committees performing medical review function were protected.
Samuelson v. Susen 576 F.2d 546 (1978).	Hospital review committee records could not be obtained for a defamation suit.	West Covina Hospital v. Superior Court of the County of Los Angeles 200 Cal.Rptr. 162 (1984).	Hospital staff committee minutes were protected.
		Young v. Gersten 381 N.E.2d 353 (1978).	Hospital review committee records were protected by statute.

paper. The state statute did not specifically protect them.

Good Samaritan Hospital Association v. Simon 370 So.2d 1174 (1979). Although a statute barred discovery of medical review committee records, there was another statute that granted immunity to members of medical review committees who did not act with malice. Therefore, the court said that records of medical review committees could be discovered when there was a question of malice on the part of some of the committee members.

Robinson v. Magovern 83 F.R.D. 79 (1979). In a federal antitrust action brought by a physician denied staff privileges at a hospital, the federal court allowed discovery of peer review activities even though protected by state statute because the need for pertinent evidence was greater than the need for protection of hospital committee records.

State of Missouri ex rel Chandra v. Sprinkle 678 S.W.2d 804 (1984). Peer review records were discoverable. The state law did not protect medical staff committee *records* but did protect *members* of medical review, peer review, utilization review, pharmacy review, and similar committees from liability to anyone subject to actions of these committees unless such actions were malicious or unsupportable.

Tucson Medical Center, Inc. v. Misevch 545 P.2d 958 (1976). This court took the position that minutes and reports of committees were not subject to disclosure by discovery to the plaintiffs by statute, but the information considered by these committees could be obtained by subpoena.

Unnamed Physician v. Commission on Medical Discipline 400 A.2d 396 (1979). The supreme court of Maryland said that records of hospital review committees were available to the state's Commission on Medical Discipline. The court held that the statute that protected these records from discovery applied only to use of these records in civil actions and did not prevent the Commission on Medical Discipline from obtaining the records. Cf. *Cocco v. Maryland Commission on Medical Discipline* 384 A.2d 766 (1978).

Wesley Medical Center v.Clark 669 P.2d 209 (1983). A Kansas court allowed discovery of peer review committee records. There is no statutory protection of such records in Kansas.

NOSOCOMIAL INFECTIONS

Table 4.3 lists cases (in alphabetical order) that involve hospital-acquired infections and related topics. Separate sections discussing cases related to AIDS, hepatitis B, herpes, *Legionella*, and toxic shock syndrome follow.

Table 4.3. Recent Law Suits Involving Various Nosocomial Infections

Case and Citation	Basis of Lawsuit	Case and Citation	Basis of Lawsuit
Adamski v. Tacoma General Hospital 579 P.2d 970 (1978).	Staphylococcal infection after trauma and emergency room suturing.	Burcl v. North Carolina Baptist Hospital 266 S.E.2d 726 (1980).	Postoperative infection.
Albersett v. Country Mutual Insurance 398 N.E.2d 611 (1979).	Gas gangrene after trauma on farm and hospitalization.	Burns v. Hartford Hospital 472 A.2d 1257 (1984).	Streptococcal infection postoperative (cutdowns).
Banton v. Marks 623 S.W.2d 113 (1981).	Septicemia possibly secondary to decubiti.	Butler v. Berkeley 25 N.C.App. 325 (1975). 213 S.E.2d 571 (1975).	Nosocomial infection.
Barrella v. Richmond Memorial Hospital 453 N.Y.S.2d 444 (1982).	Postoperative jaundice. See "Hepatitis B."	Byers v. Burleson 713 F.2d 856 (1983).	Postoperative infection. Subsequent legal malpractice case.
Bearce v. Bowers 587 S.W.2d 219 (1979).	Infected wound after trauma and emergency room treatment.	Carter v. Carr 314 S.E.2d 281 (1984).	Postoperative infection.
Bell v. Western Pennsylvania 437 A.2d 978 (1981).	Gas gangrene after trauma and hospitalization.	Cashio v. Baton Rouge General Hospital 378 So.2d 182 (1979).	Postoperative staphylococcal infection.
Belle Bonfils Memorial Blood Bank v. Hansen 579 P.2d 1158 (1978).	See "Hepatitis B."	Charles v. Meyer Medical Group, S.C. 421 N.E.2d 334 (1981).	Postoperative infection.
Berroyer v. Hertz 672 F.2d 334 (1982).	Postoperative infection.	Chavous v. Richmond County Hospital Authority 313 S.E.2d 492 (1984).	Postoperative staphylococcal infection from instruments, dressings, and sutures.
Bloskas v. Murray 646 P.2d 907 (1982). 618 P.2d 719 (1980).	Postoperative infection.	Ciprut v. Moore 540 F.Supp. 817 (1981).	Postoperative infection.
Booker v. Duke Medical Center 256 S.E.2d 189 (1979).	See "Hepatitis B."	Clark v. Hawkes Hospital of Mt. Carmel 459 N.E.2d 559 (1984).	Staphylococcal endocarditis after inappropriate hospital treatment.
Bost v. Riley 262 S.E.2d 391 (1980).	Postoperative infection.	Colton v. New York Hospital 414 N.Y.S.2d 866 (1979).	Postoperative infection.
Bowes v. International Pharmakon Laboratories, Inc. 314 N.W.2d 642 (1981).	Meningitis secondary to contaminated antiseptic.	Conklin v. Montefiore Hospital and Medical Center 421 N.Y.S.2d 159 (1979).	Postoperative infection.
Broughton v. Cutter Laboratories 622 F.2d 458 (1980).	See "Hepatitis B."		

Table 4.3.—*Continued*

Case and Citation	Basis of Lawsuit
Conrad v. St. Clair 599 P.2d 292 (1979).	Postoperative infection.
Cooley v. Carter-Wallace, Inc. 478 N.Y.S.2d 375 (1984).	Postoperative infection.
Cooper v. Edinbergh 410 N.Y.S.2d 962 (1978).	Postoperative infection.
Cordova v. Hartford Accident & Indemnity Company 378 So.2d 1088 (1979). 387 So.2d 574 (1980).	Postoperative infection.
Cornelius v. Gipe 625 S.W.2d 880 (1981).	Postoperative staphylococcal infection.
Cornfeldt v. Tongen 295 N.W.2d 638 (1980).	See "Hepatitis B."
Crain v. Allison 443 A.2d 558 (1982).	Postprocedure (joint injection) infection.
Cummings v. Fondak 474 N.Y.S.2d 356 (1983).	See "Herpes."
Cunningham v. Yankton Clinic, P.A. 262 N.W.2d 508 (1978).	Postoperative infection.
Dale Manufacturing Company v. Commonwealth of Pennsylvania, Workmen's Compensation Appeal Board 382 A.2d 1256 (1978).	Postoperative infection.
D'Angona v. County of Los Angeles 613 P.2d 238 (1980). 166 Cal.Rptr. 177 (1980).	Nosocomial meningococcemia.
DeBattista v. Argonaut-Southwest Insurance Company 410 So.2d 279 (1982).	See "Hepatitis B."
403 So.2d 26 (1981). 385 So.2d 518 (1980).	See "Hepatitis B."
Matter of DeMarco 414 A.2d 1339 (1980).	Post-lumbar puncture injuries.
District of Columbia v. Barriteau 399 A.2d 563 (1979).	Gas gangrene and osteomyelitis.
Doss v. U.S. 659 F.2d 863 (1981). 476 F.Supp. 630 (1979).	See "Hepatitis B."
Durden v. American Hospital Supply Corporation 375 So.2d 1096 (1979).	
Easter v. Lexington Memorial Hospital 271 S.E.2d 545 (1980). 278 S.E.2d 253 (1981).	Tetanus after burn treatment in emergency room.
Ellis v. International Playtex, Inc. 745 F.2d 292 (1984).	See "Toxic Shock Syndrome."
Ellis v. Springfield Women's Clinic, P.C. 678 P.2d 268 (1984).	Postpartum infection.
Evans v. Stoval 403 N.E.2d 1321 (1980).	Postoperative infection and subsequent countersuit.
Feinstein v. Massachusetts General Hospital 643 F.2d 880 (1981).	See "Hepatitis B."
Ferguson v. Lankford 374 So.2d 1205 (1979).	Postpartum infection.
Fisher v. Sibley Memorial Hospital 403 A.2d 1130 (1979).	See "Hepatitis B."

Fitzgerald v. Manning 679 F.2d 341 (1982).	Nosocomial pneumonia.
France v. St. Clare's Hospital and Health Center 441 N.Y.S.2d 79 (1981).	Positive VDRL in blood donor.
Gammill v. U.S. 727 F.2d 950 (1984).	Hepatitis. See "Historical Background of Infections and the Law."
Garza v. Keillor 623 S.W.2d 669 (1981).	Postoperative infection.
Gaston v. Hunter 588 P.2d 326 (1978).	Postoperative septicemia and meningitis.
Gaudynski v. Corbett 401 N.E.2d 1218 (1980).	Postoperative infection.
Geisel v. Flushing Hospital and Medical Center 417 N.Y.S.2d 760 (1979).	Infection after trauma and emergency room treatment.
George Bennett Motor Express Inc. v. Safeco Life Insurance Company 575 F.Supp. 449 (1983).	Infection after injection.
Gilmore v. St. Anthony Hospital 598 P.2d 1200 (1979).	See "Hepatitis B."
Goddard v. Hickman 685 P.2d 530 (1984).	Postoperative infection.
Hareng v. Blanke 279 N.W.2d 437 (1979).	Postoperative infection.
Harrington v. Cohen 374 N.E.2d 344 (1978).	Postoperative infection.
Harris v. Roberts 458 N.Y.S.2d 719 (1983).	Tuberculosis in a psychiatric center.
Harris v. State of Louisiana, through Huey P. Long Hospital 371 So.2d 1221 (1979); 378 So.2d 383 (1979).	Posttraumatic gas gangrene.
Hartman v. Cooper 474 A.2d 959 (1984).	Posttraumatic osteomyelitis.
Hardwell v. Pittman 428 So.2d 1049 (1983).	Postoperative infection.
Hensley v. Heavrin 282 S.E.2d 854 (1981).	Misdiagnosis of syphilis.
Higgins v. State of Louisiana, Department of Health & Human Resources 451 So.2d 142 (1984).	Nosocomial viral encephalitis in intern.
Jines v. Abarbanel 143 Cal.Rptr. 818 (1978).	Postoperative infection.
Johnson v. Harper Grace Hospital 284 N.W.2d 520 (1979).	Postoperative infection.
Johnson v. Podger 257 S.E.2d 684 (1979).	Postoperative infection.
Kathleen K. v. Robert B. 198 Cal.Rptr. 273 (1984).	See "Herpes."
Kehm v. Proctor & Gamble Manufacturing Company 724 F.2d 613 (1984).	See "Toxic Shock Syndrome."
Kernall v. U.S. 558 F.Supp. 280 (1982).	Postoperative infection.
Kieswetter v. Center Pavilion Hospital 662 S.W.2d 24 (1983).	Postoperative eye infection.
Kinkin v. Heupel 305 N.W.2d 589 (1981).	Postoperative infection.
Kinning v. Nelson 281 N.W.2d 849 (1979).	Postpartum osteomyelitis.
Langton v. Brown 591 S.W.2d 84 (1979).	Nosocomial urinary tract infection.
LaRocca v. Dalsheim 467 N.Y.S.2d 302 (1983).	See "AIDS."
Leahy v. Henry Ford Hospital 271 N.W.2d 34 (1978).	Postoperative infection secondary to intravenous fluids.

Table 4.3.—*Continued*

Case and Citation	Basis of Lawsuit	Case and Citation	Basis of Lawsuit
LeFever v. American Red Cross 310 N.W.2d 278 (1981).	See "Hepatitis B."	Molien v. Kaiser Foundation Hospitals 167 Cal.Rptr. 831. 616 P.2d 813 (1980). 158 Cal.Rptr. 107 (1979).	Misdiagnosis of syphilis.
Lemke v. St. Margaret Hospital 552 F.Supp. 833 (1982).	Post-trauma death.	Newell v. Corres. 466 N.E.2d 1085 (1984).	Postoperative infection.
Lennon v. U.S. 579 F.2d 12 (1978).	Post-traumatic infection. Improper antibiotics used.	New York State Association for Retarded Children, Inc. v. Carey 612 F.2d 644 (1979). 466 F.Supp. 479 (1978).	See "Hepatitis B."
Leyson v. Krause 285 N.W.2d 451 (1979).	Postoperative infection.	O'Neil v. State of Missouri 662 S.W.2d 260 (1983).	Pneumococcal meningitis in resident at state training center.
Lingquist v. Ayerst Laboratories, Inc. 607 P.2d 1339 (1980).	Postoperative infection.	Oltmans v. Orthopaedic and Fracture Clinic, P.A. 278 N.W.2d 538 (1979).	Postoperative infection.
Lipari v. Sears, Roebuck & Company 497 F.Supp. 185 (1980).	Requirement to report infections.	Osborne v. County of Los Angeles 154 Cal.Rptr. 129 (1979).	Postoperative infection.
Livingston v. Gribetz 549 F.Supp. 238 (1982).	See "Herpes."	Patten v. Milam 480 A.2d 774 (1984).	Postoperative infection.
Long v. Ponca City Hospital, Inc. 593 P.2d 1081 (1979).	Postoperative infection.	Patterson v. Kent General Hospital, Inc. 541 F.Supp. 628 (1982).	Nosocomial tuberculosis in hospital employee.
Longman v. Jasiek 414 N.E.2d 520 (1980).	Postoperative infection.	Peerman v. Sidicane 605 S.W.2d 242 (1980).	Misdiagnosis of gonorrhea.
May v. Moore 424 So.2d 596 (1982).	Postpartum meningitis.	Peters v. McCalla 461 F.Supp. 14 (1978).	Postoperative infection.
McBroom v. Zevallos 244 S.E.2d 19 (1978).	Hospital-acquired coccidioidomycosis in lab technician.	Peterson v. Hart 278 N.W.2d 133 (1979).	Postoperative infection.
McCormack v. Lindberg 352 N.W.2d 30 (1984).	See "Hepatitis B."	Pinky v. Winer 674 S.W.2d 158 (1984).	Postoperative infection.
McCormick v. Avret 267 S.E.2d 759 (1980).	Postinjection infection.		
Meeks v. Coan 302 So.2d 418 (1983).	Nosocomial infection of arteriovenous fistula.		
Mendez v. State of Oregon 669 P.2d 364 (1983).	Obstructive brain infection.		
Mercer v. Chi 282 N.W.2d 697 (1979).	Postvenogram infection.		

Plutshack v. University of Minnesota Hospitals 316 N.W.2d 1 (1982).	Postpartum meningitis.
Pommeranz v. State of Minnesota, Department of Public Welfare, Faribault State Hospital 261 N.W.2d 90 (1977).	See "Hepatitis B."
Priest v. Lindig 583 P.2d 173 (1978). 591 P.2d 1299 (1979).	Postoperative infection.
Proce v. Franklin General Hospital 442 N.Y.S.2d 147 (1981).	Postoperative infection.
Pullins v. Fentress County General Hospital 594 S.W.2d 663 (1979).	Nosocomial recluse spider bite.
Richardson v. Lutheran Hospital of Brooklyn 417 N.Y.S.2d 526 (1979).	Postoperative infection.
Roark v. St. Paul Fire and Marine Insurance Co. 415 So.2d 295 (1982).	Postoperative infection.
Robert v. Chodoff 393 A.2d 853 (1978).	Postoperative infection.
Roper v. Markle 375 N.E.2d 934 (1978).	Postoperative infection.
Ruane v. Niagara Falls Memorial Medical Center 470 N.Y.S.2d 576. 458 N.E.2d 1253 (1983).	Postoperative infection.
Sacred Heart Medical Center v. Carrado 579 P.2d 412 (1978).	See "Hepatitis B."
Sacred Heart Medical Center v. Department of Labor and Industries 600 P.2d 1015 (1979).	See "Hepatitis B."
St. Paul Fire and Marine Insurance Company v. Speerstra 666 P.2d 255 (1983).	Postoperative infection.
St. Paul Fire and Marine Insurance Company v. Prothro 590 S.W.2d 35 (1979).	Postoperative infection.
Samuels v. Health and Hospitals Corporation of the City of New York 591 F.2d 195 (1979).	See "Hepatitis B."
Sartin v. St. Paul Fire and Marine Insurance Co. 359 So.2d 649 (1978).	Postoperative infection.
Schmidt v. Intermountain Health Care 635 P.2d 99 (1981).	Postoperative infection.
Schmidt v. Heid No. MM84-IV (Morrison Cty. Dist. Ct. Minn. Jan. 17, 1984).	Misdiagnosis of bacterial endocarditis.
Shepherd v. McGinnis 257 Iowa 35. 131 N.W.2d 475 (1964).	Discussion on requirement to test presterilized equipment.
Sherrill v. McBride 603 S.W.2d 365 (1980).	Postoperative infection.
Smitherman v. New York City Department of Correction Investigation Complaint Unit 557 F.Supp. 877 (1983).	Improper treatment of syphilis.
Spadaccini v. Dolan 407 N.Y.S.2d 840 (1978).	Nosocomial pneumonia.

Table 4.3.—*Continued*

Case and Citation	Basis of Lawsuit
Stanley v. Fisher 417 N.E.2d 932 (1981).	Postoperative infection.
Steiner v. Ciba-Geigy Corporation 364 So.2d 47 (1978).	Herpes zoster.
Stewart v. City of New Orleans 418 So.2d 1389 (1982).	Nosocomial gangrene from restraints.
Tamminen v. Aetna Casualty and Surety Company 314 S.W.2d 879 (1981).	Postoperative infection.
Taylor v. Dirico 606 P.2d 3 (1980).	Postoperative infection.
Terrell v. West Paces Ferry Hospital, Inc. 292 S.E.2d 433 (1982).	Postoperative infection.
Tripp v. Pate 271 S.E.2d 407 (1980).	Postoperative infection.
Vanderdoes v. Ochsner Clinic 377 So.2d 1368 (1979).	See "Hepatitis B."
Vaughn v. North Carolina Department of Human Resources 252 S.E.2d 792 (1979). 240 S.E.2d 456 (1977).	Cytomegalovirus.
Villetto v. Weilbaecher 377 So.2d 132 (1979).	Herpes zoster.
Wade v. Thomasville Orthopedic Clinic, Inc. 306 S.E.2d 366 (1983).	Nosocomial urinary tract infection.
Waits v. U.S. 611 F.2d 550 (1980).	Postoperative infection.
Weeks v. Crow 169 Cal.Rptr. 830 (1980).	Postpartum infection.
Westphal v. Guarino 394 A.2d 377 (1978). 394 A.2d 354 (1978).	Negligence in antibiotic administration.
Whetsell v. Mutual Life Insurance Company of New York 669 F.2d 955 (1982).	Endocarditis secondary to intravenous needle.
White v. Edison 361 So.2d 1292 (1978).	Postpartum infection.
Williams v. Bennett 582 S.W.2d 577 (1979). 610 S.W.2d 144 (1980).	Postoperative infection.
Wilson v. Clark 417 N.E.2d 1322 (1981). 399 N.E.2d 651 (1980).	Postoperative infection.
Wilson v. Stilwill 309 N.W.2d 898 (1981).	Postoperative infection.
Wise v. Doctors Hospital North 455 N.E.2d 1032 (1982).	Nosocomial septicemia secondary to decubiti.
Woerth v. U.S. 714 F.2d 648 (1983).	See "Hepatitis B."

AIDS

Although most of us have heard about various transfusion-related AIDS cases that have been filed, I could find only one case involving AIDS that has been reported so far.

In a suit by prisoners in New York against the state, it was held that *if* the state congregated all prisoners with AIDS in one facility then the prisoners in that facility were entitled to a 30-day notice before that occurred. *LaRocca v. Dalsheim* 467 N.Y.S.2d 302 (1983).

Hepatitis B

In the past there were many cases involving transfusion-related hepatitis. These were clinically diagnosed as serum hepatitis. Whether these were hepatitis B or not is indeterminable. Over the last several years there have been a number of cases involving hepatitis. In some of these the disease was generic hepatitis. In others the specific hepatitis was given. In even others, like *Barrella v. Richmond Memorial Hospital* 453 N.Y.S.2d 444 (1982) jaundice occurred postoperatively and no other diagnosis was given.

In *Belle Bonfils Memorial Blood Bank v. Hansen* 579 P.2d 1158 (1978) the issue was whether supplying blood was a *sale* and the blood a *product*. As a sale there are certain implied warranties of fitness of the product sold.

In *Booker v. Duke Medical Center* 256 S.E.2d 189 (1979) a hospital laboratory technician who got blood on his fingers while testing samples contracted serum hepatitis and died. The issue was whether the hospital had to pay workmen's compensation for this illness. The court held that he had a greater risk of acquiring serum hepatitis than employees in general or members of the public.

In *Broughton v. Cutter Laboratories* 622 F.2d 458 (1980) a prisoner alleged that he contracted "infectious hepatitis" because of the blood-drawing techniques of the manufacturer (defendant).

In *Cornfeldt v. Tongen* 295 N.W.2d 638 (1980) the patient had a perforated gastric ulcer. At the time of the repair of this lesion some suspicious tissue was seen and examined by biopsy. This was diagnosed as carcinoma. She came back for surgery for this about a month later. Clinically she was well, but two tests showed liver abnormalities. Operation was performed without incident. Several days postoperatively she developed jaundice and died of liver failure. After two trials, the decision for the plaintiff's estate was reversed.

In *DeBattista v. Argonaut-Southwest Insurance*

Co. 403 So.2d 26 (1982), 410 So.2d 279 (1981), 385 So.2d 518 (1980) a patient received 3 units of blood in connection with surgery. A month later she was diagnosed as having hepatitis B. A trial court dismissed the action against the blood bank, hospital, and physicians; the appellate court affirmed. The state supreme court reversed that with respect to the blood bank and imposed strict liability on the blood bank (three judges dissenting).

Matter of DeMarco 414 A.2d 1339 (1980) must set some sort of record. A physician allegedly caused 92 cases of hepatitis among his patients by using improperly sterilized needles and syringes. His license was permanently revoked and he was fined $20,200.

Durden v. American Hospital Supply Corporation 375 So.2d 1096 (1979). In this case a regular donor was notified by a donor center that he had hepatitis antigen in his blood. He later contracted "infectious hepatitis" and he sued the donor center, alleging use of a dirty needle, failing to use a sterile needle, and failure to inspect the needle. The issue was whether the 2-year statute of limitations for medical malpractice applied or whether the 4-year statute of limitations for general negligence applied. The trial court dismissed the case, ruling that the 2-year statute of limitations had run. The appellate court reversed the trial court, holding that the 4-year statute applied because no patient care was involved.

Feinstein v. Massachusetts General Hospital 643 F.2d 880 (1981). A patient developed hepatitis after a transfusion. It was claimed that the blood was contaminated. Judgment for the hospital was affirmed on appeal.

Fisher v. Sibley Memorial Hospital 403 A.2d 1130 (1979). A patient had rectal bleeding. She received a 1-unit transfusion. Two months later she developed hepatitis. The transfused blood had been tested twice for hepatitis markers, and was negative both times. A jury verdict for the hospital was affirmed on appeal. The appellate court noted that blood transfusion was a *service* and not a *sale*; therefore, there was no warranty of fitness and no strict liability.

Gammill v. U.S. 727 F.2d 950 (1984). This case is discussed above under "Historical Background of Infections and the Law."

Gilmore v. St. Anthony Hospital 598 P.2d 1200 (1979). The patient developed hepatitis after a blood transfusion. A summary judgment in favor of the defendant hospital was reversed. It was not appropriate where there were issues of fact. The fact issue to be considered at trial was whether the hospital was negligent in screening the blood donor even though the court noted that at the time of the transfusion there was no reliable test to determine the presence of hepatitis.

LeFever v. American Red Cross 310 N.W.2d 278 (1981). In this case a patient received transfusion of platelets on February 18, 1976. That same day her physician told her that at least 1 unit of the platelets was infected with hepatitis. On July 23, 1976 she was readmitted to the hospital with what was diagnosed as serum hepatitis. The defendant raised the issue of statute of limitations; this was upheld by the trial court and affirmed on appeal.

McCormack v. Lindberg 352 N.W.2d 30 (1984). A patient had thoracic surgery and received several units of blood. Subsequently, the patient developed a chronic hepatitis with cirrhosis which was called non-A, non-B hepatitis. The issue on appeal was the jury instructions with respect to the standard of care to be followed.

New York State Association for Retarded Children, Inc. v. Carey 612 F.2d 644 (1979), 466 F.Supp. 479 (1978). This is an important case from many aspects. Mentally retarded students who were hepatitis B surface antigen positive could *not* be excluded from public school.

Pommeranz v. State of Minnesota, Department of Public Welfare, Faribault State Hospital 261 N.W.2d 90 (1977). This case involved a switchboard operator at a state hospital who contracted viral hepatitis, and then primary biliary cirrhosis. She was awarded total disability benefits, and the state appealed. The Minnesota state supreme court held that the evidence supported the finding that there was a causal connection between her employment and her illness.

Sacred Heart Medical Center v. Carrado 579 P.2d 412 (1978). A hospital employee developed hepatitis. The Board of Industrial Insurance Appeals ruled that this hepatitis was a proximate result of her employment. At a trial the jury agreed. On appeal, an appellate court reversed, holding that the employee had not established a causal relationship between her hepatitis and her employment. There was no evidence that she had come into contact with a hepatitis patient or even that there had been a patient with hepatitis in the hospital.

Sacred Heart Medical Center v. Department of Labor and Industries 600 P.2d 1015 (1979). (Same case as one supra.) The Washington state supreme court reversed the appellate court's decision and reinstated the decision of the Board of

Industrial Insurance Appeals and the trial court; there was evidence supporting the finding that the nurse acquired hepatitis in the course of her employment.

Samuels v. Health and Hospitals Corporation of the City of New York 591 F.2d 195 (1979). A patient received transfusion of whole blood and packed cells while in the hospital. Subsequently she died of hepatitis. Subsequently, her estate sued both the hospital and the blood bank. There was a jury verdict against both. The federal trial court granted a judgment in their favor. The federal appellate court reversed and granted a new trial. There was some evidence that the blood bank had not taken proper precautions in using the donor of the whole blood. There was no inquiry about whether he had had any tatoos and the donor card showed an excessive number of drawings. The donor of the packed cells was tested and no hepatitis was found. The hospital (in New York) had not checked into the blood bank (in New Jersey) and did not know of its poor quality control. The jury was deprived of the best evidence.

Vanderdoes v. Ochsner Clinic 377 So.2d 1368 (1979). While hospitalized in July 1974, a patient had blood drawn on July 10, 15, 19, and 22. Serum hepatitis was manifest on July 22, 1974. The patient eventually died in October 1975 of cancer, arteriosclerosis, and cardiac arrest. There was a summary judgment in favor of the physician and hospital.

Woerth v. U.S. 714 F.2d 648 (1983). This is another fascinating case, and it may have far-reaching applications. A woman who worked for a VA hospital contracted hepatitis. She alleged that it was as a result of the hospital's failure to follow its own prophylactic procedures. Subsequently, her husband contracted hepatitis from his wife. He then sued the hospital and the federal government for hepatitis.

Herpes

Although herpes has been around a long time, the public furor about a herpes "epidemic" has been in recent years. As one might expect this has already resulted in a few reported law suits.

In *Cummings v. Fondak* 474 N.Y.S.2d 356 (1983), the patient sued the defendant physician, alleging that the physician had not obtained informed consent for the treatment with proflavin and fluorescent light. At the trial the plaintiff (patient) got a verdict for $200,000. On appeal this was reversed, and a new trial was ordered.

In *Kathleen K. v. Robert B.* 198 Cal.Rptr. 273 (1984) the female plaintiff alleged that she had contracted genital herpes from the defendant male. She said that he was negligent because he knew or should have known that he was a carrier of venereal disease. The trial court granted a summary judgment for the defendant. (This is an area that courts have refused to enter in the past.)

On appeal, the summary judgment for the defendant was reversed. The appellate court said that she had relied on his misrepresentation that he was free of venereal disease.

In *Livingston v. Gribetz* 549 F.Supp. 238 (1982) a nurse in the newborn nursery was taking care of a child with lesions on the neck. She thought it was herpes and reported it to her supervisor. More lesions appeared and were cultured. Herpes was diagnosed, and child was transferred to the pediatric intensive care unit. Subsequently the nurse developed a herpetic lesion near her right eye.

Later she was admitted with headaches, fever, and nausea and was diagnosed as having herpes encephalitis and treated with Ara A (adenine arabinoside). The nurse sued the child's pediatrician. The case was dismissed. The court said the nurse was not a patient of the pediatrician, she was a health professional trained to handle ill patients, and there was no evidence that room placement or use of masks and gowns would have kept her face free from herpes.

Legionella

In spite of the fact that *Legionella pneumophila* was described following the outbreak in Philadelphia in July 1976 and has been described in several outbreaks since then and serologically in a couple of outbreaks earlier, there are no cases in the legal literature involving *Legionella* infection. Does that mean that there have been no claims or cases involving *Legionella*? No. You will recall from the discussion above that only cases in which opinions are rendered at the appellate level are published in the legal literature, the reports. Cases involving *Legionella* have either been settled before they got to the appellate level or the trial and appellate process is taking so long that none of the cases has reached the appellate level yet.

Toxic Shock Syndrome

Toxic shock syndrome (TSS) was first described in 1978 in children. In 1980 hundreds of cases were described in menstruating women. It is a relatively recently described clinical entity, so it is not surprising that only a few cases have reached the appellate courts and thus the legal literature.

Ellis v. International Playtex, Inc. 745 F.2d 292 (1984). A patient became ill 3 days after using tampons in May 1981. The next day she remained in bed, complaining of sore throat, aches, and a fever. She asked her son to run an errand for her to a local store. When he returned she was collapsed on the bathroom floor. An ambulance took her to a hospital where she died the following morning. The patient's estate sued the manufacturer of the tampons; at the trial, the jury found for the manufacturer. On appeal it was reversed and remanded for a new trial. The trial court had erred in refusing to admit into evidence two epidemiologic studies conducted by the Centers for Disease Control and a Tri-State Commission. The studies showed a statistically significant relationship between tampon use and TSS. The trial court had held that these studies were hearsay and not admissible. The appellate court said they were admissible because they were compilations of data by a public agency and that the groups that had collected the data were highly skilled in epidemiology and they used uniform procedures and methods widely accepted by their peers.

Kehm v. Proctor and Gamble Manufacturing Co. 724 F.2d 613 (1984) is also based on a patient who died. The award was $300,000.

References

1. Nottebart HC: Legal aspects of infection control. In Cundy KR, Ball W (eds): *Infection Control in Health Care Facilities: Microbiological Surveillance.* Baltimore, University Park Press, 1977, pp 189–200.
2. Nottebart HC: Management of medical-legal problems. In Wenzel RP (ed): *CRC Handbook of Hospital-Acquired Infections.* Boca Raton, FL, CRC Press, 1981, pp 267–300.
3. Nottebart HC: Staphylococcal infection in hospital roommates. *Infect Control* 1:105, 108, 1980.
4. Nottebart HC: Hospital-acquired staphylococcal infection transmitted by hospital personnel. *Infect Control* 1:190, 193, 1980.
5. Nottebart HC: Nosocomial infections acquired by hospital employees. *Infect Control* 1:257–259, 1980.
6. Nottebart HC: Liability of the pathology laboratory. *Medico-Legal Bull* 29:1–6, 1980.
7. Nottebart HC: Legal proof and the medical expert. *Infect Control* 1:412–413, 1980.
8. Nottebart HC: The myth of negligence. *Infect Con-*

trol 2:154–156, 1981.

9. Nottebart HC: Possible liability of a hospital for an infection acquired from a (previously) hospitalized patient. *Infect Control* 1:343, 1980.

10. Nottebart HC: Legal aspects of antibiotic audit. *Infect Control* 5:93–94, 1984.

11. Nottebart HC: Immunizations: risks and warnings about them. *Infect Control* 2:265–267, 1981.

12. Nottebart HC: Immunizations: risks and warnings about them. Part II. *Infect Control* 2:323–325, 1981.

13. Nottebart HC: Disruption of family unity. An adverse reaction to tetracycline? *Infect Control* 2:391–392, 1981.

14. Nottebart HC: Infection control committee records. *Infect Control* 1:47–49, 1980.

15. Nottebart HC: Infection control committee records—revisited. *Infect Control* 5:295–297, 1984.

Chapter 5

Hospital-Acquired Infections: Some Ethical Issues

James F. Childress, Ph.D.

Ethical issues pervade science, medicine, and health care. Rarely is it possible to draw sharp lines between ethical, technical, and other issues, including political and economic ones. Nevertheless, it is possible to highlight the ethical dimensions of certain problems, such as hospital-acquired infections.

Ethical issues or dimensions can be identified by reference to moral principles that apply to institutional and individual actions in several areas, including science, medicine, and health care. There is more agreement about the relevant moral principles than there is about their foundations (i.e., why we should affirm them) and about their implications (i.e., what they imply for institutional policies and individual acts). In this chapter the important moral principles will be identified and then some of their implications for institutional policies and professional actions regarding hospital-acquired infections will be sketched. The major focus will be on principles that are already embedded in codes of medical and nursing ethics, in institutional policies and individual judgments, and in some legal rules and decisions, without attention to the question of their ultimate foundations (1).

The rationale of medicine, nursing, and hospital care is patient benefit. For example, in the Hippocratic oath, the physician pledges to "come for the benefit of the sick" and to apply "measures for the benefit of the sick according to [his] ability and judgment." Whatever other motives are present, the fundamental purpose of the medical relationship is to benefit patients. This first principle can be called "patient benefit" (or "beneficence").

A second moral principle is captured in the maxim primum non nocere, "above all, or first, do no harm." The origins of this maxim are obscure, but in the Hippocratic corpus there is the admonition "at least do no harm," and in the Hippocratic oath there is the pledge to keep patients "from harm." In the pursuit of patient benefit, there is a duty not to harm patients and also to reduce and minimize the risks of harm. The second principle can be called "nonmaleficence."

Unfortunately, it is rarely possible to seek and to provide benefits without risks of harm. Thus, it is frequently necessary to weigh and balance risks and benefits in the care of patients. Since risk is a probabilistic term, it is more accurate to refer to balancing the probability and amount of harm against the probability and amount of benefit. The formulations of risk-benefit analysis (and, more broadly, cost-benefit analysis) are shorthand expressions for such balancing, and they are simply modern expressions for an old art that is captured in the principle of utility or proportionality—the third principle, which is required because it is impossible to do only good and to avoid all harm.

The first three moral principles focus on producing benefits, avoiding harms, and balancing benefits and harms. But these principles, unsupplemented by other principles, are not adequate. For example, they do not indicate how benefits and harms should be distributed. Balancing benefits and harms could lead to policies and actions that subject some individuals or groups to grave risks for the benefit of the society as a whole. Thus, it is essential to have a fourth principle—fairness or justice—that requires a fair or just distribution of benefits and harms.

Furthermore, the principles identified so far do not indicate whose interpretation of risks and benefits should be considered—for example, the patient's, the health care professional's, or the society's. To be sure, all three interpretations are frequently relevant, but in patient care the competent patient's judgments about what will count as harms and benefits and how much they will count should be decisive when those judgments do not put others at risk. In back of this claim is a fifth principle—respect for persons and their autonomous wishes, choices, and actions (Table 5.1). Of course, it is morally permissible to override patients' wishes, choices, and actions when they are not competent to decide (e.g., because of severe retardation) or when they impose major risks to others. Nevertheless, the principle of respect for persons establishes the rights of competent people to make their own decisions, to receive information, and to control access to information about themselves (privacy and confidentiality) as long as they do not harm others or violate their rights.

None of the above principles or others, such as keeping promises, can be considered absolute. Each of them may have to yield to other principles in some cases of conflict. One of the first tasks in making ethical judgments is to determine, in the light of the facts of the case, which moral principles apply; then emerges the more difficult task of determining which principles should have priority if they conflict. In the remainder of this chapter the implications of the five major principles—patient benefit, nonmaleficence, utility, fairness, and respect—for institutional policies and professional actions regarding hospital-acquired infections will be indicated. There will be considerable dispute about what these principles actually require and which should take priority in cases of conflict. Thus, there is room for morally sensitive people to disagree about which policies ought to be adopted and which actions ought to be undertaken in particular circumstances.

The first three principles have long been emphasized in medicine and health care, and justice and respect for persons have not been totally neglected. Even in the Hippocratic oath, there is a pledge to protect the patient from "injustice," and the virtually universal requirement to protect confidentiality relates to, and is often derived from, the principle of respect for persons. Even if these principles are widely affirmed in our society,

such factors as historical circumstances, social forces, and psychologic, orientations certainly shape how we interpret, weigh, and apply them. Two examples may be suggestive. First, in the last 25 years, the principle of respect for persons has been interpreted to require disclosure of information to patients, even though codes of medical ethics have tended to view disclosure, partial disclosure, or nondisclosure of information as part of the therapeutic art to be manipulated according to patient benefit. Second, the weighing and balancing required by the principle of utility or proportionality obviously depend on perception of risks and benefits. What counts as a harm or a benefit, how much particular harms or benefits count, and how probabilities are viewed—all depend on an individual's or society's standpoint (2). Thus, even if the same moral principles are affirmed across societies and time, how they are interpreted and applied will vary greatly, and judgments about policies and actions will differ accordingly. Yet it is important to know whether the dispute is primarily factual (e.g., about the probability of a harm's occurring) or primarily evaluational (e.g., about the acceptability of a risk in relation to a benefit).

In the prevention and control of nosocomial infections, as in several other areas, judgments about particular policies and actions do not always flow directly and smoothly from moral principles, in part because those principles sometimes conflict with each other. Often it is not possible to say definitively that a policy or an action is obligatory and ought to be undertaken. In such cases it may only be possible to claim that X is morally preferable to Y without holding that X is obligatory and Y is wrong; both X and Y may fall within the range of morally acceptable responses. Frequently, there is uncertainty, especially about the probability of a harm's occurrence.

RISKS, BENEFITS, AND UTILITIES

Regarding nosocomial infections, the first moral responsibility, derived from several of the moral principles identified earlier, is to reduce the probability of their occurrence. Both the probability and the severity of nosocomial infections are significant. As Richard Wenzel notes, of the 40 million people who are hospitalized each year in the United States, 2 to 4 million (5 to 10%) will develop nosocomial infections. In addition to morbidity and economic costs, such infections probably cause approximately 50,000 deaths each

Table 5.1. Important Moral Principles by Which Ethical Issues Can Be Framed

1. Patient benefit (beneficence)
2. At least do no harm (nonmaleficence)
3. Risk-benefit analysis (utility)
4. Fairness or justice
5. Respect for persons' wishes, choices, and actions

year (3). It is impossible to create a risk-free hospital environment. Since risks of hospital-acquired infections cannot be totally eliminated, the moral imperative might appear to be to do everything possible to reduce the risks to the lowest possible level. Yet it may not be morally obligatory or even morally preferable to do everything possible to reduce the risks to their lowest possible level. Weighing and balancing risks, costs, and benefits may be required by the principle of utility. The phrase "acceptable risks" is applied not only to risks that have to be accepted because they are unavoidable; it also includes avoidable risks that are acceptable in the pursuit of certain goals.

Not all procedures to reduce risks are worth their cost. For example, in debates about policies to reduce the risk of death from highway accidents by changes in road design, barriers, or signs, or to reduce the risk of death from heart attack by establishing mobile heart units, there are appeals to the "value of life," a somewhat misleading phrase since the issue is how much it is worth to reduce the risks of mortality. From a moral standpoint, the question is how much the society, hospitals, and professionals should do to reduce the risk of mortality and morbidity from nosocomial infections, when there are other claims on their time, energy, and resources. There is surely some limit—even if it is unclear and shifts frequently—to how much must be spent to reduce the risks of nosocomial infection as close as possible to zero. Other goods in health care and elsewhere also require resources for their realization. Thus, the society and hospitals must determine what priority the reduction of risks of nosocomial infections should have when their budgets are limited. For example, from the society's standpoint, even if there is a right to a decent minimum of health care—reflected in the metaphor of a safety net—there are debates about priorities in the allocation of resources among preventive, curative, and chronic care, among various technologies, and among various diseases. And it is not clear in the abstract what priority prevention of nosocomial infections should have in this allocation. Similar questions about priorities in the allocation of resources emerge within the hospital, for example, in designing critical care units, locating sinks, and setting nurse-patient ratios, all of which may have a significant impact on the rate of nosocomial infections.

There are other questions about the effectiveness and efficiency of procedures to reduce nosocomial infections. Some approaches to the prevention or control of hospital-acquired infections may not be cost effective and should not be implemented. Both the control and the treatment of such infections consume a significant portion of the hospital's (and the society's) budget. In some cases, significant savings could be obtained by eliminating ineffective measures or by using less expensive but equally effective measures (4). However, it is not easy to determine the effectiveness of many measures because several may interact to prevent or control nosocomial infections (5). In some cases randomized controlled trials may be useful to evaluate both old and new measures (6). At any rate more cost effectiveness studies are needed.

In both societal and hospital policies, research should have a high priority. Otherwise policies and actions will have to be undertaken on the basis of inadequate data. Only by ongoing epidemiologic surveillance is it possible to establish the nature and extent of nosocomial infections, endemic and epidemic risks, unavoidable and avoidable risks, as well as effective and efficient procedures. Nevertheless, as the controversy about AIDS (acquired immune deficiency syndrome) indicates, it is often necessary to formulate policies and to act in the face of uncertainty.

In contrast to policies that set priorities in the allocation of societal and institutional resources, other policies are more regulative: they set the rules and procedures for preventing and controlling nosocomial infections. The line between allocation and regulation is not always clear and overlap is common. For example, some regulations, such as establishing one-to-one nurse-patient ratios 24 hours a day in critical care areas, obviously entail certain allocations of resources. Nevertheless, it is useful to think about regulations as setting a societal or institutional standard of care regarding the acceptability or unacceptability of some risks and ways to prevent or control some nosocomial infections.

To take one example, there is debate about the institution's moral responsibility, to say nothing of its legal responsibility, to screen all health care providers for carriage of hepatitis B surface antigen and to transfer every exposed person to a position that does not involve patient contact. Some insist that it is not necessary for providers who are carriers to be isolated or restricted from patient contact, contending that it is sufficient for them to follow careful procedures to prevent possible infection of others (7). This debate hinges on determining an appropriate balance of risks and benefits, but it is also influenced by considerations of justice and fairness in the distribution of burdens and by considerations of liberty. Few would deny that there is a duty to protect patients even at the expense of personal liberty in many cases, but justified restrictions of liberty depend on the probability and severity of harm. And there is often disagreement about the risks involved, for example, the risks imposed by a dialysis nurse who is a hepatitis B carrier and who insists on continuing dialysis nursing (7).

A similar debate concerns the regulation of contact with patients by health care providers who have symptomatic AIDS, asymptomatic AIDS, or exposure to the HTLV-III virus that is closely linked with AIDS. The problem is the uncertainty about the transmission of the HTLV-III virus. It is morally appropriate to change regulations as evidence accumulates about risks, but the hard question is what to do when the uncertainty is great, for example, whether to err on the side of extreme caution (in view of the severity of the disease and its long incubation period) or to err on the side of permissiveness (in view of the lack of evidence that the virus is easily transmitted). A 1983 task force at the University of California, San Francisco, developed infection control guidelines for patients with AIDS and reported the sharpest differences of opinion about whether a hospital should reassign employees with asymptomatic AIDS to positions not involving patient care (8). Among the other significant issues addressed by the guidelines were the precautions that should be taken in order to protect AIDS patients from exposure to opportunistic infections and to protect other patients from exposure to AIDS patients, holding, for example, that "a private room is not necessary if the (AIDS) patient is cooperative, is not coughing, and can be adequately instructed in personal hygiene" (8).

Institutional rules and practices for screening to prevent or control nosocomial infections are not limited to screening caregivers and patients for transmissible diseases. Screening is also involved in determining whether a professional in training is ready to perform a procedure (e.g., whether a surgical resident is prepared to perform a certain operation) when the rate of nosocomial infection following that procedure may vary according to the professional's experience. Screening also covers products, such as blood, and procedures, such as scrubbing. Whether the screening is directed toward personnel, procedures, or products, the question of adequacy or sufficiency

arises, and the answer will depend, as has been suggested, on the acceptability of certain degrees and amounts of risk. Acceptability presupposes the application of all of the principles identified above. For example, utility is clearly involved in weighing and balancing risks, costs, and benefits, but justice in the distribution of benefits, costs, and risks and respect for persons also play a significant if indeterminate role.

Beyond societal and institutional regulations to reduce the risks of nosocomial infections, individual physicians, nurses, and other providers of care have certain duties or obligations. In part as a result of their assumption of their roles, which presuppose a commitment to benefit and not to harm patients, caregivers clearly have a moral duty to observe proper precautions to reduce nosocomial infections. From the time of Semmelweis, it has been known that handwashing reduces hospital infections, and Wenzel notes that "proper and frequent handwashing is the most important control measure available in preventing the transmission of infectious diseases in hospitalized patients" (3). Caregivers are guilty of "moral negligence" (if not legal negligence) when they fail to discharge or carelessly discharge this duty. Collegial chastisement or stronger responses may be appropriate when a caregiver is morally negligent.

In addition to their duty to *reduce* risks of nosocomial infections to patients, providers may also have a duty to *assume* risks in order to benefit patients. It is probably important to distinguish professionals from workers since it is plausible to argue that, by virtue of entering their professions, professionals pledge, at least implicitly, to assume some risks. Of course, workers may be informed of some risks and voluntarily assume them. But even if professionals assume a higher level of risk than others, there is a limit beyond which we do not expect them to go. We may praise them if they accept risks beyond that limit, but we do not blame them if they fail to do so. The obvious difficulty is specifying that limit in terms of the probability and severity of harm. Again, AIDS serves as a test case because the harm is so severe, but it is difficult to attach probabilities to its occurrence as a result of various contacts between professionals and AIDS patients. For example, the 1983 guidelines proposed by the task force of the University of California, San Francisco, recommended that institutions provide cardiopulmonary resuscitation (CPR) bags at the bedside of patients with AIDS or other potentially transmissible infections, such as hepatitis B or tuberculosis, in order to prevent mouth-to-mouth contact. According to these guidelines, later modified (but before the virus that is linked with AIDS was discovered in saliva), "when . . . a CPR device is available, the employee is obligated to administer CPR. The decision to withhold direct mouth-to-mouth resuscitation from a patient with AIDS when a CPR device is not available is solely that of the individual employee" (8). The task force commented, "the decision to delay or withhold mouth-to-mouth resuscitation from a patient with possible or documented AIDS in the hospital setting involves moral and ethical considerations. One must balance the universal right of all patients to be resuscitated, if they so desire, against the right of health-care workers to protect themselves from contracting a serious infectious illness, however remote that risk may be" (8). Our judgments about what is morally required, morally preferable, or morally praiseworthy will depend on our beliefs about the risks involved, in terms of both the magnitude and the probability of harm. The most recent tests of hospital employees with close contact with AIDS patients—including victims of needle-stick exposure, endoscopists, pathologists, and laboratory workers—suggest that "when current hospital isolation procedures are employed the risk of nosocomial transmission of HTLV-III is low" (9).

DISCLOSURE OF INFORMATION

The principle of respect for persons implies a patient's right to control access to information about himself or herself (the rights of privacy and confidentiality) and to receive information about procedures, their benefits, risks, and alternatives, as well as information about his or her condition. What are the limits to these rights when the subject is hospital-acquired infections and their control?

First, the rights of privacy and confidentiality are not absolute and may be overridden under some circumstances in order to protect others. It has been suggested that nosocomial infection may be considered a modern communicable disease and that health care professionals' duties may be analogous in both areas (10). Under certain circumstances professionals have a morally and legally recognized right and duty to breach privacy and confidentiality in order to protect other persons. For example, there are legal duties to report child abuse, gunshot wounds, venereal diseases, and epileptic motorists in many states. These duties may be discharged by reports to appropri-

ate authorities, but in some situations there may be a duty to warn the intended victim (e.g., of a psychiatric patient's intention to kill him or her). The question of a potential, unintended victim, such as the lover of a person with venereal disease, is more complicated. It has been argued that the traditional rule of confidentiality is now "decrepit" in the modern hospital because so many people, including those involved in infection control, have a legitimate interest in and right to information about the patient (11). Nevertheless, even when it is justified and obligatory to reveal information to others about a patient's infectious condition or susceptibility to infections in order to prevent and control nosocomial infections, this disclosure should take place within the limits of what is necessary to the parties to whom it is necessary. The ideal of confidentiality is still relevant and offers direction even when it cannot be fully realized, for example, in the collection of data as part of surveillance of nosocomial infections.

Difficult cases may arise; consider, for example, the clinician's duty to a patient who is a hepatitis B carrier, but who insists on continuing her work as a dialysis nurse and her active sexual relationships with several lovers. In discussing that case, a physician (Perkins) and an ethicist (Jonsen) argue that "the physician's responsibility to keep an immediate patient's confidences outweighs the responsibility to protect others unless there is sound evidence for a very certain, severe harm to specific others" (7). There is, however, room for major disagreements about how certain and how severe the harms have to be and how specific the potential victims have to be. In addition, there may be disagreements about the actual risks of contracting hepatitis B from a dialysis nurse. The extent to which hepatitis B already appears in dialysis patients and the availability of a safe and effective vaccine may affect the judgment about what ought to be done.

Second, it has been noted that "when a person enters a hospital, there is a baseline or minimal risk which is *accepted* as endemic or usual" (10). It is appropriate to ask, "accepted by whom?"— by patients or by institutions and caregivers for patients? The acceptance or assumption of risk presupposes *awareness* of that risk. It might be supposed that adults entering the hospital are aware of risks of nosocomial infections and that it is unnecessary to inform them of endemic and usual risks. But even if patients are aware that there are risks of hospital-acquired infections, they are probably unaware of the actual rate of endemic or background infection. It is important to consider whether it is morally obligatory or at least morally preferable to disclose information about risks of nosocomial infections from hospitalization in general, from a particular type of hospital (for example, infection rates are higher in university hospitals than in community hospitals, in part because of the university hospital's role in training professionals and in part because of the serious condition of many of its patients), from a particular area of the hospital (e.g., dialysis units and critical care areas), from certain procedures (e.g., transfusions), from certain professionals (e.g., surgical residents who have performed the procedure only a few times if at all), from certain problems, etc. Not every risk should be disclosed; whether a risk is material from the standpoint of the hypothetical reasonable person and thus should be disclosed will depend on the degree and probability of harm. For example, a pregnant woman who is given an option to have delivery by cesarean section should be informed that the risk of endometritis is 20 to 30% following cesarean sections but only 1% following vaginal delivery (12). This is a material risk even if the main negative effect is increased time in the hospital with appropriate treatment and higher costs. The risk of contracting hepatitis B or, more recently, AIDS from a blood transfusion should also be disclosed. Obviously, there will be debate about how probable and how severe the harm must be before there is an obligation to disclose it. However, the clinician's fear that the patient may refuse the treatment in question on the basis of the information does justify withholding that information. Respect for persons means respecting a competent person's informed refusal as well as his/her informed consent. One possible approach is to tell a patient that there are serious, but remote risks of a procedure and then to allow that patient to determine how much additional information he or she wants to receive about those risks (13).

A third question about the disclosure of information may be even more controversial: is there a moral duty to disclose the source of an infection after it has occurred, for example, that it was acquired in the hospital, that it was acquired during a preventable outbreak or epidemic, or that it was probably acquired as the result of negligence? There are moral arguments for and against subsequent disclosure of the source of an infection. On the one hand, the patient's right to know his or her diagnosis and prognosis seems to imply the right to information about the source

of infection, and justice may not be achieved if information about negligence is not disclosed. On the other hand, protection of the institution and professionals when there is the threat of a malpractice suit but uncertainty about the source of the infection also weighs heavily for many professionals. In one case some years ago, four infants died in an outbreak of herpes simplex virus II or Herpes hominis II (HH II) when information about it was quite inadequate. The last baby to die had been transferred to the pediatric intensive care unit from another hospital to monitor occasional apnea and weight gain. The epidemiologist discovered that this baby had used the incubator occupied by the third baby who had died and that the infection had probably resulted from inadequate cleaning of the incubator. Two recent commentators on that case have suggested, with some hesitation, that it was not morally necessary to disclose the probable source of the infection to the parents, despite their general right to know, because "it was more just, sensible, and equitable to protect the hospital from a possible suit in the presence of so few known facts about a communicable disease" (10).

In another case, a healthy 20-year-old man twisted his knee while skiing; he experienced a great deal of pain and was hospitalized for surgery on the joint. After discharge his wound failed to heal because of infection with a strain of penicillin-resistant *Staphylococcus aureus*; osteomyelitis developed and resulted in extensive tissue destruction; plastic surgery to rebuild the knee and extensive rehabilitation followed. The patient had not been at high risk for infection because of his own condition. When he asked about the cause of the infection, the nurses said that *S. aureus* is found "everywhere" and that he assumed the "usual risk" of acquiring an infection when he entered the hospital. The question has been raised whether he should have been told that the usual route of transmission is unwashed hands (10).

It is important to distinguish institutional policies from an individual professional's moral responsibility without separating them. The institution should develop a policy about the disclosure of such information on the basis of moral considerations; that policy should indicate what should be disclosed and who should make the disclosure. In general, following the principle of respect for persons, it should require liberal disclosure of information, but it should also recognize limits to that disclosure. Epidemiologists and others either involved in surveillance or aware of relevant information should disclose that information to the appropriate parties, for example, the infection control committee. Sometimes, however, they may have to face the question of their own moral responsibility to disclose information directly to patients because of their convictions about the inadequacies of the institutional policy of disclosure or about the patients' right to know in particular cases. In these situations, professionals may experience a conflict between their consciences and institutional loyalties.

Acknowledgments. This chapter was completed while the author was a Guggenheim Fellow and a Wilson Center Fellow, and he is grateful to both the Guggenheim Foundation and the Wilson Center, who are not, of course, responsible for any of the views expressed herein.

References

1. Beauchamp TL, Childress JF: *Principles of Biomedical Ethics*, ed 2. New York, Oxford University Press, 1983.
2. Douglas M, Wildavsky A: *Risk and Culture.* Berkeley, Univeristy of California Press, 1983.
3. Wenzel RP: Prevention and treatment of hospital-acquired infections. In, Wyngaarden JB, Smith LH (eds): *Cecil Text Book of Medicine.* 1985, pp 1485–1492.
4. Daschner FD: Practical aspects for cost reduction in hospital infection control. *Infect Control* 5:32–35, 1984.
5. Reber H: Rationale and testing of degerming procedures. *Infect Control* 5:28–31, 1984.
6. Burke JP: Randomized controlled trials in hospital epidemiology. *Am J Infect Control* 11:165–73, 1983.
7. Perkins HS, Jonsen AR; Conflicting duties to patients: the case of a sexually active hepatitis B carrier. *Ann Intern Med* 94 (Pt 1): 523–530, 1981.
8. Conte JE Jr, Hadley WK, Sande M, University of California, San Francisco, Task Force on the Acquired Immunodeficiency Syndrome: Infection-control guidelines for patients with the acquired immunodeficiency syndrome (AIDS). *N Engl J Med* 309:740–744, 1983.
9. Hirsch MS, Wormser GPX, Schooley RT, Ho DD, Felsenstein D, Hopkins CC, Jolline C, Duncanson F, Sarngadharan MG, Saxinger C, Gallo RC: Risk of nosocomial infection with human T-cell lymphotropic virus III (HTLV-III). *N Engl J Med* 312:1–4, 1985.
10. Chavigny KH, Helm A: Ethical dilemmas and the practice of infection control. *Law Med Health Care* 10:168–171, 174, 1982.
11. Siegler M: Confidentiality in medicine—a decrepit concept. *N Engl J Med* 307:1518–1521, 1982.
12. Donowitz LG, Wenzel RP: Endometritis following cesarean section: a controlled study of the increased duration of hospital stay and direct cost of hospitalization. *Am J Obstet Gynecol* 137:467–469, 1980.
13. Childress JF: *Who Should Decide? Paternalism in Health Care.* New York, Oxford University Press, 1982.

Chapter 6

Organizing for Infection Control

Samuel Ponce de Leon R., M.D.

"It is obvious," answered Don Quijote, "thou art not versed in matters of adventure. They are giants. And if thou art afraid, move aside and set thyself to pray because I am about to enter a fierce and uneven battle against them." And saying this, he clapped spurs to Rocinante. . . .

El Quijote de la Mancha

The organization of a nosocomial infection control program is not an easy task. The main goal of a program of this sort is to lower the risk of an infection during the time of hospitalization, a task requiring the multiple interactions of various sorts of persons, all of whom have to be convinced of a need to change their attitudes. To be able to achieve this goal, a great amount of patience, shrewdness, and hard work is needed. It is also important to be aware that each hospital has its own individuality. Every medical center is unique, even though similarities in category, number of beds, or paramedical services might exist. Thus, individual peculiarities must be considered in order to adjust the proposals for change in each hospital. Furthermore, one must avoid being in the unfortunate position of trying to change the institution in order to meet a series of preconceived regulations which may not be appropriate for the hospital. The hospital's infection control program and the hospital epidemiologist must, therefore, be dynamic yet flexible since a hospital is often very limited in such characteristics.

The three main supportive elements for the infection control program are as follows:

1. The development of an effective surveillance system;
2. The establishment of a series of regulations and policies to reduce the risk of a hospital-acquired infection;
3. The maintenance of a continuing education program for hospital personnel.

The organization of the surveillance system is the logical initial step of the program since the subsequent changes must be based on the identification of local problems which may be unique and distinctly different from those of other institutions.

The selection of a surveillance system among the multiple existent options should be made considering the special characteristics of the hospital and the expected goals. Based on the initial results of the surveillance, it is possible to have a realistic idea of the nosocomial infection rate as well as issues of morbidity, mortality, and costs. These data are essential to obtain adequate financial support for the program from the hospital administration.

The regulation of the different procedures, as well as the policy of isolation of patients, should be determined, once more, according to each hospital's possibilities. Thus, if there are no individual rooms in a given hospital, it is absurd to rule on the isolation of patients in individual rooms; other possible forms of patient isolation must be considered. Even in the United States the situation may not be so simple as to have to decide only between the two patient isolation systems proposed by the Centers for Disease Control (CDC) (category-specific isolation precautions versus disease-specific isolation precautions) (see appendix to (1) for CDC guidelines for isolation). Although, generally speaking, the safer and more practical way to initiate a program is to use the category-specific isolation precautions (2), hospital limitations might require an intermediate or alternative solution. Similarly, the acquisition of equipment or material will depend on the existing economic resources. All of the recommendations of the program should be based on the real capabilities of the hospital and its personnel. Even the proposal of a few regulations that cannot be accomplished, for any reason, is risky since the administration of the hospital might consider it unrealistic and, therefore, impracticable. The hospital's personnel will be willing to collaborate with a specific program only if they are convinced of its feasibility.

The continuing education program must first be directed to nurses. This approach has several advantages since nurses are the personnel with the greatest physical contact with patients as well as those with the greatest risk of transmission of organisms. They are, therefore, very important regarding the interruption of infection transmission.

On the other hand, nurses are one of the most receptive and enthusiastic groups in the hospital and are willing to follow control measures, as may be deduced from data obtained from handwashing studies (3). Finally, nurses are everywhere in the hospital and participate in practically every procedure within the institution. Thus, wherever a patient is exposed to a high risk procedure, it is of the utmost importance that nurses be trained for its adequate execution. If they are aware of the importance of their participation, the recommended procedures will be followed correctly and will guarantee the success of the program.

SPECIFIC RECOMMENDATIONS

There are numerous measures which may be considered as specific recommendations when an infection control program is devised. However, one of the most important measures deals with the relationship with the hospital personnel. The hospital epidemiologist or the infection control team is frequently involved with situations in which the clinical staff might feel threatened. For example, the investigation of an epidemic outbreak in a specific department will obviously affect physicians and nurses who might be fearful of being blamed for the problem. The epidemiologist must convince everybody that his work is not to judge guilt or innocence, but instead to solve a problem in the best possible way and to prevent its recurrence with their collaboration. On the contrary, if the epidemiologist has an aggressive attitude toward the personnel, not only will he not receive their support, but also he might even enhance the likelihood of their concealing future problems. The epidemiologist's goal, specifically at the beginning of a control program, must be to convince and to gain confidence, not to order.

FINANCIAL ASPECTS

The organization of an infection control program needs economic support which ideally should come from the hospital administration itself. The hospital has to be responsible for the majority of the expenses derived from the infection control department, as well as for the preventable infections contracted during hospitalization. The best way to convince the hospital administration of the advantages of supporting the program is to show morbidity and mortality rates related to nosocomial infection and to illustrate their economic impact. This information can be obtained from the experience of other hospitals or from studies from the CDC (4–6). However, it is much better to submit information about the frequency and magnitude of the problem in the same hospital, which can be derived from general data. The purpose is to show the importance of the problem in terms of human suffering as well as economic impact, emphasizing the fact that the situation is capable of being modified favorably with the proposed program (7), which will be comparatively less expensive. It is very important not to promise a drastic change in a short time, but to consider a reasonable lapse of time in order to observe favorable changes. Other sources of economic support are the industry-supported studies on the usefulness of some specific products on the control of nosocomial infections (8), such as soaps, disinfectants, or disposable devices.

POLITICAL SUPPORT

Another important aspect for the correct function and development of the program is the support of people who are politically outstanding in the hospital. The best way to obtain their support is to involve them in the program as advisors or members of the infection control committee; once they accept and participate, they become natural allies of the program. Eventually, the hospital authorities ought to be convinced of the importance of their own collaboration for the success of the program.

PERSONNEL SELECTION

The best nurses for an infection control program are those who have voluntarily expressed their interest to work in it. Otherwise, personnel who have been selected arbitrarily, without evidence of a real interest in the area, might abandon the program after receiving special training, a situation which implies a great loss of time and money. There is always a risk of abandonment, but it is reduced when people show a real interest in the program. The selected nurses should ideally be sensitive and courteous with a level of training above the average since they will establish a special nurse-physician relationship, different from the usual one, and will frequently be required to discuss or propose changes in the attitudes of hospital personnel. Alternatively, the academic status of infection control practitioners may be raised by ensuring their attendance at regional and national meetings or at local continuing education courses.

Since the infection control committee has to be a basic support for the hospital epidemiologist, its members must have a genuine interest in the activity. Even though it is useful for the infection control committee members to have relevant academic and political positions, it is more important that they be able to devote enough time to the program. Otherwise, it is better to invite very busy persons to be part time advisors than to select them as permanent members of the committee since their frequent absenteeism would obstruct the adequate progress of the program.

COMMUNICATION WITHIN THE HOSPITAL

The activities of the infection control program need to be disseminated in a comprehensible language, emphasizing the aspects that are relevant for everybody in the hospital. For example, the results of the surveillance system may be summarized for every service, with an effort to individualize as much as possible. The policies and regulations, as well as the results of achievements and difficulties, may be communicated extensively in hospital sessions and summarized in a written document.

Another important aspect is communication with the head of a department in which an epidemic has occurred or a special problem has been detected. Once the problem is confirmed, the best approach is to speak directly with the head of the affected service, before discussing the problem widely with hospital authorities and before taking any action to solve it. The personal approach is more effective than an impersonal written communication. Generally speaking, personal intervention is the best approach to any problem; however, there are situations that may be solved with a mere telephone call and many others that are routine and that may be communicated by a letter. Obviously, the media used to communicate a problem will depend upon its seriousness and the people it affects. If in doubt, however, make an appointment to meet directly with the person involved.

INTEGRATION OF THE INFECTION CONTROL PROGRAM

Probably, the greatest problem in the organization of an infection control program is the integration of its components so as to establish the supervision and feedback among its participants, with the purpose of achieving steady progress.

Figure 6.1 shows a schematic view of an infection control program where each participant is, at the same time, supervised by and supervisor of the other participants. Even though the responsibility for the maintenance of the system belongs to the hospital epidemiologist, all of its members should be considered as fundamental parts of the organization and responsible for its accomplishments. This attitude favors efficiency but will not occur spontaneously; rather, it will be necessary to create a favorable atmosphere to establish this supervision system, which will allow the evaluation of everyone's work.

The supervision system gives specific tasks to several members. The hospital epidemiologist is directly responsible for the organization and development of the surveillance activities, which are routinely carried out by infection control practitioners. He also revises and analyzes the results of the surveillance along with other members of the program, and develops a report for the infection control committee which reviews the document. In this way the commitee is supervising the job of the hospital epidemiologist and practitioners. As a result, the committee develops guidelines, regulations, or policies that have to be followed and respected not only by hospital personnel, but also by patients and visitors to the hospital. Obviously, such guidelines are designed to modify habits and attitudes and will ultimately produce changes in nosocomial infection rates. The resulting modifications in infection rates are evaluated by the epidemiologist and practitioners, who, in turn, observe the feasibility of the committee's proposals, as well as the way in which they are followed by personnel, patients, and visitors, thus closing a circle. This sequence must exist in every infection control program and emphasizes the interdependence and evaluation of each member's performance.

Within this general scheme, it is important to point out that the routine work may become uninteresting for the people who practice it. To avoid the loss of interest in weekly surveillance

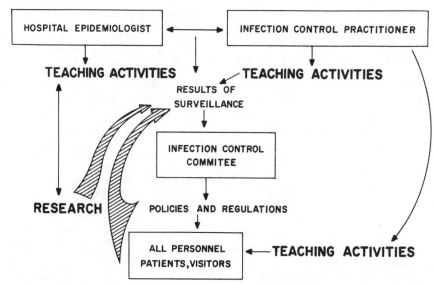

Figure 6.1. **Integrative view of assistance, research, and teaching activities of the infection control program.**

activities, certain measures need to be implemented. Surely, the routine is broken when epidemic outbreaks are detected since these imply a special and intense activity for the epidemiologist and infection control practitioners, who feel a renewed interest in their work. However, epidemic outbreaks are intermittent and should not be necessary to maintain a high interest in everyday work. Instead, it is much better to be constantly stimulated, and one of the best ways to achieve this is through education activities. In the learning process the teacher is continually challenged by his pupils to reach a higher academic level and to fulfill his responsibility in a greater fashion. The practitioner-teacher also has a higher rank in the organization and stimulates the surveillance activities while showing the pupils the best way to execute them. The involvement of practitioners in an education program provides training of newcomers and continually motivates all program members to reach a better performance level without the need of the surge of an epidemic outbreak. Figure 6.1 shows the levels where education programs should be included. Infection control practitioners may be responsible for continuing education programs for nurses and physicians interested in this work, as well as for hospital personnel; they may also be responsible for training new hospital personnel or possibly for training outsiders. The hospital epidemiologist would ideally supervise the courses and be responsible for the training of medical residents in this area. Medical residents may participate in

the infection control program, as may those in fellowship training in infectious diseases or those in an epidemiology Master of Science degree course. All involvement by local residents participating will surely enhance the value of the program.

Another aspect, which lacks relevant written information, is the development of a quality control program which will allow the objective evaluation of every member of the infection control program. There are a few reports on the sensitivity and comparative effectiveness of the various surveillance systems (9, 10) that do not contemplate the evaluation of the program itself. Once the sensitivity of a specific surveillance system is known, the program may be properly evaluated in terms of the fulfillment of its goals, such as solved problems, infection rate reductions, and alertness to detect epidemic outbreaks.

It is necessary to check the surveillance system accuracy, once or twice a year, through short prevalence studies to detect false positive or false negative reported cases, in order to improve the reliability of the program evaluation. These periodic short studies should be very easy to execute. For instance, the selection of a sample of patients hospitalized during a 1-week period would suffice. The infections detected with the Kardex system could be compared to the retrospective review (9). The sample should be designed on a sound statistical basis.

On the other hand, research projects, which are directly related to the surveillance system, are a tool for evaluating the control program, i.e., proposed regulations. An example would be the design of a research protocol to analyze the results of specialized nursing team's handling of parenteral feeding catheters in view of the high frequency of bacteremia in patients with these catheters. Research protocols should also be designed to evaluate risks, costs, and benefits of new proposals compared to existing measures. The research may be carried out by fellows in hospital epidemiology along with the infection control practitioners and under the hospital epidemiologist's supervision. These research activities enhance the work that might sometimes become routine.

In conclusion, an infection control program must perform service activities, such as surveillance and infection prevention measures, teaching, and research activities regarding infection prevention methodology. Furthermore, all activities should be supervised for the program to be optimally effective.

References

1. Garner JS, Simmons BP: CDC guidelines for isolation precautions in hospitals. *Infect Control* 4(suppl):245–325, 1983.
2. Saravolatz LD, Arking L: Isolation guidelines—A or B? Editorial. *Infect Control* 5:269–270, 1984.
3. Albert RK, Condie F: Handwashing patterns in medical intensive care units. *N Engl J Med* 304:1465–1466, 1981.
4. Wenzel RP, Osterman CA, Hunting KJ: Hospital-acquired infections. II. Infection rates by service and common procedures in a university hospital. *Am J Epidemiol* 104:645–651, 1976.
5. Rose R, Hunting KJ, Townsend TR, Wenzel RP: Morbidity/mortality and economics of hospital acquired bloodstream infections: a controlled study. *South Med J* 70:1267–1269, 1977.
6. Eickhoff TC: Hospital epidemiology: an emerging discipline. In Remington JS, Swartz MN (eds): *Current Clinical Topics in Infectious Diseases*. New York, McGraw-Hill, 1984, p 241.
7. Haley RW, Culver DH, White JW, Morgan WM, Emory TG: The nationwide nosocomial infection rate. *Am J Epidemiol* 121:159–167, 1985.
8. Wenzel RP, Schaffner W: Infection control: a progress report (editorial). *Infect Control* 6:9–10; 1985.
9. Wenzel RP, Osterman CA, Hunting KJ: Hospital-acquired infections. I. Surveillance in a university hospital. *Am J Epidemiol* 103:251–260, 1976.
10. Tager IB, Ginsberg MB, Simchen E, Miao L, Holbrook K, Faich GA: Rationale and methods for a state-wide prospective surveillance system for the identification and prevention of nosocomial infections. *Rev Infect Dis* 3:683–693, 1981.

Chapter 7

Priority Setting in Infection Control

Walter J. Hierholzer, Jr., M.D.

INTRODUCTION

During the past 25 years, infection control has become the premier risk control program in hospital care. Using variations of standard Centers for Disease Control (CDC) methodology (1), practitioners and investigators have attracted national and local support for their programs, while developing an improved scientific base and breadth in the medical literature. Throughout the course of this development, critics have raised issues concerning the efficacy of significant portions of the programs and questioned the appropriateness of the resources expended on them (2–6). Unfortunately, response to these criticisms has been lost in the perception that nosocomial infections are such a documented major hospital problem that even inefficient attempts at their control are a supportable priority.

As medical costs have increased and cost consciousness has emerged as a competing consideration in medical care, institutions and individuals have begun to re-evaluate all programs. Infection control programs are not escaping a review and should not expect to. Infection control practitioners should be prepared to defend their program priorities based on information justifying their efficacy and efficiency. Furthermore, infection control practitioners and researchers should continue to evaluate the internal components of their programs, emphasizing those portions most successfully controlling the highest risks and discarding those interventions for which scientific or applied effectiveness cannot be documented. The methods to establish priorities for an infection control program and its internal components comprise the subject of this chapter.

THE EVALUATION AND INTERVENTION PROCESS

Priorities for all intervention programs in medical care should be based on an evaluation of their effectiveness in meeting the goals of the medical institution. The usual goals of medical care may be quoted in terms of prevention and limitation of disease to the maximum benefit of the patient, while limiting the ever present potential for the side effects of these interventions, i.e., minimizing the risk. Each medical process involves a balance between the benefits it offers and the competing risks of its side effects. In the use of pharmaceutical drugs, the balance is recognized as the therapeutic index. In the consideration of larger segments of medical care, these competing forces are described as benefit to cost ratios or cost effectiveness ratios. In constructing these ratios, one estimates cost by totaling the commercial charges for care and the dollar surrogates of the mortality and morbidity side effects, or in the latter case, by using nonfinancial indicators of loss defined in terms of hospital length of stay, lost work time, lost productive years of life, or lost quality years of life.

Infection control programs and individual interventions within programs increasingly will be judged by their ability to produce positive benefit and cost effectiveness ratios and will be compared by the size of the ratios estimated.

A successful infection control program is an intervention-oriented program. The success of interventions in risk control programs is based on the following: (a) the preventability of the event (infection), (b) the efficacy of the intervention tool or process, (c) the efficiency of the intervention in terms of its cost and benefit in the average institutional situation, and (d) the compliance or acceptance by the medical worker in using the intervention or of the patient in allowing its use.

It is apparent from the literature of the experimental epidemiology of infection control that nosocomial infections at some sites and in some patients are much more preventable than others given current methodologies (7–9). When severity of infection is recorded (8, 9), a direct relationship between the severity of underlying disease and the rate of nosocomial infection is found. However, nosocomial infection in the most severely ill appeared less amenable to intervention than in other groups (9). McGowan and coauthors (10) found that less than 10% of procedure-related nosocomial bacteremias were potentially preventable in their study. Authors studying the leukemic or the transplant patient have suggested that 60 to 80% of the infections in these patients are from endogenous sources and therefore appear less amenable to prevention (11–13).

While the literature will change as new technology and methodologies appear and are reviewed, it seems obvious that the ability to prevent infection by the usual criteria varies widely by site, severity of co-morbid factors, and patient group. In situations of limited resources, cognizance of this variation will need to be included in the decision on priorities. It is equally obvious that the infection control practitioner will be a participant in the ethical discussions concerning medical practice which are of ongoing interest to other medical groups.

If the infection is potentially preventable, the next question of interest is the measured efficacy of a control program in that prevention. In the Study on the Efficacy of Nosocomial Infection Control (SENIC) (11), final evaluation suggested that approximately one-third of nosocomial infections could be prevented by full application of standard guidelines as outlined by the CDC. However, significant variation appeared between the efficacy of even the most detailed surveillance and control efforts based on site of infection. The poorest response to the surveillance and control programs was recorded with medical nosocomial pneumonias and the best response in the prevention of postoperative wound infections.

The first experiments in evaluation are frequently accomplished in carefully controlled and limited surroundings—usually the academic center or even an individual service or unit in the tertiary center. The results of the initial experiments are largely dependent on the condition of the patient and the preventability of the infection or other disease process involved and the efficacy of the intervention applied. Frequently the reports of the first phases of application appear in the literature with glowing support and offer associations which are biologically reasonable. Encouraged by the initial results, other investigators and practitioners attempt to apply the interven-

tion as a method in routine care in other units and institutions. In the second phase, results are often less promising or even negative.

While errors in experimental design or failure to control bias in the original experiment(s) may explain this lack of confirmation, several other potential changes from the original experiment may lead to the less positive, follow-up results: (*a*) poorly defined target groups of patients may be treated, with wider variation in the preventability of their disease; (*b*) the methodology may be less strictly supervised and thus less rigidly applied; (*c*) either medical personnel or patient compliance may drop, especially if the method is perceived to be cumbersome, overly detailed, or even hazardous; (*d*) finally, when stripped of the grant support of the original investigations, the cost of the intervention in time, personnel, or device expense may exceed the estimated benefit in reducing the target risk in the patients treated, either as a new or replacement technique.

Examples of these discussions are common in the infection control literature and currently include topics on control in urinary tract infections (14–17), respiratory tract infections (18–21), surgical wound infections (22, 23), intravascular site infections (24–28), and the use of protective isolation (29). In most instances, the follow-up evaluations have failed to support either the cost, the efficacy, or both and, therefore, do not allow recommendation for general application of the method. Young's discussion of the studies of the use of white cell transfusions in the immunocompromised host is an excellent example of the progression of evaluation and opinion in the application of this technique in the attempted prevention of infection in these critically ill patients (31).

The evaluation methodologies to establish productivity in programs were first developed in nonmedical fields, but have grown in their medical applications since the 1960s (30). A commonly used outline of evaluation methodology is shown in Table 7.1. It may be noted that the

Table 7.1.   The Evaluation Process

A. A question of importance
B. Criteria formation
C. Data collection and collation
D. Data evaluation
E. Intervention
F. Evaluation of intervention
G. Communication of findings

format follows the classic scientific method. The key ingredients are the formation of an appropriate and important question and criteria, data collection and evaluation, an experiment of change, another period of data collection to evaluate the results of this change, and finally communication of the results of this evaluation to those individuals and institutions interested or impacted.

A PRIORITY OBJECTIVE: THE QUALITY AND QUANTITY OF RISK

Nosocomial infections have been recognized repeatedly as medical complications of significant mortality, morbidity, and cost (32–35). The basic facts have been sufficient to convince a wide group of official and nonofficial agencies and organizations of the importance of intervention programs to attempt control (36–38). The priorities within these programs have not been so uniformly accepted (2, 6). While the classic CDC methodology (1), first developed in the 1960s, has been widely propagated, repeated criticisms have been voiced concerning their general efficacy and the philosophy of blindly promoting their routine application (3, 4). In establishing priorities in individual infection control programs, certain features may be of distinct importance.

Guidelines from the Literature

It is not always necessary to reinvent the wheel. A large and growing medical literature concerning the competing risks of various nosocomial infections in different units and services, in differing institutions is available.

Mortality Data

The infection control literature indicates an extremely high mortality rate for nosocomial infections related to primary and secondary bacteremias (43) and to nosocomial pneumonias (35, 44). High mortality rates are also reported in certain high risk units, e.g., intensive care (34, 45) and cancer chemotherapy (46).

Morbidity Data

An even larger but somewhat more diffuse literature in terms of quality reports an extensive and varied experience in measuring the morbidity of nosocomial infections. Morbidity is usually reported in terms of rates of events by site, secondary bacteremias, extended lengths of stay, and increased costs of medical care. Studies from the Hospital Infections Branch of the CDC (7, 39) and several other centers have presented comparative baseline descriptive data on nosocomial infection rates by hospital characteristics, service, site, and microorganism (8, 9, 40, 41). A vast additional literature from other sources includes both endemic and epidemic information on nosocomial risk associations and, less frequently, information on successful intervention programs with sufficient data to be convincing. High rates of morbidity reported in the literature are directly related to the severity of illness in the patient (8, 9), units where the severely ill are concentrated (33, 37, 46–48), and units where special procedures with medical devices are routine to care (49, 50). Again, pulmonary and primary bacteremias are the sites of highest morbidity, with wound infections falling intermediate between these sites and the more frequent, but less serious urinary tract infections.

In the recent literature, more sophisticated risk evaluation and stratifications have begun to appear using multivariate analysis and other statistical methods developed in chronic disease epidemiology (42, 51–54). In these analyses the host factors of age and extent of underlying disease, the presence and duration of surgery and the presence and duration of medical devices are the most consistently identified correlates of increased risk for nosocomial infection.

For the beginning practitioner or for the individual entering an unknown situation where no previous data are available, the experience in the literature points to the most prevalent problem areas found across a wide arena of studies on nosocomial infection risk.

Guidelines from Local Experience

While the reported experience in the infection control literature may provide an initial guide to identify areas of high risk requiring priority attention, the extent of variation in the literature and the less well documented experience of local practitioners would indicate that the best guidelines for developing priorities in a given institution are based on specific data identifying its nosocomial events and their associated risks. As an example, burn units are classically identified in the literature as having *Pseudomonas aeruginosa* as the most common infecting organism in the burn wound (55), but other individual reports note *Staphylococcus aureus* (56), *Enterobacter* (57), and *Providencia* species (58) as the endemic strains of importance. In another example, certain nationally renowned cancer units have extensively reported their experiences (12, 59), with *Pseudomonas* infections being most prevalent. On this basis, recommendations have been made for anti-*Pseudomonas* therapy as a routine measure in cancer patients. Generalization of the recommendation to units where other bacteria, e.g., *Legionella* or *Enterobacter*, are the prevalent infecting organisms could lead to unsatisfactory outcomes in the patients so treated.

The data generated through surveillance activities in the individual institution usually will be the best guide to developing priorities for that institution. Knowledge of the endemic experience will help to focus attention on persistent problem areas and additionally will be critical to the early identification of epidemic collections.

Recommendations for determining the significance of variations in the data from endemic experience have been published (1, 60, 61). The guidelines usually suggest using a statistically determined level to indicate a high probability that the current variation is not a chance occurrence. Trends exceeding this limiting boundary are taken as the signal to open an exploratory investigation into the potential problem area, the first step in devoting additional priority and resources.

Comparisons with past experience are difficult if significant changes have taken place in either the population studied or the medical techniques applied. Current medical experience would suggest that management of the less severely ill in ambulatory care areas is resulting in an inpatient hospital population with higher rates of severe illness, an association known to increase the risk of nosocomial infection. Therefore, if historical data are used for controls or for baselines, the potential bias of other changes must controlled.

If past data from an institution, an area, or an intervention are not available, a quick survey of current experience may be the best method of determining the priority problem areas for action. Either point prevalence or period prevalence studies are examples of rapid, low cost methods of evaluating a general risk situation (42, 62). Prevalence data may suffer the problems of the bias of the season, day, personnel rotation, holiday time, or other features which complicate generalization of the results. However, careful timing of the study, attention to the criteria, and assuring reliable methods of data collection will prevent most problems. If doubt remains concerning bias in the results, a repeat study or an augmentation by a brief incidence study in the

units under question usually will be sufficient to validate the findings.

REVIEW AND USE OF RESOURCES

In any situation of priority setting, it is important to tailor the resources to the size of the problem(s) identified. Too little resource may lead to uncontrolled risk and high infection rates with resultant legal, reputation, and financial losses. Too high a rate of resource use wastes personnel, facility, and finances, robbing other critical areas of need.

Personnel

Data from past studies, experience of practitioners in the field, and specific evaluations within the SENIC investigations (11, 60) suggest that the number and training of the personnel involved in infection control programs should be matched with the size and complexity of the medical facility. The SENIC experience would further suggest that the original CDC recommendation of one practitioner for each 250 hospital patients at risk is a valid one (11).

No information on the required background and education of the individual practitioner has been convincingly evaluated, but current guidelines of the Association for Practitioners in Infection Control for awarding credentials to infection control practitioners suggest that a background of clinical training in medicine, nursing, or laboratory practice is necessary and that a basic curriculum is important to the function and success of the program (63). These criteria have yet to be tested. In contradistinction to these criteria, some programs have made very successful use of the technical assistance of licensed practical nurses and other less highly trained individuals, especially for routine surveillance activities under the direction of a more senior nurse responsible for the education and administrative functions of the program. Such nursing extenders may increase the capability of a program at significantly lower costs (DA Rasley, S Streed, RM Massanari, and WJ Hierholzer, personal communication).

Facility and Tools

Microbiology laboratory services sufficient to the identification and routine speciation of the common bacterial and fungal organisms are a standard requirement. Routine antibiotic sensitivity testing is a minimal, additional basic requirement, important in its contribution to therapy, antibiotic use control, and epidemiologic investigation. Referral services for more extensive microbial identifications, serologies, phage typing, plasmid analysis, and other nonroutine and research techniques should be available in regional or state health department laboratories and used as needed in special investigations.

Infection control programs and other patient care evaluation programs require extensive data and information services. Therefore, data handling and information distribution systems are critical to their success. These systems range from appropriate office and secretarial services to hospital and individual program computers. Computers have become an increasingly valuable and affordable tool in increasing the efficiency of those responsible for identifying the risks important to infection control and for the information distribution and educational programs that follow (64, 65).

The educational services of the infection control unit should include book, journal, library, and audiovisual services and resources which will allow the necessary and convincing communication of the findings of surveillance and the recommendations of the infection control committee concerning procedural modification required in medical care methods to achieve control of preventable infections. Sufficient funds to provide the basic training and continuing education of the infection control practitioner are necessary for all programs and will tend to pay for themselves by allowing the institution to have the timely information necessary to the critical evaluation of the infection control impact of new methods and devices.

Time: Balancing the Process

Most infection control practitioners will find that the demands for their services routinely exceed the time available. Therefore, the question of how to budget the time for the most effective program is a common one. In the process of infection control a balance of four basic features must be found if the program is to be routinely successful: (*a*) Sufficient valid and reliable data must be generated from the institution's practice and evaluated to identify the problem areas for intervention. (*b*) Control programs based on these data must be planned and implemented. (*c*) All intervention programs initiated must themselves be evaluated for effect. (*d*) All functions of the program should be widely communicated to all levels of the medical care staff.

Failure to have activity in one or more of these areas is common in infection control programs, usually due to lack of or perceived lack of sufficient resources. Many programs "fire fight," leaping from one epidemic cluster to another without making the basic changes which would assure control of most future epidemic problems. Other programs spend excessive amounts of time in extensive hospital-wide surveillance. Data are recorded and periodically may be analyzed and presented to the infection control committee, but intervention programs are not started. No time remains to begin the necessary, but painful political process of intervention. In programs where the process is carried through to intervention, a lack of evaluation of the intervention for success or failure is the next common shortcoming. In small institutions, the data base may be insufficient to generate a timely, statistically evaluable result. Therefore, it may be reasonable to accept trends in data if comparable studies in larger centers have shown scientifically acceptable results. Finally, success in infection control is predicated on acceptance of the facts of risk and of the necessity and productivity of the interventions. Knowledge through education is basic to the acceptance and to the political support to make it work.

RATIONALIZING RISK AND RESOURCE

Having reviewed reports on nosocomial risk from the literature and having personalized the potential risks to the local environment, the infection control practitioner has the information necessary to select the most effective priorities for his/her institutional program intelligently. Having done so, he or she must recognize the personnel, facility, and resources available to the program.

Preventable death from nosocomial infection must of necessity capture a program's and the institution's highest priority. Epidemic problems leading to death mandate decisions for control at the highest level. These responses may vary from a call for outside assistance to the discontinuation of certain or all medical admissions to a service or facility. The authority of the infection control committee demanded by the Joint Commission on Accreditation of Hospitals must be exercised at its highest level in this situation, and pursuit of the problem must be carried to solution, to the exclusion of all other routine activity if necessary.

Disease of sufficient significance to lead to irreversible morbidity in patients (e.g., infection leading to septic shock and resultant stroke) commands the next level of practical priority. These problems may demand priorities near the level of those leading to preventable death, especially if they are ongoing and uncontrolled.

The lowest level of practical priority in the usual context will be in the prevention of nosocomial infection-related morbidity without obvious long term residuals, though this relative benignity may not be easily established. Attempts to reduce bacteriuria by bacteriologic monitoring during short term catheterization of patients for elective surgery may have little marginal or long term effect (66, 67). While this should not lead one to lessen the usual recommendations for prevention of such infections, the problem should demand less attention in the priorities of a program than respiratory device factors linked to uncontrolled high rates of postoperative pneumonia with its known high morbidity and mortality (44).

As a general guideline the preventable higher morbidity problems demand the priority resources. Big problems, however, may not necessarily demand the largest amounts of time and resource. If the intervention program is known to be effective and key compliance including the necessary medical leadership can be summoned, results may be impressive and timely.

The Hospital Infections Program of the Center for Infectious Diseases of the Centers for Disease Control has provided a major service by developing a manual, *Guidelines for the Prevention and Control of Nosocomial Infection* (68). The guidelines were developed by the Center's staff with the assistance of expert working groups and have been widely reviewed by practitioners and researchers in infection control. In these guidelines, each of the areas of nosocomial infection risk (urinary tract infections, intravascular infections, surgical wound infections, etc) is outlined in a brief epidemiologic review. Thereafter, a categorization scheme is presented that ranks each of the recommendations based on judgments of support for them in the literature and in experience in practice. As one might expect in such rankings and recommendations, unanimity is difficult to find, but the guidelines probably represent a current consensus.

THE POLITICS OF PRIORITY

Since infection control is a practice of communication and change, knowledge and use of the politics of support and change are critical. These interactions begin with the practitioners'

success in developing the rapport necessary to gain the assistance of the unit medical personnel in identifying infected patients. It is also essential to work effectively with the members of the infection control committee. Problems identified and presented should always be clearly and optimistically viewed as variations in practice, of concern to all, and amenable to change. Key members of the committee and the patient service studied should be involved at the earliest phases of confirmation. Self-evaluation of the data by the service or unit involved should be invited. Participation by the service in recommending guidelines for confirmation of findings and for the control interventions should be routine. Groups or services not responding to these overtures should be invited to a meeting of the infection control committee for an open and thorough discussion of the data. Refusal to participate at this level is an indication for administrative referral to the highest levels of the institution.

Staff members and services showing an ongoing interest in infection control should be strongly supported, perhaps with special program efforts to respond with enhanced details and evaluations of their data when requested. A service grand rounds sharing current local infection control data with a review of comparative data from the past and the current literature is much more effective than hours of canned nonspecific information.

Data that on evaluation survive strong biologic and statistical review and have confirming support in the literature for successful intervention should command the priority attention of the program and the committee.

When problems are recognized and given priority for intervention, the appropriate details should be communicated to the target groups. The problem(s) should be clearly defined and described, and assistance in the further evaluation of the problem, including information from the current literature, should be offered. Advice concerning the usually appropriate interventions should be provided with an option for local modifications when appropriate. Compliance with the intervention must be the responsibility of the service, but sample data on the rates of compliance may be provided by the infection control program if requested and if the infection control practitioner has sufficient time. Data should be collected on the effect of the intervention and an analysis of the results promptly provided to the committee and the service. If the intervention has not been successful, re-evaluation and modification of the control measures may be indicated. With successful intervention and control of the problem, communication of the results should be forwarded to the service with expressions of appreciation for their interest and assistance. Success should be congratulated. If new policies and procedures are the result of this process, they should be codified in the institutional manuals.

CONSOLIDATION AND CONTINUANCE: THE PROBLEM OF SUCCESS

As the infection control practitioner gains the confidence of the institution and as the first successful projects and programs are recorded, a new series of challenges based on this success may evolve. The original endemic problem areas may be consistently controlled and new epidemic collections promptly recognized and truncated. At this point a malaise of the routine may endanger the esprit de corps of the program from within and demands for continued high rates of decline in infections, backed by implications of major reductions of resource, may threaten from without. Success has its price.

It will require innovation for the practitioner to maintain the stability of the program through this "success." Fortunately, the changing technology of medicine routinely provides new challenges for infection control. New devices require evaluation before and during their addition to medical practice. They also require guidelines for disinfection and sterilization. The new procedures for disinfection and sterilization may entail new risks for breaks in technique or even new occupational risks for the medical care worker. New technologies and methodologies require structural changes in the institution. These changes provide an opportunity to review the modifications for safety, infection control risk, and other effects on patient care practice.

Medical care workers are among the most mobile in industry, especially those at the tertiary teaching center. The migration provides a seemingly endless flow of new individuals requiring orientation and instruction in infection control methodology while offering new potential interactions for risk or improvement.

Finally, the practitioner in a stable and successful program affords the institution a potential for leadership in other areas of risk control. Several authors have noted that the epidemiologic methods basic to infection control practice are common to the applications necessary for patient safety, occupational safety, and areas of nonrisk patient care evaluation (69, 70). Few practitioners in these other programs have had the support in training common to infection control. Few recognize the commonality and success of the epidemiologic techniques for their practice or have knowledge of their use in infection control. The infection control practitioner with training in applied epidemiologic methods may be the key person to assist in these other programs, increasing their level of expertise and providing the institution with an increased efficiency in meeting the requirements of these mandated efforts.

RESEARCH

For the routine practitioner of infection control, research may not appear to be a priority commitment. However, the routine process of infection control practice may open an avenue to applied research. As noted previously, many of the methods, devices, and processes used in medical care and infection control have tenuous support for their routine application. Persistent, carefully defined observations in cooperative investigations, including joint studies on a regional basis, could add much to the support of the details of infection control practice or, conversely, could identify some as ineffective and candidates for discontinuance. Studies of dressing types, catheter care details, filter effectiveness, antiseptic effectiveness, and other procedures remain open for this type of investigation.

Some program features have failed in previous investigations for unclear reasons. Given the great intellectual support for hand washing as an infection control technique, why has routine compliance remained so low? Why is compliance lowest in the senior (leadership) groups (71)? What role could the patient have in improving hand-washing compliance in the medical personnel involved in his/her care? These and other equally interesting and puzzling questions remain open to applied study by the interested infection control practitioner.

Never easy, priority setting is often controversial and always necessary. It is a part of the self-evaluation effort of each successful program. Done carefully and routinely, it establishes validity, and by example leads others to the epidemiologic tools and processes of evaluation on which quality medical care is built.

References

1. Centers for Disease Control: *Outline for Surveillance and Control of Nosocomial Infections.* Washington, DC, US Department of Health and Human Services, Public Health Service, 1972.

2. Eickhoff TC: Nosocomial infections—a 1980 view: Progress, priorities and prognosis. In Dixon RE (ed): *Nosocomial Infections.* Atlanta, Yorke Medical Books, 1981, pp 1–8.

3. Tenney JH: Nosocomial infection and the regulated hospital. *Ann Intern Med* 89 (part 2):862, 1978.

4. Jackson MM: From ritual to reason—with a rational approach to the future: an epidemiologic perspective. *Am J Infect Control* 12:213–227, 1984.

5. Schaffner W: Infection control: time to justify the costs. *Hospitals* 53:125, 1979.

6. Williams REO: Changing perspectives in hospital infection. In Brachman PS, Eickhoff TC (eds): *Proceedings of the International Congress on Nosocomial Infection.* Chicago, American Health Association, 1971, pp 1–10.

7. Haley RW, Culver DH, White JW, Morgan WM, Emori TG: The nationwide nosocomial infection rate. *Am J Epidemiol* 121:159–167, 1985.

8. Scheckler WE: Septicemia and nosocomial infection in a community hospital. *Ann Intern Med* 89 (part 2):754–756, 1978.

9. Britt MR, Schleupner CJ, Matsumiya S: Severity of underlying disease as a predictor of nosocomial infections. *JAMA* 239:1047–1051, 1978.

10. McGowan JE, Parrott PL, Duty VP: Nosocomial bacteremia: potential for prevention of procedure related cases. *JAMA* 237:2727–2729, 1977.

11. Haley RW, Culver DH, White JW, Morgan WM, Emori TG, Munn VP, Hooton TM: The efficacy of infection surveillance and control program in preventing nosocomial infection in U.S. hospitals. *Am J Epidemiol* 121:182–205, 1985.

12. Bodey GP: Infections in cancer patients. *Cancer Treat Rev* 2:89–128, 1975.

13. Pizzo PA: Infection complications in the child with cancer. III. Prevention. *J Pediatr* 98:524–530, 1981.

14. Meizels M, Schaeffer AJ: Decreased incidence of bacteriuria associated with periodic instillations of hydrogen peroxide into the urethral catheter drainage bag. *J Urol* 123:841–845, 1980.

15. Gillespie WA, Jones JE, Teasdale C, Simpson RA, Nashef L, Speller DLE: Does the addition of disinfectant to urine drainage bags prevent infection in catheterized patients? *Lancet* 1:1037–1039, 1983.

16. Thompson RL, Haley CE, Searcy MA, Guenthner SM, Kaiser DL, Groschel DM, Gillenwater JY, Wenzel RP: Catheter-associated bacteriuria: failure to reduce attack rates using periodic instillations of a disinfectant into urinary drainage system. *JAMA* 251:747–751, 1984.

17. Wassen JW, Platt R, Thomas RJ, Rosner B, Kass EH: Antibiotic irrigation and catheter-associated urinary tract infections. *N Engl J Med* 299:570–573, 1978.

18. Henry R: Moist air in the treatment of laryngotracheitis. *Arch Dis Child* 58:577, 1983.

19. Garibaldi RA, Britt MR, Webster C, Pace NL: Failure of bacterial filters to reduce the incidence of pneumonia after inhalation anesthesia. *Anesthesiology* 54:364–68, 1981.

20. Feeley TW, Hamilton WK, Xavier B, Moyers J, Eger EI: Sterile anesthesia breathing circuits do not prevent postoperative preliminary infection. *Anesthesiology* 54:369–372, 1981.

21. Mazze RI: Bacterial air filters. *Anesthesiology* 54:359–360, 1981.

22. Ravitch MM, McAuley CE: Airborne contamination of the operative wound. *Surg Gynecol Obstet* 159:177–188, 1984.

23. Alexander JW, Fischer JE, Boyajian M, Palmguest J, Morris MJ: The influence of hair-removal methods on wound infection. *Arch Surg* 118:347–352, 1983.

24. Majenfeldt MMF, Stapert J, De Jurg PCM, Soeters PB, Wesdorp RIC, Creep JM: T.P.N. catheter sepsis: lack of effect of subcutaneous tunnelling of PVC catheters on sepsis rate. *JPEN* 4:514–517, 1980.

25. Garden OJ, Sim AJW: A comparison of tunnelled and untunnelled subclavian catheters: a prospective study of complication during parenteral feeding. *Clin Nutr* 2:51–54, 1983.

26. Thompson DR, Jones GR, Sutton TW: A trial of povidone-iodine ointment for the prevention of cannula thrombophlebitis. *J Hosp Infect* 4:285–289, 1983.

27. Friedland G: Infusion-related phlebitis—is the in-line filter the solution? *N Engl J Med* 312:113–115, 1985.

28. Maki DG, Will L: Colonization and infection associated with transparent dressings for central venous, arterial and Hickman catheters—a comparative trial. An abstract presented at the 24th Interscience Conference on Antimicrobial Agents and Chemotherapy. Washington DC, American Society for Microbiology, October 8–10, 1984.

29. Nauseef WM, Maki DG: A study of the value of simple protective isolation in patients with granulocytopenia. *N Engl J Med* 304:448–453, 1981.

30. Struening EL, Guttentag M (eds): *Handbook of Evaluation Research.* Beverly Hills, CA, Sage Publications, 1976.

31. Young LS: Nosocomial infections in the immunocompromised host. *Am J Med* 70:398–404, 1981.

32. Haley RW, Schaberg DR, Von Allmen SD, McGowan JE Jr: Estimating the extra charges and prolongation of hospitalization due to nosocomial infection. A comparison of methods. *J Infect Dis* 141:248–256, 1980.

33. Goldmann DA, Freeman J, Durbin WA: Nosocomial infection and death in a neonatal intensive care unit. *J Infect Dis* 147:635–641, 1983.

34. Cross PA, Neu HA, Aswapokee P, Van Antwerpen C, Aswapokee N: Death from nosocomial infection: experience in a university and a community hospital. *Am J Med* 68:219–223, 1980.

35. Daschner F, Nadjem H, Langmaack H, Sandritter W: Surveillance, prevention and control of hospital acquired infections. *Infection* 6:261–265, 1978.

36. American Hospital Association Committee on Infection within Hospitals: *Infection Control in the Hospital,* ed 4. Chicago, American Hospital Association, 1979.

37. Joint Commission on Accreditation of Hospitals: Infection control. In *Accreditation Manual for Hospitals/84.* Chicago, Joint Commission on Accreditation of Hospitals, 1983, pp 69–76.

38. American Health Care Association: *Infection Control in Long Term Care Facilities.* Washington DC, American Health Care Association, 1983.

39. Hughes JM, Culver DH, White JW, Jarvis WR, Morgan WM, Munn VP, Mosser JL, Emori TG: Nosocomial infection surveillance, 1980–1982. *MMWR* 32:155–1655, 1984.

40. Wenzel RP, Osterman CA, Hunting KJ: Hospital acquired infection. II. Infection rates by site, service and common procedures in a university hospital. *Am J Epidemiol* 104:645–651, 1976.

41. Britt MR, Burke JP, Nordquist AG, Wilfert JN, Smith CB: Infection control in small hospitals: prevalence survey in 18 institutions. *JAMA* 236:1700–1703, 1976.

42. Freeman J, McGowan JE: Risk factors for nosocomial infections. *J Infect Dis* 138:811–819, 1978.

43. Maki DG: Nosocomial bacteremia: an epidemiologic overview. In Dixon RE (ed): *Nosocomial Infections.* New York, Yorke Medical Books, 1981, pp 183–196.

44. LaForce FM: Hospital-acquired gram-negative rod pneumonias: an overview. *Am J Med* 70:664–669, 1981.

45. Craig CP, Connelly S: Effect of intensive care unit pneumonia in duration of stay and mortality. *Am J Infect Control* 12:233–238, 1984.

46. Schimpff SC, Young VM, Green WH, Vermeulen GD, Moody MD, Wiernick PH: Origin of infection in acute nonlymphoctic leukemia. Significance of hospital acquisition of potential pathogen. *Ann Intern Med* 77:707–714, 1972.

47. Wenzel RP, Thompson RL, Landry SM, Russell BS, Miller PJ, Ponce de Leon S, Miller GB: Hospital-acquired infection in intensive care unit patients: an overview with emphasis on epidemics. *Infect Control* 4:371–375, 1983.

48. Robinson GV, Zegtmeier BR, Zara JA: Brief report: nosocomial infection rates in a cancer treatment center. *Infect Control* 5:289–294, 1984.

49. Wenzel RP, Osterman CA, Donowitz LG, Hoyt JW, Sande MA, Martone WJ, Peacock JE, Levine JI, Miller GB: Identification of procedure related nosocomial infection in high-risk patients. *Rev Infect Dis* 3:701–707, 1981.

50. Stamm WE: Infection related to medical devices. *Ann Intern Med* 89 (part 2):764–769, 1978.

51. Haley RW, Culver DH, Morgan WM, White JW, Emori TG, Hooten TM: Identifying patients at high risk of surgical wound infection: a simple multivariate index of patient susceptibility and wound contamination. *Am J Epidemiol* 121:206–215, 1985.

52. Garibaldi RA, Britt MR, Coleman ML, Reading JC, Pace NL: Risk factors for postoperative pneumonia. *Am J Med* 70:677–680, 1981.

53. Hooton TM, Haley RW, Culver DH, White JW, Morgan WM, Carroll RJ: The joint association of multiple risk factors with the occurrence of nosocomial infection. *Am J Med* 70:960–969, 1981.

54. Ehrenkranz NJ: Surgical wound infection occurrence in clean operations. Risk stratification in interhospital comparisons. *Am J Med* 70:909–914, 1981.

55. McManus WF, Goodwin CW, Mason AD, Pruitt BA: Burn wound infections. *J Trauma* 21:753–756, 1981.

56. Espersen F, Nielsen PB, Lund K, Sylvest B, Jensen K: Hospital-acquired infections in a burn unit caused by an imported strain of *Staphylococcus aureus* with unusual multi-resistance. *J Hyg Camb* 88:535–541, 1982.

57. Mayhall CG, Lamb VA, Gayle WE, Haynes BW: *Enterobacter cloacae* septicemia in a burn center: epidemiology and control of an outbreak. *J Infect Dis* 139:166–171, 1979.

58. Wenzel RP, Hunting KJ, Osterman CA, Sande MA: *Providencia stuartii*, a hospital pathogen: potential factors for its emergence and transmission. *Am J Epidemiol* 104:170–180, 1976.

59. Schimpff SC, Greene WH, Young VM, Wiernik PH: Significance of *Pseudomonas aeruginosa* in the patient with leukemia or lymphoma. *J Infect Dis* 130:5, 24–31, 1974.

60. Emori TG, Haley RW, Garner JS: Techniques and uses of nosocomial infection surveillance in U.S. hospitals, 1971–77. *Am J Med* 70:933–939, 1981.

61. Birnbaum D: Analysis of hospital infection surveillance data. *Infect Control* 5:332–338, 1984.

62. Britt MR: Infectious diseases in small hospitals. Prevalence of infections and adequacy of microbiological services. *Ann Intern Med* 89:757–760, 1978.

63. Soule BM (ed): *The APIC Curriculum for Infection Control Practice.* Association for Practitioners in Infection Control. Dubuque, Iowa, Kendall/Hunt, 1983, vols 1 and 2.

64. Etersque S, Carter MJ, Gordon KR, Sutherland JG: Computerization of a nosocomial infection system. *J Med Syst* 8:407–416, 1984.

65. Hierholzer WJ Jr, Streed SA: Two years' experience using an on-line infection data management system. Proceedings of the Sixth Annual Symposium on Computer Applications in Medical Care. Washington DC, Institute of Electrical and Electronics Engineers, October 30–November 2, 1982.

66. Jacobson JA, Burke JP, Kasworm E: Effect of bacteriologic monitoring of urinary catheters on recognition and treatment of hospital-acquired urinary tract infections. *Infect Control* 2:227–232, 1981.

67. Garibaldi RA, Mooney BR, Epstein BJ, Britt MR: An evaluation of daily bacteriologic monitoring to identify preventable episodes of catheter-associated urinary tract infection. *Infect Control* 3:466–470, 1982.

68. Simmons BP (ed): *Guidelines for the Prevention and Control of Nosocomial Infection.* Atlanta, Centers for Disease Control, 1981.

69. Elder HA: Infection control—into the next decade. *Infect Control* 5:557–558, 1984.

70. Hierholzer WJ Jr: The practice of hospital epidemiology. *Yale J Biol Med* 55:225–230, 1982.

71. Albert RK, Condie MS: Handwashing patterns in medical intensive care units. *N Engl J Med* 304:1465–1466, 1981.

Chapter 8

Surveillance and Reporting of Nosocomial Infections

Robert L. Thompson, M.D.

Confinement within hospitals has long been recognized to be associated with risks of morbidity and mortality that are in excess of the risk inherent in the illness prompting admission. Ignaz Semmelweis has come to be recognized as the father of hospital epidemiology because of his early use of surveillance techniques in documenting a hospital outbreak (1). Utilizing the same techniques, he then convincingly demonstrated the impact of a control measure on outcome in a hospital population (2). As an obstetrician at the Lying-In Hospital in Vienna in 1847, he made a series of careful clinical observations on the incidence of mortality from puerperal sepsis. Having developed an impression that mortality was more common on one obstetrical unit than another in the same institution, even though both services were plagued by similar conditions of overcrowding and poor ventilation, he made systematic observations and measurements to substantiate his hypothesis. He showed that mortality rates were, in fact, 4 times higher in the first division, which was staffed by obstetricians and medical students, than in the second division, which was staffed by midwives. After the death of a physician friend who had contracted a wound infection while performing an autopsy on a woman succumbing to childbed fever, he noted that medical students generally entered the delivery room of the first division directly from the autopsy suite. He also had recognized the odor of the autopsy room within the delivery room only when students were present. Surmising a causal association, he required all students to wash their hands in chlorinated lime prior to contact with parturients. Subsequently, he documented a dramatic decline in mortality from puerperal sepsis in the first division to a rate similar to that in the division staffed solely by midwives. Thus, even prior to an understanding of the germ theory of infectious diseases, epidemiologic methods provided both a cause and a solution to this outbreak of nosocomial infection (see Chapter 1 for a discussion of the history of nosocomial infections).

From these beginnings more than 100 years before the discovery and widespread use of antibiotics, contemporary interest in hospital epidemiology experienced a renaissance only after the failure of these antimicrobial agents to prevent epidemics of hospital-acquired infection. Antibiotics, in fact, were shown to encourage the spread of infection within hospitals during the epidemic transmission of penicillin-resistant *Staphylococcus aureus* in hospitals throughout the world in the late 1950s (3). These events rekindled a universal recognition of the need for infection control programs and the requirement for surveillance techniques to hasten the recognition and control of outbreaks of hospital-acquired infections (4, 5).

In the 1960s, infection control committees were voluntarily formed in many institutions, and various approaches to infection surveillance were advanced (6–8). Early efforts tended to emphasize extensive environmental culturing activities even though such microbiologic surveillance had not been shown to be effective in preventing infection. In 1970, the first International Conference on Nosocomial Infections encouraged the development of infection surveillance programs (9), resulting in efforts by the Centers for Disease Control to provide standard definitions of nosocomial infections and suggested methods for hospital-wide surveillance and control activities (10). Whereas only 16% of hospitals practiced infection surveillance in 1965, the proportion increased to 40% by 1970 and to 83% by 1976 (11, 12), at a time when the Joint Commission on Accreditation of Hospitals distributed its first extensive set of guidelines on infection control (13). During the same period, routine microbiologic environmental surveillance declined and now has virtually disappeared from infection surveillance programs (12).

SURVEILLANCE

The focal point for infection control activities in the hospital is a system of surveillance designed to establish and maintain a data base which describes endemic rates of nosocomial infection. Awareness of the endemic rates allows the recognition of epidemic occurrences when infection rates rise above a calculated threshold. Surveillance should ideally provide systematic and continuous observations on the occurrence and distribution of nosocomial infection within the hospital population for the purpose of prevention and control. The term surveillance implies that the observational data are regularly analyzed and reported to individuals who are in a position to take appropriate actions in order to achieve control. Surveillance activities may provide valuable epidemiologic data such as identification of epidemics, priorities for infection control activities, and the elucidation of important secular trends, such as shifts in microbial pathogens, infection rates, or outcomes of hospital-acquired infection. Surveillance activities provide the additional benefits of increasing the visibility of the infection control team in the hospital during the infection control practitioners' ward rounds, and of allowing an opportunity for informal consultation and education to unit nurses and physicians. Recent analysis of the relative effectiveness of hospital surveillance activities from the SENIC project indicated that "effective" surveillance programs were those that (a) employed an infection control nurse to perform surveillance on clinical ward rounds on a regular basis; and (b) analyzed rates of infection with at least basic epidemiologic techniques, and periodically used the data in decision making (14).

Ideally the surveillance of hospital-acquired infection should be a continuous process that consists of the following elements:

1. Definition of categories of infection;
2. Systematic case finding and data collection;
3. Tabulation of data;
4. Analysis and interpretation of data;
5. Reporting of relevant infection surveillance data to individuals and groups for appropriate action.

Interinstitutional differences limit the ability to generalize about the effects of specific surveillance and control activities and reinforce the need for each health care facility to maintain a surveillance program tailored to meet its individual requirements in achieving the ultimate goal of reducing risks of hospital-acquired infection.

DEFINITIONS

The use of consistent definitions of nosocomial infection is critical in developing background data on endemic infection rates. Definitions such as those outlined in Table 8.1 are purposely simple, requiring only clinical information or readily available laboratory data. Infections may be said to be nosocomial when they are not known to be present or incubating at the time of admission. When the incubation period is unknown, an infection is called nosocomial if it develops at any time after admission. An infection present on admission, however, may be classified as nosocomial if it is directly related to a previous admission. In a patient with a previously established nosocomial infection, a new, individual nosocomial infection should be recorded in two situations: (a) the appearance of clinical infection at a new and different site, even though associated with the same microorganism as the original infection; and (b) the appearance in culture of new and different organisms from a previously described site of nosocomial infection should be considered a new individual nosocomial infection if there is a coincident clinical continuation or deterioration in the patient's condition.

DISTRIBUTION OF NOSOCOMIAL INFECTION BY SITE

Based upon the definitions described above, it is estimated that 5 to 10% of hospitalizations are complicated by nosocomial infection. Infection rates are, of course, dependent on the type of surveillance methodology employed, the size of the institution, and the complexity of the patient population. Perhaps the most reliable estimates of the overall rates and distribution of nosocomial infection available to date from U.S. hospitals are derived from the Study on the Efficacy of Nosocomial Infection Control (SENIC). The study estimated that over a 12-month period in 1975–1976, approximately 2.1 million nosocomial infections occurred among 37.7 million admissions to the 6449 acute care hospitals in the United States (15). This results in an overall infection rate of 5.7 infections/100 admissions. The distribution of nosocomial infections and the infection rate for the major categories of infection are presented in Table 8.2. Urinary tract infections

Table 8.1.   Definitions of Nosocomial Infections Used in Performing Surveillance

Infection Site	Criteria for Infection	Comments
Postoperative wound	Pus at the incision site	Deep postoperative wounds, cellulitis, and endometritis are classified separately.
Other wounds	Presence of pus	Includes decubitis ulcer, tracheostomy site.
Blood	Positive culture	Must rule out contaminant.
Pulmonary	Infiltrate on chest X-ray not present on admission associated with new sputum production	Clinical picture must be compatible and other entities—e.g., atelectasis and pulmonary embolus with infarction—ruled out; in immunosuppressed patients, sputum production is not essential.
Urine	$\geq$ 100,000 colonies of bacteria/ml	Lower counts may be considered significant if associated with compatible symptoms and pyuria.
Intestinal	Positive culture for pathogen or unexplained diarrhea for $\geq$ 2 days	Nosocomial antibiotic-associated colitis or diarrhea may be diagnosed by presence of *Clostridium difficile* cytotoxin.
Burns	$\geq$ 10^6 microorganisms/g of burn wound biopsy tissue or new inflammation or purulence not present on admission	
Miscellaneous (hepatitis, upper respiratory infections, peritonitis, etc)	Clinical picture	

constituted 42% of all nosocomial infections, surgical wound infections 24%, pneumonia 10%, and primary and secondary bacteremia 5%. All other types of nosocomial infection accounted for the remaining 19%.

DISTRIBUTION OF NOSOCOMIAL INFECTIONS BY PATHOGEN

The distribution of pathogenic microorganisms implicated in nosocomial infection obviously varies among individual institutions. The National Nosocomial Infection Study provides descriptive data from a group of 54 hospitals across the United States which illustrate the variability of pathogens which cause nosocomial infection. Although not stratified to reflect a representative sample of U.S. hospitals, participating hospitals conduct active hospital-wide surveillance using uniform definitions (16). The most frequently isolated pathogens and their percentage distribution for each site of infection (Table 8.3) illustrate their relative prevalence as agents of nosocomial infection and their variability dependent on site of infection.

Table 8.2.   Distribution and Rates of Nosocomial Infections by Site*

Category	Proportion of Nosocomial Infections (%)	Infection rate†
Urinary tract infection	42.0	2.39
Surgical wound infection	23.8	1.35
Pneumonia	10.5	0.60
Bacteremia	4.8	0.27
All other sites	18.9	1.07
Total	100.0	5.68

* Adapted from the Study on the Efficacy of Nosocomial Infection Control (SENIC) (18).
† Number of nosocomial infections/100 admissions.

Based upon surveillance data collected in an individual institution, analyses such as these and analysis of the prevalence of antibiotic resistance among bacterial isolates associated with infections identified during routine surveillance may provide information useful to clinicians, particu-

Table 8.3. The 15 Most Frequently Isolated Pathogens and Their Percentage Distribution for Each Site of Infection, 1983*

Pathogen	UTI	SWI	LRI	BACT	CUT	Other	Total Isolates	%
Eschericola coli	31.7	11.4	7.1	12.8	7.7	7.3	5,779	18.6
Staphylococcus aureus	1.6	19.0	12.8	12.8	33.3	16.4	3,356	10.8
Enterococci	14.9	11.4	1.6	7.3	9.5	7.3	3,308	10.7
Pseudomonas aeruginosa	12.5	8.1	15.1	6.1	7.2	6.2	3,286	10.6
Klebliella sp.	7.6	4.8	12.8	9.1	4.4	4.0	2,288	7.4
Coagulase-negative staphylococci	3.7	8.4	1.1	14.2	9.5	11.1	1,892	6.1
Enterobacter sp.	4.4	6.9	10.0	6.9	4.1	4.1	1,811	5.8
Proteus sp.	7.3	5.0	4.4	1.7	3.5	3.2	1,667	5.4
Candida sp.	5.1	1.4	4.2	5.6	4.5	13.4	1,570	5.1
Serratia sp.	1.2	2.0	5.6	2.8	1.8	1.8	691	2.2
Other fungi	2.0	0.4	1.8	1.0	0.4	2.3	471	1.5
Bacteroides sp.	0.0	4.4	0.2	3.4	1.0	1.9	439	1.3
Group B *Streptococcus*	1.0	1.8	0.7	2.8	1.3	1.7	418	1.3
Citrobacter sp.	1.4	1.3	1.7	1.1	1.1	0.9	403	1.3
Other anaerobes	0.0	2.3	0.0	2.1	0.9	4.2	337	1.1
All others†	5.6	11.4	20.9	13.6	9.8	14.2	3,296	10.6
Number of isolates	13,165	6,163	4,490	2,292	1,798	3,104	31,012	100.0

* From Jarvis WR, White JW, Munn VP, Mosser JL, Emori TG, Culver DH, Thornsberry C, Hughes JM: Nosocomial infection surveillance, 1983. *MMWR* 33(suppl 255):9SS–22SS, 1984.

UTI, urinary tract infection; SWI, surgical wound infection, LRI, lower respiratory infection; BACT, bacteremia, CUT,

† No other pathogen accounted for more than 3% of the isolates at any site.

larly in decisions regarding empirical choices of therapy. Similar analyses of data collected during routine surveillance can display the distribution of pathogens by hospital service or unit. The data base can be used creatively to provide physician-specific infection rates or rates associated with specific procedures, such as invasive diagnostic interventions or surgical procedures (17). The collection of procedure-specific information allows not only the monitoring of especially high risk surgical or nonoperative procedures, but when performed on a continuing basis, provides a sensitive index for the early detection of outbreaks of infection that are very likely to be preventable (18).

SOURCES OF INFECTION SURVEILLANCE DATA

Effective surveillance programs must utilize information generated from a wide variety of sources from both within and outside the institution (Table 8.4). It is impossible for an infection control practitioner to review data from all patients on a daily or a weekly basis either prospectively or retrospectively. Sampling techniques,

Table 8.4. Sources of Surveillance Information

Clinical ward rounds
Microbiology laboratory reports
Radiology reports
Pharmacy
Admissions department
Medical records department
Operating room activity reports
Outpatient clinic
Employee health clinic
Postdischarge surveillance
Public health resources
Regional professional societies

therefore, must be developed, preferably independently by individual institutions, to identify patients who are at greatest risk for acquiring a nosocomial infection. These techniques should provide for the timely identification of infections allowing the potential for early intervention.

Clinical ward rounds provide an excellent source of information that in many institutions can be focused on specific subsets of the inpatient population known to be at high risk for acquiring infection (19). These include patients with fever or serious underlying disease, those patients on isolation precautions, those receiving antibiotics or wound care, and those who have had high risk diagnostic or therapeutic invasive procedures. Other major sources of surveillance information are microbiology laboratory reports. When laboratory line listings are available on a frequent basis, they may serve an important adjunctive role in directing clinical ward surveillance. Many hospital information systems may be capable of providing microbiologic data by specific ward location, etiologic agents, and antibiotic susceptibility profiles that will aid in outbreak identification. As advances are realized in the implementation of the automated medical record, valuable information of a similar nature will become more readily available from radiographic, ultrasound, and nuclear medicine reports, hospital pharmacy, admissions department, operating room, medical records department, and outpatient clinics. Postdischarge follow-up information may prove especially useful in selected patients, such as surgical patients and newborns, in whom infections frequently become manifest after hospital discharge. Additional sources of potentially useful information on secular trends include local, state, and national public health advisories and regional professional organizations, such as the Association of Practitioners of Infection Control.

MINIMUM DATA COLLECTION

The nature and extent of information collection in conjunction with each recognized infection is best determined independently by individual institutions and will likely vary by site of infection, service, or hospital location. Certain essential identifying data may be recommended, including name, age, sex, hospital identification number, ward location, service, date of admission, date of onset of infection, site of infection, microorganisms isolated from culture materials associated with the infection, antibiotic susceptibility profiles of suspected etiologic agents, dates and types of surgical procedures, and operating surgeon. Other invasive procedures associated with infections—such as intravascular, urinary, and respiratory tract instrumentation—should be recorded and may be analyzed periodically in outbreak surveillance.

METHODS OF CASE FINDING

Considerable controversy has surrounded direct and indirect comparisons of case-finding methods used in infection control programs. An analysis of the relative sensitivities of these methods has recently been presented by Freeman and McGowan (20). A hypothetical standard for the total number of detectable nosocomial infections was defined as those infections found by a specially trained physician who not only examined each patient, each hospital record, and all nursing care plans but also verified all microbiologic information after all results were complete. Measured against this standard, the relative sensitivities of other published methods of detecting nosocomial infections are presented in Table 8.5. Use of self-report forms submitted by individual clinicians was least sensitive. Prospective clinical surveillance for evidence of fever, antibiotic use, or both, as well as a variety of techniques of surveillance of clinical microbiology laboratory reports were only moderately sensitive. However, selective chart review of high risk patients achieved a measure of sensitivity comparable to total prospective chart review (19). Retrospective chart review as performed in the SENIC pilot project had an average sensitivity of 0.74 which was comparable to physician-epidemiologist-supervised prospective data collection (21).

Since a variety of methods of case finding may be utilized in the identification of hospital-acquired infections, the data collected may be presented as either incidence surveys or prevalence surveys. Incidence surveys are performed on con-

Table 8.5.   **Relative Sensitivity of Published Methods of Case Finding of Nososomial Infections***

Method	Reference	Sensitivity
Physician self-report forms	8	0.14–0.34
Fever	19	0.47
Antibiotic use	19	0.48
Fever plus antibiotic use	19	0.59
Microbiology reports	6, 8, 19, 21	0.33–0.65
Selected chart review using "Kardex clues"	19	0.85
Total chart review	19	0.90
SENIC pilot retrospective	21	0.66–0.80
Standard	20	1.00†

*Adapted from Freeman J, McGowan JE JR: Methodologic issues in hospital epidemiology. I. Rates, case finding and interpretation. *Rev Infect Dis* 3:658–667, 1981.

† By definition, all other sensitivities are referable to this standard.

secutive sequential hospitalizations. This usually requires retrospective record review and, therefore, is subject to considerable reporting delays. Incidence data are ideally expressed as the number of new cases of infection occurring per unit population over a specified time period of observation. Usually, however, incidence surveys of nosocomial infection do not report strict incidence as defined above, but rather as an attack rate. The attack rate is defined as the proportion of patients at risk who become infected over an entire period of exposure, such as the duration of hospitalization, and they are most commonly derived in terms of the number of nosocomial infections/100 admissions or discharges. They may be interpreted as the probability of acquiring one or more nosocomial infections during a hospitalization. Thus, an attack rate is usually independent of any unit measure of time. The second type of survey is the prevalence survey, in which either patients or their records are examined for an event at a single point in time. Prevalence is expressed as the proportion of patients with a particular characteristic at a single moment in time.

Freeman and McGowan reviewed published series of prevalence and incidence surveys of nosocomial infections (20). They report prevalence proportions ranging from 4.5 to 15.5% and attack rates from incidence series ranging from 3.1 to 14.1%. The variability in proportions and rates is due, in part, to differences in patient populations, lengths of hospital stay, and time of performance of the individual studies. In large measure, however, the differences are related to fundamental differences in the surveillance techniques used in case finding. Methods of case finding in infection control programs typically include elements of both prevalence and incidence surveys, in part because of differences in operational definitions of nosocomial infection at the varying infection sites.

IDENTIFICATION OF PATIENTS AT HIGH RISK OF NOSOCOMIAL INFECTION

No system of routine prospective surveillance is completely sensitive in the identification of nosocomial infections. Optimal use of the time available to infection control practitioners for surveillance activities requires methods to identify subsets of patients who are at highest risk. Data from the SENIC project identified a number of patient characteristics which were associated with an increased risk of acquiring a nosocomial infection (22). Patients undergoing surgical pro-

cedures, while constituting only 42% of the hospital population, experienced 71% of all nosocomial infections. This included 56% of urinary tract infections, all surgical wound infections, 74% of pneumonias, and 54% of bacteremias. Overall, the relative risk of a surgical patient developing a nosocomial infection was 3 times that of a nonsurgical patient, with ratios of infection percentage of 1.77 for urinary tract infection, 3.91 for pneumonia, 1.57 for bacteremia, and 2.93 for all four major sites combined. Whereas urinary tract infection risks were highest for neurosurgical and urologic subspecialty services, surgical wound infection percentages were highest in obstetrical patients undergoing cesarean section and lowest for gynecology services. Pneumonia rates were highest for thoracic surgery, general surgery, and neurosurgery services, while bacteremia risk was highest for thoracic surgery. Infection percentages also increased at all four major infection sites in direct relation to duration of preoperative hospitalization as well as to duration of surgery. The percentage of patients developing surgical wound infection increased linearly with the duration of the surgical procedure. There was over a 20-fold increment in risk between the shortest (1 to 30 minutes) and longest (greater than 2½ hours) categories. Similarly, infection percentages also increased for the other three sites with increasing duration of surgery, including a 49-fold increase for postoperative pneumonia, a 12-fold increase for urinary tract infections, and a 36-fold increment for bacteremia risk (15). Other patient characteristics associated with increased infection risk included indwelling urethral catheterization, continuous mechanical ventilatory support, use of immunosuppressive drug therapy during hospitalization, increasing age, and presence of a previous community-acquired or nosocomial infection (22).

Other investigations have identified patients confined within critical care units to be at high risk of nosocomial infection. Wenzel and co-workers have shown that as many as 33 to 45% of all nosocomial pulmonary infections and bacteremias occur in intensive care unit (ICU) patients who reside in only 5 to 10% of hospital beds (23). Additionally, ICUs are the most frequent focal point of recognized epidemics of nosocomial infections (24). Donowitz and associates have shown that the overall infection rate in a surgical ICU was 18% compared to a 6% rate among general ward patients (25). Although the surgical wound infection rates were similar in ward and ICU patients, rates for nosocomial urinary tract infection, pneumonia, and bacteremia were 2- to 7-fold higher in the ICU setting. These categories of infection are frequently device-related (indwelling urethral catheters, intravascular cannulation, endotracheal intubation, etc) and, therefore, are potentially preventable. While patients treated in burn units are at high risk for wound sepsis, remarkably high attack rates for nosocomial pneumonia and primary and secondary bacteremia—many of which are also device-related (26)—have also been reported in burn centers (27).

In summary, priorities for nosocomial infection surveillance must be established within each individual institution based upon the resources available and the complexity and heterogeneity of the patient population. Surveillance for nosocomial bacteremia, which may be primarily laboratory-based, is a high priority in view of the significant morbidity and mortality associated with these infections (28). Surveillance of nosocomial urinary tract infection, while perhaps of less critical importance clinically, is also efficiently accomplished via laboratory surveillance techniques. Detection of surgical wound infections and pulmonary infections is poorly suited to laboratory-based surveillance methods because of the clinical nature of the standard definitions of these infections (10).

Design of prospective clinical ward surveillance activities should be selectively focused on recognized high risk groups, with surgical patients and patients in ICUs given the highest priority. In these areas, the high incidence density of nosocomial infection generally justifies total patient surveillance at frequent intervals. Prospective clinical patient surveillance on general medical wards must be selectively focused on patients at high risk of nosocomial infection, utilizing case-finding clues available from graphic records, nursing care plans, or hospital information systems which access useful information sources (e.g., operating room or anesthesia records, pharmacy, admissions office, and medical records data banks).

The SENIC project has provided the first conclusive evidence for the effectiveness of surveillance activities in the prevention of nosocomial infection (14). Although SENIC was not able to determine precisely which methods and schedules should be used in performing surveillance, most of the study hospitals were detecting infections by a combination of ward rounds, review of laboratory records, and other clinical activities on a continuous daily basis in most areas of the hospital (14). It is not possible to infer that other techniques—such as periodic prevalence studies, focused surveillance limited to specific units and other targeted approaches—are as effective as continuous hospital-wide surveillance.

ROLE OF THE INFECTION CONTROL PRACTITIONER IN SURVEILLANCE

Specially trained practitioners have played the major role in the collection of routine infection surveillance data for over 15 years (29). Emori and co-workers have described the techniques and uses of nosocomial infection surveillance in a representative sample of 433 acute care hospitals participating in the SENIC project (30). Ninety-seven percent of hospitals were conducting some type of surveillance. Eighty-four percent performed continuous daily surveillance, while 10% exclusively performed regularly scheduled prevalence surveys and 3% performed irregular prevalence surveys. Most performed hospital-wide surveillance using active case-finding techniques (31). Ninety-three percent covered ICUs, 90% covered general surgery, pediatrics, and the newborn nursery, and 88% routinely covered general medicine and obstetric and gynecology units. On average, infection control practitioners—usually nurses—spent 46% of their time performing surveillance (30). This percentage did not vary significantly when analyzed by total number of hours/week worked in infection control activities or by hospital size.

Additionally, infection control nurses spent 23% of their time researching and developing infection control policies, 13% of their time in in-service educational programs in infection control, 10% consulting with hospital personnel, and 8% in the investigation of suspected outbreaks of infection. Hospitals with more intensive surveillance programs were significantly more likely to have used surveillance data to detect outbreaks and to look for specific ongoing infection problems (14).

Forty two percent of SENIC hospitals had at least one full time equivalent (FTE) infection control practitioner for every 300 beds (14). In analyzing the changes in infection rates between 1970 and 1975–1976, the authors showed that having a full time equivalent infection control practitioner for every 250 occupied beds was an important component of programs designated as "very effective." Reductions in infection rates in the SENIC project fell off sharply as the number of beds/full time equivalent infection control nurse increased from 250 to 400 beds (14), providing strong support for staffing at the 250 bed/full time equivalent infection control nurse level (10).

EFFICACY OF NOSOCOMIAL INFECTION SURVEILLANCE

Despite extensive clinical research into the methodology of nosocomial infection surveillance and control in the past two decades, convincing evidence of the actual effectiveness of infection control programs in reducing infection risk has been lacking due to the infinite variability of individual hospital populations, the confounding effects of multiple uncontrolled variables, changing medical technologies, incomplete identification of causal or predisposing factors, and arbitrary measurements of their quantitative effects. Several uncontrolled studies from individual institutions have reported reductions in the rates of nosocomial infection by 30 to 50% after the institution of infection surveillance and control programs (6, 32, 33), but the lack of simultaneous control observations prevented valid assessments of the efficacy and cost effectiveness of such programs (34). The need for this information resulted in the commissioning of the SENIC investigation by the CDC in 1974.

SENIC

The SENIC project had three major objectives: (*a*) to determine whether, and to what degree, implementation of infection surveillance and control programs have lowered the rate of nosocomial infection in major categories of U.S. hospitals; (*b*) to describe the current status of infection surveillance and control programs and nosocomial infection rates in a representative sample of U.S. general hospitals; and (*c*) to study the relationships among the characteristics of hospitals and patients, the components of infection surveillance and control programs, and changes in nosocomial infection rates at specific infection sites and on specific services during the time interval studied (35). The objectives also included determining whether the surveillance or the control function was more important in reducing infection risks and whether other recommended components of infection control programs, such as the infection control nurse-to-patient ratio and the characteristics of the infection surveillance and control programs supervisor, were important determinants of a program's efficacy. The project

was designed to study questions separately relating to the efficacy of infection surveillance and control programs for infections involving the surgical wound, the urinary tract, the lower respiratory tract, and the bloodstream, which together account for approximately 80% of all nosocomial infections.

Data in the SENIC project were collected in three phases (36). In phase I, a detailed questionnaire was mailed to all U.S. general hospitals which was designed to obtain the information needed to calculate two prespecified indices: a "surveillance index," which measured the extent to which each hospital conducted active surveillance of nosocomial infections and disseminated the results, and a "control index," which measured the intensity of efforts to intervene in the care of patients to reduce infection risks (35). A random sample of 338 U.S. hospitals was selected from 16 strata determined by the joint categorization of their respective surveillance and control indexes (Fig. 8.1).

In phase II, a team of interviewers visited each of the sample hospitals and interviewed the 12 hospital personnel most likely to have important duties related to infection surveillance and control as well as a random sample of staff nurses. These responses were used to corroborate and supplement the responses obtained in the phase I questionnaire.

In phase III, 500 adult general medical and surgical patients who were admitted during the 1970 calendar year and during the 12-month period April 1975 through March 1976 were randomly selected in each of the 338 sample hospitals. Thus, estimates of the nosocomial infection rates were made both before any of the sample hospitals had established infection surveillance and control programs and again at the time of the phase I survey. The study populations each contained over 169,000 patients representative of all adult general medical and surgical patients admitted to U.S. hospitals during each time period, with each population group comprising more than 1,600,000 patient-days of observation. Every patient's entire medical record was reviewed; the information abstracted included patient demographic information, all discharge diagnoses, surgical procedures, postoperative diagnoses, and selected clinical data from each hospital day (14). Specific details of the analytic strategies and statistical methods employed in analysis of the SENIC project have been published (35, 36). The salient findings of the study

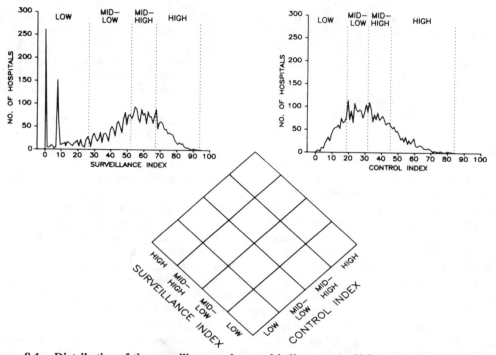

Figure 8.1. Distribution of the surveillance and control indices among U.S. hospitals and their use in the stratification and selection of the SENIC sample. (From Haley RW, Culver DH, White JW, Morgan TM, Emori TG, Munn VP, Hooten TM: The efficacy of infection surveillance and control programs in preventing nosocomial infections in U.S. hospitals. *Am J Epidemiol* 121:185, 1985.)

are summarized by the major sites of infection (Table 8.6). Findings are subcategorized by patient risk groups, assessment of the quality of the hospital's surveillance and control program, and the most important components identified in the quantitative assessment of effective programs.

Surgical Wound Infection

Among patients characterized as at high risk for development of surgical wound infection (Table 8.6), 85% underwent clean or clean-contaminated operations, while 15% were contaminated or dirty cases. Infection control and surveillance programs which were found to be "very effective" were characterized by two components: (*a*) high intensity surveillance as well as high intensity control activities which specifically included a system for reporting surgical wound infection rates back to the practicing surgeons; and (*b*) having an "effectual hospital epidemiologist," defined as an individual who had enough interest to have taken courses on the subject of infection control and who was sufficiently active in directing the infection control and surveillance program to have brought about a reduction in the hospital's level of routine environmental cultur-

ing. Five percent of U.S. hospitals were estimated to have "very effective" programs resulting in reduction of infection rates among high risk patients by 35%. Establishing one but not both of these components resulted in a "moderately effective" program that characterized infection control and surveillance programs in 51% of U.S. hospitals and was associated with a reduction in the surgical wound infection rate of 20%.

Among "low risk" surgical patients (98% of whom had clean or clean-contaminated procedures), a more stringent program model was required to achieve similar levels of protection. "Very effective" programs were characterized by two components. The first included establishment of a program with both high intensity surveillance and control activities as well as a system for reporting surgical wound infection rates back to the practicing surgeons. The second component was the presence of an effectual hospital epidemiologist as defined above. An estimated 4% of U.S. hospitals had "very effective" programs for patients at low risk of surgical wound infection, which resulted in a 41% decrease in infection risk. Having only the first of these components resulted in a "moderately effective" pro-

Table 8.6. The SENIC Project: Percentage Reduction in Nosocomial Infection Risk in Hospitals Establishing Effective Infection Surveillance and Control Programs*

Site of Infection	Patient Risk Group (% of Patients)	Quality Assessment of Hospital's Surveillance and Control Program	Important Components of Qualitative Assessment of Hospital's Surveillance and Control Program	% of U.S. Hospitals	% Reduction in Infection Risk
Surgical wound	High risk (50%)	Very effective	1) a. High intensity surveillance and control activities b. Feedback of infection rates to surgeons and 2) Effectual hospital epidemiologist†	5%	35%
		Moderately effective	Component 1 or 2 only	51%	20%
	Low risk (50%)	Very effective	1) a. High intensity surveillance and control activities b. Feedback of infection rates to surgeons and 2) Effectual hospital epidemiologist	4%	41%
		Moderately effective	Component 1 only	29%	19%
Urinary tract	High risk (27%)	Very effective	High intensity surveillance activities and ≥ 1 FTE infection control nurse/ 250 beds	7%	31%
	Low risk (73%)	Very effective	Very high intensity surveillance and control activities and ≥ 1 FTE infection control nurse/ 250 beds	4%	41%
Pneumonia	Surgical	Very effective	High intensity surveillance activities and ≥ 1 FTE infection control nurse per 250 beds	7%	27%
	Medical	Moderately effective	Moderately high intensity surveillance and control activities	47%	13%
Bacteremia All patients		Very effective	1) High intensity control activities 2) Moderately high intensity surveillance activities 3) ≥ FTE infection control nurse/ 250 beds 4) Hospital epidemiologist	4%	35%
		Moderately effective	High intensity control activities	14%	15%

* Adapted from Haley RW, Culver DH, White JW, Morgan TM, Emori TB, Munn VP, Hooten TM: The efficacy of infection surveillance and control programs in preventing nosocomial infections in U.S. hospitals. *Am J Epidemiol* 121:182–205, 1985.

† See text for definition.

gram (characterizing 29% of U.S. hospitals), which was associated with a 19% reduction in infection risk.

Urinary Tract Infections

The prevention of nosocomial urinary tract infections among high risk patients optimally required an infection control program with high intensity surveillance activities with at least a moderately low level of control activities staffed by at least one full time equivalent infection control nurse/250 occupied hospital beds. In hospitals with less than 200 beds, this level of prevention could be attained with less infection control nurse staffing if there were other staff members performing the intensive type of surveillance required. The estimated 7% of U.S. hospitals with programs meeting these requirements noted a 31% reduction in infection risk.

Optimal prevention of nosocomial urinary tract infection among the 73% of patients classified as low risk required the establishment of very intensive surveillance and very intensive control activities with at least one full time equivalent infection control nurse/250 occupied beds, or in small hospitals an equivalent staffing pattern as described above for high risk patients. The 4% of U.S. hospitals with such programs realized a 41% reduction in infection risk.

Pneumonia

Prevention of postoperative pneumonia in surgical patients required the establishment of a high intensity surveillance program as well as a full time equivalent infection control nurse for every 250 occupied hospital beds. The level of control activities did not correlate with preventive efficacy of the infection control program. In the 7% of U.S. hospitals with such a program, a 27% reduction in postoperative pneumonia rates resulted.

Evidence for the effectiveness of infection surveillance and control efforts in the prevention of nosocomial pneumonia among medical patients was less impressive. The moderately high intensity surveillance and control activities in the infection control program of 47% of U.S. hospitals resulted in only a 13% reduction in infection risk.

Bacteremia

An impressive 35% reduction in the risk of nosocomial bacteremia was demonstrated by the 4% of U.S. hospitals that had infection control programs characterized by high intensity control

activities combined with at least medium high intensity surveillance activities, at least one full time equivalent infection control nurse/250 beds, and a hospital epidemiologist. A 15% risk reduction occurred in hospital programs classified as "moderately effective" which featured at least a high intensity level of control activities.

Among the 14% of hospitals in the SENIC sample that established "very effective" programs for at least one infection site, site-specific infection rate reductions of 7 to 48% were demonstrated. The most impressive overall reductions in infection risk were documented among the 0.5% of hospitals that established infection control programs that were assessed as being "very effective" for all infection sites, where the overall infection rates decreased approximately 36% over the 6-year study interval. In contrast, site-specific infection rates increased consistently at all sites in those institutions that established an ineffective or no infection control program during this interval. Although SENIC data suggest that only 6% of nosocomial infections were being prevented by the infection control programs in place in 1975–1976, the authors estimate that nearly one-third of all nosocomial infections could have been prevented had *all* U.S. hospitals adopted the most effective programs (14). The Study on the Efficacy of Nosocomial Infection Control thus appears to have finally provided firm evidence to justify investment in the development and maintenance of infection control programs in general hospitals. The results of the SENIC project should serve as a guide in the continuing modification of infection surveillance and control activities within individual institutions to achieve the greatest reductions in rates of nosocomial infection.

REPORTING

The purpose of reporting data derived from infection surveillance activities is to inform and educate clinical and administrative personnel who are in positions to initiate appropriate actions to lower infection risks. The frequency and style of reporting should be sufficiently flexible to provide information that is relevant and understandable to groups and individuals with varying needs and backgrounds.

Reports prepared for the infection control committee membership are prepared at a frequency and level of complexity that would perhaps be inappropriate for other groups with different responsibilities in the hospital. These reports are usually prepared monthly and contain tabulated data with appropriate analyses and interpretation of overall infection rates, as well as site-specific, pathogen-specific, unit-specific, or service-specific rates. The data should provide insight into endemic rates of infection throughout the institution. It may be appropriate to establish epidemic thresholds of varying sensitivities for particularly important categories of infection, such as primary bacteremia or nosocomial pneumonia. Review of monthly infection rates is enhanced by tabular and graphic displays depicting secular trends within the institution by utilizing, for example, incidence data from the preceding 12 consecutive months.

Other reports may be routinely prepared for specific groups or individuals within the institution, such as surgeon-specific, procedure-specific, or diagnosis-specific infection rates. These reports may be designed to educate, to heighten interest in infection control, or to modify behavior. Surgical wound infection rates, especially surgeon-specific rates, should be regularly reported to the infection control committee and to individual surgeons (37, 38).

Special reports are indicated in the event of outbreaks of nosocomial infection. These reports are not only intended to call attention to the problem but also to serve as a vehicle to promote control activities. Special reports may also be useful in announcing institutional policy changes or in promoting employee health prevention programs such as hepatitis B immunization of high risk personnel.

The maintenance of an organized hospital-wide surveillance program has been shown to be an essential part of infection control programs which have effectively reduced the incidence of nosocomial infection. Each infection control committee should periodically reassess the effectiveness of its surveillance activities and creatively modify them to meet the unique requirements of the individual institution (39). The development of effective surveillance programs should recognize the impact of nosocomial infections on length of hospital stay and cost.

References

1. Miller PJ: Semmelweis. *Infect Control* 3:405–409, 1982.
2. Semmelweis IP: Classics in infectious diseases: childbed fever. *Rev Infect Dis* 3:808–811, 1981.
3. Berntsen CA, McDermott W: Increased transmissibility of staphylococci to patients receiving an antimicrobial drug. *N Engl J Med* 262:637–642, 1960.
4. Langmuir AD: The surveillance of communicable diseases of national importance. *N Engl J Med* 268:182–192, 1963.
5. Brachman PS: Surveillance of institutionally acquired infections. In *Proceedings of the National Conference on Institutionally Acquired Infections*, Minneapolis, University of Minnesota School of Public Health, September 4–6, 1963. Public Health Service Publication no. 1188. Washington, DC, US Government Printing Office, 1964, pp 138–147.
6. Thoburn R, Fekety FR, Cluff LE: Infections acquired by hospitalized patients. *Arch Intern Med* 121:1–10, 1968.
7. Wenzel K: The role of the infection control nurse. *Nurs Clin North Am* 5:89–98, 1970.
8. Eickhoff TC, Brachman PS, Bennett JV, Brown JF: Surveillance of nosocomial infections in community hospitals. I. Surveillance methods, effectiveness and initial results. *J Infect Dis* 120:305–317, 1969.
9. Garner JS, Bennett JV, Scheckler WE: Surveillance of nosocomial infections. In *Proceedings of the International Conference on Nosocomial Infections*, August 3–6, 1970. Chicago, American Hospital Association, 1971, pp 277–281.
10. Centers for Disease Control: *Outline for Surveillance and Control of Nosocomial Infections*. Atlanta, Centers for Disease Control, 1972.
11. Centers for Disease Control: Infection surveillance and control programs in U.S. hospitals: an assessment, 1976. *MMWR* 27:139–145, 1978.
12. Haley RW, Shachtman RH: The emergence of infection surveillance an control programs in U.S. hospitals: an assessment, 1976. *Am J Epidemiol* 111:574–591, 1980.
13. Joint Commission on Accreditation of Hospitals: *Accreditation Manual for Hospitals*. Chicago, Joint Commission on Accreditation of Hospitals, 1976.
14. Haley RW, Culver DH, White JW, Morgan TM, Emori TG, Munn VP, Hooten TM: The efficacy of infection surveillance and control programs in preventing nosocomial infections in U.S. hospitals. *Am J Epidemiol* 121:182–205, 1985.
15. Haley RW, Culver DH, White JW, Morgan WM, Emori TG: The nationwide nosocomial infection rate: a new need for vital statistics. *Am J Epidemiol* 121:159–167, 1985.
16. Jarvis WR, White JW, Munn VP, Mosser JL, Emori TG, Culver DH, Thornsberry C, Hughes JM: Nosocomial infection surveillance, 1983. *MMWR* 33 (suppl 255):9SS–22SS, 1984.
17. Farber BF, Kaiser DL, Wenzel RP: Relation between surgical volume and incidence of postoperative wound infection. *N Engl J Med* 305:200–204, 1981.
18. Ponce de Leon S, Critchley S, Wenzel RP: Polymicrobial bloodstream infections in ICU patients undergoing prolonged vascular catheterization. *Crit Care Med* 12:856–859, 1984.
19. Wenzel RP, Osterman CA, Hunting KJ, Gwaltney JM Jr: Hospital-acquired infections. I. Surveillance in a university hospital. *Am J Epidemiol* 103:251–260, 1976.
20. Freeman J, McGowan JE Jr: Methodologic issues in hospital epidemiology. I. Rates, case finding and interpretation. *Rev Infect Dis* 3:658–667, 1981.
21. Haley RW, Schaberg DR, McClish DK, Quade D,

Crossley KB, Culver DH, Morgan WM, McGowan JE, Shachtman RH: This accuracy of retrospective chart review in measuring nosocomial infection rates. *Am J Epidemiol* 111:516–533, 1980.

22. Haley RW, Hooten TM, Culvar DH, Stanley RC, Emori TC, Handison GD, Quade D, Shachtman RH, Schaberg DR, Shah BV, Schatz GD: Nosocomial infections in U.S. hospitals, 1975–1976: estimated frequency by selected characteristics of patients. *Am J Med* 70:947–959, 1981.

23. Wenzel RP, Osterman CA, Donowitz LG, Hoyt JW, Sande MA, Martone WJ, Peacock JE Jr, Levine JI, Miller GB: Identification of procedure-related nosocomial infections in high-risk patients. *Rev Infect Dis* 3:701–707, 1981.

24. Wenzel RP, Thompson RL, Landry SM, Russell BS, Miller PJ, Ponce de Leon S, Miller GB: Hospital-acquired infections in intensive care unit patients: an overview with emphasis on epidemics. *Infect Control* 4:371–375, 1983.

25. Donowitz LG, Wenzel RP, Hoyt JW: High risk of hospital-acquired infection in the ICU patient. *Crit Care Med* 10:355–357, 1982.

26. Wenzel RP: Surveillance and reporting of hospital acquired infections. In Wenzel RP (ed): *Handbook of Hospital Acquired Infection.* Boca Raton, FL, CRC Press, 1981, pp 35–72.

27. Mayhall CG: Infections in burn patients. In Wenzel RP (ed): *Handbook of Hospital Acquired Infection.* Boca Raton, FL, CRC Press, 1981, pp 317–339.

28. Maki DG: Epidemic nosocomial bacteremias. In Wenzel RP (ed): *Handbook of Hospital Acquired Infection.* Boca Raton, FL, CRC Press, 1981, pp 371–512.

29. Emori TG, Haley RW, Stanley RC: The infection control nurse in U.S. hospitals 1976–1977: characteristics of the position and its occupant. *Am J Epidemiol* 111:592–607, 1980.

30. Emori TG, Haley RW, Garner JS: Techniques and uses of nosocomial infection surveillance in U.S. hospitals, 1976–1977. *Am J Med* 70:933–940, 1981.

31. Haley RW, Shachtman RH: The emergence of infection surveillance and control programs in U.S. hospitals: an assessment, 1976. *Am J Epidemiol* 111:574–591, 1980.

32. Streeter S, Dunn H, Lepper M: Hospital infection—a necessary risk? *Am J Nurs* 67:526–533, 1967.

33. Shoji KT, Aznick K, Rytel MW: Infections and antibiotic use in a large municipal hospital 1970–1972: a prospective analysis of the effectiveness of a continuous surveillance program. *Health Lab Sci* 11:283–292, 1974.

34. Sencer DJ, Axnick NW: Utilization of cost-benefit analysis in planning prevention programs. *Acta Med Scand* 576(S):123–128, 1975.

35. Haley RW, Quade D, Freeman HE, Bennett JV, CDC SENIC Planning Committee: The SENIC project: summary of study design. *Am J Epidemiol* 111:472–485, 1980.

36. Quade D, Culver DH, Haley RW, Whaley FS, Kalsbeek WD, Hardison CD, Hohnson RE, Stanley RC, Shachtman RH: The SENIC sampling process: design for choosing hospitals and patients and results of sample selection. *Am J Epidemiol* 111:486–502, 1980.

37. Cowdon RE, Schalte WJ, Malangoni MA, Anderson-Teschendorf MJ: Effectiveness of a surgical wound surveillance program. *Arch Surg* 118:303–307, 1983.

38. Olson M, O'Conner M, Schwartz ML: Surgical wound infections: a 5-year prospective study of 20,193 wounds at the Minneapolis VA Medical Center. *Ann Surg* 199:253–259, 1984.

39. Haley RW: Surveillance by objective: a new priority-directed approach to the control of nosocomial infections. *Am J Infect Control* 13:78–89, 1985.

Chapter 9

Data Collection and Management for Infection Control

Donald L. Kaiser, Dr.P.H., and Richard L. Barr, M.A.

INTRODUCTION

All effective infection control programs have, as an essential part of their activities, the collection of data characterizing patients, organisms, and hospital procedures. To control infections, one must understand them by examining the cause and effect patterns which emerge from large sets of information. This approach is, obviously, the underlying thread of the scientific method. We observe, postulate, and test hypotheses in order both to understand a process and to devise an intervention to alter its course.

The amount and focus of the data collected can vary substantially from one program to another, but one common issue has emerged over the past 10 years. Virtually all programs have considered how they may use the computer to assist infection control professionals in the organization, collection, management, and analysis of their data.

This chapter will deal with the significant issues in data collection and management in infection control programs, in the context of cost and capability of computers. When designing and implementing computerized information systems for infection control, one must plan in three areas: the nature and variety of information to be collected; the mechanisms for collecting these data; and the strategies to be used in computerization (Fig. 9.1). Solutions in these areas will be proposed based on current technology, some involving the use of computers and others not. As circumstances change in the future, more and more computer-based applications will be possible.

DEFINING DATA ELEMENTS

The major data items of interest to programs which seek to identify and control hospital-acquired infections can be classified as *clinical*. That is, they provide information about the clinical circumstances of hospitalization: diagnoses, tests, test findings, clinical observations, and, occasionally, prognoses.

Patient Demographics

Information identifying the patient is certainly the most obvious component of an infection control data system. Included in this component should be name; medical record number; case identifying number (unless date of admission alone uniquely describes individual patient events); patient name (if a system includes patients' names, unauthorized access to data must be minimized; remember that data files should be considered part of the institution's medical record on the patient); sex; race; date of birth (much preferable to age, which can always be calculated).

Details of Hospitalization

Hospitalization should be viewed as an *event*, with characteristics which will be important in identifying and understanding that event, and in placing it properly in relation to other events. The event has a beginning date and an ending date. Simply knowing that a hospitalization was 5 days long may not be enough if it matters that the event occurred in the first week of September, 1984, and that the patient was admitted on a Saturday.

This issue brings up an important rule: Always provide the highest *attainable* level of precision in the data. We recognize that being too precise can cause errors, so the word attainable is an important one. The concept of precision is important because data can always be made less precise (temporarily) in subsequent use; however, it is not possible to make data more precise (without re-entering it). In other words, a hospitalization which begins on Sunday, January 13, 1985, and which ends in discharge on Friday,

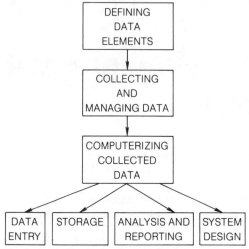

Figure 9.1.   Designing a program for data collection and management.

January 18, can be identified as being 5 days in duration and placed with all other 5-day admissions, or with all admissions with durations under 10 days and so on. However, had the person entering the data simply categorized the duration of admission as "10 days or more" and "under 10 days," the more specific information about actual date and day of admission would be unidentifiable.

Other important aspects of the hospitalization are as follows: the hospital service admitting and caring for the patient (not necessarily the same); the location of the patient's room, and any transfers of the patient from room to room; and information about surgery and other procedures—including invasive diagnostic procedures—provided to the patient.

Risk Factors and Underlying Conditions

Host factors which exist on admission or which develop later, as well as specific actions taken in the hospital which may predispose a patient to develop infection are important to include in the data. In order to do this, one must rely on prescience in anticipating etiology. There are, however, some obvious choices:

The diagnoses (conditions) present are an immediate choice. One needs to strike a balance between obtaining all potentially relevant diagnoses and burdening the data base—and those collecting the data—with excessive information management tasks. Further, it is important to identify those diagnoses regarded as pertinent for other purposes, specifically for the calculation of

the Diagnosis Related Group for the hospitalization. Currently, the Diagnosis Related Group system uses the principal discharge diagnosis, other secondary diagnoses (including the occurrence of a nosocomial infection), and the patient's age, to calculate the authorized reimbursement for the case from federal health programs. Although the authorized reimbursement differs according to type of hospital and region of the country, the fundamental classification does not.

Treatments which predispose patients to hospital-acquired infections are, for the most part, also identifiable. Surgical procedures, immunosuppression, placement of invasive monitors and prosthetic devices all compromise natural defense systems in ways which are understood to invite infection. Conditions and treatments are an area where coding can make data acceptably precise while providing some check against error and ambiguity. This aspect will be discussed below under "Data Management."

Predisposing factors are the major area where thoughtful planning and anticipation may be required in deciding what information to record. What factors other than those mentioned above may have etiologic connection to the acquisition of an infection? One can imagine quite a number of elements—some of which may offend certain readers, but which must be mentioned by way of example. The administering of certain treatments by a first-year resident may (because of excess time taken, inexperience, faulty technique, etc) cause infection. Treatment by weekend or night staff may also be related. A change in the supplier of a device or the use of a new lot of a device might also be important. In other words, one can imagine scores of data items which could be included in an infection control data base (from the examples above: name of person giving treatment, time consumed by treatment, number of prior treatments given by treatment giver, time of day treatment administered, serial or lot number of device used).

Many of these items would probably wind up consuming space and data analysis resources without ever providing additional insight into the nature of nosocomial infections. Choices have to be made when the data base is designed, since it is frequently difficult to change its design and always time consuming to go back and collect additional data on old records. There is no magic formula which can tell a hospital epidemiologist what to choose. In the beginning it is advisable to get together a group of concerned staff with the expertise to advise; be prepared to make the hard decisions after consulting with this group.

Characteristics of the Infection

An important facet of the data recorded about hospital-acquired infections is the type or nature of the infection itself. The site (urinary tract, bloodstream, pulmonary, postoperative wound, and "other" are common categories) and type of organism are obvious choices in this area. Additional information about the antibiotic susceptibility of organisms should be recorded as well. The coding of organisms and antibiotics for susceptibility should be considered. (See "Data Coding Techniques" below for some suggestions.)

Hospital practices sometimes permit troublesome ambiguity in describing infections. For example, the presence of pus at an incision site is, in many institutions, sufficient evidence for determining the presence of a postoperative wound infection. Specific information about the nature of the organism(s) involved may not be available for some time—or may never be available in some institutions. "Pus" is obviously not the name of an organism, yet if the practitioner leaves the organism section blank, the report may suggest that data were available but missed. Because of the implication for labor and cost of additional laboratory testing to identify organisms, each institution must resolve the problem individually.

Hospitals with automated laboratory data systems may want to link them to their infection control system. While it may result in the inclusion of extra, and perhaps unnecessary, information in the infection control system, it also provides for greater recording accuracy and saves data entry effort and expense.

Elements of Treatment

Hospitalized patients are provided an ever growing array of pharmacologic treatments. Many of the therapies employed either increase susceptibility (as immunosuppresives do), successfully eliminate the offending microorganism, or alter the susceptibility pattern of a family of organisms. Accordingly, we need to record such treatments in order to understand the long range implications of pharmacologic intervention. Obviously, the use of specific antibiotics may have important implications with subsequent emergence of resistant isolates.

An important aspect of this effort is standardization. As names of agents become more complex, the temptation grows to abbreviate or "mnemonicize." One approach is to fall back on the hospital's formulary as the official nomenclature for agents. (This approach may also provide a framework for coding.) Most hospitals subscribe to formulary services which could provide interinstitutional standardization as well. Generic names could be used if one were certain of equivalence. However, this technique might prove cumbersome and costly to administer.

The quantity of agents administered and the frequency of administration may prove important, especially in retrospective evaluation of treatment efficacy. Moreover, the dates and quantities should be recorded since they could provide useful data about efficacy and cost of prophylactic treatment.

Nonpharmacologic interventions (other than those mentioned under "Risk Factors and Underlying Conditions," above) may also prove significant. For example, physical therapy often involves seemingly benign substances—such as hydrotherapy tanks, lotions, bandages, and supports—which may provide transmission links and reservoirs for pathogens. Minimal information about the administration of such treatments could well produce unsuspected etiologic evidence in some cases.

Discharge and Posthospital Data

Patient status at discharge (sent home well, dead, transferred, moved to lower level of care, etc) is an important aspect of each case for evaluating the impact of hospital-acquired infections and their treatment. It would be well to include diagnoses active at discharge, separate from admission and intrastay diagnoses. This is particularly true if the data system is running well and identifies patients shortly after admission. Patients with residual infections who are readmitted within a short period of time may need special handling within the institution.

In an era of cost consciousness, outpatient treatment often is used an an alternative to prolonged hospitalization. Information from these encounters is no less important than that about the patients in acute care beds and should be added assiduously to the system to give a complete picture of patient care.

Costs

Costs (and/or charges) should at least be considered as elements of the data system. While such items are often more difficult to collect and are usually viewed as the unpleasant side of hospital care, they are critical pieces of information for effective and intelligent management of a hospital. Emphasis on costs is currently at an all-time high. In deciding what financial data to include, one should remember that infection control programs must compete for the hospital's dollar along with all other services. The more solid evidence practitioners can provide to their institution about the impact and importance of the program, the more competitive the infection control program will be. Dollars may not be as interesting to discuss as the science of our work, but they are a marvelous way of keeping score in the institutional games which all must play.

Summary

A substantial array of choices which must be made in designing and implementing an infection control data system has been discussed. While an elegant system would include everything presented, it would take a unique institution to gather all of the information suggested without also incurring massive costs. Each program must make its own decisions based on feasibility and the individual opinions of its local experts. After the difficult choices are made, one needs to decide how the information should be gathered. Some ideas are offered below about enhancing data collection, improving accuracy, and making systems more efficient. However, once again, each method must be examined for utility, practicality, reliability, and cost.

DATA MANAGEMENT

There are many methods for managing a data system, once the contents of the system have been determined. Management covers a broad range of activities, including the implementation process, and data acquisition, data entry, management and updating of stored files, and file utilization (reports and analyses).

Implementation is largely an issue that must be resolved within individual institutions. There are, however, some general principles regarding the use of information as an incentive and control mechanism (1, 2) and the mechanics of implementation (planning, time charts, vendor/production monitoring, and quality control) (3–7). Those principles go far beyond the scope of this chapter, and interested readers are referred to the references listed.

Data Collection and Reliability

Who will be the primary gatherer(s) of data for the system? This fundamental question will probably determine the ultimate success of the infection control system in any institution. Once again, there are some obvious choices. On-site (ward and bedside) providers of care and services (physicians, nurses, paraprofessionals) can be provided with forms and instructions regarding patients with nosocomial infections. Alternatively, professionals specifically identified with the infection control program and specifically trained for that role can canvass the institution on a periodic basis—perhaps when notified by on-site providers. Finally, clerical or other nonprofessional staff can be used to do the canvassing. Each of these three major strategies has advantages and disadvantages.

Collection by on-site care providers will probably provide the most accurate information (accurate taken here to mean the most precise reflection of reality). These persons are in a position to make primary observations of the patient. However, they are probably less motivated than a professional whose primary responsibility is to the infection control program. The collection of infection control data may be seen as simply one more burden added to an existing work load. In addition, they must be trained (and periodically retrained) to deal with criteria and reporting standards established by the infection control program. Further, in terms of cost, these highly paid professionals may be the most expensive and least efficient data gatherers.

At the other end of the spectrum are non-health professionals (clerical personnel, data base technicians, programmers, etc) who can be trained specifically for the infection control data system tasks, will appreciate the inherent implications of data values, coding, etc, but who will understand only very little of the clinical issues surrounding the data gathered. Such persons are probably the most cost-effective alternative, but only if one counts errors in purely objective terms. If, on the other hand, one appreciates the fact that errors are very costly in terms of the science of controlling nosocomial infections, then this alternative becomes much less appealing.

The rational middle ground is to seek out health care professionals who have an interest in hospital-acquired infections, who can be trained in the data system principles, and who will work closely with the data system personnel involved in the program. These persons (physicians, nurses, respiratory therapists, laboratory technologists, etc) will certainly cost more than the clerical persons described above, but will more than make up for increased cost with significantly improved accuracy. Further, they will find it easier to identify with, and elicit assistance from, the on-site professionals with whom they must work for truly effective data collection.

Once it is determined who will collect the data, the next decision is how the data are to be collected (i.e., on what types of forms). For primary data (that is, data generated for the first time by the staff and placed on forms) there is no problem. However, a substantial amount of information is recorded for the first time for someone else's purposes (laboratory reports, medication record, clinical observations for the patient's chart, etc). The decision to be made then is whether to re-record the data on infection control forms, or to secure a copy of the primary form and include it in the packet of information. The trade-off is between the potential translation errors of re-recording versus the inclusion in the data forms of extraneous and/or noncompatible data sheets. The appropriate decision will differ significantly from one institution to another and must be weighed using such considerations as cost and reliability of duplication, type of data entry used (see "Error Checking during Data Entry," below), and so on. In an institution with an effective information system, much of the data will be automated in its primary form. The infection control data system's implementors are then confronted with the task of interfacing one system to another. While it is rarely a trivial task, it is at least one where the decisions usually do not compromise data reliability.

Improving and Increasing Available Data

At some point in the implementation of an infection control data program one must begin to consider improving data collection procedures optimally. As mentioned before, some basic aspects of the system will influence effectiveness: who collects data and what data are collected. There are some additional implementation methods which can further improve data accuracy and can also increase the amount of data available, at virtually no increase in effort or cost.

Hospitals virtually run on information, and persons working in hospitals are asked to provide data by many different entities within the organization. Further, it is almost always the case that the best (most precise, complete, etc) data provided by an individual are those recorded for his or her own use. In seeking information for an infection control program, then, the one implementing the program should attempt to find ways to collect data which serve both the program and the individual providing the data. For example, data on the administration of antibiotics are important and represent a potentially voluminous component of information on patients with a

nosocomial infection. Requiring someone to enter those data to satisfy the needs of the infection control service, the pharmacy, and the hospital ward may not be necessary or prudent.

As an alternative, it might be possible to have the pharmacy enter the data as a part of their record keeping, have the floor merely confirm the administration (by retaining a copy of the entry for the chart), and have the infection control program enter the confirmation. While such a strategy clearly requires a coordinated data system, many hospitals are in a position to implement such an approach, which could be developed and coordinated by the infection control program staff.

Many hospitals might consider a higher level of assistance and require that each nosocomial infection be reported by someone involved with the case (often the responsible physician). If the data acquisition process for the infection control data system could be combined with the preparation of the report, one could save labor by the health professionals, provide a clearer (i.e., computer-prepared) report, and place needed data directly in the data system. There are several reputable software systems which could provide the mechanism for a physician or nurse to answer questions about the case, and which would then prepare a printed report and load the data into the infection control system.

Finally, it is always desirable to explore existing data systems within the hospital for information which could supplement or enhance the infection control data system. While a hospital may not have a central information system, it may have localized systems at work in many places within the institution. Potential sources are the billing department (for accurate patient identification, as well as cost and charge data), the clinical laboratory, the operating room (OR logs), the pharmacy (drug utilization), and central sterile supply (device and materials utilization).

Data Coding Techniques

Is it important to code information? This is not a trivial question, and there are strong arguments on each side. The negative argument often points out that the use of English words and phrases is already an encoding of observations of phenomena, and that the language makes it possible to append important modifiers (like *minor, moderate,* and *slight*) to one's descriptions. The positive argument says that, if organized comprehensively and logically (as Linnaeus did with plants and animals, or Mendeleev with elements), a coding system can provide for both aggregation and discrimination, with a minimal loss of precision. Certainly we are accustomed to using labels in medicine—witness the plethora of disease states which we have named. Furthermore, the sectors which impinge on medicine (accounting and management, government, etc) have embraced coding with few reservations. On the whole, we should be willing to accept coded data, as long as its purposes and limitations are kept in mind.

Coding systems already exist for many of the entities about which we collect data. Foremost among these systems is the *International Classification of Diseases, 9th Revision, Clinical Modification* (ICD-9-CM). In this schema one can find a numeric code for virtually any disease state, even those resulting from injury and misadventure. The virtues of this system are its ability to embrace similar conditions within numerical ranges, its comprehensiveness, and its long history of use and refinement. One would almost need to be deranged to reject this system in favor of any other numeric coding for disease.

A similarly venerable system for clinical procedures is the *Physicians' Current Procedural Terminology* (CPT), now in its 4th edition. Published by the American Medical Association, this coding system is anatomically based (excepting laboratory and radiology procedures) and probably not as rational in its aggregative aspect as the ICD-9-CM. It has the great appeal of almost universal use and should be used when coding procedures and tests.

An outgrowth of the ICD-9-CM (and government predisposition to overtaxonomize) are the Diagnosis Related Group (DRG) codes. These codes attempt to combine disease category with case severity in order to identify patients expected to have comparable resource utilization. Although the mechanism for assigning a DRG to a case is somewhat complex, this type of coding may be useful if one is interested in the role of nosocomial infections in increasing costs.

There is not any widely accepted coding strategy for the only other aspect of infection control data which might benefit from coding, organisms. However, there is some merit to the idea that organisms should be coded. It would make it possible to aggregate similar organisms (e.g., all gram negatives) within a range even though they are from varying genus designations. Antibiotic susceptibility might be embedded in the scheme, though with changing patterns it might not be a good idea. However, at the moment, no one has

devised a strategy. If a practitioner undertakes this task within an institution, he or she should make sure that the purposes of coding are fulfilled in the organizational approach.

Designing Forms

Not all data must be placed on a form; indeed, it is generally better to have data entered directly by those making observations. Still, it is not always possible, and intermediate forms must be used for recording information. To some people implementing an infection control data system, the forms may seem to be an insignificant aspect of the program; others will probably overstate their importance:

Certainly, forms and their structure can make the difference between readable data and scribbling; for instance, providing adequate space to write answers promotes legibility. Using boxes instead of lines may assure the use of a code where one is needed instead of a written entry. In addition, providing a space to stamp a plate or identification card may get more accurate patient registration data. Finally, providing a place for the name of the person gathering the data will permit the identity of the person with whom to check when data are in question (Figs. 9.2 and 9.3). All of the refinements (and a good many others) can spell the difference between good data and entries which must be constantly checked and returned to the primary source. However, forms are merely instruments within the system, not the system itself, and *it* is the critical component. One should avoid designing a system around forms.

The major issue in form design for data systems in infection control is how many forms one actually needs, or, more precisely, into how many portions are the data to be divided. The focus here is really the collection process rather than the form. One could use a single form (probably consisting of more than one piece of paper) and declare that form to be incomplete until it has been fully filled out. This means that incomplete forms may be floating around—and getting lost—until all data are available and placed on the form. On the positive side, it also means that a single person could be designated as responsible for making certain that all data are collected on a case and that the data will not be entered until they are complete.

An alternative is to declare the form to be made up of sections which consist of data generated at

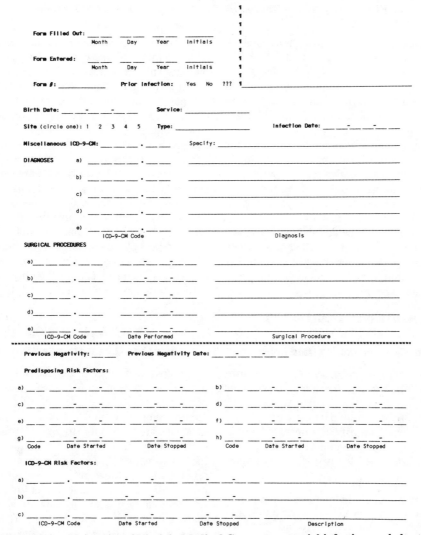

Figure 9.2.   University of Virginia Medical Center nosocomial infection worksheet.

Culture Date	Organism	Type	Description	Sensitivity Pattern								
				A A C M M B K P N	C C C E E F F P X	C C E H L R L I Y	F G M O E O X N X	N N P A I E F T N	P S S I X T P T P	S T T U E O L T B	V M A E N Z	
a)												
b)												
c)												
d)												

	Antibiotic	Treatment (circle one)				Date Administered		
a)		1	2	3	4			
b)		1	2	3	4			
c)		1	2	3	4			
d)		1	2	3	4			
e)		1 Prophyl	2 Rx Prior	3 Rx Pres.	4 No Rx	Month	Day	Year

Figure 9.3.

89

a single point in time (a single microbiology laboratory report, a single day's antibiotic treatment, the set of preinfection risk factors, the patient's registration information, etc) and which are completed at once. The advantage is that there would be no incomplete floaters; instead, there would be a potential for a better linkage to other information systems. The disadvantage is that the data system is fragmented and more difficult to control. With this alternative it is also important to provide appropriate links among the forms filled out on a single event or case (patient, date, and type of infection are obvious choices).

Form design cannot be covered completely in this context. It is sufficient to say that this activity is quite important, and one should consider every aspect very carefully before sending off the completed design to be printed.

COMPUTERIZING COLLECTED INFORMATION
Error Checking during Data Entry

Once information has been recorded on forms it must be transferred to the computer. Manual data entry introduces the possibility, indeed the inescapable *probability*, of data entry errors. As a result, data base integrity is threatened unless techniques are developed to detect erroneous information. Error checking is particularly important for epidemiology:

Many databases have in their usage an inherent feedback mechanism which may serve to maintain accuracy. If a bank account record is updated erroneously, there will eventually be a feedback from the customer ... in the case of an epidemiologic database, however, the data for the transaction will be received only after the patient has been discharged. It will be out of the hands of those who can compare the data with the case directly. In the future, the data will be dealt with only in a statistical sense (DS MacLaughlin, unpublished manuscript).

One way to avoid the feedback problem is to have data entered by the person who collected it. However, this is at best a partial solution, for even the collector is likely to make data entry errors. Another strategy is to have a second person re-enter the same data and have the computer check for inconsistencies; while double entry is a common key-punch technique, it wastes time that could be better spent if errors could be caught the first time around. In fact, software can do just that, if judiciously designed. When the data base

is developed, and whenever another element is added, one should pause to define criteria to test the reasonableness of each item collected. Generally, such criteria simply codify common sense, as when one instructs entry software to test data for *allowable range* (identifying future and long past birthdates), *valid codes* (flagging hospital locations your surveillance does not cover), and *proper data type* (rejecting numeric answers to an alphabetic question). Ideally, software would also compare related data for *compatibility*, identifying nosocomial infection dates prior to hospital admission or even questioning unexpected organisms entered for a particular infection site. While it is not possible to catch all entry errors, such strategies will prevent the most common ones, and save subsequent editing for only the most elusive mistakes (see "Editing and Correcting Data," below).

DATA BASE DESIGN
Selecting Global Storage Strategy

Perhaps the most important decision in designing an infection control computer system is data organization—a choice that will affect memory requirements (how much disk space and magnetic tape are needed for storage), software speed (how quickly information can be entered, examined, and extracted), facility for preparing datasets for analysis (how easily subsets of the data can be extracted), and capability for future expansion (how hard it is to add new kinds of information, if in fact it is possible at all). This subject will merit a good deal of research and discussion, and the discussion here is confined to the most important concepts involved.*

Organizing data means deciding how it should be stored for future reference. Office clerks typically use a series of ingenious schemes to file away important papers, and data bases emulate some of their more successful techniques. (Of course all of us have, at one time or another, inadvertently designed less successful storage strategies that preclude retrieval.) Drawing on the natural analogy with office file cabinets, *file* has been made the generic computer term for any set of related information. Basic admission data might

---

* There are several solid introductory treatments of data base design available; particularly recommended are references 8–10. Bear in mind that even the most recent article may soon be obsolete as new packages appear and old ones are enhanced.

be one set and laboratory tests another. A *data base* is merely a complicated file, one which contains several sets of the same data—and possibly several *kinds* of sets—stored in a systematic fashion.

The system chosen depends on how large and varied these sets are, and how stable their structure and size are. While there are many good storage systems to consider, just comparing two basic approaches will reveal the kinds of trade-offs each choice presents. A fundamental question in storing information is deciding how individual data items should be separated. *Fixed length sets* answer this question by applying the maxim: "a place for everything and everything in its place." In this approach, the data base is divided into uniform slots, and one dataset is stored in each slot. Since each set must be the same size, the items within it may not vary in length. For instance, if patient name were one element of a dataset, each name entered would have to be padded with spaces to a predetermined length. And any unexpectedly long name would have to be cut down to size.

Fixed length strategies thus require that one know a lot about the data in advance. Such an approach has clear strengths and weaknesses. This kind of data base needs only relatively unsophisticated software, produces neatly structured files that are easy to print and scan for errors, and readily provides the kind of "card-image" subsets that most statistical analysis packages demand. On the other hand, it is difficult to add new items to these sets or to modify items they already contain because any change alters the inviolable fixed length. At best, one can build in limited flexibility by saving dead space in each set. In large datasets, such dead space quickly adds up and makes for inefficient memory use (and costly computer storage bills).

Variable length sets avoid the storage problem at the cost of some simplicity and speed. As the name suggests, each set can have any size because its elements are defined not by physical location (e.g., patient name occupies the first 40 characters in a record), but by relative logical position (patient name is the first item, no matter how long). Such sets require more sophisticated software because they use special codes to separate individual items and the computer must parse each record to interpret it. On the other hand, the additional sophistication makes it easier to modify the contents of any set—to add new items or to expand old ones. Another drawback of this

strategy is that it adds a step to statistical analysis, since variable length sets usually must be converted to fixed length ones before they can be studied; again, though, good data base software should be able to handle the conversion simply and quickly.

Resolving Local Storage Issues

As this very basic comparison suggests, every data base technique must be evaluated in terms of how it facilitates or hinders normal epidemiologic use. The same issues are raised when one compares different ways to store individual items in a dataset. Perhaps the most common choice here is deciding whether to encode information or enter it as is. Uncoded data offer the same benefits and drawbacks as a fixed field data base. Thus, recording, entering, and editing uncoded information are straightforward because no interpretation is required; for the same reason, it is much easier to catch erroneous entries by visual inspection.

On the other hand, computers are better prepared to catch errors in *coded* data, because codes rigidly define acceptable values for each item. For this reason, codes greatly facilitate extracting, sorting, and analyzing well defined subsets on the computer; after all, in uncoded form, the same item could be described in many different ways, and it is hard to tell a computer how to decide whether such entries belong in a special subset. Coding also shrinks the overall size of a data base because it describes information succinctly; of course, a price is paid for this savings, because rigidly enforced brevity sometimes precludes subtle shadings of meaning (see "Data Coding Techniques," above). The costs and benefits of coding should be examined for each data item independently. In most cases some information is just right for coding while other facts are best handled in uncoded form; such a mixture will offer the benefits of both approaches.

Editing and Correcting Data

Although global and local information storage decisions will shape the way data are edited and corrected, some issues can be addressed independently. To begin with, mistakes are just as frequent when editing information as when entering it initially; accordingly, entry and editing software must apply the exact same error-checking controls. Once an item is edited correctly, there are several options for handling the old incorrect entry. Some data bases simply overwrite old entries with new ones; however, a safer technique is to preserve a so-called "audit trail" by marking the old entry as deleted but not physically removing it from the data base. In this way one can always recover from overzealous editing sessions. Such security, though, does require a great deal of extra storage space. When on-line disk space is a premium, one can compromise by transferring deleted data to a less convenient peripheral medium, such as magnetic tape; if needed, it can be restored to the disk without much delay.

PRODUCING REPORTS AND ANALYSES

No matter how convenient the data base packages may make data entry and editing, their utility is ultimately measured by their flexibility and speed in extracting information. This utility will be rigorously tested by the many routine and special reports that epidemiologists need. Any data base should allow users to enter commands at a terminal to retrieve any specific data item without much difficulty. Good software will let them store frequently repeated series of commands in files, which the computer will read whenever they ask; these so-called *command files* eliminate tedious, repetitive typing and thus simplify periodic extraction of data for routine reports (e.g., all patients with noscomial infections reported during the previous month). When the data base grows large, some kinds of extraction may be slow (specifically, those that run counter to the information storage structure that was selected). Many computer systems provide utilities for doing time-consuming information retrieval "off-line" and allowing one to do other work in the meantime.

So far, ways have been discussed to request reports from the data base; it would be nice if the data base could occasionally indicate when a report is needed. For instance, whenever it receives data for a new month or year, the data base could automatically extract the relevant monthly or yearly information for analysis. In addition, very clever software might be designed to analyze data as they are entered, and to produce special reports automatically whenever special events occur. For instance, the data base might look for unexpected combinations of organism and infection site—the same kind of unusual pairing an error identifier might question. Such sophisticated scrutiny would inevitably slow

the entry and editing process, and, if desired, it too should take place off-line.

COMPUTER SYSTEM DESIGN FOR EPIDEMIOLOGY

Throughout this chapter computer issues have been discussed which involve collecting and managing infection control data; we would be remiss if we did not stress that the first step in computerization is always deciding whether a computer will solve more problems than it creates. While computers help to organize and analyze data enormously more efficiently than would be possible with file cabinets and pencils, such efficiency is purchased by paying often overlooked start-up and maintenance costs. To begin with, surveillance sheets will generally need to be redesigned to facilitate computer data entry; entered data must be backed up to protect against software and hardware failures; and software and hardware must be protected by expensive support and maintenance agreements. Computer problems, then, come with computer power, and both need to be carefully weighed.

In most cases computerization will seem an attractive alternative; the problem then becomes "what kind of system best serves our needs?" People commonly approach the question from the wrong end, first choosing a good machine and then selecting adequate software. Too often this strategy ends up molding the procedures around an existing *machine*, rather than designing an overall *system* that fits them closely. Better results are achieved if the research process is reversed by breaking it into three steps: First, carefully assess current and future storage, reporting, and analysis needs. Then, decide what kind of data base and statistical software best suits them. Only then should one consider what hardware environment best serves this software. In fact, by designing a system this way, epidemiologists may well discover that their needs are best served by a hardware configuration that combines the strengths of several machines.†

Many of the common tasks for which epidemiologists need computers have already been discussed; in addition, several software alternatives for meeting their needs have been covered. How-

---

† Readers who would like a detailed assessment of optimal computer system design in these terms can consult reference 11.

ever, the most important software issue has yet to be mentioned. Regardless of the strategy selected, it is necessary to decide who should translate the strategies into program form. It is better to purchase a package, pay for a custom-designed one, or write your own? Although many epidemiologists have programming experience, few can spare the enormous amounts of time and money necessary to develop *and maintain* software of any complexity. For instance, at our Clinical Computing Laboratory, we need at least two full time programmers to look after a data base system of moderate size and sophistication. Unless its procedures are very unusual, a hospital will be better served by using commercial packages to handle its data base, statistical, graphics, and word-processing needs; and, for the infrequent task that cannot be handled this way, many headaches can be avoided by commissioning professional programmers to custom design the necessary software.

After selecting a combination of commercial packages, alternative hardware environments should be researched. Since almost all hospitals have at least one computer center which operates a mini or mainframe computer, the choice is between a self-maintained microcomputer and time sharing on a larger system. Large systems are faster for many tasks and, in an academic setting, generally cheaper because maintenance and support contracts are split among many users; on the other hand, micros may be faster during busy times of the day, and they are generally more secure and convenient because all of the equipment is at one's disposal. While financial considerations or other problems may sometimes force users to choose between these options, our own experience suggests that the best hardware configurations combine the two. Communications packages enable a micro to communicate with a mainframe by programming it to act as a terminal with some added features; with this kind of package, users can convert a free-standing micro to a terminal any time they need to access the power of the larger computer, and then switch it back to utilize the convenience of an independent unit.

CONCLUSION

The fundamental issues involved in planning and establishing an infection control data system in a hospital have been reviewed: defining data elements, planning data collection, and managing data. Any implementation of these ideas will necessarily be influenced by individual institutional realities. While common wisdom may produce only common results, conscious consideration of the principles presented above can be expected to produce better results than when systems are simply permitted to grow in an unguided manner. It is especially important to remember the unique environment of the hospital, with significant numbers of professionals, each with his or her own ideas and experiences. Any program which meaningfully involves as many of these persons as possible in the planning and implementation is much more likely to achieve its goals.

References

1. Shortell SM, Kaluzny AD (eds): *Health Care Management: A Text in Organization Theory and Behavior.* New York, John Wiley & Sons, 1983.
2. Freidson E: *Doctoring Together: A Study of Professional Social Control.* New York, Elsevier, 1975.
3. Austin CJ: *Information Systems for Hospital Administration,* ed 2. Ann Arbor, MI, Health Administration Press, 1983.
4. Thompson G, Handelman I: *Health Data and Information Management.* Boston, Butterworth, 1978.
5. Priest SL: *Managing Hospital Information Systems.* Rockville, MD, Aspen, 1982.
6. Schmitz HH: *Hospital Information Systems.* Rockville, MD, Aspen, 1979.
7. Waters KA, Murphy GF: *Medical Records in Health Information.* Rockville, MD, Aspen, 1979.
8. *Byte,* September 1984.
9. Date CJ: *An Introduction to Database Systems.* Reading, MA, Addison-Wesley, 1976.
10. Martin J: *Computer Database Organization.* Englewood Cliffs, NJ, Prentice Hall, 1977.
11. Barr R, Gerzoff R: Controlling urges and infections: computer system design for epidemiology. *Infect Control* 6:317–322, 1985.

Chapter 10

Epidemics—Identification and Management

Richard P. Wenzel, M.D.

An epidemic or outbreak of noscocomial infections is usually defined statistically: a significant increase in the rate of certain infections above that noted in the past ($p < 0.05$). The assumptions implicit in the identification of an epidemic are that neither the definition of a case, the case-finding methods, nor the laboratory identification of organisms has changed. The most common outbreaks refer to a specific pathogen at a single anatomic site such as *Serratia marcescens* bloodstream infections or *Staphylococcus aureus* postoperative wound infections. As a result, in the usual situation one seeks to identify the unique reservoir and the mode of transmission of the identified pathogen (1). Certainly, it is possible for more than one organism to reside at the same reservoir (2). In addition, if multiple organisms are involved with infections at a single site, then possibly the epidemic relates primarily to a break in technique. Such an outbreak has recently been described involving nine different species infecting the bloodstream of six criticial care unit patients whose vascular catheters remained in place longer than uninfected controls (3).

Epidemics of nosocomial infections represent an important medical problem. It has been estimated that they occur at a rate of 1/10,000 admissions, are often life threatening since they frequently involve the bloodstream, and usually occur in critical care units (1, 4). In one 5-year study of all patients who became infected after hospitalization, approximately 4% became infected as part of a major epidemic (1, 4). It has also been estimated that an additional 6% of patients are infected as part of an epidemiologic cluster which does not quite reach statistical significance ($p < 0.05$); in such clusters the cases are linked by one or more similar risk factors. Thus, as many as 10% of patients may be infected as part of a major outbreak or a cluster. Furthermore, of all patients who developed a nosocomial bloodstream infection, 8% did so as part of a major epidemic (1). Nevertheless, the most significant point medically is that, by definition, all epidemics are preventable. That fact alone makes them important.

What adds to the importance of the medical significance of outbreaks are the political, economic, and legal consequences. These additional issues become the burden of the team investigating the epidemic. Politically, most problems can be averted by maintaining communication with all leading administrators, including all heads of departments. In general, it is reasonable to assume that each wants to be totally informed of any news; and none wants to be surprised by a call from a news reporter, a colleague, or a senior administrator. In an ongoing investigation, weekly written reports should be preceded by frequent telephone calls and personal briefings. Most importantly, someone should be identified at the beginning of the investigation as the person in charge.

It costs money to perform an adequate investigation, and all reasonable costs simply must be borne by the hospital administration. Although it is obvious that the identification of an epidemic implies no wrong on the part of the hospital or specific personnel, there may be suits arising from the damages of infected patients. The hospital's director will need to be appraised of the details of the findings of the investigating team for this reason. The key point is that for medical, political, economic, and legal reasons, a detailed diary should be maintained by the investigating team. Notes in the diary might include the dates and statements of various people interviewed, including information stated but not acted on initially by the infection control team. The analogy of the epidemiologist-investigator with a supersleuth begins with the purchase and use of a diary.

RECENT TRENDS

A reasonable estimation of the major epidemics being reported was constructed after a computer search of published articles which have focused on epidemics of nosocomial infections (5–167) (Figs. 10.1 to 10.4). The time period surveyed was the 6-year period between January 1979 and the end October 1984. There has been a striking change since 1981 in the number of reported epidemics in which gram-positive cocci were implicated as the offending pathogen (5–36) (Fig. 10.1). In 1979 and 1980, only two and three epidemics caused by gram-positive cocci were noted, respectively. However, since 1981 at least five epidemics each year were reported. Furthermore, of the 27 epidemics reported between 1981 and the end of 1984, 17 (63%) were caused by methicillin-resistant *S. aureus*. During the same period only two outbreaks caused by sensitive *S. aureus* strains were reported.

Of the 75 epidemics which were identified with the computer search to have been caused by gram-negative rods (37–111), 51 (68%) were caused by one of four genera: *Serratia* species, *Salmonella* species, *Klebsiella* species, or *Pseudomonas* species (Fig. 10.2). There appear to have been fewer reports of outbreaks with gram-negative rods in 1983 and 1984 compared to the earlier 4 years.

Of particular interest is the recognition of at least 38 outbreaks of nosocomial viral infections (112–149) (Fig. 10.3). The various agents of viral hepatitis caused seven (18%), and the other important agents included both rotavirus (causing gastrointestinal infections) and respiratory syncytial virus (causing respiratory infections in newborns). In six outbreaks, varicella-zoster virus was identified as the offending pathogen.

Of the less common agents causing outbreaks of nosocomial infection in the 6-year period selected (150–167), *Legionella pneumophilia* was noted to have caused five of the outbreaks (Fig. 10.4). Other outbreaks involved the agents of atypical mycobacteria, diphtheria, scabies, *Nocardia*, and *Clostridium difficile*.

The patients who are particularly susceptible to infections as part of the epidemic are the immune-suppressed, including the neonate and those in critical care units. The vast majority of outbreaks caused by methicillin-resistant *S. aureus* or nosocomial bloodstream infections caused by aerobic gram-negative rods occur in the intensive care units (ICUs). The beds in the ICUs comprise 5 to 10% of all hospital beds; thus, it has been suggested that routine surveillance ought to be carried out at least in critical care units in order to identify most life-threatening outbreaks (1, 4).

With respect to the immune-suppressed hos-

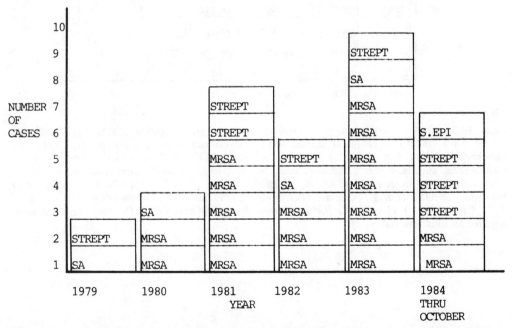

Figure 10.1.   Outbreaks of infections in hospitals caused by gram-positive cocci and identified via MEDLINE computer search. There appears to have been an increase in outbreaks caused by gram-positive cocci since 1981, the vast majority of which were caused by methicillin-resistant *S. aureus*. *STREPT*, streptococcus; *SA*, methicillin-sensitive *S. aureus*; *MRSA*, methicillin-resistant *S. aureus*; *S. EPI*, *S. epidermidis*.

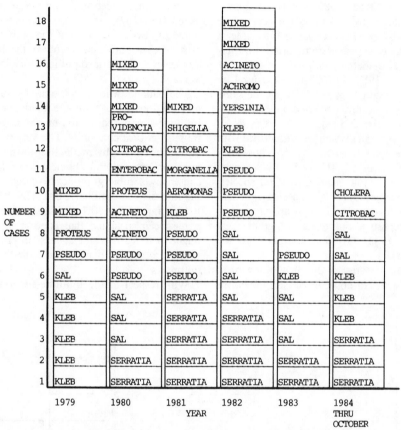

Figure 10.2.   Outbreaks of infections in hospitals caused by gram-negative rods. Of the 75 outbreaks identified via MEDLINE computer search, 16 (21%) were caused by *Serratia* species, 13 (17%) by *Salmonella* species, and 12 (16%) by *Klebsiella* species. Ten outbreaks (13%) were caused by *Pseudomonas* species. Fewer outbreaks caused by gram-negative bacilli were reported in 1983 and 1984 compared to previous years. *KLEB, Klebsiella* species; *PSEUDO, Pseudomonas* species; *SAL, Salmonella* species; *ACINETO, Acinetobacter* species; *ENTEROBAC, Enterobacter* species; *CITRO-BAC, Citrobacter* species; *ACHROMO, Achromobacter* species; *MIXED*, more than one gram-negative bacillus involved.

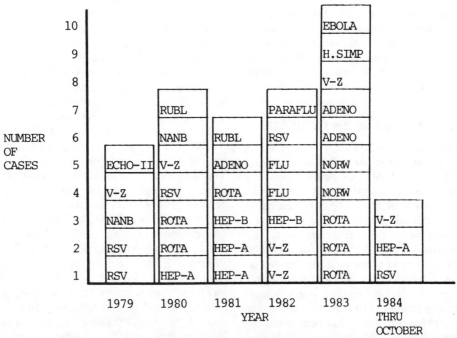

Figure 10.3.   Of the 38 outbreaks of infections in hospitals caused by viral agents and identified via MEDLINE computer search, six were caused by rotavirus (*ROTA*), five by respiratory syncytial virus (*RSV*) , and seven by various agents causing hepatitis (*ADENO*, adenovirus; *HEP-A*, hepatitis A; *HEP-B*, hepatitis B; *H. SIMP*, H. simplex; *NANB*, non-A, non-B hepatitis; *NORW*, Norwalk; *PARAFLU*, parainfluenza virus; *V-Z*, varicella-zoster; *RUBL*, rubella.

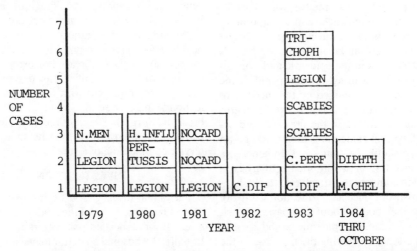

Figure 10.4.   Outbreaks of infection caused by less commonly encountered organisms. Of the 18 outbreaks identified via MEDLINE computer search, five were caused by *Legionella pneumophila*. *LEGION, L. pneumophila; N. MEN, Neisseria meningitidis; H. INFLU, H. influenzae; NOCARD, Nocardia species; C. DIF, Clostridium difficile; C. PERF, Clostridium perfringens; TRICHOPH, Trichophyton species; DIPHTH, diphtheroids; M. CHEL, Mycobacterium cheloni.*

pitalized patients, prominent outbreaks include those due to *L. pneumophila*, varicella-zoster virus, *Nocardia* species, and JK diphtheroids. Patients on renal transplant wards and those on hematology-oncology services are the ones often affected. The nursery and pediatric wards are the locations from which outbreaks of *Salmonella*, rotavirus, *Streptococcus pyogenes*, and respiratory syncytial virus have been reported frequently.

IDENTIFICATION OF AN OUTBREAK

Outbreaks are extremely labor intense, but for medical and ethical reasons all must be investigated. At the same time, it should be obvious that the investigation of a nonepidemic is grossly inefficient, a waste of time. The first step before proceeding to a full scale study is to determine if, in fact, an epidemic exists. If prospective surveillance is being performed routinely, it is possible that routine reviews of the data may suggest an outbreak. Alternatively, it is possible that notification by a concerned clinician, microbiologist or nurse may prompt an initial investigation. Use of an algorithm (Fig. 10.5) may help to prevent an extensive investigation's being launched before a true epidemic is identified.

Once a potential epidemic comes to the attention of the infection control team, it is important that the epidemic and pre-epidemic periods be defined. Thereafter, one can ask if any of the following were different in the two time periods: case definition, surveillance, and/or laboratory techniques to identify the infecting agent. Only if all three have been similar in both time periods can the attack rates in the epidemic and nonepidemic periods be meaningfully compared. If the number of infections divided by the number of patients at risk in the epidemic period is significantly greater than that in the pre-epidemic period ($p < 0.05$), an epidemic is identified and an investigation should be conducted. In general, a Fisher's exact test or a chi square analysis is performed to compare the attack rates (see Chapter 32, Statistical Concepts in Infection Control).

Some further points about comparing attack rates may be useful. The epidemic period is easily defined as that time covering the first case to the current ones under investigation. The pre-epidemic period is arbitrarily defined in part depending on the number of cases. For example, it may require up to 12 months of data in the pre-epidemic time to gather sufficient numbers for comparison in a low frequency event. Furthermore, use of 12 months will avoid any seasonal bias. In any outbreak, however, it is wise to examine at least 6 months of surveillance data prior to the presumed outbreak in order to calculate attack rates. The attack rates may be calculated with either the number of patients or the number of infections (more commonly) in the numerator and the number of patients at risk in the denominator. Initially, the denominator may simply be the number of patients admitted to the service(s) with cases. However, with postoperative wound infections or procedure-related infections, it is better to use the number of patients undergoing the type of surgery or procedure involved. The definition of a case may change as new information is gathered. For example, the initial case definition of a postoperative wound infection may be pus at the incision site. Later, however, it may be obvious that all infections being investigated are on the same service, such as thoracic surgery. Still later the definition might be pus at the incision site following mitral valve replacement. Eventually, it may be *Staphylococcus epidermidis* sternal wound infections after mitral valve replacement. Similarly, as new cases are identified there may be a further refinement in the definition of the epidemic and pre-epidemic periods.

Early communication with the microbiology laboratory is important because it is essential to identify the organism as completely as possible: genus, species, subtype, antibiogram, etc. Most importantly, *all isolates must be saved.*

An early communication with the employee health service may also provide an initial clue to the solution of an outbreak. For example, in an outbreak of *S. aureus* infections, one might note the visits of employees with dermatitis, skin infections, boils, or styes. Similarly, with an outbreak of *S. pyogenes* wound infections, one might review all employees with visits to the health service complaining of a sore throat.

INVESTIGATION

The actual investigation begins with a review of the literature, a plot of the epidemic curve, and a search for associated risk factors for infection. Initially, the hospital epidemiology team needs to think about the offending organism. Specifically, what is its usual reservoir, and what is the usual mode of transmission? Has it been incriminated in previous outbreaks? Is the organism virulent, or does it affect only hosts with altered defense mechanisms? All of this is to say that there is no substitute for experience, and an immediate re-

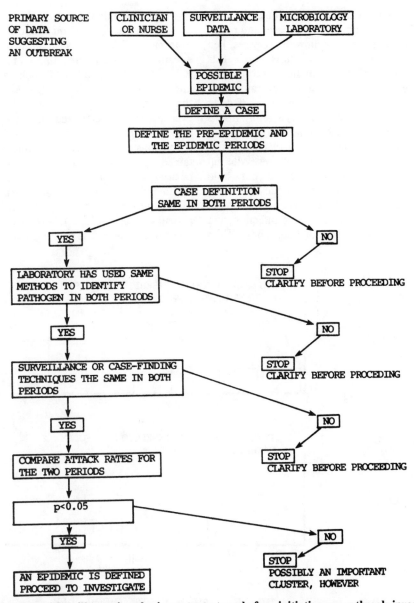

Figure 10.5. Algorithm illustrating the important steps before initiating an outbreak investigation for nosocomial infections. The pre-epidemic and epidemic periods must be defined, and then there must have been uniform case definitions, surveillance, and laboratory techniques utilized to identify the infection in both periods. Thereafter, the attack rates can be meaningfully compared.

view of the literature is warranted (see Chapter 33, Using the Literature). Key pharasing for the librarian might be as follows: *epidemics of [organism] [site]—infections.* The literature search may yield valuable clues as to reservoir, mode of transmission, host population affected, prognosis for infected patients, and effective control measures.

The outbreak should be defined graphically with the epidemic curve: on the X-axis is time (days, weeks or, months), and on the Y-axis is the number of cases adhering to the existing case definition. If possible, plot all of the cases for the 6- to 12-month pre-epidemic period as well.

The next phase of the investigation is the search for risk factors; it begins with detailed line lists of all cases, their admission and infection dates, their demographic data, underlying diseases and preinfection exposures to the following: services, bed assignments, personnel, and tests. Line lists should be made of all information, and the data should be summarized: number of cases with exposure A/number of cases; number of cases with exposure B/number of cases; etc. At this point it may be obvious what the likely risk factor is, and one can then proceed to verify the putative risk factors by microbiologic cultures. Alternatively, it may not be so obvious, and then it would be helpful to present the data graphically: on the X-axis is the interval time (days or weeks) between exposure to a risk factor and infection, and on the Y-axis is the number of cases. The graphics

may yield not only the clues to the risk factor but also the range for the incubation period. For example, if five cases with nosocomial bloodstream infection all were admitted to the medical ICU, all had Foley catheters, Hickman catheters, and arterial catheters, it might be helpful to know that there was no consistent interval between exposure to risk factors and infection except with respect to arterial catheters (Fig. 10.6). It should be obvious also that as new information is obtained, updated changes in control measures may be needed. For example, in an outbreak of bloodstream infections due to *S. aureus*, it is reasonable initially to emphasize hand washing between all patient contacts. If later it is discovered that the infections are related to prolonged usage of Swan-

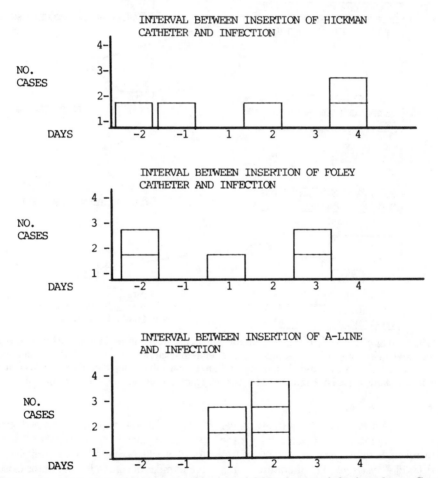

Figure 10.6.   Hypothetical graphic analysis of nosocomial bloodstream infections due to *S. marcescens*. Two patients developed infection *prior to* insertion of the Hickman catheter and two developed infection *prior to* insertion of a Foley catheter. All five, however, developed a bloodstream infection after insertion of an arterial catheter and all within **48** hours of its insertion, suggesting a possible association.

Ganz catheters, still new recommendations regarding deviation of indwelling vascular lines are needed.

Hypothesis and Case Control Study

The review of charts, line lists, and associated graphics may give a clue regarding reservoir and mode of transmission. At this point a hypothesis regarding probable cause-effect relationships is generated. These relationships can be strengthened by performing a case control study in which cases are matched to controls and the proportions in each group exposed to various risk factors can be compared. The question is whether there is a high association of a risk factor in cases which is not seen in controls, and whether that association with cases is statistically strong ($p < 0.05$).

In the comparison of cases and controls, several points should be underscored:
1. If there are a small number of cases (<10), it may be useful to have two to four controls for each patient.
2. Controls need to be selected from the population of uninfected patients in the hospital during the epidemic period.
3. Controls should not be tightly matched to cases since the important risk factor would not be identified in very close matches. For example, if the risk factor for infection was insertion of an arterial catheter, and if cases were matched to controls with arterial catheters, the risk factor could not be identified. Initially, it is wise to match only for age, sex, and service.

Table 10.1 illustrates some of the points and refers to an outbreak of *Salmonella* bacteremia from platelet transfusions in immunologically compromised patients (168). Eventually the epidemic was traced to a hematogenous carrier of *Salmonella cholerae-suis*. The reader should note the larger number of controls than cases and the fact that within the confines of the analysis the *p* was obviously small (0.10), not statistically significant but clinically important. The authors correctly did not ignore the association with platelets and eventually proved that all patients received platelets, but only four of five received them within 1 week of bacteremia.

At this point in the investigation, control measures may again need to be updated. Once epidemiologic and/or statistical evidence points to a specific reservoir and mode of transmission, the next step is to confirm the hypothesis microbiologically. Microbiologic confirmation is usually easy; but if cultures of solutions are needed, one may need the help of a experienced microbiologist to insure a sensitive and accurate test. Similarly, if antiseptic agents need to be cultured, one needs to ask if neutralizers need to be added before culturing in order to remove any residual effect of the material. Failure to use neutralizers can lead to false negative culture results.

Last, the steps of an investigation include documentation of control measures, a written report, and development of new guidelines as a result of the outbreak. Obviously, the more often that outbreaks are reported in the general scientific literature, the better.

In summary (Table 10.2), the investigation of an epidemic involves epidemiologic, microbiologic, political, and administrative skills. It requires a knowledge of the existing literature, attention to detail, and accurate recording of the facts. Only then can one proceed with the analysis and control of the problem.

Table 10.1. Exposure of Infected Patients with *Salmonella cholerae-suis* Bacteremia and Control Patients to Selected Therapeutic Agents*

Therapeutic Agent	Bacteremic Patients ($N = 5$)		Controls ($N = 22$)		P (Fisher's Exact Test)
	No.	(%)	No.	(%)	
Platelets	4	(80)	8	(36)	0.10
Allopurinol	4	(80)	12	(55)	0.29
Antacid	3	(60)	4	(18)	0.19
Nystatin	3	(60)	6	(27)	
Gentamicin	3	(60)	8	(36)	
Erythrocytes	3	(60)	9	(41)	
Narcotic	2	(40)	8	(36)	
Prednisone	2	(40)	15	(68)	

* Bacteremic patients in week before first positive blood culture; control patients in week before investigation. Modified from Rhame et al (168).

Table 10.2.   Summary—Investigation of an Outbreak

1. Provide a case definition. Prove that an epidemic exists: show statistically that current rates are higher than pre-epidemic rates.
2. Perform a literature review.
3. Open lines of communication. Include department heads, microbiology director, administrators, employee health director.
4. Purchase a diary and keep detailed notes of interviews.
5. Plot the epidemic curve.
6. Review charts of infected patients and perform line lists of all potential risk factors.
7. Formulate a hypothesis about likely reservoir and mode of transmission. Institute temporary control measures.
8. Perform case control study to develop epidemiologic evidence to confirm hypothesis.
9. Update control measures.
10. Document the reservoir and mode of transmission microbiologically.
11. Document efficacy of control measures by continued surveillance.
12. Write a report for the hospital's infection control committee. Change policies and procedures if necessary.

PREVENTION AND CONTROL

The control measures utilized routinely for endemic infections are thought to be useful in the prevention and control of epidemic infections: strict hand washing between patients, limitation of the use and duration of devices, proper isolation of infected patients, and aseptic technique and use of strict protocols for all procedures. Data are limited or absent which would show the specific contribution of each item listed, however. Nevertheless, they are based on reason and are frequently associated with control of problems. What follows are selected comments—gleaned from outbreak reports—which the reader may find useful.

In an investigation of recurrent staphylococcal infections in a neonatal special care unit, Haley and Bregman highlighted the important risk factors of understaffing and overcrowding (24). Specifically, the incidence of clusters was 16 times higher after periods when the infant:nurse ratio exceeded 7 and 7 times higher after periods when the infant census exceeded 33.

With respect to methicillin-resistant *S. aureus*, Peacock and colleagues studied bed assignments to determine the bed to next bed movement of the epidemic strain (34), and Thompson et al showed the importance of isolation as a control measure (169). In the latter study the importance of isolating colonized patients, not only infected cases, was emphasized; and case finding improved when cultural surveys were employed to identify patient carriers.

The study by Boyce and his colleagues showed that the occurrence of methicillin-resistant *S. aureus* infections in burn units may lead to increased transmission of the organism to nonburn patients, and therefore control of such infections in burn units may control spread to other patients (19). Importantly, Archer and Mayhall investigated epidemiologic markers as tools for case finding and emphasized the poor reproducibility of phage typing and conversely the utility of plasmid pattern analysis (14).

Outbreaks of *S. pyogenes* have occurred in surgical, neonatal, and geriatric wards; and it is now generally recognized that organism carriage may be pharyngeal, anal, and/or vaginal. Effective control measures include strict hand washing, cohorting and treatment of carriers and cases. In some cases more extraordinary measures may be needed. For example, in an outbreak in a maternity unit in Sweden, control was achieved only after the unit was closed for a week (17). In a report of an outbreak in a geriatric hospital, the usual methods of isolation and treatment of cases and carrier failed to stop the epidemic. Only after "mass treatment" of all 32 patients on the wards was the outbreak controlled (25).

Recently, the special problem of nosocomial meningitis due to *Citrobacter diversus* has been recognized. This is a devastating illness in part because the organism has an unusually high rate of brain abscess formation (83, 170). In general, environmental sources have not been found, but hand and rectal carriers have been identified. Although control of the epidemics has been linked to elimination of carrier (37), most of the epidemiology of this infection remains unknown.

An unusual outbreak of *Pasteurella multocida* infections in seven patients in a chronic disease hospital in New York has been reported (92). All seven patients were bedridden, had tracheostomia, and required mechanical ventilation. Six were febrile, two had positive blood cultures, and the other five had positive sputum cultures. Of interest was the finding that one of the cats owned by an inhalation therapist was found to have the identical serotype of *P. multocida* as the patients. The clusters of infection were linked temporally to the rotation assignment of the therapist who owned the carrier cat, and coincident with his resignation from the hospital, no further cases were reported (92). Hand carriage of the organism was suspected but not confirmed.

An outbreak of norcardiosis in seven renal transplant patients suggested that perhaps respiratory isolation may be indicated for this organism (158). Stevens and colleagues isolated *N. asteroides* from the air and dust inside the unit and elsewhere in the hospital. Extensive bacteriologic investigation of isolates indicated that those from patients were identical with those from the unit's environment yet different from those outside of the unit.

Legionella pneumophila is regarded as a waterborne agent, and chlorination of hospital water and elevation of the hot water temperature have been utilized as control measures in epidemics (161). More recently, Helms and his colleagues at the University of Iowa restricted water use by patients in the hematology-oncology unit until the water was free of *Legionella* (152). Furthermore, the authors suggested that hospitalization of immunocompromised patients in facilities served by *L. pneumophila*-containing water be avoided.

Two recent outbreaks of varicella, in which the authors used tracer gases to demonstrate airflow patterns, have suggested that in the hospital nosocomial spread may be airborne (129, 171). The authors have suggested that patients hospitalized with varicella be placed in strict isolation in negative pressure rooms to reduce the risk of transmission.

Although infection with enteroviruses is usually mild, an outbreak in a special care neonatal unit indicated the potentially lethal aspect of echovirus 11. Nagington and colleagues reported an outbreak involving nine babies, three of whom died within 36 hours of the onset of symptoms (172). The virus was introduced by the mother of the first case, transmitted to two hospital workers, and thereafter spread by the latter two to the other babies. The histologic findings had not been reported earlier for fatal echo 11 infections: small vessel thrombi confined to the medulla, hemorrhagic infarction in the medulla and inner cortex of the adrenals, and renal hemorrhage (172). A subsequent report described another outbreak, and the authors described closing the unit to all new admissions for a 3-week period as a control measure (148).

The 27-NM Norwalk virus has been identified with numerous outbreaks of infectious gastroenteritis. In a recent outbreak, it was concluded that the agent was transmitted on chicken sandwiches prepared by a member of the kitchen staff excreting the virus (117). The paper by Pether and Caul described an outbreak on an orthopaedic ward which was subsequently transferred to a geriatric ward. In a similar outbreak in a chronic care hospital in Tennessee, Gustafson and his colleagues showed an attack rate of 61% in nursing employees on one ward and 55% in the elderly psychiatric patients. Of interest was the finding that anticholinergic drugs appeared to mask the symptoms, and psyllium (Metamucil) may have prevented infection in some patients (116).

Ebola virus, first identified in 1976, has been associated with outbreaks of hemorrhagic fever in southern Sudan and northeastern Zaire. In the early reports 55% of cases in Sudan and 8% in Zaire were fatal. In a recent report from Sudan, Baron and his colleagues describe hospital dissemination and intrafamilial spread (115). The importance of close contact for transmission was emphasized since those family members providing nursing care had a 5-fold increased risk of infection. However, the absence of infection among close contacts who had no physical contact confirmed earlier impressions that there is no risk of airborne transmission (115). The authors point out that outbreaks of ebola virus, Lassa fever, Marburg virus disease, and Crimean-Congo hemorrhagic fever have resulted from nosocomial spread, and they underscore the importance of prompt recognition and isolation. With rapid air travel it is prudent to isolate foreign patients with febrile illnesses which are consistent with the above infections. Unfortunately, early symptoms may mimic typhoid fever or malaria, and the virulence of the true infecting agent may not be appreciated initially.

References

1. Wenzel RP, Thompson RL, Landry SM, Russell BS, Miller PJ, Ponce de Leon S, Miller GB Jr: Hospital-acquired infections in intensive care unit patients: an overview with emphasis on epidemics. *Infect Control* 4:371–375, 1983.
2. Donowitz LG, Marsik FJ, Fisher KA, Wenzel RP: Contaminated breast milk: a source of *Klebsiella* bacteremia in a newborn intensive care unit. *Rev Infect Dis* 3:716–720, 1981.
3. Ponce de Leon S, Critchley S, Wenzel PR: Polymicrobial bloodstream infections related to prolonged vascular catheterization. *Crit Care Med* 12:856–859, 1984
4. Wenzel RP, Osterman CA, Donowitz LG, Hoyt JW, Sande MA, Martone WJ, Peacock JE Jr, Levine JJ, Miller GB Jr: Identification of procedure-related nosocomial infections in high-risk patients. *Rev Infect Dis* 3:701–707, 1981.
5. Collins JK, Smith JS, Kelly MT: Comparison of

phage typing, plasmid mapping, and antibiotic resistance patterns as epidemiologic markers in a nosocomial outbreak of methicillin-resistant *Staphylococcus aureus* infections. *Diagn Microbiol Infect Dis* 2:233–245, 1984.

6. Pemberton LB, Lyman B, Mandal J: Outbreak of *Staphylococcus epidermidis* nosocomial infections in patients receiving total parenteral nutrition (letter). *JPEN* 8:325–326, 1984.

7. Wiesenthal AM: A maternal neonatal outbreak of infections due to an unusual group A beta-hemolytic streptococcus. *Infect Control* 5:271–174, 1984.

8. Whitby M, Sleigh JD, Reid W, McGregor I, Colman G: Streptococcal infection in a regional burns centre and a plastic surgery unit. *J Hosp Infect* 5:63–69, 1984.

9. Hill SF, Ferguson D: Multiply resistant *Staphylococcus aureus* (bacteriophage type 90) in a special care baby unit. *J Hosp Infect* 5:56–52, 1984.

10. Isenberg HD, Tucci V, Lipsitz P, Facklam RR: Clinical laboratory and epidemiological investigations of a *Streptococcus pyogenes* cluster epidemic in a newborn nursery. *J Clin Microbiol* 19:366–370, 1984.

11. Scopetti F, Orefici G, Biondi F, Benini F: *Staphylococcus aureus* resistant to methicillin and gentamicin as a cause of outbreak of epidemic enteritis in a hospital. *Boll Ist Sieroter Milan* 62:406–411, 1983.

12. Gordts B: Epidemic of multiresistant *Staphylococcus aureus* in an intensive care unit. *Acta Anaesthesiol Belg* 34:175–178, 1983.

13. Rutala WA, Katz EBS, Sherertz RJ, Sarubbi FA Jr: Environmental study of a methicillin-resistant *Staphylococcus aureus* epidemic in a burn unit. *J Clin Microbiol* 18:683–688, 1983.

14. Archer GL, Mayhall CG: Comparison of epidemiological markers used in the investigation of an outbreak of methicillin-resistant *Staphylococcus aureus* infections. *J Clin Microbiol* 18:395–399, 1983.

15. Reid RI, Briggs RS, Seal DV, Pearson AD: Virulent *Streptococcus pyogenes*: outbreak and spread within a geriatric unit. *J Infect* 6:219–225, 1983

16. Gerken MV: An outbreak of methicillin resistant *Staphylococcus aureus* in a large medical center. *Am Surg* 49:179–81, 1983

17. Berg U, Bygdeman S, Henningsson A, Kystrom B, Tunnell R: An outbreak of group A streptococcal infection in a maternity unit. *J Hosp Infect* 3:333–339, 1982.

18. Hamoudi AC, Palmer RN, King TL: Nafcillin resistant *Staphylococcus aureus*: a possible community origin. *Infect Control* 4:153–157, 1983.

19. Boyce JM, White RL, Causey WA, Lockwood WR: Burn units as a source of methicillin-resistant *Staphylococcus aureus* infections. *JAMA* 249:2803–2807, 1983.

20. Cross AS, Zierdt CH, Roup B, Almazan R, Swan JC: A hospital wide outbreak of septicemia due to a few strains of *Staphyococcus aureus*. *Am J Clin Pathol* 79:598–603, 1983.

21. Price EH, Brain A, Dickson JAS: An outbreak of infection with a gentamicin and methicillin-resistant *Staphylococcus aureus* in a neonatal unit. *J Hosp Infect* 1:221–228, 1980.

22. Saravolatz LD, Pohlod DJ, Arking LM: Community acquired methicillin resistant *Staphylococcus aureus* infections: a new source for nosocomial outbreaks. *Ann Intern Med* 97:325–329, 1982.

23. Pavillard R, Harvey K, Douglas D, Hewstone A, Andrew J, Collopy B, Asche V, Carson P, Davidson A, Gilbert G, Spicer J, Tosolini F: Epidemic of hospital acquired infection due to methicillin-resistant *Staphylococus aureus* in major Victorian hospitals. *Med J Aust* 1:451–454, 1982.

24. Haley RW, Bregman DA: The role of understaffing and overcrowding in recurrent outbreaks of staphylococcal infection in a neonatal special care unit. *J Infect Dis* 145:875–885, 1982.

25. Rahman M: Outbreak of *Streptococcus pyogenes* infections in a geriatric hospital and control by mass treatment. *J Hosp Infect* 2:63–69, 1981.

26. Mulhern B, Griffin E: An epidemic of gentamicin/cloxacillin resistant staphylococcal infection in a neonatal unit. *Ir Med J* 74:228–229, 1981.

27. Ward TT, Winn RE, Hartstein AI, Sewell DL: Observations relating to an interhospital outbreak of methicillin-resistant *Staphylococcus aureus*: role of antimicrobial therapy in infection control. *Infect Control* 2:453–459, 1981.

28. Saravolatz LD, Markowitz N, Arking L, Pohlod D, Fisher E: Methicillin resistant *Staphylococcus aureus*. Epidemiologic observation during a community acquired outbreak. *Ann Intern Med* 96:11–16, 1982.

29. Boyce JM, Landry M, Deetz TR, DuPont HL: Epidemiologic studies of an outbreak of nosocomial methicillin resistant *Staphylococcus aureus* infections. *Infect Control* 2:110–116, 1981.

30. Craven DE, Reed C, Kollisch N, DeMaria A, Lichtenberg D, Shen K, McCabe WR: A large outbreak of infections caused by a strain of *Staphylococcus aureus* resistance of oxacillin and aminoglycosides. *Am J Med* 71:53–58, 1981.

31. Ayton M: An outbreak of streptococcal infection in a children's ward. *Nurs Times* 77:1–8, 1981.

32. Dunkle LM, Naqvi SH, McCallum R, Lofgren JP: Eradication of epidemic methicillin-gentamicin-resistant *Staphylococcus aureus* in an intensive care nursery. *Am J Med* 70:455–458, 1981.

33. Tanner EI, Bullin J, Bullin CH, Gamble DR: An outbreak of post-operative sepsis due to a staphylococcal disperser. *J Hyg* 85:219–225, 1980.

34. Peacock JE, Jr, Marsik FJ, Wenzel RP: Methicillin resistant *Staphylococcus aureus*: introduction and spread within a hospital. *Ann Intern Med* 93:526–532, 1980.

35. Forse RA, Dixon C, Bernard K, Martinez L, McLean APH, Meakins JL: *Staphylococcus epidermidis*: an important pathogen. *Surgery* 86:507–514, 1979.

36. Greenhood GP, Hill DL, Dixon RE, Carter MJ, Kanto WP: Changing phage typing patterns of epidemic gentamicin resistant *Staphylococcus aureus*. Evidence for transmission of gentamicin resistance. *Lancet* 1:289–291, 1979.

37. Williams WW, Mariano J, Spurrier M, Donnel HD Jr, Breckenridge RL Jr, Anderson RL, Wachsmuth IK, Thornsberry C, Graham DR, Thibeault DW, Allen JR: Noscomial meningitis due to *Citrobacter diversus* in neonates: new aspects of the epidemiology. *J Infect Dis* 150:229–235, 1984.

38. Facinelli B, Calegari L: A hospital epidemic caused by a multiple antibiotic resistant *Klebsiella pneumoniae*: implication of a conjugative R plasmid. *Boll Ist Sieroter Milan* 63:111–117, 1984.

39. Montanaro D, Grasso GM, Annino I, De Ruggiero N, Scarcella A, Schioppa F: Epidemiological and bacteriological investigation of *Serratia marcescens* epidemic in a nursery and in a neonatal intensive care unit. *J Hyg* 93:67–78, 1984.

40. Horan MA, Gulati RS, Fox RA, Glew E, Ganguli L, Kaeney M: Outbreak of *Shigella sonei* dysentery on a geriatric assessment ward. *J Hosp Infect* 5:210–212, 1984.

41. Mhalu FS, Mtango FDE, Msengi AE: Hospital outbreaks of cholera transmitted through close person to person contact. *Lancet* 2:82–84, 1984.

42. Echols RM, Palmer DL, King RM, Long GW: Multidrug resistant *Serratia marcescens* bacteriuria related to urologic instrumentation. *South Med J* 77:173–177, 1984.

43. Spitalny KC, Okowitz EN, Vogt RL: Salmonellosis outbreak at a Vermont hospital. *South Med J* 77:168–172, 1984.

44. Saravolatz LD, Arking L, Pohlod D, Fisher EJ, Borer R: An outbreak of gentamicin resistant *Klebsiella pneumoniae*: analysis of control measures. *Infect Control* 5:79–84, 1984.

45. Svenninggen NW, Bekassy AN, Christensen P, Kamme C: Nosocomial *Klebsiella pneumoniae* infection: clinical and hygienic measures in a neonatal intensive care unit. *Scand J Infect Dis* 16:29–35, 1984.

46. Muhlbauer B, Fattal A, Siegman Igra Y: A small outbreak of *Serratia marcescens* sepsis and meningitis. *Isr J Med Sci* 19:980–981, 1983.

47. Smith PJ, Brookfield DSK, Shaw DA, Gray J: An outbreak of *Serratia marcescens* infections in a neonatal unit. *Lancet* 1:151–153, 1984.

48. Bhujwala RA, Shriniwas, Dutta S: Epidemiological study of *Serratia marcescens* infection in a hospital. *Indian J Med Res* 78:29–36, 1983.

49. Seals JE, Parrott PL, McGowan JE Jr, Feldman RA: Nursery salmonellosis: delayed recognition due to unusually long incubation period. *Infect Control* 4:205–208, 1983.

50. Perinpanoyagam RM, Grundy HC: Outbreak of gentamicin resistant *Pseudomonas aeruginosa* infection in a burns unit. *J Hosp Infect* 4:71–73, 1983.

51. Kumarasinghe G, Hamilton WJ, Gould JDM, Palmer SR, Dudgeon JA, CBE, Marshall WC: An outbreak of Salmonella muenchen infection in a specialist paediatric hospital. *J Hosp Infect* 3:341–344, 1982.

52. John JF Jr, McKee KT Jr, Twitty JA, Schaffner W: Molecular epidemiology of sequential nursery epidemics caused by multiresistant *Klebsiella pneumoniae. J Pediatr* 102:825–830, 1983.

53. Robins-Browne RM, Rowe B, Ramsaroop R, Naran AD, Threlfall EJ, Ward LR, Lloyd DA, Mickel RE: A hospital outbreak of multiresistant *Salmonella typhimurium* belonging to phage type 193. *J Infect Dis* 147:210–216, 1983.

54. Murray SA, Snydman DR: Investigation of an epidemic of multidrug resistant *Pseudomonas aeruginosa. Infect Control* 3:456–460, 1982.

55. Rangnekar VM, Banker DD, Jhala HI: R-plas-mids in *Salmonella oranienburg* isolated from hospital outbreak. *Indian J Med Res* 76:353–357, 1982.

56. Bullock DW, Bidwell JL, Reeves DS, White LO, Turner A, Speller DCE, Wilkinson PJ: Outbreaks of hospital infection in southwest England caused by gentamicin resistant *Serratia marcescens. J Hosp Infect* 3:263–273, 1982.

57. Scheidt A, Drusin LM, Krauss AN, Machalek SG: Noscomial outbreak of resistant *Serratia* in a neonatal intensive care unit. *NY State J Med* 82:1188–1191, 1982.

58. French GL, Casewell MW, Roncoroni AJ, Knight S, Phillips I: A hospital outbreak of antibiotic resistant *Acinetobacter anitratus*: epidemiology and control. *J Hosp Infect* 1:125–131, 1980.

59. Shanson DC: Outbreaks of *Pseudomonas aeruginosa* infection in a nursery (letter). *J Hosp Infect* 1:83–86, 1980.

60. Alkan M, Soffer S: Emergence of resistance to antibiotics during an outbreak of hospital acquired salmonellosis. *J Hosp Infect* 3:185–187, 1982.

61. Blenkharn JI, Hughes VM: Suction apparatus and hospital infection due to multiply resistant *Klebsiella aerogenes. J Hosp Infect* 3:173–178, 1982.

62. Hart CA: Nosocomial gentamicin and multiply resistant enterobacteria at one hospital. Factors associated with carriage. *J Hosp Infect* 3:165–172, 1982.

63. Farmer JJ 3d, Weinstein RA, Zierdt CH, Brokopp CD: Hospital outbreaks caused by *Pseudomonas aeruginosa*: importance of serogroup O11. *J Clin Microbiol* 16:266–270, 1982.

64. Strand CL, Bryant JK, Morgan JW, Foster JG Jr, McDonald HP Jr, Morganstern SL: Nosocomial *Pseudomonas aeruginosa* urinary tract infections. *JAMA* 248:1615–1618, 1982.

65. Mehta G, Prakash K, Sharma KB: *Salmonella oranienburg* infection in a neonatal unit in New Delhi. *Indian J Med Res* 75:480–484, 1982.

66. Makarem EH: Outbreak of multiple drug resistant *Salmonella havana* originating in pediatric wards of two hospitals in Shiraz, Iran—in vitro susceptibility patterns. *J Trop Pediatr* 28:14–19, 1982.

67. Hart CA: Nosocomial gentamicin and multiply resistant enterobacteria at one hospital. I. Description of an outbreak. *J Hosp Infect* 3:15–28, 1982.

68. Carlquist JF, Conti M, Burke JP: Progressive resistance in a single strain of *Acinetobacter calcoaceticus* recovered during a nosocomial outbreak. *Am J Infect Control* 10:43–48, 1982.

69. McGuckin MB, Thorpe RJ, Koch KM, Alavi A, Staum M, Abrutyn E: An outbreak of *Achromobacter xylosoxidans* related to diagnostic tracer procedures. *Am J Epidemiol* 115:785–793, 1982.

70. Mutton JK, Brady LM, Harkness JL: *Serratia* cross infection in an intensive therapy unit. *J Hosp Infect* 2:85–91, 1981.

71. Smith PW, Rusnak PG: Aminoglycoside resistant *Pseudomonas aeruginosa* urinary tract infection: study of an outbreak. *J Hosp Infect* 2:71–75, 1981.

72. Hughes VM, Henderson WG, Datta N: Discriminating between multiply resistant *Klebsiella* strains during a hospital outbreak: use of klebecin typing and a screening test for plasmids. *J Hosp Infect* 2:45–54, 1981.

73. McKee KT Jr, Cotton RB, Stratton CW, Lavely

GB, Wright PF, Shenai JP, Evans ME, Melly MA, Farmer JJ, Karzon DT, Schaffner W: Nursery epidemic due to multiply resistant *Klebsiella pneumoniae*: epidemiologic setting and impact on perinatal health care delivery. *Infect Control* 3:150–156, 1982.

74. Christensen GD, Korones SB, Reed L, Bulley R, McLaughlin B, Bisno AL: Epidemic *Serratia marcescens* in a neonatal intensive care unit: importance of the gastrointestinal tract as a reservoir. *Infect Control* 3:127–133, 1982.

75. Martone WJ, Osterman CA, Fisher KA, Wenzel RP: *Pseudomonas cepacia*: implications and control of epidemic nosocomial colonization. *Rev Infect Dis* 3:708–715, 1981.

76. Geiseler PJ, Harris B, Andersen BR: Nosocomial outbreak of nitrate negative *Serratia marcescens* infections. *J Clin Microbiol* 15:728–730, 1982.

77. Ratnam S, Mercer E, Picco B, Parsons S, Butler R: A nosocomial outbreak of diarrheal disease due to *Yersinia entercolitica* serotype 0:5, biotype 1. *J Infect Dis* 145:242–247, 1982.

78. Cookson BD, Houang EC, Lee JV: Clustering of *Aeromonas hydrophila* septicaemia (letter). *Lancet* 2:1232, 1981.

79. Tucci V, Isenberg HD: Hospital cluster epidemic with *Morganella morganii*. *J Clin Microbiol* 14:563–566, 1981.

80. Chakravarti A, Mandal A, Sharma KB: An outbreak due to multiple drug resistant *Serratia marcescens* in a children's hospital. *Indian J Med Res* 74:196–201, 1981.

81. Arroyo JC, Milligan WL, Postic B, Northey J, Parker E, Bryan CS: Clinical epidemiologic and microbiologic features of a persistent outbreak of amikacin resistant *Serratia marcescens*. *Infect Control* 2:367–372, 191.

82. Fisher MC, Long SS, Roberts EM, Dunn JM, Balsara RK: *Pseudomonas maltophilia* bacteremia in children undergoing open heart surgery. *JAMA* 246:1571–1574, 1981.

83. Graham DR, Anderson RL, Ariel FE, Ehrenkranz NJ, Rowe B, Boer HR, Dixon RE: Epidemic nosocomial meningitis due to *Citrobacter diversus* in neonates. *J Infect Dis* 144:203–209, 1981.

84. Anagnostakis D, Fitsialos J, Koutsia C, Messaritakis J, Matsaniotis N: A nursery outbreak of *Serratia marcescens* infection. Evidence of a single source of contamination. *Am J Dis Child* 135:413–414, 1981.

85. Adair FW: Nosocomial *Serratia* outbreak: guilt by association or scientific investigation? (letter). *Lancet* 1:563, 1981.

86. Rubens CE, Farrar WE Jr, McGee ZA, Schaffner W: Evolution of a plasmid mediating resistance to multiple antimicrobial agents during a prolonged epidemic of nosocomial infections. *J Infect Dis* 143:170–181, 1981.

87. Parida SN, Verma IC, Deb M, Bhujwala RA: An outbreak of diarrhea due to *Citrobacter freundii* in a neonatal special care nursery. *Ind J Pediatr* 47:81–84, 1980.

88. Bachrach SJ: Successful treatment of an institutional outbreak of shigellosis. *Clin Pediatr (Phila)* 20:127–131, 1981.

89. Powell J, Bureau MA, Pare C, Gaildry ML, Cabana D, Patriquin H: Necrotizing enterocolitis. Epidemic following an outbreak of *Enterobacter cloacae* type 3305723 in a neonatal intensive care unit. *Am J Dis Child* 134:1152–1154, 1980.

90. Schaberg DR, Haley RW, Highsmith AK, Anderson RL, McGowan JE Jr: Nosocomial bacteriuria: a prospective study of case clustering and antimicrobial resistance. *Ann Intern Med* 93:420–424, 1980.

91. Puri V, Thirupuram S, Khalil A, Vergheese A, Gupta S: Nosocomial *Salmonella typhimurium* epidemic in a neonatal special care. *Indian Pediatr* 17:233–239, 1980.

92. Itoh M, Tierno PM Jr, Milstoc M, Berger AR: A unique outbreak of *Pasteurella multocida* in a chronic disease hospital. *Am J Public Health* 70:1170–1173, 1980.

93. Krieger JN, Levy Zombek E, Scheidt A, Drusin LM: A nosocomial epidemic of antibiotic resistant *Serratia marcescens* urinary tract infections. *J Urol* 124:498–502, 1980.

94. Bettelheim KA: Colony incompatibility among strains of *Escherichia coli* isolated during an outbreak of gastroenteritis in one ward. *J Med Microbiol* 13:463–468, 1980.

95. Kumari S, Gupta R, Bhargava SK: A nursery outbreak with *Salmonella newport*. *Indian Pediatr* 17:11–16, 1980.

96. Cunha BA, Klimek JJ, Gracewski J, McLaughlin JC, Quintillani R: A common source outbreak of *Acinetobacter* pulmonary infections traced to Wright respirometers. *Postgrad Med J* 56:169–172, 1980.

97. Parry MF, Hutchinson JH, Brown NA, Wu CH, Estreller L: Gram negative sepsis in neonates: a nursery outbreak due to hand carriage of *Citrobacter diversus*. *Pediatrics* 65:1105–1109, 1980.

98. Montgomerie JZ: Epidemiology of *Klebsiella* and hospital-associated infections. *Rev Infect Dis* 736–753, 1979.

99. Pitt TL, Erdman YJ, Bucher C: The epidemiological type identification of *Serratia marcescens* from outbreaks of infection in hospitals. *J Hyg* 84:269–283, 1980.

100. Kocka FE, Srinivasan S, Mowjood M, Kantor HS: Nosocomial multiply resistant *Providencia stuartii*: a long-term outbreak with multiple biotypes and serotypes at one hospital. *J Clin Microbiol* 11:167–169, 1980.

101. Cook LN, Davis RS, Stover BH: Outbreak of amikacin resistant *Enterobacteriaceae* in an intensive care nursery. *Pediatrics* 65:264–268, 1980.

102. Lyons RW, Samples CL, DeSilva HN, Ross KA, Julian EM, Checko PJ: An epidemic of resistant *Salmonella* in a nursery. Animal to human spread. *JAMA* 243:546–547, 1980.

103. Falkiner FR, Keene CT: *Pseudomonas* infection—recent outbreaks in some Dublin hospitals. *Ir Med J* 72:321–326, 1979.

104. Houang ET, Evans MAL, Simpson CN: Control of hospital epidemic of gentamicin resistant *Klebsiella aerogenes* (letter). *Lancet* 2:205, 1979.

105. Gruneberg RN, Bendall MJ: Hospital outbreak of trimethoprim resistance in pathogenic coliform bacteria. *Br Med J* 2:7–9, 1979.

106. Sadowski PL, Peterson BC, Gerding DN, Cleary PP: Physical characterization of ten R plasmids obtained from an outbreak of nosocomial *Kleb-*

siella pneumonia infections. *Antimicrob Agents Chemother* 15:616–624, 1979.

107. Gerding DN, Buxton AE, Hughes RA, Cleary PP, Arbaczawski J, Stamm WE: Nosocomial multiply resistant *Klebsiella* pneumonia: epidemiology of an outbreak of apparent index case origin. *Antimicrob Agents Chemother* 15:608–615, 1979.

108. Chow AW, Taylor PR, Yoshikawa TT, Guze LB: A nosocomial outbreak of infections due to multiply resistant *Proteus mirabilis*: role of intestinal colonization as a major reservoir. *J Infect Dis* 139:621–627, 1979.

109. Singh M, Singhi S, Kalra V, Deb M: Nosocomial *Klebsiella pneumoniae* epidemic in a neonatal special care unit. *Indian Pediatr* 15:635–639, 1978.

110. French GL, Lowry MF: An outbreak of *Salmonella heidelberg* infection in Jamaica. *West Indian Med J* 18:40–44, 1979.

111. Taylor MR, Keane CT, Kerrison IM, Sronge JL. Simple and effective measures for control of enteric cross infection in a children's hospital. *Lancet* 1:865–867, 1979.

112. Krober MS, Bass JW, Brown JD, Lemon SM, Rupert KJ: Hospital outbreak of hepatitis A: risk factors for spread. *Pediatr Infect Dis* 3:296–299, 1984.

113. Eckstein R, Loy A, Jehn U: A spell of chicken pox on a cancer patients' ward. *Klin Wochenschr* 62:387–389, 1984.

114. Meissner HC, Murray SA, Kiernan MA, Snydman DR, McIntosh K: A simultaneous outbreak of respiratory syncytial virus and parainfluenza virus type 3 in a newborn nursery. *J Pediatr* 104:680–684, 1984.

115. Baron RC, McCormick JB, Zubeir OA: Ebola virus disease in southern Sudan: hospital dissemination and intrafamilial spread. *Bull WHO* 61:997–1003, 1983.

116. Gustafson TL, Kobylik B, Hutcheson RH, Schaffner W: Protective effect of anticholinergic drugs and psyllium in a nosocomial outbreak of Norwalk gastroenteritis. *J Hosp Infect* 4:367–374, 1983.

117. Pether JVS, Caul EO: An outbreak of food borne gastroenteritis in two hospitals associated with a Norwalk like virus. *J Hyg* 91:343–350, 1983.

118. Ono IP, Machado RD, Couceiro JN: Outbreak of parainfluenza virus in a hospital in Rio de Janeiro. *Rev Latinoam Microbiol* 24:19–23, 1982.

119. McCarrol CJ, Vogel HL: Rotavirus outbreak in a newborn nursery: report of cases. *J Am Osteopath Assoc* 82:914–916, 1983.

120. Hammerberg O, Watts J, Chernesky M, Luchsinger I, Rawls W: An outbreak of herpes simplex virus type 1 in an intensive care nursery. *Pediatr Infect Dis* 2:290–294, 1983.

121. Rodriguez WJ, Kim HW, Brandt CD, Gardner MK, Parrott RH: Use of electrophoresis of RNA from human rotavirus to establish the identity of strains involved in outbreaks in a tertiary care nursery. *J Infect Dis* 148:38–40, 1983.

122. Holzel H, Cubitt DW, McSwiggan DA, Sanderson PJ, Church J: An outbreak of rotavirus infection among adults in a cardiology ward. *J Infect* 2:33–37, 1980.

123. Chapin M, Yatabe J, Cherry JD: An outbreak of

rotavirus gastroenteritis on a pediatric unit. *Am J Infect Control* 11:88–91, 1983.

124. Straube RC, Thompson MA, Van Dyke RB, Wadell G, Connor JD, Wingard D, Spector SA: Adenovirus type 7b in a children's hospital. *J Infect Dis* 147:814–819, 1983.

125. Keenlyside RA, Hierholzer JC, D'Angelo LJ: Keratoconjunctivitis associated with adenovirus type 37: an extended outbreak in an ophthalmologists's office. *J Infect Dis* 147:191–198, 1983.

126. Juel Jensen BE: Outbreak of chickenpox from a patient with immunosuppressed herpes zoster in hospital (letter). *Br Med J* [Clin Res] 286:60, 1983.

127. Rivera M, Gonzalez N: An influenza outbreak in a hospital. *Am J Nurs* 82:1836–1838, 1982.

128. Faizallah R, Green HT, Krasner N, Walker RJ: Outbreak of chickenpox from a patient with immunosuppressed herpes zoster in hospital. *Br Med J* [Clin Res] 285:1022–1023, 1982.

129. Gustafson TL, Lavely GB, Brawner ER Jr, Hutcheson RH Jr, Wright PF, Schaffner W: An outbreak of airborne nosocomial varicella. *Pediatrics* 70:550–556, 1982.

130. Carl M, Blakey DL, Francis DP, Maynard JE: Interruption of hepatitis B transmission by modification of a gynaecologist's surgical technique. *Lancet* 1:731–733, 1982.

131. Valenti WM, Clarke TA, Hall CB, Menegus MA, Shapiro DL: Concurrent outbreaks of rhinovirus and respiratory syncytial virus in an intensive care nursery: epidemiology and associated risk factors. *J Pediatr* 100:722–726, 1982.

132. Van Voris LP, Belshe RB, Shaffer JL: Nosocomial influenza B virus infection in the elderly. *Ann Intern Med* 96:153–158, 1982.

133. Moss AL: Hospital outbreak of hepatitis B (letter). *NZ Med J* 94:65–66, 1981.

134. Orenstein WA, Wu E, Wilkins J, Robinson K, Francis DP, Timko N, Wayne R: Hospital acquired hepatitis A: report of an outbreak. *Pediatrics* 67:494–497, 1981.

135. Seeberg S, Brandberg A, Hermodsson S, Larsson P, Lundgren S: Hospital outbreak of hepatitis A secondary to blood exchange in a baby (letter). *Lancet* 1:1155–1156, 1981.

136. Levandowski RA, Rubenis M: Nosocomial conjunctivitis caused by adenovirus type 4. *J Infect Dis* 143:28–31, 1981.

137. Strassburg MA, Imagawa DT, Fannin SL, Turner JA, Chow AW, Murrary RA, Cherry JD: Rubella outbreak among hospital employees. *Obstet Gynecol* 57:283–288, 1981.

138. Hildreth C, Thomas M, Ridgway GL: Rotavirus infection in an obstetric unit. *Br Med J* [Clin Res] 282:231, 1981.

139. Garvie DG, Gray J: Outbreak of respiratory syncytial virus infection in the elderly. *Br Med J* 281:1253–1254, 1980.

140. Benenson MW, Takafuji ET, Bancroft WH, Lemon SM, Callahan MC, Leach DA: A military community outbreak of hepatitis type A related transmission in a child care facility. *Am J Epidemiol* 112:471–481, 1980.

141. Polk BF, White JA, DeGirolami PC, Modlin JF: An outbreak of rubella among hospital personnel. *N Engl J Med* 303:541–545, 1980.

142. Cubitt WD, Holzel H: An outbreak of rotavirus

infection in a long stay ward of a geriatric hospital. *J Clin Pathol* 33:306–308, 1980.

143. Helmsing PJ, Duermeyer W, Van Hattem GCAM, Wielaard F: An outbreak of hepatitis A in an institution for the mentally retarded. *J Med Virol* 5:143–150, 1980.

144. Goldson EJ, McCarthy JT, Welling MA, Todd JK: A respiratory syncytial virus outbreak in a transitional care nursery. *Am J Dis Child* 133:1280–1282, 1979.

145. Mintz L, Ballard RA, Sniderman SH, Roth RS, Drew WL: Nosocomial respiratory syncytial virus infections in an intensive care nursery: rapid diagnosis by direct immunofluorescence. *Pediatrics* 64:149–153, 1979.

146. Galbraith RM, Diestag JL, Purcell RH, Gower PH, Zuckerman AJ, Williams R: Non-A non-B hepatitis associated with chronic liver disease in a haemodialysis unit. *Lancet* 1:951–953, 1979.

147. Meyers JD, MacQuarrie MB, Merigan TC, Jennison MH: Nosocomial varicella. Part I: outbreak in oncology patients at a children's hospital. *West J Med* 130:196–199, 1979.

148. Davies DP, Hughes CA, MacVicar J, Hawkes P, Mair HJ: Echovirus-11 infection in a special care baby unit (letter). *Lancet* 1:96, 1979.

149. Quinn JP, Arnow PM, Weil D, Rosenbluth J: Outbreak of JK diphtheroid infections associated with environmental contamination. *J Clin Microbiol* 19:668–671, 1984.

150. Newman PE, Goodman RA, Waring GO 3rd, Finton RJ, Wilson LA, Wright J, Cavanagh HD: A cluster of cases of *Mycobacterium chelonei* keratitis associated with outpatient office procedures. *Am J Ophthalmol* 97:344–348, 1984.

151. Reported by Pancoast SJ, Kis JJ: Leads from the MMWR. Patient source scabies among hospital personnel—Pennsylvania. *JAMA* 250:1817–1818, 1983.

152. Helms CM, Massanari RM, Zeitler R, Streed S, Gilchrist MJR, Hall N, Hausler WJ Jr, Sywassink J, Johnson W, Wintermeyer L, Hierholzer WJ Jr: Legionnaires' disease associated with a hospital water system: a cluster of 24 nosocomial cases. *Ann Intern Med* 99:171–178, 1983.

153. Yamagishi T, Sakamoto K, Sakurai S, Konishi K, Daimon Y, Matsuda M, Gyobu Y, Kubo Y, Kodama H: A nosocomial outbreak of food poisoning caused by enterotoxigenic *Clostridium perfringens*. *Microbiol Immunol* 27:291–296, 1983.

154. Lerche NW, Currier RW, Juranek DD, Baer W, Dubay NJ: Atypical crusted "Norwegian" scabies: report of nosocomial transmission in a community hospital and an approach to control. *Cutis* 31:637–642, 668, 684, 1983

155. Faergemann J, Fredriksson T, Herczka D, Krupicka O, Bjorklund KN, Sjokvist M: Tinea incognito as a source of an epidemic of *Trichophyton violaceum* infections in a dermatologic ward. *Int J Dermatol* 22:39–40, 1983.

156. Kim K, DuPont HL, Pickering LK: Outbreaks of diarrhea associated with *Clostridium difficile* and its toxin in day-care centers: evidence of person-to-person spread. *J Pediatr* 102:376–382, 1983.

157. Mehtar S, Law CA: An outbreak of beta lactamase producing *Haemophilus influenzae* (biotype III) on a geriatric ward. *J Hosp Infect* 1:357–358, 1980.

158. Stevens DA, Pier AC, Beaman BL, Morozumi PA, Lovett IS, Houang ET: Laboratory evaluation of an outbreak of nocardiosis in immunocompromised hosts. *Am J Med* 71:928–934, 1981.

159. Lovett, IS, Houang ET, Burge S, Turner Warwick M, Thompson FD, Harrison AR, Joekes AM, Parkinson MC: An outbreak of *Nocardia asteroides* infection in a renal transplant unit. *Q J Med* 50:123–135, 1981.

160. Brown A, Yu VL, Elder EM, Magnussen MH, Kroboth F: Nosocomial outbreak of Legionnaire's disease at the Pittsburgh Veterans Administration Medical Center. *Trans Assoc Am Physicians* 93:52–59, 1980.

161. Fisher Hoch SP, Bartlett CLR, Tobin JO'H, Gillett MB, Nelson AM, Pritchard JE, Smith MG, Swann RA, Talbot JM, Thomas JA: Investigation and control of an outbreak of Legionnaires' disease in a district general hospital. *Lancet* 1:932–936, 1981.

162. England AC 3rd, Fraser DW: Sporadic and epidemic nosocomial legionellosis in the United States. Epidemiologic features. *Am J Med* 70:707–711, 1981.

163. Valenti WM, Pincus PH, Messner MK: Nosocomial pertussis: possible spread by a hospital visitor. *Am J Dis Child* 134:520–521, 1980.

164. Cohen MS, Steere AC, Baltimore R, Von Graevenitz A, Pantelick E, Camp B, Root RK: Possible nosocomial transmission of group Y *Neisseria meningitidis* among oncology patients. *Ann Intern Med* 91:7–12, 1979.

165. Marks JS, Tsai TF, Martone WJ, Baron RC, Kennicott J, Holtzhauer FJ, Baird I, Fay D, Feeley JC, Mallison GF, Fraser DW, Halpin TJ: Nosocomial Legionnaires' disease in Columbus, Ohio. *Ann Intern Med* 90:565–569, 1979.

166. Belle EA, DSouza TJ, Zarzour JY, Lemieux M, Wong CC: Hospital epidemic of scabies: diagnosis and control. *Can J Public Health* 70:133–135, 1979.

167. Haley CE, Cohen ML, Halter J, Meyer RD: Nosocomial Legionnaires' disease: a continuing common source epidemic at Wadsworth Medical Center. *Ann Intern Med* 90:583–586, 1979.

168. Rhame FS, Root RK, MacLowry JO, Dadisman TA, Bennett JV: Salmonella septicemia from platelet transfusions. Study of an outbreak traced to a hematogenous carrier of *Salmonella choleraesuis*. *Ann Intern Med* 78:633–641, 1973.

169. Thompson RL, Cabezudo I, Wenzel RP: Epidemiology of nosocomial infections caused by methicillin-resistant *Staphylococcus aureus*. *Ann Intern Med* 97:309–317, 1982.

170. Graham DR, Band JD: *Citrobacter diversus* brain abscess and meningitis in neonates. *JAMA* 245:1923–1925, 1981.

171. Leclair JM, Zaia JA, Levin MJ, Congdon RG, Goldmann DA: Airborne transmission of chickenpox in a hospital. *N Engl J Med* 302:450–453, 1980.

172. Nagington J, Wreghitt TG, Gandy G, Roberton NRC, Berry PJ: Fatal echovirus 11 infections in outbreak in special-care baby unit. *Lancet* 2:725–728, 1978.

Chapter 11

The Infection Control Committee

Richard P. Wenzel, M.D.

Politically and administratively, the most important hour in the month is the one set aside for the meeting of the infection control committee. It is surprising, therefore, that so little preparation is made by so many intelligent and industrious practitioners of infection control. This fact is generally evidenced by a review of the last year's minutes from the meetings: the same topic is discussed for months on end, no significant decisions are made, and little is accomplished.

It is the purpose of this chapter to suggest that the committee meetings are important and deserve a great deal of effort, and that they can be stimulating, informative, and politically rewarding. What is required is some insight into decision making, a commitment to planning, and realistic expectations as to who will do most of the work.

MEMBERSHIP QUALIFICATIONS

If the author could choose ideal members of the committee, they would have the following attributes (listed in order of importance):

1. Interest in the committee and its duties;
2. Representative of a large group within the hospital;
3. Authoritative figures (experts) in their specialty within the hospital;
4. Tactful and communicative;
5. Charismatic.

At first glance, it may seem unlikely that such an array of characteristics can easily be found. Nevertheless, the ideal needs to be stated so that when choices for replacement are being made, the candidates can be compared. It needs to be emphasized continually that interest is the only essential qualification.

At this point, it is worth stating that in the author's opinion, the purpose of the committee is to ratify the ideas of the thoughtful infection control team, to disseminate the information discussed in the meeting, and to give political and administrative support. Although new ideas and new perspectives are welcomed, it is not realistic for the hospital epidemiologist or infection control practitioner to assume that a major function of the infection control committee is to generate new ideas or to perform any serious amount of work for the infection control team. Instead, not only will ideas be generated but also the day-to-day work will be carried out by the "nucleus" of the infection control committee: the hospital epidemiologist, the infection control practitioners, the clinical microbiologist, and the employee health director. In fact, some major conflicts may arise, as well as ill will and inertia from the practitioners' false expectations that those members outside of the "nucleus" will contribute their time significantly to the solution of routine infection control problems.

COMMITTEE COMPOSITION

It seems reasonable that all members of the "nucleus" be members of the committee. For an effective committee, however, it is also obvious that other representatives from the following large and important groups be invited members: hospital administration, nursing service, internal medicine, surgery, pharmacy, pediatrics, and central sterile supply.

Although it may be desirable in some institutions to have members on the committee from housekeeping, dietary services, respiratory therapy, and other services, they may not be essential. Whether or not a hospital chooses to invite members outside of those suggested initially depends primarily on the level of enthusiasm for the committee and the commitment to infection control.

THE CHAIRMAN

The major qualification of the chairman is that he or she have a special interest in hospital epidemiology and infection control. Expertise is required, and attendance at all or almost all meetings should be a prerequisite. The most effective chairmen will be those who can easily communicate with clinicians, and for all of the above reasons, the author suggests that a clinician be chairman. Ideally, he or she would be trained in infection control but certainly should have had training in infectious diseases.

The statement above may be construed as solely a bias since many effective programs have a pathologist as chairman of the committee (1). However, with the numerous issues that arise related (*a*) to clusters of infections in patients, implications of ill employees for patient management, and preventive medicine programs and (*b*) to the political consequences of an outbreak, it seems reasonable to expect that communication will be more credible to the hospital staff and thus more effective if the committee is directed by a clinician-epidemiologist or an infectious diseases clinician.

In academic institutions the chairman tends to be a member of the Infectious Diseases Division. In a survey of 121 infectious diseases programs in the United States in 1980, 83% had a division member who acted as head of the infection control committee (2).

It has also been suggested that there be continuity in committee leadership and that the effective chairman remain in position for long periods rather than rotate out of office after only 1 or 2 years (3).

MEETING TIMES AND FREQUENCY

The Joint Commission for the Accreditation of Hospitals (JCAH) recommends that hospital infection control committees meet at least every other month (4). Nevertheless, the majority of committees meet 10 to 12 times annually, with some institutions postponing meetings during the summer months when vacations preclude adequate attendance.

The most common and presumably effective scheduling arrangement is one with an assigned week of the month, day of the week, and hour of the day. For example, at the University of Virginia Hospital, meetings are held at 12 o'clock noon on the second Wednesday of the month with lunch provided by the hospital. In many hospitals, breakfast or luncheon meetings are preferred with the meal provided by the administration. However, government hospitals are not permitted to provide free meals for committee members.

An effective committee chairman will contact the secretaries of the members directly to be sure that the meeting times are noted on the members' respective calendars. In addition, it is useful if the meeting location does not change, has comfortable seating, and is in a room only slightly larger than necessary. The main goal is to create an informal atmosphere in which all members feel free to express their opinions.

MINUTES OF THE COMMITTEE

The minutes of the meeting of the infection control committee are very important documents for medical, administrative, political, legal, and ethical reasons. Their importance should not be underestimated, and care should be taken to record the events accurately, concisely, and tactfully. As with any task, the recording of minutes should be assigned to an interested party and be reviewed carefully before they are finally approved and sent to the executive committee. Examples of minutes of the committee at the University of Virginia Hospital are included in the Appendix to this chapter.

THE AGENDA

There should be no "old business." New items should be discussed at each meeting after a brief summary of surveillance data. Since criteria for nosocomial infections should have been developed, it is not the purpose of the summary to review each case but instead to highlight the trends and announce new problems. In general, the following format has worked well in many hospitals in Virginia:

1. Overall infection rate.
2. Presence or absence of any clusters.
3. Summary of the patients with bloodstream infections.
4. Specific review of the antibiogram of nosocomial bloodstream pathogens with emphasis on:
   a. The percentage of unique isolates of *Staphylococcus aureus* and *Staphylococcus epidermidis* strains resistant to methicillin;
   b. The percentage of gram-negative rods resistant to aminoglycosides and second and third generation cephalosporins used at the hospital.

It should be emphasized that in the antibiogram report, each patient-isolate should be counted only once even if the patient had numerous positive cultures. Such a report is most helpful to the clinician who can estimate the probability that a specific nosocomial pathogen will be resistant to antibiotics available. He can then make an optimal and rational choice for initial therapy of life-threatening nosocomial infections based on epidemiologic data gathered by the infection control team.

In general, the members of the committee can be briefed in 5 to 10 minutes regarding the general infection rate, the presence or absence of any clusters, and current trends in nosocomial pathogens and in antibiotic resistance to drugs on the formulary. Most of the remaining 50 minutes should be devoted to decision making.

DECISION MAKING

A modest but generally unachieved goal is to approve one policy or one procedure at each meeting. One might respond by stating that this is setting the goals too low, but experience suggests that it is a good starting point. The policies or procedures should be of major import, such as the following:

1. What will be the hospital's policy on hepatitis B vaccination of employees?
2. How should AIDS patients be managed in the hospital?
3. How should the hospital react to the diagnosis of AIDS in an employee?
4. Which employees of the hospital should be vaccinated for rubella?
5. How should endoscopes be disinfected or sterilized?
6. What procedures should be followed in management of a patient with Jakob-Creutzfeldt disease who goes to surgery for a brain biopsy?
7. How long should various vascular catheters remain in place before rotation to another site?

Once a topic is selected, it is most important that it not be presented to the committee until all background information has been obtained and analyzed. A premature presentation will only postpone decision making. Obviously, if there is a cluster of infections or a true epidemic, this problem should be the high priority topic for discussion by the committee.

The most important theme is that "all of the homework must be done" for effective committee function. This means that a literature search must have been made on the topic under discussion, all pertinent literature read, and, if necessary, all national experts called on the telephone. When a topic is chosen and the infection control team is ready to present its ideas to the committee, the use of a one- to two-page handout is often useful. Whenever possible, important information should be presented in a graphic fashion or in simple tables. On top of the handout in bold lettering is the issue to be discussed. The chairman can point to the headline if conversation strays from the main theme.

The current issues and controversies must be clearly stated and referenced in the handout.

Then, the well designed studies which have addressed the questions at hand should be summarized and the major data supporting the conclusions succinctly stated. After all available data have been summarized, expert testimony should be presented: opinions from the Centers for Disease Control (CDC), JCAH, and other national experts. Thereafter, it is politically wise to invite the local expert in the hospital to present his opinion of the data and his conclusions. The chairman or a member of the infection control nucleus could then present a list of options for the hospital and the preferred choice. Time should then be available for general discussion by other members of the committee with the understanding by all that diverse opinions have the respect of the committee (5). At the end of the general discussion, a vote should be made before adjournment. Lastly, the minutes of the infection control committee should be forwarded to the executive committee for approval (Table 11.1). If all works well, the members of the infection control committee will not only support the proposals but will disseminate the information to their respective colleagues. This is more likely to occur after the nucleus group gains the respect of the other committee members. In turn, respect is more likely as people get to know each other, and the wise practitioner will quickly develop a working relationship with other committee members. The respect will be maintained when the members know that the physician-epidemiologist or practitioner can be trusted.

BEFORE THE MEETING

Although the discussion above and Table 11.1 appear straightforward, the question may arise as to how easy or difficult it is to accomplish these goals in one meeting. In large part, the answer lies in some political maneuvering prior to the meeting. It would be unwise to "spring" a new topic on the committee members, overburden them with facts for 50 minutes, and ask them to vote on an important issue. They may feel that they are being misled or that their opinions are not respected. Their concerns can be alleviated by a series of briefings on a one-to-one basis prior to the meeting.

Essentially, in the premeeting briefing, the facts must be summarized for the committee members, opinions of the infection control team presented, and a request made to elicit the opinion of the individual committee member. Generally, if the practitioner or physician-epidemiologist has

Table 11.1.   Outline of the General Approach to Decision Making for the Infection Control Committee

Choose a topic.

↓

Do all necessary literature review, and analysis.
Perform telephone survey with regional or national authorities.

↓

Write the question on top of a 1–2-page handout.

↓

Present the literature concisely, give data on
current issues and controversies, and provide
references and citations on handout.

↓

Give conclusions of studies which address the major issue.

↓

List testimony from JCAH, CDC, and experts
who have written in literature.

↓

Have local expert in the hospital give his
review of issue and opinion.

↓

A member of infection control committee's "nucleus"
presents decision options and the preferred option.

↓

General discussion.

↓

Vote—decision.

↓

Minutes presented to executive committee for approval.

been thorough and thoughtful, the other member will either agree with his decisions or present cogent arguments for an alternate recommendation. This statement presupposes a critical review of the literature which could be made available to the individual members. In the quiet and security of his office, the committee member can feel free to express his opinion without concern that a committee of his peers will inhibit his presentation or react negatively.

Many practitioners express concerns that even if the agenda goes well, certain members of the committee have a propensity to block progress because they have negative attitudes toward change. There is no simple solution to this problem, but one approach is to anticipate the comments prior to the open discussion and plan to have the negative opinions neutralized by a thoughtful ally. It is important that the ally be briefed, understand the issues clearly, and have an opinion favoring change. The assistance from the ally avoids the perception that the "nucleus" group is unsupported in its ideas. Furthermore, it avoids the unwanted and unpleasant situation of the practioner's or clinician-epidemiologist's appearing to defend a purely personal position. Instead, it is consistent with the goal that all decisions be based on data derived from well designed studies published in peer-reviewed journals, on expert opinions, and on the special needs and resources of the institution.

SECULAR TRENDS IN ACCOMPLISHMENT

It is helpful to review the last year's minutes of the committee on an annual basis, to identify its

accomplishments, and to note the number of months required for each major decision. If fewer than one decision each month was accomplished or if it required 2 or more months for others, then goals can be generated for the new year.

The accomplishments of the committee can thereafter be measured annually and secular trends can be identified.

References

1. Haley RW: The "hospital epidemiologist" in U.S. hospitals, 1976–1977: a description of the need of the infection surveillance and control program. *Infect Control* 1:21–32, 1980.
2. Shands JW Jr, Wenzel RP, Wolff SM, Eickhoff TC, Fields BN, Jackson GG: Hospital epidemiology and infection control: the changing role of the specialist in infectious diseases. *J Infect Dis* 144:609–613, 1982.
3. Schaffner W: The effective physician epidemiologist. In Wenzel RP (ed): *Handbook of Hospital Acquired Infections.* Boca Raton, FL, CRC Press, 1981, pp 13–18.
4. *Accreditation Manual for Hospitals.* Chicago, Joint Commission on Accreditation of Hospitals, 1983, p 72.
5. Cargenie D: *How to Win Friends and Influence People.* New York, Pocket Books, 1970.

Appendix

INFECTION CONTROL COMMITTEE MEETING
SEPTEMBER 12, 1984

Minutes

Surveillance Data

    1a. Surveillance data for June, July, and August 1984 were reviewed. The hospital's infection rate remains within the 95% confidence limits (Fig. 11.1). In June, there were four coagulase-negative staphylococcal bloodstream isolates with two further identified as *S. epidermidis.* All were sensitive to methicillin.

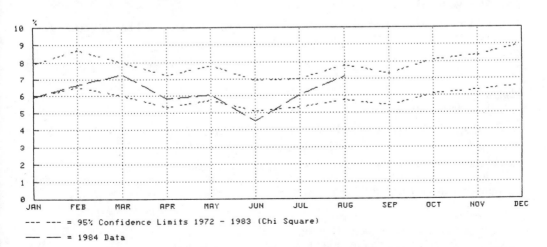

Figure 11.1.   The University of Virginia Medical Center nosocomial infection rate, August 1984.

b. Five *S. aureus* bloodstream infections were identified which were all sensitive to methicillin. In 1984, we have not had any nosocomial methicillin-resistant *S. aureus* blood isolates.

c. In July, there was one *Pseudomonas maltophilia* bloodstream isolate on N3 resistant to gentamicin, and a *P. aeruginosa* bloodstream isolate resistant to gentamicin and intermediate to amikacin. There were eight coagulase-negative bloodstream isolates, and five were resistant to methicillin. There were six bloodstream infections in the newborn intensive care unit (NICU).

d. In August, there were five coagulase-negative staphylococcal isolates and five *S. aureus* isolates. The NICU had six bloodstream isolates.

Major Topic for Discussion
2. The increase of bloodstream infections in NICU patients during July and August was discussed (see below). There was no common organism, and no common source of infection could be identified. The NICU has had a higher daily census than usual as well as more ill, lower birth weight infants who have required more indwelling lines. Although a statistically significant increase in infections was documented (Fig. 11.2), it was the opinion of the committee at this time that the higher rate was due to a higher admission rate of low birth weight babies.
3. The NICU director asked the committee to review the possible traffic flow problem in the new NICU prior to the September 28 opening. The hospital epidemiologist will tour the new unit and make recommendations.

Other Items Briefly Discussed
4. A recent case of chickenpox exposure in the hospital was reviewed. On July 18, 1984, a pediatric resident presented at work and went on rounds with a few vesicular lesions which had erupted the previous evening. The total number of patients exposed was 84. Twelve susceptible patients remained in-house on July 25th and were isolated. One hundred fifty-one employees were exposed. Fourteen had a negative chickenpox history, and titers were drawn on these persons. Of these, nine had true negative serology and six were sent home from July 25th to August 9th. The remaining three were allowed to work under restricted conditions. There were no secondary cases.

The direct costs involved in this current episode are as follows:

Lost salaries	$4,453.00
Cost of blood titers	$536.00
Employee health staff time	$186.00
Epidemiology staff time	$430.86
ZIG	$3,026.40
Total	$8,632.26

The representative from the hospital administration said he would re-evaluate the hospital's policy regarding costs of drugs and services administered to patients for the prevention of nosocomial infections.

5. Committee membership was discussed. The chairman of surgery will be contacted regarding new representation from the surgery department.

6. The employee health nurse briefly reviewed our current rubella screening policy. This will be the major topic discussed at the October meeting.

Adjournment
7. Meeting adjourned at 1 p.m.

INCREASE IN NEWBORN INTENSIVE CARE UNIT NOSOCOMIAL BLOODSTREAM INFECTIONS

Surveillance definition of bloodstream infection (BSI) in a neonate:
1. New clinical picture consistent with sepsis in a patient with a positive culture. The clinical picture may have included the following:
   a. New onset of apena and bradycardia;
   b. Increased O_2 requirement;
   c. Sudden deterioration in condition;
   d. Fever or temperature instability;
   e. Increased peripheral white blood cell count with left shift.

$$\frac{\text{No. Positive}}{\text{No. admissions}}$$ 5/29   1/33   1/23   1/30   1/40   4/38   6/32   6/37

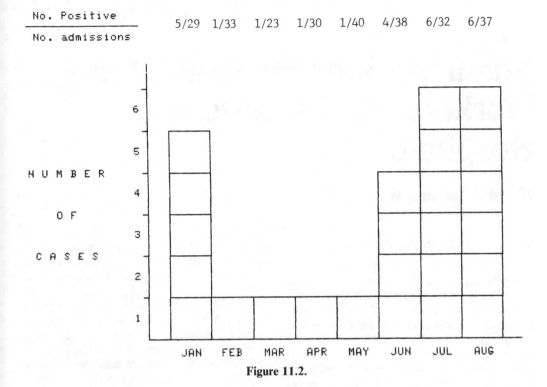

Figure 11.2.

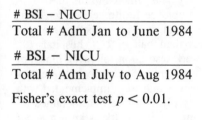

$$\frac{\text{\# BSI} - \text{NICU}}{\text{Total \# Adm Jan to June 1984}} \quad \frac{13}{193}$$

$$\frac{\text{\# BSI} - \text{NICU}}{\text{Total \# Adm July to Aug 1984}} \quad \frac{12}{69}$$

Fisher's exact test $p < 0.01$.

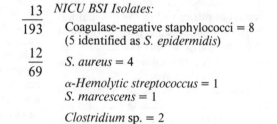

NICU BSI Isolates:

Coagulase-negative staphylococci = 8
(5 identified as *S. epidermidis*)

S. aureus = 4

α-Hemolytic streptococcus = 1
S. marcescens = 1

Clostridium sp. = 2

Chapter 12

Immunizations for Health Care Workers and Patients in Hospitals

David S. Fedson, M.D.

INTRODUCTION

The prevention and control of infections within hospitals require that careful attention be given to the essential role of immunizations for health care workers and patients (1–3). A number of preventable infections can be transmitted from patients to personnel, from personnel to patients, or among patients and hospital employees themselves. Adequate immunization of hospital staff assures that preventable diseases will not be acquired in the hospital or community and subsequently spread to others within the hospital setting. Likewise, immunization of patients provides vital protection against serious preventable diseases that may be acquired either in the hospital or following hospital discharge.

As with hospital infection control programs in general, programs for immunizing staff and patients require (a) an effective employee health service, (b) sound employee education, (c) rigorous pre- and postemployment screening and immunization, and (d) comprehensive policies for specific infections, hospital areas, and certain employees at special risk, particularly pregnant women (4, 5). A close working relationship between infection control practitioners and the employee health service is essential. Common guidelines for screening and immunization must be established (1–3). For employees, these policies must stipulate not only who should be screened for susceptibility to preventable diseases and immunized, but also which procedures should be followed when unimmunized staff are exposed to preventable disease. The latter include the definition of who has authority and responsibility for implementing employee work restrictions, and what policies exist for compensating staff during periods of work absence (6). The issues of employee noncompliance with hospital guidelines for screening and immunization also must be addressed. Legal and ethical questions raised in this process may require expert opinion and guidance.

Approximately half of all visits to the employee health service are for pre-employment evaluation, health maintenance, or evaluation of acute illness or exposure to infectious diseases (7). Screening and immunization are common features of these important employee health service activities. However, survey data gathered in the mid-1970s showed that employee health service screening programs for hepatitis B and rubella were conducted in less than half of U.S. hospitals (8). Policies for work restriction following illness or exposure often were at variance with recommended guidelines and were implemented with great variability (9). No data were obtained on employee immunization. Little is known about the overall status of immunization policies and practices for hospital personnel, although most hospitals, regardless of size, consider pre-employment screening and immunization to be important (10). Such screening programs have shown that substantial numbers of new staff lack adequate immunity to preventable diseases (11, 12).

In addition to health care workers, patients receiving care in hospitals often should be considered for immunization against preventable diseases. However, nothing is known about the extent of hospital screening and immunization programs for hospital patients, nor about the impact of such programs for both employees and patients on the prevention and control of nosocomial infections (13).

IMMUNIZATION IN THE HOSPITAL SETTING

This chapter focuses on preventable infectious diseases that are encountered in the hospital setting, and their frequency and seriousness for both health care workers and patients. For each disease, the rationale for and use of vaccines, toxoids, and/or immune globulins are discussed. The various serologic tests used in screening for susceptibility are not discussed in detail; more complete information should be obtained elsewhere. Infection control practitioners and employee health service personnel responsible for hospital immunization programs should be fully familiar with general guidelines (14) and recent recommendations on adult immunization (15, 16). More detailed guidance on the use of individual immunobiologic agents can be found in the specific recommendations of the Immunization Practices Advisory Committee (ACIP) which are published in *Morbidity and Mortality Weekly Report*. In addition, instructions in the package insert for each product should be followed closely.

Hepatitis B

Hepatitis B Virus and HBV Infections in the United States

Hepatitis B virus (HBV) is a major cause of acute and chronic hepatitis in the United States (17–20). The average person has a 5% lifetime risk of HBV infection. Each year approximately 200,000 persons, mostly young adults, are infected. Of these, 25% become jaundiced, 10,000 are hospitalized, and 250 die of fulminant disease. A reservoir of infection is maintained because 6 to 10% of young adults with acute infection become chronic carriers of HBV. There currently are an estimated 500,000 to 1,000,000 infectious carriers in the U.S., more than 25% of whom develop chronic active hepatitis. Annually, approximately 4,000 persons die from HBV-related cirrhosis. In addition, HBV infection is causally related to hepatocellular carcinoma, a disease that claims more than 800 lives in the U.S. each year.

Hepatitis B virus is a 42-nm DNA virus. Three major antigens have been identified: (*a*) hepatitis B surface antigen (HbsAg), which is detectable in large amounts in the serum of persons with both acute and chronic HBV infection (several subtypes (d-y, a-w) have been identified); (*b*) hepatitis B e antigen (HBeAg), which is a soluble antigen associated with HBV replication, a high titer of HBsAg in serum, and increased infectivity; and (*c*) hepatitis B core antigen (HBcAg). Antibody to HBsAg (anti-HBs) indicates past infection with HBV and is associated with long-lasting immunity. Antibody to HBcAg (anti-HBc) indicates previous infection with HBV. It persists indefinitely, and is found both in persons who have

recovered from HBV infection (anti-HBs positive) and in those who have become chronic carriers (persistent HBsAg positivity for 6 months or more). Immunoglobulin M (IgM) anti-HBc is a sensitive and reliable indicator of acute or recent (i.e., less than 6 months) HBV infection. Antibody to HBeAg (anti-HBe) often is found in the serum of carriers who have a low titer of HBsAg (20).

The incubation period for hepatitis B generally is 60 to 120 days. A large number of HBV infections are subclinical; in patients with illness, the onset is insidious. Fatality rates in reported cases are less than 2%. In chronic carriers who develop cirrhosis, there are no clinical characteristics of the acute (21) or chronic illness (22) that distinguish chronic hepatitis B from chronic hepatitis due to other causes. Although concomitant exposure to other hepatotoxins may worsen the prognosis, the effect of immunosuppressive or anti-inflammatory agents on the outcome of disease is uncertain (23, 24). On the other hand, prognosis can be altered by coinfection with δ agent, an independently transmissible RNA virus that infects and causes illness only in the presence of active HBV infection (25). It is unclear whether simultaneous co-primary infection with HBV and δ agent is associated with greater mortality (26, 27), but δ superinfection of chronic HBV carriers appears to increase the risk of developing chronic active hepatitis (28). No therapeutic agents have been discovered that successfully eradicate the chronic HBV carrier state.

The HBV carrier is central to the epidemiology of HBV transmission in the U. S. (20). Persons who are carriers or who are acutely infected have highest concentrations of HBV in blood and serous fluids, with lower amounts in other body fluids. Transmission can occur by the percutaneous (e.g., contaminated needles) or permucosal (e.g., sexual contact) route. Intimate contact within the household or in institutional settings also is associated with infection, although not by the fecal-oral route. The prevalence of HBsAg positivity in the general population is low (0.3%), but is markedly increased in certain high risk groups. Approximately 6 to 7% of homosexually active men and parenteral drug abusers are HBsAg-positive, and eventually the majority acquire HBV infection. Other high risk groups include sexual and household contacts of HBV carriers, patients of hemodialysis units and others who frequently receive blood products (e.g., hemophiliacs), residents of some mental institutions, and immigrants and refugees from areas of high HBV endemicity, particularly east Asia.

Male prisoners and staff of institutions for the mentally retarded are at moderately increased risk. Because of their frequent contact with these HBV carriers groups, health care workers also are at substantially increased risk of HBV infection.

HBV Infection in Health Care Workers

Surveys conducted in the 1970s determined that 0.9 to 1.5% of all patients admitted to teaching hospitals were HBsAg-positive, a rate substantially above that of the general population (29–31). Although many of these patients had underlying high risk conditions, the majority were asymptomatic, and without active serologic surveillance up to 90% would have escaped detection. During the same period reported rates for viral hepatitis among hospital personnel ranged from 21 cases/100,000 employees/year in rural hospitals without dialysis units to 542 cases/100,000 employees/year in urban hospitals with dialysis units (32). Staff in some special care units experienced particularly high attack rates (approximately 100 cases/1,000 employees/year; 32, 33). In most instances, viral hepatitis was caused by occupationally acquired HBV infection.

Transmission of HBV infection in the hospital is primarily from patients to staff, and in clinical settings is closely related to the incidence of accidental exposures to blood, the majority of which are needlestick injuries. In teaching hospitals rates for needlestick injuries among nursing, laboratory, and housekeeping personnel range from 75 to 150/1000 employees/year (34–36), although rates for all exposure incidents can be substantially higher in groups such as phlebotomists (37). The frequency of such accidental exposures generally is lower in smaller and rural hospitals (37, 38).

Because of the frequency of admission of HBsAg-positive patients and of exposure incidents, many health care workers show evidence of previous HBV infection (Table 12.1). Numerous surveys have demonstrated prevalence rates for HBV markers of between 5 and 30% or more for hospital-based physicians and other clinical and laboratory personnel (33, 39–55). Other reports have shown high rates of marker positivity among surgeons (56), anesthesiologists (57), phlebotomists (58), oncology staff personnel (59–61), and emergency medicine technicians and paramedics (62). Dentists, particularly oral surgeons, also are at greater risk of HBV infection (63–66). In general, these studies demonstrate that the risk of developing HBV marker positivity is associated with the frequency and intensity of contact with blood or patient secretions, especially in settings which have large numbers of HBsAg-positive patients (59, 67, 68). In addition, duration of employment is a prominent factor, although the rate of acquisition of HBV markers is greater during the initial years of employment (51). In rural hospitals the frequency of marker positivity can be lower than what is observed in urban settings (52). Also, not all marker-positive health care workers necessarily have had previous HBV infections. In some of those with less intense exposure to blood, an anti-HBs-positive but anti-HBc-negative serologic picture may indicate natural immunization with HBsAg alone, rather than infection with HBV (47).

Although the direction of HBV transmission in hospitals is overwhelmingly from patients to staff, approximately 1% of health care workers are HBsAg-positive. This suggests that health care workers who are chronic carriers are at risk for transmitting HBV infection to patients. Although the observed risk for such transmission is low (69–71), nosocomial infection of patients has been observed in relation to open heart surgery (72), gynecologic surgery (73, 74), and dental procedures or oral surgery (75–80). HBV infection has been transmitted in hospitals through carelessness or accidental tears in surgeons' gloves. Among dentists, contact with HBsAg-containing patient blood or gingival crevicular fluid during procedures can cause infection through minor skin abrasions or trauma to fingernails which are impacted with occult blood (81–83). There are approximately 3000 dentists in the U.S. who are chronic HBV carriers (77). Because fewer than 20% of dentists wear gloves when they work, those who are HBsAg-positive can infect their patients. In some instances when this has occurred, gloving during dental procedures has been sufficient to halt further transmission of HBV infection.

Successful efforts to prevent HBV transmission in hospitals have included screening blood donors (84) (approximately 1 in every 1000 units is HBsAg-positive) and active surveillance and isolation of HBsAg-positive patients in high risk settings such as dialysis units (85–87). Strict adherence to guidelines for the care of patients hospitalized with hepatitis B, particularly blood precautions, also has been helpful (88). Nonetheless, current prevention of HBV infections in hospitals is centered on passive immunization with hepatitis B immune globulin and active immunization with hepatitis B vaccine (89).

Hepatitis B Immune Globulin (HBIG)

Of the two agents available for immunization against HBV infection, immune globulin preparations were the first to become available. HBIG is prepared from plasma known to contain anti-HBs antibody in a titer > 1:100,000 by radioimmunoassay (RIA) and to be free of HBsAg (20). Immune globulin (IG) preparations are not preselected for anti-HBs content, but they generally contain anti-HBs titers of ≥ 1:100 by RIA. Neither HBIG nor IG transmits HBV infection. Both should be administered intramuscularly (0.06 ml/kg), not intravenously. Neither one is contraindicated in pregnant women. Although HBIG and IG cause few adverse reactions, approximately 3% of recipients can experience an allergic reaction with rash or fever.

Hepatitis B Vaccine: Antigenicity and Safety

Hepatitis B (HB) vaccine is prepared from plasma obtained from asymptomatic, high titer HBsAg carriers, many of whom are homosexual men (20). Vaccine production includes purification by ultracentrifugation and a three-step inactivation process (pepsin at pH 2, 8 M urea, and 1:4000 formalin). This process inactivates all classes of viruses found in human blood. In its final form HB vaccine is a suspension of inactivated alum-adsorbed 22-nm HBsAg particles, in a concentration of 20 μg/ml of HBsAg protein. The vaccine should be stored at 2 to 8°C; freezing destroys its potency.

Because HB vaccine contains only HBsAg particles, immunization elicits an anti-HBs response without anti-HBc. In immunocompetent adults and older children a series of three intramuscular doses (20 μg) given at 0, 1, and 6 months is followed by protective titers of anti-HBs in 91 to 100% of vaccinees (20, 89). Relatively few persons seroconvert from negative to positive with the third dose, which is given primarily to increase the anti-HBs titer. Somewhat lower seroconversion rates and titers are observed in persons aged 50 years and older, but anti-HBs responses are excellent in neonates, infants, and children up to 9 years of age who are given three 10-μg doses. HB vaccine is less antigenic in patients undergoing hemodialysis (90, 91), and in those with renal transplants and other conditions associated with immunocompromise (89); in these patients three 40-μg (2.0-ml) doses should be used. However, other groups of high risk patients, including homosexual men and hemophiliacs, respond as do normal adults to the recommended 20-μg doses. Approximately 10 to 15% of persons vaccinated with HB vaccine will lose detectable levels of anti-HBs after four to five years (89), although in such persons a booster dose of vaccine is followed by a prompt anamnestic response (92). Because such a high proportion of recipients respond to HB vaccination, it is unnecessary to confirm this response serologically except in hemodialysis and other patients who respond less well, and in certain groups of health care workers (e.g., dialysis staff) who are continuously exposed to HBsAg.

A small number of immunocompetent persons fail to respond as expected to a properly administered three-dose series of HB vaccine. Genetic factors may be partially responsible for this (89). However, field experience with the use of HB vaccine has shown surprisingly low seroconversion rates among staff in some hospitals (93). Retrospective surveys indicate that poor antibody responses are associated with giving the vaccine in the buttock and not in the arm, a route of administration more likely to deliver vaccine into fat instead of muscle (84, 95). These findings emphasize the importance of administering HB vaccine intramuscularly, as recommended. They also suggest that, although routine postvaccination serologic testing is not recommended, it may be advisable to test persons who were vaccinated in the buttock. Those failing to show an anti-HBs response should receive a booster dose of HB vaccine in the arm.

The safety of HB vaccine is firmly established (20). Up to 10% of vaccine recipients can experience minor local reactions, but these are self-limited. Since its licensure in the U.S., approximately 100 severe reactions, including Guillain-Barré syndrome, have been reported following HB vaccination. None appears to have occurred at a rate exceeding that expected in the general population. HB vaccine produces no adverse reactions when given to HBsAg carriers, nor is it therapeutic. When given simultaneously with HBIG or IG it is fully immunogenic and without adverse effects (96). Although there are no data on the safety of HB vaccine for the developing fetus, there should be no risk because the vaccine contains only noninfectious HBsAg particles. For pregnant women who are at increased risk for HBV infection, HB vaccine is not contraindicated.

The major concern regarding the safety of HB vaccine has been the theoretical possibility that, because it is derived from the plasma of human donors (many of whom are homosexual men), it

Table 12.1   Prevalence of HBV Markers in Health Care Workers*

Title or Service	HBsAg		Anti-HBs		Either HBsAg or anti-HBs	
	%	References	%	References†	%	References†
Occupational title						
All physicians	1–5	(45, 65, 84)	10–18	(45, 48, 49, 55, 65)	12–18	(40, 45, 51, 65)
Internal medicine			18	(43)		
Surgeon			23–28	(43, 56)		
Pathologist			27	(43)	16	(42)
Radiologist					2	(42)
Obstetrician/gynecologist			16	(43)		
Anesthesiologist			17	(43)		
Pediatrician			21	(43)		
Family practitioner			16	(43)		
Houseofficer			6	(49)		
Medical	0	(47)	8	(47)	8–20	(44, 47)
Surgical	0	(47)	14–15	(47, 54)	14–25	(44, 47)
Medical student	4	(45)	5–7	(45, 143)	11	(45)
All nurses	1–3	(45, 84)	14–18	(41, 45)	12–21	(40, 45, 51)
Practical nurse/aide					20–22	(40)
Housekeeper	1–8	(45, 84)	18	(45)	13–33	(40, 42, 45)
Food services					21	(40)
Clerical					8	(40)
Administrator	0–1	(45, 47)	6–16	(41, 45, 47)	9–16	(40, 45, 47)
Dentist	1–2	(63–66)	12–15	(64–66)	13–15	(64–66)
Dental students			6	(143)		

Clinical service						
Intensive care unit			7–17	(33, 41, 145)	12–28	(50, 53)
Nurses only	2	(47)	3–13	(47, 49, 54)	10	(47)
Dialysis unit	2–3	(84, 86)	6–32	(48, 54, 67)	17	(50)
Nurses only	1–2	(55)	31	(55)	32	(55)
General medicine	1–2	(45)	6–19	(33, 45, 48)	12–20	(40, 45, 53)
Nurses only	0	(47)	5–15	(47, 49)	5	(47)
Intravenous therapy technicians	0	(47)	8–22	(47, 54)	22	(47)
Surgery	3	(45)	14–21	(45, 48, 145)	9–24	(40, 45, 51, 53)
Operating room			5–26	(49, 54, 145)	25–29	(40, 50)
Emergency room			6–27	(47, 54)	5–28	(40, 53, 86)
Nurses only	4	(47)	16	(62)	30	(47)
Emergency medical technicians	1	(62)	23	(47)	17	(62)
Pathology	4	(47)			9–27	(47, 51)
Radiology	5	(45)	6–13	(45, 49)	12	(45)
Anesthesiology	2–10	(45, 57)	12–21	(45, 53, 57)	12–31	(45, 51, 57)
Oncology	6	(60)	10	(60)	16	(60)
Obstetrics/gynecology			0–5	(33, 54)	4–20	(41, 53)
Pediatrics	3	(45)	0–5	(33, 45)	5–18	(45, 53)
Dental	0	(55)	2–5	(54, 55)	2–15	(50, 51, 55)
All laboratories	1–3	(45–47)	9–23	(41, 45–49, 54, 145)	11–31	(33, 40, 42, 45–47, 51)
Clinical chemistry	1–2	(45, 84)	9–40	(41, 45, 67)	10–18	(42, 45)
Hematology	2	(84)	21–32	(41, 67)	13	(42)
Blood bank	0–1	(47, 84)	24–26	(47, 67)	6–26	(42, 47)
Microbiology	0–1	(84)	7–21	(41,67)	8	(42)
Phlebotomy	3	(58)	25	(58)	12–28	(42, 58)
Volunteer blood donors	0–1	(63, 65, 84)	4	(65)	4	(65)

* Excludes serologic studies of groups with less than 20 health care workers.
† Data from reference 47 include subjects with anti-HBs and/or anti-HBc.

may contain and transmit human T cell lymphotrophic virus type III (HTLV-III) which is the causative agent for acquired immune deficiency syndrome (AIDS) (97, 98). However, studies indicate that (a) persons vaccinated with HB vaccine do not develop antibodies to HTLV-III; (b) AIDS has not been observed in health care workers and others who have received HB vaccine and are at low risk for AIDS; (c) the incidence of AIDS is no higher in homosexual men who received HB vaccine compared with those who did not; (d) pepsin, urea, and formalin inactivation used in the production of HB vaccine also inactivates HTLV-III and other related retroviruses; and (e) HB vaccine contains no HTLV-III-related nucleic acid sequences (99–103). Considered together, these findings demonstrate that there is no increased risk of acquiring AIDS from HB vaccine.

Efficacy of Pre-exposure Hepatitis B Vaccination

Numerous randomized, double-blind, placebo-controlled clinical trials have demonstrated a high degree of efficacy for HB vaccine when given to dialysis staff, dialysis patients, and homosexual men (89). In dialysis staff, low dose (3 to 5 μg) vaccination regimens in European trials (104, 105) as well as routine doses in the U.S. (106) have been shown to be highly protective. Of the few infections that occurred in vaccine recipients, most were regarded as having been contracted before vaccine was given and were mild (104). In dialysis patients, the European vaccines were 53% (91) and 78% (105) protective. However, in the U.S., a study that used three 40-μg doses failed to demonstrate protection (107). This disappointing result reflected not only a low rate of antibody response among vaccinees, but also a low overall attack rate of HBV infection that rendered the size of the study population too small to permit clear interpretation of the results.

The most definitive studies of the efficacy of HB vaccine have been conducted in homosexual men. In one study which used three 40-μg doses, vaccine efficacy was 71.5% for anti-HBc conversion alone, and 92.1% for biochemically evident hepatitis B (108, 109). Furthermore, HB vaccine was nearly 100% protective in persons who developed an antibody response, and probably was partially effective in modifying the severity of infection in early cases of hepatitis that were incubating at the time the first dose was given. Similar results were obtained using a 20 μg/dose

regimen (110). Another clinical trial of HB vaccine in health care workers was terminated too soon to show protective efficacy when all hepatitis B events were considered, although a definite trend in this direction was observed (111).

It is important to recognize that, although there is no vaccine to prevent δ hepatitis, immunization with HB vaccine should prevent δ infection because this agent is dependent on HBV infection for its replication.

Guidelines for Pre-exposure Prophylaxis with HB Vaccine

The results of these clinical trials provide the basis for current recommendations for pre-exposure prophylaxis against HBV infection (20, 112, 113), guidelines for which are shown in Table 12.2. Health care workers constitute one of the

Table 12.2. Pre-exposure Prophylaxis for Hepatitis B*

Health care workers†
Special patient groups
  Hemodialysis patients‡
  Recipients of certain blood products (e.g., factor concentrates for hemophiliacs)§
Life style factors
  Homosexually active men
  Illicit injectable drug abusers
  Heterosexually active persons with multiple sexual partners
Environmental factors
  Household and sexual contacts of HBV carriers
  Inmates of long term correctional facilities
  Clients and staff of some institutions for the mentally retarded
  Special high risk populations (e.g., immigrants and refugees from countries with high rates of endemic HBV infection)
  Certain international travelers at increased risk of acquiring HBV infection.

* Three doses (20 μg each) of hepatitis B vaccine should be given intramuscularly (in the deltoid muscle not the buttock) at 0, 1, and 6 months.
† The risk of HBV infection for health care workers varies both among hospitals and within hospitals. In developing immunization strategies hospitals should consider published information (see Table 12.1). In addition, hospitals may wish to evaluate their own clinical experience with HBV infection, and develop screening programs for certain groups of high risk health care workers.
‡ Hemodialysis patients should receive three 40-μg doses of HB vaccine.
§ Patients with hemophilia should be immunized subcutaneously not intramuscularly.

largest target groups and have received the most attention. Patient groups include those requiring hemodialysis and renal transplantation, and those with clotting disorders and other conditions who require frequent blood component therapy. Persons whose life styles place them at greater risk of HBV infection, and household and sexual contacts of HBsAg carriers should be immunized. In general, patients and staff of institutions for the mentally retarded should be considered candidates for HB vaccine, although in some settings this may not be warranted (114, 115). Inmates of correctional facilities also are at increased risk. Depending on the circumstances, certain population groups (e.g., immigrants and refugees from highly endemic areas (116, 117) and Alaskan Eskimos) may require extensive vaccination programs. Finally, international travelers who plan to live in areas of high endemicity for more than 6 months, or who on short term travel anticipate contact with blood from or sexual contact with residents in such areas, also should receive HB vaccine.

Efficacy of Postexposure Prophylaxis with HBIG and Hepatitis B Vaccine

Perinatal transmission from carrier mothers to their infants is the single most important determinant of the prevalence of HBV infection in many countries and accounts for close to half of the chronic HBsAg carriers worldwide (118, 119). In highly endemic areas maternal infectivity is directly related to the titer of HBsAg; in the presence of HBeAg, 90% or more of newborn infants can be infected, and most who are infected become chronic carriers. Although the risk of perinatal infection is greatest with HBeAg-positive mothers, severe or even fatal infections have been observed in the U.S. in infants born of HBsAg-positive but anti-HBe-positive mothers (120, 121). In addition, acute HBV infection during the third trimester of pregnancy or within 2 months of delivery can be transmitted to 70% of infants. In spite of high levels of HBsAg in maternal blood, *in utero* infections are infrequent, accounting for fewer than 5% of all perinatal infections.

Clinical trials in Taiwan have shown that multiple doses of HBIG starting at birth can reduce by 75% the number of infections in infants born of HBeAg-positive mothers. However, passive immunity only postpones childhood infection; by the second or third year of life more than half of children who are HBsAg-negative at 12 months

of age have become infected (122). For this reason, combined passive-active immunization with HBIG and HB vaccine has been studied and shown to be more than 90% protective (123, 124). These studies also suggest that there is little to be gained from more than one dose of HBIG, and that HB vaccine is effective when delayed up to 7 days after birth. In the U.S., HBIG and a three-dose (20 μg) regimen of HB vaccine administered to infants born of HBeAg-positive Asian-American mothers was 85% effective in preventing the development of the chronic carrier state (125). Among infants who were immunized and still became infected, most were infected either before birth or within the next few months. These findings are the basis for current recommendations regarding prophylaxis against perinatal HBV infections. All infants born of HBsAg-positive mothers, not just those whose mothers also are HBeAg-positive, qualify for combined passive-active prophylaxis (20).

There is a substantial risk of HBV transmission to sexual contacts of persons with acute (126) and chronic (127) infection, but few data support the efficacy of postexposure prophylaxis in this setting. In the only controlled trial, a single dose of HBIG given to the spouses of persons with acute infection appeared to protect against both clinical disease and subclinical infection (128), but the design and interpretation of this study have been criticized (89). More recently, both HBIG and IG given to sexual contacts of persons with acute HBV infection have been shown to be similarly protective when compared to historical controls (129). There are no reports of the efficacy of postexposure prophylaxis with HB vaccine, although the results from clinical trials conducted in homosexual men suggest that HB vaccine could be partially protective when given to sexual contacts during the incubation period (130). Similarly, no studies have been reported on the efficacy of passive-active prophylaxis with HBIG and HB vaccine. In the absence of more definitive information, current recommendations for prophylaxis of sexual contacts are of necessity based on extrapolations from experience in other settings.

In hospitals postexposure prophylaxis is considered most frequently for employees following needlestick injuries or other accidental percutaneous exposures to blood. Because a large number of such incidents go unreported (34–36), and not all that are reported are followed by testing the source for HBsAg, the precise risk of acquiring

HBV infection following such exposures is indeterminate. However, in one clinical study, if the source was HBsAg-positive, there was a 5.9% risk of acquiring clinical hepatitis following needlestick injury (131). Two doses of HBIG reduced this risk to 1.4% and brought about a 3-fold reduction in all HBV events, both clinical and serologic. Uncontrolled observations (132) also have suggested protection, but elsewhere HBIG only prolonged the incubation period and did not prevent or modify HBV infection (133). One reason for this failure may have been the diminished potency of the HBIG that was used (89). HBIG also may fail to protect if the source of exposure has a very high titer of HBsAg, as indicated by sensitive techniques for measuring HBeAg and other markers of infectivity (134).

Guidelines for Postexposure Prophylaxis with HBIG and HB Vaccine

Guidelines for HBIG and HB vaccine prophylaxis following perinatal, sexual, and percutaneous exposure are shown in Table 12.3 (20, 135). To be effective, perinatal prophylaxis requires that HBsAg-positive mothers be identified before delivery. Prenatal testing should be routine for pregnant women who (*a*) are of Asian, Pacific Island, or Alsakan Eskimo descent or were born in Haiti or sub-Saharan Africa; (*b*) have acute or chronic liver disease; (*c*) work in or are patients in a hemodialysis unit or institution for the mentally retarded; (*d*) are health care workers with frequent exposure to blood; (*e*) have household contact with an HBV carrier or hemodialysis patient; (*f*) have been repeatedly transfused or rejected as a blood donor; (*g*) have had multiple episodes of sexually transmitted disease; or (*h*) are known to be parenteral drug abusers. If the mother's HBsAg status is not known, it should be determined as soon as possible after delivery, because HBIG is less effective in neonates when delayed beyond 48 hours. If the mother is discovered to be HBsAg-positive later on, the child still should receive prophylaxis if a venous blood sample is HBsAg-negative. Three doses of HB vaccine should be given. Testing for HBsAg (not HBcAg) at 6 months is optional (it will detect a therapeutic failure and the third dose of vaccine can be omitted), but should be undertaken at 12 to 15 months to determine whether treatment has been successful. If anti-HBs is found, the child is protected. Neither HBIG nor HB vaccine should affect responses to routine pediatric vaccinations.

For persons with sexual exposure to someone who is HBsAg-positive, HBIG always should be given. Close follow-up of the HBsAg-positive contact is required to determine whether a second dose of HBIG is needed because of prolonged HBsAg positivity, or whether HB vaccine should be given because the contact has become a chronic carrier. Homosexual men and regular sexual contacts of known carriers should receive HB vaccine from the outset unless serologic tests show that they already have been infected. Other household contacts of persons with acute HBV infections are at little risk and do not need HBIG (126), but HBIG and HB vaccine should be given to other household contacts of chronic carriers.

The schedule for prophylaxis following percutaneous exposure is complex (Table 12.3). The choice of treatment depends on both the vaccination status of the person exposed and the HBsAg status of the source of exposure. For unvaccinated health care workers treatment always should include HB vaccine because repeated blood exposure is likely. Health care workers who already have been vaccinated will need HBIG if they have low titers of anti-HBs or have not responded to the vaccine.

Implementing Programs for the Control of Hepatitis B in Hospitals

Many factors affect the administrative decision as to whether a hospital should modify its program for hepatitis B control by offering HB vaccine to its employees (136). To some extent the decision will depend on the reported incidence of infection in the community, the types of patients served and the services offered by the hospital, and the frequency with which hepatitis patients are admitted. In general, the need will be greater for larger urban than for smaller rural hospitals (52). In addition, the frequency of exposure incidents should be considered, although differences in rates among hospitals of different size are not great, and estimates of exposures are imprecise because many go unreported (34–36).

In developing a new strategy each hospital's infection control practitioners and administrators must assess their current policies and practices for postexposure prophylaxis. Unfortunately, many hospitals do not have or disregard recommended control guidelines (137). Problems include the lack of ready availability of HBIG or a delay in its administration, inadequate evaluation of the extent of exposures, delays in receiving the results of serologic tests and implementing blood precautions, and poor communication among

Table 12.3. Postexposure Prophylaxis for Hepatitis B

Exposure	HBIG	HB vaccine
Perinatal	0.5 ml IM within 12 hours of birth	0.5 ml (10 μg) IM within 12 hours of birth (no later than 7 days), and at 1 and 6 months*; test for HBsAg and anti-HBs at 12 to 15 months
Sexual	0.06 ml/kg IM within 14 days of sexual contact; a second dose should be given if the index patient remains HBAg-positive after 3 months	1.0 ml (20 μg) IM at 0, 1, and 6 months for homosexual men and regular sexual contacts of HBV carriers
Percutaneous; exposed person unvaccinated		
Source known HBsAg-positive	0.06 ml/kg IM within 24 hours	1.0 ml (20 μg) IM within 7 days, and at 1 and 6 months†
Source known, possibly HBsAg-positive	Test source for HBsAg; if positive give exposed person 0.06 ml/kg IM once within 7 days	1.0 ml (20 μg) IM within 7 days, and at 1 and 6 months†
Source known, unlikely HBsAg-positive	Testing source for HBsAg is not necessary; HBIG is not required	1.0 ml (20 μg) IM within 7 days, and at 1 and 6 months
Source unknown	Nothing required	1.0 ml (20 μg) IM within 7 days, and at 1 and 6 months
Percutaneous; exposed person vaccinated		
Source known HBsAg-positive	Test exposed person for anti-HBs; if titer is <10 SRU by RIA or negative by EIA give 0.06 ml/kg within 24 hours and 1 month later‡	Nothing required§
Source known, possibly HBsAg-positive	If vaccinated person is a known nonresponder, test source for HBsAg; if source is positive give exposed person 0.06 ml/kg IM within 24 hours and 1 month later	Nothing required
Source known, unlikely HBsAg-positive	Nothing required	Nothing required
Source unknown	Nothing required	Nothing required

* If HBIG and HB vaccine are given simultaneously, they should be given at separate sites. If HBIG is unavailable, IG should be given in the same dose.

† If HB vaccine is not given, a second dose of HBIG should be given 1 month later.

‡ Anti-HBs titers < 10 standard ratio units (SRU) by radioimmunoassay (RIA) or negative by enzyme immunoassay (EIA) indicate lack of protection. Testing the exposed person for anti-HBs is not necessary if a protective level of antibody has been demonstrated within the previous 12 months.

§ If the exposed person has not completed a three-dose series of HB vaccine, the series should be completed. If an adequate antibody response in the past is shown on retesting to have declined to an inadequate level, a booster dose (1.0 ml) of HB vaccine should be given.

staff and with the employee health service. All of these factors contribute to the inadequate and often inappropriate postexposure prophylaxis received by health care workers. Even where programs are adequate the average cost per incident for blood tests, treatments, and working time lost can approach $100 (138). The cost of HBIG (up to $500 for two doses) alone can account for 80% of a hospital's overall costs for its hepatitis B control program. In addition, expenses related to cases of occupationally acquired HBV infection in persons who develop clinical illness, become chronic carriers, or die of fulminant hepatitis can reach several thousand dollars (138–141).

Although HB vaccine also is expensive (approximately $100 for three doses), it is less costly to provide postexposure prophylaxis to an immunized health care worker than to one who has not been vaccinated. Administrative decisions to undertake vaccination programs must take into consideration the cost of vaccination, the cost of screening for susceptibility, and the prevalance of already immune health care workers. The screening of groups with a high prevalence (i.e., more than 20%) of anti-HBs is likely to be cost effective, but screening is not justified for health care workers during their training years (48, 140, 142, 143). Simple nomograms have been published to help guide decisions on whether to undertake screening before vaccination or to vaccinate all employees (20, 140). Regardless of which approach is taken, HB vaccination programs targeted to recognized groups of high risk employees can fail to reach 50% or more of those who require postexposure prophylaxis after an exposure incident (138). In addition, it may take many years before they become cost saving to the hospital (141).

Acceptance of HB vaccination by health care workers generally has been similar across occupational groups in spite of differences in perceived risks of exposure (144, 145). Effective in-service educational programs, discussions with co-workers, and provision of vaccine at no cost to employees have been important factors in the success of some programs. Concern about adverse effects, especially the potential risk of AIDS, accounts for the refusal of many health care workers to be immunized. In spite of elaborate decision strategies that justify vaccination (98, 146), the evidence that AIDS cannot be contracted from HB vaccine is more likely to persuade reluctant health care workers to be immunized.

Future Directions for HB Vaccination Programs for Health Care Workers

In the 3 years following licensure of HB vaccine in 1982, an estimated 750,000 persons had been immunized, and 80% or more of these were health care workers (20). Thus, only a small proportion (probably fewer than 20%) of health care workers at increased risk has benefited from this protection. Vaccine policies and usage in hospitals have varied widely. In some areas vaccination

rates have been greater in smaller community hospitals with lower prevalence rates for HBV markers than they have been in larger urban and teaching hospitals where the risks of acquiring HBV infection are greater (54). Whether concern over safety issues alone explains these differences is unknown, but as the question of vaccine safety becomes relatively less important it will be necessary to discover other factors that are important determinants for the success of hospital-based HB vaccination programs.

The stimulus to develop a more active approach to immunizing health care workers may arise from a number of external sources. Momentum is increasing toward acceptance of a health care industry-wide standard of practice requiring hospitals to offer voluntary, cost-free HB vaccination to their employees (147). Occupational safety and health laws, collective bargaining negotiations, worker's compensation statutes, and recommendations issued by professional organizations all will play a greater role in the hospital's decision to implement more active programs. Legal concerns regarding liability for negligence toward employees and patients, and the risks of litigation that can follow also will be important (147, 148). Progress initially may be slow as hospitals adapt to increasing financial constraints. However, some relief from the cost burden of paying for HB vaccine may come as newer, less expensive vaccines become available. Recently a vaccine has been produced by recombinant DNA techniques which permit expression of HBsAg in yeast. It has been tested in man and shown to be antigenic and free of short term adverse reactions (149, 150). As the cost of HB vaccine declines, it should become possible to devote greater efforts to immunizing health care workers during their years of training. Given the greater risk of acquiring HBV infection during the early years of employment, in the long run this approach offers the greatest promise of success in preventing HBV infection among hospital staff.

Hepatitis A

Hepatitis A Virus and HAV Infections in the United States

Hepatitis A virus (HAV) infection is caused by a 27-nm picornavirus that is transmitted primarily by the fecal-oral route (20, 151). In the United States, HAV accounts for approximately 40% of all cases of hepatitis (152). The incubation period is short, averaging 28 to 30 days. Approximately two-thirds of persons infected with HAV are asymptomatic (151). In those with clinical illness the onset is abrupt, and fever, malaise, gastrointestinal symptoms, and jaundice are the predominant features. Adults usually experience more severe illness when compared with children, but recovery is the rule. In contrast to the situation with hepatitis B, only 50 deaths from fulminant hepatitis A are estimated to occur in the U.S. each year (151).

Clinical and epidemiologic studies have become more precise because of newer methods for detecting HAV in stool (153) and more sensitive and specific techniques for measuring IgM-anti-HAV and total anti-HAV in serum (20, 154). The risk of transmitting HAV infection is greatest during the 2 weeks preceding the onset of jaundice, when persons excrete large amounts of virus in their stools and are, for a short period, viremic. Once illness appears, virus titers decline; HAV can be found in the stools of only 50% of patients hospitalized with hepatitis A. Risk factors for infection include exposure in common source outbreaks caused by contaminated food or water, and previous contact with patients with hepatitis (152). In recent years HAV transmission in day care centers (155) and among homosexual men (156, 157) has become more widely appreciated (152). Although the overall incidence of hepatitis A has declined in the U.S., it is still a common disease. More than half of the population 40 years of age and older has serologic evidence of previous infection.

Prevention of Hepatitis A with Immune Globulin

Recent experience in natural outbreaks has confirmed the efficacy of immune globulin (IG) in preventing transmission of HAV to contacts of infected patients (20, 158, 159). When given within 2 weeks of exposure IG can be 80 to 90% protective. Although anti-HAV levels in IG have declined in recent years (due to a decreased incidence of infection in the general population of donors), titers are generally adequate for protection (160, 161). The dose of IG is 0.02 ml/kg intramuscularly.

Recommendations for pre-exposure prophylaxis against hepatitis A generally are limited to persons traveling to developing countries with poor sanitation (20). The usual dose is sufficient to provide protection for 2 months. For longer periods of travel 0.06 mg/kg should be given every 5 months. Screening these persons for anti-

HAV can detect those who already are immune and who, therefore, do not need IG. When considering postexposure prophylaxis, the diagnosis of hepatitis A first should be confirmed by testing the index case for IgM-anti-HAV (20, 135). Screening numerous contacts is unnecessary because it is more costly than giving IG. Postexposure prophylaxis is indicated for household, sexual, and day care center contacts, and sometimes for those in outbreaks in schools, work sites, and institutions for custodial care. Immune globulin often is not helpful in common source outbreaks once cases are diagnosed because exposure already has occurred more than 2 weeks previously.

Hepatitis A and Its Control in Hospitals

Until recently nosocomial hepatitis A was rarely reported (162). However, HAV transmission among hospital patients and employees may not be an uncommon event (163–170). Infection often spreads from an index case that is asymptomatic but fecally incontinent. Many reported outbreaks have occurred in neonatal care units. Transmission to nursing staff and other personnel, to other patients, and to family contacts of both is frequent, and in some instances extensive. Attack rates among susceptible employees can be 10% or greater (165, 168). The overall costs of one outbreak were reported to be $60,000 (165).

Routine pre-exposure prophylaxis with IG is not recommended for hospital personnel. The major factor responsible for the spread of HAV infection in reported outbreaks has been inattention to basic principles of patient care, including prudent handling of stools (which should be common practice with all patients) and careful hand washing (170). In many of the reported outbreaks there was no opportunity to use IG for postexposure prophylaxis because transmission already had occurred. However, in a few instances IG was given to staff, other patients, and family contacts with some apparent effect in curbing HAV transmission (166, 168, 169).

Earlier seroepidemiologic studies of patients receiving frequent blood transfusions failed to show any increased risk for acquiring hepatitis A (171, 172). More recently, however, HAV transmission has been documented following transfusion with blood or blood products (173–179). Careful investigation has shown that the donor usually developed clinical hepatitis A soon after donating blood. In some instances the donor had just returned from foreign travel to a country where HAV infections are common (173, 177).

In one notable outbreak a single unit of HAV-containing blood transfused to 11 neonates led to secondary fecal-oral transmission involving 55 nurses, physicians, parents, and relatives scattered over a wide area (178). Occasionally IG has been given to contacts, although its role in controlling the spread of infection has been difficult to assess (173, 178).

These experiences with nosocomial hepatitis A emphasize that good patient care techniques and a high index of suspicion are of primary importance if nosocomial HAV transmission is to be prevented or controlled. Although IG has a role to play, and should be used among contacts once an outbreak is recognized, its contribution to control efforts usually will not be great. The eventual development and clinical use of a hepatitis A vaccine may be of help in the control of hospital outbreaks (180). Pre-exposure vaccine prophylaxis for high risk employees could prevent infection among hospital staff, but would have less impact on its spread to unvaccinated patients and family contacts.

Rubella

The Changing Pattern of Rubella Virus Infections

The devasting effects of rubella virus infection of pregnant women were demonstrated in the 1964–1965 epidemic in the United States. There were an estimated 12.5 million cases of rubella, 11,000 fetal deaths by miscarriage or abortion, and 20,000 cases of congenital rubella syndrome (CRS) (181, 182). The long term manifestations of CRS include (a) a variety of endocrine disorders, (b) deafness, (c) ocular damage, (d) vascular disease, and (e) progressive rubella panencephalitis (183). Today there are more than 6000 students with hearing impairments who require special education programs as a result of this epidemic. The average lifetime cost of each CRS child is estimated to be more than $220,000. In addition, the current costs of providing round-the-clock supervision for 3000 persons severely affected by the 1964–1965 epidemic approach $90 million/year (184).

The frequency of CRS after confirmed maternal rubella is more than 80% when it occurs during the first 12 weeks of pregnancy, and 54% at 13 and 14 weeks (185). Most women who discover that they have been infected with rubella virus early in pregnancy elect therapeutic abortion. Thus, the primary goal of rubella immunization policy has been the elimination of CRS (186).

Since the licensure of live, attenuated rubella virus vaccines in 1969 there have been dramatic declines in the occurrence of epidemic rubella and CRS in the U.S. (187). Initially, rubella immunization policy focused on vaccination of preschool children and those in the early grades of school. Although epidemic rubella and CRS were controlled, the policy had little effect on the incidence of endemic CRS as long as immunization rates in the primary target groups were 80% or less (188–191). Since 1977, intensified efforts to immunize all school children have brought further declines in reported cases of rubella and, since 1980, reports of CRS (192). Provisional data for 1984 showed only 745 reported cases of rubella and two cases of CRS (193). Whether the decline in CRS is due primarily to the rigorous enforcement of school immunization laws (with childhood immunization rates currently approaching 100%), or to the widespread use of therapeutic abortion by pregnant women exposed to or infected with rubella virus, is unknown (194, 195).

Over the past decade numerous studies have demonstrated that approximately 10 to 20% of older adolescents and younger adults remain susceptible to rubella (196–209). In general, at any given age, women and men are equally susceptible. Surveys of military recruits have demonstrated minor geographic variability in susceptibility, with slightly higher rates for California (202), and rates of 30 to 55% among small groups of Asian women (202, 207). Similar rates of seronegativity have been observed among adolescent and younger adult males in the United Kingdom; fewer young women are susceptible because in the U.K. primary attention is given to immunizing adolescent girls but not boys (210, 211).

The rubella susceptibility rates for older adolescents and younger adults explain why 70% or more of reported cases now affect persons 15 years of age and older. In recent years rubella outbreaks have arisen on military bases (201, 202), college campuses (212, 213), in night clubs (214), and in office buildings (215). When extensive they have been associated with cases of congenital rubella syndrome (216, 217).

Rubella Vaccine

Since 1979, RA27/3 live rubella virus vaccine has been the only preparation licensed for use in the U.S., replacing earlier live virus vaccines (186). Numerous clinical trials have shown that 95% or more of susceptible persons immunized after 12 months of age develop antibody after a single dose (187). In a high proportion antibody remains detectable for up to 16 years (218–224). Other data suggest that rubella vaccine affords lifelong protection against clinical rubella and asymptomatic viremia in almost all recipients. In a small proportion of vaccinees, rubella antibodies measured by the standard hemagglutination-inhibition (HI) test can fall to undetectable levels. However, more sensitive serologic techniques show that antibody still is present, and the response of such persons to revaccination is characteristic of a secondary rather than a primary antibody response (219, 222, 223). In a recent case-control study among high school students immunzied an average of more than 8 years previously, the clinical efficacy of rubella vaccine was 90% (225). Near universal immunization of military recruits has virtually eliminated rubella on military bases (201).

Rubella vaccine is administered as a single 0.5-ml dose subcutaneously, either as monovalent vaccine or in combination with measles and/or mumps vaccines. Care must be taken to store the vaccine at 2 to 8°C and to avoid exposure to light. Reconstituted vaccine must be used within 8 hours or discarded.

Rubella vaccine is recommended for all persons 12 months of age or older, unless there is evidence of pre-existing immunity as shown by laboratory testing or a firmly documented history of rubella immunization. A clinical history of rubella itself or an undocumented history of rubella immunization are unreliable indicators of protection; such persons should be regarded as nonimmune until tested serologically or vaccinated.

Rubella Immunization during Pregnancy

Because of the great risk of CRS in infants born to mothers infected with rubella virus during the early weeks of pregnancy, there has been justifiable concern about the risks associated with exposure of pregnant women to rubella vaccine virus (226). Although a small amount of virus may be shed by vaccine recipients, it is not transmitted to others. Thus, vaccinated children whose mothers are pregnant pose no risk (186). Pregnant women should not be given rubella vaccine because of the theoretical risk of teratogenicity. However, occasionally vaccine has been given inadvertently, and intrauterine infection has been demonstrated serologically and by virus isolation in some instances (227–230). In this respect, RA27/3 vaccine causes far fewer (3%) intrauterine infections than earlier rubella vaccines. More importantly, careful observation over a 12-year period of 1096 women vaccinated from 3 months before to 3 months after conception, including approximately 300 known to be susceptible to rubella, has shown that none of their infants was born with congenital abnormalities compatible with CRS (231). It should be added that occasional reinfections with rubella virus have been documented in persons with minimal levels of detectable antibody; in rare instances CRS has been observed in infants born of mothers who previously had been successfully immunized (232–234). Although the theoretical maximum risk of CRS following inadvertent RA27/3 immunization is 3%, it is no greater than the risk of birth defects occurring in the absence of rubella immunization. These data provide the basis for the current recommendation that inadvertent rubella immunization of women during early pregnancy should not be considered reason for therapeutic abortion (186).

For the unimmunized pregnant woman who is exposed to natural rubella, assessing the risks of fetal infection and the potential for CRS in the infant is a complex problem, requiring serologic follow-up and careful interpretation of often imprecise test results (235). This can be avoided by assuring that women of childbearing age are immunized before their first pregnancy. In general, routine serologic testing of women of childbearing age is expensive and unnecessary. If a woman is considered susceptible and is not known to be pregnant, rubella vaccine should be given without serologic study beforehand. However, care should be take to avoid pregnancy for 3 months following immunization.

Side Effects, Adverse Reactions, Precautions, and Contraindications to Rubella Immunization

Side effects to rubella vaccine, including constitutional symptoms, rash, and lymphadenopathy, are infrequent and mild (186). In children arthralgias and arthritis also are infrequent, but in young women joint symptoms can occur in 10 to 15% or more of vaccine recipients. These reactions have been less severe following RA27/3 vaccine compared with earlier rubella vaccines (236). Immunologic studies indicate that they are more likely to occur or to be more severe in vaccinees with pre-existing antibodies, suggesting an immune-mediated response following secondary rather than primary exposure to the virus (236–238).

As noted above, rubella vaccine is contraindicated in pregnant women. The vaccine can be given after exposure to rubella, not with the expectation that it will prevent illness, but that it will provide future protection. Immune globulin (IG) can modify illness, but will not prevent maternal infection, viremia, fetal infection, or CRS. Recent recipients of IG should postpone rubella immunization for at least 3 months. Acute febrile illness, unless severe, is not a contraindication to rubella immunization. Hypersensitivity reactions to rubella vaccine are rare. Anaphylactic reactions to eggs are a contraindication only if rubella vaccine is given in combination with measles and mumps vaccines which, unlike rubella vaccine, are produced in chick embryo cell cultures. Persons with anaphylactic reactions to neomycin should not be given rubella vaccine because it may contain trace amounts of this antimicrobial agent (186). Persons with immune deficiencies, either congenital or associated with neoplastic diseases or immunosuppressive therapy, should not receive rubella vaccine. Both a short course (less than 2 weeks) of systemic corticosteroid therapy, and topical or local steroid treatment are exceptions to this rule.

Rubella Susceptibility and Outbreaks in Hospitals

The general susceptibility of young adults to rubella virus infection also is seen among hospital employees; between 11 and 21% have been seronegative in recent surveys (Table 12.4) (239–246). Not surprisingly, numerous outbreaks of rubella have been reported in hospitals (Table 12.5) (240–245, 247–252). Many of these outbreaks have begun in obstetrical clinics, but elsewhere they have spread from other health care workers or from infants with CRS. In some re-

ports substantial numbers of pregnant women in their first trimester have been exposed. Staff-to-patient transmission has been documented in three outbreaks (241–243), and both pregnant staff and patients who were infected have chosen therapeutic abortions. Fortunately, no instance of CRS has been observed to date as a result of nosocomial rubella.

Control and Prevention of Rubella in Hospitals

Efforts to prevent nosocomial rubella begin with maintaining high levels of rubella immunization in all children, together with increased immunization of adolescents and younger adults, especially women of childbearing age who previously have not received vaccine (181, 182, 186, 193). Rubella immunization should be considered during all routine visits for medical, gynecologic, or family planning care. Premarital screening for rubella susceptibility should be extended, but success will require follow-up immunization rates in susceptibles greater than the 37 to 41% reported (196, 205, 253). In the immediate postpartum or postabortion setting, the need for rubella vaccine should be reviewed. Because one-third to one-half of mothers who give birth to a child with CRS previously have been pregnant, the benefits would be substantial. Many programs for postpartum rubella immunization have had limited success (181, 217), although in one report 83% of seronegative women received vaccine (254). Transmission of rubella vaccine virus to the mother's infant rarely may occur, but causes only mild disease (255, 256). Greater efforts to give rubella vaccine before college entry and in work sites also are needed (186).

In addition to these general measures, the ACIP

Table 12.4.   Rubella Susceptibility and Vaccine Acceptance among Hospital Employees

Year	No. Screened		Percent Susceptible*	No. of Susceptibles Offered Vaccine†	Percent Immunized	Reference
	Female Only	Both Sexes				
1976–1977	1225		17.7	193	65.3	239
1978		163	20.0			240
1978		410	18.5			241
1978		1600	21.0			242
1979		114	11.4			243
1979	1246‡		11.8	2983	66.2	244
1979		2456	14.0	197	53.3	245
1979–1980		771	16.0	121	63.6	246
1981				2496	29.0	262

* Susceptibility defined by a hemagglutination-inhibition (HI) antibody titer < 1:8, < 1:10, or an equivalent titer with a passive hemagglutination test.
† All immunization programs were voluntary, not mandatory.
‡ Females only were screened; all employees were offered vaccine.

Table 12.5.   Rubella Outbreaks in Health Care Settings, United States, 1977–1982

Year	Index Case(s)	No. Exposed			No. of Additional Rubella Cases			No. of Therapeutic Abortions		Cases of CRS	Reference
		Staff	Pregnant Patients		Staff	Pregnant Patients		Staff	Patients		
			All	Seronegative		All	Seronegative				
1977	Obstetric clinic nurse	44	151	2*	1	0		0	0	0	247
1977	Five OB/GYN clinic staff		200†								245
1978	Male OB/GYN resident	170	11	4	0	0		0	0	0	240
1978	Male OB/GYN resident	13‡	231	35	4	1				0	241
1978	Male obstetrician			56	2§		1			0	242
1979					7	¶					243
1979	Dietary worker		0		46	0		1		0	244
1979	CRS infant				2	0		0		0	248
1979	CRS infant				1	0		0		0	248
1979	Four CRS infants				3	0		0		0	248
1980	Male obstetrician										249
1982	Dental student	329			16						250
1982	16 hospital outbreaks	31	77		56	0	0	3	1	0	252

* Two of 14 patients in the first trimester of pregnancy screened for susceptibility.
† All patients in the first trimester of pregnancy.
‡ Staff in the first trimester of pregnancy.
§ One clinic assistant in her third trimester.
¶ Two male inpatients were infected.

and the Advisory Committee on Infections within Hospitals of the American Hospital Association have established guidelines for the control and prevention of rubella outbreaks in hospitals (186, 257–261). Control measures should include respiratory isolation for all patients admitted with or who contract rubella in the hospital. This should last for 5 days after the onset of rash. Infants with CRS should be isolated at any time during their first year of life because they may be shedding virus. Only personnel immune to rubella should participate in their care. Employees not known to be immune to rubella who develop fever and rash should be excluded from work until 5 days after the onset of rash. Acute and convalescent sera should be tested to determine whether rubella virus infection has occurred. Contacts of infectious patients and staff should be identified and closely followed for clinical signs of rubella. Exposed susceptible personnel should be excluded from work during the period from 8 to 21 days after exposure, with serologic follow-up for rubella if it is suspected. Pregnant women exposed in their first trimester should have paired sera tested for rubella antibody, and the results should be carefully assessed (235). Susceptible pregnant employees should be excluded from work for the duration of the outbreak. Other nonpregnant personnel should be immunized as rapidly as possible. Serologic screening beforehand is not necessary because rubella vaccine is not harmful to those already immune.

Preventing rubella outbreaks in hospitals is preferable to controlling them when they occur. This can be accomplished by insuring that all staff are immune, and vaccinating all who are considered susceptible (186, 257). However, acceptance of rubella vaccine by hospital staff in voluntary programs has been disappointing (Table 12.4) (239, 244–246, 262). Participation by physicians has been especially poor; only 12 to 16% of senior staff have been immunized, although rates have been higher for medical than for surgical residents (244, 262). Large numbers of hospital employees, including up to two-thirds of physicians, have declined rubella vaccine because they assumed that they already were protected as a result of a previous history of clinical rubella (262). This reason is a notoriously unreliable indicator of immunity. A fair number of employees experience mild side effects including joint symptoms following immunization, but work absence due to adverse reactions has not been a problem, averaging only 0.2 to 0.3 day/vaccinee (243–245, 262). Concern over side effects has not been an important reason for employee nonparticipation in hospital immunization programs.

Hospital Policies for Rubella Control and Prevention, and Their Implementation

Policy statements regarding rubella immunization of hospital employees have suggested that documentation of rubella immunity should be a requirement for new employment, and that staff refusing to be screened or vaccinated should be transferred from areas frequented by pregnant patients, or terminated (186, 259). Mandatory programs have been favored over those that are voluntary. These policies are based on assumptions that (a) rubella immunization will be accepted by health care workers even if no personal benefit is derived from the vaccine; (b) health care workers are at significant risk of exposing pregnant patients to rubella; and (c) mandatory policies for screening and immunization are appropriate from a moral, ethical, and legal point of view.

There continues to be considerable debate over these issues (261), and strict policies for rubella immunization of health care workers have come under strong criticism (246). Acceptance of rubella vaccine has been greatest among female health care workers of childbearing age, the one group other than children for whom rubella vaccine is most necessary. Although health care workers with rubella are at risk of exposing pregnant hospital employees as well as patients, published reports document small numbers of cases in exposed pregnant women, with few therapeutic abortions and no cases of CRS (Table 12.5). Furthermore, it has been argued that most cases of rubella occur in the community, and that pregnant women spend little time in health care settings (246). While this is undeniably true, extensive community-wide outbreaks of rubella may be associated with cases among pregnant staff and patients in many hospitals (252). The cost effectiveness of hospital-based programs for rubella screening and immunization has not been thoroughly examined; reports show that they can be very expensive (244, 246, 262). Finally, the moral, ethical, and legal issues related to mandatory programs have not been resolved.

For many of the reasons cited above, and in spite of firm guidelines from experts, the implementation of rubella screening and immunization programs by hospitals has been extremely variable. A state-wide survey of hospitals conducted 1 year after voluntary guidelines for screening were established revealed several problems (263). Although approximately 50% of hospitals had voluntary or mandatory screening policies, in many they were restricted to selected groups, such as women, those who worked in high risk areas, or those who had direct patient contact. Very few hospitals included physicians, students, and volunteers in their programs, in spite of many reports of outbreaks arising from physicians who had been infected with rubella virus. Furthermore, very few hospitals imposed sanctions on physicians and other personnel who failed to comply with screening and immunization policies. When they did, sanctions often were limited to counseling, signing waivers, or documenting noncompliance in employee health records. Hospitals without screening policies cited as reasons their high cost, the high turnover of hospital personnel, concern over liability, and the absence of any (recognized) cases of rubella in employees.

The questions raised by the current debate over the guidelines for control and prevention of rubella in hospitals require further study. If they remain unresolved for the next 20 to 30 years, they will no longer be pertinent. Continued success with universal childhood immunization should eliminate the threat of rubella in hospitals, and with it the possibility that it could lead to congenital rubella syndrome.

Measles

The Changing Pattern of Measles Virus Infections

The incidence of measles has declined dramatically in recent years, but it remains a serious disease, with complications including otitis media, pneumonia, and encephalitis (264–267). Up to 25% of persons with measles encephalitis develop serious neurologic sequelae. Infection during pregnancy can be associated with prematurity, spontaneous abortion, or low birth weight infants. During the 1970s, 10 to 20% of reported cases of measles required hospitalization (268). Approximately 1 of every 3000 reported cases died, with the risk of death being greater in infants and adults than in older children and adolescents.

The remarkable decline in the incidence of measles is directly attributable to widespread implementation of earlier vaccination programs, the Childhood Immunization Initiative of 1977, and the Measles Elimination Program begun in 1978 (265, 267). As a result, only 1000 to 3000 cases are reported each year. Reports of subacute sclerosing panencephalitis (SSPE), which usually becomes evident approximately 7 years after measles virus infection, also have declined; the incidence of SSPE now is less than 100 cases/year (269). Thus, the strategy of achieving high immunization levels through enforcement of laws requiring proof of measles immunity as a condition for school attendance has been notably effective (270). In addition, active surveillance and vigorous response to reported cases have resulted in the near elimination of endemic measles, and the occurrence of relatively few and usually limited outbreaks of epidemic disease. However, efforts to eliminate indigenous measles have been hampered by the occurrence of cases in children too young (< 15 months of age) to be vaccinated. Also, importations of measles from other countries where measles remains endemic have assumed greater prominence; in 1981 cases directly or indirectly attributable to importations accounted for almost 20% of all cases reported (271). An increasing proportion has affected returning U. S. citizens. Although approximately half of all importations have been traced to children less than 5 years of age, almost 10% have affected young adults.

Within the past few years, increased attention has focused on the problem of measles occurring in young adults, particularly those on college campuses (272–276). Serologic studies indicate that 5 to 15% of college-aged persons remain susceptible to measles. Reasons for this include (a) failure to be immunized as children in the mid-1960s during the early years following licensure of measles vaccine in 1963; (b) ineffective vaccination with either "killed" vaccine (which was given to 600,000 to 900,000 persons from 1963 to 1967), or vaccination with live virus vaccine before 12 months of age; (c) failure to acquire natural infection because of decreased virus transmission caused by widespread vaccine use; and (d) the inability of "herd immunity" to protect against infection with such a highly communicable virus (277). In 1983 college or college-associated cases accounted for 38% of all cases reported nationwide (275). Many of these outbreaks were due to importations by students. Because of the extended case-to-case interval (generally 2 weeks), many outbreaks became widespread before they were recognized, and as a result were difficult and expensive to control (273, 275). College outbreaks have been of particular concern because of the greater severity of measles in adults compared to school children, including complications such as pneumonia (278), hepatitis (279), and more severe illness in those who previously have received killed-virus vaccine (280, 281). Deaths among students have been reported (276).

Measles Transmission in Medical Facilities

The importance of measles on college campuses has been paralleled by increasing recognition of measles transmission in medical facilities (282–288). Among 241 cases occurring in the U.S. between 1980 and 1984, 47% were acquired in hospitals (often in emergency rooms) and 35% in physicians' offices (288). Children less than 5 years in age accounted for 54% of cases. However, 24% affected medical personnel, most often nurses, but also physicians (particularly house officers) as well as other health care personnel. In instances where the pattern of transmission of infection could be determined, 50% were associated with patient-to-patient spread, and 37% from patients to staff; staff-to-patient transmission was very infrequent (284, 288). Face-to-face contact was not the only mode of spread; well studied outbreaks clearly showed that airborne transmission can occur. In some instances infection spread to susceptible persons who entered a medical facility as long as 75 minutes after the index case had left (285, 287).

Although measles transmission in medical facilities is uncommon, it does occur, and often plays a major role in perpetuating measles outbreaks in the community. Recent studies indicate that 16 to 39% of cases in community outbreaks have been contracted in medical facilities (288). There have been occasional cases of measles acquired by hospital inpatients, but no reports of sustained outbreaks occurring within hospitals. Nonetheless, the potential for such outbreaks can be expected to increase over the next decade, as increasing numbers of susceptible adolescents enter the work force, many of them in health care settings.

Measles Vaccine

Persons can be considered immune to measles if they can document (a) a history of physician-diagnosed measles, (b) laboratory evidence of immunity, or (c) receipt of live measles vaccine on or after their first birthday (264). In addition, persons born before 1957 are likely to have been infected with measles virus and can be considered naturally immune. Anyone not meeting these criteria should be considered susceptible, and should be immunized unless there are specific contraindications. Even these strict criteria may be inadequate in situations where historical documentation of natural or vaccine-acquired immunity is incomplete (203, 289).

The current, further-attenuated live measles vaccine should be administered as a single dose subcutaneously, regardless of whether the monovalent or combination (with rubella or rubella and mumps) vaccine is used (264). Over 95% of persons aged 15 months or older will develop levels of antibody that should afford lifelong protection. Measles vaccine produces a mild or inapparent infection that is noncommunicable. Approximately 5 to 15% of recipients develop fever ($\geq 39.4°C$), beginning on day 6 following vaccination and lasting up to 5 days. Transient rashes are infrequent (5%), and central nervous system reactions are decidedly rare. Concern that measles vaccine itself may cause SSPE has been mitigated by its clear-cut protection against SSPE due to natural infection (269). In the few instances when SSPE has developed in persons without a history of natural measles who have received measles vaccine, it is likely that an unrecognized measles virus infection occurred before vaccination (264, 290).

Although a few cases of measles have been observed in persons who have been vaccinated properly, they are not epidemiologically important. In the general population there is no reason for serologic screening to uncover the few persons who still might be susceptible, nor for giving booster doses of vaccine (264, 291). However, revaccination with live measles vaccine is indicated for persons who previously received killed vaccine between 1963 and 1967, or who received live vaccine before 12 months of age (292). Persons previously given killed vaccine can experience frequent local or systemic adverse effects following live measles vaccination, and rarely may require hospitalization (264, 293). However, the risk is far lower than that of developing atypical measles with natural infection following earlier receipt of killed vaccine. In contrast, there is no increased risk of side effects from live measles vaccine in those who previously have had natural measles or received live vaccine.

Measles vaccine is contraindicated in women known to be pregnant because of the theoretical but still unsubstantiated risk of fetal infection with live vaccine virus. Vaccination should be postponed in those with serious febrile but not minor illnesses. Serious hypersensitivity reactions are extremely rare, having been reported in persons with anaphylactoid reactions to egg ingestion (the vaccine is produced in chick embryo cell culture) or neomycin (but not penicillin, which is not present in the vaccine). A protocol has been developed that should be followed in persons with serious egg allergy (294). Measles vaccine also is contraindicated in persons with tuberculosis and

in those with immunocompromise due to any cause. Vaccination should be postponed if persons have received immune globulin within 3 months (264).

Control of Measles in the Hospital

The strategy for the control of measles in hospitals and in other medical facilities reflects the same principles as those followed in the national measles elimination program. Control among health care workers is best guaranteed by having a fully immunized staff. Vaccination of all susceptible health care workers should be routine, and is best undertaken in conjunction with rubella immunization. As on college campuses, compliance is likely to be far better with mandatory than with voluntary programs (295). The general guidelines for measles vaccination issued by the ACIP regard persons born before 1957 to be immune as a result of natural infection. However, approximately two-thirds of all health care workers contracting measles in medical facilities have been in this supposedly immune older age group (288). For this reason, consideration of measles vaccine for susceptible older health care workers may be appropriate in some settings (e.g., emergency rooms).

Any patient appearing in a medical facility with a clinical illness compatible with measles should be isolated. Where possible care should be taken to ventilate the isolation area externally. Cases should be reported immediately to local health authorities, before serologic or virologic confirmation is obtained, in order not to delay the recognition of a possible outbreak. Measles patients requiring hospital admission should be placed on respiratory isolation in private rooms for 7 days following the onset of rash, and cared for only by staff with documented immunity. Susceptible inpatients should be separately cohorted for 18 days following exposure, or discharged if possible. If not contraindicated, measles vaccine can afford some protection to contacts if given within 3 days of exposure. Immune globulin (0.25 ml/kg; maximum dose 15 ml) also may prevent or modify measles if given within 6 days of exposure, and should be used in all patients for whom measles vaccine is contraindicated (264, 288, 296). However, immune globulin should not be used to control measles outbreaks in medical facilities or anywhere else. Other procedures to control measles transmission to health care workers include vaccination programs which, given the infectivity of measles virus, often require vaccinating large numbers of staff. Alternatively, exclusion of workers who have had contact with infected patients and cannot provide documentation of immunity has been used (297). Either measure theoretically may be helpful in controlling or preventing the spread of measles virus infection, but both disrupt the usual work routine and are quite expensive. Neither one is likely to be as effective as having a staff fully immunized against measles.

Tetanus and Diphtheria

Patterns of Susceptibility to Tetanus and Diphtheria

The occurrence of tetanus and diphtheria has declined dramatically in the United States, primarily as a result of widespread childhood immunization. In spite of its low incidence, two-thirds of the 90 to 100 cases of tetanus reported each year affect persons 50 years of age or older (298). Similarly, very few cases of diphtheria are reported (fewer than 5 to 10/year) (298). The majority affect adults of lower socioeconomic status (299). For both diseases almost all cases occur in persons who are unimmunized or inadequately immunized. Recent serologic surveys show that approximately 11% of younger adults, 40% of older adults, and 46 to 70% of the elderly lack protective levels of tetanus antitoxin (300–302). For diphtheria, 62% of younger adults, and 40 to 90% of older and elderly persons may not be adequately protected. In general, women are more likely than men to have inadequate protection.

There is no evidence that health care workers are at any greater risk from tetanus and diphtheria than the general population. Nonetheless, the case fatality rate for tetanus has remained constant at 45 to 55%, and many cases occur following wounds not considered to be tetanus-prone (298). In past years mortality from diphtheria was 5 to 10%, with higher rates among the elderly. For these reasons, health care workers, like all other adults, should be assured the complete protection which follows immunization with tetanus and diphtheria toxoids. At the time of employment, the immunization history of every health care worker should be reviewed; if indicated, a primary series or booster dose of tetanus and diphtheria toxoids should be given. In addition, health care providers should take measures to include immunization against tetanus and diphtheria as part of the overall care they provide to patients seen in the hospital setting. Rarely,

cases of tetanus may arise postoperatively after surgical procedures (303), and a few cases of neonatal tetanus are reported in the U.S. each year (298). Also, patients recovering from tetanus and diphtheria require vaccination; infection alone does not lead to the development of circulating antitoxins.

Tetanus and Diphtheria Toxoids and Their Use

Tetanus and diphtheria toxoids are formalin-treated preparations of their respective toxins and are available as (*a*) single antigen preparations; (*b*) combined tetanus-diphtheria (Td) toxoid adsorbed for adult use (persons 7 years of age or older); and (*c*) in combination with pertussis vaccine (DTP) (298). For adults combined Td toxoid should be used whenever either individual toxoid is indicated, unless there is a specific reason not to do so. Compared with DTP, combined Td toxoid contains a lower dose of diphtheria toxoid, the lower dose being associated with fewer side effects when used in adults.

For older children (≥ 7 years in age) and adults who have never been immunized, a primary series of combined Td toxoid should be given (two 0.5-ml doses intramuscularly at 0 and at 4 to 8 weeks, followed by a third dose at 6 to 12 months). This schedule produces adequate protection in virtually all recipients (304). If primary immunization is delayed or interrupted, there is no need to restart the series; the remaining doses should be given. Following a primary series, protective levels of antitoxin generally persist for 10 or more years; however, booster doses of combined Td toxoid should be given every 10 years, most conveniently on the mid-decade birthday (e.g., 25, 35, 45 years, etc). In younger adults, a single booster dose of tetanus toxoid is sufficient to produce adequate levels of antitoxin (305). Among elderly persons, two doses of combined Td toxoid generally are necessary to produce protective levels of antitoxins (300). In this group antitoxin levels occasionally may fall below levels considered protective after 4 years, and a third dose may be considered (306).

Tetanus Prophylaxis in Wound Management

Proper cleansing and debridement are essential in the management of all wounds. Chemoprophylaxis against tetanus is not useful. The use of combined Td toxoid and tetanus immune globulin (TIG) in wound management is outlined in Table 12.6 (298). Persons with clean, minor wounds who have had a complete primary series

Table 12.6. Tetanus Prophylaxis in Routine Wound Management

History of Tetanus Immunization	Clean, Minor Wounds		All Other Wounds	
	Td*	TIG†	Td	TIG
Unknown, uncertain, 0–2 doses	Yes	No	Yes	Yes‡
Three or more doses§	No¶	No	No‖	No

* Combined tetanus-diphtheria (Td) toxoid. For children less than 7 years of age, DTP (DT if pertussis vaccine is contraindicated) is preferred to tetanus toxoid alone. For persons 7 years of age or older, Td is preferred to tetanus toxoid alone.
† Tetanus immune globulin.
‡ When Td and TIG are given simultaneously, adsorbed and not fluid tetanus toxoid should be used.
§ If only three doses of fluid toxoid have been received, a fourth dose of adsorbed toxoid should be given.
¶ Td should be given if more than 10 years since the last dose.
‖ Td should be given if more than 5 years since the last dose. More frequent boosters may increase side effects and are unnecessary.

or a booster dose within 10 years are adequately protected; otherwise a booster dose of combined Td toxoid should be given, but TIG is unnecessary. For more severe wounds, combined Td toxoid should be given if more than 5 years have elapsed since the last dose. If the history of tetanus immunization is unknown, uncertain, or if less than three doses of toxoid have been given previously, or if the wound is more than 24 hours old, TIG (250 units intramuscularly) also should be given. When TIG is given along with combined Td toxoid, separate sites and syringes and adsorbed rather than fluid toxoid should be used. The use of combined Td toxoid rather than tetanus toxoid alone provides the opportunity to increase protection against diphtheria as well.

Diphtheria Prophylaxis for Contacts

All household contacts of patients with diphtheria, and all health care personnel in contact with patients hospitalized with diphtheria should be given combined Td toxoid if they have not received a booster dose within 5 years (298). This should be followed by the remaining doses of a full primary series if indicated. For contacts who lack up-to-date protection, chemoprophylaxis also should be given. Oral erythromycin (adults, 1 g/day; children 40 mg/kg/day) should be taken for 7 to 10 days; intramuscular benzathine penicillin (1.2 million uints for adults; 600,000 units for children < 6 years of age) may be slightly less effective, but is preferable if noncompliance with oral therapy is anticipated. If bacteriologic surveillance is undertaken, culture-positive carriers of toxigenic *Corynebacterium diphtheriae* should receive chemoprophylaxis. Close contacts of cases of cutaneous diphtheria also should be treated; although it is more likely that strains associated with cutaneous infection are nontoxigenic, cutaneous infection can be more contagious than respiratory infection.

Side Effects and Adverse Reactions to Td Toxoid

Immunization with combined Td toxoid is not associated with a rate of adverse reactions greater than that seen with either toxoid given alone (298). Local reactions are frequent but are mild and self-limited (304, 307, 308). Constitutional reactions are far less frequent and rarely require a physician visit. The only contraindication to combined Td toxoid is a severe hypersensitivity or neurologic reaction following a previous dose. If there is a history suggesting an anaphylactic reaction to a previous dose of tetanus toxoid, intradermal skin testing with serial dilutions of toxoid can be helpful in deciding whether to proceed with immunization; all but 1 to 2% of subjects will be nonreactive and will tolerate a full dose (308). If tetanus toxoid cannot be given, TIG may be required. Persons who have experienced severe, local Arthus-type hypersensitivity reactions to tetanus toxoid usually have very high levels of antitoxin; they can be immunized, but care should be taken not to give booster doses more frequently than every 10 years.

Tetanus and Diphtheria Immunization in Hospitals

There has been only one report of a long term program to vaccinate hospital patients with tetanus and diphtheria toxoids, but no data were provided on immunization rates (309). In all likelihood most of the tetanus toxoid currently used in hospitals is given as part of wound management in emergency rooms. However, a recent study of the tetanus prophylaxis in the emergency room management of open soft tissue injuries has shown that 23% of patients were treated incorrectly (310). Overtreatment was more common than undertreatment, but treatment errors were most likely to occur in incompletely immunized persons with tetanus-prone wounds; only 27% were properly treated with both tetanus toxoid and TIG.

There are no figures on the hospital use of combined Td toxoid in routine practice. Because so many older adults lack adequate levels of both antitoxins, a strong case can be made for incorporating tetanus and diphtheria immunization into the routine care of patients seen anywhere in the hospital setting.

Pertussis

With the exception of the use of DTP in routine childhood immunization, there rarely is any need for health care workers to consider using pertussis vaccine in hospitals. However, the controversy surrounding its safety has become a matter of serious public concern, with implications that affect policies for the use of all vaccines (311).

Pertussis in the United States

Pertussis was once a major cause of morbidity and mortality in childhood, but nearly universal immunization with DTP has resulted in a dramatic decline in its occurrence in the United States. Over the past 10 years approximately 1000 to 2000 cases, and 5 to 10 deaths have been reported each year (298, 312–315). More than half of all cases and almost all deaths have occurred in children less than one year in age. Pertussis infection undoubtedly is more widespread, but clinically it often is unrecognized. Laboratory confirmation of *Bordetella pertussis* infection by culture or direct fluorescent antibody techniques may be unreliable, and confirmed cases often go unreported. Undiagnosed pertussis may be particularly common in adults, with cases occurring even in those with histories of previous immunization or infection (316, 317). Within families an index case can infect 90% or more of unimmunized household contacts. On occasion adults as well as older siblings are the source of infection for infants (318). Recent use of enzyme-linked immunosorbent assays for antibodies to *B. pertussis* has been helpful in defining intrafamilial spread of infection, often uncovering many asymptomatic cases (319). However, the role of these asymptomatic persons in the household transmission of pertussis remains ill defined.

In other countries concern over the safety of pertussis vaccine has resulted in a steep decline in immunization rates. This has been most notable in the U.K., where epidemic pertussis reappeared in 1977 (320, 321). This experience, in contrast to persistent low rates for disease in the U.S., reflects the maintenance of very high levels of DTP immunization in the U.S. (313). Careful estimates of the costs and benefits of pertussis immunization indicate that current policies and practice in the U.S. are responsible for an approximately 10-fold reduction in the annual number of cases, hospital days, and deaths due to pertussis compared to what would be expected without an immunization program (322). In spite of the occurrence of vaccine-associated complications, pertussis immunization continues to confer impressive economic and disease reduction benefits.

Pertussis Vaccination, Adverse Reactions, and Contraindications

Pertussis vaccine is a suspension of killed *B. pertussis* organisms (298). It almost always is used in combination with diphtheria and tetanus toxoids (DTP) in an aluminum salt adsorbed preparation. DTP (unlike combined Td toxoid) is indicated only for children less than 7 years of age. The full five-dose series begins with three doses (0.5 ml each intramuscularly) given at 4- to 8-week intervals, starting when the child is 6 to 8 weeks old. A fourth dose is given 6 to 12 months after the third, and a fifth dose before entering school. Vaccination leads to the development of measurable levels of circulating pertussis-specific agglutinins; however, their correlation with levels of clinical protection is not precise. In clinical studies pertussis vaccine has had an efficacy of 70 to 90% in preventing acquisition of disease (298, 311, 313) and has shown similar efficacy in reducing disease severity in those infected (314). Full 0.5-ml doses should be used; reduced doses can be associated with fewer local reactions but are likely to be less protective (298).

Local reactions following DTP immunization are common but self-limited, and require no treatment. They occur more frequently with increasing numbers of doses of DTP (323, 324). Mild systemic reactions, including fever, drowsiness, irritability, and anorexia, are not uncommon. More severe systemic reactions, such as persistent or unusual crying, collapse, or seizures, are very uncommon and occur less frequently with increasing numbers of doses of DTP. Anaphylaxis is extremely rare.

The major concern with the safety of pertussis vaccine has centered on its possible role in causing acute encephalopathy with or without permanent brain damage, seizures, and death, including sudden infant death syndrome (SIDS). Epidemiologic assessment of the risks for these adverse events is difficult because DTP is given at a time in infancy when neurologic conditions due to other causes become clinically evident. The most extensive examination of the risks of DTP-related CNS adverse events has been the National Childhood Encephalopathy Study in the U.K. (320, 325). This case-control study concluded that DTP was associated with a greater frequency of acute neurologic reactions than would be expected by chance alone, although the majority of children appeared to recover completely, and most such illnesses were not temporally related to receipt of DTP. The attributable risk of a serious neurologic event occurring within 7 days of DTP vaccination was 1 in 110,000 doses, and for permanent neurologic sequelae was 1 in 310,000 doses. Other reports of an association between DTP vaccination and recurrent seizures have had serious methodologic problems that preclude any determination that the two were causally related (326). Similarly, in spite of earlier reports of an association between DTP vaccination and SIDS, a more definitive multicenter case-control study has demonstrated that fewer SIDS cases had received pertussis vaccine when compared to healthy controls (327).

The still unsettled public concern and persistent scientific uncertainty regarding pertussis vaccine safety has led to a reassessment of the contraindications to DTP vaccination (298). Table 12.7 summarizes the clinical conditions that require a decision as to whether DTP can be given, should be delayed, or is contraindicated. In children for whom DTP is contraindicated, further immunization should be undertaken with diphtheria and tetanus (DT not Td) toxoids. A decision on whether to complete a primary series of three doses with either DTP or DT should be made no later than the child's first birthday.

It is hoped that replacement of the current pertussis vaccine with a new acellular component vaccine might be associated with fewer neurologic reactions (328). However, since most of the reactions temporally related to DTP administration are due to other causes, clinical and epidemiologic assessment of the assumed greater safety of an acellular vaccine will be extremely difficult. The best that might be hoped for may be that the fewer and less severe minor reactions observed with the acellular vaccine will prompt investigators to search for other causes to explain the neurologic events occurring in association with DTP immunization (326).

Pertussis in the Hospital Setting

Although infants with pertussis frequently require hospital admission, the surprisingly few reports of nosocomial pertussis emphasize the general failure to consider the diagnosis or to obtain laboratory confirmation of suspected cases (329–331). Each of the reports of hospital-acquired pertussis demonstrates the susceptibility of young adults to reinfection in spite of previously documented immunization, and the spread of infection from staff to other patients and to household contacts. Control measures in these outbreaks have included (a) postexposure passive immunization of nonimmunized infants with pertussis immune globulin (329) (this product is no longer available in the U.S.); (b) vaccination of 25% of all hospital employees with single-antigen pertussis vaccine (330—this is the only published report of its use); (c) exclusion from work of employees with respiratory symptoms; (d) closure of wards to elective admissions; and (e) administration of antimicrobial agents to pertussis cases and their patient and staff contacts.

There are no data to support routine pertussis immunization of hospital personnel. In the one nosocomial outbreak in which single-antigen vaccine was used, side effects, including one neurologic reaction, were disturbing (330). Control measures to prevent pertussis transmission in hospitals focus on decreasing the infectivity of the patient and protecting all close contacts (298). Patients should be given oral erythromycin (children 40 mg/kg/day) or trimethoprim-sulfamethoxazole (children 8 mg/kg/day and 40 mg/kg/day, respectively), with the expectation of reducing infectivity rather than the duration or severity of disease. A 14-day course is necessary; shorter courses often are associated with failure to eradicate the organism or bacteriologic relapse (332, 333). A similar course of antimicrobial prophylaxis should be considered for close contacts under 1 year of age and for unimmunized contacts less than 7 years of age. It also should be considered for exposed hospital personnel, recognizing that there are no data from a large scale clinical trial that demonstrate the efficacy of antimicrobial chemoprophylaxis in this setting. In all likelihood, early recognition of infection among pa-

Table 12.7. Conditions Requiring Decision on Whether DTP Can Be Given, Should Be Delayed, or Is Contraindicated*

Condition	Decision
Unimmunized but suspected of having underlying (latent) neurologic disease	Delay†
Neurologic or systemic event temporally associated with DTP	Contraindicated
Collapse or shock-like state (hypotonic-hyporesponsive episode)	
Convulsion(s) with or without fever occurring within 3 days‡	
Encephalopathy (e.g., alterations in consciousness including excessive somnolence and/or generalized or focal neurologic signs) occurring within 7 days§	
Persistent crying lasting ≥ 3 hours or unusual, high pitched cry	
High fever (≥ 40.5°C)	
Hypersensitivity to a vaccine component	
Incompletely immunized, neurologic event occurring between doses	Delay
Stable neurologic condition (e.g., well controlled seizures)	Give DTP
Resolved or corrected neurologic disorder	Give DTP
Family history of convulsions or other neurologic disorder	Give DTP

* Decision also applies to the use of single-antigen pertussis vaccine.

† Decision should be made on an individual basis, delaying DTP until the condition is clarified or has stabilized. Decision to use DTP or DT to complete a primary series of three doses should be made no later than the first birthday.

‡ All children with convulsions, especially those occurring within 7 days of DTP vaccination, should be fully evaluated to clarify their medical and neurologic status before deciding whether to initiate or continue DTP vaccination.

§ A small but significant increased risk of encephalopathy has been shown only within the 3-day period following DTP vaccination. However, most authorities believe that encephalopathy occurring within 7 days of DTP vaccination should be considered a contraindication to further doses of DTP.

tients and staff, and respiratory isolation and work exclusion are of equal if not greater importance in the control of pertussis in hospitals.

Influenza

The Impact of Influenza in the United States

Influenza virus infections regularly cause pronounced increases in serious morbidity, hospitization, and mortality throughout the United States (334, 335). The impact is greatest among the elderly and in persons with serious underlying medical conditions that place them at increased risk. In 1980–1981 the A/Bangkok/79 (H3N2) epidemic caused an estimated 52,200 excess deaths nationwide (336). Since 1977 there has been co-circulation of H3N2 and H1N1 subtypes. Although H1N1 variants have caused widespread infection in children and younger adults, and occasionally severe disease among the elderly (337), they have not been associated with extensive mortality. Younger persons are the usual targets for influenza type B virus infection; however, in 1979–1980 influenza B/Singapore/79 caused severe disease among older adults (338, 339) and was associated with almost 44,000 ex-

cess deaths (336). Children also can be seriously affected; approximately 60 to 70% of cases of Reye's syndrome have been associated with influenza (340).

Recent longitudinal studies have shown that the overall impact of influenza is more severe than was previously suggested by estimates of excess mortality based on national surveillance data (334, 341–344). Each year (not just every 2 or 3 years) influenza viruses can be isolated from the community, and this is followed by increases in hospital admissions and deaths from acute respiratory disease (334, 341). The risk for hospitalization among persons aged 65 years and older has been approximately 1:100, and 40% of all adult admissions for respiratory infections have been concerntrated in the 10-week period each year when influenza viruses circulate. Influenza viruses can be isolated with surprising frequency from patients hospitalized with pneumonia at times when there has been little influenza activity recognized in the community (345).

The economic impact of annual influenza epidemics is substantial. Conservative estimates for the 1970s suggest that excess hospital admissions for pneumonia and influenza in epidemic years averaged $300 million (346). The overall economic burden of influenza exceeds several billion dollars each year (347).

Influenza in Hospitals and Nursing Homes

Influenza viruses have been known to cause nosocomial infections for many years (348). No report better illustrates the seriousness of nosocomial influenza than the classic study of an outbreak caused by Asian influenza virus (349); the admission of one patient with influenza quickly was followed by infection of almost half of the patients and staff on one hospital ward. The importance of Asian influenza in the spread of nosocomial staphylococcal infection also was well documented (350).

In recent years there have been surprisingly few reports of nosocomial influenza on the adult (345, 351–355) and pediatric (356–361) wards of acute care hospitals. Very few cases have been detected as a result of systematic virologic surveillance (353, 357–359). Both type A (H3N2 and H1N1) and type B influenza viruses have been incriminated. The patterns of transmission have not been discerned in all instances, but it is clear that patient-to-patient, patient-to-staff, and staff-to-patient spread have occurred. Often there has been delayed recognition that illness was due to influenza. Among adults almost all infections have involved older persons with serious underlying medical conditions who have not been immunized with influenza vaccine. Attack rates among patients on the same ward often have been 30% (351, 355). Many patients have died (345, 351, 352), and the length of stay for those who have survived has been prolonged (353, 355). On pediatric services hospital-acquired infection accounted for 21% of all cases of influenza in one report (357). In other studies, assessment of hospital-acquired influenza has been limited only to those children who were hospitalized 7 days or more. In one report only 2% of patients studied over a 4-month period developed nosocomial influenza (359), but in another, 71% of children with influenza who were studied during a community outbreak acquired their infections in the hospital (358). A high proportion of these children had underlying high risk conditions. The high rate of employee absenteeism observed in many of these outbreaks emphasizes the importance of health care workers as transmitters of nosocomial influenza virus infections to patients (362).

In addition to outbreaks in acute care hospitals, nosocomial influenza has been a serious problem in chronic disease hospitals (337, 363–367) and in nursing homes (336, 368–375). In both settings attack rates among patients have ranged from 25 to 50% or more (363, 372), and substantial numbers of staff also have been infected. Many patients have required acute hospital care (363, 370, 372, 373), and case-fatality rates have been high, in one instance reaching 30% (370).

The reports from hospitals and nursing homes illustrate the difficulties of preventing and controlling nosocomial influenza. Measures often undertaken to limit the spread of influenza include (*a*) not admitting elective patients, (*b*) separating patients with influenza-like illness from other noninfected patients, and (*c*) prohibiting persons with respiratory symptoms from visiting high risk patients. The effectiveness of these recommended procedures remains uncertain (375–377). Amantadine rarely is given to patients and staff (337, 374). Few hospitalized patients have been immunized previously with influenza vaccine. However, in some nursing homes large numbers have been immunized (368, 369, 371–374). Nonetheless, influenza has occurred in vaccine recipients, and occasionally has caused deaths (373, 374).

Influenza Vaccine: Antigenicity and Safety

Influenza vaccine contains the antigens of influenza viruses that are most likely to cause outbreaks of disease (378). Current vaccines are trivalent, containing antigens from two type A influenza viruses (H3N2 and H1N2) and one type B virus. Vaccine viruses are grown in embryonated eggs, inactivated with formalin, and made available as either whole virus or ether-disrupted ("split" or subunit) vaccine. A single 0.5-ml dose contains 15 μg of each hemagglutinin (H) antigen. For persons 12 years of age and older, one dose of whole or split virus vaccine should be administered intramuscularly. Children from 3 to 12 years of age require two 0.5-ml doses of split virus vaccine, and those from 6 months to 3 years of age require two 0.25-ml doses. The two doses should be separated by 4 weeks. Children who have received at least one dose of split virus vaccine at any time since 1978–1979 require only one dose. Split virus vaccine should be used in chidren because it causes fewer febrile reactions; either vaccine can be used in adults.

Influenza vaccination leads to the development of serum and secretory antihemagglutinin and antineuraminidase antibodies. Protection generally is best correlated with serum antihemagglutinin titers $\geq$ 1:40. In the most recently published assessment of vaccine antigenicity (1978–1979 vaccine) one dose ($\sim$20 μg) given to persons aged 65 years and older produced antihemagglutinin titers $\geq$ 1:40 in 88% (A/Texas/77 (H3N2)), 80% (A/USSR/77 (H1N1)), and 69% (B/Hong Kong/72), respectively (379). Similar results were observed in another study (380). Comparable if not better antibody responses can be seen in younger adults, although two doses of vaccine often are necessary to achieve antihemagglutinin titers $\geq$ 1:40 against H1N1 viruses (379).

Local adverse reactions to influenza vaccine are uncommon, and rates differ little from those observed in placebo recipients (378). Fever, malaise, myalgia, and other systemic symptoms are very rare in adults, although they can occur more frequently in children who have had little or no previous experience with influenza virus infections or influenza vaccines. The reactions usually begin 6 to 12 hours after immunization and last 1 to 2 days. Immediate, presumably allergic, reactions are extremely rare. They consist of a local flare and wheal or as respiratory symptoms of hypersensitivity and are believed to be due to sensitivity to a component of the vaccine, presumably residual egg protein. For this reason persons with known anaphylactic hypersensitivity to eggs (i.e., those who develop swelling of the lips or tongue or any evidence of acute respiratory distress or circulatory collapse) should not be given influenza vaccine.

The safety of influenza vaccine has been the subject of intense scrutiny since 1976, when swine influenza vaccine was shown to be associated with an increased risk of developing Guillain-Barré syndrome (GBS) (381, 382). Careful epidemiologic surveillance since then has shown that recipients of later influenza vaccines have not been at any increased risk for GBS (383). The reason for the swine influenza vaccine-GBS association remains unknown. More recently, influenza vaccine has been shown to affect the hepatic cytochrome P-450-linked monooxygenase system, depressing the metabolic clearance of several drugs, including warfarin, theophylline, and phenytoin. Not all pharmacokinetic studies have demonstrated these effects (384), and regardless of whether they occur, they rarely are of any clinical significance (385, 386).

Clinical Efficacy of Influenza Vaccine

There are no randomized, double-blind, placebo-controlled clinical trials that demonstrate the efficacy of influenza vaccines in older and high risk persons for whom they are recommended, although numerous reports document efficacy in healthy young adults. However, among elderly persons, uncontrolled studies have shown influenza vaccines to be approximately 70% or more protective against serious clinical illness (337, 364, 387, 388), hospitalization (389), and death (370, 374, 387–389). In contrast, other reports have shown relatively poor protection against influenza-like illness caused by type A (24 to 43%) (370, 372, 373, 375) and type B (27 to 35%) (371) influenza viruses. A number of reasons have been invoked to explain these observations. In some instances, an antigenic difference between the vaccine strain and the subtype variant causing infection was the most obvious cause (373). In one notable example, A/Hong Kong/68 vaccine was only 5% protective against febrile illness caused by the A/England/72 variant (368). The lack of efficacy against type B influenza virus infections (358, 371) can be partially accounted for by the lower degree of antigenicity of type B compared with type A hemagglutinins (379, 380). Host factors, including declining B-cell function in the elderly, also can play a role (390). Finally, persons who previously have received influenza vaccines may show minimal antibody responses to subsequent vaccination (380, 391). Repeated vaccination usually boosts antibody titers to earlier strains of influenza virus, but often has little effect on titers to the most current vaccine strain. This may account for the clinically observed "Hoskins' effect," in which annual vaccination eventually fails to provide protection (392). Unfortunately, there has been no study of the serial antibody responses of older and high risk persons who have been vaccinated annually for a number of years with conventional influenza vaccines.

In spite of experience showing varying degrees of efficacy for influenza vaccines among elderly persons, it is reasonable to conclude from the available data that immunization generally is effective. Although vaccine may be only partially protective in preventing influenza-like illness, it affords greater protection against such serious complications as pneumonia, hospitalization, and death.

Target Groups for Influenza Vaccination

Annual influenza vaccination continues to be the single most important measure for the prevention and control of influenza (378, 393). The

ACIP has established priorities for classifying high risk groups that should be targeted for immunization. First priority is given to (a) adults and children with chronic cardiopulmonary disorders that are severe enough to have required regular outpatient care or hospitalization within the preceding year, and (b) residents of nursing homes and other chronic care facilities. Second priority is given to vaccinating physicians, nurses, and other health care workers who have extensive contact with elderly persons, patients with cardiopulmonary disorders and conditions associated with immunocompromise, and infants in neonatal intensive care units. Third priority is given to vaccinating otherwise healthy adults aged 65 years and older, and younger adults and children who require regular medical care for chronic metabolic diseases (including diabetes mellitus), renal dysfunction, anemia, immunosuppression, and asthma. Although patients with some of these conditions may not respond optimally to influenza vaccine (e.g., patients with lymphoma), in most the antibody responses are similar to those seen in otherwise healthy persons (394, 395).

In addition to these high priority groups, influenza vaccine can be given to persons who wish to reduce their risks of infection, particularly those who provide essential community services. Pregnant women and their fetuses are not at increased risk for serious complications of influenza. The vaccine is considered safe for pregnant women, although it is reasonable to delay immunization until after the first trimester. Vaccination also should be delayed until recovery from acute febrile illnesses. Influenza vaccine is contraindicated in persons with anaphylactic hypersensitivity to eggs and in those with previous anaphylactic reactions to influenza vaccine. Most patients who are targets for influenza vaccine also should be immunized once with pneumococcal vaccine. The two vaccines can be given simultaneously at different sites, with good antibody responses to both, and without increased side effects (378).

Antiviral Prophylaxis and Therapy with Amantadine

The antiviral agent amantadine interferes with the uncoating of type A influenza viruses during the replication cycle and reduces virus shedding from persons who are infected (378). When given prophylactically it can be 70 to 90% protective against type A infection, but it has no activity against type B influenza viruses. Also, amanta-dine can be effective when given as therapy within 24 to 48 hours of the onset of illness, reducing the duration of fever and other symptoms, and permitting a more rapid return to normal activity. In this respect amantadine can be more effective than aspirin (396). Amantadine may not completely prevent infection, but it also does not interfere with the antibody response to either infection or influenza vaccination. In fact, the protection afforded by amantadine and vaccine-induced antibody together can be greater than that from either one alone.

The usual dose of amantadine is 200 mg/day (378). Side effects, including insomnia, lightheadedness, irritability, and difficulty concentrating, can affect 5 to 10% of healthy adults. The drug is not metabolized and is dependent on normal renal function for its clearance (397). For this reason, toxic levels can develop in persons with underlying renal dysfunction. Side effects can be reduced by giving amantadine in divided doses. Persons aged 65 years and older (who generally have some degree of reduced renal function even in the absence of recognized renal disease) should be given only 100 mg/day. This dose also should be used in persons with active seizure disorders because they may be at increased risk of seizures when taking the usual dosage. Children 1 to 9 years of age should be given 4.4 to 8.8 mg/kg/day, preferably in two divided doses, not to exceed 150 mg/day. If essential, the lower dose can be used cautiously in children less than 1 year of age, although this regimen has not been adequately evaluated. All patients receiving amantadine should be monitored closely for side effects, and the dosage reduced or the drug withheld should they appear. For persons with recognized renal disease, a protocol based on the creatinine clearance has been developed to guide reductions in the dose of amantadine (378). The related antiviral agent, rimantadine, has an efficacy comparable to that of amantadine, but appears to cause fewer side effects (398). Although it is not yet licensed for use in the U.S., rimantadine is safe when given prophylactically to elderly persons for prolonged periods (399).

Amantadine prophylaxis is recommended in the following circumstances: (a) as prophylaxis throughout the course of presumed outbreaks of influenza A virus infections, particularly when the vaccine may be less effective because there have been major antigenic changes in the virus; (b) as a short term adjunct to the late immunization of high risk patients, giving amantadine during the 2-week interval from the time of vaccination until a protective antibody response should develop; (*c*) to reduce disruption of medical services and the spread of infection to high risk patients by treating physicians, nurses, and other health care workers who have not yet received influenza vaccine, giving it for 2 weeks to those who accept vaccine and throughout the course of the outbreak to those who refuse vaccination; (*d*) to supplement protection in immunocompromised patients who respond poorly to influenza vaccine; and (*e*) as chemoprophylaxis for the duration of an outbreak in those for whom influenza vaccine is contraindicated. Problems with compliance should be anticipated among both patients and health care workers. This emphasizes the primary importance of vaccination rather than antiviral chemoprophylaxis in the prevention and control of influenza.

Prevention and Control of Influenza in Hospitals

Nosocomial influenza remains a major threat in hospitals primarily because most patients who should receive influenza vaccine have not been immunized. For the past 15 years (not including 1976) only 20% of the elderly and younger persons with high risk conditions have received influenza vaccine (378). Equally important, only 2 to 3% of all medical patients hospitalized during influenza outbreaks can be expected to have been immunized with influenza vaccine prior to hospital admission (400, 401). Furthermore, numerous reports of nosocomial influenza involving health care workers mention that few or none had been vaccinated. In addition, very few hospitals appear to conduct active programs to immunize hospital employees (402). These limited data stand in striking contrast to the more extensive information gathered on the immunization of hospital employees against hepatitis B and rubella. Thus, it is reasonable to assume that virtually all hospitalized patients and the staff who care for them remain susceptible (i.e., unvaccinated) to infection during community outbreaks of influenza.

Supplementary measures, including respiratory isolation, cohorting of patients and personnel, avoiding elective admissions, and restricting visitors, have been recommended and should be used in attempts to limit the transmission of nosocomial influenza virus infection (376–378). Great care must be taken to avoid the use of aspirin in treating children and adolescents with

suspected influenza because of its association with Reye's syndrome (403). Although the efficacy of amantadine in treating seriously ill influenza patients has not been determined, available data strongly suggest that the drug should be given to patients and staff to reduce the risk of influenza. In the only study that has been reported, amantadine was 80% effective in preventing nosocomial infection (400). Limited data show that practicing physicians have prescribed amantadine more frequently in recent years, albeit more for younger than for older patients, and in years when type B influenza viruses (which are not affected by amantadine) have predominated (404). However, there are no figures on the extent to which amantadine has been used for the treatment and prevention of influenza in hospitals.

Current recommendations for influenza vaccination give high priority to immunizing health care workers who have the greatest potential for introducing influenza viruses into high risk hospital settings (378). To be successful, immunization programs need to be planned well in advance and implemented aggressively. It would be helpful to have descriptive information on the experience of hospitals with employee immunization, including vaccination rates for personnel working in high risk areas, and details on the voluntary or mandatory nature of such programs, the nature of sanctions or job reassignments (if any) for workers who refuse vaccine, and the legal issues encountered. Unfortunately, no such studies have been reported, and they are badly needed.

There is limited information on influenza immunization of patients who receive their care in the hospital setting. Two reports have shown that approximately 30 to 40% of patients hospitalized with pneumonia, influenza, and related respiratory conditions have been discharged from hospital within the previous year (343, 401). This suggests that hospitals should undertake organized programs for immunizing discharged patients. One attempt to do so was only modestly successful; most patients were not offered influenza vaccine; and overall only 25% were vaccinated (401). However, among patients who actually were offered vaccine, 56% were immunized. Greater success has been achieved in hospital outpatient clinics, where a variety of approaches, including active participation by nurses and computer-generated reminders, have resulted in immunization rates of 40 to 50% or greater among high risk patients (401, 402, 405–407). These programs can be simple to organize, inexpensive to operate, and can become self-sustaining from year to year (408).

The crucial importance of organizational factors to the success of an institution's immunization program has been clearly shown in a report on influenza vaccination in nursing homes (409). Almost all nursing homes studied usually offered influenza vaccine to their residents on a voluntary basis, and overall, 62% were immunized. The most significant finding was that lower rates of immunization were found in nursing homes that required written consent from relatives, compared with homes that did not have this requirement (median 57% and 90%, respectively). Furthermore, nursing homes with high immunization rates ($\geq$ 80%) characteristically had sporadic cases of influenza, whereas outbreaks were observed in homes that immunized fewer residents (375). These studies represent the first assessment of the microepidemiology of influenza immunization practices in health care institutions, and their effects on the prevention and control of nosocomial influenza. They highlight the need for similar studies of immunization practices within hospitals.

Annual influenza vaccination of all persons aged 65 years or older and younger persons aged 45 to 64 years has been shown to be cost effective (410). The failure to immunize all but a small proportion (20%) of the high risk population cannot solely be ascribed to the lack of knowledge and negative attitudes of physicians and their patients; in fact, most physicians favor influenza vaccine, and most patients are inclined to accept it (401). The ACIP has established the goal of immunizing no less than 80% of residents of institutions for the aged and chronically ill, patients with severe cardiopulmonary disorders, and health care personnel who can transmit influenza in high risk hospital settings (378). This goal can be reached only by establishing administrative guidelines and procedures for immunization programs, and seeing to it that they are vigorously implemented by hospital infection control personnel.

Pneumococcal Infections

The Unchanging Pattern of Pneumococcal Infections

Pneumococcal infections are considered the leading cause of community-acquired bacterial pneumonia requiring hospital care, accounting for 26 to 78% of all cases (411). Recent experience documents their continued importance (412, 413). In one report in which diagnostic studies included counterimmunoelectrophoresis as well as culture, pneumococcal infections were responsible for 76% of adult community-acquired pneumonias admitted to hospital (414). Mortality rates for pneumococcal bacteremia in adults remain 20 to 30%; among the elderly they can reach 40 to 65%, in spite of prompt antimicrobial therapy and intensive care support (412, 415, 416). Most deaths from pneumococcal pneumonia, with or without bacteremia, occur among the elderly and in those with underlying medical conditions. Approximately two-thirds occur within the first 5 days of illness. More than 50,000 deaths are reported each year with pneumonia as the underlying cause, and close to 100,000 deaths occur with pneumonia mentioned in any diagnostic position on the death certificate. Thus, it is clear that at least several tens of thousands of deaths each year are caused by pneumococcal infections. The economic impact of pneumococcal pneumonia also is substantial; hospital care accounts for 90% of all costs associated with its treatment (412). In addition, pneumococcal infections rank third among the causes of bacterial meningitis in the United States, and they are the most common cause in persons 60 years of age and older (417).

Although less well studied than community-acquired infections, hospital-acquired pneumonia and bacteremia frequently are caused by pneumococcal organisms. In a few instances infection can develop as a result of person-to-person transmission (418), but most illnesses occur in persons who already are carriers. Pneumococcal infection has accounted for 10% of cases of nosocomial pneumonia (419) and 12.5% of cases of bacteremic nosocomial pneunomia (420). Among patients with pneumococcal bacteremia, nosocomial infections have caused from 10 to 59% of cases (421–423); mortality rates also have varied widely. Previous antimicrobial therapy has been cited as a contributing cause in some though not all studies, but there is common agreement that most patients with nosocomial pneumococcal bacteremia and pneumonia have serious underlying illnesses that ultimately will be fatal (422–424). A surprising number of cases develop 2 or more weeks after hospital admission.

Health care workers are not at increased risk for pneumococcal infection. Nonetheless, they are in a unique position to prevent these infections in the patients for whom they care.

Pneumococcal Vaccine

The currently available, second generation pneumococcal vaccine contains purified capsular polysaccharides of 23 types of Streptococcus pneu-

moniae known to cause 87% of bacteremic pneumococcal infections in the United States (425, 426). Each 0.5-ml dose contains 575 μg of polysaccharide; 25 μg each of types 1, 2, 3, 4, 5, 6B, 7F, 8, 9N, 9V, 10A, 11A, 12F, 14, 15B, 17F, 18C, 19F, 19A, 20, 22F, 23F, and 33F. Most healthy adults, including the elderly, develop a 2-fold rise in type-specific antibody titer to most of these antigens within 2 to 3 weeks of immunization (425, 427). Limited data suggest that levels of 100 to 300 ng of antibody nitrogen/ml as measured by radioimmunoassay are protective (428). Although levels decline over time, in immunocompetent adults and older children, elevated antibody titers generally persist for 3 to 5 years, if not longer.

The efficacy of earlier pneumococcal vaccines was demonstrated in randomized controlled trials in healthy young adults, but data from similar trials in elderly and high risk persons have been inconclusive (429). In these latter groups casecontrol and quasi-cohort studies have estimated the efficacy of the first generation, 14-valent pneumococcal vaccine to be approximately 60 to 80% (430, 431).

Pneumococcal vaccine is recommended for (*a*) all adults with chronic cardiopulmonary conditions in whom respiratory conditions cause increased morbidity; (*b*) adults with conditions known to be associated with increased risk of pneumococcal infection and its complications, specifically splenic dysfunction or anatomic asplenia (432–434), sickle cell anemia (435–437), alcoholism, cirrhosis (438), diabetes mellitus (439), chronic renal failure (including dialysis and transplantation) (440, 441), Hodgkin's disease and lymphoma (442, 443), multiple myeloma (444), other conditions or therapies associated with immunocompromise (445–447), and cerebrospinal fluid fistulas; and (*c*) all persons, healthy or otherwise, who are 65 years of age or older (426). The response to immunization can be suboptimal or shorter lasting in many patients with immune deficiencies, but vaccine should be given with the expectation that some patients will benefit. For these patients penicillin prophylaxis also should be considered. However, it should be noted that 80 to 90% of patients with pneumococcal bacteremia do not have any of the conditions associated with immunocompromise and should respond well to pneumococcal vaccine (421). Children under 2 years of age respond poorly to pneumococcal capsular polysaccharides and should not be immunized.

Mild local side effects have been observed in up to half of vaccine recipients, but fever and constitutional symptoms affect fewer than 1% (426). Severe adverse reactions have been extremely rare. Pregnant women can be immunized if vaccine is indicated by the presence of a high risk condition, but vaccine should be deferred until the second trimester to allay any concern about the theoretical risk to the fetus. Pneumococcal and influenza vaccines can be given at the same time but in different sites, with no increase in side effects. Current recommendations state that persons who previously have received pneumococcal vaccine (usually 14-valent) should not be reimmunized with 23-valent vaccine. Whether the local Arthus-type reactions and the systemic reactions observed following reimmunization in earlier studies occur with unacceptable frequency following a second dose of 23-valent vaccine is unknown, and this question merits further study (436, 437, 448).

Pneumococcal Immunization in Hospitals

In the first 5 years following its licensure, approximately 11.1 million doses of pneumococcal vaccine were distributed in the United States (449). Surveys of generalist physicians indicate that most believe the vaccine should be used in the groups for which it has been recommended (450, 451). In spite of these attitudes, the distribution figures suggest that no more than 20 to 25% of persons who should receive pneumococcal vaccine have been immunized (412). Recent retrospective population-based and hospital-based studies in England and the United States have shown that high proportions of patients with pneumonia and pneumococcal infections have been discharged from hospital at least once within the previous 3 to 5 years, including almost two-thirds of those with pneumococcal bacteremia (Table 12.8) (412, 421, 423, 452–455). Furthermore, cohort analysis in the population-based studies has shown that relatively few (approximately 50 to 100) older and high risk patients would need to be immunized at the time of hospital discharge to prevent within the next 5 years one readmission with preventable pneumococcal pneumonia (412, 452). These studies provide a strong rationale for hospital-based pneumococcal immunization.

To date, there has been limited experience with hospital-based pneumococcal immunization. Less than 3% of the vaccine distributed has been sold to hospitals (449). Equally important, very few hospitalized medical patients have received pneumococcal vaccine prior to admission (454, 456). However, in programs designed to promote pneumococcal immunization of high risk dis-

Table 12.8.   Previous Hospital Care in Patients with Pneumococcal Bacteremia

Location	Period	No. of Patients	Previous Hospital Care		Reference
			%	Years*	
Chicago	1970–1980	166	63	5	421
Cooperstown	1974–1982	39	59	5	421
Pittsburgh	1975–1980	58†	53	1	423
Huntington	1978–1981	59‡	58	3	453
New York	1980–1982	56§	59	5	454

* Number of years prior to admission with pneumococcal bacteremia.
† Excludes 14 patients for whom information on previous hospital care was not available.
‡ Excludes 12 patients who were not considered candidates for pneumococcal vaccine.
§ Excludes five patients for whom information on previous hospital care was not available.

charged patients, up to 78% have received the vaccine (454, 456). High immunization rates also have been achieved in hospital outpatient clinics (405, 406, 408, 412, 457). Each of these studies demonstrates that rates for pneumococcal immunization improve markedly wherever there is an organized program for vaccine delivery.

Pneumococcal immunization of all elderly persons and younger persons with high risk conditions is cost effective (458) and is partially reimbursed under the Medicare program. Because the majority of persons destined to be hospitalized or to die of pneumococcal infections have had previous hospital care, physicians and other health care workers in hospitals have a unique opportunity to assure that elderly and high risk patients receive adequate protection. If widely implemented, hospital-based pneumococcal immunization could reduce by up to 10% the number of hospital admissions caused by all pneumonias (412).

Meningococcal Infections

In the United States there are approximately 3000 to 4000 cases of meningitis caused by *Neisseria meningitidis* each year, accounting for 20% of all cases (459). No major epidemic of meningococcal disease has occurred since 1946; cases generally occur singly or in clusters among close contacts. The peak incidence occurs in late winter and early spring. Attack rates are highest in infants less than 1 year of age and lowest in persons 20 years of age and older (14.6 and 0.3 cases/100,000 population, respectively). The overall case-fatality rate for meningococcal meningitis and bacteremia is 19%. In 1980, the most recent year reported, serogroup B accounted for 50 to 55% of all cases, followed by serogroup W135 (21%), serogroup C (18%), serogroup Y (7% to 8%), and serogroup A (3%).

Persons with anatomic and functional asplenia probably are at increased risk of developing meningococcal infection, for reasons analogous to their susceptibility to pneumococcal infections (460). In addition, those with component deficiencies of the final complement pathway can develop serious, often multiple infections (461). Small outbreaks of nosocomial meningococcal meningitis and pneumonia have been reported, without spread to health care workers caring for infected patients (363, 462, 463).

Meningococcal Vaccines

Two meningococcal vaccines are available for use; bivalent A-C and quadrivalent A, C, Y, W135 vaccines (464). They contain 50 μg of purified capsular polysaccharide of each of their component serogroups. Each polysaccharide antigen independently induces serogroup-specific immunity (465), although antibody titers are low in children less than 18 to 24 months in age and decline more rapidly when compared with titers in adults. In school children and adults, protective levels of antibody probably persist for 3 years.

Routine vaccination with either of the two meningococcal vaccines is not recommended for civilians in the United States, including health care workers. This is because the overall incidence of the disease is low, no vaccine is available for serogroup B which is the major cause of disease, and much of the disease occurs in children too young to benefit from immunization. Quadrivalent meningococcal vaccine is routinely given to military recruits. Among civilians it should be reserved for persons with terminal complement component deficiencies and those with splenic disorders. Antibody responses to serogroup A and C polysaccharides are normal in persons who have undergone splenectomy for trauma or nonlymphoid tumors, but are greatly reduced in asplenic patients who have had prior chemotherapy and radiation therapy for hematologic malignancies (466).

Meningococcal vaccines are administered as a single dose, 0.5 ml subcutaneously. Side effects following immunization are infrequent and mild. The safety of the vaccines for pregnant women has not been established, and they should be used only for those with high risk conditions. The need for revaccination is unknown, although children given their first dose when less than 4 years of age might benefit from another dose 2 to 3 years later.

When sporadic cases of meningococcal infection occur in the hospital setting or in households, antimicrobial chemoprophylaxis of intimate contacts remains the primary preventive measure for eradicating nasopharyngeal carriage of the organism. Rifampin is the agent most commonly used and should be given twice daily for 2 days (600 mg for adults, 10 mg/kg for children over 1 year in age, and 5 mg/kg for those younger). It should not be given to pregnant women because of its known teratogenicity in laboratory animals. Rifampin colors tears orange, so contact lenses should not be worn during treatment to avoid staining. In recent years fewer than 10% of serogroup B, Y, and W135 isolates have been resistant to sulfonamides; thus, the use of a sulfonamide in the chemoprophylaxis of contacts can be justified if the organisms isolated are known to be sensitive (459). In addition, rifampin or a sulfonamide has been recommended for patients being treated for meningococcal disease, because systemic antimicrobial therapy with other agents does not always eradicate nasopharyngeal carriage (467). Although immunization of close contacts with either bivalent or quadrivalent vaccine might be considered as an adjunct to chemoprophylaxis, it offers very little in the way of additional benefit.

Varicella-Zoster

Varicella-Zoster Virus Infections

Varicella-zoster virus (VZV) infection is a highly contagious childhood disease, with more than 90% of the three million cases each year affecting children less than 15 years of age (468–470). The clinical illness usually is benign, although in infants less than 1 year of age and in adults (3% of all cases) there is a greater risk of pneumonia, encephalitis, and death (471, 472). Among the elderly, latent VZV can reactivate, causing localized or occasionally generalized disease. Again, the risk of mortality in immunocompetent patients generally is low, even in those who disseminate (473). Each year an estimated 100 deaths are caused by VZV infections (469).

In certain groups VZV infections can be life threatening. In one study of children aged 11 days to 14 years with severe illness requiring hospitalization, 27% had secondary bacterial infections (7% pneumonia), 25% had encephalitis, and 21% had Reye's syndrome (471). Although only a small proportion (6 to 16%) of children hospitalized with VZV infections are immunocompromised, they have a greater mortality rate (7%) when compared with children who are immunocompetent (0.4%) (469). Maternal infection during the first 16 weeks of pregnancy rarely may lead to varicella embryopathy (474). Infants born of mothers in whom clinical varicella has developed during the period from 5 days before to 48 hours after delivery have a 17% risk of infection, and a case-fatality rate of 31% (469).

Varicella-Zoster Virus Infections in Hospitals

It is estimated that 6500 persons with VZV infections are hospitalized each year (469). Their presence on hospital wards poses a serious threat to other patients who are immunocompromised. In addition, they can infect physicians, nurses, and other health care workers (475–483). Nosocomial outbreaks can spread by person-to-person contact, although airborne dissemination of virus has been documented and may be more common than currently is recognized (478, 479). Secondary VZV infections in immunocompromised patients can be fatal (475, 478, 480). In some institutions approximately 10 to 20% of patient care staff may be susceptible (477, 481, 484). Even when none becomes infected, the costs to hospitals when nosocomial varicella disrupts services can be considerable (482).

Varicella-Zoster Immune Globulin

Specific zoster immune globulin (ZIG), derived from the plasma of patients recovering from herpes zoster, has been shown to prevent clinical infection in normal children if administered within 6 days of exposure (468). When administered to immunodeficient susceptible high risk children after household exposure to varicella, one study showed that clinical illness developed in 36% of cases, a rate of infection far lower than the 61 to 89% rate expected in normal susceptible children following similar exposure (485). Most children who were infected developed only mild illness. In 1981, varicella-zoster immune globulin (VZIG) became available for clinical use. It is prepared from blood donor plasma found by routine screening to have high titers of antibody to VZV. In a clinical trial in immunocompromised children comparing VZIG with ZIG, clinical or serologically confirmed varicella developed in 60% of the recipients of VZIG and 69% of the recipients of ZIG (486). These rates were lower than would have been expected without such protection. When clinical illness occurred it usually was mild; only 10 to 16% of subjects developed more than 100 lesions.

VZIG in the Management of Varicella-Zoster Infections in Hospitals

The decision to administer VZIG requires determination of (a) whether the patient is likely to be susceptible to varicella; (b) whether the exposure is likely to lead to infection; and (c) whether there is an increased risk of serious complications if infection occurs (468, 487). Immunocompromised children (< 15 years of age) with no history of prior varicella, or an unknown history of varicella, should be regarded as susceptible. If a similar history is obtained from normal adolescents and adults, they generally can be considered to be immune, unless demonstrated to be susceptible by reliable antibody testing. However, older persons with no history of, or an unknown history of, varicella should be considered susceptible. Once susceptibility has been established, the exposure criteria for which VZIG is indicated must be established. These criteria include (a) continuous household contact; (b) close indoor contact greater than 1 hour in duration; (c) hospital contact in adjacent beds or in the same two- to four-bed room, or prolonged face-to-face contact with an infectious staff member or patient; and (d) an infant born of a mother who developed clinical varicella in the period from 5 days before to 2 days after delivery. In all instances, the time elapsed from exposure to administering VZIG should be no more than 96 hours.

Once susceptibility and exposure have been determined, VZIG should be given to patients at increased risk for serious disease. The most important group is immunocompromised children, including those with leukemia or lymphoma, congenital or acquired immunodeficiency, and immunosuppressive treatment. Newborn infants who meet the above criteria should receive VZIG; those born of mothers who developed varicella more than 5 days before delivery should be protected by maternal antibody. Newborns are at much less risk of serious illness or death if their mothers develop varicella more than 48 hours after delivery. VZIG also should be considered for premature infants (≥ 28 weeks' gestation) whose mothers have no previous history of varicella, and for infants of less than 28 weeks' gestation or whose birth weight is less than 1000 g. Even if there is a positive maternal history of varicella, these infants may not yet have acquired maternal antibody. Immunocompromised adults who are susceptible and have had significant exposure should receive VZIG, but normal adults should be evaluated on an individual basis. Although the risk of death from varicella in normal adults may be 25 times greater than that in normal children, supplies of VZIG are limited. It should always be available to protect immunocompromised children and high risk newborns, whose risks of death exceed that in adults by factors of 140 and 620, respectively. Pregnant women should be evaluated no differently than normal adults. The risk of varicella embryopathy is low to begin with, and there is no evidence that VZIG would prevent this condition if given.

In addition to administering VZIG to patients at high risk, the management of varicella outbreaks in the hospital setting requires strict isolation precautions, cohorting of exposed patients, and early discharge (468, 488). Children and adolescents should not be given salicylates because of their known association with Reye's syndrome (340, 403). Ideally, staff caring for patients with VZV infections or those who have been exposed and may be incubating the disease should be known to be immune, either through a definite prior history or serologic testing. Susceptible staff with significant exposure should be excluded from direct patient contact from days 10 through 21 after exposure, during which time varicella may be expected to occur. This period should be extended to 28 days if the staff member was exposed to an immunocompromised VZIG-treated patient. In these patients, VZV infections can have a more prolonged incubation period, and thus extend the period of exposure for hospital personnel. No studies demonstrate that giving VZIG prophylactically to hospital staff is effective in controlling nosocomial outbreaks of VZV infection. In all likelihood, large numbers of health care workers would have to be immunized. Because VZIG is in limited supply, it should be reserved for patients at high risk.

Varicella-zoster immune globulin should be administered no later than 96 hours after exposure. The recommended dose is 125 units/10 kg (1 vial) up to 625 units (5 vials; $375). It should be given intramuscularly and should never be administered intravenously. Local discomfort at the injection site is infrequent, and systemic and serious hypersensitivity reactions are rare. It is not known whether VZIG is useful in treating clinical varicella, or localized or generalized zoster; it should not be used for these conditions. VZIG is available through selected American Red Cross Blood Centers (468).

Live Attenuated Varicella Vaccine

Although as yet unlicensed in the United States, live attenuated varicella vaccine has been shown to be antigenic, safe, and highly effective in preventing clinical disease in healthy children who have had household exposure to varicella (489, 490). Similar effectiveness has been shown in children with acute lymphocytic leukemia in remission (491, 492). In the latter instance, varicella vaccine was 80% effective in preventing clinical varicella and completely protective against severe illness. Within the next few years this vaccine will provide another means of preventing serious VZV infections in immunocompromised patients who receive their care in hospitals. In addition, it may be useful for immunizing seronegative hospital personnel whose duties bring them in direct contact with patients at high risk for serious VZV infections.

Rabies

Human and Animal Rabies

Human rabies is a rare disease in the United States; no more than five cases a year have been reported since 1960 (493–495). In recent years, the majority of cases have been imported, following bites by rabid dogs outside the U.S. Active control programs have markedly reduced the incidence of rabies among domestic animals, mainly dogs and cats. Wild animals, principally skunks, foxes, bats, and (increasingly in recent years) raccoons, are now the most likely sources of infection for humans and domestic animals (496). Almost all fatal cases occur after bites by rabid animals, but transmission by aerosol in the laboratory and by corneal transplantation from donors subsequently shown to have had rabies have been reported (493, 497). When human rabies occurs, the diagnosis often is not considered early in the course of illness. In almost all instances treatment is delayed, suboptimal, or not given at all (494, 495).

Each year approximately 25,000 persons in the U.S. receive prophylaxis against rabies (493, 498).

The vast majority are given postexposure prophylaxis following bites or exposure to animals proven to have or suspected of having rabies. When exposed to patients with rabies, many health care workers in hospitals and other settings require postexposure prophylaxis. In addition, pre-exposure prophylaxis is given to persons whose work or outside activities place them at increased risk of infection. Although rabies prophylaxis is costly, and in many instances given when not required, the extent of its use is understandable, since human rabies remains almost 100% fatal.

Human Diploid Cell Rabies Vaccine and Rabies Immune Globulin

The prevention of rabies is accomplished with two products (493). Human diploid cell rabies vaccine (HDCV) was licensed for use in the U.S. in 1980. It is an inactivated preparation of rabies virus grown in human diploid cell cultures, and is supplied in 1.0-ml single-dose vials of lyophilized vaccine. Unlike the earlier duck embryo vaccine which it replaced, HDCV produces an excellent antibody response in virtually all persons when administrered according to recommended schedules. Only one HDCV product currently is available in the United States. In 1985, Wyeth (WI-38) HDCV was withdrawn from the market because antibody titers in some persons given postexposure prophylaxis (see below) were inadequate (499). The reasons for this are unknown; they may have been caused by factors intrinsic to the vaccine itself or by improper administration (e.g., injection in the buttock) (95, 499). Merieux HDCV, which is produced in MRC-5 cell cultures, has continued to produce excellent antibody responses and is the only HDCV that should be used until the uncertainties regarding the Wyeth vaccine are resolved.

Rabies immune globulin (RIG) is prepared from the plasma of hyperimmunized human donors, and contains 150 international units/ml of rabies neutralizing antibody. It has replaced equine antirabies serum in the U.S., although the equine preparation still is used in some parts of the world.

Pre-exposure Immunization with HDCV

Pre-exposure immunization with HDCV is indicated for (*a*) veterinarians, animal handlers (including those in medical research centers), and laboratory workers who can come in contact with the virus; (*b*) certain travelers who may be at risk of exposure to rabid animals when traveling abroad; and (*c*) others whose activities bring them in contact with potentially rabid animals (493). Pre-exposure prophylaxis provides protection against future inapparent exposure to rabies, ensures protection when postexposure prophylaxis is delayed, and simplifies the usual postexposure treatment regimen. Three 1.0-ml doses of HDCV should be given intramuscularly on days 0, 7, and 28. The uniformly good antibody response with this regimen makes routine postvaccination serologic testing unnecessary. Persons with continuous exposure to rabies virus (e.g., vaccine production workers) should have serologic testing every 6 months, and receive booster doses of HDCV if indicated. Those with frequent exposure (e.g., wildlife workers in epizootic areas) should be considered for booster immunization or have serologic confirmation of continued protection every 2 years.

Efforts to reduce the costs of pre-exposure prophylaxis have led to the widespread use of smaller (0.1 ml) intradermal doses of HDCV. Studies with the Merieux preparation in the U.S. indicate that this alternative route of administration results in adequate levels of protective antibody (500), although field experience abroad has shown that many recipients did not develop a satisfactory antibody response (501). Although mean titers and the duration of the antibody response following intradermal administration can be somewhat lower when compared with those following the intramuscular route, pre-exposure intradermal immunization is an acceptable alternative.

Postexposure Immunization with HDCV and RIG

The decision to embark on a course of postexposure prophylaxis involves consideration of three factors: (*a*) type of exposure—transmission is primarily by the bite of a rabid animal, although virus also may be introduced from saliva into open wounds or, rarely, may be transmitted by aerosol; (*b*) species of biting animal—wild carnivores are more likely to be rabid, whereas rodents and lagomorphs are rarely infected and have not been associated with human disease; and (*c*) circumstances of the biting incident—an unprovoked attack is more likely than a provoked attack to indicate that the animal is rabid (493). Postexposure prophylaxis may be unnecessary if the biting animal, usually a dog or cat, is healthy and can be observed to remain so for 10 days. If

the animal is unavailable, postexposure prophylaxis may be indicated. Bites by wild carnivores require postexposure prophylaxis unless laboratory tests prove the animal is nonrabid.

The first step in postexposure prophylaxis is immediate and thorough washing of all wounds and scratches with soap and water. The importance of this simple measure should not be underestimated. Next, RIG should be administered, 20 IU/kg, with half the dose infiltrated into the wound area, and the other half given intramuscularly. The only exceptions to the use of RIG are persons who previously have received the recommended pre-exposure or postexposure regimens of HDCV, or who have a protective antibody titer known from serologic testing. RIG can be given up to the eighth day after beginning a course of HDCV. All persons require a course of HDCV for postexposure prophylaxis. If there is a past history of pre-exposure prophylaxis with HDCV, or if the antibody titer is known, only two doses of HDCV, 1.0 ml intramuscularly on days 0 and 3, are required. All other persons should be given five doses of HDCV, 1.0 ml intramuscularly on days 0, 3, 7, 14, and 28. The vaccine must not be injected into the same site that was used for RIG. The intradermal route has not been evaluated in postexposure prophylaxis and should not be used.

The combination of RIG and HDCV for postexposure prophylaxis provides immediate as well as sustained levels of protective antibody (493, 502). Experience in the U.S. and in other countries has shown that none of the persons bitten by rabid animals has developed rabies when this regimen was followed. On the other hand, postexposure prophylaxis with HDCV alone, without RIG and in the absence of pre-exposure prophylaxis, has been associated with fatal rabies (503). Postexposure prophylaxis should begin as soon as possible after exposure, but still should be undertaken even when there has been long delay (e.g., 6 months) in recognizing that exposure to rabies has occurred.

Adverse Reactions and Precautions with Rabies Prophylaxis

Local reactions to HDCV are fairly common, and a variety of mild systemic reactions affect 20% of vaccinees (493). Rare cases of neurologic illness have been reported, but no conclusions can be drawn regarding their relationship to HDCV (504). More recently, two types of systemic allergic reactions have been noted: (*a*) a

Type I (IgE-mediated) immediate hypersensitivity reaction (1/10,000 vaccinees), and (*b*) a Type III (IgG- or IgM-mediated) immune-complex disease (9/10,000 vaccinees) (505). Few patients have required hospitalization, and no deaths have occurred. Over 90% of the reported Type III hypersensitivity reactions occurred after 2-year booster doses of HDCV, and they affected 13.5% of HDCV recipients. Until there is more experience with booster immunizations, they should be reserved only for persons at risk for inapparent or unavoidable exposure to rabies virus. In those with a history of Type III reactions, HDCV should be given under close medical supervision.

Local pain and occasionally low grade fever can occur following administration of RIG, but these reactions have caused no serious problems. When equine antirabies serum must be used, serum sickness can be expected in up to 40% of recipients.

Pregnancy is not a contraindication to preexposure and postexposure prophylaxis if the risk of rabies warrants the use of inactivated HDCV. Treatment with corticosteroids and other immunosuppressive agents should be avoided unless essential for other reasons; if given, an adequate antibody response should be documented by serologic testing.

Patterns of Rabies Postexposure Prophylaxis

Epidemiologic monitoring in the U.S. has shown that 88% of persons receiving postexposure prophylaxis have been treated according to recommended guidelines (498). Approximately two-thirds of these have been treated after exposure to domestic animals, although these sources account for a much smaller proportion of proved animal rabies. Available evidence indicates a considerable amount of overtreatment of persons whose exposures carry little if any risk of infection. A single course of postexposure prophylaxis costs more than $400 for HDCV and RIG alone. Statewide consultation programs have been shown to be cost effective, and have substantially reduced the number of persons who require postexposure prophylaxis (506).

When patients with rabies are hospitalized, many of the staff, particularly intensive care unit nurses, physicians, and respiratory therapists, are given and should be given HDCV and RIG. Although there has been no documentation of human-to-human transmission in this setting, experimental evidence of transmission by contact with rabies-infected secretions justifies this precaution.

Poliovirus Infections

Poliomyelitis in the United States

Since the introduction of poliovirus vaccines in the United States in 1955, the occurrence of poliomyelitis has declined dramatically (507–509). Inactivated poliovirus vaccine (IPV) was used at first, but was replaced in 1963 by live attenuated oral poliovirus vaccines (OPV). Approximately 24 million doses of OPV are now distributed in the U.S. each year, and more than 97% of children entering school have completed a primary series of vaccination. The last outbreak of poliomyelitis occurred in 1979, and involved 10 persons who had not been vaccinated. No indigenous wild-type poliovirus has been isolated from a person with poliomyelitis since 1981, evidence that the disease has been virtually eliminated in the United States (508). However, clinicians recently have begun to see patients with late postpoliomyelitis muscular atrophy, a condition which affects middle-aged adults who have recovered from a previous episode of acute paralytic disease (510). This further emphasizes the need to maintain universal immunization against poliovirus infections.

Poliovirus Vaccines

Both OPV and IPV are trivalent vaccines that include type 1, type 2, and type 3 polioviruses (511). A complete primary series with either vaccine induces long-lasting protection in more than 95% of recipients. OPV currently is the vaccine of choice in the U.S. because it induces intestinal immunity, is simple to give, is well accepted by patients, and can induce immunity in contacts. IPV can induce comparable levels of neutralizing antibodies in vaccine recipients (512), and its use in other countries has eradicated indigenous poliomyelitis. However, in countries with high rates of childhood immunization with either OPV or IPV, outbreaks of paralytic poliomyelitis have occurred in subpopulations that have not been vaccinated (513, 514).

For children, a primary series of OPV consists of three doses, with a supplementary dose at the time of school entry (511). If IPV is used, four primary doses plus the supplementary dose are required. Additional supplementary doses of IPV every 5 years until 18 years of age have been suggested (511), although there may be little need for these extra doses. In one recent report 6% of persons aged 21 to 29 years lacked detectable neutralizing antibodies to one of the serotypes of poliovirus (515). However, the absence of detectable neutralizing antibodies in persons who previously have been immunized does not necessarily indicate the absence of immunity; challenge with IPV elicits a brisk, high titer anamnestic antibody response, indicating solid immunologic memory (516).

Serious adverse reactions have not been reported with IPV. With OPV, vaccine-induced paralytic disease can occur in healthy recipients and in their close contacts (1 in 8.7 million, and 1 in 5.1 million doses distributed, respectively) (508). During the period from 1978 to 1983 an average of 12 cases of poliomyelitis was reported each year in the U.S., almost two-thirds of which were epidemiologically classified as vaccine-associated. More precise laboratory strain characterization, including oligonucleotide fingerprinting, confirmed the epidemiologic classification in most instances.

The occurrence of rare cases of OPV-related paralytic disease underlies the policy debate in the U.S. over whether IPV should be used in place of OPV (507–509, 511, 516). Current research indicates that it may be possible to develop a totally safe OPV in which the regions of the viral genome associated with neurovirulence have been deleted or altered (517). On the other hand, more potent and less expensive inactivated vaccines are being developed, and it is possible that recombinant DNA techniques can be used to produce subunit vaccines that induce long-lasting immunity with reduced vaccination schedules (518). Any change in policy will be based on the results of clinial trials of these newer vaccines, together with continued assessment of the ability of current vaccination programs to maintain high levels of immunity.

The Use of Poliovirus Vaccines in Hospitals

The use of poliovirus vaccine (OPV) in hospitals is largely confined to routine immunization in pediatric clinics. In general, persons 18 years of age or older do not require poliovirus vaccine; most already are immune and have little risk of exposure to wild-type poliovirus infection (511–515). However, certain health care workers may be at increased risk of exposure to vaccine strain or rarely wild-type polioviruses. Laboratory personnel and others who frequently handle stool specimens or have close contact with patients who

may be excreting polioviruses, the staff of pediatric clinics and inpatients units, and emergency room personnel should be fully immunized.

Previously unvaccinated health care workers should be given a primary series of three doses of IPV at 1- to 2-month intervals, followed by a fourth dose at 6 to 12 months (511). OPV should not be used because of the slightly higher risk of vaccine-associated paralysis in adults compared with children. The one exception to this is the need for immediate protection; in this instance an initial dose of OPV should be given; followed by the remaining doses of vaccine. Incompletely immunized adults who risk exposure to polioviruses should complete their full primary series with OPV or IPV. Those with a complete primary series can be given a booster dose of OPV if they are at increased risk of exposure. It is advisable on theoretical grounds to avoid giving OPV or IPV to pregnant women, although there is no evidence that either vaccine will harm the mother or the fetus. However, OPV can be given if there is a strong need for immediate protection.

Health care workers also must be aware of the potential risks of OPV for patients with immune deficiency, regardless of its cause. IPV not OPV should be used to immunize these patients and, equally important, their household contacts. If OPV is given inadvertently to a household contact of an immunodeficient patient, close contact between the two must be avoided for 1 month to reduce the risk of exposing the patient to vaccine virus. Unfortunately, in most cases of OPV-associated paralysis occurring in patients with immunodeficiency, the immunodeficiency state is diagnosed only after poliomyelitis occurs (508). However, in families of immunodeficient patients, other family members should not receive OPV until their immune status is determined. Finally, health care workers must always be aware that in certain groups of patients (e.g., children of migrant workers, immigrants, or members of certain religious sects) immunization against poliovirus infections is not widespread. Paralytic poliomyelitis occurs because of the failure to vacciate, not vaccine failure. Thus, all patients must be assured the protection provided by poliovirus vaccination.

Mumps

Mumps Virus Infections

Since the introduction of live mumps virus vaccine in 1967 there has been a 97% decline in the annual number of cases reported in the

United States (519). Fewer than 10 cases of mumps-associated encephalitis and death are now reported each year. With widespread vaccination of children entering school, an increasing proportion of reported cases now occurs in adolescents. Mumps infection of younger men can cause unilateral orchitis, and in the first trimester of pregnancy it can increase the risk of spontaneous abortion (520). However, most adults have experienced natural infection with mumps virus (30% subclinical) and can be considered immune.

Mumps Vaccine

Live mumps vaccine induces protective levels of antibody that last 15 years or more (520, 521). It usually is given in combination with measles and rubella (MMR) vaccines. Parotitis, mild allergic reactions, and transient neurologic problems have been observed following receipt of mumps vaccine. Vaccination is contraindicated in anyone with a history of an anaphylactic reaction to egg ingestion or neomycin, and in persons with immune deficiency disorders. Vaccination should be postponed during pregnancy, and for 3 months if immune globulin has been given.

Health care workers are not at any greater risk for mumps than the general population and need not be considered for mumps vaccination alone. However, whenever measles or rubella vaccine is indicated, advantage should be taken of this opportunity to assure protection against mumps by administering MMR. Mumps vaccine should not be given to immune-deficient patients, although vaccination of their susceptible close contacts can and should be carried out in order to reduce their risk of acquiring natural infection (520). Although mumps virus infections are clinically and epidemiologically less important than measles and rubella, community outbreaks of mumps can be costly, and mumps vaccination (given as MMR) is important; it has a benefit-cost ratio of almost 40:1 (522).

Haemophilus influenzae Type b

H. influenzae Type b Infections

In the United States the leading cause of bacterial meningitis in children under 5 years of age is *H. influenzae* type b (Hib) infection (523, 524). Approximately 12,000 cases occur annually, with residual neurologic deficits affecting 25 to 35% and death occurring in 5% of cases. Systemic Hib infections involving other organs also occur, but those that cause otitis media and bronchitis are usually caused by nontypeable strains, not Hib. Available data suggest that every child has an 0.5% risk of developing systemic Hib disease at some time within the first 5 years of life. Although most infections develop during the first year, 35 to 40% occur after 18 months of age, and 25% occur above 24 months of age. There is an increased risk of infection among children enrolled in day care centers and among the socioeconomically disadvantaged. Children with sickle cell disease (525), splenic dysfunction or asplenia, Hodgkin's disease and other hematologic malignancies (526), and antibody deficiency syndromes appear to be at increased risk of acquiring systemic Hib infections (523, 524). In addition, secondary cases of Hib infection occur in younger children who are close household or day care center contacts of primary cases.

H. influenzae Type b (Hib) Vaccine

In 1985 a capsular polysaccharide vaccine against Hib infections was licensed for use in the United States (524). Following vaccination, levels of serum antibody that correlate with clinical protection (1 μg/ml) are achieved in 90% of children 24 to 35 months old, and in 75% of children 18 to 23 months old (524, 527). Mild local reactions and low grade fever are common among vaccinees, but more serious systemic reactions have been extremely rare. A randomized controlled clinical trial has shown that Hib vaccine was approximately 90% protective against systemic disease in children from 2 to 5 years of age (527). Protection was demonstrated over a 4-year follow-up period. Data from this trial were insufficient to demonstrate vaccine efficacy in children 18 to 23 months in age, but protection was not shown in children younger than 18 months of age.

These data provide the basis for the current recommendation that Hib vaccine be given to all children at 24 months of age (524). Although only 25% of systemic Hib infections occur in children above this age, vaccination still is likely to be cost effective (523). Simultaneous vaccination with DTP does not alter the immune response to Hib or DTP antigens. The demonstrated antigenicity (but still uncertain clinical efficacy) of Hib vaccine in children 18 to 23 months of age suggests that vaccination also should be considered for particular groups of high risk children (e.g., day care center attendees). Because of their increased risk of infection, children with sickle cell disease, splenic disorders, and hematologic malignancies also should be vaccinated, although there are few data on the antibody response to Hib vaccine in these patients. As yet, there is no information on which to base a recommendation for revaccination, nor for vaccination of older children and adults with high risk conditions. Hib vaccine is not indicated for older persons with recurrent upper respiratory tract infections, most of which are caused by nontypeable strains of *H. influenzae*. Hib vaccine also is not recommended for children less than 18 months of age. Future development of a more highly antigenic Hib polysaccharide-protein conjugate vaccine may extend the benefits of vaccination to younger children who experience most of the morbidity and mortality from Hib infections.

Tuberculosis and BCG Vaccination

Tuberculosis in the United States

Epidemiologic surveillance continues to show declining rates for tuberculosis in the United States (528, 529). However, more than 20,000 new cases and approximately 1,800 deaths still occur each year. Only 3 to 4% of reported cases affect children less than 5 years old, although children from Hispanic and Indochinese refugee families have a much greater risk for tuberculosis than children in the general population (530). In recent years Indochinese refugees alone have accounted for more than 5% of all reported cases (531). Relatively few cases represent primary infection; more than 90% are due to reactivation of previous tuberculosis (532). An increasing proportion (approximately 30%) of cases now occurs among persons aged 65 years and older.

The steady decline in tuberculosis reflects the success of chemotherapy in newly diagnosed cases, and the effectiveness of screening their contacts and instituting isoniazid (INH) prophylaxis, where indicated. Among children less than 4 years old INH prophylaxis of subclinical infection has been completely effective in preventing clinical disease, and treatment of pulmonary tuberculosis during childhood has been similarly successful in preventing reactivation in later years (533). Nonetheless, approximately 10 million persons currently are infected with tubercle bacilli, and each is at risk for future reactivation (528). Because the care of patients with tuberculosis has shifted from specialized facilities to general hospitals (534), health care workers are at risk of acquiring infection. Yet, in as many as half of cases of reactivation pulmonary tuberculosis the diagnosis is not suspected or not made at the time of hospital admission (535, 536). Often it is not made until postmortem examination (537). In addition to the risk of transmission in hospitals, tuberculosis recently has been recognized as an endemic and nosocomial infection in nursing homes (538, 539).

BCG Vaccines

Current BCG vaccines are derived from a strain of *Mycobacterium bovis* that has been attenuated through serial passage in many laboratories throughout the world (540, 541). When given to tuberculin (purified protein derivative (PPD))-negative individuals BCG vaccine produces an attenuated infection that is believed to confer resistance against subsequent infection with *M. tuberculosis*. BCG vaccine is very safe; although local ulceration and lymphadenitis can occur in up to 10% of vaccinees, disseminated infection is very rare. Severe or fatal BCG infections almost always affect persons with underlying immune deficiencies. In clinical trials conducted over many decades, the efficacy of BCG vaccines for both children and adults has varied from 0 to 80% (540, 542, 543), although in larger studies that were methodologically sound, vaccine efficacy has been firmly established (544).

Current recommendations for BCG vaccine in the United States restrict consideration for its use to selected individuals (e.g., infants in a household) who are PPD-negative and have repeated exposure to untreated or ineffectively treated sputum-positive pulmonary tuberculosis (541). In other groups (e.g., persons without a regular source of medical care) BCG vaccine should be considered if there is a high rate of tuberculosis that cannot be controlled by the usual surveillance and treatment programs.

BCG vaccine is not recommended for routine use among health care workers. However, current guidelines state that it should be considered for certain groups (especially those working in major urban hospitals with a high community prevalence of tuberculosis) if the risk of repeated exposure to tuberculosis is high, and the frequency of PPD conversions indicating new infection exceeds 1% annually (541). Thus, the question of whether to administer BCG vaccine to health care workers is dependent on (*a*) the annual rate of skin test conversion that results from exposure to patients with active pulmonary tuberculosis, and (*b*) the adequacy of alternate measures to control tuberculosis in the hospital setting.

Transmission and Control of Tuberculosis in Hospitals

The undiagnosed patient hospitalized with pulmonary tuberculosis can be a source of transmission to health care workers. Some studies have reported that the average case exposes 35 hospital employees, and that as many as 30 to 45% of contacts of such patients develop tuberculin sensitivity, suggesting nosocomial infection (545, 546). In addition, earlier studies among medical students, physicians, and other health care workers reported annual PPD conversion rates varying from 1 to almost 8% (545, 547), suggesting that these groups should be considered for BCG vaccination.

It appears that these high rates of skin test conversion may overestimate the risk to health care workers of nosocomial tuberculosis. Careful studies have shown that PPD conversion rates have been similar in groups of hospital employees at high and low risk for acquiring infection, and that conversion rates increase with age (547, 548). These findings most likely reflect the "booster effect" that is seen in persons who are repeatedly skin tested (548–550). When a modified two-step approach is taken to skin testing to eliminate the booster effect, annual PPD conversion rates have been much lower; in one study they fell from a range of 4.5 to 5.1% using the conventional approach to as low as 0.59% with the modified two-step approach (551). A recent study also has shown conversion rates among medical students of only 0.13%/year (552). Furthermore, prospective surveillance of hospital personnel and medical students exposed to persons with unsuspected tuberculosis has demonstrated that only 1.65% developed a positive skin test (553), a rate far lower than those reported in other studies (30 to 45%) (545, 546). When cases of unsuspected tuberculosis are hospitalized, employees are exposed for relatively few days; when the diagnosis is suspected at the time of admission and the patient is placed on respiratory isolation, the risk of exposure is minimal (536). Considered together, these data indicate that health care workers caring for patients with known tuberculosis are not at increased risk for acquiring infection. Even when the diagnosis is unsuspected, the risk probably is lower than previously estimated.

It should be noted that the problem of nosocomial tuberculosis is not one which affects only health care workers; patients can acquire infection from health care workers, and in some institutions patients have been at greater risk than hospital employees for nosocomial infection (548, 554). Unlike hospital personnel exposed to patients with tuberculosis, patient contacts of infected health care workers rarely receive adequate follow-up care. However, when they do, nosocomial transmission of tuberculosis from staff to patients is not always the rule (555).

Current guidelines for surveillance and control of tuberculosis among health care workers include skin testing at the time of initial employment. Some experts advocate that persons who are PPD-negative should be retested within 1 to 3 weeks (the two-step approach), although there still is some disagreement as to whether this approach is necessary (550, 551). For health care workers who are PPD-positive, a chest roentgenogram should be obtained. Careful clinical follow-up for 2 to 3 years is necessary, but there now is general agreement that annual chest films are of no value as part of a tuberculosis control program for hospital employees (556–558). However, follow-up chest films may be indicated for employees with high risk factors who have not completed 1 year of INH prophylaxis or an adequate course of chemotherapy. These conditions include a history of inadequately treated tuberculosis, a negative tuberculin test in the past 2 years (with a highly positive recent conversion), immune deficiency disorders and immunosuppressive therapy, diabetes, alcoholism, silicosis, and previous gastrectomy (547). INH prophylaxis generally is indicated for recent PPD converters under 35 years of age (559, 560). Other control measures include limited or widespread investigation of contacts of unsuspected but later diagnosed cases of pulmonary tuberculosis (551, 553). Also, a centralized tuberculosis registry has been helpful in improving communication between hospital personnel and health department staff and practicing physicians who care for patients with tuberculosis (551).

Coordinated efforts are required to control tuberculosis in hospitals and to prevent nosocomial transmission to health care workers and to patients. Infection control practitioners must choose one of two approaches: ongoing surveillance with chemoprophylaxis and chemotherapy of persons who become infected or develop disease, or primary prevention with BCG vaccine. The two approaches are approximately equivalent in their costs, and both are more expensive than simply treating disease when it occurs (561). Current practice seems uniformly to favor surveillance and antituberculous therapy. In settings such as nursing homes, INH chemoprophylaxis can be effective in preventing cases of nosocomial tuberculosis among the elderly (539). In younger adults who are compliant, it also is efficacious, although the potential for INH-associated hepatotoxicity must be recognized (559, 560). However, noncompliance perhaps is a greater problem; among physicians given INH prophylaxis, up to 75% have failed to begin or to complete their course of therapy (545). Yet, the protection afforded by BCG vaccination also is incomplete; tuberculosis has developed in some physicians who have been vaccinated (545). BCG vaccine is used in hospitals as an immunotherapeutic agent for patients with neoplastic diseases (562). However, there are no published reports that it currently is being used to prevent tuberculosis among health care workers.

Vaccines for International Travel

Health care workers, and the patients they care for, frequently travel abroad. Before departure it is important to assess each person's need for protection against hepatitis A, measles, rubella, poliomyelitis, tetanus, and diphtheria. In certain instances, vaccination against rabies, hepatitis B, influenza, and pneumococcal and meningococcal infections also may be indicated.

Typhoid Vaccine

Typhoid fever is an uncommon disease in the United States, with only 500 to 750 cases reported each year. Approximately 40% are indigenously acquired, usually as a result of contact with a chronic carrier or exposure to contaminated food or water (563, 564). In recent years a number of cases have involved health care workers in hospital microbiology laboratories, and in some instances infection has been transmitted to family members, often with serious consequences (565). More than 60% of cases have been acquired during travel abroad, and half of these have been imported from Mexico (563). Overall mortality rates have been 1 to 2%.

Currently available typhoid vaccine contains killed *Salmonella typhosa* organisms (566). Two 0.5-ml doses given subcutaneously at least 4 weeks apart can be 70% or more protective. Its use is confined largely to persons who travel to typhoid-endemic areas. Because of the low incidence of typhoid fever, typhoid vaccine is not recommended for health care workers. However, typhoid fever is a severe disease that often results in hospitalization. Strict adherence to stool precautions and careful handling of laboratory specimens from typhoid patients are mandatory. Laboratory workers who routinely handle *S. typhosa* organisms should be considered for typhoid vaccination. Clinical trials of an orally administered live typhoid vaccine have been promising, and oral vaccine should replace the current killed vaccine in the near future (567).

Yellow Fever Vaccine

Countries in tropical Africa and South America continue to report cases of yellow fever, and the extent of disease in most areas is greater than what officially is reported. Yellow fever vaccine may be indicated for protection against endemic disease, and can be required for entry into some countries. A single dose (0.5 ml subcutaneously) of live attenuated yellow fever vaccine produces effective, long-lasting protection (568, 569). It can be given simultaneously with immune globulin. Local adverse reactions generally are mild. Constitutional symptoms can occur 5 to 10 days after vaccination, but affect no more than 5% of recipients. Yellow fever vaccine is contraindicated in persons with immune deficiencies and anaphylactic reactions to egg ingestion. Because of the theoretical risk to the fetus, the vaccine should not be given to pregnant women unless thay must travel to an endemic area where the risk of yellow fever is high. The vaccine is given only in approved vaccination centers whose locations can be identified by contacting local or state health authorities.

Cholera Vaccine

Currently available cholera vaccines are considered to be no more than 50% effective in reducing the severity of clinical illness, and protection lasts no more than 3 to 6 months (570). However, many countries still require documentation of cholera vaccination for travelers entering from cholera-endemic areas. Two doses, given 1 week to 1 month apart, are recommended for persons who will be exposed to unsanitary conditions in cholera-endemic areas, but one dose will satisfy travel requirements. Serious reactions are very uncommon. Cholera vaccine does not interfere with the response to yellow fever vaccine.

Smallpox Vaccine

With the global eradication of smallpox (571) there no longer is any indication or requirement to administer smallpox vaccine to travelers, and it now is unavailable for civilian use in the U.S.

(572). Smallpox vaccine is reserved for laboratory workers who work with smallpox or closely related orthopox (e.g., monkeypox and vaccinia) viruses. It should never be used for the prevention or treatment of herpes simplex virus infections or any other condition.

Health care workers must be aware that smallpox vaccine continues to be used in the military, and disseminated vaccinia, vaccinia necrosum, and vaccinia encephalitis can develop in vaccine recipients or their close contacts (573, 574). Vaccinia can be a serious or life-threatening illness in children less than 1 year old and in persons with immune deficiencies and eczema. Admission of such patients to hospitals poses a significant risk to health care workers (an increasing proportion of whom will not have received smallpox vaccine) and to other patients. Strict isolation precautions must be observed with vaccinia patients, and if possible only health care workers who have received smallpox vaccine in the past should be given responsibility for their care. In patients with serious complications, vaccinia immune globulin (VIG) may be indicated; it can be obtained by contacting the Centers for Disease Control (572).

Prospects for the Future

There is little doubt that the number of immunizing agents currently available in hospitals will be augmented in the future by newer, more potent, and less expensive vaccines (575). A recent report of an expert committee of the Institute of Medicine of the National Academy of Sciences has provided direction for new vaccine development in the United States (576). Vaccines against five diseases have been singled out for top priority - hepatitis B, influenza (live attenuated or subunit vaccine), varicella, *H. influenzae* type b, and respiratory syncytial virus (live attenuated vaccine). Substantial progress already has been reported for a number of these vaccines (149, 150, 489–492, 519, 577). However, the development of these and other new vaccines alone will not guarantee that patients will be benefited. Efforts must be made to increase public awareness of the importance of current and future vaccines. The problem of developing an equitable system of compensation for vaccine-associated injuries must be solved (578). Provision of pertinent information to physicians and other health care providers about the indications for and use of vaccines must be improved. Finally, there must be greater understanding of the organizational factors that often determine whether vaccines are effectively delivered (575, 579).

The considerable achievements of immunization have come about largely as a result of vaccine delivery in the office practice setting or in publicly funded clinics and programs. To date, the contribution of hospitals to this effort has been marginal. Nonetheless, infection control practitioners have a major responsibility to assure that vaccines, toxoids, and immune globulin preparations are effectively used to prevent the nosocomial transmission of many preventable diseases. Equally important, they must recognize that one of the most effective ways to control the nosocomial transmission of these infections is to immunize patients cared for in hospitals, thereby preventing the acquisition of disease in the community (580).

References

1. Williams WW: Guideline for infection control in hospital personnel. *Infect Control* 4 (Suppl):326–349, 1983.
2. Klein JO: Management of infections in hospital employees. *Am J Med* 70:919–923, 1981.
3. Brown TC, Kreider SD, Lange WR: Guidelines for employee health services in hospitals, clinics and medical research institutions. *J Occupat Med* 25:771–773, 1983.
4. Votra EM, Rutala WA, Sarubbi FA: Recommendations for pregnant employee interaction with patients having communicable infectious diseases. *Am J Infect Control* 11:10–19, 1983.
5. Gurevich I, Tafuro P: Caring for the infectious patient: risk factors during pregnancy. *Infect Control* 5:482–487, 1984.
6. Valenti WM: Employee work restrictions for infection control. *Infect Control* 5:583–584, 1984.
7. Valenti WM, Dorn MR, Andrews BP, Presley BA, Reifler CB: Infection control and employee health: epidemiology and priorities for program development. *Am J Infect Control* 10:149–153, 1982.
8. Haley RW, Emori TG: The employee health service and infection control in U.S. hospitals, 1976–77. I. Screening procedures. *JAMA* 246:844–847, 1981.
9. Haley RW, Emori TG: The employee health service and infection control in U.S. hospitals, 1976–77. II. Managing employee illness. *JAMA* 246:962–966, 1981.
10. Pugliese G, McArthur BJ, Weinstein S, Shannon R, Jackson MM, Lynch P, Tsinzo M, Serkey J, McGuire N: A national task analysis of infection control practitioners, 1982. Part three: the relationship between hospital size and tasks performed. *Am J Infect Control* 12:221–227, 1984.
11. Schneider E, Dykan M: The preplacement medical evaluation of hospital personnel. *J Occupat Med* 20:741–749, 1980.
12. Lewy RM: Occupational health programs for housestaff physicians: preemployment medical examination. *JAMA* 246:1432–1434, 1981.
13. Haley RW, Culver DH, White JW, Morgan WM, Emori TG, Munn VP, Hooton TM: The efficacy

of infection surveillance and control programs in preventing nosocomial infections in US hospitals. *Am J Epidemiol* 121:182–205, 1985.

14. Centers for Disease Control: Recommendation of the Immunization Practices Advisory Committee (ACIP): general recommendations on immunization. *MMWR* 32:1–17, 1983.

15. Centers for Disease Control: Immunization Practices Advisory Committee: adult immunization. *MMWR* 33 (Suppl):S1–S68, 1984.

16. Committee on Immunization: *Guide for Adult Immunization.* Philadelphia, American College of Physicians, 1985.

17. Krugman S: The newly licensed hepatitis B vaccine. Characteristics and indications for use. *JAMA* 247:2012–2015, 1982.

18. Alter HJ: The evolution, implications, and applications of the hepatitis B vaccine. *JAMA* 247:2272–2275, 1982.

19. Centers for Disease Control: Recommendation of the Immunization Practices Advisory Committee. Inactivated hepatitis B vaccine. *MMWR* 31:317–322, 327–328, 1982.

20. Centers for Disease Control: Recommendation of the Immunization Practices Advisory Committee: recommendations for protection against viral hepatitis. *MMWR* 34:313–324, 329–335, 1985.

21. Shah N, Ostrow D, Altman N, Baker AL: Evolution of acute hepatitis B in homosexual men to chronic hepatitis B. Prospective study of placebo recipients in a hepatitis B vaccine trial. *Arch Intern Med* 145:881–882, 1985.

22. Weissberg JT, Andres LI, Smith CI, Weick S, Nichols JE, Garcia G, Robinson WS, Merigan TC, Gregory PB: Survival in chronic hepatitis B: an analysis of 379 patients. *Ann Intern Med* 101:613–616, 1984.

23. de la Monte SM, Hutchins GM, Moore GW: Risk factors for development of lethal sequelae after hepatitis B virus infection in humans. *Am J Med* 77:482–488, 1984.

24. Nowicki MJ, Tong MJ, Nair PV, Stevenson D: Detection of anti-HBc IgM following prednisone treatment in patients with chronic active hepatitis B virus infection. *Hepatology* 4:1129–1133, 1984.

25. Rizzetto M: The delta agent. *Hepatology* 3:729–737, 1983.

26. Govindarajan S, Chin KP, Redeker AG, Peters RL: Fulminant B viral hepatitis: role of delta agent. *Gastroenterology* 86:1417–1420, 1984.

27. Centers for Disease Control: Delta hepatitis—Massachusetts. *MMWR* 33:493–494, 1984.

28. Carreda F, Rossi E, Monforte A d'A, Zampini L, Re T, Meroni B, Moroni M: Hepatitis B virus-associated coinfection and superinfection with δ agent: indistinguishable disease with different outcome. *J Infect Dis* 151:925–928, 1985.

29. Linnemann CC Jr, Hegg ME, Ramundo N, Schiff GM: Screening hospital patients for hepatitis B surface antigen. *Am J Clin Pathol* 67:257–259, 1977.

30. Mahoney JP, Richman AV, Teague PO: Admission screening for hepatitis B surface antigen in a university hospital. *South Med J* 71:624–629, 1978.

31. Maynard JE: Nosocomial viral hepatitis. *Am J Med* 70:439–444, 1981.

32. Osterholm M, Andrews JS Jr: Viral hepatitis in hospital personnel in Minnesota: report of a statewide survey. *Minn Med* 62: 683–689, 1979.

33. Levy BS, Harris JC, Smith JL, Washburn JW, Mature J, Davis A, Crosson JT, Polesky H, Hanson M: Hepatitis B in ward and clinical laboratory employees of a general hospital. *Am J Epidemiol* 106:330–335, 1977.

34. McCormick RD, Maki D: Epidemiology of needle-stick injuries in hospital personnel. *Am J Med* 70:928–932, 1981.

35. Jacobson JT, Burke JP, Conti MT: Injuries of hospital personnel from needles and sharp objects. *Infect Control* 4:100–102, 1983.

36. Neuberger JS, Harris JA, Kundin WD, Bischone A, Chin TDY: Incidence of needlestick injuries in hospital personnel: implications for prevention. *Am J Infect Control* 12:171–176, 1984.

37. Dandoy SE, Kirkman-Liff B, Krakowski FM: Hepatitis B exposure incidents in community hospitals. *Am J Public Health* 74:804–807, 1984.

38. Dandoy S, Kirkman-Liff B: Hepatitis B prevention in small rural hospitals. *West J Med* 141:627–630, 1984.

39. Lewis TL, Alter HJ, Chalmers TC, Holland PV, Purcell RH, Alling DW, Young D, Frenkel LD, Lee SL, Lamson ME: A comparison of the frequency of hepatitis-B antigen and antibody in hospital and nonhospital personnel. *N Engl J Med* 289:647–651, 1973.

40. Pattison CP, Maynard E, Berquist KR, Webster HM: Epidemiology of hepatitis B in hospital personnel. *Am J Epidemiol* 101:59–64, 1975.

41. Leers WD, Kouroupis GM: Prevalence of hepatitis B antibodies in hospital personnel. *Can Med Assoc J* 113:844–847, 1975.

42. Wruble LD, Masi AT, Levinson MJ, Rightsell WA, Bale GF, Bertram P, Blackwell CF: Hepatitis B surface antigen (HBsAg) and antibody (anti-HBs), prevalence among laboratory and non-laboratory hospital personnel. *South Med J* 70:1075–1079, 1977.

43. Denes AE, Smith JL, Maynard JE, Doto IL, Berquist KR, Finkel AJ: Hepatitis B infection in physicians: results of a nationwide seroepidemiologic survey. *JAMA* 239:210–212, 1978.

44. Parry MF, Brown AE, Dobbs LG, Gocke DJ, Neu HC: The epidemiology of hepatitis-B infection in housestaff. *Infection* 6:204–206, 1978.

45. Janzen J, Tripatzis I, Wagner U, Schlieter M, Muller-Dethard E, Wolters E: Epidemiology of hepatitis B surface antigen (HBsAg) and antibody to HBsAg in hospital personnel. *J Infect Dis* 137:261–265, 1978.

46. Hirschowitz BA, Dasher CA, Whitt FJ, Cole GW: Hepatitis B antigen and antibody and tests of liver function—a prospective study of 310 hospital laboratory workers. *Am J Clin Pathol* 73:63–68, 1980.

47. Dienstag JL, Ryan DM: Occupational exposure to hepatitis B virus in hospital personnel: infection or immunization? *Am J Epidemiol* 115:26–39, 1982.

48. Grady GF: Hepatitis B immunity in hospital staff targeted for vaccination: role of screening tests in immunization programs. *JAMA* 248:2266–2269, 1982.

49. Palmer DL, Barash M, King R, Neil F: Hepatitis among hospital employees. *West J Med* 138:519–523, 1983.

50. Jovanovich JF, Saravolatz LD, Arking LM: The risk of hepatitis B among select employee groups in an urban hospital. *JAMA* 250:1893–1894, 1983.

51. Snydman DR, Munoz A, Werner BG, Polk BF, Craven DE, Platt R, Crumpacker C, Ouellet-Hellstrom R, Nash B, Grady G, Dienstag JL: A multivariate analysis of risk factors for hepatitis B infection among hospital employees screened for vaccination. *Am J Epidemiol* 120:684–693, 1984.

52. Harris JR, Finger RF, Kobayashi JM, Hadler SC, Murphy BL, Berkelman RL, Bussell KE: The low risk of hepatitis B in rural hospitals: results of a seroepidemiologic survey. *JAMA* 252:3270–3272, 1984.

53. Hadler SC, Doto IL, Maynard JE, Smith J, Clark B, Mosley J, Eickhoff T, Himmelsbach CK, Cole WR: Occupational risk of hepatitis B infection in hospital workers. *Infect Control* 6:24–31, 1985.

54. Klimek JJ, Brettman L, Neuhaus E, Garibaldi RA: A multi-hospital hepatitis B vaccine program: prevalence of antibody and acceptance of vaccination among high-risk hospital employees. *Infect Control* 6:32–34, 1985.

55. West DJ: The risk of hepatitis B infection among health professionals in the United States: a review. *Am J Med Sci* 287:26–33, 1984.

56. Hardt F, Aldershvile J, Dietrichson O, Juhl E, Nielson JO, Schlichting P, Skinhoj P, Tage-Jensen U: Hepatitis B virus infections among Danish surgeons. *J Infect Dis* 140:972–974, 1979.

57. Berry AJ, Isaacson IJ, Hunt D, Kane MA: The prevalence of hepatitis B viral markers in anesthesia personnel. *Anesthesiology* 60:6–9, 1984.

58. Craig CP, Gribble C, Suarez K: Risk of hepatitis B among phlebotomists. *Am J Infect Control* 9:11–14, 1981.

59. Wands JR, Walker JA, Davis TT, Waterbury LA, Owens AH, Carpenter CCJ: Hepatitis B in an oncology unit. *N Engl J Med* 291:1371–1375, 1974.

60. Tabor E, Gerety RJ, Mott M, Wilbur J: Prevalence of hepatitis B in a high-risk setting: a serologic study of patients and staff in a pediatric oncology unit. *Pediatrics* 61:711–715, 1978.

61. Williams BG, Pruitt B: Natural and induced immunity to hepatitis B virus among the staff of a pediatric oncology center. *Am J Infect Control* 12:261–265, 1984.

62. Kunches LM, Craven DE, Werner BG, Jacobs LM: Hepatitis B exposure in emergency medical personnel: prevalence of serologic markers and need for immunization. *Am J Med* 75:269–272, 1983.

63. Feldman RE, Schiff ER: Hepatitis B in dental professionals. *JAMA* 232:1228–1230, 1975.

64. Mosley JW, Edwards VM, Casey G, Redeker AG, White E: Hepatitis B virus infection in dentists. *N Engl J Med* 293:729–734, 1975.

65. Smith JL, Maynard JE, Berquist KR, Doto IL, Webster HM, Sheller MJ: Comparative risk of hepatitis B among physicians and dentists. *J Infect Dis* 133:705–706, 1976.

66. Berris B, Feinman SV, Sinclair JC, Wrobel D: Hepatitis and hepatitis B surface antigen and antibody in dentists. *Can Med Assoc J* 119:1040–1043, 1978.

67. Williams SV, Huff JC, Feinglass EJ, Gregg MB, Hatch MH, Matsen JM: Epidemic viral hepatitis, type B, in hospital personnel. *Am J Med* 57:904–911, 1974.

68. Mayor GH, Hourani MR, Greenbaum DS, Patterson MJ: Prevalence of hepatitis B in 27 Michigan hemodialysis centers. *Am J Public Health* 69:581–584, 1979.

69. Alter HJ, Chalmers TC, Freeman BM, Lunceford JL, Lewis TL, Holland PV, Pizzo PA, Plotz PH, Meyer WJ III: Health-care workers positive for hepatitis B surface antigen: are their contacts at risk? *N Engl J Med* 292:454–457, 1975.

70. Williams SV, Pattison CP, Berquist KR: Dental infection with hepatitis B. *JAMA* 232:1231–1233, 1975.

71. Alter HJ, Chalmers TC: The HBsAg positive health worker revisited. *Hepatology* 1:467–470, 1981.

72. Snydman DR, Hindman SH, Wineland MD, Bryan JA, Maynard JE: Nosocomial viral hepatitis B: a cluster among staff with subsequent transmission to patients. *Ann Intern Med* 85:573–577, 1975.

73. Collaborative study by Central Public Health Laboratories: Acute hepatitis B associated with gynecologic surgery. *Lancet* 1:1–6, 1980.

74. Carl M, Blakey DL, Francis DP, Maynard JE: Interruption of hepatitis B transmission by modification of a gynecologist's surgical technique. *Lancet* 1:731–733, 1982.

75. Levin ML, Maddrey WC, Wands JR, Mendeloff AI: Hepatitis B transmission by dentists. *JAMA* 228:1139–1140, 1974.

76. Rimland D, Parken WE, Miller GB Jr, Schrack WD: Hepatitis B outbreak traced to an oral surgeon. *N Engl J Med* 296:953–958, 1977.

77. Hadler SC, Sorley DL, Acree KH, Webster HM, Schable CA, Francis DP, Maynard JE: An outbreak of hepatitis B in a dental practice. *Ann Intern Med* 95:133–138, 1981.

78. Reingold AL, Kane MA, Murphy BL, Checko P, Francis DP, Maynard JE: Transmission of hepatitis B by an oral surgeon. *J Infect Dis* 145:262–268, 1982.

79. Goodman RA, Ahtone JL, Finton RJ: Hepatitis B transmission from dental personnel to patients: unfinished business. *Ann Intern Med* 96:119, 1982.

80. Centers for Disease Control: Hepatitis B among dental patients—Indiana. *MMWR* 34:73–75, 1985.

81. Rothstein SS, Goldman HS, Arcomano A: Methods of hepatitis B virus transfer in oral surgery. *J Oral Surg* 39:754–756, 1981.

82. Allen AL, Organ RJ: Occult blood accumulation under the fingernails: a mechanism for the spread of blood-borne infection. *J Am Dent Assoc* 105:455–459, 1982.

83. Ahtone J, Goodman RA: Hepatitis B and dental personnel: transmission to patients and prevention issues. *J Am Dent Assoc* 106:219–222, 1983.

84. Polesky HF, Hanson M: AABB-CAP survey data on hepatitis—incidence, surveillance, and preven-

tion. *Am J Clin Pathol* 74:565–568, 1980.

85. Najem GR, Louria DB, Thind IS, Lavenhar MA, Gocke DJ, Baskin SE, Miller AM, Frankel HJ, Notkin J, Jacobs MG, Weiner B: Control of hepatitis B infection: the role of surveillance and an isolation hemodialysis center. *JAMA* 245:153–157, 1981.
86. Favero MS, Deane N, Leger RT, Sosin AE: Effect of multiple use of dialyzers on hepatitis B incidence in patients and staff. *JAMA* 245:166–167, 1981.
87. Alter MJ, Ahtone J, Maynard JE: Hepatitis B virus transmission associated with a multiple-dose vial in a hemodialysis unit. *Ann Intern Med* 99:330–333, 1983.
88. Favero MS, Maynard JE, Leger RT, Graham DR, Dixon RE: Guidelines for the care of patients hospitalized with viral hepatitis. *Ann Intern Med* 91:872–876, 1979.
89. Seeff LB, Koff RS: Passive and active immunoprophylaxis of hepatitis B. *Gastroenterology* 86:958–981, 1984.
90. Stevens CE, Szmuness W, Goodman AI, Weseley SA, Fotino M: Hepatitis B vaccine: immune responses in haemodialysis patients. *Lancet* 2:1211–1213, 1980.
91. Crosnier J, Jungers P, Couroucé AM, Laplanche A, Benhamon E, Degos F, Lacour B, Prunet P, Cerisier Y, Guesry P: Randomized placebo controlled trial of hepatitis B surface antigen vaccine in French haemodialysis units. II. Haemodialysis patients. *Lancet* 1:797–800, 1981.
92. McLean AA, Hilleman MR, McAleer WJ, Buynak EB: Summary of world-wide experience with H-B-vax (B,MSD). *J Infect* 7:95–104, 1983.
93. Schaaff DM, Lender M, Snedeker P, Graham LA: Hepatitis B vaccine in a hospital. *Ann Intern Med* 101:720–721, 1984.
94. Centers for Disease Control: Suboptimal response to hepatitis B vaccine given by injection into the buttock. *MMWR* 34:105–108, 113, 1985.
95. Cockshott WP, Thompson GT, Howlett LJ, Seeley ET: Intramuscular or intralipomatous injections? *N Engl J Med* 307:356–358, 1982.
96. Szmuness W, Stevens CE, Oleszko WR, Goodman A: Passive active immunization against hepatitis B: immunogenicity studies in adult Americans. *Lancet* 1:575–577, 1981.
97. Gerety RJ, Tabor E: Newly licensed hepatitis B vaccine: known safety and unknown risks. *JAMA* 249:745–746, 1983.
98. Sacks HS, Rose DN, Chalmers TC: Should the risk of acquired immunodeficiency syndrome deter hepatitis B vaccination? A decision analysis. *JAMA* 252:3375–3377, 1984.
99. Stevens CE: No increased incidence of AIDS in recipients of hepatitis B vaccine. *N Engl J Med* 308:1163–1164, 1983.
100. Centers for Disease Control: Hepatitis B vaccine: evidence confirming lack of AIDS transmission. *MMWR* 33:685–687, 1984.
101. Gerberding JL, Hopewell PC, Karinsky LS, Sande MA: Transmission of hepatitis B without transmission of AIDS by accidental needlestick. *N Engl J Med* 312:56–57, 1985.
102. Stevens CE, Taylor PE, Rubenstein P, Ting RCY, Bodner AJ, Sarngadharan MG, Gallo RC: Safety of hepatitis B vaccine. *N Engl J Med* 312:375–376, 1985.
103. Papaevangelou G, Kallinikos G, Roumeliotou A, Politou K: Risk of AIDS in recipients of hepatitis B vaccine. *N Engl J Med* 312:376–377, 1985.
104. Crosnier J, Jungers P, Couroucé AM, Laplanche A, Benhamon E, Degos F, Lacour B, Prunet P, Cerisier Y, Guesry P: Randomized placebo-controlled trial of hepatitis B surface antigen vaccine in French haemodialysis units. I. Medical staff. *Lancet* 1:455–459, 1981.
105. Desmeyer J, Colaert J, de Groote G, Reynders M, Reerink-Brongers EE, Lelie PN, Dees PJ, Reesink HW: Efficacy of heat-inactivated hepatitis B vaccine in haemodialysis patients and staff: double-blind, placebo-controlled trial. *Lancet* 2:1323–1328, 1983.
106. Szmuness W, Stevens CE, Harley EJ, Zang EA, Alter HJ, Taylor PE, DeVera A, Chen GTS, Kellner S, and the Dialysis Vaccine Trial Study Group: Hepatitis B vaccine in medical staff of hemodialysis units: efficacy and subtype cross-protection. *N Engl J Med* 307:1481–1486, 1982.
107. Stevens CE, Alter HJ, Taylor PE, Zang EA, Harley EJ, Szmuness W, and the Dialysis Vaccine Trial Study Group: Hepatitis B vaccine in patients receiving hemodialysis: immunogenicity and efficacy. *N Engl J Med* 311:496–501, 1984.
108. Szmuness W, Stevens CE, Harley EJ, Zang EA, Oleszko WR, William DC, Sadovsky R, Morrison JM, Kellner A: Hepatitis B vaccine: demonstration of efficacy in a controlled clinical trial in a high-risk population in the United States. *N Engl J Med* 303:833–841, 1980.
109. Szmuness W, Stevens CE, Zang EA, Harley EA, Kellner A: A controlled clinical trial of the efficacy of hepatitis B vaccine (Heptavax B): a final report. *Hepatology* 1:377–388, 1981.
110. Francis DP, Hadler SC, Thompson SE, Maynard JE, Ostrow DG, Altman N, Braff EH, O'Malley P, Hawkins D, Judson FN, Penley K, Nylund T, Christie G, Meyers F, Moore JN, Gardner A, Doto IL, Miller JH, Reynolds GH, Murphy BL, Schable CA, Clark BT, Curran JW, Redeker AG: The prevention of hepatitis B with vaccine: report of the Centers for Disease Control multi-center efficacy trial among homosexual men. *Ann Intern Med* 97:362–366, 1982.
111. Dienstag JL, Werner BG, Polk BG, Snydman DR, Craven DE, Platt R, Crumpacker CS, Ouellet-Hellstrom R, Grady GF: Hepatitis B vaccine in health care personnel: safety, immunogenicity, and indications of efficacy. *Ann Intern Med* 101:35–40, 1984.
112. Directive on Hepatitis B vaccine. Veterans Administration Professional Services Letter. June 28, 1982. *Infect Control* 3:430, 432, 1982.
113. American Hospital Association: Hepatitis B vaccine recommendations for hospital employees. October 1982. *Infect Control* 4:41–43, 1983.
114. Mann JM, Babb CJ, Hull HG, Ball FD, Brown GW, Steece RS: Low prevalence of hepatitis B infections among residents of an institution for the mentally retarded in New Mexico. *West J Med* 141:339–341, 1984.
115. Lohiya G, Lohiya S, Caires S, Reesal MR: Occupational exposure to hepatitis B virus. Analysis of

indications for hepatitis B vaccine. *J Occupat Med* 26:189–196, 1984.

116. Skinhoj JP, Aldershvile J, Kjersem M, Black FM: Hepatitis B infection in Vietnamese families. *J Med Virol* 11:125–129, 1983.

117. Nichols ES, Chaudhary RK, Kennedy DA, Jung J, Davies JW, Gill P: Hepatitis B followup among Indochinese refugees. *Can Med Assoc J* 131:1073–1076, 1984.

118. Zuckerman AJ: Perinatal transmission of hepatitis B. *Arch Dis Child* 59:1007–1009, 1984.

119. Prevention of perinatally transmitted hepatitis B infection. *Lancet* 1:939–941, 1984.

120. Sinatra FR, Shah P, Weissman JY, Thomas DW, Merritt RJ, Tong MJ: Perinatal transmitted acute icteric hepatitis B in infants born to hepatitis B surface antigen-positive and anti-hepatitis Be positive carrier mothers. *Pediatrics* 70:557–559, 1983.

121. Delaplane D, Yogev R, Crussi F, Shulman ST: Fatal hepatitis B in early infancy: the importance of identifying HBsAg-positive pregnant women and providing immunoprophylaxis to their newborns. *Pediatrics* 72:176–180, 1983.

122. Beasley RP, Hwang LY: Postnatal infectivity of hepatitis B surface antigen-carrier mothers. *J Infect Dis* 147:185–190, 1983.

123. Beasley RP, Hwang LY, Lee GC, Lan CC, Roan CH, Huang FY, Chen CL: Prevention of perinatally transmitted hepatitis B virus infection with hepatitis B immune globulin and hepatitis B vaccine. *Lancet* 2:1099–1102, 1983.

124. Wong VCW, Ip HMH, Reesink HW, Lelie PN, Reerink-Brongers EE, Yeung CY, Ma HK: Prevention of the HBsAg carrier states in newborn infants in mothers who are chronic carriers of HBsAg and HBeAg by administration of hepatitis B vaccine and hepatitis B immune globulin: double-blind randomized placebo-controlled study. *Lancet* 1:921–926, 1984.

125. Stevens CE, Toy PT, Tong MJ, Taylor PE, Vyas GN, Nair PV, Gudavalli M, Krugman S: Perinatal hepatitis B virus transmission in the United States. *JAMA* 253:1740–1745, 1985.

126. Koff RS, Slavin MM, Connelly LJD, Rosen DR: Contagiousness of acute hepatitis B: secondary attack rates in household contacts. *Gastroenterology* 72:297–300, 1977.

127. Perrillo RP, Gelb L, Campbell C, Wellinghoff W, Ellis FR, Overby L, Aach RD: Hepatitis B e antigen, DNA polymerase activity, and infection of household contacts with hepatitis B virus. *Gastroenterology* 76:1319–1325, 1979.

128. Redeker AG, Mosley JW, Gocke DJ, McKee AP, Pollack W: Hepatitis B immune globulin as a prophylactic measure for spouses exposed to acute type B hepatitis. *N Engl J Med* 293:1055–1059, 1975.

129. Perrillo RP, Campbell CR, Strang S, Bodicky CJ, Costigan DJ: Immune globulin and hepatitis B immune globulin: prophylactic measures for intimate contacts exposed to acute type B hepatitis. *Arch Intern Med* 144:81–85, 1984.

130. Papaevangelou G, Roumeliotou-Karayannis A, Tassopoulos N, Kolaitis N, Contoyannis P, Krugman S: Post-exposure hepatitis B vaccination of sexual partners of acute viral hepatitis patients. *J Infect* 7 (Suppl):63–67, 1983.

131. Seeff LB, Wright EC, Zimmerman HJ, Alter HJ, Dietz AA, Felsher BF, Finkelstein JD, Garcia-Pont P, Gerin JL, Greenlee HB, Hamilton J, Holland PV, Kaplan PM, Kiernan T, Koff RS, Leevy CM, McAuliffe VJ, Nath N, Purcell RH, Schiff ER, Schwartz CC, Tamburro CH, Vlahcevic Z, Zemel R, Zimmon DS: Type B hepatitis after needle-stick exposure: prevention with hepatitis B immune globulin. Final report of the Veterans Administration Cooperative Study. *Ann Intern Med* 88:285–293, 1978.

132. A Combined Medical Research Council and Public Health Laboratory Service Report: The incidence of hepatitis B infection after antecedent exposure and anti-HBs immunoglobulin prophylaxis. *Lancet* 1:6–8, 1980.

133. Grady GF, Lee VA, Prince AM, Gitnick GL, Fawaz KA, Vyas GN, Levitt MD, Senior JR, Galambos JT, Bynum TE, Singleton JW, Clowdus BF, Akdamar K, Aach RD, Winkelman EI, Schiff GM, Hersh T: Hepatitis B immune globulin for accidental exposures among medical personnel: final report of a multicenter controlled trial. *J Infect Dis* 138:625–637, 1978.

134. Masuko K, Mitsui T, Iwano K, Yamazaki C, Aihara S, Baba K, Takai E, Tsuda F, Nakamura T, Miyakawa Y, Mayumi M: Factors influencing postexposure immunoprophylaxis of hepatitis B virus infection with hepatitis B immune globulin. High deoxyribonucleic acid polymerase activity in the inocula of unsuccessful cases. *Gastroenterology* 88:151–155, 1985.

135. Centers for Disease Control: Postexposure prophylaxis of hepatitis. *MMWR* 33:285–290, 1984.

136. Dandoy S, Kirkman-Liff B: Should your hospital's employees receive hepatitis B vaccine? *Am J Infect Control* 12:297–300, 1984.

137. Dandoy S, Kirkman-Liff BL, Krakowski FM: Hepatitis B exposure of multiple hospital employees: five case studies. *Arch Intern Med* 144:720–723, 1984.

138. Kirkman-Liff B, Dandoy S: Cost of hepatitis B prevention in hospital employees: post-exposure prophylaxis. *Infect Control* 5:385–389, 1984.

139. Pantelick EL, Steere AC, Lewis HD, Miller DJ: Hepatitis B infection in hospital personnel during an eight year period: policies for screening and pregnancy in high risk areas. *Am J Med* 70:924–927, 1981.

140. Mulley AG, Silverstein MD, Dienstag JL: Indications for use of hepatitis B vaccine, based on cost-effectiveness analysis. *N Engl J Med* 307:644–652, 1982.

141. Hamilton JD: Hepatitis B virus vaccine: an analysis of its potential use in medical workers. *JAMA* 250:2145–2150, 1983.

142. Hanson M, Polesky JF: Prevalence of anti-HBc in anti-HBs positive individuals: implications for selecting vaccine candidates. *Am J Clin Pathol* 82:716–719, 1984.

143. Perrillo RP, Parker ML, Campbell C, Sanders GE, Strang SP, Regenstein F: Prevaccination screening of medical and dental students. Should low levels of antibody to hepatitis B surface antigen preclude vaccination? *JAMA* 250:2481–2484, 1983.

144. Palmer DL, King DL: Attitude toward hepatitis

vaccination among high-risk hospital employees. *J Infect Dis* 147:1120–1121, 1983.

145. Anderson AC, Hodges GR: Acceptance of hepatitis B vaccine among high-risk health workers. *Am J Infect Control* 11:207–211, 1983.

146. Littenberg B, Ransohoff DF: Hepatitis B vaccination: three decision strategies for the individual. *Am J Med* 77:1023–1026, 1984.

147. Baker CH, Brennan JM: Keeping health care workers healthy: legal aspects of hepatitis B immunization programs. *N Engl J Med* 311:684–688, 1984.

148. Sachs HL: Dentistry and hepatitis B: the legal risks. *J Am Dent Assoc* 102:177–180, 1981.

149. Scolnick EM, McLean AA, West DJ, McAleer WJ, Miller WJ, Buynack EB: Clinical evaluation in healthy adults of a hepatitis B vaccine made by recombinant DNA. *JAMA* 251:2812–2815, 1984.

150. Jilg W, Lorbeer B, Schmidt M, Wilske B, Zoulek G, Deinhardt F: Clinical evaluation of a recombinant hepatitis B vaccine. *Lancet* 2:1174–1175, 1984.

151. Francis DP, Maynard JE: The transmission and outcome of hepatitis A, B, and non-A, non-B: a review. *Epidemiol Rev* 1:17–31, 1979.

152. Francis DP, Hadler SC, Prendergast TJ, Peterson E, Ginsberg MM, Lookabaugh C, Holmes JR, Maynard JE: Occurrence of hepatitis A, B, and non-A/non-B in the United States. CDC Sentinel County Hepatitis Study I. *Am J Med* 76:69–74, 1984.

153. Carl M, Kantor RJ, Webster HM, Fields HA, Maynard JE: Excretion of hepatitis A virus in the stools of hospitalized hepatitis patients. *J Med Virol* 9:125–129, 1982.

154. Snydman DR, Dienstag JL, Stedt B, Brink EW, Ryan DM, Fawaz KA: Use of IgM-hepatitis A antibody testing. Investigating a common source, food-borne outbreak. *JAMA* 245:827–830, 1981.

155. Hadler SC, Webster HM, Erben JJ, Swanson JE, Maynard JE: Hepatitis A in day-care centers: a community-wide assessment. *N Engl J Med* 302:1222–1227, 1980.

156. Corey L, Holmes KK: Sexual transmission of hepatitis A in homosexual men: incidence and mechanism. *N Engl J Med* 302:435–438, 1980.

157. Christenson B, Brostrom C, Bottinger M, Hermanson J, Weiland O, Ryd G, Berg JVR, Sjoblom R: An epidemic outbreak of hepatitis A among homosexual men in Stockholm. Hepatitis A, a special hazard for the male homosexual subpopulation in Sweden. *Am J Epidemiol* 116:599–607, 1982.

158. Hall WT, Madden DL, Mundon FK, Brandt DEL, Clarke NA: Protective effect of immune serum globulin (ISG) against hepatitis A infection in a natural epidemic. *Am J Epidemiol* 106:72–75, 1977.

159. Hadler SC, Erben JJ, Matthews D, Starko K, Francis DP, Maynard JE: Effect of immunoglobulin on hepatitis A in day-care centers. *JAMA* 249:48–53, 1983.

160. Smallwood LA, Tabor E, Finlayson JS, Gerety RJ: Antibodies to hepatitis A virus in immune serum globulin. *Lancet* 2:482–483, 1980.

161. Mortimer PP, Parry JV: Anti-hepatitis-A-virus potency of immunoglobulin. *Lancet* 1:1364–1365, 1981.

162. Meyers JD, Romm FJ, Tiken WS, Bryan JA: Food-borne hepatitis A in a general hospital: epidemiologic study of an outbreak attributed to sandwiches. *JAMA* 231:1049–1053, 1975.

163. Orenstein WA, Wu E, Wilkins J, Robinson K, Francis DP, Timko N, Wayne R: Hospital-acquired hepatitis A: report of an outbreak. *Pediatrics* 67:494–497, 1981.

164. Williams G, Murray-Lyon I: Surgical transmission of hepatitis A. *Lancet* 1:848, 1981.

165. Goodman RA, Carder CC, Allen JR, Orenstein WA, Finton RJ: Nosocomial hepatitis A transmission by an adult patient with diarrhea. *Am J Med* 73:220–226, 1982.

166. Ebisawa I, Kurosu Y, Hatashita T: Nursery-associated hepatitis A traced to a male nurse. *J Hyg Lond* 92:251–254, 1984.

167. Klein BS, Michaels JA, Rytel MW, Berg KG, Davis JP: Nosocomial hepatitis A. A multinursery outbreak in Wisconsin. *JAMA* 252:2716–2721, 1984.

168. Krober MS, Bass JW, Brown JD, Lemon SM, Rupert KJ: Hospital outbreak of hepatitis A: risk factors for spread. *Pediatr Infect Dis* 3:296–299, 1984.

169. Reed CM, Gustafson TL, Siegel J, Duer P: Nosocomial transmission of hepatitis A from a hospital-acquired case. *Pediatr Infect Dis* 3:300–303, 1984.

170. Alter MJ: Nosocomial hepatitis A infection: can we wash our hands of it? *Pediatr Infect Dis* 3:294–295, 1984.

171. Szmuness W, Dienstag JL, Purcell RH, Prince AM, Stevens CE, Levine RW: Hepatitis type A and hemodialysis. A seroepidemiologic study in 15 U.S. centers. *Ann Intern Med* 87:8–12, 1977.

172. Mayor GH, Klein AM, Kelly TJ, Patterson MJ: Antibody to hepatitis A and hemodialysis. *Am J Epidemiol* 116:821–827, 1982.

173. Seeberg S, Brandberg A, Hermodsson S, Larsson P, Lundgren S: Hospital outbreak of hepatitis A secondary to blood exchange in a baby. *Lancet* 1:1155–1156, 1981.

174. Barbara JAJ, Howell DR, Briggs M, Parry JV: Post-transfusion hepatitis A. *Lancet* 1:738, 1982.

175. Skidmore S, Boxall E, Ala F: A case report of post-transfusion hepatitis A. *J Med Virol* 10:223, 1982.

176. Hollinger FB, Khan NC, Oefinger PE, Yawn DH, Schmulen AC, Dreesman GR, Melnick JL: Post-transfusion hepatitis type A. *JAMA* 250:2313–2317, 1983.

177. Sherertz RJ, Russell BA, Reuman PD: Transmission of hepatitis A by transfusion of blood products. *Arch Intern Med* 144:1579–1580, 1984.

178. Noble RC, Kane MA, Reeves SA, Roeckel I: Posttransfusion hepatitis A in a neonatal intensive care unit. *JAMA* 252:2711–2715, 1984.

179. Grady GF: Hepatitis A in neonatal care units: not rare enough? *JAMA* 252:2755, 1984.

180. Anderson BN, Coulepsis AG, Gust ID: Towards a hepatitis A vaccine. A review. *J Hyg Lond* 93:269–276, 1984.

181. Orenstein WA, Bart KJ, Hinman AR, Preblud

SR, Greaves WL, Doster SW, Stetler HC, Sirotkin B: The opportunity and obligation to eliminate rubella from the United States. *JAMA* 251:1988–1994, 1984.

182. Hinman AR, Orenstein WA, Bart KJ, Preblud SR: Rational strategy for rubella vaccination. *Lancet* 1:39–41, 1983.

183. Sever JL, South MA, Shaver KA: Delayed manifestations of congenital rubella. *Rev Infect Dis* 7 (Suppl):S164–S169, 1985.

184. Appel MW: The multihandicapped child with congenital rubella: impact on family and community. *Rev Infect Dis* 7 (Suppl):S17–S21, 1985.

185. Miller E, Cradock-Watson JE, Pollock TM: Consequences of confirmed maternal rubella at successive stages of pregnancy. *Lancet* 2:781–784, 1982.

186. Centers for Disease Control: Recommendation of the Immunization Practices Advisory Committee (ACIP): rubella prevention. *MMWR* 33:301–310, 315–318, 1984.

187. Preblud SR, Serdula MK, Frank FA Jr, Brandling-Bennett AD, Hinman AR: Rubella vaccination in the United States: a ten year review. *Epidemiol Rev* 2:171–194, 1980.

188. Schoenbaum SC, Hyde JN, Bartoshesky L, Crampton K: Benefit cost of rubella vaccination policy. *N Engl J Med* 294:306–310, 1976.

189. Anderson RM, May RM: Vaccination against rubella and measles: quantitative investigations of different policies. *J Hyg Camb* 90:259–325, 1983.

190. Hethcote HW: Measles and rubella in the United States. *Am J Epidemiol* 117:2–13, 1983.

191. Schoenbaum SC: Benefit-cost aspects of rubella immunization. *Rev Infect Dis* 7 (Suppl):S210–S211, 1985.

192. Centers for Disease Control: Rubella and congenital rubella—United States, 1983. *MMWR* 33:237–242, 247, 1984.

193. Centers for Disease Control: Elimination of rubella and congenital rubella syndrome—United States. *MMWR* 34:65–66, 1985.

194. Nelson DB, Layde MM, Chatton TB: Rubella susceptibility in inner-city adolescents: the effect of a school immunization law. *Am J Public Health* 72:710–713, 1982.

195. Serdula MK, Marks JS, Herrmann KL, Orenstein WA, Hall AD, Bomgaars MR: Therapeutic abortions following rubella infections in pregnancy: the potential impact on the incidence of congenital rubella syndrome. *Am J Public Health* 74:1249–1251, 1984.

196. Judson FN, Shaw BS, Vernon TM: Mandatory premarital rubella screening in Colorado. *JAMA* 229:1200–1202, 1974.

197. Falvo CE, Weiss KE, Liss SM: A rubella screening and immunization program in an adolescent clinic. *Am J Public Health* 69:283–285, 1979.

198. Vaeth SJ: A rubella vaccination program for women entering the U.S. Army. *Public Health Rep* 94:564–567, 1979.

199. Shilian DM: Screening and immunization of rubella-susceptible women: experience in a large, prepaid medical group. *JAMA* 240:662–663, 1978.

200. Chappell JA, Taylor MAH: Implications of rubella susceptibility in young adults. *Am J Public Health* 69:279–281, 1979.

201. Crawford GE, Gremillion DH: Epidemic measles in Air Force recruits: impact of immunization. *J Infect Dis* 144:403–410, 1981.

202. Blouse LE, Lathrop GD, Dupuy HJ, Ball RJ: Rubella screening and vaccination program for U.S. Air Force trainees: an analysis of findings. *Am J Public Health* 72:280–283, 1982.

203. Preblud SR, Gross F, Halsey NA, Hinman AR, Herrmann KL, Koplan JP: Assessment of susceptibility to measles and rubella. *JAMA* 247:1134–1137, 1982.

204. Dales LG, Chin J: Public health implications of rubella antibody levels in California. *Am J Public Health* 72:167–172, 1982.

205. Lieberman E, Faich GA, Simon PR, Mullan RJ: Premarital rubella screening in Rhode Island. *JAMA* 245:1333–1335, 1981.

206. Robinson RG, Dudenhoeffer FE, Holyroyd HJ, Baker LR, Bernstein DI, Cherry JD: Rubella immunity in older children, teenagers, and young adults: a comparison of immunity in those immunized with those unimmunized. *J Pediatr* 101:188–191, 1982.

207. Birdsong WM, Harris RE: Rubella susceptibility and syphilis in Asian pregnancies: *Am J Obstet Gynecol* 142:705–706, 1982.

208. Miller KA, Zager TD: Rubella susceptibility in an adolescent female population. *Mayo Clin Proc* 59:31–34, 1984.

209. Hunter K, Stagno S, Capps E, Smith RJ: Prenatal screening of pregnant women for infections caused by cytomegalovirus, Epstein-Barr virus, herpesvirus, rubella, and *Toxoplasma gondii*. *Am J Obstet Gynecol* 145:269–273, 1983.

210. Hambling MH: Changes in the distribution of rubella antibodies in women of childbearing age during the first eight years of a rubella vaccination programme. *J Infect* 2:341–346, 1980.

211. Clarke M, Schild GC, Miller C, Seagroatt V, Pollock TM, Finlay SE, Barbara JAJ: Surveys of rubella antibodies in young adults and children. *Lancet* 1:667–669, 1983.

212. Chretien JH, Esswein JG, McGarvey MA, de-Stwolinski A: Rubella: pattern of outbreak in a university. *South Med J* 69:1042–1044, 1976.

213. Centers for Disease Control: Rubella in universities—Washington, California. *MMWR* 31:394–395, 1982.

214. Marks JS, Serdula MK, Halsey NA, Gunaratne MVH, Craven RB, Murphy KA, Kobayashi GY, Wiebenga NH: Saturday night fever: a common source outbreak of rubella among adults in Hawaii. *Am J Epidemiol* 114:574–583, 1981.

215. Centers for Disease Control: Rubella outbreak among office workers—New York City. *MMWR* 32:349–352, 1983.

216. Dales LG, Chin J: An outbreak of congenital rubella. *West J Med* 135:266–270, 1981.

217. Lamprecht C, Schauf V, Warren D, Nelson K, Northrop R, Christiansen M: An outbreak of congenital rubella in Chicago. *JAMA* 247:1129–1133, 1982.

218. Hillary IB, Griffith AH: Persistence of antibody 10 years after vaccination with Wistar RA27/3

strain live attenuated rubella vaccine. *Br Med J* 280:1580–1581, 1980.

219. Balfour HH Jr, Groth KE, Edelman CK, Amren DP, Best JM, Banatvala JE: Rubella viraemia and antibody responses after rubella vaccination and reimmunisation. *Lancet* 1:1078–1080, 1981.

220. Herrmann KL, Halstead SB, Wiebenga NH: Rubella antibody persistence after immunization. *JAMA* 247:193–196, 1982.

221. O'Shea S, Best JM, Banatvala JE, Marshall WC, Dudgeon JA: Rubella vaccination: persistence of antibodies for up to 16 years. *Br Med J* 285:253–255, 1982.

222. O'Shea S, Best JM, Banatvala JE: Viremia, virus excretion, and antibody responses after challenge in volunteers with low levels of antibody to rubella virus. *J Infect Dis* 148:639–647, 1983.

223. Serdula MK, Halstead SB, Wiebenga NH, Herrmann KL: Serological response to rubella revaccination. *JAMA* 251:1974–1977, 1984.

224. Horstmann DM, Schlueuderberg A, Emmons JE, Evans BK, Randolph MF, Andiman WA: Persistence of vaccine-induced immune responses to rubella: comparison with natural infection. *Rev Infect Dis* 7 (Suppl):S80–S85, 1985.

225. Greaves WL, Orenstein WA, Hinman AR, Nersesian WS: Clinical efficacy of rubella vaccine. *Pediatr Infect Dis* 2:284–286, 1983.

226. Bart SW, Stetler HC, Preblud SC, Williams NR, Orenstein WA, Bart KJ, Hinman AR, Herrmann KL: Fetal risk associated with rubella vaccine: an update. *Rev Infect Dis* 7 (Suppl):S95–S102, 1985.

227. Hayden GF, Herrmann KL, Buimovici-Klein E, Weiss KE, Neiburg PI, Mitchell JE: Subclinical congenital rubella infection associated with maternal rubella vaccination in early pregnancy. *J Pediatr* 96:869–872, 1980.

228. Bernstein DI, Ogra PL: Fetomaternal aspects of immunization with RA27/3 live attenuated rubella virus vaccine during pregnancy. *J Pediatr* 97:467–470, 1980.

229. Banatvala JE, O'Shea S, Best JM, Nicholls MV, Cooper K: Transmission of RA27/3 rubella vaccine strain to products of conception. *Lancet* 1:392, 1981.

230. Preblud SR, Stetler HC, Frank FA Jr, Greaves WL, Hinman AR, Herrmann KL: Fetal risk associated with rubella vaccine. *JAMA* 246:1413–1417, 1981.

231. Centers for Disease Control: Rubella vaccination during pregnancy—United States, 1971–1983. *MMWR* 33:365–368, 373, 1984.

232. Partridge JW, Flewett TH, Whitehead JEM: Congenital rubella affecting an infant whose mother had rubella antibodies before conception. *Br Med J* 282:187–188, 1981.

233. Bott LM, Eizenberg DH: Congenital rubella after successful vaccination. *Med J Aust* 1:514–515, 1982.

234. Enders G, Calm A, Schaub J: Rubella embryopathy after previous maternal rubella vaccination. *Infection* 12:96–98, 1984.

235. Mann JM, Preblud SR, Hoffman RD, Brandling-Bennett AD, Hinman AR, Herrmann KL: Assessing risks of rubella infection during pregnancy: a standardized approach. *JAMA* 245:1647–1652, 1981.

236. Polk BF, Modlin JF, White JA, DeGirolami PC: A controlled comparison of joint reactions among women receiving one of two rubella vaccines. *Am J Epidemiol* 115:19–25, 1982.

237. Tingle AJ, Yang T, Allen M, Kettyls RP, Larke B, Schulzer M: Prospective immunological assessment of arthritis induced by rubella vaccine. *Infect Immun* 40:22–28, 1983.

238. Tingle AJ, Pot CH, Chantler JK: Prolonged arthritis, viraemia hypogammaglobulinemia, and failed seroconversion following rubella immunisation. *Lancet* 1:1475–1476, 1984.

239. Weiss KE, Falvo CE, Buimovici-Klein E, Magill JW, Cooper LZ: Evaluation of an employee health service as a setting for a rubella screening and immunization program. *Am J Public Health* 69:281–283, 1979.

240. McLaughlin MC, Gold LH: The New York rubella incident: a case for changing hospital policy regarding rubella testing and immunization. *Am J Public Health* 69:287–289, 1979.

241. Strassburg MA, Imagawa DT, Fannin SL, Turner JA, Chow AW, Murray RA, Cherry JD: Rubella outbreak among hospital employees. *Obstet Gynecol* 57:283–288, 1981.

242. Fliegel PE, Weinstein WM: Rubella outbreak in a prenatal clinic: management and prevention. *Am J Infect Control* 10:29–33, 1982.

243. Centers for Disease Control: Rubella in hospital personnel and patients—Colorado. *MMWR* 28:325–327, 1979.

244. Polk BF, White JA, DeGirolami PC, Modlin JF: An outbreak of rubella among hospital personnel. *N Engl J Med* 303:541–545, 1980.

245. Orenstein WA, Heseltine PNR, LeGagnoux SJ, Portnoy B: Rubella vaccine and susceptible hospital employees. Poor physician participation. *JAMA* 245:711–713, 1981.

246. Hartstein AI, Quan MA, Williams ML, Osterud HT, Foster LR: Rubella screening and immunization of health care personnel: critical appraisal of a voluntary program. *Am J Infect Control* 11:1–9, 1983.

247. Gladstone JL, Millian SJ: Rubella exposure in an obstetric clinic. *Obstet Gynecol* 57:182–186, 1981.

248. Centers for Disease Control: Nosocomial rubella infection—North Dakota, Alabama, Ohio. *MMWR* 29:629–631, 1981.

249. McCubbin JH, Smith JS: Rubella in a practicing obstetrician: a preventable problem. *Am J Obstet Gynecol* 136:1087, 1980.

250. Elvin-Lewis M, Storch GA, Parker M: Control of a rubella outbreak in a dental school population. *J Am Dent Assoc* 108:783–785, 1984.

251. Centers for Disease Control: Rubella in hospitals—California. *MMWR* 32:37–39, 1983.

252. Strassburg MA, Stephenson TG, Habel LA, Fannin SL: Rubella in hospital employees. *Infect Control* 5:123–126, 1984.

253. Povar GJ, Maloney M, Watson WN, McBean AM, Giguere G: Rubella screening and follow-up immunization in Vermont. *Am J Public Health* 69:285–286, 1979.

254. Griffiths PD, Baboonian C: Is postpartum rubella vaccination worthwhile? *J Clin Pathol* 35:1340–1344, 1982.

255. Landes RD, Bass JW, Millunchick EW, Oetgen

WJ: Neonatal rubella following postpartum maternal immunization. *J Pediatr* 97:465–467, 1980.

256. Klein EB, Byrne T, Cooper LZ: Neonatal rubella in a breast-fed infant after postpartum maternal infection. *J Pediatr* 97:774–775, 1980.

257. Preblud SR, Hinman AR: Rubella vaccination of hospital employees. *JAMA* 245:736–737, 1981.

258. Greaves WL, Orenstein WA, Stetler HC, Preblud SR, Hinman AR, Bart KJ: Prevention of rubella transmission in medical facilities. *JAMA* 248:861–864, 1982.

259. The Advisory Committee on Infections within Hospitals of the American Hospital Association: Recommendations for the control of rubella within hospitals. *Infect Control* 2:410–411, 424, 1981.

260. Schoenbaum SC: Rubella policies for hospitals and health workers. *Infect Control* 2:366, 416–417, 1981.

261. Evans ME, Schaffner W: Rubella immunization of hospital personnel: a debate. *Infect Control* 2:387–390, 1981.

262. Fischer DL, Jungkind HD, Nieman RE: Factors influencing participation in a rubella vaccination program. *Am J Infect Control* 10:121–127, 1982.

263. Sacks JJ, Olson B, Soter J, Clark C: Employee rubella screening programs in Arizona hospitals. *JAMA* 249:2675–2678, 1983.

264. Centers for Disease Control: Recommendation of the Immunization Practices Advisory Committee (ACIP): measles prevention. *MMWR* 31:217–224, 229–231, 1982.

265. Hinman AR, Eddins DL, Kirby CD, Orenstein WA, Bernier RH, Turner PM, Bloch AB: Progress in measles elimination. *JAMA* 247:1592–1595, 1982.

266. Hinman AR, Orenstein WA, Bloch AB, Bart KJ, Eddins DL, Amler RW, Kirby CD: Impact of measles in the United States. *Rev Infect Dis* 5:439–444, 1983.

267. Hinman AR, Kirby CD, Eddins DL, Orenstein WA, Bernier RH, Turner PM, Bart KJ: Elimination of indigenous measles from the United States. *Rev Infect Dis* 5:538–545, 1983.

268. Nolan TF Jr, Goodman RA, Patriarca PA, Hinman AR: Hospitalizations for measles, 1970–78. *Am J Public Health* 72:1037–1039, 1982.

269. Centers for Disease Control: Subacute sclerosing panencephalitis surveillance—United States. *MMWR* 31:585–588, 1982.

270. Robbins KB, Brandling-Bennett AD, Hinman AR: Low measles incidence: association with enforcement of school immunization laws. *Am J Public Health* 71:270–274, 1981.

271. Amler RW, Bloch AB, Orenstein WA, Bart KJ, Turner PM, Hinman AR: Imported measles in the United States. *JAMA* 248:2129–2133, 1982.

272. Krause PS, Cherry JD, Desada-Tous S, Champion JG, Strassburg M, Sullivan C, Spencer MJ, Bryson YJ, Welliver RC, Boyer KM: Epidemic measles in young adults: clinical, epidemiologic, and serologic studies. *Ann Intern Med* 90:873–876, 1979.

273. Amler RW, Kim-Farley RJ, Orenstein WA, Doster SW, Bart KJ: Measles on campus. *J Am Coll Health* 32:53–57, 1983.

274. Amler RW, Orenstein WA: Measles: current status and outbreak control on campus. *J Am Coll Health* 33:64–66, 1984.

275. Centers for Disease Control: Measles—New Hampshire. *MMWR* 33:549–554, 559, 1984.

276. Centers for Disease Control: Multiple measles outbreaks on college campuses—Ohio, Massachusetts, Illinois. *MMWR* 34:129–130, 1985.

277. Fox JP: Herd immunity and measles. *Rev Infect Dis* 5:463–466, 1983.

278. Gremillion DH, Crawford GE: Measles pneumonia in young adults: an analysis of 106 cases. *Am J Med* 71:539–542, 1981.

279. Gavish D, Kleinman Y, Morag A, Chajek-Shaul T: Hepatitis and jaundice associated with measles in young adults: an analysis of 65 cases. *Arch Intern Med* 143:674–677, 1983.

280. Martin DB, Weiner LB, Nieburg PI, Blair DC: Atypical measles in adolescents and young adults. *Ann Intern Med* 90:877–881, 1979.

281. Hinman AR, Koplan JP: Public health policy toward atypical measles syndrome in the United States. *Med Decis Making* 2:71–77, 1982.

282. Centers for Disease Control: Measles in medical settings—United States. *MMWR* 30:125–126, 1981.

283. Foulon G, Klein-Zablan ML, Guansou-Nezzi L, Martin-Bouyer G: Preventing the spread of measles in childrens' clinics. *Lancet* 2:1498–1499, 1983.

284. Seavy D, Moloy M, Dasco C, Anderson D, Feigen R: Nosocomial measles in a children's hospital transmitted by adult health care personnel (abstract). *Am J Infect Control* 10:111–112, 1984.

285. Remington PL, Hall WN, Davis IH, Herald A, Gunn RA: Airborne transmission of measles in a physician's office. *JAMA* 253:1574–1577, 1985.

286. Dales LG, Kizer KW: Measles transmission in medical facilities. *West J Med* 142:415–416, 1985.

287. Bloch AB, Orenstein WA, Ewing WM, Spain WH, Mallison GF, Herrmann KL, Hinman AR: Measles outbreak in a pediatric practice: airborne transmission in an office setting. *Pediatrics* 75:676–683, 1985.

288. Davis RM, Orenstein WA, Frank JA Jr, Sacks JJ, Dales LG, Preblud SR, Bart KJ, Williams NM, Hinman AR: Transmission of measles in medical settings, 1980 through 1984. *JAMA* 255:1295–1298, 1986.

289. Scott RM, Butler AB, Schydlower M, Rawlings P: Ineffectiveness of historical data in predicting measles susceptibility. *Pediatrics* 73:777–780, 1984.

290. Zilber N, Rannon L, Alter M, Kahana E: Measles, measles vaccination, and risk of subacute sclerosing panencephalitis (SSPE). *Neurology* 33:1558–1564, 1983.

291. Smith FL, Curran AS, Raciti KA, Black FL: Reported measles in persons immunlogically primed by prior vaccination. *J Pediatr* 101:391–393, 1982.

292. Yeager AS, Harvey B, Crosson FJ Jr, Davis JH, Ross LA, Halonen PE: Need for measles revaccination in adolescents: correlation with birth date prior to 1972. *J Pediatr* 102:191–195, 1983.

293. Stetler HC, Gens RD, Seastrom GR: Severe local reactions to live measles virus vaccine following an immunization program. *Am J Public Health* 73:899–900, 1983.

294. Herman JJ, Radin R, Schneiderman R: Allergic reactions to measles (rubeola) vaccine in patients hypersensitive to egg protein. *J Pediatr* 102:196–199, 1983.

295. Hopkins RA, DeMartin KE, Reifler CB: Process and results of an immunization requirement at the University of Rochester. *J Am Coll Health* 33:76–80, 1984.

296. Kay HEM, Rankin A: Immunoglobulin prophylaxis of measles in acute lymphoblastic leukemia. *Lancet* 1:901–902, 1984.

297. Centers for Disease Control: Transmission of measles across state lines—Kentucky, New Hampshire, Tennessee, Virginia. *MMWR* 31:123–126, 1982.

298. Centers for Disease Control: Recommendation of the Immunization Practices Advisory Committee (ACIP): diphtheria, tetanus, pertussis: guidelines for vaccine prophylaxis and other preventive measures. *MMWR* 34:405–414, 419–426, 1985.

299. Dixon JMS: Diphtheria in North America. *J Hyg Camb* 93:419–432, 1984.

300. Rubin FL, Nagel J, Fireman P: Antitoxin responses in the elderly to tetanus-diphtheria (Td) immunization. *Am J Epidemiol* 108:145–149,1978.

301. Crossley K, Irvine P, Warren JB, Lee BK, Meade K: Tetanus and diphtheria immunity in urban Minnesota adults. *JAMA* 242:2298–2300, 1979.

302. Weiss BP, Strassburg MA, Feeley JC: Tetanus and diphtheria immunity in an elderly population in Los Angeles County. *Am J Public Health* 73:802–804, 1983.

303. Myers K, Heppell J, Bode WE, Culp CE, Thurber DL, van Scoy RE: Tetanus after anorectal abscess. *Mayo Clin Proc* 59:429–430, 1984.

304. Myers MG, Beckman CW, Vosdingh RA, Hankins WA: Primary immunization with tetanus and diphtheria toxoids: reaction rates and immunogenicity in older children and adults. *JAMA* 248:2478–2480, 1982.

305. Simonsen O, Kjeldsen K, Heron I: Immunity against tetanus and effect of revaccination 25–30 years after primary vaccination. *Lancet* 2:1240–1242, 1984.

306. Rubin FL, Fireman P: Follow-up study: protective immunization in the elderly. *Am J Public Health* 73:1330, 1983.

307. Middaugh J: Side effects of diphtheria-tetanus toxoid. *Am J Public Health* 69:246–249, 1979.

308. Jacobs RL, Lowe RS, Lanier BQ: Adverse reactions to tetanus toxoid. *JAMA* 247:40–42, 1982.

309. Thorley JD, Holmes RK, Sanford JP: Tetanus and diphtheria antitoxin levels following a hospital based adult immunization program. *Am J Epidemiol* 101:438–443, 1975.

310. Brand DA, Acampora D, Gottlieb LD, Glancy KE, Frazier WH: Adequacy of antitetanus prophylaxis in six hospital emergency rooms. *N Engl J Med* 309:636–640, 1983.

311. Hinman AR: The pertussis vaccine controversy. *Public Health Rep* 99:255–259, 1984.

312. Broome CV, Preblud SR, Bruner B, McGowan JE, Hayes PS, Harris PP, Elsea W, Fraser DW: Epidemiology of pertussis, Atlanta, 1977. *J Pediatr* 98:362–367, 1981.

313. Centers for Disease Control: Pertussis—United States, 1982 and 1983. *MMWR* 33:573–575, 1984.

314. Cherry J: The epidemiology of pertussis and pertussis immunization in the United Kingdom and in the United States: a comparative study. *Curr Probl Pediatr* 9:1–56, 1984.

315. Geller RJ: The pertussis syndrome: a persistent problem. *Pediatr Infect Dis* 3:182–186, 1984.

316. Trollfors B, Rabo E: Whooping cough in adults. *Br Med J* 283:696–697, 1981.

317. MacLean DW: Adults with pertussis. *J R Coll Gen Pract* 32:298–300, 1982.

318. Nelson JD: The changing epidemiology of pertussis in young infants. The role of adults as reservoirs of infection. *Am J Dis Child* 132:371–373, 1978.

319. Mertsola J, Ruuskanen O, Eerola E, Viljanen MK: Intrafamilial spread of pertussis. *J Pediatr* 103:359–363, 1983.

320. Miller DL, Alderslade R, Ross EM: Whooping cough and whooping cough vaccine: the risks and benefits debate. *Epidemiol Rev* 4:1–24, 1982.

321. Pollock TM, Miller E, Lobb J: Severity of whooping cough in England before and after the decline in pertussis immunisation. *Arch Dis Child* 59:162–165, 1984.

322. Hinman AR, Koplan JP: Pertussis and pertussis vaccine: reanalysis of benefits, risks and costs. *JAMA* 251:3109–3113, 1984.

323. Cody CL, Baroff LJ, Cherry JD, Marcy SM, Manclark CR: The nature and rate of adverse reactions associated with DTP and DT immunization in infants and children. *Pediatrics* 68:650–660, 1981.

324. Pollock TM, Mortimer JY, Miller E, Smith G: Symptoms after primary immunization with DTP and DT vaccine. *Lancet* 2:146–149, 1984.

325. Miller DL, Ross EM, Alderslade R, Bellman MH, Rawson NSB: Pertussis immunisation and serious acute neurological illness in children. *Br Med J* 282:1595–1599, 1981.

326. Cherry J, Shields WD: Recurrent seizures after diphtheria, tetanus and pertussis immunization. Cause and effect v. temporal association. *Am J Dis Child* 138:904–907, 1984.

327. Hoffman JH, Hunter JC, Hasslemeyer EG: SIDS and DTP. In *Proceedings of the 17th Immunization Conference.* Atlanta, Centers for Disease Control, 1982, pp 79–88.

328. Sato Y, Kimura M, Fukumi H: Development of a pertussis component vaccine in Japan. *Lancet* 1:122–126, 1984.

329. Kurt TL, Yeager AS, Guenette S, Dunlop S: Spread of pertussis by hospital staff. *JAMA* 221:264–267, 1972.

330. Linnemann CC Jr, Ramundo N, Perlstein PH, Minton SD, Englender GS, McCormick JB, Hayes PS: Use of pertussis vaccine in an epidemic involving hospital staff. *Lancet* 2:540–543, 1975.

331. Valenti WM, Pincus PH, Messner MK: Nosocomial pertussis: possible spread by a hospital visitor. *Am J Dis Child* 134:520–521, 1980.

332. Halsey NA, Welling MA, Lehman RM: Nosocomial pertussis: a failure of erythromycin treatment and prophylaxis. *Am J Dis Child* 134:521–522, 1980.

333. Henry RL, Dorman DC, Skinner JA, Mellis CM:

Antimicrobial therapy in whopping cough. *Med J Aust* 2:27–28, 1981.

334. Glezen WP: Serious morbidity and mortality associated with influenza epidemics. *Epidemiol Rev* 4:25–44, 1982.

335. Alling DW, Blackwelder WC, Stuart-Harris CW: A study of excess mortality during influenza epidemics in the United States, 1968–1976. *Am J Epidemiol* 113:30–43, 1981.

336. Centers for Disease Control: *Influenza Surveillance: Summary: July 1979–June 1981.* Report no. 94. Atlanta, Centers for Disease Control, June 1984.

337. Mathur U, Bentley DW, Hall CB, Roth FK, Douglas RG Jr: Influenza A/Brazil/78 (H1N1) infection in the elderly. *Am Rev Respir Dis* 123:633–635, 1981.

338. Baine WB, Luby JP, Martin SM: Severe illness with influenza B. *Am J Med* 68:181–189, 1980.

339. Nolan TF, Goodman RA, Hinman AR, Noble GR, Kendall AP, Thacker SB: Morbidity and mortality associated with influenza B in the United States, 1979–1980. A report from the Centers for Disease Control. *J Infect Dis* 142:360–362, 1982.

340. Hurwitz ES, Nelson DB, Davis C, Morens D, Schonberger LB: National surveillance for Reye syndrome: a five year review. *Pediatrics* 70:895–900, 1982.

341. Glezen WP: Viral pneumonia as a cause and result of hospitalization. *J Infect Dis* 147:765–770, 1983.

342. Barker WH, Mullooly JP: Impact of epidemic type A influenza in a defined adult population. *Am J Epidemiol* 112:798–811, 1980.

343. Barker WH, Mullooly JP: Pneumonia and influenza deaths during epidemics: implications for prevention. *Arch Intern Med* 142:85–89, 1982.

344. Foy HM, Cooney MK, Allen I, Kenny GE: Rates of pneumonia during influenza epidemics in Seattle, 1964–1975. *JAMA* 241:253–258, 1979.

345. Kimball AM, Foy HM, Cooney MK, Allen ID, Matlock M, Plorde JJ: Isolation of respiratory syncytial and influenza viruses from the sputum of patients hospitalized with pneumonia. *J Infect Dis* 147:181–184, 1983.

346. Barker WH: Excess pneumonia and influenza associated hospitalization during influenza epidemics in the U.S., 1970–78. *Am J Public Health*, 76:761–764, 1986.

347. Kavet J: A perspective on the significance of pandemic influenza. *Am J Public Health* 67:1067–1070, 1977.

348. Douglas RG Jr, Betts RF, Hruska J, Hall CB: Epidemiology of nosocomial viral infections. In Weinstein L, Remington J (eds): *Seminars in Infectious Diseases.* New York, Stratton, 1979, pp 98–144.

349. Blumenfeld HL, Kilbourne ED, Louria DB, Rogers DE: Studies on influenza in the pandemic of 1957–1958. I. An epidemiologic, clinical, and serologic investigation in an intrahospital epidemic, with a note on vaccination efficacy. *J Clin Invest* 38:199–212, 1959.

350. Vogel RA, Trotter YJ, Shinaberger JH, McCroan JE: The genesis and spread of a hospital staphylococcal epidemic on an adult medical ward. *N Engl J Med* 261:1301–1309, 1959.

351. Kapila R, Lintz DI, Tecson FT, Ziskin L, Louria DB: A nosocomial outbreak of influenza A. *Chest* 71:576–579, 1977.

352. McDougal BA, Hodges GR, Lewis HD, Davis JW, Caldwell SA: Nosocomial influenza A infection. *South Med J* 70:1023–1024, 1977.

353. Valenti WM, Menegus MA, Hall CB, Pincus PH, Douglas RG Jr: Nosocomial viral infections. I. Epidemiology and significance. *Infect Control* 1:33–37, 1979.

354. Balkovic ES, Goodman RA, Rose FB, Borel CO: Nosocomial influenza A (H1N1) infection. *Am J Med Technol* 46:318–320, 1980.

355. Van Voris LP, Belshe RB, Shaffer JL: Nosocomial influenza B virus infection in the elderly. *Ann Intern Med* 96:153–158, 1982.

356. Bauer CR, Elie K, Spence L, Stein L: Hong Kong influenza in a neonatal intensive care unit. *JAMA* 223:1233–1235, 1973.

357. Gardner PS, Court SDM, Brocklebank JT, Downham MAPS, Weightman D: Virus cross-infection in paediatric wards. *Br Med J* 2:571–575, 1973.

358. Hall CB, Douglas RG Jr: Nosocomial influenza as a cause of intercurrent fever in infants. *Pediatrics* 55:673–677, 1975.

359. Wenzel RP, Deal EC, Hendley JO: Hospital-acquired viral respiratory illness on a pediatric ward. *Pediatrics* 60:367–371, 1977.

360. Meibalane R, Sedmak GV, Sasidharan P, Garg P, Grausz JP: Outbreak of influenza in a neonatal intensive care unit. *J Pediatr* 91:974–976, 1977.

361. Hall CB: Nosocomial viral respiratory infections: perennial weeds on pediatric wards. *Am J Med* 70:670–676, 1981.

362. Hammond GW, Cheang M: Absenteeism among hospital staff during an influenza epidemic: implications for immunoprophylaxis. *Can Med Assoc J* 131:449–452, 1984.

363. Young LS, LaForce FM, Head JJ, Feeley JC, Bennett JV: A simultaneous outbreak of meningococcal and influenza infections. *N Engl J Med* 287:5–9, 1972.

364. Serie C, Barme M, Hannoun C, Thibon M, Beck H, Aquino JP: Effects of vaccination on an influenza epidemic in a geriatric hospital. *Dev Biol Stand* 39:317–321, 1977.

365. Gowda HT: Influenza in a geriatric unit. *Postgrad Med J* 55:188–191, 1979.

366. Mathur U, Bentley DW, Hall CB: Concurrent respiratory syncytial virus and influenza A infections in the institutionalized elderly and chronically ill. *Ann Intern Med* 93:49–52, 1980.

367. Centers for Disease Control: Influenza A in a hospital—Illinois. *MMWR* 30:79–80, 85, 1981.

368. Rubin FL, Johnston F, Streiff EJ: Influenza in a partially immunized aged population: effectiveness of killed Hong Kong vaccine against infection with the England strain. *JAMA* 230:863–866, 1974.

369. Hall WN, Goodman RA, Noble GR, Kendal AP, Steece RS: An outbreak of influenza B in an elderly population. *J Infect Dis* 144:297–302, 1981.

370. Goodman RA, Orenstein WA, Munro TF, Smith SC, Sikes RK: Impact of influenza A in a nursing

home. *JAMA* 247:1451–1453, 1982.

371. Centers for Disease Control: Influenza vaccine efficacy in nursing home outbreaks reported during 1981–1982. *MMWR* 31:190, 195, 1982.

372. Budnick LD, Stricof RL, Ellis F: An outbreak of influenza A (H3N2) in a nursing home, 1982. *NY State J Med* 84:235–238, 1984.

373. Arroyo JC, Postic B, Brown A, Harrison K, Birgenheier R, Dowda H: Influenza A/Philippines/ 2/82 outbreak in a nursing home: limitations of influenza vaccination in the aged. *Am J Infect Control* 12:329–334, 1984.

373. Patriarca PA, Weber JA, Parker RA, Hall WN, Kendall AP, Bregman DJ, Schonberger LB: Efficacy of influenza vaccine in nursing homes: reduction in illness and complications during an influenza A(H3N2) epidemic. *JAMA* 253:1136– 1139, 1985.

375. Patriarca PA, Weber JA, Parker RA, Orenstein WA, Hall WN, Kendal AP, Schonberger LB: Risk factors for outbreaks of influenza in nursing homes: a case-control study. *Am J Epidemiol* 124:114–119, 1986.

376. Hoffman PC, Dixon RE: Control of influenza in the hospital. *Ann Intern Med* 87:725–728, 1977.

377. Valenti WM, Betts RF, Hall CB, Hruska JF, Douglas RG Jr: Nosocomial viral infections. II. Guidelines for prevention and control of respiratory viruses, herpesviruses, and hepatitis viruses. *Infect Control* 1:165–178, 1979.

378. Centers for Disease Control: Recommendation of the Immunization Practices Advisory Committee (ACIP): prevention and control of influenza. *MMWR* 34:261–268, 273–275, 1985.

379. LaMontagne JR, Noble GR, Quinnan GV, Curlin GT, Blackwelder WC, Smith JI, Ennis FI, Bozeman FM: Summary of clinical trials of inactivated influenza vaccine—1978. *Rev Infect Dis* 5:723– 736, 1983.

380. Brandriss MW, Betts RF, Mathur U, Douglas RG Jr: Response of elderly subjects to monovalent A/ USSR/77 (H1N1) and trivalent A/USSR/77 (H1N1) - A/Texas/77 (H3N2) - B/Hong Kong/ 72 vaccines. *Am Rev Respir Dis* 121:681–684, 1981.

381. Langmuir AD, Bregman DJ, Kurland LT, Nathanson N, Victor M: An epidemiologic and clinical evaluation of Guillain-Barré syndrome reported in association with the administration of swine influenza vaccines. *Am J Epidemiol* 119:841–879, 1984.

382. Kaplan JE, Katona P, Hurwitz ES, Schonberger LB: Guillain-Barré syndrome in the United States, 1979–1980 and 1980–1981. Lack of association with influenza vaccination. *JAMA* 248:698–700, 1982.

383. Brenner JG, Hayner NS: Guillain Barré syndrome and its relationship to swine influenza vaccination in Michigan, 1976–1977. *Am J Epidemiol* 119:880–889, 1984.

384. Stults BM, Hashisaki PA: Influenza vaccination and theophylline pharmacokinetics in patients with chronic obstructive lung disease. *West J Med* 139:651–654, 1983.

385. Patriarca PA, Kendal AP, Stricof RL, Weber JA, Meissner MK, Dateno B: Influenza vaccination

and warfarin or theophylline toxicity in nursing home residents. *N Engl J Med* 308:1601–1602, 1983.

386. Lipsky BA, Pecoraro RE, Roben NJ, de Blaquiere P, Delaney CJ: Influenza vaccination and warfarin anticoagulation. *Ann Intern Med* 100:835–837, 1984.

387. Howells CHL, Vesselinova-Jenkins CK, Evans AD, James J: Influenza vaccination and mortality from bronchopneumonia in the elderly. *Lancet* 1:381–383, 1975.

388. Aymard M, Bentejac MC, Larbaigt G, Michaut D, Triau R: Efficacy of the anti-influenza A vaccination during epidemics due to A/Vic/3/75 and A/Texas/1/77 viruses. *Dev Biol Stand* 43:231– 239, 1979.

389. Barker WH, Mullooly JP: Influenza vaccination of elderly persons: reduction in pneumonia and influenza hospitalizations and deaths. *JAMA* 244:2547–2549, 1980.

390. Phair J, Kauffman CA, Bjornson A, Adams L, Linneman C Jr: Failure to respond to influenza vaccine in the aged: correlation with B-cell number and function. *J Lab Clin Med* 92:882–888, 1978.

391. Powers RD, Hayden FG, Samuelson J, Gwaltney JM Jr: Immune response of adults to sequential influenza vaccination. *J Med Virol* 14:169–175, 1984.

392. Hoskins TW, Davies JR, Smith AJ, Miller CL, Allchin A: Assessment of inactivated influenza A vaccine after three outbreaks of influenza A at Christ's Hospital. *Lancet* 1:33–35, 1979.

393. Ruben FL: Prevention of influenza in the elderly. *J Am Geriatr Soc* 30:577–580, 1982.

394. Schildt RA, Luedke DW, Kaiser G, El-Beheri S, Laham MN: Antibody response to influenza immunization in adult patients with malignant disease. *Cancer* 44:1629–1635, 1979.

395. Nikoskelainen J, Vaananen P, Forsstrom J, Kasanen A: Influenza vaccination in patients with chronic renal failure. *Scand J Infect Dis* 14:245– 251, 1982.

396. Younkin SW, Betts RF, Roth FK, Douglas RG Jr: Reduction in fever and symptoms in young adults with influenza A/Brazil/78 H1N1 infection after treatment with aspirin or amantadine. *Antimocrob Agents Chemother* 23:577–582, 1983.

397. Horadam VW, Sharp JG, Smilack JD, McAnalley BH, Garriott JC, Stephens MK, Prati RC, Brater DC: Pharmacokinetics of amantadine hydrochloride in subjects with normal and impaired renal function. *Ann Intern Med* 94:454–458, 1981.

398. Dolin R, Reichman RC, Madore HP, Maynard R, Linton PN, Webber-Jones J: A controlled trial of amantadine and rimantadine in the prophylaxis of influenza A infection. *N Engl J Med* 307:580– 584, 1982.

399. Patriarca PA, Kater NA, Kendal AP, Bregman DJ, Smith JD, Sikes RK: Safety of prolonged administration of rimantadine hydrochloride in the prophylaxis of influenza A virus infections in nursing homes. *Antimicrob Agents Chemother* 26:101–103, 1984.

400. O'Donoghue JM, Ray CG, Terry DW Jr, Beaty HN: Prevention of nosocomial influenza infection

with amantadine. *Am J Epidemiol* 97:276–282, 1973.

401. Fedson DS, Kessler HA: A hospital-based influenza immunization program, 1977–78. *Am J Public Health* 73:442–445, 1983.
402. Fedson DS: Influenza: the continuing need and justification for immunization. *Primary Care* 4:761–779, 1977.
403. Centers for Disease Control: Reye syndrome—United States, 1984. *MMWR* 34:13–16, 1985.
404. Bailowitz A, Kaslow RA: Use of amantadine in the United States, 1977–1982. *J Infect Dis* 151:372–373, 1985.
405. Ratner ER, Fedson DS: Influenza and pneumococcal immunization in medical clinics, 1978–1980. *Arch Intern Med* 143:2066–2069, 1983.
406. McDonald CJ, Hui SL, Smith DM, Tierney WM, Cohen SJ, Weinberger M, McCabe GP: Reminders to physicians from an introspective computer medical record: a two-year randomized trial. *Ann Intern Med* 100:130–138, 1984.
407. Davidson RA, Fletcher SW, Retchin S, Duh S: A nurse-initiated reminder system for the periodic health examination: implementation and evaluation. *Arch Intern Med* 144:2167–2170, 1984.
408. Fedson DS: Influenza and pneumococcal immunization in medical clinics, 1971–1983. *J Infect Dis* 149:817–818, 1984.
409. Patriarca PA, Weber JA, Meissner MK, Stricof RL, Dateno B, Braun JE, Arden NH, Kendal AP: Use of influenza vaccine in nursing homes. *J Am Geriatr Soc* 33:463–466, 1985.
410. Riddiough MA, Sisk JE, Bell JC: Influenza vaccination: cost-effectiveness and public policy. *JAMA* 249:3189–3195, 1983.
411. Mufson MA: Pneumococcal infections. *JAMA* 246:1942–1948, 1981.
412. Fedson DS: Improving the use of pneumococcal vaccine through a strategy of hospital-based immunization: a review of its rationale and implications. *J Am Geriatr Soc* 33:142–150, 1985.
413. Burman LA, Norrby R, Trollfors B: Invasive pneumococcal infections: incidence, predisposing factors, and prognosis. *Rev Infect Dis* 7:133–142, 1985.
414. MacFarlane JT, Finch RG, Ward MJ, Macrae AD: Hospital study of adult community-acquired pneumonia. *Lancet* 2:255–258, 1982.
415. Hook EW III, Horton CA, Shaberg DR: Failure of intensive care unit support to influence mortality from pneumococcal bacteremia. *JAMA* 249:1055–1057, 1983.
416. Lamonthe F, Delage G, Laverdiere M, Saint-Antoine P: Serogroups and serotypes of pneumococci in Montreal: correlations with age, outcome and indications for vaccination. *Can Med Assn J* 130:737–740, 1984.
417. Schlech WF, Ward JI, Band JD, Hightower A, Fraser DW, Broome CV: Bacterial meningitis in the United States, 1978 through 1981. *JAMA* 253:1749–1754, 1985.
418. Davies AJ, Hawkey PM, Simpson RA, O'Connor KM: Pneumococcal cross infection in hospital. *Br Med J* 288:1195, 1984.
419. Graybill JR, Marshall LW, Charache P, Wallace CK, Melvin VB: Nosocomial pneumonia: a continuing major problem. *Am Rev Respir Dis* 108:1130–1140, 1973.
420. Bryan C, Reynolds KL: Bacteremic nosocomial pneumonia: analysis of 172 episodes from a single metropolitan area. *Am Rev Respir Dis* 129:668–671, 1984.
421. Fedson DS, Chiarello LA: Previous hospital care and pneumococcal bacteremia: importance for pneumococcal immunization. *Arch Intern Med* 143:885–889, 1983.
422. Mylotte JM, Beam TR Jr: Comparison of community-acquired and nosocomial pneumococcal bacteremia. *Am Rev Respir Dis* 124:265–268, 1981.
423. Ruben FL, Norden CW, Kornica Y: Pneumococcal bacteremia at a medical/surgical hospital for adults between 1975 and 1980. *Am J Med* 77:1091–1094, 1984.
424. Berk SL, Gallemore GM, Smith JK: Nosocomial pneumococcal pneumonia in the elderly. *J Am Geriatr Soc* 29:319–321, 1981.
425. Robbins JB, Austrian R, Lee CJ, Rastogi SC, Schiffman G, Henrichsen J, Makela PH, Broome CV, Facklam RR, Tiesjema RH, Parke JC Jr: Considerations for formulating the second generation pneumococcal capsular polysaccharide vaccine with emphasis on cross-reactive types within groups. *J Infect Dis* 148:1136–1159, 1983.
426. Centers for Disease Control: Recommendations of the Immunization Practices Advisory Committee (ACIP): update: pneumococcal polysaccharide vaccine usage—United States. *MMWR* 33:273–276, 281, 1984.
427. Ruben FL, Uhrin M: Specific immunoglobulin-class antibody responses in the elderly before and after 14-valent pneumococcal vaccine. *J Infect Dis* 151:845–849, 1985.
428. Katz MA, Landesman SH, Schiffman G: A comparison of antibody concentration measured by mouse protection assay and radioimmunoassay in sera from patients at high risk of developing pneumococcal disease. *Mol Immunol* 21:1061–1065, 1984.
429. Schwartz JS: Pneumococcal vaccine: clinical efficacy and effectiveness. *Ann Intern Med* 96:208–220, 1982.
430. Shapiro ED, Clemens JD: A controlled evaluation of the protective efficacy of pneumococcal vaccine for patients at high risk of serious pneumococcal infections. *Ann Intern Med* 101:325–330, 1984.
431. Bolan G, Broome CV, Facklam RR, Plikaytis BD, Fraser DW, Schlech WF: Pneumococcal vaccine efficacy in selected populations in the United States. *Ann Intern Med* 104:1–6, 1986.
432. Zarrabi MH, Rosner F: Serious infections in adults following splenectomy for trauma. *Arch Intern Med* 144:1421–1424, 1984.
433. Caplan ES, Boltansky H, Snyder MJ, Rooney J, Hoyt NJ, Schiffman G, Cowley RA: Response of traumatized splenectomized patients to immediate vaccination with polyvalent pneumococcal vaccine. *J Trauma* 23:801–805, 1983.
434. Giebink GS, Le CT, Schiffman G: Decline of serum antibody in splenectomized children after vaccination with pneumococcal capsular polysaccharides. *J Pediatr* 105:576–582, 1984.

435. Chudwin DS, Wara DW, Matthay KK, Caulfield MH, Schiffman G, Mentzer WC, Ammann AJ: Increased serum opsonic activity and antibody concentration in patients with sickle cell disease after pneumococcal polysaccharide immunization. *J Pediatr* 102:51–54, 1983.

436. Rigau-Perez JG, Overturf GD, Chan LS, Weiss J, Powars D: Reactions to booster pneumococcal vaccination in patients with sickle cell disease. *Pediatr Infect Dis* 2:199–202, 1983.

437. Weintrub PS, Schiffman G, Addiego JE Jr, Matthay KK, Vichinsky E, Johnson R, Lubin B, Mentzer WC, Ammann AJ: Long-term follow-up and booster immunization with polyvalent pneumococcal polysaccharide in patients with sickle cell anemia. *J Pediatr* 105:261–263, 1984.

438. Pirovino M, Lydick E, Grob PJ, Arrenbrecht S, Altorfer J, Schmid M: Pneumococcal vaccination: the response of patients with alcoholic liver cirrhosis. *Hepatology* 4:946–949, 1984.

439. Lederman MM, Schiffman G, Rodman HM: Pneumococcal immunization in adult diabetics. *Diabetes* 30:119–121, 1981.

440. Linnemann CC Jr, First MR, Schiffman G: Response to pneumococcal vaccine in renal transplant and hemodialysis patients. *Arch Intern Med* 141:363–370, 1981.

441. Tejani A, Fikrig S, Schiffman G, Gurumurthy K: Persistence of protective pneumococcal antibody following vaccination in patients with nephrotic syndrome. *Am J Nephrol* 4:32–37, 1984.

442. Chou MY, Brown AE, Blevins A, Armstrong D: Severe pneumococcal infection in patients with neoplastic disease. *Cancer* 51:1546–1550, 1983.

443. Shildt RA, Boyd JF, McCracken JD, Schiffman G, Giolma JP: Antibody response to pneumococcal vaccine in patients with solid tumors and lymphomas. *Med Pediatr Oncol* 11:305–309, 1983.

444. Birgens HS, Espersen F, Hertz JB, Pedersen FK, Drivsholm A: Antibody response to pneumococcal vaccination in patients with myelomatosis. *Scand J Haematol* 30:324–330, 1983.

445. Winston DJ, Ho WG, Schiffman G, Champlin RE, Feig SA, Gale RP: Pneumococcal vaccination of recipients of bone marrow transplants. *Arch Intern Med* 143:1735–1737, 1983.

446. Simberkoff MS, El Sadr W, Schiffman G, Rahal JJ Jr: *Streptococcus pneumoniae* infections and bacteremia in patients with acquired immunodeficiency syndrome, with report of a pneumococcal vaccine failure. *Am Rev Respir Dis* 130:1174–1176, 1984.

447. McDonald E, Jarrett MP, Schiffman G, Grayzel AI: Persistence of pneumococcal antibodies after immunization in patients with systemic lupus erythematosus. *J Rheumotol* 11:306–308, 1984.

448. Mufson MA, Krause HE, Schiffman G: Reactivity and antibody responses of volunteers given two or three doses of pneumococcal vaccine. *Proc Soc Exp Biol Med* 117:220–225, 1984.

449. Sisk JE, Pickar E, Locke KE: *Update of Federal Activities Regarding the Use of Pneumococcal Vaccine.* Washington, DC, US Congress Office of Technology Assessment, March 1984.

450. Patriarca PA, Schlech WF, Hinman AR, Conn JM, Gunn WJ: Pneumococcal vaccination practices among private physicians. *Public Health Rep* 97:406–408, 1982.

451. Berk SL, Verghese A, Berk ML, Dison C, Smith JK: Survey of physician acceptance of the pneumococcal vaccine. *South Med J* 77:450–454, 1984.

452. Fedson DS, Baldwin JA: Previous hospital care as a risk factor for pneumonia: implications for immunization with pneumococcal vaccine. *JAMA* 248:1989–1995, 1982.

453. Mufson MA, Oley G, Hughey D: Pneumococcal disease in a medium-sized community in the United States. *JAMA* 248:1486–1489, 1982.

454. Klein RS, Adachi N: Pneumococcal vaccine in the hospital: improved use and implications for high-risk patients. *Arch Intern Med* 143:1878–1881, 1983.

455. Magnussen CR, Valenti WM, Mushlin AI: Pneumococcal vaccine strategy: feasibility of a vaccination program directed at hospitalized and ambulatory patients. *Arch Intern Med* 144:1755–1757, 1984.

456. Klein RS, Adachi N: An effective hospital-based pneumococcal immunization program. *Arch Intern Med* 146:327–329, 1986.

457. Siebers MJ, Hunt VB: Increasing the pneumococcal vaccination rate of elderly patients in a general internal medicine clinic. *J Am Geriatr Soc* 33:175–178, 1985.

458. Willems JS, Sanders CR, Riddiough MA, Bell JC: Cost effectiveness of vaccination against pneumococcal pneumonia. *N Engl J Med* 303:553–559, 1980.

459. Band JL, Chamberland ME, Platt T, Weaver RE, Thornsberry C, Fraser DW: Trends in meningococcal disease in the United States, 1975–1980. *J Infect Dis* 148:754–758, 1983.

460. Holmes FF, Weyandt T, Glazier J, Cuppage FE, Moral LA, Lindsey NJ: Fulminant meningococcemia after splenectomy. *JAMA* 246:1119–1120, 1981.

461. Ross SC, Densen P: Complement deficiency states and infection: epidemiology, pathogenesis and consequences of neisserial and other infections in an immune deficiency. *Medicine* 63:243–273, 1984.

462. Cohen MS, Steere AC, Baltimore R, von Graevenitz A, Pantelick E, Camp B, Root RK: Possible nosocomial transmission of group Y *Neisseria meningitidis* among oncology patients. *Ann Intern Med* 91:7–12, 1979.

463. Rose HD, Lenz IE, Sheth NK: Meningococcal pneumonia: a source of nosocomial infection. *Arch Intern Med* 141:575–577, 1981.

464. Centers for Disease Control: Recommendation of the Immunization Practices Advisory Committee (ACIP): meningococcal polysaccharide vaccines. *MMWR* 34:255–259, 1985.

465. Hankins WA, Gwaltney JM, Hendley JO, Farquhar JD, Samuelson JS: Clinical and serologic evaluation of a meningococcal polysaccharide vaccine groups A, C, Y, and W135. *Proc Soc Exp Biol Med* 169:54–57, 1982.

466. Ruben FL, Hankins WA, Zeigler Z, Norden CW, Harrison A, Winkelstein A, Herrmann DJ: Anti-

body responses to meningococcal polysaccharide vaccine in adults without a spleen. *Am J Med* 76:115–121, 1984.

467. Abramson JS, Spika JS: Persistence of *Neisseria meningitidis* in the upper respiratory tract after intravenous antibiotic therapy for systemic meningococcal disease. *J Infect Dis* 151:370–371, 1985.

468. Centers for Disease Control: Recommendations of the Immunization Practices Advisory Committee (ACIP): varicella-zoster immune globulin for the prevention of chickenpox. *MMWR* 33:84–90, 95–100, 1984.

469. Preblud SR, Orenstein WA, Bart KJ: Varicella: clinical manifestations, epidemiology and health impact in children. *Pediatr Infect Dis* 3:505–509, 1984.

470. Weller TH: Varicella and herpes zoster: changing concepts of the natural history, control, and importance of a not-so-benign virus. *New Engl J Med* 309:1362–1368, 1434–1440, 1983.

471. Fleisher G, Henry W, McSorley M, Arbeter A, Plotkin S: Life-threatening complications of varicella. *Am J Dis Child* 135:896–899, 1982.

472. Preblud SR: Age-specific risks of varicella complications. *Pediatrics* 68:14–17, 1981.

473. Dolin R, Reichman RC, Mazur MH, Whitley RJ: Herpes zoster-varicella infections in immuno-suppressed patients. *Ann Intern Med* 89:375–388, 1978.

474. Brunnel PA: Fetal and neonatal varicella-zoster infections. *Sem Perinatol* 7:47–56, 1983.

475. Meyers JD, MacQuarrie MB, Merigan TC, Jennison MH: Nosocomial varicella—Part 1. Outbreak in oncology patients at a children's hospital. *West J Med* 130:196–199, 1979.

476. Morens DM, Bergman DJ, West CM, Greene MH, Mazur MH, Dolin R, Fisher RI: An outbreak of varicella-zoster virus infection among cancer patients. *Ann Intern Med* 93:414–419, 1980.

477. Hastie IR: Varicella-zoster virus affecting immigrant nurses. *Lancet* 2:154–155, 1980.

478. LeClair JM, Zaia JA, Levin MJ, Congdon RG, Goldmann DA: Airborne transmission of chickenpox in a hospital. *N Engl J Med* 302:450–453, 1980.

479. Gustafson TL, Lavely GB, Brawner ER Jr, Hutcheson RH Jr, Wright PF, Schaffner W. An outbreak of airborne nosocomial varicella. *Pediatrics* 70:550–555, 1982.

480. Faizallah R, Green HT, Krasner N, Walker RJ: Outbreak of chickenpox from a patient with immunosuppressed herpes zoster in hospital. *Br Med J* 285:1022–1023, 1982.

481. Steele RW, Coleman MA, Fiser M, Bradsher RW: Varicella zoster in hospital personnel: skin test reactivity to monitor susceptibility. *Pediatrics* 70:604–608, 1982.

482. Hyams PJ, Stuewe MCS, Heitzer V: Herpes zoster causing varicella (chickenpox) in hospital employees: cost of a casual attitude. *Am J Infect Control* 12:2–5, 1984.

483. Gustafson TL, Shehab Z, Brunell PA: Outbreak of varicella in a newborn intensive care nursery. *Am J Dis Child* 138:548–550, 1984.

484. Hyams PJ, Vernon S, Eckert D: Susceptibility to varicella virus of certain adults in the southeastern United States. *Am J Infect Control* 12:6–9, 1984.

485. Orenstein WA, Heymann DL, Ellis RJ, Rosenberg RL, Nakano J, Halsey NA, Overturf GD, Hayden GF, Witte JJ: Prophylaxis of varicella in high-risk children: dose-response effect of zoster immune globulin. *J Pediatr* 98:368–373, 1981.

486. Zaia JA, Levin MJ, Preblud SJ, Leszcynski J, Wright GG, Ellis RJ, Curtis AC, Valerio MA, LeGore J: Evaluation of varicella-zoster immune globulin: protection of immunosuppressed children after household exposure to varicella. *J Infect Dis* 147:737–743, 1983.

487. Committee on Infectious Diseases: Expanded guideline for use of varicella-zoster immune globulin. *Pediatrics* 72:886–889, 1983.

488. Myers MG, Rasley DA, Hierholzer WJ: Hospital infection control for varicella zoster virus infection. *Pediatrics* 70:199–202, 1982.

489. Arbeter AM, Starr SE, Preblud SR, Ihara T, Paciorek PM, Miller DS, Zelson CM, Proctor EA, Plotkin SA: Varicella vaccine trials in healthy children: a summary of comparative and followup studies. *Am J Dis Child* 138:434–438, 1984.

490. Weibel RE, Neff BJ, Kuter BJ, Guess HA, Rothenberger CA, Fitzgerald AJ, Connor KA, McLean AA, Hilleman MR, Buynak EB, Scolnick EM: Live attenuated varicella virus vaccine: efficacy trial in healthy children. *N Engl J Med* 310:1409–1415, 1984.

491. Brunell PA, Geiser C, Shehab Z, Waugh JE: Administration of live varicella vaccine to children with leukemia. *Lancet* 2:1069–1073, 1982.

492. Gershon AA, Steinberg SP, Gelb L, Galasso G, Borkowsky W, LaRussa P, Ferrara A, the National Institute of Allergy and Infectious Diseases Varicella Vaccine Collaborative Study Group: Live attenuated varicella vaccine: efficacy for children with leukemia in remission. *JAMA* 252:355–362, 1984.

493. Centers for Disease Control: Recommendation of the Immunization Practices Advisory Committee (ACIP): rabies prevention—United States, 1984. *MMWR* 33:393–402, 407–408, 1984.

494. Anderson LJ, Nicholson KG, Tauxe RV, Winkler WG: Human rabies in the United States, 1960 to 1979: epidemiology, diagnosis and prevention. *Ann Intern Med* 100:728–735, 1984.

495. Centers for Disease Control: Human rabies acquired outside the United States. *MMWR* 34:235–236, 1985.

496. Centers for Disease Control: Update: raccoon rabies—Mid-Atlantic states. *MMWR* 32:97–98, 1983.

497. Anderson LJ, Williams LP, Layde JB, Dixon FR, Winkler WG: Nosocomial rabies: investigation of contacts of human rabies cases associated with a corneal transplant. *Am J Public Health* 74:370–372, 1984.

498. Helmick CG: The epidemiology of human rabies postexposure prophylaxis, 1980–1981. *JAMA* 250:1990–1996, 1983.

499. Centers for Disease Control: Rabies postexposure prophylaxis with human diploid cell vaccine: lower neutralizing antibody titers with Wyeth vaccine. *MMWR* 34:90–92, 1985.

500. Bernard KW, Roberts MA, Sumner J, Winkley WG, Mallonee J, Baer GM, Chaney R: Human diploid cell rabies vaccine: effectiveness of immunization with small intradermal or subcutaneous doses. *JAMA* 247:1138–1142, 1982.
501. Centers for Disease Control: Field evaluations of pre-exposure use of human diploid cell rabies vaccine. *MMWR* 32:601–603, 1983.
502. Anderson LJ, Sikes RK, Langkop CW, Mann JM, Smith JS, Winkler WG, Deitch MW: Postexposure trial of a human diploid cell strain of rabies vaccine. *J Infect Dis* 142:133–138, 1980.
503. Devriendt J, Staroukine M, Costy F, Vanderhaeghen JJ: Fatal encephalitis apparently due to rabies: occurrence after treatment with human diploid cell vaccine but not rabies immune globulin. *JAMA* 248:2304–2306, 1982.
504. Bernard KW, Smith PW, Kader FJ, Moran MJ: Neuroparalytic illness and human diploid cell rabies vaccine. *JAMA* 248:3136–3138, 1982.
505. Centers for Disease Control: Systemic allergic reactions following immunization with human diploid cell rabies vaccine. *MMWR* 33:185–187, 1984.
506. Mann JM, Burkhart MJ, Rollag OJ: Anti-rabies treatments in New Mexico: impact of a comprehensive consultation-biologics system. *Am J Public Health* 70:128–132, 1980.
507. Nathanson N: Eradication of poliomyelitis in the United States. *Rev Infect Dis* 4:940–950, 1982.
508. Kim-Farley RJ, Bart KJ, Schonberger LB, Orenstein WA, Nkowane BM, Hinman AR, Kew OM, Hatch MH, Kaplan JE: Poliomyelitis in the USA: virtual elimination of disease caused by wild virus. *Lancet* 2:1315–1317, 1984.
509. Schonberger LB, Kaplan J, Kim-Farley R, Moore M, Eddins DL, Hatch M: Control of paralytic poliomyelitis in the United States. *Rev Infect Dis* 6 (suppl): S424–S426, 1984.
510. Dalakas MC, Sever JL, Madden DL, Papadopoulos NM, Shekarchi IC, Albrecht P, Krezlewicz A: Late postpoliomyelitis muscular atrophy: clinical, virologic, and immunologic studies. *Rev Infect Dis* 6 (suppl):S562–S567, 1984.
511. Centers for Disease Control: Recommendation of the Immunization Practices Advisory Committee (ACIP): poliomyelitis prevention. *MMWR* 31:22–26, 31–34, 1982.
512. McBean AM, Thoms ML, Johnson RH, Gadless BR, MacDonald B, Nerhood L, Cummins P, Hughes J, Kinnear J, Watts C, Kraft M, Albrecht P, Boone EJ, Moore M, Frank JA Jr, Bernier R: A comparison of the serologic responses to oral and injectable trivalent poliovirus vaccines. *Rev Infect Dis* 6 (suppl):S552–S555, 1984.
513. Kim-Farley RJ, Rutherford G, Litchfield P, Hsu ST, Orenstein WA, Schonberger LB, Bart KJ, Lin KJ, Lin CC: Outbreak of paralytic poliomyelitis, Taiwan. *Lancet* 2:1322–1324, 1984.
514. Centers for Disease Control: Poliomyelitis—Finland. *MMWR* 34:5–6, 1985.
515. Mayer TR, Balfour HH: Prevalence of poliovirus neutralizing antibodies in young adult women. *JAMA* 1207–1209, 1981.
516. Salk D, van Wezel AL, Salk J: Induction of long-term immunity to paralytic poliomyelitis by use of non-infectious vaccine. *Lancet* 2:1317–1321, 1984.
517. Melnick JL: Live attenuated oral poliovirus vaccine. *Rev Infect Dis* 6 (suppl): S323–S327, 1984.
518. van Wezel AL, van Steenis G, van der Marel P, Osterhaus ADME: Inactivated poliovirus vaccine: current production methods and new developments. *Rev Infect Dis* 6 (suppl): S335–S340, 1984.
519. Centers for Disease Control: Mumps—United States, 1980–1983. *MMWR* 32:545–547, 1983.
520. Centers for Disease Control: Recommendation of the Immunization Practices Advisory Committee (ACIP): mumps vaccine. *MMWR* 31:617–620, 1982.
521. Weible RE, Buynak EB, McClean AA, Roehm RR, Hilleman MR: Persistence of antibody in human subjects for 7 to 10 years following administration of combined live attenuated measles, mumps, and rubella virus vaccines. *Proc Soc Exp Biol Med* 165:260–263, 1980.
522. Koplan JP, Preblud S: A benefit-cost analysis of mumps vaccine. *Am J Dis Child* 136:362–364, 1982.
523. Cochi SL, Broome CV, Hightower AW: Immunization of US children with *Hemophilus influenzae* type b polysaccharide vaccine: a cost-effectiveness model of strategy assessment. *JAMA* 253:521–529, 1985.
524. Centers for Disease Control: Recommendation of the Immunization Practices Advisory Committee (ACIP): polysaccharide vaccine for prevention of *Haemophilus influenzae* type b disease. *MMWR* 34:201–205, 1985.
525. Ward J, Smith AL: *Haemophilus influenzae* bacteremia in children with sickle cell disease. *J Pediatr* 88:261–263, 1976.
526. Siber GR: Bacteremias due to *Haemophilus influenzae* and *Streptococcus pneumoniae:* their occurrence and course in children with cancer. *Am J Dis Child* 134:668–672, 1980.
527. Peltola H, Kayhty H, Virtanen M, Makela PH: Prevention of *Hemophilus influenzae* type B bacteremic infections with the capsular polysaccharide vaccine. *N Engl J Med* 310:1561–1566, 1984.
528. Centers for Disease Control: Tuberculosis—United States, 1984. *MMWR* 34:299–302, 307, 1985.
529. Grzybowski S: Epidemiology of tuberculosis and the role of BCG. *Clin Chest Med* 1:175–187, 1980.
530. Powell KE, Meador MP, Farer LS: Recent trends in tuberculosis in children. *JAMA* 251:1289–1292, 1984.
531. Powell KE, Brown ED, Farer LS: Tuberculosis among Indochinese refugees in the United States. *JAMA* 249:1455–1460, 1983.
532. Nagami PH, Yoshikawa TT: Tuberculosis in the geriatric patient. *J Am Geriatr Soc* 31:356–363, 1983.
533. Hsu KHK: Thirty years after isoniazid. Its impact on tuberculosis in children and adolescents. *JAMA* 251:1283–1285, 1984.
534. Dandoy S: Current status of general hospital use for patients with tuberculosis in the United States. Eight-year update. *Am Rev Respir Dis* 126:270–273, 1982.
535. Greenbaum M, Beyt BE, Murray PR: The accuracy of diagnosing pulmonary tuberculosis at a teaching hospital. *Am Rev Respir Dis* 121:477–

481, 1980.

536. Brabender W, Hodges GR: Current problems in the recognition and management of patients with tuberculosis in a general hospital. *Am J Infect Control* 11:130–132, 1983.

537. Bobrowitz ID: Active tuberculosis undiagnosed until autopsy. *Am J Med* 72:650–658, 1982.

538. Narain JP, Lofgren JP, Warren E, Stead WW: Epidemic of tuberculosis in a nursing home: a retrospective cohort study. *J Am Geriatr Soc* 3:258–263, 1985.

539. Stead WW, Lofgren JP, Warren E, Thomas C: Tuberculosis as an endemic and nosocomial infection among the elderly in nursing homes. *N Engl J Med* 312:1483–1487, 1985.

540. Eickhoff TC: The current status of BCG immunization against tuberculosis. *Annu Rev Med* 28:411–422, 1977.

541. Centers for Disease Control: Recommendation of the Immunization Practices Advisory Committee (ACIP): BCG vaccines. *MMWR* 28:241–244, 1979.

542. Tuberculosis Prevention Trial, Madras: Trial of BCG vaccine in South India. *Indian J Med Res* 72 (suppl):1–74, 1980.

543. Curtis HM, Leck I, Bamford FN: Incidence of childhood tuberculosis after neonatal BCG vaccination. *Lancet* 1:145–148, 1984.

544. Clemens JD, Chuong JJH, Feinstein AR: The BCG controversy. A methodological and statistical appraisal. *JAMA* 249:2362–2369, 1983.

545. Barrett-Connor E: The epidemiology of tuberculosis in physicians. *JAMA* 241:33–38, 1979.

546. Cantanzaro A: Nosocomial tuberculosis. *Am Rev Respir Dis* 125:559–562, 1982.

547. Berman J, Levin ML, Orr ST, Desi L: Tuberculosis risk for hospital employees: analysis of a five-year tuberculin skin testing program. *Am J Public Health* 71:1217–1222, 1981.

548. Ruben FL, Norden CW, Schuster N: Analysis of a community hospital employee tuberculosis screening program 31 months after its inception. *Am Rev Respir Dis* 115:23–28, 1977.

549. Thompson NJ, Glassroth JL, Snider DE, Farer LS: The booster phenomenon in serial tuberculin testing. *Am Rev Respir Dis* 119:587–597, 1979.

550. McGowan JE Jr: The booster effect—a problem for surveillance of tuberculosis in hospital employees. *Infect Control* 1:147–149, 1980.

551. Bryan CS: The hospital tuberculosis registry: an aid to infection control. *Am J Infect Control* 11:57–62, 1983.

552. Weinstein RS, Oshins J, Sacks HS: Tuberculosis infection in Mount Sinai medical students: 1974–1982. *Mt Sinai J Med* 51:283–286, 1984.

553. Craven RB, Wenzel RP, Atuk NO: Minimizing tuberculosis risk to hospital personnel and students exposed to unsuspected disease. *Ann Intern Med* 82:628–632, 1975.

554. Ashley MJ, Wigle WD: The epidemiology of active tuberculosis in hospital employees in Ontario, 1966–1969. *Am Rev Respir Dis* 104:851–860, 1971.

555. Burk JR, Bahar D, Wolf FS, Greene J, Bailey WC: Nursery exposure of 528 newborns to a nurse with pulmonary tuberculosis. *South Med J* 71:7–10, 1978.

556. Barrett-Connor E: The periodic chest roentgenogram for the control of tuberculosis in health care personnel. *Am Rev Respir Dis* 122:153–155, 1980.

557. Cope R, Hartstein AI: The annual chest roentgenogram for the control of tuberculosis in hospital employees: recent changes and their implications. *Am Rev Respir Dis* 125:106–107, 1982.

558. Reeves SA, Noble RC: Ineffectiveness of annual chest roentgenograms in tuberculin skin-test positive hospital employees. *Am J Infect Control* 11:212–216, 1983.

559. Taylor WC, Aronson MD, Delbanco TL: Should young adults with a positive tuberculin test take isoniazid? *Ann Intern Med* 94:808–813, 1981.

560. Comstock GW: Evaluating isoniazid preventive therapy: the need for more data. *Ann Intern Med* 94:817–819, 1981.

561. Barrett-Connor E: Nososomial tuberculosis in physicians: an analysis of direct costs of prevention and disease. *Prev Med* 10:69–76, 1981.

562. Clemens JD, Stanton BF: BCG prophylaxis against cancer: methodological evaluation of a continuing controversy. *J Chronic Dis* 37:45–54, 1984.

563. Taylor DN, Pollard RA, Blake PA: Typhoid in the United States and the risk to the international traveller. *J Infect Dis* 148:599–602, 1983.

564. Taylor JP, Shandera WX, Betz TG, Schraitle K, Chaffee L, Lopez L, Henley R, Rothe CN, Bell RF, Blake PA: Typhoid fever in San Antonio, Texas: an outbreak traced to a continuing source. *J Infect Dis* 149:553–557, 1984.

565. Blaser MJ, Hickman FW, Farmer JJ III, Brenner DJ, Balows A, Feldman RA: *Salmonella typhii:* the laboratory as a reservoir of infection. *J Infect Dis* 142:934–938, 1980.

566. Centers for Disease Control: Recommendation of the Immunization Practices Advisory Committee (ACIP): typhoid vaccine. *MMWR* 27:231–233, 1978.

567. Wahden MH, Serie C, Cerisier Y, Sallam S, Germanier R: A controlled field trial of live *Salmonella typhii* strain Ty 21a oral vaccine against typhoid: three-year results. *J Infect Dis* 145:292–295, 1982.

568. Centers for Disease Control: Recommendation of the Immunization Practices Advisory Committee (ACIP): yellow fever vaccine. *MMWR* 27:268–270, 1978.

569. Poland JD, Calisher CH, Monath TP, Downs WG, Murphy K: Persistence of neutralizing antibodies 30–35 years after immunization with 17D yellow fever vaccine. *Bull WHO* 59:895–900, 1981.

570. Centers for Disease Control: Recommendation of the Immunization Practices Advisory Committee (ACIP): cholera vaccine. *MMWR* 27:173–174, 1978.

571. Fenner F: Global eradication of smallpox. *Rev Infect Dis* 4:916–922, 1982.

572. Centers for Disease Control: Recommendation of the Immunization Practices Advisory Committee (ACIP): smallpox vaccine. *MMWR* 34:341–342, 1985.

573. Centers for Disease Control: Vaccinia outbreak—Nevada. *MMWR* 32:403–404, 1983.

574. Centers for Disease Control: Contact spread of

vaccinia from a recently vaccinated marine—Louisiana. *MMWR* 33:37–38, 1984.

575. Hilleman MR: Newer directions in vaccine development and utilization. *J Infect Dis* 151:407–419, 1985.

576. Committee on Issues and Priorities for New Vaccine Development: *New Vaccine Development. Establishing Priorities.* Vol. I: *Diseases of Importance in the United States.* Washington, DC, National Academy Press, 1985.

577. Clements ML, Betts RF, Murphy BR: Advantage of live attenuated cold-adapted influenza A virus over inactivated vaccine for A/Washington/80 (H3N2) wild-type virus infection. *Lancet* 1:705–708, 1984.

578. Peter G: Vaccine crisis: an emerging societal problem. *J Infect Dis* 151:981–983, 1985.

579. Riddiough MA, Willems JS, Sanders CR, Kemp K: Factors affecting the use of vaccines: considerations for immunization program planners. *Public Health Rep* 96:528–535, 1981.

580. Fedson DS, Tarlov AR: Pneumococcal immunization: strategies for implementation. *Infect Control* 3:293–294, 1982.

Chapter 13

Infection Control Aspects of Hospital Employee Health

Robert J. Sherertz, M.D., and A. Lex Hampton, M.D.

Hospital employee health (HEH) programs have been in existence for many years, yet the services they provide have received very little critical attention. A review of the medical literature between 1966 and October 1984 produced 246 English language citations dealing with HEH, yet among these articles there was only a single institution that has published its experience with an HEH program (1). A number of attempts have been made to provide guidelines for practitioners of HEH. The first significant publication on HEH was found in *Infection Control in the Hospital* by the American Hospital Association (2). It provided a general overview and largely emphasized immunizations. Several similar works were subsequently published (3–7). Haley and Emori provided the first assessment of the standard of practice of HEH in the United States through an analysis of the Study on the Efficacy of Nosocomial Infection Control (SENIC) project data (8, 9). They found that in 1976 a significant proportion of their 433 sample hospitals did not have employee health programs (32%), failed to employ recommended screening tests, or continued unnecessary, expensive ones (8). In general, they discovered that staff nurses were unfamiliar with published recommendations about when an illness or infection exposure should exclude them from patient contact (9). In 1979, Kaslow and Garner developed the first detailed disease-specific recommendations for a hospital employee health service (10). In the same year Atuk et al provided the first in-depth look at the needs of a comprehensive HEH program (11). Not only were subjects covered in greater depth than by previous authors, but they presented detailed information about their experience with needle sticks, hepatitis B, and tuberculosis. The book chapter by Atuk et al (11) and a report by Valenti et al in 1982 (1) represent the only two attempts to summarize a single institution's experience

with an HEH program. The only book on the subject was published in 1982 and contains the proceedings of the First National Conference on Hospital Employee Health (12). The final important publication about HEH came from the Centers for Disease Control (CDC) (13). This document represents a consensus of more than 28 experts in the area of infection control. They make extensive recommendations about the content of an HEH program, but more importantly they emphasize for the first time which infectious diseases are likely to be transmitted to patients, to personnel, or to both.

In spite of the more recent comprehensive works about HEH programs, more research is needed to answer a number of questions. Can the acquired immune deficiency syndrome (AIDS) be transmitted to hospital employees, and if so how can the transmission be prevented? Has the hepatitis B vaccine had an impact on preventing hepatitis B in hospital employees? What is the optimal way to prevent employees from being vectors of viral diseases on pediatric wards? Although many of these and other questions are being investigated, few if any HEH programs are systematically studying how hospital employee health care should be delivered. In order to appreciate HEH one must reach some understanding of the problems with which such a service must deal.

SHANDS HOSPITAL EMPLOYEE HEALTH PROGRAM

In 1982, the commitment was made by Shands Hospital (a 450-bed university hospital in Gainesville, Florida) to develop a comprehensive employee health program. Initially, approximately 3500 employees would be cared for including (665) doctors, (1283) nurses, (485) paramedical personnel, and (911) clerical staff. The following services were offered:

1. Management of all employee infection exposures;
2. Surveillance for tuberculosis infections by skin test;
3. Vaccination of high risk employees—hepatitis B vaccine, measles-mumps-rubella (MMR), influenza, and diphtheria/tetanus;
4. Management of minor intercurrent illnesses and triage of more serious medical problems;
5. Continuing education of employees to reduce on-the-job injuries and other medical problems.

During a 1-year period two nurse practitioners and a secretary were hired and the services of a medical director with training in infectious diseases and hospital epidemiology were obtained. Because the program was to be administered and run by the two nurse practitioners, a series of medical protocols was written to define precisely which medical problems could be handled in employee health and which problems should be triaged elsewhere. To develop a better understanding of the program and to facilitate the delivery of medical care we also developed a computer data base for employee health which consisted of certain demographic information, a record of significant medical problems, details of each employee's immunization status, and details of each employee visit. After 1 year we examined the data base to determine the nature of our HEH program.

By design, the majority of our employee visits (57%) were related to infection prevention or surveillance efforts (Table 13.1). During the first year of tuberculosis monitoring it was possible to skin test over 90% of the nonphysician patient care personnel; 2.4% of them were positive. MMR vaccinations were administered to all personnel not already known to be seropositive. Serology for varicella was performed during this time period only because of personnel exposures to chickenpox or zoster for individuals who had a negative history of chickenpox; 95% were seropositive. Most rubella serologic testing was carried out as mandatory policy on personnel working with pediatric or obstetric patients without a prior history of vaccination or positive serology. An additional large number of rubella tests resulted from a pseudo-outbreak due to false positive serology (14). Ninety percent of those tested for rubella had antibodies.

Of the remaining 43% of personnel visits, half were due to noninfectious problems (Table 13.2). Skin complaints occurred most frequently. Hand dermatitis, the most common skin problem, was usually related to or exacerbated by the frequent hand washing required in many patient units. An occasional individual with severe hand dermatitis and patient care responsibilities was sent home due to the risk of becoming a source of nosocomial infections (15). Back pain was a common problem, and it occurred most frequently in individuals working in the operating room who were required to lift patients on and off the tables. Although uncommon, serious problems, including cardiopulmonary arrest, did occur.

Table 13.1. Employee Health Visits— Infection Prevention or Surveillance, Shands Hospital, July 1983 to June 1984

Health Maintenance Activity	No.	Percentage of Total Visits
Tuberculosis PPD surveillance (36 were positive)	1522*	26.9
Immunizations—MMR† (411), hepatitis B vaccine (346), diphtheria/tetanus (267), influenza (200)	1224*	21.6
Surveillance serology—rubella (271), varicella (182), other (4)	457	8.1
Total	3203	56.6

* Number of employees (i.e., application of and reading a PPD constitute a single visit; the full hepatavax-B series is counted as one visit).

† MMR, measles- mumps-rubella.

Table 13.2. Employee Health Visits— Noninfectious Medical Problems, Shands Hospital, July 1983 to June 1984

Medical Problem	No.	Percentage of Total Visits
Skin—contact dermatitis (49), scabies (17), other (160)	226	4.0
Blood pressure check	218	3.9
Orthopedic—low back pain, other	199	3.5
Return to work approval	54	1.0
Suspected pregnancy	54	1.0
Stress	27	0.5
Eye	27	0.5
Headache	21	0.4
Ears, sinuses	20	0.4
Miscellaneous—chest pain (14), asthma (3), cardiopulmonary arrest (2), seizure (1), anaphylaxis (1)	282	5.0
Total	1128	19.9

The other half of the unscheduled personnel visits were due to infectious diseases (Table 13.3) or exposures to infectious diseases (Table 13.4). Nearly one-quarter of all such visits were secondary to upper respiratory tract infections. Only 10.5% of the 294 employees with pharyngitis had group A streptococcal infection. The remainder were probably viral infections and often occurred in small clusters in intensive care unit and pediatric personnel. Diarrhea, gastroenteritis, and impetigo occurred most commonly in pediatric personnel. Ten cases of herpes simplex were diagnosed; eight were cold sores, and both of the other two cases presented with clusters of vesicles on the chest wall that could easily have been confused with varicella-zoster. Of the nine documented cases of hepatitis, seven were hepatitis B (Table 13.5) and two were non-A, non-B hepatitis. None of these individuals received immunoglobulin prophylaxis, and only one of them had a history of an unequivocal exposure to a patient with hepatitis. In the six cases of chickenpox, two were due to patient exposures (one chickenpox and one zoster) and the other four were believed

Table 13.3. Employee Health Visits—Infectious Diseases or Syndromes, Shands Hospital, July 1983 to June 1984

Infectious Illness	No.	Percentage of Total Visits
Respiratory tract—pharyngitis (294), upper respiratory infection (213), bronchitis (28), pneumonia (3)	538	9.5
Gastrointestinal—diarrhea (46), gastroenteritis (28), nausea/vomiting (19)	93	1.6
Urinary tract infection	91	1.6
Ears, sinuses—otitis media (55), otitis externa (16), sinusitis (16)	87	1.5
Skin—miscellaneous soft tissue infections (28), impetigo (18), herpes simplex (10), carbuncle (2)	58	1.0
Conjunctivitis	56	1.0
Miscellaneous viral*—viral syndrome (30), hepatitis B (7), chickenpox (6), influenza (2), infectious mononucleosis (2), cytomegalovirus (2), non-A, non-B hepatitis (2), hepatitis A (1)	52	0.9
Total	975	17.2

* Specific infections were serologically diagnosed except influenza, which was diagnosed clinically.

Table 13.4. Employee Health Visits—Infectious Disease Exposures, Shands Hospital, July 1983 to June 1984

Infectious Exposure	No.	Percentage of Total Visits
Needles sticks*	116	2.1
Tuberculosis	(90)†	(1.6)†
Varicella	89	1.6
Hepatitis exposure (other)*—B (21), A (19), non-A, non-B (13)	53	0.9
Syphilis‡	53	0.9
Miscellaneous—mumps (13), AIDS (4), cytomegalovirus (4), influenza (2), animal/human bite (2), measles (2), meningococcus (2), other (14)	44	0.8
Total	355	6.3

* Of 94 documented hepatitis exposures (hepatitis B (51), non-A, non-B (24), A (19)), all received immunoprophylaxis and no symptomatic disease developed.
† Already counted in Table 13.1.
‡ Virtually all exposures resulted from a single case of laryngeal syphilis in a patient requiring intubation.

Table 13.5.   Hepatitis B in Shands Hospital Personnel, April 1983 to April 1984

Job	Type of Exposure	Received Prophylaxis
Physician		
Surgical housestaff	Needle stick	no
Medical housestaff	"Blood"*	no
Nurses		
Obstetrics	"Blood"	no
Hemodialysis	"Blood"	no
Intensive care unit	"Blood"	no
Cardiac catheterization lab	Needle stick	no
Other		
Dietary	Unknown	no

* "Blood"—without any known break in their skin, these individuals' hands came in contact with blood from patient who was HBsAg-positive.

to have been acquired in the community related to a school-associated outbreak. No secondary cases occurred. Conjunctivitis was usually sporadic and never bacterial on initial presentation. Notably, two small clusters of conjunctivitis did occur, resulting in significant loss of personnel time. All four cases of mumps were acquired due to community exposures.

Of the 355 documented infection exposures, only the two secondary cases of chickenpox mentioned above developed. With the hepatitis exposures this is most likely due to immunoprophylaxis. With tuberculosis and chickenpox, the information suggests that the exposures were minimal, but it also reflects the difficulty associated with handling infection exposures. Patients with hepatitis B, tuberculosis, chickenpox, AIDS, and meningococcal infection produce hysterical responses in many hospital personnel regardless of whether they were actually exposed to the index case. Exposure histories obtained from such individuals may be inaccurate.

In summary, our HEH service was largely self-defined. Thus, the amount of preventive health maintenance that each institution decides to offer will be a major factor affecting the size of an HEH program. The unscheduled visits, the part of the program over which one has little control, were divided equally between miscellaneous medical problems and infections or exposures to infections. How general medical problems are handled will depend upon the extent to which each hospital wants to provide outpatient clinic services to its employees. The core of each HEH program must deal directly with infection control-related problems.

THE CONTROL OF INFECTION TRANSMISSION TO AND FROM HOSPITAL PERSONNEL

The following sections provide background information necessary to decide what employee health services will best meet the needs of each institution. We will discuss those infectious diseases which have been found to impact on hospital employees through our own experience and that of others. In each disease category current and past medical literature will be summarized and an interpretation of its importance provided when possible. For each disease, emphasis will also be placed on whether an employee is more likely to be a vector or a recipient of the infection. This information is summarized in Table 13.6. If more detailed recommendations are desired, those offered by the CDC (13) or one of the other references cited in the introductory discussion are recommended.

Acquired Immune Deficiency Syndrome

As of January 1985 the number of AIDS cases was still increasing, with over 7000 cases reported in the United States since the CDC first initiated surveillance in 1981 (16). Epidemiologic evidence suggests that it is transmitted by sexual activity, parenteral injection, or from mother to child before, during, or after the time of birth (17). There is no evidence to suggest that it can spread by casual contact (17). The incubation period for the clinical manifestations of AIDS is thought to range from about 4 to 57 months (18, 19). Existing evidence suggests that HTLV-3 is the

Table 13.6.   Risk of Infection Transmission between Patients and Hospital Personnel

Disease	Transmission Route	
	Patient to Employee	Employee to Patient
AIDS	?*	?
Chickenpox/disseminated zoster	High	High
Localized zoster	Low	Low
Conjunctivitis/viral	High	High
Cytomegalovirus	Low	?
Hepatitis A	Low	Rare
Hepatitis B	Low	Rare
Hepatitis non-A, non-B	Low	?
Herpes simplex	Low	Rare
Influenza	Intermediate	Intermediate
Measles	High	High
Meningococcal infection	Rare	?
Mumps	Intermediate	Intermediate
Pertussis	Intermediate	Intermediate
Respiratory syncytial virus	Intermediate	Intermediate
Rotavirus	Intermediate	Intermediate
Rubella	Intermediate	Intermediate
Salmonella/Shigella	Low	Low
Scabies	Low	Low
S. aureus	?	Rare
Streptococcus, group A	?	Rare
Syphilis	Low	?
Tuberculosis	Low to high	Low to high

* ?, Insufficient data available to comment.

cause of AIDS. HTLV-3 has been isolated from lymphocytes, saliva, semen, and the blood of patients with AIDS or in high risk groups (20). Serologic surveys have shown that 68 to 100% of AIDS patients have antibodies to the HTLV-3 virus (17). Other groups with high prevalence rates to this antibody include homosexual men (22 to 65%), intravenous drug abusers admitted to a detoxification program in New York City (86%), persons with hemophilia A (56 to 72%), and sexual partners of men with AIDS (35%) (20).

Due to the limited duration of follow-up available on individuals with documented exposures and the long incubation period of the disease, the risk of this infection to hospital employees is yet to be determined. With an average of 14 months of observation, no cases of AIDS developed in 27 hospital employees with parenteral exposure to blood from AIDS patients; 24 were needle sticks (21). Through December 31, 1984 the CDC had received reports on 361 health care workers who had been exposed to blood, or body fluids from AIDS patients. The types of exposures included needle stick injuries (68%), mucosal exposures

(13%), cuts with sharp instruments (10%), and contamination of open skin lesions with potentially infected body fluids (9%). None of these workers has developed AIDS; 143 have been followed for 12 months or longer (22). In another recent publication, 85 hospital employees exposed to AIDS patients (30 by needle stick) were tested for antibodies to HTLV-3 with a mean elapsed time of 8 months since their exposure; none of them was seropositive (23). The only worrisome report to date appeared in the December 15, 1984 issue of *Lancet* in which a nurse seroconverted to HTLV-3 49 days after a needle stick associated with an AIDS patient (24). Another concern raised by hospital employees is that they might acquire AIDS by receiving the hepatitis B vaccine. Recent data bearing on this subject include the demonstration of inactivation of HTLV by the vaccine preparation process, the lack of HTLV-3 in vaccine lots, and the finding that after more than 700,000 individuals have received the vaccine no cases of AIDS have occurred in persons not in high risk groups (25). The data make it extremely unlikely that AIDS can be acquired by this route. Finally, there is no information at this time about whether any kind of postexposure prophylaxis is worth considering.

Chickenpox/Zoster

The varicella-zoster virus is particularly well suited to cause difficulties in the hospital setting because a high proportion of children are susceptible to infection, and it is highly contagious. Chickenpox is known to become infectious as early as 4 days before the onset of rash, but it is more likely to be infectious 1 or 2 days prior to onset (26). The limits of communicability in noncompromised hosts were elegantly demonstrated by Thomson et al in a 12-bed children's infectious disease ward by a series of studies between 1912 and 1919 (27–29). In these studies each child with chickenpox was introduced to the ward one at a time, and all of the exposed children were observed for secondary cases. When stringent efforts were made to prevent contact transmission (i.e., attempting to focus on airborne transmission), cross-infection ceased to occur after the third day of vesicular eruption (Table 13.7). If no efforts were made to prevent contact transmission, then secondary cases did not occur after the fifth day of eruption (Table 13.7). Notice that the rate of what is presumed to be airborne transmission is relatively low in comparison to the transmission

Table 13.7. Attack Rates in Children for the Transmission of Chickenpox by Day of Rash*

No. of Days after Rash Onset	Attack Rate (No. Infected/No. Exposed) × 100%	
	Isolation Efforts Employed to Prevent Contact Transmission	No Isolation Efforts
1	11.8 (2/17)	
2	14.3 (3/21)	
3	1.7 (3/175)	
4	0 (0/24)	
5	0 (0/13)	13.0 (3/23)
6	0 (0/24)	0 (0/10)
7	0 (0/7)	0 (0/12)
8	0 (0/10)	0 (0/23)
9		0 (0/15)
10	0 (0/3)	0 (0/12)
11		0 (0/5)
12		0 (0/9)
16		0 (0/5)

* Derived from Thomson FH, Price C: The aerial conveyance of infection. *Lancet* 1:1669–1673, 1914; Thomson FH: The aerial conveyance of infection. With a note on the contact infection of chicken-pox. *Lancet* 1:341–344, 1916; and Thomson FH: Contact infection of chicken-pox. Lancet 1:397, 1919.

rate among susceptible household contacts where 90% of those exposed develop chickenpox (30, 31). The duration of exposure required to transmit chickenpox is not clearly known, but exposures as short as 2 hours to an individual incubating chickenpox have been shown to be adequate (32). Thus, the risk of transmission varies considerably with the extent, duration, and type of exposure.

Ninety-nine percent of chickenpox cases develop skin lesions between 11 and 20 days after exposure (33). In noncompromised hosts the virus can be isolated from skin lesions during the first 3 days, occasionally on the fourth day, but never thereafter (30). This correlates well with the data on the risk of transmission generated by Thomson. However, with immunocompromised hosts the virus can be easily isolated from skin lesions for up to 10 days (34), and reports exist of lesions persisting for as long as 24 weeks (35).

The infectivity of the zoster manifestation (shingles) of varicella infection is not nearly as well understood as that of chickenpox, but there is general agreement that its localized form is much less infectious (13, 32). In a study reported by Seiler, 10 of 184 patients with dermatomal zoster gave rise to cases of chickenpox—9 of 10 were children (36). This probably reflects a lower likelihood of an adult with zoster coming in contact with a child in comparison to a child with chickenpox exposing another child. No good evidence exists to suggest that dermatomal zoster can be transmitted by an airborne route. However, patients with disseminated zoster appear quite infectious and capable of causing outbreaks (37–39). These studies strongly suggest that disseminated zoster is transmissible by the aerosol route.

The importance of varicella in the hospital setting derives from the significant morbidity and mortality that a hospital outbreak can produce in immunocompromised hosts (40–43). Bone marrow transplant patients appear to be at greatest risk (43). Information obtained from reports of nosocomial varicella outbreaks can be used to understand how to protect such patients from exposure to varicella. At least 10 outbreaks of hospital-acquired varicella infection have been described since 1970, and they are summarized in Table 13.8 (37–39, 44–50). They have occurred in different hospital locations, including a medical ward, 1; pediatric burn unit, 1; newborn nursery, 1; cancer wards, 2; and pediatric wards, 3. On pediatric wards the index case always had chickenpox, whereas on adult wards it was either

Table 13.8. Summary of 10 Nosocomial Varicella Outbreaks Reported in the Literature

Reference	Year of Report	Hospital Location	Index Case Varicella Presentation	Secondary Cases— Patient/Employee	Death
37	1970	Medical ward	Disseminated zoster	0/1	0
44	1974	Pediatric burn unit	Chickenpox	6/0	0
45	1979	Pediatric ward	Chickenpox	20/0	1
46	1980	Cancer ward	Unclear	8/1	1
47	1980	Pediatric ward	Chickenpox	13/1	0
48	1982	Pediatric ward	Chickenpox	8/1	0
38	1983	Adult ward	Disseminated zoster	1/4	0
49	1984	Neonatal ICU	Chickenpox	2/2	0
50	1984	Medical ward	Chickenpox, zoster	3/0	0
39	1984	Adult ward	Disseminated zoster	0/2	0

disseminated zoster, 3; zoster, 1; or chickenpox, 1. One notable finding in these 10 reports is that more secondary cases involving employees occurred on adult wards (eight cases) than on pediatric wards (four cases). Although the explanation for this difference is not clear, it may be because cases of chickenpox are isolated properly, but cases of disseminated zoster may not be. In the three reports where the index case had disseminated zoster and the single report where one index case had dermatomal zoster it is stated clearly that isolation was either not employed or ignored (37–39, 50). Of significance, there is only one outbreak which was attributed to dermatomal zoster (50). Only a single secondary case developed in this report involving the patient's roommate. This information further amplifies the impression of others that dermatomal zoster is much less infectious than the other two manifestations of varicella. Other important factors contributing to the development of varicella in these outbreaks include the impossibility of isolating an airborne transmissible agent if the patient's room has positive air pressure relative to the hall outside (47, 48) and the known ability of chickenpox transmission to occur before vesicles appear (26). The economic impact of such outbreaks may be significant. Hyams et al estimated the cost of their outbreak in 1980 at $19,000 (39), and Boyce et al reported spending $20,100 in 1982 (38).

The approach to managing hospital employees with an exposure to a case of chickenpox or zoster is straightforward. First the details of the suspected index case must be verified to ensure the correct diagnosis of chickenpox or zoster and to be certain a case described as dermatomal zoster is not a disseminated case with its much greater risk of transmission. Then the exposed employees should be evaluated to determine if they have a history of prior infection or positive varicella serology. A history of an individual exposed in a home setting to children with chickenpox cannot be relied upon as indicative of immunity (39). However, a positive history of chickenpox is essentially 100% reliable (51–53). For those individuals whose status is uncertain or unknown, blood should be drawn for immediate serologic testing. Either an indirect fluorescent antibody test or enzyme-linked immunosorbent assay can be used, but not a complement fixation test because it is too insensitive (30). The majority of these individuals (72 to 96%) will show serologic evidence of prior varicella infection (51–53). Those who are seronegative should be sent home starting 10 days after the first day of possible exposure (13). Those who do not develop chickenpox by day 21 should be allowed to return to work. Each case of chickenpox in an employee should be evaluated individually. The CDC recommends that employees remain home until all lesions are crusted and dry, although data provided by Thomson (Table 13.7) suggest that some individuals may be able to return to work sooner (27–29).

Conjunctivitis

Conjunctivitis occurs uncommonly in hospital personnel (1% of our HEH visits). Although bacteria are reported to be the most common cause of conjunctivitis in adults (54), in our experience this presentation is uncommon in hospital employees. Only a few of the 56 cases of conjunctivitis seen during the 1-year study period had purulence associated with their conjunctivitis. Although we cannot determine the number of viral cases because routine viral cultures were not done, two small clusters of severe conjunctivitis were determined to be due to adenovirus infection. Since this organism is the predominant cause of epidemic keratoconjunctivitis, we will focus on its epidemiology.

The incubation period for adenovirus keratoconjunctivitis ranges from 4 to 24 days, and the conjunctivitis may last from 1 to 4 weeks (55). Outbreaks of this disease commonly involve medical personnel (56–69), occurring in ophthalmologists' offices (56, 58, 65, 67), factory dispensaries (59, 61), and hospitals (57, 60, 62–64, 68, 69). Both inanimate reservoirs (ophthalmic solutions, tonometry equipment, and a linen roll towel dispenser) (58, 59, 61, 65, 67) and person-to-person contact (57, 62, 66, 69) have been implicated as mechanisms of transmission. This highly contagious form of adenovirus infection has been documented to spread from patient to staff and from staff to patient. If not recognized quickly, massive outbreaks may occur. Straube et al reported an outbreak of adenovirus that developed in a children's hospital where 78% of 383 personnel questioned became ill during the epidemic period (69). Significantly, most of these individuals had either upper respiratory tract symptoms (72%) or diarrhea (28%); only 15% of the involved personnel had conjunctivitis. The most reliable method for interrupting disease transmission is to identify and eliminate any environmental reservoirs, isolate infected patients appropriately, send home involved personnel, and emphasize strict hand washing (58, 66, 69).

Cytomegalovirus

Cytomegalovirus (CMV) infection occurs throughout the world, especially in less developed areas. Even in the United States reported prevalence rates range from 45 to 79% (70). Significantly, a number of distinct patient populations have a high prevalence of CMV infection and organism shedding, particularly young children, organ transplant patients, and AIDS patients (70–76). Children constitute the greatest patient source of CMV in the hospital setting (72–73). In the second year of life CMV excretion rates in saliva and urine may exceed 80% (71). Higher excretion rates are found in children raised in day care centers compared to those raised at home (72). Transmission of CMV occurs by several routes—direct contact, sexual contact, breast feeding, congenital transmission, and transfusion (70).

Its clinical manifestation in adults is most commonly a mononucleosis-like illness which may be protracted and result in significant time lost from work (70). Of greater concern is that a primary CMV infection may develop in a pregnant employee. Such infections may have devastating consequences, as 25% of these infants may have congenital CMV infection at the time of birth (70).

Much controversy exists over the risk of a hospital employee acquiring CMV infection from a patient. Several studies examining pediatric personnel have found a greater risk of CMV infection comparing those with frequent versus infrequent patient contact (77, 78) or pediatric versus nonpediatric personnel (78). In contrast, other investigators studying similar groups found no clear differences (79–81). None of the six cited studies matched the populations for socioeconomic status, age, sexual activity, marital status, or exposure to young children. While it may not be possible to carry out a study controlling for all important variables, the failure to control for the presence of young children may explain the extreme variations in study outcome.

Presently, the best evidence suggesting a low risk of acquiring CMV infection by hospital personnel from patients is provided by studies employing restriction endonuclease analysis. If personnel acquire CMV infections from patients, this is probably due to poor technique, such as inadequate hand washing. This would also transmit CMV to other susceptible patients and culminate in clusters of infection due to the same virus. Recent studies by Spector et al using restriction enzyme analysis have demonstrated that almost all of these clusters are coincidental because the isolated viruses in each cluster are usually different (82, 83). The risk of drawing erroneous conclusions based on coincidental infections is further substantiated by three additional case studies. In each case a woman who had worked with congenitally CMV-infected infants subsequently developed an active CMV infection and assumed that it came from her patients (84–86). Yet, restriction enzyme analysis clearly showed that the viruses from the hospitalized children were different from those of the health care workers. No similar evidence has been provided suggesting that employees are transmitting CMV infections to patients.

The existing data do not support unusual means to prevent the transmission of CMV to pregnant personnel. It seems reasonable to emphasize hand washing as part of pregnancy counseling, but it does not seem warranted to institute serologic screening or to move personnel to "low risk" areas.

Hepatitis A

Hepatitis A is uncommon in the hospital because it is rarely severe enough to require hospitalization (87). Since it commonly presents without symptoms (87), a cluster of secondary cases may be the earliest evidence of hepatitis A. Transmitted most commonly by the fecal-oral route, the peak of infectivity occurs about the time jaundice begins (87). The virus can be detected in the stool from 2 to 3 weeks prior to 8 days after the onset of jaundice (87). Due to recently available test methods for measuring IgM antibody to hepatitis A (88, 89), nosocomial hepatitis A is being described with increasing frequency (90–102). Significantly, hepatitis A is usually introduced into a hospital by blood transfusion (94–101), a route of transmission once thought to be nonexistent (100). Hospital outbreaks have occurred in the following locations: cafeteria, 1; surgery ward, 1; pediatric ward, 2; medicine ward, 2; and neonatal care units, 4. In all but one of these outbreaks a patient was the index case. At least one report exists of an outbreak in a nursery attributed to a nurse (102).

Limiting the spread of hepatitis A in the hospital setting depends upon the immediate use of serum immune globulin prophylaxis (0.02 ml/kg) for exposed patients, hospital personnel, and family members (101). Whether an outbreak occurs and how big it becomes will be determined by how quickly the first case of hepatitis A is identified. In one report of transfusion-related hepatitis A, early diagnosis of the blood donor followed by the institution of globulin prophylaxis limited the outbreak to two secondary cases in addition to the index nosocomial case (100). In a similar situation where the information was not available on the blood donor, 55 cases of nosocomial hepatitis A developed—over half of them symptomatic (101).

Hepatitis B

Hepatitis B occurs frequently in hospital employees (103–106). During a 1-year monitoring of employee health visits we found hepatitis B to be the most common infectious cause of prolonged work absence; time lost ranged from 3 weeks to 2 months (Table 13.5). Persons in those occupations with the greatest exposure to blood or patient tissue specimens have the greatest risk (107). Groups at highest risk include surgeons, anesthesiologists, pathologists, hemodialysis personnel, surgical intensive care unit personnel, and laboratory workers who handle or draw blood specimens (103–106). These groups have serologic hepatitis B prevalence rates of 10 to 30%. Similarly, dentists represent another high risk group working in hospitals and outpatient areas (108). The prevalence of past hepatitis B infection in any of these populations increases with the duration of exposure (104, 106). Although hepatitis B in hospital staff most commonly occurs sporadically, outbreaks have been described involving an oncology unit (109), dialysis units (110, 111) and operating room staff (112–114).

Among hospital personnel who develop symptomatic hepatitis B, there is an impressive lack of concrete exposures. For our seven personnel who became ill with hepatitis B, only two of them had an unequivocal exposure (a needle stick). The findings of other investigators have been even more worrisome. Hansen et al found that only 4 of 27 employees who developed hepatitis B reported an exposure (115), and Schneider reported that only 4 of 30 employees related any hepatitis B exposure prior to disease onset (116). Similarly, in four of the six cited hepatitis B outbreaks involving employees there were no identified needle stick or other clearly documented exposures (109, 110, 113, 114). While some of these data may be explained by underreporting, this information is the strongest argument for the use of the hepatitis B vaccine. A detailed discussion of this vaccine is presented in Chapter 12.

For hospital employees with identifiable exposures to hepatitis B the most common type is a needle puncture or sharp instrument injury (88%), followed by blood in cuts (7%), or miscellaneous other accidents (5%) (115). Even these more definitive exposures are underreported (117, 118), particularly by new employees (117), by nurses or laboratory personnel (118), and, in our experience, by physicians. Hospital personnel with the greatest risk for acquiring a needle stick exposure are nurses, housekeepers, and clinical laboratory workers (117–120). Practices increasing the risk of needle stick exposures include improper disposal of objects in needle boxes or trash baskets in patient rooms (the latter affecting housekeeping personnel) and recapping needles. These risks are amplified for part time and night shift personnel (118, 120).

Conversely, what is the risk of an HBsAg-positive hospital staff member's transmitting the virus to a patient? A prospective study examining this question followed contacts of three chronic carriers (two physicians and a nurse) and two individuals with acute hepatitis B (a physician and a food handler) (121). Of 228 identified contacts followed for 6 months, none developed serologic evidence of hepatitis B infection. Studies examining the contacts of two dentists (122) and an orthopaedic surgeon (123) incubating acute hepatitis B found similar results. Subsequently, a number of reports have demonstrated the transmission of hepatitis B from employee to patient. Clusters of hepatitis B infection have been associated with a nurse (124), a respiratory therapist (112), a cardiac perfusion pump technician (125), a general practitioner (126), a thoracic surgeon (125), gynecologic surgeons (127–129), and dentists/oral surgeons (130–133). Proposed mechanisms of transmission in these outbreaks include exudative dermatitis and arterial cannula manipulation, 1; bleeding warts, 1; unknown, 2; and intraoperative field instrument of needle pricks. Since personnel hands appear to be the source of hepatitis B in each of these outbreaks, such individuals are recommended either to start wearing gloves or to use a double-glove technique. While this has been successful with some individuals (128, 131), it does not always work (125). Thus, the decision about whether a carrier of HBsAg can work must be determined individually. Fortunately, this route of transmission is uncommon.

The management of hepatitis B employee exposures hinges upon an understanding of hepatitis B serology. As a general rule, any individual with a positive test for HBsAg, anti-HBs, and/or anti-core antibody can be considered to have had a hepatitis B infection. Individuals who are chronically HBsAg-positive should be considered immune related to subsequent exposures to this virus. Those with antibody to HBs and/or core antigen also appear to be protected from such exposures (134). Two uncommon exceptions include individuals who make subtype-specific antibody (135) and individuals who make antibody without any specificity (136). The latter occurs in approximately 2% of blood donors with anti-HBs antibodies (135). The first situation cannot be detected outside of a reference laboratory, but the second can be suspected if the individual is anti-HBs-positive and anti-core antibody-negative and has not received the hepatitis B vaccine. If screening for core antibody is not already done routinely, then each institution must decide if the extra cost of measuring core antibody is worthwhile. It is also important to be aware that false positive HBsAg tests may occur if the test is performed incorrectly, and this should be sus-

pected if test results are inconsistent with clinical findings (137).

Once serologic testing has demonstrated that an exposed employee is susceptible to hepatitis B or if such testing is not available, then consideration must be given to immunoglobulin administration. This has been discussed elsewhere in detail (13, 134, 138). The CDC recommends the immediate administration of 0.06 ml/kg of hepatitis B immune globulin (13) for individuals with parenteral or mucosal exposures to blood, that is HBsAg-positive or is from a high risk patient (drug addict, etc) or hospital area (dialysis ward, etc). For susceptible individuals it is further recommended that the first injection be followed by either the immediate administration of the hepatitis B vaccine (139) or in 1 month by a second dose of globulin. When hepatitis B immune globulin is administered in this fashion, the risk of developing symptomatic infection can be reduced to approximately 2% (140). Unfortunately, there are no compelling data justifying the second dose of globulin (134), which is unfortunate because its elimination would save millions of dollars every year nationwide. The time interval from exposure to globulin administration is quite important, for when it is given within 48 hours the incidence of hepatitis B infection is more than 2-fold less than when it is given later (141). Although the CDC suggests that globulin prophylaxis for needle sticks may not be effective later than 7 days after the exposure (13), the actual time limit is unknown. For spouses of individuals with hepatitis B, protection has been shown up to several weeks after the initial exposure (142).

Hepatitis Non-A, Non-B

Due to the lack of serologic markers for diagnosing non-A, non-B (NANB) hepatitis, the true magnitude of the problem as a cause of nosocomial infection is unknown. Although data from India show the transmission of a variety of NANB by the fecal-oral route (143), in the United States no data exist to suggest that NANB hepatitis transmission occurs any differently than hepatitis B. For hepatitis cases requiring admission to referral hospitals in the United States, 25% were due to NANB hepatitis (144). Ninety percent of post-transfusion hepatitis cases have been attributed to NANB hepatitis (145). At least one outbreak of nosocomial NANB hepatitis has occurred involving an oncology unit (146), as well as transmission from patient to personnel via needle stick (147). All information on the prophylaxis of NANB infection originates from studies on the prevention of post-transfusion hepatitis. Serum immune globulin has been reported to decrease the incidence of NANB infection (144, 148); other similar studies fail to demonstrate any protection (149, 150). Although controversial, it seems reasonable to suggest that significant personnel exposures to blood or body fluids from a patient with NANB hepatitis should be treated with serum immune globulin.

Herpes Simplex

Herpes simplex infections are of importance to hospital personnel for two reasons: herpetic whitlow and other localized infections develop from occupational exposures, and health care personnel are capable of transmitting herpes simplex infections.

First described in hospital personnel in 1959 (151), herpetic whitlows can occur in any health care person frequently exposed to oropharyngeal secretions—nurses, dentists, or dental assistants, respiratory therapists, and anesthesiologists (152–156). Herpetic whitlows are caused both by type 1 and type 2 herpes simplex viruses (157, 158), and either type may be recurrent (159). Employees with herpes whitlows frequently lose 2 to 3 weeks from work, and absence of up to 7 weeks has been reported (154). The current availability of oral acyclovir may significantly reduce the time lost. Some authorities recommend the use of gloves on both hands while performing any type of oral care or suctioning (160). However, after 70,000 general anesthetic administrations, Orkin identified only one definite and one suspected case of herpetic whitlow among the employees (161). He thought the costs to prevent these two cases would be excessive; in 1976 wearing a glove on each hand would have cost an additional $5,600. It has been recommended that personnel with herpes whitlows can work if they wear gloves (154); however, this suggestion has not been adequately tested.

Recent outbreaks of herpes simplex infection have demonstrated the significant role that employees may play in the transmission of the virus. In one investigation by Adams et al three nurses in a pediatric intensive care unit developed whitlows, and one developed a herpes simplex pharyngitis after exposure to two infants with herpes simplex infections (162). Subsequently, restriction endonuclease mapping demonstrated that these nurses transmitted herpes simplex to another child and the husband of one of the nurses.

The question of whether herpes labialis can be transmitted to a child has been raised because individuals with fever blisters can usually be demonstrated to have the virus on their hands, and the virus can persist there for up to 2 hours (163). More definitively, by use of endonuclease mapping, herpes labialis has been demonstrated to be transmitted from parent to infant (164, 165). Thus, neither parents nor employees with herpes labialis should kiss a newborn infant. It has been recommended that employees with such infections should be kept from working with infants and other immunocompromised hosts (13); however, no data exist to show that wearing a mask is not sufficient to prevent cross-infection.

Influenza

Nationwide outbreaks of influenza A are more common than influenza B, a phenomenon attributed to the more frequent antigenic shifts that occur with influenza A (166, 167). For influenza A the same mechanism has also been used to explain the relative lack of long-lasting immunity and the more severe illness that occurs in comparison with influenza B (166, 167). Influenza is predominantly transmitted by small particle aerosols; a single individual can transmit the infection to many others (167). Viral secretion begins about 1 day before symptoms, maximizes at 24 to 48 hours, and then declines rapidly with a total duration of 5 to 10 days, although it may be prolonged in young children (167).

In parallel to the nationwide occurrence of influenza, nosocomial outbreaks are more frequently due to type A (168–181) than type B (166, 182, 183). This is because nosocomial outbreaks are preceded by community outbreaks. Thus, hospital employees risk acquiring the infection from at least two routes—their own children and hospitalized patients (167). Control of nosocomial influenza infections depends upon recognizing that the problem exists. Except when a major and unpredicted antigenic shift occurs, the influenza vaccine minimizes the impact of an outbreak on hospital personnel (see Chapter 12). However, even when the appropriate vaccine is used, compliance problems with personnel leave a substantial nonimmune population. Knowing this is very important when considering outbreak interventions, including vaccination and amantadine prophylaxis (184). Simultaneous administration of both the vaccine and amantadine is recommended to stop an influenza A outbreak (167, 184). This allows immunity to develop, while amantadine prevents infections from occurring. When administered in this fashion, amantadine needs to be given for only 2 weeks (167). Otherwise it may need to be continued until the outbreak subsides (167). Its major drawback is a high frequency of central nervous system side effects (insomnia, jitteriness, and difficulty concentrating). The recommended dose of amantadine is 200 mg/day, although 100 mg/day has been used successfully with a lower incidence of side effects (185). Also, rimantadine, if available, is just as effective as amantadine with a lower incidence of side effects (167). No drug is currently available for the prophylaxis of influenza B infections.

Measles

Measles is one of the most communicable infectious diseases, because transmission is largely by aerosol and may occur over very long distances (186–189). Viral shedding begins approximately 9 or 10 days after exposure and lasts for 7 to 10 days (190, 191). The introduction of the measles vaccine in 1962 markedly decreased the number of cases and changed the principal age groups in which the disease occurs to adolescents and young adults (190). Recent studies among young adults have found that from 4 to 20% are seronegative (192–194). This level of susceptibility appears sufficient to support "mini-epidemics" (186, 187, 192, 194–198). These have occurred among military recruits, on college campuses, at summer camps, in pediatric clinics, and in elementary schools. The transmission of measles has been reported in the hospital setting (199); most of the cases have involved nurses or clerical staff, and the majority of reports cite only one case each (range—one to six). It is likely that hospitals have not had any sizeable outbreaks because the susceptible individuals are scattered among a predominantly immune population, unlike the situation in military recruits and on college campuses where susceptibles exist in high density. Of note, the most common source of recent outbreaks has been foreign importation (200). Because foreign visitors and immigrants still come in large numbers to the United States, the risk of a case of measles presenting in a hospital is ever present. The best method for preventing outbreaks or terminating an existing outbreak is through the use of the measles vaccine (192, 193, 196, 197). This is covered in detail in Chapter 12. For individuals in whom a live virus vaccine is contraindicated, immunoglobulin will attenuate the infection if given within 3 days of exposure (190, 191).

Meningococcal Infection

Because of the explosive nature of meningococcal disease, exposure of hospital personnel to such patients produces a great deal of anxiety. However, the risk of an employee's becoming colonized appears to be quite low (less than 5%) in the setting of the usual patient with meningitis (201). Prior to antibiotic therapy certain factors are likely to increase this risk, including mouth-to-mouth resuscitation; mucosal contact with oral secretions; sharing food, drink, or eating utensils; suctioning the patient; or exposure to a patient with meningococcal pneumonia (202–205). Although patients with pneumonia would appear much more infectious, a recent study by Cohen et al found only 1 of 349 hospital personnel working in or near an area where a patient with meningococcal pneumonia resided had a positive throat swab for the organism (204). The data indicate that the organism is predominantly transmitted by direct contact and suggest that hospital personnel should receive antibiotic prophylaxis only if they fall into one of the above high risk groups. Such individuals should receive rifampin, 600 mg twice a day for 2 days (203). There is no evidence to suggest that any surveillance cultures should be performed on employees.

Mumps

The incidence of mumps has declined substantially since the introduction of a live vaccine in 1967 (206). Since that time it has been a very uncommon problem in the hospital setting with only two outbreaks reported—one on a pediatric ward in the United States in 1968 and the other in an infant nursery in Japan in 1971 (207, 208). This is fortunate because such outbreaks are almost impossible to control until all susceptibles are infected, due to the asymptomatic viral shedding that begins up to 9 days prior to the appearance of parotitis (209). Currently, mumps is an unlikely problem from the standpoint of employee health.

Pertussis

The incidence of pertussis infection in the United States is low due to the widespread use of the vaccine (210). Recently the lay press has produced a great deal of concern in the general public about vaccine-related complications. As a result there is a significant impression among pediatricians that the use of the vaccine has declined substantially. If the trend continues, the rate of pertussis infection may rise.

Even currently there is a continuing risk of transmitting this infection from children to hospital personnel. Lasting immunity does not occur with natural infection, and up to 50% of individuals who are at least 12 years from their vaccination are susceptible (210, 211). Nosocomial transmission has been documented in at least two reports (212, 213). One outbreak involved eight physicians and five nurses (213). Transmission in these circumstances often occurs before an individual develops a cough (213). Thus, once an outbreak is recognized it may be necessary to remove heavily exposed individuals from work at the first sign of any respiratory infection. Erythromycin prophylaxis effectively prevents exposed cases from developing clinical pertussis, and the vaccine may prevent secondary cases (212). Control is important because the disease in adults may be severe (213).

Respiratory Syncytial Virus (RSV)

RSV is the most common cause of lower respiratory tract infection in infants (214). With primary infection in this age group, 40 to 70% of infants develop pneumonia or bronchiolitis (214). Potentially fatal in normal infants, RSV has an even higher associated death rate in infants with cardiopulmonary disease, congenital disorders, or immunocompromised states (214–217). As protective immunity develops infrequently after primary infection, virtually any age group is susceptible and may contribute to the spread of the disease (214). About half of normal adults become infected after exposure to RSV, and these individuals usually manifest upper respiratory tract symptoms (214). However, in older patients, particularly those who are hospitalized, bronchopneumonia is frequent (214, 218, 219).

Nosocomial outbreaks of RSV infection are well described (214, 215, 220–229) and occur in association with community outbreaks during the winter months (214). The transmission of nosocomial RSV infection has been carefully examined in a series of studies by Hall. Viral shedding by infected infants was found to be quite high and to persist throughout hospitalization (223, 224). The virus was capable of surviving on countertops for up to 6 hours (230). In the outbreak setting about half of the medical staff caring for the infants developed an RSV infection (214, 221, 229). The wearing of gowns and masks did not prevent viral transmission (228). Cohorting of infected infants and staff was the only measure found to decrease the incidence of viral transmission to other infants (227). Unfortunately, this measure did not have any influence on the incidence of RSV disease in the staff (226). Thus, due to the high attack rate among hospital staff in an outbreak setting, it will be impossible to send employees home when they become ill.

Rotavirus

Rotaviruses are the most common cause of diarrhea in industrialized regions of the world (231). Predominantly a disease of young children (232, 233), it also occurs in adults, particularly contacts of infected children (234–236). Although the illness may be quite severe (237), deaths occur uncommonly, affecting the very young (238, 239) and the very old (240, 241). A previous infection does not produce immunity, but subsequent infections are generally milder (242). Asymptomatic viral shedding may be seen in 50 to 70% of children under 6 months old (243, 244). Thought to be transmitted by the fecal-oral route (245), some evidence suggests that respiratory secretions may play a role (246).

Nosocomial infection with this virus is well recognized (240, 241, 247–251). Outbreaks have been described on pediatric, maternity and geriatric wards. Striking features of some of these outbreaks include short incubation periods (1 to 2 days), large numbers of infected patients (241, 251), infected personnel (250), a temporal association of the outbreak with an ongoing community outbreak (249, 251), and great difficulty in controlling the outbreak (249, 251). Viral transmission is hard to prevent because viral shedding can occur in asymptomatic individuals (244, 247) and can persist for more than 3 weeks in normal hosts (248) and indefinitely in immunocompromised hosts (R. Sherertz, P. Reumen, B. Russell, and M. Sullivan, unpublished data). Strict cohorting of patients and personnel is the best method of managing these outbreaks.

Rubella

Rubella infections continue to occur and have an important medical and economic impact because of the catastrophic effect of the virus on a fetus in the first trimester (252). Since 1969 when the live rubella vaccine was put into use, there have been no major outbreaks of rubella in the United States (252). However, minor outbreaks continue to occur, because about 20% of young adults are seronegative for rubella (252–256). A number of outbreaks have occurred in the hospital setting (254–259). Significantly, the index cases in these outbreaks have been hospital employees, not inpatients. In four well characterized outbreaks the index cases were obstetricians, an obstetrical nurse, and a dietary worker (254, 256, 258, 259). Such outbreaks have resulted in therapeutic abortions (255) as well as substantial expenditures of time and money. Polk et al, at the end of their 1979 hospital rubella outbreak, estimated that laboratory tests, lost work time, and extra wages paid to personnel involved in the immunization cost about $50,000 (258).

The prevention of a hospital rubella outbreak is relatively straightforward. It must be recognized that a history of rubella is an unreliable indicator of immunity (260), infected individuals begin shedding virus up to 7 days before the characteristic rash appears, and subclinical cases may transmit the illness (252). At present the CDC recommends that hospital personnel working in areas at high risk for contacting patients with rubella and/or pregnant females should be immune to rubella (13). Serologic screening followed by vaccination of seronegative individuals is an obvious approach to this problem (193). However, two significant considerations hinder this solution. Some institutions feel they cannot legally mandate rubella vaccinations (255, 258). This is further complicated by the poor compliance of physicians in voluntary vaccine programs (258, 261). Thus, success in decreasing the likelihood of a rubella outbreak depends upon one's ability to execute a vaccine program (see Chapter 12).

Salmonella/Shigella

Nosocomial *Salmonella* infections in hospitals and other health care institutions are well recognized and quite common (262–269). In a 10-year period in the United States the CDC received information on 112 *Salmonella* outbreaks (270), and in a 2-year period their counterpart in England, the Communicable Disease Surveillance Centre, tabulated information on 55 outbreaks (271). Both found similar patterns of outbreaks with relevance to hospital employee health. Outbreaks most commonly involved pediatric patients (36.6%) who were either admitted with the infection or who acquired the organism from their mother during birth. Cross-infection by personnel was the mechanism responsible for the largest number of outbreaks. Foodborne outbreaks were relatively uncommon. These outbreaks involve hospital personnel in several ways. Most of the time employees serve as a vector probably by forgetting to wash their hands be-

tween patient contacts. However, they may participate primarily if their gastrointestinal tract becomes colonized with *Salmonella*. The surveillance group in London found that in outbreak investigations where all at-risk individuals were cultured, one-third of infected patients and three-quarters of infected personnel were asymptomatic (271). In four hospital outbreaks of *Salmonella* infections where screening cultures of personnel were reported, asymptomatic personnel secretors (range—2 to 10) were found in each case (262–265).

Some infected personnel will become chronic carriers and continue to be a risk for the nosocomial transmission of *Salmonella*. With *S. typhi* the risk is 1 to 3%; for nontyphoidal salmonellas the risk is less than 1% (272). Although the risk of nontyphoidal infections leading to a carrier state is less than with *S. typhi*, in the United States these infections are much more common (46:1). Thus, nontyphoidal carriers may exist in greater numbers than *S. typhi* carriers (266). Nontyphoidal carriers are most commonly *S. paratyphi* B (37%) or *S. typhimurium* (20%), and overall about 20% of these carriers have been associated with outbreaks (273). Most states have public health laws that prohibit any *Salmonella* carriers from working as food preparers or hospital employee with patient contact.

The existing data on *Salmonella* infections suggest the following considerations for the management of hospital personnel. If an outbreak of *Salmonella* infections occurs in a hospital, stool cultures should be performed on all individuals with contact exposure to infected patients or implicated fomites. Personnel with positive stool cultures for *Salmonella*, asymptomatic or not, should be followed up with serial cultures every month or two until negative or until they are established as chronic carriers—positive for more than 1 year (272). State laws may mandate that certain employees, such as food handlers, not be allowed to work until culture-negative. Chronic carriers implicated as the cause of an outbreak should be removed from their jobs until either the carrier state can be eliminated or they can be reassigned to low risk occupations. Employees with acute infections should be job restricted until asymptomatic. If state laws permit, asymptomatic individuals with positive cultures may be allowed to work if they avoid contact with high risk patients (13).

The nosocomial transmission of *Shigella* occurs but has been documented much less frequently than *Salmonella* (274). This may relate to the much lower frequency of a long term *Shigella* carrier state (275). Management of employees with *Shigella* should be similar to that for those with *Salmonella*. However, unlike *Salmonella* infections in which antibiotics prolong the carrier state (262), a course of antibiotics will shorten the duration of the carrier state of *Shigella* and thus decrease the time lost from work by the employee (276).

Scabies

Our experience suggests that the acquisition of scabies by hospital personnel is not uncommon despite the small number of reports in the literature (277–280). Those developing the infection usually have a history of skin-to-skin contact with the index case. The incubation period ranges from about 1 to 4 weeks. Lerche et al provided an extensive discussion of the management of an outbreak involving patients and hospital staff (280). Control measures involve cohorting of staff and personnel; mass cleaning of patient bedding, clothing, food trays, etc; and treatment of all employees or patients with direct patient contact or contact with likely fomites (280). The usual treatment for adults is lindane, a pesticide.

Staphylococcus aureus

Although *S. aureus* is one of the most important nosocomial pathogens, the relationship of hospital personnel to the development of such infections is not totally understood. *S. aureus* nasal carriage in the general population ranges from 20 to 40% and in hospital personnel it is 50%, 70%, and 90% among physicians, nurses, and ward attendants, respectively (281, 282). In spite of high staphylococcal carrier rates, relatively few point source outbreaks have been demonstrated to be due to hospital personnel (283–287). This may be true for several reasons. Finding this organism on an individual's skin appears to correlate better with nasal carriage than with other conditions, such as a skin boil or pustule (288, 289). Nasal carriage of *S. aureus* also seems to be a prerequisite for an individual's being able to disperse (shed) the organism into the air (288). Not all nasal carriers shed the organism—only those with large numbers of staphylococci detectable by quantitative culture (289). Interestingly, shedding staphylococci into the air occurs in 10% of male carriers but in only 1% of female carriers (288, 290, 291). Males not only shed organisms

more frequently but in greater numbers (290, 291). Little objective evidence exists to support the notion that patients with *S. aureus* infections or carrier states are a risk to hospital personnel.

Studies of individuals implicated as the source of staphylococcal outbreaks provide further understanding. In two outbreaks of staphylococcal skin disease in nurseries where a single nurse was found to be the source, both were controlled by the successful eradication of the individuals' staphylococcal carrier states (283, 284). In another outbreak associated with an operating room technician, the carrier state could not be eliminated (285). In an intensive 4-year study, he was found to disperse up to six colony-forming units of *S. aureus* per cubic foot of air sampled during 2-minute exercise periods. Shedding could be suppressed temporarily but not eliminated by oral antibiotics (cloxacillin, erythromycin, and tetracycline). Daily povidone-iodine baths were ineffective, but daily bathing with chlorhexidine detergent markedly reduced the airborne dispersal of staphylococci. Significantly, although his dispersal was actively suppressed, his nasal carriage of the organism remained intact, suggesting that his skin, not his nose, was the source. The converse may also be possible. As described by Eichenwald et al, the so-called "cloud babies" shed their organisms from their nose only during an active upper respiratory viral infection (292). In a recent outbreak that we evaluated (284) infections were documented only during two time periods when the implicated nurse had an upper respiratory tract infection. Thus, an individual who is not a chronic staphylococcal disperser may become one when a viral upper respiratory tract infection is superimposed upon the nasal carriage of *S. aureus.*

The weight of evidence suggests that when a point source outbreak occurs, nasal carriers of *S. aureus* should be sought and treated if found. Various approaches have been tried to modify or eliminate the carrier state. Attempts using oral antibiotics have almost uniformly failed. Topical antibiotics applied nasally have produced variable results. Early work demonstrated gentamicin to be slightly more effective than vancomycin or chlorhexidine (293). A recent study indicated that vancomycin and bacitracin were not significantly different from placebo (294). The most encouraging antibiotic for this purpose has turned out to be rifampin. In two studies it has decreased the number of carriers significantly in comparison to controls, and no evidence of resistance was found post-treatment (295, 296). Of significance, the addition of a second antibiotic in combination with rifampin to prevent the development of resistance either did no better than rifampin alone (295) or reduced the effectiveness of rifampin (296). Overall the data suggest that the carrier state is unlikely to be eradicated in many individuals, and the concept of suppression is more viable. If one employee continues to be linked with *S. aureus* infections in spite of attempts to suppress nasal carriage in combination with other modalities, such as daily antiseptic baths, then consideration should be given to relocating the employee to another job (285).

Streptococcus, Group A

The group A streptococcus, *Streptococcus pyogenes*, was first demonstrated to be a cause of nosocomial infections by Semmelweis (297). Employees are most commonly affected by this organism in the form of sore throats. It is unclear if many of the infections result from patient exposures. Outbreaks of infections linked to employees have been well described. Interestingly, none of them were associated with employees with sore throats. Implicated sites of employee colonization have included the nose, perirectal area, and vagina (298–307). In one unusual outbreak an anesthesiologist was determined to be a rectal carrier, and the data suggested that the organism was spread by the airborne route (300). Unlike the staphylococcal carrier state, the group A streptococcus carrier has been easy to treat. Implicated individuals should have their pharynx, rectum, and vagina cultured. If the throat culture only is positive, then 1.2 million units of benzathine penicillin should be employed (11). For anal and vaginal carriers penicillin has also been effective (11), and vancomycin has been shown to work for anal carriers (298).

Syphilis

The risk of a hospital employee's developing syphilis after any kind of nosocomial exposure is not entirely clear. Inoculation studies in volunteers have shown that the 50% infecting dose (ID50) is approximately 57 organisms when given by injection (308), and as few as 4 organisms can cause infection (309). Since primary and secondary syphilitic lesions, unlike tertiary lesions, have large numbers of organisms in them (up to 10,000,000/g of tissue with primary lesions) it seems reasonable that transmission could occur (309). Whitney summarized 10 physician cases

of syphilis that were believed to be acquired from patients (310). Nine of these physicians had lesions on their fingers. Seven were able to identify exposures, including a scalpel wound, changing dressings of a suppurative node, examining a perirectal secondary syphilis lesion, performing a tonsillectomy and adenoidectomy on a child with active syphilis, and performing bare-handed vaginal examinations. Essentially all of these could have been prevented by wearing gloves. Although in patients with tertiary syphilis spirochetes have been found in the aqueous humor, cerebrospinal fluid, and gummas (311, 312), there are no documented cases of transmission occurring in this setting. Since this disease and a possible exposure to it often incite hysteria, each "exposure" needs to be evaluated individually to determine if therapy is necessary.

Tuberculosis

Tuberculosis will be a continual problem for employee health services as long as patients with this disease are admitted to the hospital. The current acquisition rate of tuberculosis for hospital employees (as judged by purified protein derivative (PPD) conversion) is about 1 to 2%/year (313–319). Employee groups within the hospital at greatest risk for developing tuberculosis include nurses, physicians, radiology technicians, laboratory technicians working with *Mycobacterium tuberculosis*, housekeeping, laundry workers, maintenance and engineering personnel (313, 315, 317). Some of these groups, such as housekeeping, laundry workers, etc, have very little patient exposure and most likely acquire their tuberculosis outside of the hospital (317). For those with patient contact the greatest risk of infection results from exposure to an undiagnosed patient (320). Such patients are the cause of virtually all outbreaks of tuberculosis in the hospital setting (321–325).

Most authorities agree that employees should be screened for tuberculosis by yearly skin test (11, 13), but not by annual chest X-ray because the latter approach is ineffective (13, 326). The Mantoux skin test using 5 tuberculin units (TU) of PPD is the accepted method for performing this screening (327). There is no reason to use PPD in concentrations of 100 TU or higher, since they will not allow one to distinguish controls from individuals infected with tuberculosis (328). Although some groups have used multipuncture techniques to screen large numbers of people rapidly and have found certain tests to be satisfactory (329), it is generally thought that such tests should be avoided (13).

A controversial aspect of skin testing is the routine employment of the two-step method advocated by the CDC (330). The approach involves the application of a second Mantoux skin test at least 1 week after the first to individuals with negative or nonsignificant initial tests. An increase in the amount of skin test induration by greater than 6 mm from a baseline of less than 10 mm to a final value of greater than 10 mm represents a positive booster response. It is thought to be caused by a remote tuberculous infection or sensitization to a nontuberculous *Mycobacterium* (331). Incremental yields above the PPD rate with a single Mantoux test have included 0%, Rochester, NY (332); 0.4%, Sacramento, CA (333); 4.5%, 10 different states (331); 7.4%, Dayton, OH (334); and 8.3%, Mobile, AL (335). The data suggest that this approach to skin testing will have to be evaluated individually by each hospital to decide if the cost of the added effort is worthwhile.

Who should be skin tested? This question always arises after any documented tuberculosis exposure. The actual question is, how infectious was the patient? Although many factors affect the infectivity of a patient, only a few are practical to consider. Young children with nonprogressive primary tuberculosis are unlikely to be contagious unless they have a cough and a cavitary infiltrate (336). If available, the most useful information is the presence or absence of acid-fast bacilli (AFB) on the sputum smear (337, 338). Smear-positive individuals have a 20-fold greater risk of transmitting infection than those with negative smears. A second important variable is the duration of chemotherapy. Although many studies suggest that a population of individuals being treated for tuberculosis rapidly becomes noninfectious (339–341), for an individual patient it is impossible to say when this will occur (341). The Public Health Service has recommended that 2 to 3 weeks of treatment should be adequate (341). Is this appropriate for a neutropenic, bone marrow transplant patient with a very positive sputum smear? Or, at the other extreme, what about a young asymptomatic adult without a cough or sputum production who has a single AFB found by bronchoscopy of a 3- to 4-cm nodular infiltrate? Rather than adopt a rigid policy about when a patient or employee should be considered noninfectious, it seems prudent to evaluate each case individually (338, 342, 343).

For contacts of smear-negative individuals, the investigation should be limited only to those with close contact (nurses, physicians, medical students caring directly for the patient). For smear-positive individuals, it is probably reasonable to consider two approaches. For those with just a few organisms seen on smear, an initial investigation of only close contacts seems appropriate. If many of these are positive, then consideration should be given to casual contacts, etc. When the sputum smear is very positive and the patient has other risk factors for being infectious, such as an active cough or a cavitary infiltrate, close as well as casual contacts should be looked at initially. Such individuals occasionally produce very high infection rates transmitting the organism to individuals who had no known exposure to the index patient (322).

The use of isoniazid (INH) chemoprophylaxis in the management of tuberculosis-infected employees has stirred much controversy. Data from prospective controlled studies of tuberculosis household contacts clearly demonstrate the effectiveness of 1 year of INH in decreasing the subsequent number of cases of tuberculosis (344). Equally solid is the documentation that INH causes hepatitis which may be fatal (345, 346). The disagreement arises over the interpretation of this information. The CDC recommends that HEH programs should initiate INH prophylaxis for individuals who are new infections, significant reactors with abnormal chest roentgenograms and negative bacteriologic findings, persons with special clinical conditions (on steroids, etc), significant reactors under age 35 years even in the absence of additional risk factors, and household members of persons with newly discovered tuberculosis (13). One aspect of this has been aggressively challenged by Taylor et al (347). They believe that these recommendations are too aggressive for individuals whose only risk factor is a positive tuberculin skin test. They felt that the original data analysis overestimated the long term risk of developing tuberculosis and the long term effectiveness of INH. Comstock's rebuttal of this challenge (348) strongly disagrees with most of the major suppositions upon which Taylor et al base their decision analysis. Both sides of this argument make debatable assumptions. Until more data are available it seems reasonable to follow the CDC recommendations except that each individual hospital should make its own decision concerning the administration of INH to employees under 35 with a positive PPD as the only risk factor for tuberculosis.

The method of monitoring individuals receiving INH has also been a subject for disagreement. The CDC and the American Thoracic Society discourage the use of liver function tests to monitor INH therapy because their elevation does not correlate with subsequent development of hepatitis (13, 349). Recently, several investigators have recommended that routine monthly liver function tests should be performed (350, 351). The first study by Byrd et al was a prospective randomized evaluation of liver function tests comparing INH to placebo during a 3-month period (350). They found that abnormal SGOT values occurred significantly more often on INH than placebo and reported no differences in symptoms between the groups and no relationship between elevated symptoms and SGOT. While we are essentially in agreement with their findings, our analysis of their data demonstrated a relationship between increased SGOT and "flu"-like symptoms in the INH group ($p < 0.05$, Fisher's exact test). Their study demonstrates that symptoms associated with isoniazid toxicity are nonspecific, but it does not show that checking an individual's transaminases provides any additional help. In fact it could be argued that measuring serum enzymes only on a monthly basis might allow a case of hepatitis that became active right after a monitoring visit to become quite significant before the next monitoring visit (345). The existing recommendations for monitoring only with symptoms still seem to be the best approach.

AREAS OF SPECIAL CONCERN
Day Care Nurseries

Many hospitals make infant day care available to assist the efforts of their working parents. Day care centers offer unique opportunities for the transmission of infectious diseases due to the sustained close contact maintained by young children. Diseases which have caused outbreaks in this setting include cryptosporidia (352), *Giardia* (353, 354), *Haemophilis influenzae* (355), hepatitis A (356–363), influenza (364), meningococcal infection (365), rotavirus (366), *Salmonella* (367), and *Shigella* (368–372). Recent information even suggests that hepatitis B is transmissible in this setting (373). Due to their frequency and ease of spread, hepatitis A and *Shigella* are the most likely diseases to impact on hospital staff. Good discussions exist elsewhere on the management of infections in this setting (374–377). A hospital employee health service may decrease the likelihood of such outbreaks by making nursery personnel aware that they can occur.

Laboratory Personnel

A detailed discussion of laboratory-acquired infections is beyond the scope of this chapter and unnecessary since the subject has been covered quite well by other authors (378–381). Individuals working in hospital laboratories have unique risks for developing infections due to continuous contact with patient specimens. Employees at highest risk are those who handle blood (hepatitis B, non-A, non-B hepatitis) and those who work in diagnostic microbiology. In over 80% of the cases no accident can be identified as the source of an infection (378). When an accident does occur the most likely causes in descending order of frequency are needle and syringe, spills or sprays, injury with a sharp object, and pipette aspiration (378). The most important causes of infection in this setting are *S. typhi*, *Brucella*, *M. tuberculosis*, arboviruses, hepatitis B, and fungal infections (coccidioidomycosis, histoplasmosis) (378). It is likely that virtually all of these infections are due to poor technique. The significance of this cannot be overemphasized because even such routine matters as laboratory proficiency examinations have had a fatal outcome (382). Education of personnel may play an important role in decreasing the likelihood of a laboratory-acquired infection.

Pregnant Personnel

The concern is that pregnant personnel may acquire a work-related infection which results in congenital infection of their child. Those infections with the greatest risk of producing congenital infection have been discussed in great detail elsewhere (383, 384). A summary of this information is provided in Table 13.9. Rubella, undoubtedly, has the greatest potential to affect the developing fetus adversely. Other infections with a high risk of adversely affecting the fetus include enterovirus infections (mainly ECHO viruses) at the time of delivery, hepatitis B in the third trimester, syphilis at any time during the pregnancy, toxoplasmosis in the third trimester, and varicella infection in the week prior to delivery. Lower risk infections include cytomegalovirus, herpes simplex, measles, mumps, and tuberculosis. The risk of acquiring these infections in the hospital setting greatly affects these considerations. For example, toxoplasmosis is rarely acquired under these circumstances (385). The risks of hospital personnel acquiring these infections have largely been discussed in previous sections and are summarized in Table 13.6. Based on these two sets of risks a policy has been developed at our institution for the management of pregnant employees (Table 13.10). For further details on this subject the reader is referred to Votra et al (383) and Remington and Klein (384).

COST OF AN EMPLOYEE HEALTH PROGRAM

As discussed in the introduction, the size of a hospital's employee health program is to a significant extent determined by the services offered. This same factor has direct bearing on the cost of the program to the hospital. The more services that are offered, the more personnel who are required to deliver them and the greater the cost. To give a frame of reference, the approximate costs of the major expenditures in our program are listed in Table 13.11. This is roughly $38/ employee examined/year. Additional hidden costs exist, such as time lost when an employee must be sent home after a chickenpox exposure. This example is particularly appropriate because the manner in which it is handled may have a

Table 13.9. Risk of Congenital Transmission for Pregnant Employees Exposed to Patients with Infectious Diseases

Disease	Risk of Congenital Transmission (383, 384)
Cytomegalovirus	Low risk of symptomatic disease transmission
Enterovirus	High risk of ECHO viruses at time of delivery, lower for coxsackie viruses
Hepatitis B	High risk with third trimester infection of mother
Herpes simplex	Low risk, infection during delivery is more likely
Influenza	Low risk
Measles	Low risk
Mumps	Undefined
Rubella	Very high risk during first 3 months
Syphilis	High risk at any time during pregnancy
Toxoplasmosis	Highest in third trimester
Tuberculosis	Rare, insufficient data to quantify risk
Varicella	High risk if rash appears within 7 days of delivery

Table 13.10. Recommendations for Pregnant Employee Interaction with Patients Having Communicable Infectious Diseases

Patient Disease	Employee Susceptibility*	Recommendations†
Chickenpox/zoster	S	A
	I	C
Cytomegalovirus	S	B
	I	C
Enterovirus	S	‡
Hepatitis B	S	B, D
	I	C
Herpes simplex	S	C or A
Influenza	S	A
Measles	S	A
	I	C
Mumps	S	A
	I	C
Polio virus	S	A
	I	C
Rubella	S or I	A
Syphilis	S	C
Toxoplasmosis	S	C
Tuberculosis	S or I	A

* S, Susceptible; I, immune.
† A, do not enter patient's room;
   B, no direct patient care;
   C, direct patient care using appropriate isolation precautions;
   D, seronegative pregnant women may wish to transfer out of a high risk area for the duration of pregnancy.
‡ During third trimester follow recommendation B.

Table 13.11. Approximate Costs for a 1-Year Period of an Employee Health Program in a 450-Bed University Hospital

Salaries: nurse practitioner, 2 additional RNs, secretary, clerk, medical director	$120,000
Pre-employment physical examinations (done by family practitioners on a contract basis)	$45,000
Drugs (90% is due to either hepatitis B immune globulin or Heptavax-B)	$50,000
Computer data base	$5,000
Miscellaneous	$15,000
Total	$235,000

large effect on compliance with work restrictions. / If an employee knows that he will not be paid when he is sent home because of an infectious illness, he is not likely to report his illness. Since the cost of an outbreak is always considerably more than the cost of the time lost to a single employee, this is not beneficial. Other costs can be reduced by employee education. For example, if significant employee time is being lost due to back injuries, then teaching the correct lifting technique may save a lot of money. The same is true with needle sticks and globulin prophylaxis. Additional cost savings can be gained by having housestaff (if available) do physical exams or by not doing them at all (13). Also, a computer data base for a hospital employee health program can be maintained very inexpensively on a microcomputer rather than on a mainframe. Once the program is set up and running, other ways to reduce costs will be found in addition to those mentioned.

Acknowledgments. We are indebted to the library research and editorial efforts of Carol Brown. We would also like to thank Janie Cusick for her efforts in setting up our employee health program and the Shands Hospital Administration for their continuing support.

References

1. Valenti WM, Dorn MR, Andrews BP, Presley BA, Reifler CB: Infection control and employee health: epidemiology and priorities for program development. *Am J Infect Control* 10:149–153, 1982.
2. *Infection Control in the Hospital,* ed 1, Chicago, American Hospital Association, 1968, p 30.
3. Gardner P, Oxman MN, Breton S: Hospital management of patients and personnel exposed to communicable diseases. *Pediatrics* 56:700–709, 1975.
4. Werdegar D: Guidelines for infection control aspects of employee health. *J Assoc Pract Infect Control* 5 (Sept):17–22, 1977.
5. Werdegar D: Guidelines for infection control aspects of employee health. *J Assoc Pract Infect Control* 5 (Dec):15–22, 1977.
6. *Infection Control in the Hospital,* ed 4. Chicago, American Hospital Association, 1979, p 30.
7. Klein JO: Management of infections in hospital employees. *Am J Med* 70:919–23, 1981.
8. Haley RW, Emori TG: The employee health service and infection control in US hospitals, 1976–1977, I. Screening procedures. *JAMA* 246:844–847, 1981.
9. Haley RW, Emori TG: The employee health service and infection control in US hospitals, 1976–1977. II. Managing employee illness. *JAMA* 246:962–966, 1981.
10. Kaslow RA, Garner JS: Hospital personnel. In Bennett JV, Brachman PS (eds): *Hospital Infections,* Boston, Little, Brown, and Co, 1979, p 27.
11. Atuk NO, Townsend TR, Hunt EH, Wenzel RP: An employee health service for infection control. In Wenzel RP (ed): *Handbook of Hospital Acquired Infections.* Boca Raton, FL, CRC Press, 1981, p 211.
12. *Hospital Employee Health,* Atlanta, American Health Consultants, 1982.
13. Williams WW: Guideline for infection control in hospital personnel, *Infect Control* 4:326–349, 1983.
14. Sullivan ML, Sherertz RJ, Russell BA, Rand KH, Hermann K, Gutekunst RR: Pseudo-outbreak of nosocomial rubella due to false positive IgM serology. 83rd Meeting of the American Society for Microbiology, New Orleans, 1983, abstract L28.
15. Buxton AE, Anderson RL, Werdegar D, Atlas E: Nosocomial respiratory tract infection and colonization with *Acinetobacter calcoaceticus. Am J Med* 65:507–513, 1978.
16. AIDS Surveillance Centers for Disease Control, Atlanta, December 18, 1984.
17. Centers for Disease Control; Food and Drug Administration; Alcohol, Drug Abuse, and Mental Health Administration; National Institutes of Health; Health Resources and Services Administration: Provisional Public Health Service interagency recommendations for screening donated blood and plasma for antibody to the virus causing acquired immunodeficiency syndrome. *MMWR* 34:1–5, 1985.
18. Ammann AJ, Cowan MJ, Wara DW, Weintrub P, Dritz S, Goldman H, Perkins HA: Acquired immunodeficiency in an infant: possible transmission by means of blood products. *Lancet* 1:956–958, 1983.
19. Curran JW, Lawrence DN, Jaffe H, Kaplan JE, Zyla LD, Chamberland M, Weinstein R, Lui K-J, Schonberger LB, Spira TJ, Alexander WJ, Swinger G, Amman A, Solomon S, Auerbach D, Mildvan D, Stoneburner R, Jason JM, Haverkos HW, Evatt BL: Acquired immunodeficiency syndrome (AIDS) associated with transfusions. *N Engl J Med* 310:69–75, 1984.
20. Broder S, Gallo RC: A pathogenic retrovirus (HTLV-III) linked to AIDS, *N Engl J Med* 311:1292–1297, 1984.
21. Wormser GP, Joline C, Duncanson F, Cunningham-Rundles S: Needle-stick injuries during the care of patients with AIDS. *N Engl J Med* 310:1461–1462, 1984.
22. Thomas GA, Talbot G, Jahre J, Legaspi C, Silverman D, Gold J, Grieco M, Lange M, Vieira J, Matkovic C, Laporta A, Stricof R, Jacobson JA, Sanchez MA, Luce HD, McCutchan JA, Thrupp L, Jacobson N, Buggy BP, Eberenz M, Dennehy P, Everhart AH: Prospective evaluation of healthcare workers exposed via parenteral or mucous-membrane routes to blood and body fluids of patients with acquired immunodeficiency syndrome. *MMWR* 33:181–182, 1984.
23. Hirsch MS, Wormser GP, Schooley RT, Ho DD, Felsenstein D, Hopkins CC, Joline C, Duncanson F, Sarngadharan MG, Saxinger C, Gallo RC: Risk of nosocomial infection with human T-cell lym-

photropic virus 3 (HTLV-III). *N Engl J Med* 312:1–4, 1985.

24. Needlestick transmission of HTLV-III from a patient infected in Africa. *Lancet* 2:1376–1377, 1984.

25. Poiesz B, Tomar R, Lehr B, Moore J: Hepatitis B vaccine: evidence confirming lack of AIDS transmission. *MMWR* 33:685–687, 1984.

26. Evans P: An epidemic of chickenpox. *Lancet* 2:339–340, 1940.

27. Thomson FH, Price C: The aerial conveyance of infection. *Lancet* 1:1669–1673, 1914.

28. Thomson FH: The aerial conveyance of infection. With a note on the contact infection of chickenpox. *Lancet* 1:341–344, 1916.

29. Thomson FH: Contact infection of chicken-pox. *Lancet* 1:397, 1919.

30. Brunell PA: Varicella-zoster virus. In Mandell GL, Douglas RG Jr, Bennett JE (eds): *Principles and Practice of Infectious Diseases.* New York, John Wiley & Sons, 1985, p 952.

31. Ross AJ: Modification of chickenpox in family contacts by administration of gamma globulin. *N Engl J Med* 267:369–376, 1962.

32. Henderson DK: Nososcomial herpesvirus infections. In Mandell GL, Douglas RG Jr, Bennett JE (eds): *Principles and Practice of Infectious Diseases.* New York, John Wiley & Sons, 1985, p 1630.

33. Gordon JE, Meader FM: The period of infectivity and serum prevention of chickenpox. *JAMA* 93:2013–2015, 1929.

34. Whitley RJ, Soong S-J, Dolin R, Betts R, Linnemann C, Alford CA, and the NIAID Collaborative Antiviral Study Group: Early vidarabine therapy to control the complications of herpes zoster in immunosuppressed patients. *N Engl J Med* 307:971–975, 1982.

35. Gallagher JG, Merigan TC: Prolonged herpes-zoster infection associated with immunosuppressive therapy. *Ann Intern Med* 91:842–846, 1979.

36. Seiler HE: A study of herpes zoster particularly in its relationship to chickenpox. *J Hyg* 47:253–262, 1949.

37. Berlin BS, Campbell T: Hospital-acquired herpes zoster following exposure to chickenpox. *JAMA* 211:1831–1833, 1970.

38. Boyce JM, Spruill EY, White RL: Outbreak of nosocomial varicella among personnel exposed to herpes zoster. 83rd Annual Meeting of the American Society for Microbiology, New Orleans, 1983, abstract L27.

39. Hyams PJ, Stuewe MCS, Heitzer V: Herpes zoster causing varicella (chickenpox) in hospital employees: cost of a casual attitude. *Am J Infect Control* 12:2–5, 1984.

40. Feldman S, Hughes WT, Daniel CB: Varicella in children with cancer: seventy-seven cases. *Pediatrics* 56:388–397, 1975.

41. Myers MG: Viremia caused by varicella-zoster virus: association with malignant progressive varicella. *J Infect Dis* 140:229–233, 1979.

42. Dolin R, Reichman RC, Mazur MH, Whitley RJ: Herpes zoster-varicella infections in immunosuppressed patients. *Ann Intern Med* 89:375–388, 1978.

43. Schimpff S, Serpick A, Stoler B, Rumack B, Mellin H, Joseph JM, Block J: Varicella-zoster infection in patients with cancer. *Ann Intern Med* 76:241–254, 1972.

44. Weintraub WH, Lilly JR, Randolph JG: A chickenpox epidemic in a pediatric burn unit. *Surgery* 76:490–494, 1974.

45. Meyers JD, MacQuarrie MB, Merigan TC, Jennison MH: Nosocomial varicella. Part I. Outbreak in oncology patients at a children's hospital. *West J Med* 130:196–199, 1979.

46. Morens DM, Bregman DJ, West CM, Greene MH, Mazur MH, Dolin R, Fisher RI: An outbreak of varicella-zoster virus infection among cancer patients. *Ann Intern Med* 93:414–419, 1980.

47. Leclair JM, Zaia JA, Levin MJ, Congdon RG, Goldmann DA: Airborne transmission of chickenpox in a hospital. *N Engl J Med* 302:450–453, 1980.

48. Gustafson TL, Lavely GB, Brawner ER Jr, Hutcheson RH Jr, Wright PF, Schaffner W: An outbreak of airborne nosocomial varicella. *Pediatrics* 70:550–556, 1982.

49. Gustafson TL, Shehab Z, Brunell PA: Outbreak of varicella in a newborn intensive care nursery. *Am J Dis Child* 138:548–550, 1984.

50. Eckstein R, Jehn U, Loy A: Endemic chickenpox infection on a cancer ward. *J Infect Dis* 149:829–830, 1984.

51. Hyams PJ, Vernon S, Eckert D: Susceptibility to varicella virus of certain adults in the southeastern United States. *Am J Infect Control* 12:6–9, 1984.

52. Steele RW, Coleman MA, Fiser M, Bradsher RW: Varicella zoster in hospital personnel: skin test reactivity to monitor susceptibility. *Pediatrics* 70:604–608, 1982.

53. Shehab ZM Brunell PA: Susceptibility of hospital personnel to varicella-zoster virus. *J Infect Dis* 150:786, 1984.

54. Hirst LW, Thomas JV, Green WR: Conjunctivitis. In Mandell GL, Douglas RG Jr, Bennett JE (eds): *Principles and Practice of Infectious Diseases.* New York, John Wiley & Sons, 1985, p 749.

55. Baum SG: Adenovirus. In Mandell GL, Douglas RG Jr, Bennett JE (eds): *Principles and Practice of Infectious Diseases.* New York, John Wiley & Sons, 1985, p 991.

56. Dawson C, Darrell R: Infections due to adenovirus type 8 in the United States. I. An outbreak of epidemic keratoconjunctivitis originating in a physician's office. *N Engl J Med* 268:1031–1034, 1963.

57. Laibson PR, Ortolan G, Dupre-Strachan S: Community and hospital outbreak of epidemic keratoconjunctivitis. *Arch Ophthalmol* 80:467–473, 1968.

58. Wegman DH, Guinee VF, Millian SJ: Epidemic keratoconjunctivitis. *Am J Public Health* 60:1230–1237, 1970.

59. Sprague JB, Hierholzer JC, Currier RW, Hattwick MAW, Smith MD: Epidemic keratoconjunctivitis. A severe industrial outbreak due to adenovirus type 8. *N Engl J Med* 289:1341–1346, 1973.

60. Faden H, Gallagher M, Ogra P, Laughlin SM: Nosocomial outbreak of pharyngoconjunctival fe-

ver due to adenovirus, type 4—New York. *MMWR* 27:49, 1978.

61. Guyer B, O'Day DM, Hierholzer JC, Schaffner W: Epidemic keratoconjunctivitis: a community outbreak of mixed adenovirus type 8 and type 19 infection. *J Infect Dis* 132:142–150, 1975.

62. Harrison HR, Howe P, Minnich L, Ray CG: A cluster of adenovirus 19 infection with multiple clinical manifestations. *J Pediatr* 94:917–919, 1979.

63. Tullo AB, Higgins PG: An outbreak of adenovirus keratoconjunctivitis in Bristol. *Br J Ophthalmol* 63:621–626, 1979.

64. Tullo AB, Higgins PG: An outbreak of adenovirus type 4 conjunctivitis. *Br J Ophthalmol* 64:489–493, 1980.

65. D'Angelo LJ, Hierholzer JC, Holman RC, Smith JD: Epidemic keratoconjunctivitis caused by adenovirus type 8: epidemiologic and laboratory aspects of a large outbreak. *Am J Epidemiol* 113:44–49, 1981.

66. Levandowski RA, Rubenis M: Nosocomial conjunctivitis caused by adenovirus type 4. *J Infect Dis* 143:28–31, 1981.

67. Keenlyside RA, Hierholzer JC, D'Angelo LJ: Keratoconjunctivitis associated with adenovirus type 37: an extended outbreak in an ophthalmologist's office. *J Infect Dis* 147:191–198, 1983.

68. Darougar S, Grey RHB, Thaker U, McSwiggan DA: Clinical and epidemiological features of adenovirus keratoconjunctivitis in London. *Br J Ophthalmol* 67:1–7, 1983.

69. Straube RC, Thompson MA, Van Dyke RB, Wadell G, Connor JD, Wingard D, Spector SA: Adenovirus type 7b in a children's hospital. *J Infect Dis* 147:814–819, 1983.

70. Ho M: Cytomegalovirus. In Mandell GL, Douglas RG Jr, Bennett JE: *Principles and Practice of Infectious Diseases.* New York, John Wiley & Sons, 1985, p 960.

71. Pass RF, August AM, Dworsky M, Reynolds DW: Cytomegalovirus infection in a day-care center. *N Engl J Med* 307:477–479, 1982.

72. Pass RF, Hutto SC, Reynolds DW, Polhill RB: Increased frequency of cytomegalovirus infection in children in group day care. *Pediatrics* 74:121–126, 1984.

73. Stagno S, Reynolds DW, Tsiantos A, Fuccillo DA, Long W, Alford CA: Comparative serial virologic and serologic studies of symptomatic and subclinical congenitally and natally acquired cytomegalovirus infections. *J Infect Dis* 132:568–577, 1975.

74. Fiala M, Payne JE, Berne TV, Moore TC, Henle W, Montgomerie JZ, Chatterjee JN, Guze LB: Epidemiology of cytomegalovirus infection after transplantation and immunosuppression. *J Infect Dis* 132:421–433, 1975.

75. Quinnan GV Jr, Kirmani N, Esber E, Saral R, Manischewitz JF, Rogers JL, Rook AH, Santos GW, Burns WH: HLA-restricted cytotoxic T lymphocyte and nonthymic cytotoxic lymphocyte responses to cytomegalovirus infection of bone marrow transplant recipients. *J Immunol* 126:2036–2041, 1981.

76. Drew WL, Conant MA, Miner RC, Huang E-S, Ziegler JL, Groundwater JR, Gullett JH, Volberd-ing P, Abrams DI, Mintz L: Cytomegalovirus and Kaposi's sarcoma in young homosexual men. *Lancet* 2:125–127, 1982.

77. Haneberg B, Bertnes E, Haukenes G: Antibodies to cytomegalovirus among personnel at a children's hospital. *Acta Paediatr Scand* 69:407–409, 1980.

78. Friedman HM, Lewis MR, Nemerofsky DM, Plotkin SA: Acquisition of cytomegalovirus infection among female employees at a pediatric hospital. *Pediatr Infect Dis* 3:233–235, 1984.

79. Yeager AS: Longitudinal, serological study of cytomegalovirus infections in nurses and in personnel without patient contact. *J Clin Microbiol* 2:448–452, 1975.

80. Ahlfors K, Ivarsson S-A, Johnsson T, Renmarker K: Risk of cytomegalovirus infection in nurses and congenital infection in their offspring. *Acta Paediatr Scand* 70:819–823, 1981.

81. Dworsky ME, Welch K, Cassady G, Stagno S: Occupational risk for primary cytomegalovirus infection among pediatric health-care workers. *N Engl J Med* 309:950–953, 1983.

82. Spector SA: Molecular analysis of cytomegalovirus infections in hospitalized infants. *Pediatr Res* 15:621, abstract 1073, 1981.

83. Spector SA: Transmission of cytomegalovirus among infants in hospital documented by restriction-endonuclease-digestion analysis. *Lancet* 1:378–381, 1983.

84. Yow MD, Lakeman AD, Stagno S, Reynolds RB, Plavidal FJ: Use of restriction enzymes to investigate the source of a primary cytomegalovirus infection in a pediatric nurse. *Pediatrics* 70:713–716, 1982.

85. Wilfert CM, Huang E-S, Stagno S: Restriction endonuclease analysis of cytomegalovirus deoxyribonucleic acid as an epidemiologic tool. *Pediatrics* 70:717–721, 1982.

86. Dworsky M, Lakeman A, Stagno S: Cytomegalovirus transmission within a family. *Pediatr Infect Dis* 3:236–238, 1984.

87. Robinson WS: Hepatitis A virus. In Mandell GL, Douglas RG Jr, Bennett JE (eds): *Principles and Practice of Infectious Diseases.* New York, John Wiley & Sons, 1985, p 829.

88. Bradley DW, Fields HA, McCaustland KA, Maynard JE, Decker RH, Whittington R, Overby LR: Serodiagnosis of hepatitis A by a modified competitive binding radioimmunoassay for immunoglobulin M anti-hepatitis A virus. *J Clin Microbiol* 9:120–127, 1979.

89. Lacarnini SA, Ferris AA, Lehmann NI, Gust ID: The antibody response following hepatitis A infection. *Intervirology* 8:309–318, 1977.

90. Meyers JD, Romm FJ, Tihen WS, Bryan JA: Food-borne hepatitis A in a general hospital. Epidemiologic study of an outbreak attributed to sandwiches. *JAMA* 231:1049–1053, 1975.

91. Orenstein WA, Wu E, Wilkins J, Robinson K, Francis DP, Timko N, Wayne R: Hospital-acquired hepatitis A: report of an outbreak. *Pediatrics* 67:494–497, 1981.

92. Goodman RA, Carder CC, Allen JR, Orenstein WA, Finton RJ: Nosocomial hepatitis A transmission by an adult patient with diarrhea. *Am J*

Med 73:220–226, 1982.
93. Klein BS, Michaels JA, Rytel MW, Berg KG, Davis JP: Nosocomial hepatitis A. A multinursery outbreak in Wisconsin. *JAMA* 252:2716–2721, 1984.
94. Skidmore SJ, Boxall EH, Ala F: A case report of post-transfusion hepatitis A. *J Med Virol* 10:223, 1982.
95. Seeberg S, Brandberg A, Hermodsson S, Larsson P, Lundgren S: Hospital outbreak of hepatitis A secondary to blood exchange in a baby. *Lancet* 1:1155–1156, 1981.
96. Barbara JAJ, Howell DR, Briggs M, Parry JV: Post-transfusion hepatitis A. *Lancet* 1:738, 1982.
97. Azimi PH, Roberto RR, Guralnik J, Livermore T, Hoag S, Hagens S, Lugo N: Transfusion acquired hepatitis A in a premature infant with secondary nosocomial spread in an intensive care nursery. Presented at the 23rd Interscience Conference on Antimicrobial Agents and Chemotherapy, Las Vegas, October 24–26, 1983, abstract 1.
98. Khanchit L, Dayton L, Plank S: Transfusion-transmited hepatitis A with subsequent nosocomial and community spread, California. Presented at 32nd Annual Epidemic Intelligence Conference, Centers for Disease Control, Atlanta, April 18–22, 1983.
99. Hollinger FB, Khan NC, Oefinger PE, Yawn DH, Schmulen AC, Dreesman GR, Melmck JL: Post-transfusion hepatitis type A. *JAMA* 250:2313–2317, 1983.
100. Sherertz RJ, Russell BA, Reuman PD: Transmission of hepatitis A by transfusion of blood products. *Arch Intern Med* 144:1579–1580, 1984.
101. Noble RC, Kane MA, Reeves SA, Roeckel I: Posttransfusion hepatitis A in a neonatal intensive care unit. *JAMA* 252:2711–2715, 1984.
102. Ebisawa I, Kurosu Y, Hatashita T: Nursery-associated hepatitis A traced to a male nurse. *J Hyg* 92:251–254, 1984.
103. Levy BS, Harris JC, Smith JL, Washburn JW, Mature J, Davis A, Crosson JT, Polesky H, Hanson M: Hepatitis B in ward and clinical laboratory employees of a general hospital. *Am J Epidemiol* 106:330–335, 1977.
104. Denes AE, Smith JL, Maynard JE, Doto IL, Berquist KR, Finkel AJ: Hepatitis B infection in physicians. Results of a nationwide seroepidemiologic survey. *JAMA* 239:210–212, 1978.
105. Janzen J, Tripatzis I, Wagner U, Schlieter M, Muller-Dethard E, Wolters E: Epidemiology of hepatitis B surface antigen (HBsAg) and antibody to HBsAg in hospital personnel. *J Infect Dis* 137:261–265, 1978.
106. Scheiermann N, Kuwert EK, Pieringer E, Dermietzel R: High risk groups for hepatitis B virus infection in a university hospital staff as determined by detection of HB antigens, antibodies and Dane particles. *Med Microbiol Immunol* 166:241–247, 1978.
107. Hadler SC, Doto IL, Maynard JE, Smith J, Clark B, Mosley J, Eickhoff T, Himmelsbach CK, Cole WR: Occupational risk of hepatitis B infection in hospital workers. *Infect Control* 6:24–31, 1985.
108. Mosley JW, Edwards VM, Casey G, Redeker AG, White E: Hepatitis B virus infection in dentists. *N*

Engl J Med 293:729–734, 1975.
109. Wands JR, Walker JA, Davis TT, Waterbury LA, Owens AH, Carpenter CCJ: Hepatitis B in an oncology unit. *N Engl J Med* 291:1371–1375, 1974.
110. Spector D: Hepatitis B miniepidemic in a peritoneal dialysis unit. *Arch Intern Med* 137:1030–1031, 1977.
111. Snydman DR, Bryan JA, Macon EJ, Gregg MB: Hemodialysis-associated hepatitis: report of an epidemic with further evidence on mechanisms of transmission. *Am J Epidemiol* 104:563–570, 1976.
112. Snydman DR, Hindman SH, Wineland MD, Bryan JA, Maynard JE: Nosocomial viral hepatitis B. A cluster among staff with subsequent transmission to patients. *Ann Intern Med* 85:573–577, 1976.
113. Shanson DC: Hepatitis B outbreak in operating-theatre and intensive care staff. *Lancet* 2:596, 1980.
114. Moss ALH: Hospital outbreak of hepatitis B. *N Z Med J* 94:65–66, 1981.
115. Hansen JP, Falconer JA, Hamilton JD, Herpok FJ: Hepatitis B in a medical center. *J Occup Med* 23:338–342, 1981.
116. Schneider WJ: Hepatitis B: an occupational hazard of health care facilities. *J Occup Med* 21:807–810, 1979.
117. Hamory BH: Underreporting of needlestick injuries in a university hospital. *Infect Control* 11:174–177, 1983.
118. Jacobson JT, Burke JP, Conti MT: Injuries of hospital employees from needles and sharp objects. *Infect Control* 4:100–102, 1983.
119. McCormick RD, Maki DG: Epidemiology of needle-stick injuries in hospital personnel. *Am J Med* 70:928–932, 1981.
120. Neuberger JS, Harris J-A, Kundin WD, Bischone A, Chin TDY: Incidence of needlestick injuries in hospital personnel: implications for prevention. *Am J Infect Control* 12:171–176, 1984.
121. Alter HJ, Chalmers TC, Freeman BM, Lunceford JL, Lewis TL, Holland PV, Pizzo PA, Plotz PH, Meyer WJ: Health-care workers positive for hepatitis B surface antigen. Are their contacts at risk? *N Engl J Med* 292:454–457, 1973.
122. Williams SV, Pattison CP, Berquist KR: Dental infection with hepatitis B, *JAMA* 232:1231–1233, 1975.
123. Meyers JD, Stamm WE, Kerr MM, Counts GW: Lack of transmission of hepatitis B after surgical exposure. *JAMA* 240:1725–1727, 1978.
124. Garibaldi RA, Rasmussen CM, Holmes AW, Gregg MB: Hospital-acquired serum hepatitis. *JAMA* 219:1577–1580, 1972.
125. Coutinho RA, Albrecht-Van Lent P, Stoutjesdijk L, Meerburg-Snarenberg P, Courouce-Pauty AM, Van Dijk BA, Kloek J: Hepatitis B from doctors. *Lancet* 1:345–346, 1982.
126. Grob PJ, Bischof B, Naeff F: Cluster of hepatitis B transmitted by a physician. *Lancet* 2:1218–1220, 1981.
127. Epidemiological Research Laboratory, London: Acute hepatitis B associated with gynaecological surgery. *Lancet* 1:1–6, 1980.

128. Carl M, Blakey DL, Francis DP, Maynard JE: Interruption of hepatitis B transmission by modification of a gynaecologist's surgical technique. *Lancet* 1:731–733, 1982.

129. Lettau LA, Smith JD, Williams D, Lundquist WD, Sikes RK, Hadler SC: Nosocomial transmission of hepatitis B by an Ob-Gyn surgeon. 24th Interscience Conference on Antimicrobial Agents and Chemotherapy, Washington DC, 1984, abstract 519.

130. Rimland D, Parkin WE, Miller GB Jr, Schrack WD: Hepatitis B outbreak traced to an oral surgeon. *N Engl J Med* 296:953–958, 1977.

131. Hadler SC, Sorley DL, Acree KH, Webster HM, Schable CA, Francis DP, Maynard JE: An outbreak of hepatitis B in a dental practice. *Ann Intern Med* 95:133–138, 1981.

132. Reingold AL, Kane MA, Murphy BL, Checko P, Francis DP, Maynard JE: Transmission of hepatitis B by an oral surgeon. *J Infect Dis* 145:262–268, 1982.

133. Hamm RH, Peare RB, Painter WL, Allman KC, Hamilton M, Cutting K, Barrett CL, Centers for Disease Control: Hepatitis B among dental patients—Indiana. *MMWR* 34:73–75, 1985.

134. Robinson WS: Hepatitis B virus and the delta agent. In Mandell GL, Douglas RG Jr, Bennett JE (eds.): *Principles and Practice of Infectious Diseases.* New York, John Wiley & Sons, 1985, p 1002.

135. Hoofnagle JH, Schafer DF, Waggoner JG: Antibody to hepatitis B surface antigen in dog and man. *Gastroenterology* 86:1001, 1984.

136. Sherertz RJ, Spindel E, Hoofnagle JH: Antibody to hepatitis B surface antigen may not always indicate immunity to hepatitis B virus infection. *N Engl J Med* 309:1519, 1983.

137. Schultz AL, Laxson L, Hopkins RS, Centers for Disease Control: Hepatitis B contamination in a clinical laboratory—Colorado. *MMWR* 29:459–465, 1980.

138. Wenzel RP: Nosocomial viral hepatitis. In Mandell GL, Douglas RG Jr, Bennett JE (eds): *Principles and Practice of Infectious Diseases.* New York, John Wiley & Sons, 1985, p 1627.

139. Immunization Practices Advisory Committee: Postexposure prophylaxis of hepatitis B. *MMWR* 33:285–290, 1984.

140. Hoofnagle JH, Seeff LB, Bales ZB,Wright EC, Zimmerman HJ, The Veterans Administration Cooperative Study Group: Passive-active immunity from hepatitis B immune globulin. Reanalysis of a Veterans Administration Cooperative Study of needle-stick hepatitis. *Ann Intern Med* 91:813–818, 1979.

141. Grady GF: Viral hepatitis: passive prophylaxis with globulins—state of the art in 1978. In Vyas GN, Cohen SN, Schmidt R (eds): *Viral Hepatitis: A Contemporary Assessment.* Philadelphia, Franklin Institute Press, 1978, p 467.

142. Redeker AG, Mosley JW, Gocke DJ, McKee AP, Pollack W: Hepatitis B immune globulin as a prophylactic measure for spouses exposed to acute type B hepatitis. *N Engl J Med* 293:1055–1059, 1975.

143. Khuroo MS: Study of an epidemic of nonA, nonB hepatitis: possibility of another human hepatitis virus distinct from post-transfusion non-A, non-B type. *Am J Med* 68:818–824, 1980.

144. Dienstag JL, Allaama A, Mosley JW, Redeker AG, Purcell RH: Etiology of sporadic hepatitis B surface antigen negative hepatitis. *Ann Intern Med* 87:1–6, 1977.

145. Robinson WS: Non-A, non-B hepatitis. In Mandell GL, Douglas RG Jr, Bennett JE (eds): *Principles and Practice of Infectious Diseases.* New York, John Wiley & Sons, 1985, p 1029.

146. Meyers JD, Dienstag JL, Purcell RH, Thomas ED, Holmes KK: Parenterally transmitted non-A, non-B hepatitis: an epidemic reassessed. *Ann Intern Med* 87:57–59, 1977.

147. Herron W, Peterson E, Taylor JW: Non-A, non-B hepatitis infection transmitted via a needle—Washington. *MMWR* 28:157–158, 1979.

148. Seeff LB, Zimmerman HJ, Wright EC, Finkelstein JD, Garcia-Pont P, Greenlee HB, Dietz AA, Leevy CM, Tamburro CH, Schiff ER, Schimmel EM, Zemel R, Zimmon DS, McCollom RW: A randomized double blind controlled trial of the efficacy of immune serum globulin for the prevention of post-transfusion hepatitis. *Gastroenterology* 72:111–121, 1977.

149. Knodell RG, Conrad ME, Ginsberg AL, Bell CJ, Flannery EP: Efficacy of prophylactic gammaglobulin in preventing non A, non B post-transfusion hepatitis. *Lancet* 1:557–561, 1976.

150. Kuhns WJ, Prince AM, Brotman B, Hazzi C, Grady GF: A clinical and laboratory evaluation of immune serum globulin from donors with a history of hepatitis: attempted prevention of post-transfusion hepatitis. *Am J Med Sci* 272:255–261, 1976.

151. Stern H, Elek SD, Millar DM, Anderson HF: Herpetic whitlow. A form of cross-infection in hospitals. *Lancet* 2:871–874, 1959.

152. Hambrick GW Jr, Cox RP, Senior JR: Primary herpes simplex infection of fingers of medical personnel. *Arch Dermatol* 85:583–589, 1962.

153. Orkin FK: Herpetic whitlow—occupational hazard to the anesthesiologist. *Anesthesiology* 33:671–673, 1970.

154. Greaves WL, Kaiser AB, Alford RH, Schaffner W: The problem of herpetic whitlow among hospital personnel. *Infect Control* 1:381–385, 1980.

155. Rowe NH, Heine CS, Kowalski CJ: Herpetic whitlow: an occupational disease of practicing dentists. *J Am Dent Assoc* 105:471–473, 1982.

156. Manzella J, McConville J, Menegus M, Valenti W, Swierkosz E, Arens M: An outbreak of herpes simplex virus gingivostomatitis in a dental practice. 22nd Interscience Conference on Antimicrobial Agents and Chemotherapy. Miami, 1982, abstract 451.

157. Glogau R, Hanna L, Jawetz E: Herpetic whitlow as part of genital virus infection. *J Infect Dis* 136:689–692, 1977.

158. Haburchak DR: Recurrent herpetic whitlow due to herpes simplex virus type 2. *Arch Intern Med* 138:1418–1419, 1978.

159. Chang T-W, Gorbach SL: Primary and recurrent herpetic whitlow. *Int J Dermatol* 16:752–754, 1977.

160. Hamory BH, Osterman CA, Wenzel RP: Herpetic whitlow. *N Engl J Med* 292:268, 1975.
161. Orkin FK: Herpetic whitlow (cont.). *N Engl J Med* 292:648, 1975.
162. Adams G, Stover BH, Keenlyside RA, Hooton TM, Buchman TG, Roizman B, Stewart JA: Nosocomial herpetic infections in a pediatric intensive care unit. *Am J Epidemiol* 113:126–132, 1981.
163. Turner R, Shehab Z, Osborne K, Hendley JO: Shedding and survival of herpes simplex virus from "fever blisters." *Pediatrics* 70:547–549, 1982.
164. Douglas J, Schmidt O, Corey L: Acquisition of neonatal HSV-1 infection from a paternal source contact. *J Pediatr* 103:908–910, 1983.
165. Yeager AS, Ashley RL, Corey L: Transmission of herpes simplex virus from father to neonate. *Pediatrics* 103:905–907, 1983.
166. Van Voris LP, Belshe RB, Shaffer JL: Nosocomial influenza B virus infection in the elderly. *Ann Intern Med* 96:153–158, 1982.
167. Douglas RG Jr, Betts RF: Influenza virus. In Mandell GL, Douglas RG Jr, Bennett JE (eds): *Principles and Practice of Infectious Diseases.* New York, John Wiley & Sons, 1985, p 846.
168. Blumenfeld HL, Kilbourne ED, Louria DB, Rogers DE: Studies on influenza in the pandemic of 1957—58. I. An epidemiological, clinical and serologic investigation of an intrahospital epidemic, with a note on vaccination efficacy. *J Clin Invest* 38:199–212, 1959.
169. Muchmore HG, Felton FG, Scott LV: A confirmed hospital epidemic of Asian influenza. *J Okla State Med Assoc* 53:142–145, 1960.
170. Brocklebank JT, Court SDM, McQuillan J, Gardner PS: Influenza-A infection in children. *Lancet* 2:497–500, 1972.
171. O'Donoghue JM, Ray CG, Terry DW Jr, Beaty HN: Prevention of nosocomial influenza infection with amantadine. *Am J Epidemiol* 97:276–282, 1973.
172. Bauer DR, Elie K, Spence L, Stern L: Hong Kong influenza in a neonatal unit. *JAMA* 223:1233–1235, 1973.
173. Hall CB, Douglas RG Jr: Nosocomial influenza infections as a cause of intercurrent fevers in infants. *Pediatrics* 55:673–677, 1975.
174. McDougal BA, Hodges GR, Lewis HD, Davis JW, Caldwell SA: Nosocomial influenza A infection. *South Med J* 70:1023–1024, 1977.
175. Meibalane R, Sedmak GV, Sasidharan P, Garg P, Grausz JP: Outbreak of influenza in a neonatal intensive care unit. *J Pediatr* 91:974–976, 1977.
176. Kapila R, Lintz DI, Tecson FT, Ziskin L, Louria DB: A nosocomial outbreak of influenza A. *Chest* 71:576–579, 1977.
177. Balkovic ES, Goodman RA, Rose FB, Borel CO: Nosocomial influenza A (H1N1) infection. *Am J Med Technol* 46:318–320, 1980.
178. Mathur U, Bentley DW, Hall CB: Concurrent respiratory syncytial virus and influenza A infections in the institutionalized elderly and chronically ill. *Ann Intern Med* 93:49–52, 1980.
179. Centers for Disease Control: Influenza A in a hospital—Illinois. *MMWR* 30:79–85, 1981.
180. Goodman RA, Orenstein WA, Munro TF, Smith SC, Sikes RK: Impact of influenza A in a nursing home. *JAMA* 247:1451–1453, 1982.
181. Stricof R, Morse D, Rothenberg R, Johnson M, Weaver D, Luft W, Pidcoe V, Centers for Disease Control: Impact of influenza on a nursing home population—New York. *MMWR* 32:32–34, 1983.
182. Wenzel RP, Deal EC, Hendley JO: Hospital-acquired viral respiratory illness on a pediatric ward. *Pediatrics* 60:367–371, 1977.
183. Hall WN, Goodman RA, Noble GR, Kendal AP, Steece RS: An outbreak of influenza B in an elderly population. *J Infect Dis* 144:297–302, 1981.
184. Hoffman PC, Dixon RE: Control of influenza in the hospital. *Ann Intern Med* 87:725–728, 1977.
185. Payler DK, Purdham PA: Influenza A prophylaxis with amantadine in a boarding school. *Lancet* 1:502–504, 1984.
186. Riley RC: The role of ventilation in the spread of measles in an elementary school. *Ann NY Acad Sci* 353:25–34, 1980.
187. Centers for Disease Control: Imported measles with subsequent airborne transmission in a pediatrician's office—Michigan. *MMWR* 32:401–402, 1983.
188. Langmuir AD: Changing concepts of airborne infection of acute contagious diseases: a reconsideration of classic epidemiologic theories. *Ann NY Acad Sci* 353:35–44, 1980.
189. Riley EC, Murphy G, Riley RL: Airborne spread of measles in a suburban elementary school. *Am J Epidemiol* 107:421–432, 1978.
190. Gershon AA: Measles virus. In Mandell GL, Douglas RG Jr, Bennett JE (eds): *Principles and Practice of Infectious Diseases.* New York, John Wiley & Sons, 1985, p 889.
191. Benenson AS (ed): *Control of Communicable Diseases in Man.* Washington, DC, American Public Health Association, 1981, p 211.
192. Krause PJ, Cherry JD, Deseda-Tous J, Champion JG, Strassburg M, Sullivan C, Spencer MJ, Bryson YJ, Welliver RC, Boyer KM: Epidemic measles in young adults. Clinical, epidemiologic, and serologic studies. *Ann Intern Med* 90:873–876, 1979.
193. Crawford GE, Gremillion DH: Epidemic measles and rubella in Air Force recruits: impact of immunization. *J Infect Dis* 144:403–410, 1981.
194. Preblud SR, Gross F, Halsey NA, Hinman AR, Herrmann KL, Koplan JP: Assessment of susceptibility to measles and rubella. *JAMA* 247:1134–1137, 1982.
195. Yangco BG: Epidemic measles in a summer camp. *Ann Intern Med* 92:440, 1980.
196. Poi KM: Measles: the epidemiology and control of an outbreak. *J Am Coll Health* 31:158–161, 1983.
197. Bridgewater SC, Lotz DI: Measles (rubeola): the control of an outbreak at a large university. *J Am Coll Health* 32:201–204, 1984.
198. Lotz D, Hongen R, Sharp TW, Blankenbaker RG, Chastain G, Barrett CL, Freund E Jr, Halpin TJ, Buu C, Key M, Bopp J, Brownstein B, Gurd B, Hicks R, Osborn G, Smith BJ, Wallace C, Whitehurst JR, Alexander CE, Webb CR: Measles outbreaks on university campuses—Indiana, Ohio, Texas. *MMWR* 32:193–195, 1983.

199. Centers for Disease Control: Measles in medical settings—United States. *MMWR* 30:125–126, 1981.

200. Centers for Disease Control: Chains of measles transmission—United States, 1982. *MMWR* 32:282–284, 1983.

201. Artenstein MS, Ellis RE: The risk of exposure to a patient with meningococcal meningitis. *Milit Med* 133:474–477, 1968.

202. Feldman HA: Meningococcal infections. *Adv Intern Med* 18:117–140, 1972.

203. Baker CJ, Feigin RD, Lampe RM, Baird J, Buv C, Craven J, Huber T, MacLean RA, Jensen F, Poindexter M, Williams DW, Hafkin B, Webb LR, Enriquez MB, Maled A, Morgan RA, Gunn RA, Centers for Disease Control: Meningococcal disease—United States, 1981. *MMWR* 30:113–115, 1981.

204. Cohen MS, Steere AC, Baltimore R, von Graevenitz A, Pantelick E, Camp B, Root RK: Possible nosocomial transmission of group Y *Neisseria meningitidis* among oncology patients. *Ann Intern Med* 91:7–12, 1979.

205. Rose HD, Lenz IE, Sheth NK: Meningococcal pneumonia. A source of nosocomial infection. *Arch Intern Med* 141:575–577, 1981.

206. Baum SG, Litman N: Mumps virus. In Mandell GL, Douglas RG Jr, Bennett JE (eds): *Principles and Practice of Infectious Diseases*. New York, John Wiley & Sons, 1985, p 871.

207. Brunell PA, Brickman A, O'Hare D, Steinberg S: Ineffectiveness of isolation of patients as a method of preventing the spread of mumps. *N Engl J Med* 279:1357–1361, 1968.

208. Ikeda S, Chiba S, Chiba Y, Nakao T, Fukui S: Epidemiological, clinical and serological studies on epidemic of mumps in an infant nursery. *Tohoku J Exp Med* 105:327–337, 1971.

209. Benenson AS (ed): *Control of Communicable Diseases in Man*. Washington, DC, American Public Health Association, 1981, p 232.

210. Wilkins J, Wehrle PF: *Bordetella* species (including whooping cough). In Mandell GL, Douglas RG Jr, Bennett JE (eds): *Principles and Practice of Infectious Diseases*. New York, John Wiley & Sons, 1985, p 1301.

211. Lambert HJ: Epidemiology of a small pertussis outbreak in Kent County, Mich. *Public Health Rep* 80:365–369, 1965.

212. Linnemann CC Jr, Ramundo N, Perlstein PH, Minton SD, Englender GS, McComick JB, Hayes PS: Use of pertussis vaccine in an epidemic involving hospital staff. *Lancet* 2:540–543, 1975.

213. Kurt TL, Yeager AS, Guenette S, Dunlop S: Spread of pertussis by hospital staff. *JAMA* 221:264–267, 1972.

214. Hall CB: Respiratory syncytial virus. In Mandell GL, Douglas RG Jr, Bennett JE: *Principles and Practice of Infectious Diseases*. New York, John Wiley & Sons, 1985, p 877.

215. Ditchburn RK, McQuillin J, Gardner PS, Court SDM: Respiratory syncytial virus in hospital cross-infection. *Br Med J* 3:671–673, 1971.

216. MacDonald NE, Hall CB, Suffin SC, Alexson C, Harris PJ, Manning JA: Respiratory syncytial viral infection in infants with congenital heart disease. *N Engl J Med* 307:397–400, 1982.

217. Hall CB, MacDonald NE, Klemperer MR, Ettinger LJ: Respiratory syncytial virus in immunosuppressed children. *Pediatr Res* 15:613, abstract 1021, 1981.

218. Mathur U, Bentley DW, Hall CB: Concurrent respiratory syncytial virus and influenza A infection in the institutionalized elderly and chronically ill. *Ann Intern Med* 93 (Part 1):49–52, 1980.

219. Garvie DG, Gray J: Outbreak of respiratory syncytial virus infection in the elderly. *Br Med J* 281:1253–1254, 1980.

220. Gardner PS, Court SDM, Brocklebank JT, Downham MAPS, Weightman D: Virus cross-infection in paediatric wards. *Br Med J* 2:571–575, 1973.

221. Hall CB, Douglas RG Jr, Geiman JM, Messner MK: Nosocomial respiratory syncytial virus infections. *N Engl J Med* 293:1343–1346, 1975.

222. Sims DG, Downham MAPS, Webb JKG, Gardner PS, Weightman D: Hospital cross-infection on children's wards with respiratory syncytial virus and the role of adult carriage. *Acta Paediatr Scand* 64:541–545, 1975.

223. Hall CB, Douglas RG Jr, Geiman JM: Quantitative shedding patterns of respiratory syncytial virus in infants. *J Infect Dis* 132:151–156, 1975.

224. Hall CB, Douglas RG Jr, Geiman JM: Respiratory syncytial virus infections in infants: quantitation and duration of shedding. *Pediatrics* 89:11–15, 1976.

225. Hall CB: The shedding and spreading of respiratory syncytial virus. *Pediatr Res* 11:236–239, 1977.

226. Hall CB: Geiman JM, Douglas RG Jr, Meagher MP: Control of nosocomial respiratory syncytial viral infections. *Pediatrics* 62:728–732, 1978.

227. Hall CB, Douglas RG Jr: Modes of transmission of respiratory syncytial virus. *J Pediatr* 99:100–103, 1981.

228. Hall CB, Douglas RG Jr: Nosocomial respiratory syncytial viral infections. Should gowns and masks be used? *Am J Dis Child* 135:512–515, 1981.

229. Hall CB: The nosocomial spread of respiratory syncytial viral infections. *Annu Rev Med* 34:311–319, 1983.

230. Hall CB, Douglas RG Jr, Geiman JM: Possible transmission by fomites of respiratory syncytial virus. *J Infect Dis* 141:98–102, 1980.

231. DuPont HL: Rotaviral gastroenteritis—some recent developments. *J Infect Dis* 149:663–666, 1984.

232. Gurwith M, Wenman W, Hinde D, Feltham S, Greenberg H: A prospective study of rotavirus infection in infants and young children. *J Infect Dis* 144:218–224, 1981.

233. Kapikian AZ, Kim HW, Wyatt RG, Cline WL, Arrobio JO, Brandt CD, Rodriguez WJ, Sack DA, Chanock RM, Parrott RH: Human reovirus-like (HRVL) agent as the major pathogen associated with "winter" gastroenteritis—etiologic, epidemiologic studies in infants, young children and their contacts. *N Engl J Med* 294:965–972, 1976.

234. Kim HW, Brandt CD, Kapikian AZ, Wyatt RG, Arrobio JO, Rodriguez WJ, Chanock RM, Parrott RH: Human reovirus-like agent infection. Occurrence in adult contacts of pediatric patients with gastroenteritis. *JAMA* 238:404–407, 1977.

235. Rodriguez WJ, Hyun WK, Brandt CD, Yolken

RH, Richard M, Arrobio JO, Schwartz RH, Kapikian AZ, Chanock RM, Parrott RH: Common exposure outbreak of gastroenteritis due to type 2 rotavirus with high secondary attack rate within families. *J Infect Dis* 140:353–357, 1979.

236. Echeverria P, Blacklow NR, Cukor GG, Vibulbandhitkit S, Changchawalit S, Boonthai P: Rotavirus as a cause of severe gastroenteritis in adults. *J Clin Microbiol* 18:663–667, 1983.

237. Rodriguez WJ, Kim HW, Arrobio JO, Brandt CD, Chanock RM, Kapikian AZ, Wyatt RG, Parrott RH: Clinical features of acute gastroenteritis associated with human reovirus-like agent in infants and young children. *Pediatrics* 91:188–193, 1977.

238. Foster SO, Palmer EL, Gary GW Jr, Martin ML, Herrmann KL, Beasley P, Sampson J: Gastroenteritis due to rotavirus in an isolated Pacific island group: an epidemic of 3,439 cases. *J Infect Dis* 141:32–39, 1980.

239. Carlson JAK, Middleton PJ, Szymanski MT, Huber J, Petric M: Fatal rotavirus gastroenteritis. An analysis of 21 cases. *Am J Dis Child* 132:477–479, 1978.

240. Cubitt WD, Holzel H: An outbreak of rotavirus infection in a long-stay ward of a geriatric hospital. *J Clin Pathol* 33:306–308, 1980.

241. Halvorsrud J, Orstavik I: An epidemic of rotavirus-associated gastroenteritis in a nursing home for the elderly. *Scand J Infect Dis* 12:161–164, 1980.

242. Bishop RF, Barnes GL, Cipriani E, Lund JS: Clinical immunity after neonatal rotavirus infection. A prospective longitudinal study in young children. *N Engl J Med* 309:72–76, 1983.

243. Murphy AM, Albrey MB, Crewe EB: Rotavirus infections of neonates. *Lancet* 2:1149–1150, 1977.

244. Champsaur H, Questiaux E, Prevot J, Henry-Amar M, Goldszmidt D, Bourjouane M, Bach C: Rotavirus carriage, asymptomatic infection, and disease in the first two years of life. I. Virus shedding. *J Infect Dis* 149:667–674, 1984.

245. Kapikian AZ, Yolken RH: Rotavirus. In Mandell GL, Douglas RG Jr, Bennett JE (eds): *Principles and Practice of Infectious Diseases.* New York, John Wiley & Sons, 1985, p 933.

246. Santosham M, Yolken RH, Quiroz E, Dillman L, Oro G, Reeves WC, Sack RB: Detection of rotavirus in respiratory secretions of children with pneumonia. *J Pediatr* 103:583–585, 1983.

247. Chrystie IL, Totterdell B, Baker MJ, Scopes JW, Banatvala JE: Rotavirus infections in a maternity unit. *Lancet* 2:79, 1975.

248. Flewett TH, Bryden AS, Davies H, Morris CA: Epidemic viral enteritis in a long-stay children's ward. *Lancet* 1:4–5, 1975.

249. Ryder RW, McGowan JE Jr, Hatch MH, Palmer EL: Reovirus-like agent as a cause of nosocomial diarrhea in infants. *J Pediatr* 90:698–702, 1977.

250. Hildreth C, Thomas M, Ridgway GL: Rotavirus infection in an obstetric unit. *Br Med J* 282:231, 1981.

251. Russell B, Sherertz R, Reuman P, Sullivan M: Nosocomial rotavirus outbreak parallels community infections. Presented at the 11th Annual Meeting of the Association for the Practioners of Infection Control, Washington, DC, 1984.

252. Gershon AA: Rubella virus (German measles). In

253. Mclaughlin MC, Gold LH: The New York rubella incident: a case for changing hospital policy regarding rubella testing and immunization. *Amer J Public Health* 69:287–289, 1979.

254. Strassburg MA, Imagawa DT, Fannin SL, Turner JA, Chow AW, Murray RA, Cherry JD: Rubella outbreak among hospital employees. *Obstet Gynecol* 57:283–288, 1981.

255. Strassburg MA, Stephenson TG, Habel LA, Fannin SL: Rubella in hospital employees. *Infect Control* 5:123–126, 1984.

256. Fliegel PE, Weinstein WM: Rubella outbreak in a prenatal clinic: management and prevention. *Am J Infect Control* 10:29–33, 1982.

257. Carne S, Dewhurst CJ, Hurley R: Rubella epidemic in a maternity unit. *Br Med J* 1:444–446, 1973.

258. Polk BF, White JA, DeGirolami PC, Modlin JF: An outbreak of rubella among hospital personnel. *N Engl J Med* 303:541–545, 1980.

259. Gladstone JL, Millian SJ: Rubella exposure in an obstetric clinic. *Obstet Gynecol* 57:182–186, 1981.

260. Lerman SJ, Lerman LM, Nankervis GA, Gold E: Accuracy of rubella history. *Ann Intern Med* 74:97–98, 1971.

261. Orenstein WA, Heseltine PNR, LeGagnoux SJ, Portnoy B: Rubella vaccine and susceptible hospital employees. Poor physician participation. *JAMA* 245:711–713, 1981.

262. Datta N, Pridie RB, Anderson ES: An outbreak of infection with *Salmonella typhimurium* in a general hospital. *J Hyg* 58:229–241, 1960.

263. Rice PA, Craven PC, Wells JG: *Salmonella heidelberg* enteritis and bacteremia. An epidemic on two pediatric wards. *Am J Med* 60:509–516, 1976.

264. Lintz D, Kapila R, Pilgrim E, Tecson F, Dorn R, Louria D: Nosocomial *Salmonella* epidemic. *Arch Intern Med* 136:968–973, 1976.

265. Anand CM, Finlayson MC, Garson JZ, Larson ML: An institutional outbreak of salmonellosis due to a lactose-fermenting *Salmonella newport*. *Amer J Clin Pathol* 74:657–659, 1980.

266. Steere AC, Craven PJ, Hall WJ III, Leotsakis N, Wells JG, Farmer JJ III, Gangarosa EJ: Person-to-person spread of *Salmonella typhimurium* after a hospital common-source outbreak. *Lancet* 1:319–322, 1975.

267. Chmel H, Armstrong D: *Salmonella oslo*. A focal outbreak in a hospital. *Am J Med* 60:203–208, 1976.

268. Ryder RW, Crosby-Ritchie A, McDonough B, Hall WJ III: Human milk contaminated with *Salmonella kottbus*. A cause of nosocomial illness in infants. *JAMA* 238:1533–1534, 1977.

269. Ayliffe GAJ, Geddes AM, Pearson JE, Williams TC: Spread of *Salmonella typhi* in a maternity hospital. *J Hyg* 82:353–359, 1979.

270. Baine WB, Gangarosa EJ, Bennett JV, Barker WH Jr, Centers for Disease Control: Institutional salmonellosis. *J Infect Dis* 128:357–360, 1973.

271. Palmer SR, Rowe B: Investigation of outbreaks of *Salmonella* in hospitals. *Br Med J* 287:891–893, 1983.

272. Hook EW: *Salmonella* species (including typhoid

fever). In Mandell GL, Douglas RG Jr, Bennett JE (eds): *Principles and Practice of Infectious Diseases.* New York, John Wiley & Sons, 1985, p 1256.

273. Musher DM, Rubenstein AD: Permanent carriers of nontyphosa salmonellae. *Arch Intern Med* 132:869–872, 1973.

274. Bachrach SJ: Successful treatment of an institutional outbreak of shigellosis. *Clin Pediatr* 20:127–131, 1981.

275. Levine MM, DuPont HL, Khodabandelou M, Hornick RB: Long-term *Shigella*-carrier state. *N Engl J Med* 288:1169–1171, 1973.

276. DuPont HL: *Shigella* species (bacillary dysentery). In Mandell GL, Douglas RG Jr, Bennett JE (eds): *Principles and Practice of Infectious Diseases.* New York, John Wiley & Sons, 1985, p 182.

277. Gooch JJ, Strasius SR, Beamer B, Reiter MD, Correll GW: Nosocomial outbreak of scabies. *Arch Dermatol* 114:897–898, 1978.

278. Belle EA, D'Souza TJ, Zarzour JY, Lemieux M, Wong CC: Hospital epidemic of scabies: diagnosis and control. *Can J Public Health* 70:133–135, 1979.

279. Pancoast SJ, Kisher JJ, Centers for Disease Control: Patient-source scabies among hospital personnel—Pennsylvania. *MMWR* 32:489–490, 1983.

280. Lerche NW, Currier RW, Juranek DD, Baer W, Dubay NJ: Atypical crusted "Norwegian" scabies: report of nosocomial transmission in a community hospital and an approach to control. *Cutis* 31:637–684, 1983.

281. Fekety FR Jr: The epidemiology and prevention of staphylococcal infection. *Medicine* 43:593–613, 1964.

282. Godfrey ME, Smith IM: Hospital hazards of staphylococcal sepsis. *JAMA* 166:1197–1201, 1958.

283. Nakashima AK, Allen JR, Martone WJ, Plikaytis BD, Storer B, Cook LM, Wright SP: Epidemic bullous impetigo in a nursery due to a nasal carrier of *Staphylococcus aureus*: role of epidemiology and control measures. *Infect Control* 5:326–331, 1984.

284. Sullivan M, Sherertz R, Reuman P, Russell B: Simultaneous *Staphylococcus aureus* nursery outbreaks in a community and a university teaching hospital traced to one nurse. Presented at the 11th Annual Meeting of the Association for Practitioners of Infection Control, Washington, DC, May 1984.

285. Tanner EI, Bullin J, Bullin CH, Gamble DR: An outbreak of post-operative sepsis due to a staphylococcal disperser. *J Hyg* 85:219–225, 1980.

286. Ayliffe GAJ, Collins BJ: Wound infections acquired from a disperser of an unusual strain of *Staphylococcus aureus. J Clin Pathol* 20:195–198, 1967.

287. Payne RW: Severe outbreak of surgical sepsis due to *Staphylococcus aureus* of unusual type and origin. *Br Med J* 2:17–20, 1966.

288. Hare R, Thomas CGA: The transmission of *Staphylococcus aureus. Br Med J* 2:840–844, 1956.

289. White A: Relation between quantitative nasal cultures and dissemination of staphylococci. *J Lab Clin Med* 58:273–277, 1961.

290. Bethune DW, Blowers R, Parker M, Pask EA: Dispersal of *Staphylococcus aureus* by patients and surgical staff. *Lancet* 1:480–483, 1965.

291. Hill J, Howell A, Blowers R: Effect of clothing on dispersal of *Staphylococcus aureus* by males and females. *Lancet* 2:1131–1133, 1974.

292. Eichenwald HF, Kotsevalov O, Fasso LA: The "cloud-baby": an example of bacterial-viral interaction. *Am J Dis Child* 100:161–173, 1960.

293. Williams JD, Waltho CA, Ayliffe GAJ, Lowbury EJL: Trials of five antibacterial creams in the control of nasal carriage of *Staphylococcus aureus. Lancet* 2:390–392, 1967.

294. Bryan CS, Wilson RS, Meade P, Sill LG: Topical antibiotic ointments for staphylococcal nasal carriers: survey of current practices and comparison of bacitracin and vancomycin ointments. *Infect Control* 1:153–156, 1980.

295. Wheat LJ, Kohler RB, White AL, White A: Effect of rifampin on nasal carriers of coagulase-positive staphylococci. *J Infect Dis* 144:177, 1981.

296. McAnally TP, Lewis MR, Brown DR: Effect of rifampin and bacitracin on nasal carriers of *Staphylococcus aureus. Antimicrob Agents Chemother* 25:422–426, 1984.

297. Semmelweis IF: *The Etiology, the Concept and the Prophylaxis of Childbed Fever.* Birmingham, AL, Classics of Medicine Library, 1981.

298. McKee WM, Di Caprio JM, Roberts CE Jr, Sherris JC: Anal carriage as the probable source of streptococcal epidemic. *Lancet* 2:1007–1009, 1966.

299. McIntyre DM: An epidemic of *Streptococcus pyogenes* puerperal and postoperative sepsis with an unusual carrier site—the anus. *Am J Obstet Gynecol* 101:308–314, 1968.

300. Schaffner W, Lefkowitz LB Jr, Goodman JS, Koenig MG: Hospital outbreak of infections with group A streptococci traced to an asymptomatic anal carrier. *N Engl J Med* 280:1224–1225, 1969.

301. Gryska PF, O'Dea AE: Postoperative streptococcal wound infection—the anatomy of an epidemic. *JAMA* 213:1189–1191, 1970.

302. Decker J, Hammond H, MacArthur M, Bailey J, Fukushima T, Centers for Disease Control: Hospital outbreak of streptococcal wound infection—Utah. *MMWR* 25:141, 1976.

303. Richman DD, Breton SJ, Goldmann DA: Scarlet fever and group A streptococcal surgical wound infection tracted to an anal carrier. *J Pediatr* 90:387–390, 1977.

304. Stamm WE, Feeley JC, Facklam RR: Wound infections due to group A *Streptococcus* traced to a vaginal carrier. *J Infect Dis* 138:287–292, 1978.

305. Quinn RW, Hillman JW: An epidemic of streptococcal wound infections. *Arch Environ Health* 11:28–33, 1965.

306. Hamburger M Jr, Green MJ, Hamburger VG: The problem of the "dangerous carrier" of hemolytic streptococci. II. Spread of infection by individuals with positive nose cultures who expelled large numbers of hemolytic streptococci. *J Infect Dis* 77:96–108, 1945.

307. Schrack WD Jr, Miller GB, Parkin WE, Fontana DB: Four streptococcal infections traced to an anal carrier. *Pa Med* 82:35–36, 1979.

308. Magnuson HJ, Thomas FW, Olansky S, Kaplan BI, DeMello L, Cutler JC: Inoculation syphilis in

human volunteers. *Medicine* 35:33–82, 1956.
309. Tramont EC: *Treponema pallidum* (syphilis). In Mandell GL, Douglas RG Jr, Bennett JE (eds): *Principles and Practice of Infectious Diseases.* New York, John Wiley & Sons, 1985, p 1323.
310. Whitney CM: The physician's danger in treating patients who have syphilis. *Am J Syph* 12:1–12, 1928.
311. Smith JL, Israel CW: The presence of spriochetes in late seronegative syphilis. *JAMA* 199:980–984, 1967.
312. Handsfield H, Lukehart SA, Sell S, Norris SJ, Holmes KK: Demonstration of *Treponema pallidum* in a cutaneous gumma by indirect immunofluorscence. *Arch Dermatol* 119:677–680, 1983.
313. Ashley MJ, Wigle WD: The epidemiology of active tuberculosis in hospital employees in Ontario, 1966–1969. *Am Rev Respir Dis* 104: 851–860, 1971.
314. Atuk NO, Hunt EH: Serial tuberculin testing and isoniazid therapy in general hospital employees. *JAMA* 218:1795–1798, 1971.
315. Ruben FL, Norden CW, Schuster N: Analysis of a community hospital employee tuberculosis screening program 31 months after its inception. *Am Rev Respir Dis* 115:23–28, 1977.
316. Barrett-Connor E: The epidemiology of tuberculosis in physicians. *JAMA* 241:33–38, 1979.
317. Berman J, Levin ML, Tangerose S, Desi L: Tuberculosis risk for hospital employees: analysis of a five-year tuberculin skin testing program. *Am J Public Health* 71:1217–1222, 1981.
318. Barrett T, Renteln HA, Centers for Disease Control: Tuberculous infection associated with tissue processing—California. *MMWR* 30:73–74, 1981.
319. Levine I: Tuberculosis risk in students of nursing. *Arch Intern Med* 121:545–548, 1968.
320. Craven RB, Wenzel RP, Atuk NO: Minimizing tuberculosis risk to hospital personnel and students exposed to unsuspected disease. *Ann Intern Med* 82:628–632, 1975.
321. Alpert ME, Levison ME: An epidemic of tuberculosis in a medical school. *N Engl J Med* 272:718–721, 1965.
322. Ehrenkranz NJ, Kicklighter JL: Tuberculosis outbreak in a general hospital: evidence for airborne spread of infection. *Ann Intern Med* 77:377–382, 1972.
323. Catlin BJ, Hanson F, Iseman MD, Sbarbaro JA, Hopkins RS: Tuberculosis in a drug rehabilitation center—Colorado. *MMWR* 29:543–544, 1980.
324. Catanzaro A: Nosocomial tuberculosis. *Am Rev Respir Dis* 125:559–562, 1982.
325. Munger R, Anderson K, Leahy R, Allard J, Kobayashi JM, Centers for Disease Control: Tuberculosis in a nursing care facility—Washington. *MMWR* 32:121–128, 1983.
326. Reeves SA, Noble RC: Ineffectiveness of annual chest roentgenograms in tuberculin skin test-positive hospital employees. *Am J Infect Control* 11:212–216, 1983.
327. American Thoracic Society: The tuberculin skin test. *Am Rev Respir Dis* 104:769–775, 1971.
328. Comstock GW: Frost revisited: the modern epidemiology of tuberculosis. *Am J Hyg* 101:363–382, 1975.
329. Donaldson JC, Elliott RC: A study of co-positivity of three multipunture techniques with intradermal

PPD tuberculin. *Am Rev Respir Dis* 118:843–846, 1978.
330. Centers for Disease Control: *Guidelines for Prevention of TB Transmission in Hospitals,* revised ed. (HEW Publication (CDC) 79–8371), Atlanta, Centers for Disease Control, 1979.
331. Thompson NJ, Glassroth JL, Snider DE, Farer LS: The booster phenomenon in serial tuberculin testing. *Am Rev Respir Dis* 119:587–597, 1979.
332. Valenti WM, Andrews BA, Presley BA, Reifler CB: Absence of the booster phenomenon in serial tuberculin skin testing. *Am Rev Respir Dis* 125:323–325, 1982.
333. Le CT: Cost-effectiveness of the two-step skin test for tuberculosis screening of employees in a community hospital. *Infect Control* 5:570–572, 1984.
334. Simon JA, McVicker SJ, Ferrell CR, Payne CB Jr: Two-step tuberculin testing in a veterans domiciliary population. *South Med J* 76:866–872, 1983.
335. Bass JB Jr, Serio RA: The use of repeat skin tests to eliminate the booster phenomenon in serial tuberculin testing. *Am Rev Respir Dis* 123:394–396, 1981.
336. Lincoln EM, Sewell EM: *Tuberculosis in Children.* New York, McGraw-Hill, 1963, p 14.
337. Rouillon A, Perdrizet S., Parrot R: Transmission of tubercle bacilli: the effects of chemotherapy. *Tubercle* 57:275–299, 1976.
338. Rose CE, Zerbe GO, Lantz SO, Bailey WC: Establishing priority during investigation of tuberculosis contacts. *Am Rev Respir Dis* 119:603–609, 1979.
339. Riley RL, Mills CC, O'Grady F, Sultan LU, Wittstadt F, Shivpuri DN: Infectiousness of air from a tuberculosis ward. Ultraviolet irradiation of infected air: comparative infectiousness of different patients. *Am Rev Respir Dis* 85:511–525, 1962.
340. Kamat SR, Dawson JJY, Devadatta S, Fox W, Janardhanam B, Radhakrishna S, Ramakrishnan CV, Somasundaram PR, Stott H, Velu S: A controlled study of the influence of segregation of tuberculous patients for one year on the attack rate of tuberculosis in a 5-year period in close family contacts in south India. *Bull WHO* 34:517–532, 1966.
341. Noble RC: Infectiousness of pulmonary tuberculosis after starting chemotherapy. Review of the available data on an unresolved question. *Am J Infect Control* 9:6–10, 1981.
342. American Thoracic Society: Guidelines for the investigation and management of tuberculosis contacts. *Am Rev Respir Dis* 114:459–463, 1976.
343. American Thoracic Society: Guidelines for work for patients with tuberculosis. *Am Rev Respir Dis* 108:160–161, 1973.
344. Ferebee SH: Controlled chemoprophylaxis trials in tuberculosis: a general review. *Adv Tuberc Res* 17:28–106, 1970.
345. Maddrey WC, Boitnott JK: Isoniazid hepatitis. *Ann Intern Med* 79:1–12, 1973.
346. Mitchell JR, Zimmerman HJ, Ishak KG, Thorgeirsson UP, Timbrell JA, Snodgrass WR, Nelson SD: Isoniazid liver injury: clinical spectrum, pathology, and probable pathogenesis. *Ann Intern Med* 84:181–192, 1976.
347. Taylor WC, Aronson MD, Delbanco TL: Should young adults with a positive tuberculin test take isoniazid? *Ann Intern Med* 94:808–813, 1981.

348. Comstock GW: Evaluating isoniazid preventive therapy: the need for more data. *Ann Intern Med* 94:817–819, 1981.

349. American Thoracic Society: Preventive therapy of tuberculous infection. *Am Rev Respir Dis* 110:371–374, 1974.

350. Byrd RB, Horn BR, Griggs GA, Solomon DA: Isoniazid chemoprophylaxis. Association with detection and incidence of liver toxicity. *Arch Intern Med* 137:1130–1133, 1977.

351. Byrd RB, Horn BR, Solomon DA, Griggs GA: Toxic effects of isoniazid in tuberculosis chemoprophylaxis. Role of biochemical monitoring in 1,000 patients. *JAMA* 241:1239–1241, 1979.

352. Centers for Disease Control: Cryptosporidiosis among children attending day-care centers—Georgia, Pennsylvania, Michigan, California, New Mexico. *MMWR* 33:599–601, 1984.

353. Black RE, Dykes AC, Sinclair SP, Wells JG: Giardiasis in day-care centers: evidence of person-to-person transmission. *Pediatrics* 60:486–491, 1977.

354. Pickering LK, Woodward WE, DuPont HL, Sullivan P: Occurrence of *Giardia lamblia* in children in day care centers. *J Pediatr* 104:522–526, 1984.

355. Ward JI, Gorman G, Phillips C, Fraser DW: *Haemophilus influenzae* type b disease in a day-care center. Report of an outbreak. *J Pediatr* 92:713–717, 1978.

356. Storch G, McFarland LM, Kelso K, Heilman CJ, Caraway CT: Viral hepatitis associated with day-care centers. *JAMA* 242:1514–1518, 1979.

357. Hadler SC, Webster HM, Erben JJ, Swanson JE, Maynard JE: Hepatitis A in day-care centers. A community-wide assessment. *N Engl J Med* 302:1222–1227, 1980.

358. Benenson MW, Takafuji ET, Bancroft WH, Lemon SM, Callahan MC, Leach DA: A military community outbreak of hepatitis type A related to transmission in a child care facility. *Am J Epidemiol* 112:471–481, 1980.

359. Rosenblum BF, Wren R, Ornelas E Jr, Adeogba B, Hafkin B, Webb CR Jr, Centers for Disease Control: Hepatitis A outbreak in a day-care center—Texas. *MMWR* 29:565–567, 1980.

360. Hadler SC, Erden JJ, Francis DP, Webster HM, Maynard JE: Risk factors for hepatitis A in day-care centers. *J Infect Dis* 145:255–261, 1982.

361. Vernon AA, Schable C, Francis D: A large outbreak of hepatitis A in a day-care center: association with non-toilet-trained children and persistence of IgM antibody to hepatitis A virus. *Am J Epidemol* 115:325–331, 1982.

362. Hammack C, Ochoa A, Henderson C, Fullilove P, Fondren G: Hepatitis A outbreak related to a day care center in Forrest County, Mississippi. *J Miss State Med Assoc* 23:40–43, 1982.

363. Gingrich GA, Hadler SC, Elder HA, Ash KO: Serologic investigation of an outbreak of hepatitis A in a rural day-care center. *Am J Public Health* 73:1190–1193, 1983.

364. Klein JD, Collier Am, Glezen WP: An influenza B epidemic among children in day-care. *Pediatrics* 58:340–345, 1976.

365. Saez-Nieto JA, Perucha M, Casamayor H, Marcen JJ, Llacer A, Garcia-Barreno B, Casal J: Outbreak of infection caused by *Neisseria meningitidis* group C type 2 in a nursery. *J Infect* 8:49–55, 1984.

366. Chiba S, Akihara M, Kogasaka R, Horino K, Nakao T, Urasawa T, Urasawa S, Fukui S: An out-break of acute gastroenteritis due to rotavirus in an infant home. *Tohoku J Exp Med* 127:265–271, 1979.

367. Lieb S, Gunn RA, Taylor DN: Salmonellosis in a day-care center. *J Pediatr* 100:1004–1005, 1982.

368. Weissman JB, Gangorosa EJ, Schmerler A, Marier RL, Lewis JN: Shigellosis in day-care centres. *Lancet* 1:88–90, 1975.

369. Rosenberg ML, Weissman JB, Gangarosa EJ, Reller LB, Beasley RP: Shigellosis in the United States: ten-year review of nationwide surveillance, 1964–1973. *Am J Epidemiol* 104:543–551, 1976.

370. Pickering LK, Evans DG, DuPont DL, Vollett JJ 3rd, Evans DJ Jr: Diarrhea caused by *Shigella*, rotavirus, and *Giardia* in day-care centers: prospective study. *J Pediatr* 99:51–56, 1981.

371. Tacket CO, Cohen ML: Shigellosis in day care centers: use of plasmid analysis to assess control measures. *Pediatr Infect Dis* 2:127–130, 1983.

372. Johnson K, Boase J, Helgerson SD, Kobayashi JM, Centers for Disease Control: Shigellosis in day-care centers—Washington, 1983. *MMWR* 33:250–251, 1984.

373. Leichtner AM, Leclair J, Goldman DA, Schumacher RT, Gewolb IH, Katz AJ: Horizontal nonparenteral spread of hepatitis B among children. *Ann Intern Med* 94:346–349, 1981.

374. Black RE, Dykes AC, Anderson KE, Wells JG, Sinclair SP, Gary GW Jr, Hatch MH, Gangarosa EJ: Handwashing to prevent diarrhea in day-care centers. *Am J Epidemiol* 113:445–451, 1981.

375. Hadler SC, Erben JJ, Matthews D, Starko K, Francis DP, Maynard JE: Effect of immunoglobulin on hepatitis A in day-care centers. *JAMA* 249:48–53, 1983.

376. Trumpp CE, Karasic R: Management of communicable diseases in day care centers. *Pediatr Ann* 12:219–229, 1983.

377. Lemp GF, Woodward WE, Pickering LK, Sullivan PS, DuPont HL: The relationship of staff to the incidence of diarrhea in day-care centers. *Am J Epidemiol* 120:750–758, 1984.

378. Pike RM: Laboratory-associated infections: incidence, fatalities, causes, and prevention. *Annu Rev Microbiol* 33:41–66, 1979.

379. Sulkin SE, Pike RM: Survey of laboratory-acquired infections. *Am J Public Health* 41:769–781, 1951.

380. Long ER: The hazard of acquiring tuberculosis in the laboratory. *Am J Public Health* 41:782–787, 1951.

381. Collins CH: Laboratory-acquired tuberculosis. *Tubercle* 63:151–155, 1982.

382. Blaser MJ, Lofgren JP: Fatal salmonellosis originating in a clinical micorbiology laboratory. *J Clin Microbiol* 13:855–858, 1981.

383. Votra EM, Rutala WA, Sarubbi FA: Recommendations for pregnant employee interaction with patients having communicable infectious diseases. *Am J Infect Control* 11:10–19, 1983.

384. Remington JS, Klein JO: *Infectious Disease of the Fetus and Newborn.* Philadelphia, WB Saunders, 1984.

385. Markvart K, Rehnov'a M, Ostrovsk'a A: Laboratory epidemic of toxoplasmosis. *J Hyg Epidemiol Microbiol Immunol* 22:477–484, 1978.

Chapter 14

Microbiologic Aspects of Infection Control

Patricia A. Ristuccia, M.S., and Burke A. Cunha, M.D.

SURVEILLANCE
Environmental Surveillance

The hospital environment is closely related to and plays a prominent role in nosocomially acquired infections. However, routine microbiologic sampling of the environment has been shown to contribute little to the prevention of nosocomial infections (1), and has proven to be a costly and time-consuming practice. Therefore, with few exceptions, environmental cultures should be employed only during the investigation of an outbreak (2, 3). Routine monitoring of the inanimate environment is still necessary for steam, gas, and dry heat sterilizers and for water used for the preparation of dialysis fluid (4).

Sterilizers

The overall performance of sterilization units is essential in assuring the adequacy of the sterilization process. Proper loading of all types of sterilizers is of primary importance for the correct operation of these instruments. In order to check the effectiveness of sterilization, quality control measures are employed. These include physical, chemical, and biologic indicators, process controls, and daily function test sheets (vacuum autoclaves). All steam and dry heat sterilizers should be equipped with accurate recording thermometers, timers, and pressure gauges which will monitor these parameters during the processing of each load. Physical indicators, such as autoclave tape, which is attached to the outside of each package being sterilized, will indicate that the load was exposed to the appropriate sterilization process. Chemical indicators such as color strips, bars, or pellets that melt are placed in the center of each load verifying steam penetration. Daily function test sheets (formerly the Bowie-Dick test) are processed daily in the first sterilization cycle of all vacuum autoclaves to verify complete

removal of air, even distribution of steam, and no leakage of air back into the chamber (5, 6).

However, none of the above control measures is used as an absolute indication that sterilization has occurred. For this reason, the most reliable test of sterilization is the combination of the above indicators along with a biologic spore challenge test. Commercially prepared spore tests, available as spores sealed in glass ampules containing media, in double-walled plastic ampules containing spores in one section and growth media in another, or paper strips impregnated with spores, are used to check that sterilization has actually occurred (7). For steam autoclaves, spores of *Bacillus stearothermophilus* should be used at least once a week to confirm sterilization. Performance of ethylene oxide sterilizers should be checked at least once a week, utilizing spores of *B. subtilis* var. *niger* (*globigii*). Biologic indicators should be placed along with each load of implantable objects sterilized by the above methods, to assure high level disinfection with each load (4, 7). Dry heat sterilizers should be checked at least once a month with spores of *B. subtilis* var *niger* (*globigii*). All indicators should be processed according to the manufacturers' recommendations. Strict quality control checks of all media used by the microbiology laboratory are essential for assuring the reliability of spore test results. A previous report of presumed autoclave failure was traced to the use of contaminated trypticase soy broth for the culture of the processed spore strips (8). The contaminant, identified as *Bacillus coagulans*, was detected when the broth was incubated at 55°C, resulting in the misinterpretation of the spore test. The organism remained undetected when the uninoculated broth was incubated at 37°C as a quality control measure. Recommendations by the Centers for Disease Control (CDC) state that quality control tests for medium sterility should be performed at the temperature at which the inoculated medium is incubated.

Hemodialysis fluid

The risk of infection caused by gram-negative water bacteria is high in those individuals undergoing hemodialysis. Although the water used to prepare the dialysis fluid, as well as the dialysis fluid itself, need not be sterile, these organisms multiply relatively fast. This may lead to possible serious consequences. It is recommended that routine monitoring of these fluids be performed at least once a month to quantitate the concentration of viable organisms present (4). Commercially prepared colony count samplers (Total-Count and Coli-Count Samplers; Millipore Corporation, Bedford, MA) are used to culture these fluids. The concentration of organisms present in the water used to prepare the dialysis fluid should not exceed 200 colonies/ml. Dialysis fluid should be sampled at the end of dialysis and should contain no more than 2000 colonies/ml (9). If these quantitative microbiologic guidelines are exceeded, appropriate steps must be taken to correct the problem.

Significance of Microorganisms in the Hospital

It is difficult for microbiology laboratory personnel to determine the significance of microorganisms in the hospital setting. Instead, their significance depends upon the clinical setting, which is usually not known to laboratory personnel. The site from which the microorganism is recovered, the frequency with which it is recovered, and its susceptibility pattern are all factors of clinical importance. The laboratory usually receives cultures of body fluids or cultures from various sites in the body. Such information provides infection rates for various organisms as well as their susceptibility patterns. It is the role of the laboratory to provide accurate identification of the organisms and reliable statistics for the infection control team. Proper specimen collection and processing are essential to providing meaningful information from laboratory results. Accurate laboratory data provide the background information necessary for the recognition of change in the incidence or prevalence of nosocomial pathogens and are useful in outbreak investigation. The main dilemma from the laboratory's standpoint is deciding how far and how fast to process various clinical specimens. For example, it is of no microbiologic, infection control,

or clinical value to speciate multiple organisms cultured from an uncomplicated open wound. In contradistinction, it may be very important to speciate $< 10^5$ organisms/ml in the urine of a patient who is catheterized and receiving antimicrobial therapy. The microbiology laboratory must be aware of the potential significance of nosocomial pathogens so that particular attention is paid to their accurate identification, incidence, and susceptibility patterns (10–16). In an outbreak investigation, the resources of the microbiology laboratory are indispensable in determining the nature and extent of the outbreak. In such situations the microbiology laboratory is frequently overwhelmed with a large number of specimens from patients, medical personnel, and environmental sources. The infection control team needs to coordinate the collection of such specimens to minimize the work of the microbiology laboratory and to direct the culturing of sources that are most likely to be associated with the pathogen involved with the outbreak. Data from the microbiology laboratory are particularly useful in providing the initial information differentiating pseudoinfection or pseudo-outbreak from their real counterparts. Ultimately, infection control personnel must determine the significance of the organism with respect to the patient and the institution (12, 16).

Most gram-negative organisms exist in the hospital environment in fluids. Common environmental sources for gram-negative organisms include respiratory support equipment, irrigation fluids, intravenous fluids, and disinfectants. Some organisms, such as the atypical mycobacteria, are present in tap water. The association of *Legionella* with water/air cooling systems is well known. *Clostridium difficile* is unique, and it may survive in spore form on the floor or on fomites for months. Certain organisms, such as staphylococci and JK diphtheroids, have no environmental source. In reviewing the human sources of these organisms, one realizes that hands are important in the transmission of virtually all nosocomial pathogens. The importance of hand washing and controlling the spread of infection from person to person has been emphasized. Depending upon the organism, either respiratory secretions, feces, or urine may provide human sources for the organism within the institution (Table 14.1). Such information provides laboratory personnel with the framework for determining the significance of the isolate for the individual patient (16–20). Person-to-person spread of

Table 14.1. Sources of Nosocomial Pathogens*

Microorganism	Environmental Source	Human Source	Type of Infection
Klebsiella	Respiratory support equipment	Pharynx, stool, urine	Respiratory, wound, UTI, bacteremia, diarrhea
Enterobacter	Intravenous fluids, water	Hands, stool, urine	UTI, pneumonia, bacteremia
Serratia	Respiratory support equipment	Hands, urine	UTI, bacteremia, pneumonia, wound infections
P. aeruginosa	Water, disinfectants, respiratory support equipment	Hands, pharynx, stool, urine	UTI, wound infections, pneumonia
P. cepacia	Water reservoirs, contaminated equipment	Hands	Wound infections, bacteremia, UTI
P. maltophilia	Water	Hands	Meningitis, septicemia, wound infections
Proteus/Morganella/ Providencia	Water	Hands, urine	Bacteremia, UTI, wound infections
Flavobacterium	Water, intravenous fluids	Hands	Septicemia, meningitis
Citrobacter	Water	Hands	Bacteremia, meningitis, UTI, wound infections
Acinetobacter	Respiratory support equipment	Hands	Pneumonia, bacteremia, wound infections
Staphylococcus aureus/ S. epidermidis/MRSA	None	Hands, nares	Bacteremia, wound infections, infected devices
JK diphtheroids	None	Hands	Bacteremia, infected devices
C. difficile	Surfaces near infected patients and utility rooms	Hands, stool	Diarrhea, colitis
Legionella	Water/air-cooling systems	Respiratory secretions	Pneumonia, wound infections
Atypical mycobacteria	Tap water, contaminated respirators	Respiratory secretions	Wound infections

* UTI, urinary tract infection; MRSA, methicillin-resistant *S. aureus.*

certain microorganisms within an institution is usually readily apparent by studies employing epidemiologic methods. However, certain organisms, because of their ubiquitous nature or fastidious growth requirements, may be difficult to incriminate in person-to-person spread (Table 14.2). These organisms are not part of the usual microbiologic or infection control statistics and therefore deserve special awareness of their potential for person-to-person transmission (18).

ANTIBIOGRAMS

Sensitivity Testing

Antimicrobial susceptibility testing is one of the most important procedures performed in the

Table 14.2. Nosocomial Organisms Which Have Not Been Clearly Linked to Person-to-Person Spread

Proteus mirabilis
Haemophilus influenzae
Legionella pneumophila
Chlamydia psittaci
Pneumocystis carinii
Clostridium difficile
Cryptosporidium

microbiology laboratory. It is directed toward correlating the in vitro susceptibility of the infecting organism with the pharmacokinetic characteristic of antimicrobial agents. Various considerations are necessary when selecting an appropriate antimicrobial agent for the treatment of an infectious disease. These include the knowledge of the in vitro susceptibility of the infecting pathogen; the pharmacokinetic characteristics of antibiotics, including absorption, distribution, metabolism, excretion, protein binding, tissue penetration, and toxicity; the natural history and pathology of the infectious process; and the immune status of the patient. If performed carefully and interpreted correctly, the results obtained from in vitro testing will provide valuable guidance for appropriate and optimal in vivo response. Antimicrobial susceptibility tests may also be used as a means of providing accurate and reproducible epidemiologic markers for determining the relatedness of microorganisms found in the hospital environment as well as monitoring changes in the populations of those organisms.

The most widely used method of performing susceptibility tests has been, until recently, the Kirby-Bauer disk diffusion method (21). Described in 1966, this procedure is performed by inoculating a standardized concentration of microorganism onto the surface of Mueller-Hinton agar and placing paper disks impregnated with known concentrations of antibiotics on the agar. The plates are incubated under controlled conditions, and after overnight incubation (16–18 hours), the zone of inhibited growth around the disks is measured. Zone sizes have been standardized for different organisms which translate millimeters into categories: sensitive, intermediate, or resistant (21–23). The zone size "breakpoints" may relate to clinically achievable serum concentrations of antibiotics.

The reliability of results obtained from disk diffusion testing depends upon the awareness of several factors influencing performance. These include inoculum density; constituents or ionic content, pH and depth of the test medium; rate of diffusion of the antibiotics through the test medium; growth rates of the organisms being tested; incubation temperature and time. Standardization procedures have been developed to keep the influence of these factors on test results to a minimum; and when strictly controlled, adequate reproducibility is assured in clinical and epidemiologic studies.

The most important variable which will affect the overall outcome of the susceptibility test is inoculum size. A light inoculum will cause organisms with the ability to produce antibiotic inactivating enzymes (e.g., β-lactamases) to act in-

effectively on the diffused antibiotic, resulting in large zones of inhibition and false susceptibility. Likewise, heavy inocula undermine the critical drug diffusion/cell mass ratio, resulting in very small zones of inhibition and, therefore, false resistance (24).

Temperature has also been shown to play a large role in the reliability of susceptibility data. Variations in temperature have affected both the activity of antibiotics as well as the growth rates of various organisms (25–27). These variations in temperature have been shown to have strong influence on the detection of methicillin resistance among strains of *S. aureus* (28, 29). The resistant strains grow more slowly at 37°C and therefore require longer incubation periods ($\geq$ 48 hours) before detection is possible. The initial recommendation for the detection of methicillin-resistant *S. aureus* (MRSA) was to use 30°C, a temperature at which the organisms grew faster. The use of the standardized 35°C is adequate for the detection of MRSA; however, a longer incubation period ($\geq$ 24 hours instead of 16–18 hours) has been suggested.

The extent to which the test medium affects susceptibility results has led to the recommendation that only Mueller-Hinton medium be used for susceptibility testing. This medium has been chosen because it has the nutritive capacity to support the growth of most organisms, it is an isotonic medium, and with the addition of blood allows the growth of fastidious organisms. This medium has the buffering capacity sufficient to prevent pH shifts due to bacterial growth, which may affect the activity of various antibiotics.

One of the major problems with Mueller-Hinton medium has been the inconsistency of susceptibility data due to the lot-to-lot and manufacturer-to-manufacturer variability in the concentration of the divalent cations, calcium and magnesium. Most reports have been on the effect of these free cations on the activity of polymyxins, aminoglycosides, and tetracyclines against *Pseudomonas* sp (30–33). Calcium and magnesium incorporate themselves into the cell wall of *Pseudomonas*, making it less permeable and more stable to the aminoglycosides. Therefore, as the cation concentration in the test medium increases, the less active the antibiotic will appear. A different mechanism of "resistance" is seen with the tetracyclines and polymyxins, in which case the antibiotic is inactivated by chelation with calcium or magnesium. It has been recommended that Mueller-Hinton medium be supplemented to achieve and maintain approximately 50 mg/liter of calcium and 25 mg/liter of magnesium to assure reliability and reproducibility of susceptibility results (34). With alterations in the media supplementation, the associated changes in susceptibility reports may have serious clinical and epidemiologic implications. It is important, therefore, that the performance of the media be assessed by appropriate quality control means. This involves the daily testing of the control strains *Staphylococcus aureus* ATCC 25923, *Escherichia coli* ATCC 25922, and *Pseudomonas aeruginosa* ATCC 27853.

Although there has been overwhelming acceptance and application of the standardized disk diffusion method, a major disadvantage of the procedure is the qualitative data it generates. Recent reports (35, 36) show a trend toward dilution procedures for susceptibility testing. The dilution tests, using either agar or broth media, provide quantitative data by determining the minimal concentration of antimicrobic necessary to inhibit or kill a particular organism. The procedure involves the serial dilution of antibiotic in the test medium followed by inoculation with a standardized suspension of the test organism. After overnight incubation, under controlled conditions, the lowest dilution of antibiotic which inhibits the growth of the organism is considered the minimal inhibitory concentration (MIC), which can be correlated with concentrations of antimicrobial agents found in any body fluid.

The generation of quantitative rather than qualitative data may be of greater help to the epidemiologist in the determination of the relatedness of organisms during an outbreak investigation. Organisms considered resistant by the disk diffusion method may be regarded as similar when in fact more than one strain may exist. A limiting factor of disk diffusion procedures is that zone diameters less than 6 mm are not detectable. Therefore, organisms moderately resistant will not be differentiated from ones with higher degrees of resistance. This may lead to erroneous conclusions on the part of the epidemiologist as to the differences among organisms (37).

Agar dilution procedures are inexpensive to perform when large numbers of organisms are being tested. However, a disadvantage which is not found with the broth dilution procedure is the inability to determine minimal bactericidal concentrations (MBC) of antibiotics. Using broth dilution tests, tubes showing inhibition of growth may be subcultured to antibiotic free medium, allowing for the determination of MBCs. This is of clinical importance, especially in cases of endocarditis where "tolerant" strains of *S. aureus* may be involved.

Over the past few years, broth dilution procedures have been modified and miniaturized into microdilution methods. These microdilution tests are performed as the macro method. However, the final volume of broth is one-tenth that of the conventional method. Many commercially prepared microdilution trays are available which consist of dried stabilized antibiotic dilutions which are rehydrated with a suspension of the test organism. These prediluted trays may be stored conveniently, and they have eliminated the need for laboratory preparation of media or antibiotic solutions.

One of the advantages of both the macro and microdilution methods has been their easy adaptation to mechanization. Systems which have been developed include the Autobac 1, MTS and IDX systems (General Diagnostics, Morris Plains, NJ), MS-2 and Advantage Systems (Abbott Laboratories, Irving, TX), and the Vitek AMS system (Vitek Systems, Inc., St. Louis, MO). Microdilution methods include Sensititre (Gibco Diagnostics, Lawrence, MA), Sceptor (Becton Dickinson, Cockeysville, MD), Micro-Media (Micro-Media Systems, Potomac, MD), and API UniScept (Analytab Products Inc., Plainview, NY) systems. Many of these systems are fully automated, and all have the ability to generate quantitative or semiquantitative data. The Autobac, MS-2, and AMS systems are capable of producing susceptibility results in 3 to 10 hours, while the microdilution procedures require 15 to 20 hours for completion of the test.

Although these methods have been readily incorporated into the microbiology laboratory and have been shown to correlate well with other methods (38–41), problems have appeared which are found to affect these methods and antibiotic susceptibility testing in general. Some problem areas include testing of *Enterobacter/Serratia* sp. possessing inducible β-lactamases, *P. aeruginosa/enterococci* and false susceptibility results, and the detection of methicillin resistance associated with *S. aureus*. These problems may have significant impact on the care of patients infected or colonized with these organisms as well as on the data derived from surveillance studies for these organisms.

A major problem which is inherent to all microdilution methods is the small volumes used to

Table 14.3.   Organism-Antibiotic Combinations Producing Unreliable Susceptibility Results by Broth Dilution Methods (38, 40, 42–46, 49, 50)

Organism	Antibiotic
Staphylococcus sp.	Erythromycin
	Penicillin G
	Methicillin
Enterobacter sp.	Ampicillin
	Cephalothin
	Cefamandole
Serratia sp.	Aminoglycosides
	Polymyxins
P. aeruginosa	Aminoglycosides
	Moxalactam
	Cefoperazone
	Ceftizoxime
	Cefotaxime

reconstitute the antimicrobial dilutions. This problem is most evident when testing penicillin and methicillin against *S. aureus*, and cefamandole against *Enterobacter* and *Serratia sp.* (Table 14.3). Although the initial inoculum density is adjusted to $\sim 10^5$ colony forming units (CFU)/ml, the fact that only 0.1 ml is being used as the final volume decreases the actual cell density tested by at least one log. Within a given population of cells, the percentage of resistant cells can be extremely small. Also, the mutational frequency is approximately 10^{-5}. Therefore, it is obvious that the bacterial inoculum must contain $\geq 10^5$ CFU/ml in order to detect emerging resistant strains. Studies have indicated that most of the newer dilution procedures do, in fact, have this problem of underestimating resistance (38, 42–46). To overcome this, the use of higher inoculum densities may be used. However, this may create a problem of false resistance (47). The problem of underestimating resistance also arises with automated systems, not because of the miniaturization of test volumes, but simply because the test is not run long enough for expression of resistance to occur (36).

Due to the nature of the test, automated dilution susceptibility systems have problems recognizing resistance among certain organisms, as well as producing variability in test results. Most automated systems monitor the growth (or death) of bacterial cells in the presence of antibiotics compared to that of the control containing bacterial cells only. It is obvious that it would be difficult for the instrument to differentiate between dying cells and a few replicating (resistant) cells within the concentrated test area.

One other factor affecting the reproducibility of the automated systems is the effect which subinhibitory concentrations have on the morphology and ultrastructure of bacterial cells (43, 48). Exposing microorganisms to antibiotic concentrations lower than the MIC produces elongation and swelling of the cells, which may affect light scattering or turbidimetric readings of the instruments. These erratic readings may lead to misinformation regarding the susceptibility of various organisms and contribute to the inability of these automated systems to provide reproducible results under certain circumstances.

Results obtained from susceptibility tests help the infection control practitioner to distinguish potential pathogens from other less significant environmental microorganisms. It is essential, therefore, that the methodology implemented by the microbiology laboratory to determine the susceptibility patterns of these organisms be accurate and reproducible. All of the available procedures used for determining the activity of antibiotics to microorganisms have both advantages and disadvantages. If chosen wisely and used correctly, the method will produce antibiograms helpful to the clinician in determining patient therapy, as well as to the epidemiologist as a tool to recognize and control potential nosocomial infections.

Strain Identification

Determining whether a single bacterial strain is the sole cause of "cluster" infections among hospitalized patients is of great concern to the epidemiologist during an outbreak investigation. The microbiology laboratory plays a major role in the recognition and evaluation of this problem. Since methicillin-resistant *S. aureus* and gram-negative bacilli, mainly the Enterobacteriaceae and Pseudomonadaceae, are more frequently associated with nosocomial infections, the laboratory should be able to isolate as well as accurately and consistently identify, at least to the species level, the responsible pathogen. However, determining the species identification should not be the only means of recognizing similarities among these isolates. Additional procedures—such as antibiotic susceptibility testing, serologic typing, bacteriophage or bacteriocin typing, DNA hydridization and plasmid analysis, along with the biochemical characteristics of the organism (biotype)—are necessary to establish a more meaningful and detailed epidemiologic marker (Table

Table 14.4.   Epidemiologic Typing Systems Useful for Evaluating Nosocomial Microorganisms*

Typing System	Microorganism
Biotyping	Enterobacteriaceae, *Pseudomonas, Neisseria, Haemophilus, S. epidermidis*
Antibiotic susceptibility	Staphylococci, Enterobacteriaceae, *Pseudomonas*, other nonfermentative bacteria
Serotyping	Enterobacteriaceae, *P. aeruginosa*, streptococci, viruses
Bacteriophage typing	Staphylococci, *Salmonella*, other gram-negative aerobic bacilli

* Adapted from references 7, 10, 11, and 71.

14.4). The data are compiled, the likelihood of a true nosocomial outbreak can be determined and appropriate steps taken to eliminate the problem.

The biochemical profile (biotype) of a particular organism may prove to be a valuable piece of information useful in identifying and differentiating the gram-negative bacilli isolated by the microbiology laboratory. Most hospitals are now using one of the commercially prepared biochemical test "kits" (e.g., API-20E, Analytab Products, Inc., Plainview, NY) or automated systems (e.g., Advantage Systems, Abbott Diagnostics, Irving, TX) for the identification of these organisms. These systems utilize lyophilized biochemical substrates which are reconstituted with a standardized bacterial inoculum. The rapid systems detect the presence of constitutive enzymes and metabolic products and, therefore, are able to yield identification within 4 hours. The others require the growth of the organism, and although they can be read after 5 hours, are best read after 18 to 24 hours of incubation.

Most systems are used in conjunction with a computer data bank which has been programmed to contain the various biochemical profiles of numerous bacterial strains. All "positive" reactions are assigned a numerical value, and the octal number generated determines the identity of the organism. The great advantage of this system is that it provides a rapid and simple means of differentiating organisms that may be of epidemiologic importance. For example, a laboratory which usually isolates a bacterial strain with a particular biotype number that now has a "cluster" of isolates of the same genus and species but with a different biotype number may alert the epidemiologist to the possible emergence of an organism of epidemiologic significance. However, the sole reliance on changes in biotype numbers for determining differences between organisms may not be as safe a practice as once thought. Even though these tests may be extremely reliable in determining genus and species

identification, the degree of reproducibility of the individual biochemical reactions is suspect. Butler and colleagues (51) studied the reproducibility of the API-20E system for the identification of Enterobacteriaceae and found the system capable of producing identical biotype numbers in only 55.5% of the 110 strains tested. The reproducibility of each of 20 biochemical reactions was reviewed and found to range from 80% (for citrate) to 100% (for H_2S, indole, mannitol, tryptophan diaminase). When the same technologist performed and interpreted the biochemical reactions, increases in both inoculum size and incubation time affected the reproducibility of the system. Incubation time, increased from 15 hours to 22 hours, resulted in a change in percent agreement from 67.5% to 75.8%. Higher inoculum sizes, from 10^3 CFU/ml to 10^7 CFU/ml, resulted in a change in percent agreement from 65% to 77.5%.

Sneath and Johnson (52) evaluated methods used for the identification of *Pseudomonas* and reported a disagreement of almost 3% with results obtained within laboratory, and interlaboratory disagreement was as high as 15%. It was suggested that serious errors in identification are not significant as long as the probability of an erroneous result is maintained below 10%.

Barry and co-workers (53), in a collaborative study, looked at the accuracy and precision of the Autobac system, compared with a conventional method, for identification of gram-negative bacilli. The overall precision of the conventional method ranged from 93.5% to 99.2%. The reproducibility of each of the biochemical reactions varied from 74.9% (for growth on triple sugar agar at 42°C) when testing glucose nonfermenters, to 99.4% (oxidase spot test) when testing glucose fermenters.

It is evident that biotyping of organisms can be a valuable epidemiologic tool. However, one should keep in mind the inherent variability of each system and the organism as well. Therefore, one must recognize the limitations in biotyping as a sole means of providing epidemiologic information and perform additional procedures to determine the existence of true similarities among microorganisms.

Antimicrobial susceptibility testing is another useful marker system for determining the epidemiologic relatedness of microorganisms. Agar disk diffusion methods (Kirby-Bauer) or broth dilution procedures to determine the susceptibility pattern (antibiogram) of the organism to various antibiotics may be used. There is some variability between methods which may have to be taken into account to compare dissimilar results for two different laboratories.

Serologic typing of various organisms may also be useful as an epidemiologic marker, although its greatest use is as an aid in the diagnosis of an infectious disease. Serodiagnosis is based on the principle that an antigen and antibody specific for it (or vice versa) when mixed together will produce a detectable reaction. Traditional serologic procedures include agglutination, complement fixation, and precipitation. Agglutination and precipitation procedures have been used for years in the microbiology laboratory for the rapid identification of many pathogenic organisms. These include the slide agglutination procedures for serotyping *Salmonella, Shigella, E. coli* and other members of Enterobacteriaceae (54), and the Lancefield precipitin procedure of grouping β-hemolytic streptococci (55).

Coagglutination is used for the identification of groups A, B, C, and G β-hemolytic streptococci as well as *Haemophilus influenzae* type b, *Neisseria* and *Salmonella* species. This procedure is based on the ability of *S. aureus* (Cowan strain), rich in protein A, to bind the Fc portion of IgG subclasses 2 and 4. The unbound Fab portion of the immunoglobulin is left free to react with antibody molecules specific for the organism being tested. Olcen and colleagues (56) showed this procedure to have less autoagglutination and more specificity than the traditional agglutination procedures for the detection of *Neisseria meningitidis* in cerebrospinal fluid.

Another agglutination procedure, using sensitized latex particles, has gained widespread use as a serologic technique. These techniques can identify *H. influenzae* type b, *N. meningitidis* groups A, B, and C, and groups A, B, C, D, and G β-hemolytic streptococci. Nonspecific agglutination of latex particles seems less common than with coagglutination procedures, making latex agglutination procedures more reliable.

Immunologic methods for the detection and typing of various organisms have gained acceptance in the microbiology laboratory. These procedures include counterimmunoelectrophoresis (CIE), immunofluorescence (IF), radioimmunoassay (RIA), and enzyme-linked immunosorbent assays (ELISA). CIE is based on the principle of immunodiffusion with the migration of antigen and antibody toward one another, an event driven by the application of an electrical current to the test system. This procedure is most widely used for the direct detection of antigens in CSF and is capable of detecting *H. influenzae* type b, *N. meningitidis* groups A, B, C, X, Y, Z, W135, and groups B and D β-hemolytic streptococci. The system is capable of detecting small quantities of organisms ($\approx 10^5$ CFU/ml). However, cross-reactivity may occur if a larger antigenic load ($> 10^8$ CFU/ml) is present (57). Some cross-reactions occur which are not related to the amount of antigen present. Examples include *H. influenzae* type b and *N. meningitidis* group B antisera with *E. coli* Kl antigens and *E. coli* and *H. influenzae* type b with *S. aureus* (58).

Immunofluorescence has received widest application in the microbiology laboratory for the direct detection of group A streptococci in clinical specimens. However, this technique may be used for the detection of a variety of pathogens. Antibodies against specific pathogens are harvested from laboratory animals and labeled with a fluorescent dye, usually fluorescein. When these antibodies are reacted with the specific antigen, the organisms are detectable when viewed under ultraviolet light. Other applications of the technique include diagnosis of syphilis (FTA-ABS), rabies, and pertussis.

Radioimmunoassays are based on the classic antigen-antibody reaction, but a radioactive isotope is used as the marker to detect the reaction. These techniques have not been used to any great extent in microbiology, but they have found major applications in the screening of blood for hepatitis B virus antigens and antibodies.

Enzyme-linked immunosorbent assays are similar in principle to RIA but have many advantages over RIA. In place of radioactive isotopes, ELISA methods utilize enzymes as the "label," which eliminates the hazards of radioactivity and decreases the cost per test for reagents. ELISA is capable of detecting *H. influenzae* type b, *N. meningitidis* groups A and C, as well as hepatitis B, rotavirus, herpes simplex, Ebstein-Barr virus (EBV), *Candida albicans, Cryptococcus neoformans,* and *Toxoplasma gondii.*

Grouping and typing of various microorganisms by serologic methods have undergone major changes and improvements over the past 10 years. These changes are largely due to a process initiated by Kohler and Milstein in 1975 called somatic cell hybridization technology (59). The process utilizes the fusing of two different cell types to form hybrid cells which contain a mixture of nuclear material from both parent cells. Many methods are available for producing these hybrid cells (60–63), which, once produced, may be grown in continuous cell culture in an appropriate medium. Those hybrid cells found to be producing antibodies against the original antigen may then be cloned. If these clones are found to be producing antibodies, they may be preserved in cell cultures, grown in vivo in ascitic fluid in mice, or frozen indefinitely for future use. There are many advantages to the technology (64). Because antibody produced is from a "single" source, there will be no lot-to-lot variability in the activity of that antibody. Furthermore, since the hybridomas may be frozen, as well as cloned, there is the potential for a limitless supply of antibodies. Third, pure antibodies may be produced using nonpurified antigens. However, the production of nonpurified antibodies will not substantially hamper activity (there are no antispecies antibodies interfering). In fact, it may have higher titers than those produced by conventional methods.

Problems with the technology include the difficulty in obtaining hybrids that produce antibodies; instability of the clones, which results in failure to produce antibodies; fixed affinity of antibodies, which may affect activity; and antibodies lacking agglutination and precipitating activity (65).

The field of monoclonal antibody production is fairly new; however, its potential impact on microbiology and epidemiology is rapidly being recognized. It has already been utilized for the diagnosis of rabies virus infection (65), as well as for its differentiation from rabies-related viruses. Monoclonal antibodies are also being used for the detection of various bacterial infections (66–68), and their use in epidemiologic studies has begun (69).

The serologic techniques described above are useful in the detection of specific microorganisms; however, each has its own advantages, disadvantages, and limitations. The advantage of all of the techniques is that they may be performed in the hospital microbiology laboratory, a fact which will allow for rapid reporting of results. The major disadvantage with each technique is the lack of standardization and the presence of variables that will influence the outcome of the test. These variables include the specificity of the harvested antibodies, the possibility of nonspecific reactions, and the instability of the antibody over time. However, with the advent of monoclonal antibodies these factors may be eliminated. The major limiting factor of all of these procedures is that, although the antisera available commercially will cover a large range of organisms and serotypes, it is impossible to have all serotypes available to the routine microbiology laboratory.

Serotyping seems to be a stable epidemiologic marking system and in certain cases may provide helpful information to the epidemiologist. However, due to the limitations of the techniques, the use of serotyping as a major epidemiologic tool is losing prominence at this time.

Bacteriophage and bacteriocin typing are primarily used as epidemiologic tools and are rarely performed in the routine microbiology laboratory for diagnostic purposes. Both procedures are capable of detecting differences among strains that are considered identical by other epidemiologic tests. Bacteriophages are viruses that parasitize bacteria. These viruses incorporate themselves within the bacterial cell, multiply, and eventually destroy that cell. Bacteriophage typing for epidemiologic purposes has been particularly successful in staphylococcal and *Salmonella* infections and in pseudomonal infections to some degree (70, 71).

Bacteriocins are defined as a class of antibiotic proteins produced by a variety of bacterial species. These bacteriocins are active only against species of bacteria closely related to the strain of bacteria producing it. They are similar to bacteriophages except for the inability of bacteriocin to replicate. Bacteriocins are identified by the production of areas of inhibited bacterial growth similar to that seen with bacteriophage plaques, and they exhibit a great deal of specificity. The bacteriocins are designated according to the organisms responsible for production (e.g., colicin—*E.* coli; vibriocins—*Vibrio cholerae*; pesticines, *Yersinia pestis*).

Pyocine typing of *P. aeruginosa* is probably the single most useful typing procedure for the organism. The assay procedure is similar to that of phage typing, and the lytic reactions are graded +/−. Each reaction is given a numerical designation and this determines the bacteriocin type.

Both bacteriophage and bacteriocin typing of

important nosocomial pathogens are very useful epidemiologic tools. However, both procedures have major limiting factors (71, 72). Standardization of the procedure and reproducibility of results over time are two such factors. These are influenced by changes of bacterial genotype and phenotype, or by the transfer of plasmids. Another limiting factor is the availability of both virus phages and bacteriocins to accommodate the typing of all test organisms. Additionally, both procedures are time consuming and labor intensive and are, therefore, feasible only in research laboratories.

Plasmid analysis has been used as an epidemiological tool for "finger printing" bacterial isolates associated with nosocomial outbreaks. Plasmids are extrachromosomal DNA elements which may be transferred from one bacterial cell to another either through conjugation (self-transmissible) or transduction (nonself-transmissible). These plasmids contain useful genetic information which enables their bacterial host to adapt better to the environment. When these plasmids confer antibiotic resistance they are referred to as R plasmids or R factors. The size of plasmids carrying resistance information is widely variable (73) and has become the basis for the separation and identification of different plasmids by agarose gel electrophoresis (74). Bacterial cells are lysed, and the released DNA is specially treated and collected. The DNA collected then undergoes electrophoresis on agarose gel for approximately 2 hours. After this time the gel is stained in ethidium bromide, and the DNA is visualized under ultraviolet light.

Although this procedure is simple, somewhat inexpensive, and easily adaptable to the routine hospital laboratory, its role in the epidemiologic typing of nosocomial pathogens may not be as significant as hoped. R plasmids vary in their stability in growing cultures, and, therefore, the reproducibility of procedures is questionable. Furthermore, some plasmids are unable to migrate through the agarose gel, thus hampering their detection and identification. The most important drawback to the use of gel electrophoresis for plasmid analysis is that plasmids of similar molecular weights may have different DNA compositions which will go undetected (75). For this reason, restriction endonuclease analysis of plasmid DNA has been suggested. Restriction endonucleases are enzymes which make double-stranded breaks in DNA at specific sequences. The resultant fragments can be separated by elec-

trophoresis in agarose or polyacrylamide gels. Plasmids with the same electrophoretic pattern are considered identical or very similar. The sensitivity of this procedure is determined by the number of enzymes used and the number of electrophoretically distinct fragments of DNA produced. There are a limited number of commercially available endonucleases; and because of this, the technique may not be applicable for use in the routine laboratory.

Two newer procedures for determining the relatedness of microorganisms are flow cytometry and nucleic acid hybridization. In a recent report by Van Dilla and co-workers (76) the use of flow cytometry for the characterization of bacteria was described. This procedure utilizes fluorescent dyes which bind preferentially to DNA rich in guanine-cytosine and adenine-thymine. Fluorescence from the doubly stained bacteria is measured with a dual-beam fluorocytometer which provides information on the guanine-cytosine portion of total DNA content, cell concentration, and proliferation state of the population. Flow cytometry provides a sensitive and specific method for identification of bacteria in culture or clinical specimens, which may prove to be an extremely helpful epidemiologic tool.

Nucleic acid (DNA) hybridization is another helpful procedure for the detection and identification of microorganisms. Hybridization measures the degree of genetic relatedness of organisms by indirectly measuring the similarities of nucleotide sequences in different species. The first step involved is defining a portion of DNA that is unique to the organism under investigation. The DNA is released by the addition of enzymes and detergent and fixed to nitrocellulose filters. Similarly, DNA from an "indicator" organism is released and labeled with radioactive isotope (DNA probe). The DNA from the organisms is dissociated into single strands and combined. The degree of association between the two strands is directly dependent upon the sequences of complimentary nucleotides in the two strands. Detection is accomplished by autoradiography.

The majority of DNA probes described have been radiolabeled with β-^{32}P-labeled nucleotides. However, Langer and co-workers (77) described the use of biotin (formely designated as vitamin H) and avidin (a glycoprotein) as an alternative to the use of radiolabels. The biotin binds with the DNA probe which in turn binds the test DNA. The addition of the biotin does not significantly hinder the probe's binding ability. The next step is the addition of the avidin which has been fluorescently labeled. The avidin has a strong affinity for biotin and, therefore, will bind to the probe. Detection is accomplished utilizing ultraviolet light. The use of this type of system eliminates the use of biohazardous materials and the short shelf life of the reagent.

DNA hydridization has been used exclusively in the research setting for the detection of herpes simplex virus (78, 79), cytomegalovirus (80), hepatitis B virus (81), enterotoxigenic *E. coli* (82), and *Neisseria gonorrheae* (83). However, probes are commercially available for herpes simplex virus, cytomegalovirus, and *Chlamydia trachomatis*.

Although flow cytometry and DNA hybridization are not yet practical for use in the routine microbiology laboratory, these procedures have the potential for providing rapid, sensitive, and accurate epidemiologic finger-printing of significant pathogens with a degree of stability lacking in plasmid analysis.

In summary there are many techniques available to determine strain similarity in an outbreak of nosocomial infections. It is clear that no single technique is useful in all outbreaks of nosocomial infections. It is suggested that several techniques be used concurrently in the investigation of an outbreak to identify the responsible bacterial strain. If multiple typing methods are used for strain identification, related strains will be identified using several different techniques. In contradistinction, if unrelated strains are typed by more than one method, many different types will be identified. In an outbreak investigation (84), the strain should be identified by a single method, and subsequently several typing methods might be used to improve the accuracy and reproducibility of strain identification. The typing of a particular organism from a patient involved in an outbreak should only be done on a single clinical isolate per patient involving the offending strain of organism. It has been shown that there is no advantage to typing multiple strains from the same individual (85).

OUTBREAK INVESTIGATION
Culture Techniques
Respiratory Support Equipment

Cultures of the exhalation valve, spirometer, mouthpiece, or other surfaces may be obtained by swabbing with a cotton swab which was premoistened in brain heart infusion broth, followed by incubation (86).

Intravascular Monitoring Devices

Intravascular monitoring devices have been shown to be a cause of nosocomial infections (87). Cultures may be obtained by swabbing the transducer diaphragm with a cotton swab premoistened in brain heart infusion broth (88). Flush solution may be collected and inoculated directly into blood culture medium.

Intravenous Catheters

When a cluster of bacteremias caused by a specific organism is encountered, the epidemiologist may consider the intravenous fluid as a possible reservoir for infection. However, the first step in this type of investigation should involve culturing the catheter tip to determine whether this is the source of infection. Spread of infection from one patient to another due to poor hand washing techniques on the part of hospital personnel is a known factor, and breakdown in aseptic technique when starting an intravenous is a contributing cause of nosocomial bacteremia. Qualitative or semiquantitative procedures may be performed to determine the causative agent and the probable source of infection.

Qualitative cultures are performed by placing the catheter tip into a tube of nutrient broth followed by vigorous shaking. A portion of this broth is then inoculated onto a blood agar plate and into a tube of thioglycollate broth. The plate is incubated at 35°C in 5 to 10% CO_2 for 2 days and the thioglycollate broth at 35°C for 7 days (89).

A semiquantitative procedure (89, 90) is performed by rolling the catheter tip back and forth on a blood agar plate using sterile forceps, followed by incubation of the plate at 35°C in 5 to 10% CO_2 for 2 days. Guidelines are suggested regarding growth and its significance; the presence of 15 or more colonies/agar surface is considered significant catheter colonization, and fewer than 15 colonies/agar surface is considered negative or catheter contamination (90).

Intravenous Fluids

Intravenous fluids suspected of being contaminated may be cultured in a variety of ways. The fluid may be inoculated into two blood culture bottles (10 ml each) which are vented after inoculation. One bottle is incubated at 35°C, and the second is incubated at 22 to 25°C.

A semiquantitative procedure for estimating the level of intravenous fluid contamination is performed by withdrawing calibrated amounts (0.01 or 0.001 ml) of fluid and inoculating sets of nutrient agar or blood agar plates. One plate should be incubated at 35°C and the second at 22 to 25°C. The results are reported as the number of colonies per milliliter of fluid.

Other Solutions

Any fluids, medications, or additives administered to the patients during the 24 hours prior to onset of fever should also be retrieved and cultured as possible sources of contamination. Since there will be smaller volumes present, the entire portion of fluid remaining may be cultured by addition to an equal volume of brain heart infusion broth enriched with 0.5% beef extract and incubated at 35°C. Empty containers may be cultured by adding a small volume of broth and swirling the media in the container. Aseptic technique is important to avoid contamination.

Documentation is important in cases of suspected fluid contamination. The product's name, manufacturer, lot number, date and hour of preparation or administration, and listing of additive should be recorded, along with a description of the appearance of the fluid or container (91).

All Other Objects

A complete discussion of environmental sampling of objects which may be implicated in nosocomial infections may be found in Gradwohl's manual of methods (92).

Colonization versus Infection

One of the main problems in clinical infectious disease is to differentiate colonization from infection. The clinical microbiology laboratory may be of assistance by providing ancillary information, i.e., the presence of an inflammatory exudate that will permit the clinician to determine the role of the organism recovered. Recovery of an organism from a body site does not indicate pathogenicity and frequently indicates colonization. For example, bacteriuria without pyuria would suggest colonization rather than infection. A gram stain of the throat to determine the inflammatory response in the patient with pharyngitis due to infectious mononucleosis would show a paucity of polymorphonuclear neutrophils and indicate colonization rather than infection of group A streptococci grown from the patient's throat.

Unfortunately, exact knowledge of the relationship between colonization and infection is minimal. It is not well understood why in some patients known pathogens—e.g., *H. influenzae*, the meningococcus, and group A streptococci—are "colonizers" while in other patients they are clearly pathogenic. The carriage rate of these organisms varies according to the season and is maximal during the winter months. Other organisms, such as *Citrobacter*, are almost always "colonizers" and are only pathogenic under unusual circumstances. It is also generally known that colonization precedes infection as a general rule. However, in many situations an increase in colonization rates is not followed by an increase in infection rates. Colonization rates also vary according to an institution's biologic floras competing for a given niche. For example, if *Serratia* and *Pseudomonas* compete for the same environmental sites within the hospital, then an increase in *Pseudomonas* colonization would be accompanied by a decrease in *Serratia* colonization rates, and vice versa. What needs to be emphasized is that colonization is important in that it represents a potential reservoir for nosocomial pathogens and may herald a forthcoming outbreak (93–95).

Colonization of individuals with gram-negative or gram-positive organisms is normally transient. Colonization or "carriage" of an organism may be prolonged with the use of antibiotics. This is a well studied and understood phenomenon in treating patients with *Salmonella* and *Shigella* with certain antibiotics, e.g., ampicillin. Colonization is strongly associated with hospital stay as well as with the use of antibiotics. Antibiotics exert selective pressures on the patient's flora, thus selecting for potential colonizers and pathogens. Again, it is not just the volume of antibiotic usage that best correlates with colonization but rather specifically which antibiotics are being used within the institution. Furthermore, prolonged usage of antibiotics is another important factor in promoting colonization of the patient. Invasive devices, e.g., intravenous polyethylene catheters, may additionally provide a nidus for colonization of the organism within the patient (96, 97).

Colonization also is affected, in part, by the location of the patient in the hospital. Critically ill patients in intensive care units are more likely to be colonized then those on open wards. This is probably related to the fact that intensive care unit patients have impaired host defenses, usually have multiple invasive monitoring devices in place, and are those more likely to be on prolonged antibiotic therapy. Disruption of normal pharyngeal and bowel flora clearly promotes colonization. Some species of streptococci in the pharynx and *Bacteroides fragilis* in the colon are clearly present in a protective role with respect to preventing colonization by other organisms. Therefore every attempt should be made to maintain the protective value of the patient's normal flora in preventing colonization (Table 14.5) (98).

The oropharynx, gastrointestinal tract, and urinary tract are the most important reservoirs for most nosocomial colonizers. *Klebsiella*, *Enterobacter*, *Serratia*, and *Pseudomonas* species have been commonly associated with these three areas. *Citrobacter* colonization usually occurs in the gastrointestinal tract, and *Acinetobacter* may be transiently carried on the hands. Gram-positive organisms— i.e., group B streptococci, staphylococci, and JK diphtheroids—may colonize the hands of patients/medical personnel. Colonization of the lower gastrointestinal tract by *Candida* usually precedes colonization of the urine. Knowledge of the likely reservoir associated with nosocomial colonizers/pathogens is important to surveillance of the organisms as well as to control of outbreaks. The reservoirs for common nosocomial pathogens are illustrated in Table 14.6 (93, 96).

Since the process of colonization is poorly

Table 14.5. Factors Promoting Colonization with Hospital Pathogens

1. Duration of hospitalization
2. Prolonged antibiotic therapy
3. Location in hospital
4. Disruption of normal pharyngeal or bowel flora
5. Invasive devices

Table 14.6. Nosocomial Colonization of Individuals

Organism	Human Reservoir
Klebsiella	Pharynx, bowel, urine
Enterobacter	Bowel, urine
Serratia	Urine
Pseudomonas	Pharynx, bowel, urine
Citrobacter	Hands
Acinetobacter	Hands
Group B streptococcus	Vagina, hands
Staphylococcus/MRSA*	Nares, hands
JK diphtheroids	Nares, hands
Candida	Bowel, urine

* MRSA, methicillin-resistant *S. aureus.*

understood, colonization control measures are also not well understood. In spite of the best infection control efforts, colonization may continue without apparent reason. Although it is thought that infection control procedures minimize colonization, there are limited data in the literature in this regard (99, 100). Restoration of normal flora is important on a theoretical basis, but aside from discontinuing antimicrobial therapy, little can be done. Unusual increases in the carriage of certain organisms may be correlated with the use of particular antibiotics. If such an association is noted, then the restriction of the responsible antibiotics may be useful. Patients colonized with multiresistant organisms may require therapy with cefoperazone or amikacin to minimize spread of resistant organisms (101). Last, the most logical approach to colonization control relates to the recently appreciated and well described phenomenon of bacterial adherence. It has been well shown that pathogenic organisms unable to adhere to respiratory, gastrointestinal, or urogenital epithelial cells do not cause disease. A decrease in adherence may be accomplished with a variety of chemicals but is easily altered by the presence of a variety of antibiotics. Certain antibiotics actually promote infection by increasing the adherence between the bacterial cell and the host. In contradistinction, other antibiotics, e.g., tetracycline, may have the opposite effect in decreasing bacterial adherence. Limited data available suggest that adherence is important in the step between colonization and infection. Subinhibitory concentrations of antibiotic have been shown to increase the incidence of certain nosocomial infections. No good data exist with respect to the effect of specific antibiotic use as it influences adherence and colonization in a general hospital setting. Clearly, colonization control measures will probably depend upon the utilization of this principle. Furthermore, restoration of the normal flora by bacterial interference may be developed in the future. Avirulent strains of normal flora could be introduced at the appropriate body sites to displace all normal flora of colonizers/pathogens as a future control method (Table 14.7) (102, 103).

Antibiotic Resistance

Many factors are related to the development of antibiotic resistance in the community and in the hospital. Antibiotic resistance may be on the basis of one or more mechanisms. These have been well summarized in recent review articles (104–107). Chromosomal-mediated resistance, plas-

Table 14.7.   Potential Colonization Control Measures

1. Infection control procedures
2. Restoration of normal flora of the host
3. Decrease in adherence of pathogens to respiratory, gastrointestinal, and urogenital epithelial cells
4. Restriction of the use of antibiotics causing the increase in colonization
5. Use of antibiotics not associated with resistance problems and that do not readily disrupt the normal flora

mid-mediated resistance, and permeability-mediated resistance are the three forms of antibiotic resistance encountered in clinical practice. In terms of nosocomial infections, plasmid-mediated resistance is clearly the most common and important, but chromosomal resistance to certain antibiotics is also important. Permeability-mediated resistance has not been associated with widespread resistance problems to date (105).

Chromosome-mediated resistance is detected in the microbiology laboratory by noting a sudden change in the susceptibility pattern of (usually) one antibiotic to one or more organisms. Several antibiotics have been classically associated with one or more resistance patterns. Examples of chromosome-mediated resistance include the resistance of *Klebsiella* species to carbenicillin, of enterococci to streptomycin, of staphylococci to chloramphenicol, of gram-positive cocci and *Neisseria* to sulfonamides, of streptococci to the aminoglycosides, and of methicillin-resistant *S. aureus* to tetracyclines. Plasmid-mediated resistance may be detected by the infection control personnel or the microbiology laboratory by noting a gradual change in the susceptibility pattern of one or more antibiotics to multiple organisms (107).

There are many examples of plasmid-mediated resistance. Common examples include the association of *Enterobacter* resistance with cefamandole use, and *P. aeruginosa* resistance with gentamicin or tobramycin usage (108, 109). The resistance of the Enterobacteriaceae, in general, to first, second, and third generation cephalosporins has clearly been shown to be plasmid-mediated. Interestingly, R factor resistance has not been associated with cefoxitin or cefoperazone when used alone. Other organisms encountered less commonly, such as *Citrobacter*, *Providencia*, *Moraxella*, and *Acinetobacter*, have been shown to develop resistance to a wide variety of antibiotics, including cephalosporins and aminogly-

cosides, on a plasmid-mediated basis (110). Permeability-mediated resistance is characterized by a sudden or gradual change noted in the cross-resistance patterns of two antibiotics to a single organism. This type of resistance has been historically associated with the use of an aminoglycoside plus a β-lactam antibiotic in treating *Serratia* or *P. aeruginosa* infections (105) (Table 14.8). Tetracyclines have also been associated with both plasmid- and permeability-mediated resistance.

Factors which determine the type and extent of antibiotic-resistant patterns are incompletely understood. The largest pool of resistant organisms exists in nature in the livestock and poultry populations. Antibiotic-supplemented feeds are used in the United States. It has been shown that this huge animal reservoir makes its way into the human population and provides a chronic human reservoir of resistant organisms. Antibiotic resistance in animals and man has been related to the organisms being exposed to low concentrations of drug over long periods of time. This is the situation with the animal reservoir where small amounts of antibiotics are used as growth-promoting substances (111). It is a popular misconception that antibiotic use is the primary determinant of antibiotic resistance. The total volume of antibiotic use in an institution, i.e., "antibiotic tonnage," is only loosely related to the development of resistance. While it is true that a "large" hospital is more likely to have resistance problems than a "small" hospital, hospitals of similar size, in the same general geographical area, have very different resistance problems using approximately the same amount of "antimicrobial tonnage." A more important determinant of antibiotic resistance is related to the kinds of antibiotics used in a given institution rather than simply the volume of antibiotics used. The use of certain antibiotics has been associated with resistance problems even if they are used in low volume. The development of plasmid-mediated resistance has been frequently associated with ampicillin, the antipseudomonal penicillins (if used alone), and third generation cephalosporins (112). The widespread use of sulfonamides and conventional tetracyclines has also been associated with plasmid-mediated resistance problems. Widespread use of gentamicin and tobramycin has been associated with enzymatic inactivation of these antibiotics. Institutions with "resistance problems" should not only analyze total antibiotic use, but also look at the critically important factor—which antibiotics are being used. Another factor, which is not well understood, is the pro-

Table 14.8. Mechanisms and Recognition of Antibiotic Resistance Patterns

Resistance Mechanism	Resistance Pattern	Common Associations	
		Antibiotics	Microorganisms
Chromosomal resistance	Sudden change in susceptibility pattern by *one/more* organisms to *one* antibiotic	Carbenicillin Streptomycin Chloramphenicol Aminoglycosides Sulfonamides Tetracycline	*Klebsiella* Enterococci *Pseudomonas* Streptococci *Neisseria* Staphylococci Staphylococcus/ MRSA*
Plasmid resistance	Gradual change in susceptibility pattern of multiple organisms to one/ more antibiotics	Tetracycline Ampicillin 1st, 2nd, and 3rd generation cephalosporins	Enterobacteriaceae and *Acinetobacter* *Pseudomonas* *H. influenzae*
Permeability resistance	*Sudden/gradual* change in *cross-resistance* pattern of *one* organism to *two* antibiotics	Aminoglycoside + β-lactam Tetracycline Aminoglycosides	*Pseudomonas* *Serratia* Staphylococci Enterococci

* MRSA, methicillin-resistant *S. aureus.*

portion of antibiotics being used for prophylaxis versus therapy. Most prophylactic antibiotics in the hospital are used by the obstetrics, gynecology, and surgical services. If appropriate prophylaxis is used, i.e., a well timed single preoperative dose continued for no longer than 24 hours, then the likelihood of inducing resistant organisms in the patient's fecal flora is minimized. The likelihood of resistance increases with duration of therapy, particularly in association with the antibiotics mentioned above. Therefore, single dose or short term prophylactic regimens may have the benefit of minimizing resistance and thereby maintaining the usefulness of antibiotics in an institution. Although unusual, there are some reports in the literature of resistance developing even after short term prophylaxis (112, 113). As a general rule, monotherapy is preferred to combination therapy with respect to minimizing the development of resistance, with a few notable exceptions. It is well known that certain drugs should not be given alone because of the rapid development of plasmid-mediated resistance. Therefore, it has been common practice to combine trimethroprim with sulfonamides, as trimethoprim-sulfamethoxazole (TMP-SMX). Resistance to the trimethoprim component and the sulfonamide component are significant when used alone, but when used in combination, resistance is minimized. Similarly, antipseudomonal penicillins are combined with aminogly-

cosides, not only for extended spectrum and for antipseudomonal synergy, but importantly, to delay the development of plasmid-mediated resistance to the penicillin component. The antifungal/antimicrobial, 5-flucytocine (5-FC), is always used in conjunction with another antifungal/antimicrobial, e.g., amphotericin to minimize the development or resistance to 5-FC. Rifampin is another good example of a drug which should always be used in combination to minimize the development of resistance (104–105, 113). In contradistinction, certain drug combinations may be disadvantageous. Cefoxitin is a potent β-lactamase inducer, and this tendency is increased if another drug is added to a cefoxitin regimen, i.e., ampicillin/aminoglycoside. Therefore, resistance problems may be minimized if cefoxitin is used alone in prophylaxis and therapy (110). Interestingly, but very importantly, are the infection control practices of an institution. The presence of an infection control team with an active in-service education program cannot eliminate the problem of antibiotic resistance, but it can clearly minimize the nosocomial spread of resistant organisms (Table 14.9).

All third generation cephalosporins have been associated with resistance problems even when used in low volume (110, 113). Amikacin has been used in institutions where gentamicin/tobramycin resistance has been prevalent to "clean up" the aminoglycoside-resistant reservoir. This

Table 14.9.   Factors Influencing Antibiotic Resistance in the Hospital

1. Volume of antibiotic use—"antibiotic tonnage"
2. Excessive use of certain antibiotics:
   a. Sulfonamides
   b. Ampicillin
   c. Gentamicin/tobramycin
   d. Antipseudomonal penicillin (except mezlocillin)
   e. Tetracyclines (except doxycycline and minocycline)
   f. Third-generation cephalosporins
3. Proportion of prophylactic to therapeutic antibiotic usage
4. Proportion of monotherapy to combination therapy
5. Infection control procedures

has been well demonstrated in a variety of studies and has resulted in a return of sensitivity to gentamicin/tobramycin in institutions using amikacin as the primary aminoglycoside. Other institutions have utilized amikacin as the primary aminoglycoside in an attempt to keep the hospital environment free of resistant strains; this approach has been successful as well (114–117). Resistance to amikacin is usually on the basis of a permeability barrier and is infrequently on the basis of inactivating enzymes (105, 106).

The microbiology laboratory has an important role in infection control by its antibiotics surveillance, monitoring the effectiveness of the approach of the infectious disease/infection control team. It is important to appreciate that the laboratories utilizing semiautomated or automated rapid method susceptibility testing often yield falsely low resistance data. Therefore, the amount of antibiotic resistance in an institution may be underestimated, making identification of the problem and assessment of the control measures difficult (49, 118). Scrupulous infection control practices are the cornerstones limiting the spread of resistant organisms within the institution. During an outbreak, antibiotic use in general should be restricted (119). The restriction should be selective and involve only those antibiotics involved in the outbreak. The ultimate use of other antibiotics not associated with resistance problems should be encouraged, in general to prevent problems, and specifically to be used during an outbreak (Table 14.10) (104, 106, 112).

Pseudoepidemics

A pseudoepidemic may be defined as increased recovery of common/uncommon organisms by smear or culture from a body fluid/tissue that does not correlate clinically with disease usually associated with the organism. Since the late 1960s pseudoinfections and pseudo-outbreaks have been described in the literature. Pseudobacteremias remain the most frequent type of pseudoinfection described, followed by pseudopneumonias and pseudomeningitis (Tables 14.11 to 14.13). There have been sporadic reports of other pseudoinfections in various other body sites (Tables 14.14 and 14.15) (120, 121).

Pseudobacteremias are perhaps the most interesting type of pseudoepidemic (Table 14.11). A wide variety of organisms have been implicated, and a large number of patients have been infected in individual outbreaks. Of great interest are the number of patients who were infected as the result of the pseudobacteremia. In such situations, reflux of contaminated blood into the patient resulted in a small but important number of patients being actually infected in association with the pseudobacteremia. Between 1969 and 1984, 16 patients were infected as part of a related cluster of pseudobacteremias. Also of interest regarding the effect of the clinician's response to the laboratory data was the institution of unnecessary antimicrobial therapy based upon the laboratory report. With respect to pseudobacteremias from 1969 to 1984, inappropriate therapy was initiated in 67 patients. In most pseudoepidemics the recovery of an unusual organism suggests pseudoinfection. Therefore, the greatest diagnostic confusion occurs when known pathogens are recovered as the organism responsible for the pseudoepidemic, e.g., *E. coli*, *S. aureus*, *Klebsiella*, and *Pseudomonas* sp. In such cases, antimicrobial therapy was initiated in a high percentage of these pseudobacteremias. Pseudobacteremias have most frequently been associated

Table 14.10.   Resistance Control Measures

1. Optimize infection control practices.
2. Restrict antibiotics associated with resistance problem—microbiology laboratory to determine mechanism of resistance.
3. Encourage use of certain antibiotics that are not associated with resistance problems.
   a. Doxycycline/minocycline
   b. Amoxicillin/bacampicillin
   c. Trimethoprim-sulfamethoxazole
   d. Amodocillin
   e. Nitrofurantoin
   f. Vancomycin
   g. Amikacin
   h. Imipenem

with contaminated blood culture collecting or processing systems. Occasionally contaminated disinfectant solutions have been implicated, and most recently contaminated automated blood culture analyzers have been implicated in a variety of pseudobacteremias (122–148).

Pseudopneumonias have been reported from 1973 to the present time and have involved 10 separate reports of pseudoinfection involving the lungs. Although it is difficult to obtain accurate figures, at least one patient was infected by a contaminated fiberoptic bronchoscope. Considering the frequency of contaminated anesthetic solutions and fiberoptic bronchoscopes, it is remarkable that only one patient was actually infected as a result of being instrumented by contaminated fluids/instruments. In contrast to pseudobacteremias, pseudopneumonias are infrequently reported to have resulted in inappropriate antimicrobial therapy. and only two such cases could be found in the literature (Table 14.12) (148–158).

Pseudomeningitis continues to be an infrequent but serious problem. Although a smaller number of patients have been affected when compared to pseudopneumonias or pseudobacteremias, the number of patients actually begun on inappropriate antimicrobial therapy is proportionally higher than for any other form of suprainfection. A review of the literature indicates that 14 of 27 patients were begun on empiric therapy based on false positive gram stain or false positive culture results of cerebrospinal fluid. Pseudomeningitis is most frequently associated with contaminated specimen tubes or transport media (Table 14.13) (159–164).

Pseudoendocarditis was initially described in 1976, and the largest outbreak was reported by Aber in 1980. In that report three patients were affected, and inappropriate therapy was started on one patient. Interestingly, nonviable gram-positive cocci were present in contaminated broth used to macerate a tissue specimen obtained during open heart surgery. Endocarditis was assumed since gram-positive cocci are the most frequent cause of infections following open heart surgery, and therefore antibiotic therapy was begun (Table 14.14) (127, 165). Various other pseudoepidemics have been described since the mid-1970s. Pseudohepatitis, pseudoadenitis, pseudobacteriuria, and pseudowound infections have all been described. They are infrequent occurrences, but are noteworthy and suggest that more and varied pseudoinfections will continue to occur in the future. The hyperendemic incidence of the pathogen or the isolation of an unusual organism that does not correlate well with the clinical setting suggests this problem. No patients were infected in this group of pseudoinfections, and inappropriate therapy was started in three patients. Various mechanisms for the pseudoepidemics are described in Table 14.15 (127, 159, 162, 163, 166–168).

Microbiologic Approach to Pseudoepidemics

Recognition that there is a problem is fundamental in analyzing and solving the problem with respect to pseudoepidemics. Infection control personnel and laboratory personnel must be alert to unusual increases in the recovery of any microorganism from a certain body site or location in the hospital. The recovery of unusual organisms in greater than expected frequency should also alert everyone concerned that the possibility of an outbreak or pseudoepidemic exists. Methods for outbreak investigation have been well described, but the approach to pseudoepidemics has not been described to date. Therefore, guidelines are provided in Tables 14.16 and 14.17 (12, 120, 121). After it has been determined that an outbreak is not real and represents a pseudoepidemic, then efforts should be made to determine the source of the pseudoepidemic by culturing individuals or objects in the environment associated with the pseudo-outbreak.

In the laboratory investigation of a pseudobacteremia, the environment provides the most likely source for blood culture contamination. Therefore, the culture of any materials related to skin preparation, blood culture collection, or processing should be carefully performed and analyzed. If an automated blood culture analyzer is used, then the machine needs to be checked for adequate needle sterilization and contamination of the needle by spores or debris. Culture of laboratory and medical personnel is not warranted unless *S. aureus* is the organism responsible for the bacteremia.

Guidelines for pseudomeningitis, pseudoendocarditis, and pseudopneumonia investigations are provided in Table 14.17. Once again, culture of laboratory personnel is usually unrewarding and therefore unnecessary. Only rarely in the case of pseudopneumonias have laboratory personnel been incriminated in the outbreak.

In summary, the microbiology laboratory and infection control personnel must constantly be on alert for the possibility of pseudoinfections. Outbreaks are more common and more easily

Table 14.11. Pseudobacteremia

Author (Year)	Reference	Organisms	Patients Affected	Patients Infected	Therapy Affected	Problem
Norden (1969)	122	Escherichia coli	7	0	7	Contaminated penicillinase in blood culture media
Faris and Sparling (1972)	123	Acinetobacter lwoffi	27	3	4	Contaminated penicillinase in blood culture media
DuClos et al (1973)	124	Moraxella nonliquefaciens	8	1	1	Contaminated blood tube holders of blood culture tubes
Noble and Reeves (1974)	125	Bacillus sp.	26	0	0	Contaminated blood culture media
Kaslow et al (1976)	126	Pseudomonas cepacia	79	3	4	Contaminated benzalkonium chloride used for venipuncture
Coyle-Gilchrist et al (1976)	127	Flavobacterium meningosepticum	6	0	0	Contaminated chlorhexidine solution used for venipuncture
Hoffman et al (1976)	128	Serratia marcescens	40	0	0	Cross-contamination of blood cultures with bacteria from nonsterile blood collection tubes
Snydman et al (1977)	129	Acinetobacter lwoffi	11	0	2	Improper blood culture technique in a mist tent heavily contaminated with bacteria
Semel et al (1978)	130	Pseudomonas maltophilia	25	1	3	Cross-contamination of blood cultures with bacteria from nonsterile blood collection tubes
CDC et al (1979)	131	Staphylococcus aureus	11	0	5	Blood cultures contaminated by a colonized (nasopharynx) laboratory technician
Lynch et al (1980)	132	Clostridium sordellii	11	0	0	Contaminated thimerosal solution/diaphragms of blood culture media
Jones et al (1980)	133	Acinetobacter lwoffi	22	0	0	Blood cultures contaminated by humidified incubator
Spivack et al (1980)	134	Staphylococcus aureus	5	0	0	Blood culture media contaminated by physician
CDC et al (1980)	135	Aerococcus viridans	7	0	0	Inadequately disinfected blood culture bottle stoppers

Reference	No.	Organism				Source
Berkelman et al (1981)	138	*Pseudomonas cepacia*	30	0	0	Contaminated povidone-iodine solution used for venipuncture/disinfect blood culture bottle stoppers
Graham et al (1981)	137	*Enterobacter cloacae*	7	0	1	Contaminated thrombin in blood culture collection vials
Greenhood et al (1982)	139	*Klebsiella pneumoniae*	13	7*	6	Contaminated sampling needle in automated blood culture analyzer
Griffin et al (1982)	140	*Klebsiella pneumoniae* *Streptococcus pyogenes* *Staphylococcus epidermidis*	2 1 1	0	1	Inadequate needle sterilization in automated blood culture analyzer
MacDonald (1982)	141	*Bacillus* sp.	36	0	0	Contaminated syringes
Berger (1983)	142	*Bacillus* sp.	15	0	0	Contaminated cotton swabs used to disinfect blood culture bottles in automated blood culture analyzer
Keys et al (1983)	143	*Pseudomonas stutzeri*	24	1	21	Contaminated green soap solution
Whiteside et al (1983)	144	*Streptococcus faecalis* (Enterococcus)	8	0	2	Cross-contamination in automated blood culture analyzer
Crowley et al (1983)	145	*Bacillus* sp.	15	0	0	Contaminated brain-heart infusion broth
Craven et al (1984)	146	*Staphylococcus aureus* *Staphylococcus epidermidis* *Streptococcus* sp. *Escherichia coli*	11 10 1 1	0	3	Inadequate needle sterilization in automated blood culture analyzer
Donowitz and Schwartman (1984)	147	*Streptococcus bovis*	1	0	1	Inadequate cleaning of needle in automated blood culture analyzer
Gurevich et al (1984)	148	*Bacillus* sp.	26	0	1	Spore contamination of needle in automated blood culture analyzer

* Possibly infected by authors' criteria.

Table 14.12. Pseudopneumonia

Author (Year)	Reference	Organisms	Patients Affected	Patients Infected	Therapy Affected	Problem
Schaffner et al (1973)	149	*Pseudomonas cepacia*	22	0	0	Contamination of topical anesthetic used during fiberoptic bronchoscopy
Gangadarma et al (1976)	150	*Mycobacterium gordonae*	7	0	0	Sputum contaminated tap water from patients rinsing their mouths prior to specimen collection
Surratt et al (1977)	151	*Pseudomonas aeruginosa*	103	0	0	Contaminated fiberbronchoscope
Kellerhals (1978)	152	*Serratia marcescens*	8	1	0	Contaminated fiberbronchoscope
Steere et al (1979)	153	*Mycobacterium gordonae*	52	0	1	Bronchoscopy specimens contaminated with topical anesthetic dye
Schleupner and Hamilton (1980)	154	*Penicillium/Trichosporon* sp.	8	0	0	Contamination of bronchial washings with topical anesthetic (cocaine)
Nunez et al (1982)	155	*Coccidioides immitis*	7	0	0	Spore contaminated slides
Schanbacher et al (1983)	156	*Mycobacterium gordonae* *Mycobacterium avium*	>100	0	0	Bronchoscope contaminated by water/glutaraldehyde
Vogel and Neu (1983)	157	*Penicillium* sp.	21	0	0	Contaminated bronchscopy biopsy forceps
Goodman et al (1984)	158	*Mycobacterium marinum*	5	0	1	Specimens contaminated by laboratory personnel

Table 14.13. Pseudomeningitis

Author (Year)	Reference	Organisms	Patients Affected	Patients Infected	Therapy Affected	Problem
Musher and Schell (1973)	159	Gram-negative cocci	4	0	0	Contaminated glass specimen tubes
Weinstein et al (1975)	160	Gram-negative bacilli Gram-positive cocci	5	0	1	Contaminated specimen tubes in dispensary LP tray
Coyle-Gilchrist et al (1976)	127	*Flavobacterium meningosepticum*	1	1	1	Contaminated soap solution used for skin preparation
Ericsson et al (1978)	161	Gram-negative bacilli	11	0	8	Contamination of alcohol bottle/slides
Hoke et al (1979)	162	Gram-negative bacilli	2	0	2	Contaminated transport media
CDC et al (1983)	163	Gram-negative bacilli	1	0	1	Contaminated transport media
Harris et al (1983)	164	*Salmonella typhimurium*	3	0	1	Contaminated pipette bulb

Table 14.14. Pseudoendocarditis

Author (Year)	Reference	Organisms	Patients Affected	Patients Infected	Therapy Affected	Problem
Coyle-Gilchrist et al (1976)	127	*Flavobacterium meningosepticum*	1	0	0	Contaminated soap solution used for skin prep in placement of intracardiac catheter
Aber and Appelbaum (1983)	165	Gram-positive cocci	3	0	1	Broth contamination with nonviable gram-positive cocci

Table 14.15. Pseudoepidemics

Author (Year)	Reference	Organisms	Patients Affected	Patients Infected	Therapy Affected	Problem
PSEUDOHEPATITIS Weinstein et al (1975)	160	Acid-fast bacilli	2	0	0	Acid-fast bacilli specimen contaminated by laboratory personnel
Laxon et al (1981)	167	Hepatitis B virus	7	0	0	Contamination of automated pipette diluter
PSEUDOADENITIS Goodman et al (1984)	158	Mycobacterium marinum	2	0	0	Acid-fast bacilli culture contaminated by laboratory technician
PSEUDOBACTERIURIA John and Twitty (1982)	168	Pseudomonas cepacia	44	0	0	Contaminated disinfectant solution
PSEUDO-WOUND INFECTION Coyle-Gilchrist et al (1976)	127	Flavobacterium meningosepticum	3	0	0	Contaminated soap solution used for skin prep
CDC et al (1978)	163	Gram-negative bacilli	4	0	1	Contaminated transport media
Hoke et al (1979)	162	Gram-negative bacilli	2	0	2	Contaminated transport media

Table 14.16. Pseudobacteremia

Environment
1. Culture antibiotic neutralization materials, and anticoagulants used in blood culture bottles.
2. Culture blood culture bottle stoppers, diaphragms, and caps.
3. Smear/culture the blood culture media for intrinsic viable/nonviable bacterial contamination. Culture after venting blood culture bottles.
4. Culture all disinfectant solutions used on blood culture bottles, or on skin in preparation for venipuncture. Check to verify there is no cross-contamination of blood culture tubes/bottles from nonsterile items.
5. If using an automated blood culture analyzer, check needle for gross debris contamination, and for adequate needle temperature of sterilization. Check for "spore-laden" dust contamination of inside of analyzer.

Personnel
Culture laboratory/medical personnel involved in outbreak only if organism is *S. aureus.*

Table 14.17. Guidelines for Investigation of Pseudo-outbreaks

PSEUDOMENINGITIS
Environment
Compare smear/culture results of tubes, pipettes, glass slides, and water used in processing cerebrospinal fluid.
Personnel
No need to culture laboratory personnel processing specimens.
PSEUDOENDOCARDITIS
Environment
Culture any material added to cardiac biopsy/tissue specimen by microbiology laboratory/pathology laboratory.
Personnel
No need to culture laboratory personnel processing specimens.
PSEUDOPNEUMONIA
Environment
Culture all disinfectant, anesthetic, dye solutions, associated with bronchoscopy procedure.
Culture bronchoscope/biopsy forceps for inadequate disinfectant procedures/postdisinfectant contamination.
Personnel
Culture laboratory personnel processing specimens, only if all other investigations are negative.

recognized, but pseudoepidemics are important because they have been related to true infection, to inappropriate antimicrobial therapy in some, and to prolonged hospitalization in many patients. Furthermore, pseudo-outbreaks provide a better understanding of potential shortcomings of much of the equipment used in clinical medicine. Early recognition and termination of a pseudoepidemic are important not only for the patient but also to the institution in terms of expense. Thousands of dollars and countless hours of investigations are expended on an outbreak. The information provided in Tables 14.11 to 14.17 should provide the necessary background for an accurate and efficient approach to commonly encountered pseudoepidemics.

References

1. Mallison GF: Monitoring of sterility and environmental sampling in programs for the control of nosocomial infections. In Cundy KR, Ball W (eds): *Infection Control in Health Care Facilities: Microbiological Surveillance.* Baltimore, University Park Press, 1977, pp 23–31.
2. American Hospital Association, Committee on Infections within Hospitals: Statement on microbiologic sampling in the hospital. *Hospitals* 48:125–126, 1974.
3. Joint Commission on Accreditation of Hospitals: *Infection Control—Standards Adopted by Board of Commissioners.* Chicago, Joint Commission on Accreditation of Hospitals, December, 1975.
4. Simmons BP: Centers for Disease Control guidelines for hospital environmental control—microbiologic surveillance of the environment and of personnel in the hospital. *Infect Control* 2:145–146, 1981.
5. Branson D: In Balows A (ed): *Methods in Clinical Bacteriology: A Manual of Tests and Procedures,* Springfield, IL, Charles C Thomas, 1972, pp 93–94.
6. McGuckin MB, Kaplan L: The central service department. In Gurevich I, Tafuro P, Cunha BA (eds): *The Theory & Practice of Infection Control.* New York, Praeger, 1984, pp 117–129.
7. Goldmann DA: Laboratory procedures for infection control. In Lennette EH, Balows A, Hausler, WJ Jr., Truant JP (eds): *Manual of Clinical Microbiology,* ed 3. Washington, DC, American Society for Microbiology, 1980, pp 939–951.
8. Gurevich I, Holmes JE, Cunha BA: Presumed autoclave failure due to false-positive spore strip tests. *Infect Control* 3:388–392, 1982.
9. Favero MS, Peterson NJ: Microbiologic guidelines for hemodialysis systems. *Dialysis Transplant* 6:34–36, 1977.
10. Bartlett RC, Bennett JV, Weinstein RA, Mallison GF: The microbiology laboratory: its role in surveillance, investigation and control. In Bennett JV, Brachman PS (eds): *Hospital Infections.* Boston, Little, Brown, and Co., 1979, p 147.

11. Centers for Disease Control: The role of the microbiology laboratory in surveillance and control of nosocomial infections. *National Nosocomial Infections Study Report, Annual Summary, 1974.* Atlanta, Centers for Disease Control, 1977, p 27.

12. Dixon RE: Investigation of endemic and epidemic infections. In Bennett JV, Brachman PA (eds): *Hospital Infections.* Boston, Little, Brown, and Co., 1979, p 63.

13. MacGregor RB, Beaty HN: Evaluation of positive blood cultures: guidelines for early differentiation of contamination from valid positive cultures. *Arch Intern Med* 130:84–87, 1972.

14. Tafuro P, Ristuccia P: Recognition and control of outbreaks of nosocomial infections in the intensive care setting. *Heart Lung* 13:486–494, 1984.

15. Gurevich I: Appropriate collection of specimens for culture and sensitivity. *Am J Infect Control* 8:113–119, 1980.

16. Bartlett RC: *Medical Microbiology.* New York, John Wiley & Sons, 1974.

17. Tafuro P, Ristuccia P: Recognition and control of outbreaks of nosocomial infections in the intensive care setting. *Heart Lung* 13:486–94, 1984.

18. Neu HC: Unusual nosocomial infections. *DM* 30:3–68, 1984.

19. Stamm WE, Weinstein RA, Dixon RE: Comparison of endemic and epidemic nosocomial infections. *Am J Med* 70:393–397, 1981.

20. McGowan JE: The role of the laboratory in control of nosocomial infection. *Infect Control* 5:144–148, 1984.

21. Bauer AW, Kirby WMM, Sherris JC, Turck M: Antibiotic susceptibility testing by a standardized single disc method. *Am J Clin Pathol* 45:493–496, 1966.

22. Federal Register: Rules and regulations: antibiotic susceptibility disks. *Fed Regist* 37:20525–20529, 1972.

23. National Committee for Clinical Laboratory Standards: Performance standards for antimicrobic disk susceptibility tests. In *Approved Standards ASM-2,* ed 2. Villanova, PA., National Committee for Clinical Laboratory Standards, 1979.

24. Brown D, Blowers R: Disc methods of sensitivity testing and other semiquantitative methods. In Reeves DS, Phillips I, Williams JD, Wise R (eds): *Laboratory Methods in Antimicrobial Chemotherapy.* New York, Churchill Livingstone, 1978, pp 8–30.

25. Mackowiak PA: Direct effects of hyperthermia on pathogenic microorganisms: teleologic implications with regard to fever. *Rev Infect Dis* 3:508–520, 1981.

26. Mackowiak PA, Rudeman AE, Martin RM, Many WJ, Smith JW, Luby JP: Effects of physiologic variations in temperature on the rate of antibiotic-induced bacterial killing. *Am J Clin Pathol* 76:57–62, 1981.

27. Mackowiak PA, Marling-Cason U, Cohen RL: Effects of temperature on antimicrobial susceptibility of bacteria. *J Infect Dis* 145:550–553, 1982.

28. Annear DI: The effect of temperature on resistance of *Staphylococcus aureus* to methicillin and some other antibiotics. *Med J Aust* 1:444–446, 1968.

29. Thornsberry C: Methicillin-resistant (heteroresistant) staphylococci. *Antimicrob Newslett* 1:43–47, 1984.

30. Reller LB, Schoenknecht FD, Kenny MA, Sherris JC: Antibiotic susceptibility testing of *Pseudomonas aeruginosa*: selection of control strain and criteria for magnesium and calcium content in media. *J Infect Dis* 130:454–463, 1974.

31. D'Amato RF, Thornsberry C, Baker CN, Kirven LA: Effect of calcium and magnesium ions on the susceptibility of *Pseudomonas* species to tetracycline, gentamicin, polymyxin B and carbenicillin. *Antimicrob Agents Chemother* 7:596–600, 1975.

32. Pollock HM, Minshew BH, Kenny MA, Schoenknecht FD: Effect of different lots of Mueller-Hinton agar on the interpretation of the gentamicin susceptibility of *Pseudomonas aeruginosa*. *Antimicrob Agents Chemother* 14:360–367, 1978.

33. Washington JA, Snyder RJ, Kohner PC, Wiltse GG, Ilstrup DM, McCall JT: Effect of cation content of agar on the activity of gentamicin, tobramycin and amikacin against *Pseudomonas aeruginosa*. *J Infect Dis* 137:103–111, 1978.

34. Thornsberry C, Gavan TL, Gerlach EH: New developments in antimicrobial agent susceptibility testing. In Sherris JC (ed): *Cumitech 6.* Washington, DC, American Society for Microbiology, 1977.

35. Jones RN: The status of the art: a look at the past, present and antimicrobial susceptibility testing trends as monitored by the College of American Pathologists Laboratory Proficiency Survey. 1979 Aspen Conference. Skokie, IL, College of American Pathologists, 1981.

36. Sanders CC: Failure to detect resistance in antimicrobial susceptibility tests. *Antimicrob Newslett* 1:27–31, 1984.

37. Thiemke WA, Nathan DM: Simultaneous nosocomial outbreaks caused by multiply resistant *Klebsiella pneumoniae* types 2 and 30. *J Clin Microbiol* 8:769–771, 1978.

38. Thornsberry C, Gavan TL, Sherris JC, Balows A, Matsen JM, Sabath LD, Schoenknecht F, Thrupp LD, Washington JA: Laboratory evaluation of a rapid, automated susceptibility testing system: report of a collaborative study. *Antimicrob Agents Chemother* 7:466–480, 1975.

39. Kelly MT, Latimer JM, Balfour LC: Comparison of three automated systems for antimicrobial susceptibility testing of gram-negative bacilli. *J Clin Microbiol* 15:902–905, 1982.

40. Thornsberry C, Anhalt JP, Washington JA, McCarthy LR, Schoenknecht FD, Sherris JC, Spencer JH: Clinical laboratory evaluation of the Abbott MS-2 automated antimicrobial susceptibility testing system: report of a collaborative study. *J Clin Microbiol* 12:375–390, 1980.

41. Isenberg HD, D'Amato RF, McKinley GA, Hochstein L, Sampson-Scherer J: Collaborative evaluation of the UniScept quantitative antimicrobial susceptibility test. *J Clin Microbiol* 19:733–735, 1984.

42. Sherris JC, Ryan KJ: Evaluation of automated and rapid methods. In Tilton RC (ed): *Rapid Methods and Automation in Microbiology—1981.* Washington, DC, American Society for Microbi-

ology, 1982, p 1.

43. Boyce JM, White RL, Bonner MC, Lockwood WR: Reliability of the MS-2 system in detecting methicillin-resistant *Staphylococcus aureus. J Clin Microbiol* 15:220–225, 1982.

44. Cleary TJ, Maurer D: Methicillin-resistant *Staphylococcus aureus* susceptibility testing by an automated system, Autobac 1. *Antimicrob Agents Chemother* 13:837–841, 1978.

45. Mayo JB, Kiehn TE, Wong B, Bernard EM, Armstrong D: Examination of *Pseudomonas aeruginosa*-gentamicin discrepancies encountered in an Autobac 1-disc diffusion comparison. *Antimicrob Agents Chemother* 21:312–415, 1982.

46. Hanson SL, Freedy PK: Concurrent comparability of automated systems and commercially prepared microdilution trays for susceptibility testing. *J Clin Microbiol* 17:878–886, 1983.

47. Tilton RC, Isenberg HD: Evaluation of the performance parameters of a prediluted quantitative antibiotic susceptibility test device. *Antimicrob Agents Chemother* 11:271–276, 1977.

48. Lorian V: Effects of subminimum inhibitory concentrations of antibiotics on bacteria. In Lorian V (ed): *Antibiotics in Laboratory Medicine.* Baltimore, Williams & Wilkins, 1980, p 342.

49. Stone LL, Junkind DL: False-susceptible results from the MS-2 system used for testing resistant *Pseudomonas aeruginosa* against two third-generation cephalosporins, moxalactam and cefotaxime. *J Clin Microbiol* 18:389–394, 1983.

50. Schoenknecht FD, Sherris JC: Recent trends in antimicrobial susceptibility testing. *Lab Med* 11:824–832, 1980.

51. Butler DA, Lobregat CM, Gavan TL: Reproducibility of the Analytab (API 20E) system. *J Clin Microbiol* 2:322–326, 1975.

52. Sneath PHA, Johnson R: The influence on numerical taxonomic similarities of errors in microbiological tests. *J Gen Microbiol* 72:377–392, 1972.

53. Barry AL, Gavan TL, Smith PB, Matsen JM, Morello JA, Sielaff BH: Accuracy and precision of the Autobac system for rapid identification of gram-negative bacilli: a collaborative evaluation. *J Clin Microbiol* 15:1111–1119, 1982.

54. Edward PR, Ewing WH: *Identification of Enterobacteriaceae,* ed 4. Minneapolis, Burgess, 1972.

55. Finegold SM, Martin WJ (eds): *Diagnostic Microbiology,* ed 6. St Louis, CV Mosby, 1982, p 560.

56. Olcen P, Danielsson D, Kjellander J: The use of protein A-containing staphylococci sensitized with anti-meningococcal antibodies for grouping *Niesseria meningitidis* and demonstration of meningococcal antigen in cerebrospinal fluid. *Acta Pathol Microbiol Scand (B)* 83:387–396, 1975.

57. Feldman WE: Relation of concentrations of bacteria and bacterial antigen in cerebrospinal fluid to prognosis in patients with bacterial meningitis. *N Engl J Med* 296:433–435, 1977.

58. Finch CA, Wilkinson HW: Practical considerations in using counterimmunoelectrophoresis to identify the principle causative agents of bacterial meningitis. *J Clin Microbiol* 10:519–524, 1979.

59. Kohler G, Milstein C: Continuous cultures of fused cells secreting antibody of predefined specificity. *Nature* 256:495–497, 1975.

60. Blann AD: Cell hybrids: an important new source of antibody production. *Clin Lab Sci* 36:329–338, 1979.

61. Kennett RH: Monoclonal antibodies. Hybrid myelomas—a revolution in serology and immunogenics. *Am J Hum Genet* 31:539–547, 1979.

62. Goding JW: Antibody production by hybridomas. *J Immunol Methods* 39:285–308, 1980.

63. Milstein C: Monoclonal antibodies. *Sci Am* 243:66–74, 1980.

64. Fike DJ: Hybridomas: their role in the clinical and research laboratories. *Am J Med Technol* 47:891–896, 1981.

65. Koprowski H: Monoclonal hybridoma antibodies in the diagnosis of rabies. In Nakamura RM, Dito WR, Tucker ES, (eds): *Immunologic Analysis: Recent Progress in Diagnostic Laboratory Immunology.* New York, Masson, 1982, pp 87–90.

66. Bibb WF, Arnow PM, Thacker L, McKinney RM: Detection of soluble *Legionella pneumophila* antigens in serum and urine specimens by enzyme-linked immunosorbent assay with monoclonal and polyclonal antibodies. *J Clin Microbiol* 20:478–472, 1984.

67. Norgard MV, Selland CK, Kettman JR, Miller JN: Sensitivity and specificity of monoclonal antibodies directed against antigenic determinants of *Treponema pallidum* nichols in the diagnosis of syphilis. *J Clin Microbiol* 20:711–717, 1984.

68. Lyerly DM, Phelps CJ, Wilkins TD: Monoclonal and specific polyclonal antibodies for immunoassay of *Clostridium difficile* toxin A. *J Clin Microbiol* 21:12–14, 1985.

69. Brown SL, Bibb WF, McKinney RM: Use of monoclonal antibody in an epidemiologic marker system: a retrospective study of lung specimens from the 1976 outbreak of Legionnaires' disease in Philadelphia by indirect fluorescent antibody and enzyme linked immunosorbent assay methods. *J Clin Microbiol* 21:15–19, 1985.

70. Anderson ES, Williams REO: Bacteriophage typing of enteric pathogens and staphylococci and its use in epidemiology. *J Clin Pathol* 9:94–127, 1956.

71. Aber RC, Mackel DC: Epidemiologic typing of nosocomial microorganisms. *Am J Med* 70:899–905, 1981.

72. Smith PB: Bacteriophage typing. In Hoeprich PD (ed): *Infectious Diseases,* ed 2. New York, Harper & Row, 1977, p 118.

73. Bryan LE: Genetics of resistance to antimicrobial agents. In *Bacterial Resistance and Susceptibility to Chemotherapeutic Agents.* New York, Cambridge University Press, 1982, p 104.

74. Meyers J, Sanchez D, Elwell LP, Falkow S: A simple agarose gel electrophoretic method for the identification and characterization of plasmid deoxyribonucleic acid. *J Bacteriol* 127:1529–1537, 1976.

75. Goldmann DA, Macone AB: A microbiologic approach to the investigation of bacterial nosocomial infection outbreaks. *Infect Control* 1:391–400, 1980.

76. Van Dilla MA, Langlois RG, Pinkel D, Yajko D,

Hadley WK: Bacterial characterization by flow cytometry. *Science* 220:620–622, 1983.

77. Langer PR, Waldrop AA, Ward DC: Enzymatic synthesis of biotin labelled polynucleotides: novel nucleic acid affinity probes. *Proc Natl Acad Sci USA* 70:6633–6637, 1981.

78. Brautigan AR, Richman DD, Oxman MN: Rapid typing of herpes simplex virus isolates by deoxyribonucleic acid, deoxyribonucleic acid hybridization. *J Clin Microbiol* 12:226–234, 1980.

79. Stalhandske P, Petterson U: Identification of DNA viruses by membrane filter hybridization. *J Clin Microbiol* 15:744–747, 1982.

80. Chou S, Merigan TC: Rapid detection and quantitation of cytomegalovirus in clinical urine via DNA hybridization. *N Engl J Med* 308:921–925, 1983.

81. Berninger M, Hammer M, Hoyer B, Gerin JL: An assay for the detection of the DNA genome of hepatitis B virus in serum. *J Med Virol* 9:57–68, 1982.

82. Echeverria P, Leksomboon U, Chaicumpa W, Seriwatana J, Tirapat C, Rowe B: Identification by DNA hybridization of enterotoxigenic *Escherichia coli* in homes of children with diarrhea. *Lancet* 1:63–66, 1984.

83. Totten PA, Holmes KK, Handsfield HH, Knapp JS, Perine PL, Falkow S: DNA hybridization technique for the detection of *Neisseria gonorrhoeae* in men with urethritis. *J Infect Dis* 148:462–471, 1983.

84. Rubin SJ: *Klebsiella* marker systems. *Infect Control* 6:59–63, 1985.

85. Bennett WP, O'Connor ML. Wasilauskas BL: A comparison of antibiotic susceptibility profiles using single and multiple isolates per patient. *Infect Control* 6:157–160, 1985.

86. Keys TF: Optimal use of the laboratory for infection control. In Wenzel RP (ed): *Handbook of Hospital Acquired Infections*. Boca Raton, FL, CRC Press, 1981, p 91.

87. Donowitz LG, Marsik FJ, Hoyt JW, Wenzel RP: *Serratia marcescens* bacteremia from contaminated pressure transducers. *JAMA* 242:1749–1751, 1979.

88. Centers for Disease Control: *National Nosocomial Infections Study Report, The Infectious Hazards of Pressure Monitoring Devices*. US Department of Health, Education, and Welfare, Annual Summary 1974, March 1977.

89. Washington JA: Initial processing for cultures of specimens. In Washington JA (ed): *Laboratory Procedures in Clinical Microbiology*. New York, Springer-Verlag, 1981, p 91.

90. Maki DG, Weise CE, Sarafin HU: A semiquantitative culture method for identifying intravenous catheter-related infection. *N Engl J Med* 296:1305–1309, 1977.

91. National Coordinating Committee on Large Volume Parenterals: Recommended procedures for in-use testing of large volume parenterals suspected of contamination or of producing a reaction in a patient. *Am J Hosp Pharm* 35:678–682, 1978.

92. Weissfeld AS: Nosocomial infections and hospital epidemiology. In Sonnenwirth AC, Jarett L (eds): *Gradwohl's Clinical Laboratory Methods and Diagnosis*, ed 8. St Louis, CV Mosby, 1980, p 1971.

93. Hawkey PM, Penner JL, Potten MR, Stephens M, Barton LJ, Speller DC: Prospective survey of fecal, urinary tract, and environmental colonization by *Providencia stuartii* in two geriatric wards. *J Clin Microbiol* 16:422–426, 1982.

94. Goldmann DA: Bacterial colonization and infection in the neonate. *Am J Med* 70:417–422, 1981.

95. Tafuro P, Cunha BA: Hospital-acquired pneumonias: current concepts on prevention and control. *Asepsis* 3:2–4, 1981.

96. Maki DG: Control of colonization and transmission of pathogenic bacteria in the hospital. *Ann Intern Med* 89:777–780, 1978.

97. Sprunt K, Leidy G, Redman W: Abnormal colonization of neonates in an intensive care unit: means of identifying neonates at risk of infection. *Pediatr Res* 12:998–1002, 1978.

98. Haverkorn ML, Michel MF: Nosocomial klebsiellas. I. Colonization of hospitalized patients. *J Hyg (Lond)* 82:177–193, 1979.

99. Chow AW, Taylor PR, Yoshikawa TT, Guze LB: A nosocomial outbreak of infections due to multiply resistant *Proteus mirabilis*: role of intestinal colonization as a major reservoir. *J Infect Dis* 139:621–627, 1979.

100. Saravolatz LD, Arking L, Pohlod D, Fisher EJ, Borer R: An outbreak of gentamicin-resistant *Klebsiella pneumoniae*: analysis of control measures. *Infect Control* 5:79–84, 1984.

101. Wielunsky E, Durcker M, Cohen T, Reisner SH: Replacement of gentamicin by amikacin as a means of decreasing gentamicin resistance of gram-negative rods in a neonatal intensive care unit. *Isr J Med Sci* 19:1006–1008, 1983.

102. Johanson WG: Prevention of respiratory tract infection. *Am J Med* 76:69–77, 1984.

103. Shibl AM: Effect of antibiotics on adherence of microorganisms to epithelial cell surfaces. *Rev Infect Dis* 7:51–65, 1985.

104. Murray BE, Moellering RC Jr: Patterns and mechanisms of antibiotic resistance. *Med Clin North Am* 62:899–919, 1978.

105. Neu HC: Changing mechanisms of bacterial resistance. *Am J Med* 77:11–23, 1984.

106. Davies J: Microbial resistance to antimicrobial agents. In Ristuccia AM, Cunha BA (eds): *Antimicrobial Therapy*. New York, Raven Press, 1984, p 11.

107. Sherris JC, Minshew BH: Mutational antibiotic resistance. In Lorian V (ed): *Antibiotics in Laboratory Medicine*. Baltimore, Williams & Wilkins, 1980, p 418.

108. Sanders CC: Inducible β-lactamases and non-hydrolytic resistance mechanisms. *J Antimicrob Chemother* 13:1–3, 1984.

109. Sanders CC, Moellering RC Jr, Martin RR, Perkins RL, Strike DG, Gootz TD, Sanders WE Jr: Resistance to cefamandole: a collaborative study of emerging clinical problems. *J Infect Dis* 145:118–125, 1982.

110. Sanders CC, Sanders WE Jr: Emergence of resistance during therapy with the newer β-lactam antibiotics: role of inducible β-lactamases and implications for the future. *Rev Infect Dis* 5:639–648, 1983.

111. Levy SB: Man, animals and antibiotic resistance.

Pediatr Infect Dis 4:3–5, 1985.

112. Sanders CC, Sanders WE: Microbial resistance to newer generation β-lactam antibiotics: clinical and laboratory implications. *J Infect Dis* 151:399–406, 1985.

113. Jones RN: Changing patterns of resistance to new beta-lactam antibiotics. *Am J Med* 77:29–34, 1984.

114. Price KE, Kresel PA, Farchione LA, Siskin SB, Karpow SA: Epidemiological studies of aminoglycoside resistance in the U.S.A. *J Antimicrob Chemother* 8(S-A);89–105, 1981.

115. Yurasek MC, Wang WL, Mostow SR: Reduction in gentamicin resistance among gram-negative bacilli with the exclusive use of amikacin (abstract). *Clin Res* 29:92A, 1981.

116. Moody M, deJongh CA, Schimpff SC, Tillman GL: Long-term amikacin use: effects on aminoglycoside susceptibility patterns of gram-negative bacilli. *JAMA* 248:1199–1202, 1982.

117. Betts RF, Valenti WM, Chapman SW, Chonmaitree T, Mowrer G, Pincus P, Messner M, Robertson R: Five-year surveillance of aminoglycoside usage in a university hospital. *Ann Intern Med* 100:219–222, 1984.

118. Sanders CC: Failure to detect resistance in antimicrobial susceptibility tests: a "very major" error of increasing concern. *Antimicrob Newslett* 1:27–31, 1984.

119. Schaberg DR, Haley RW, Highsmith AK, Anderson RL, McGowan JE: Nosocomial bacteriuria: a prospective study of case clustering and antimicrobial resistance. *Ann Intern Med* 93:420–424, 1980.

120. Maki DG: Through a glass darkly. Nosocomial pseudoepidemics and pseudobacteremias. *Arch Intern Med* 140:26–28, 1980.

121. Weinstein RA, Stamm WE: Pseudoepidemics in hospital. *Lancet* 2:862–864, 1977.

122. Norden CW: Pseudosepticemia. *Ann Intern Med* 71:789–790, 1969.

123. Faris HM, Sparling FF: *Mima polymorpha* bacteremia. False-positive cultures due to contaminated penicillinase. *JAMA* 219:76–77, 1972.

124. DuClos TW, Hodges GR, Killian JE: Bacterial contamination of blood-drawing equipment; a cause of false-positive blood cultures. *Am J Med Sci* 266:459–463, 1973.

125. Noble RC, Reeves SA: *Bacillus* species pseudosepsis caused by contaminated commercial blood culture media. *JAMA* 230:1002–1004, 1974.

126. Kaslow RA, Machel DC, Mallison GF: Nosocomial pseudobacteremia. Positive blood cultures due to contaminated benzalkonium antiseptic. *JAMA* 236:2407–2409, 1976.

127. Coyle-Gilchrist MM, Crewe P, Roberts G: *Flavobacterium meningosepticum* in the hospital environment. *J Clin Pathol* 29:824–826, 1976.

128. Hoffman PC, Arnow PM, Goldmann DA, Parrott PL, Stamm WE, McGowan JE: False positive blood cultures—association with nonsterile blood collection tubes. *JAMA* 236:2073–2075, 1976.

129. Snydman DR, Maloy MF, Brock SM, Lyons RW, Rubin SJ: Pseudobacteremia: false-positive blood cultures from mist tent contamination. *Am J Epidemiol* 106:154–159, 1977.

130. Semel JD, Trenholme GM, Harris AA, Jupa JE,

Levin S: *Pseudomonas maltophilia* pseudosepticemia. *Am J Med* 64:403–406, 1978.

131. Centers for Disease Control, Dolan J, Joachim GR: Pseudobacteremia due to *Staphylococcus aureus*—New York. *MMWR* 28:82–83, 1979.

132. Lynch JM, Anderson A, Camacho FR, Winters AK, Hodges GR, Barnes WG: Pseudobacteremia caused by *Clostridium sordellii*. *Arch Intern Med* 140:65–68, 1980.

133. Jones BC, Stark FR, Reordan R, Lancaster M: Pseudo-positive blood cultures caused by contamination in a humidified incubator. *Infect Control* 5:109–110, 1984.

134. Spivack ML, Shannon R, Natsios GA, Wood J: Two epidemics of pseudobacteremia due to *Staphylococcus aureus* and *Aerococcus viridans*. *Infect Control* 1:321–323, 1980.

135. Centers for Disease Control, Spivack ML, Shannon R, Natsios G, Wood J: Nosocomial pseudobacteremia. *MMWR* 29:243–249, 1980.

136. Lewin S, Nicholas P, Soldeviero R, Holtzman R, Florman A, Freilich H, Craven D, Moody B, Connolly M, Stottmeier K, McCabe W, Miranda N, Friedman S, Budnick L, Shapiro S, Lyon L, Fiumara N: Contaminated povidone-iodine solution—Northeastern United States. *MMWR* 29:553–555, 1980.

137. Graham DR, Wu E, Highsmith AK, Ginsburg ML: An outbreak of pseudobacteremia caused by *Enterobacter cloacae* from a phlebotomist's vial of thrombin. *Ann Intern Med* 95:585–588, 1981.

138. Berkelman RL, Lewin S, Allen JR, Anderson RL, Budnick LD, Shapiro S, Friedman SM, Nicholas P, Holzman RS, Haley RW: Pseudobacteremia attributed to contamination of povidone-iodine with *Pseudomonas cepacia*. *Ann Intern Med* 95:32–36, 1981.

139. Greenhood GP, Highsmith AK, Allen JR, Causey WA, West MC, Dixon RE: *Klebsiella pneumoniae* pseudobactermia due to cross-contamination of a radiometric blood culture analyzer. *Infect Control* 2:460–465, 1981.

140. Griffin MR, Miller AD, Davis AC: Blood culture cross-contamination associated with radiometric analyzer. *J Clin Microbiol* 15:567–570, 1982.

141. MacDonald N: Investigation of an outbreak of pseudobacteremia attributed to *Bacillus* species in a general hospital. Abstracts, 82nd Annual Meeting of the American Society for Microbiology, Atlanta, March 7–12, 1982, p 83

142. Berger SA: Pseudobacteremia due to contaminated alcohol swabs. *J Clin Microbiol* 18:974–975, 1983.

143. Keys TF, Melton J, Maker MD, Lstrup DM: A suspected hospital outbreak of pseudobacteremia due to *Pseudomonas stutzeri*. *J Infect Dis* 147:489–493, 1983.

144. Whiteside M, Moore J, Ratzan K: An investigation of enterococcal bacteremia. *Am J Infect Control* 11:125–129, 1983.

145. Crowley MM, Shannon R, Spivack M, Natsios GH, Buetow B: Pseudobacteremia due to intrinsic contamination of blood culture media by *Bacillus* species (abstract). *Am J Infect Control* 11:150, 1983.

146. Craven DE, Lichtenberg DA, Browne KF, Coffey D, Treadwell TL, McCabe WR: Pseudobactere-

mia traced to cross-contamination by an automated blood culture analyzer. *Infect Control* 5:75–78, 1984.

147. Donowitz LG, Schwartzman JD: Pseudobacteremia and use of the radiometric blood culture analyzer (letter) *Infect Control* 5:266, 1984.

148. Gurevich I, Tafuro P, Krystofiak S, Kalter R, Cunha BA: Three clusters of *Bacillus* pseudobacteremia related to a radiometric blood culture analyzer. *Infect Control* 5:71–74, 1984.

149. Schaffner W, Reisig G, Verrall RA: Outbreak of *Pseudomonas cepacia* infection infection due to contaminated anaesthetics. *Lancet* 1:1050–1051, 1973.

150. Gangadarma PRJ, Lockhart JA, Awe RJ, Jenkins DE: Mycobacterial contamination through tap water (letter). *Am Rev Respir Dis* 113:894, 1976.

151. Suratt PM, Gruber B, Wellons HA, Wenzel RP: Absence of clinical pneumonia following bronchoscopy with contaminated and clean bronchofiberscopes. *Chest* 71:52–54, 1977.

152. Kellerhals S: A pseudo-outbreak of *Serratia marcescens* from a contaminated fiberbronchoscope. *Assoc Practitioners Infect Control J* 6:5–7, 1978.

153. Steere AC, Corrales J, Von Graevenitz A: A cluster of *Mycobacterium gordonae* isolates from bronchoscopy specimens. *Am Rev Respir Dis* 120:214–216, 1979.

154. Schleupner CJ, Hamilton JR: A pseudoepidemic of pulmonary fungal infections related to fiberoptic bronchoscopy. *Infect Control* 1:38–42, 1980.

155. Nunez D, Stanley C, Robertstad GW, Drwo DL: Pseudoepidemic of coccidioidomycosis. *Am J Infect Control* 10:68–71, 1982.

156. Schanbacher KJ, Stieritz DD, LeFrock JL, Gorodetzer MA: A pseudoepidemic of nontubercular mycobacteriosis. (abstract). *Am J Infect Control* 11:150, 1983.

157. Vogel R, Neu HC: A pseudoepidemic of *Penicillium* of fiberoptic bronchoscopy patients (abstract). *Am J Infect Control* 11:149, 1983.

158. Goodman RA, Smith JD, Kubica GP, Dougherty EM, Sikes RK: Nosocomial mycobacterial pseudoinfection in a Georgia Hospital. *Infect Control* 5:573–576, 1984.

159. Musher DM, Schell RF: False-positive gram stains of cerebrospinal fluid (letter). *Ann Intern Med* 79:603–604, 1973.

160. Weinstein RA, Stamm WE, Anderson RL: Early detection of false-positive acid-fast smears. An epidemiological approach. *Lancet* 2:173–174, 1975.

161. Ericsson CD, Carmichael M, Pickering LK, Mussett R, Kohl S: Erroneous diagnosis of meningitis due to false-positive gram stains. *South Med J* 71:1524–1525, 1978.

162. Hoke CH, Batt JM, Mirrett S, Cox RL, Reller B: False-positive gram-stained smears. *JAMA* 241:478–480, 1979.

163. Centers for Disease Control, Batt JM, Reller LB: False-positive Gram stain due to nonviable organisms in sterile commercial transport medium. *MMWR* 27:23, 1978.

164. Harris A, Pottage JC, Fliegelman R, Goodman LJ, Levin S, Vetter M, Kaplan R: A pseudoepidemic due to *Salmonella typhimurium*. *Diagn Microbiol Infect Dis* 1:335–337, 1983.

165. Aber RC, Appelbaum RC: Pseudoepidemic of endocarditis in patients undergoing open-heart surgery. *Infect Control* 1:97–99, 1983.

166. Weinstein RA, Stamm WE: Pseudoepidemics in hospitals. *Lancet* 2:862–864, 1977.

167. Laxon L, Schultz A, Kane M: Pseudo outbreak of hepatitis B in a transplant unit may answer transient positive question (abstract). Annual Conference, Association for Practitioners in Infection Control, 1981, pp 88–89.

168. John JF, Twitty JA: Pseudo-bacteriuria with plasmid-containing *Pseudomonas cepacia*: contamination of rayon balls in benzalkonium chloride (abstract). American Society for Microbiology 1982 Clinical Meeting, p 83.

Chapter 15

Selecting an Antibiotic for the Hospital Formulary

Thomas F. Keys, M.D.

INTRODUCTION

At least $2 billion are spent annually for antibiotics on hospitalized patients. While no one questions the enormous benefits that antibiotics have provided to improve patient care, especially within the last several decades, all are painfully aware that excess and inappropriate antibiotic prescribing continues, perhaps at an accelerated pace. It has been estimated that at least 50% of hospitalized patients are receiving antibiotics needlessly (1). They are either ineffective, over-kill, or simply not indicated at all. Cephalosporins and aminoglycosides account for approximately 70% of the antibiotic budget for the hospital formulary. We are presently witnessing an explosion of cephalosporin and cephalosporin-like antibiotics that will, no doubt, stretch the budget of pharmacies already being trimmed to reduce operating costs. A significant portion of antibiotic prescribing is done by well meaning physicians who order antibiotics without precise laboratory confirmation of the clinical problem. In one study from Great Britain, 50% of patients were receiving antibiotics for no apparent bacterial etiology (2). In the same series, only 7% of patients who received antibiotic prophylaxis for surgery had appropriate prescribing, with the most frequent error being prolongation of prophylaxis after operation. Similar problems were noted in patients being treated with antibiotics for lower respiratory and urinary tract infections, with therapy considered unjustified in 54% and 49% of cases, respectively (3, 4). One does not have to look at Great Britain to observe inappropriate antibiotic prescribing. Studies have amply documented the problem also in the United States. A review of antibiotic prescribing patterns for patients in 20 hospitals in Pennsylvania noted that one-third of all hospitalized patients received antibiotics— 70% for therapy and 30% for prophylaxis (5). Prophylaxis duration was excessive, with 93 cents of every prophylaxis dollar going to patients who received prophylaxis beyond 48 hours after surgery. To make matters worse, the complications of suprainfection or adverse drug reactions are destined to be more frequent in patients who receive needless antibiotics.

With ever mounting pressures from second- and third-party payers, hospitals are now forced to reduce all possible excess expenditures. Cost cutting on antibiotic use has a natural appeal. Their abuse has been well documented; their visibility in patient care is high, not only by physicians, but by infection control practitioners and pharmacists as well. It sometimes seems that everyone on the medical team wants to prescribe an antibiotic! On the other hand, it is likely that there would be few volunteers willing to prescribe cancer chemotherapy or potent cardiovascular drugs unless they had a certain expertise. Furthermore, one must not forget that, usually, antibiotic costs do not represent a large portion of a hospital bill, particularly for patients who have had elective surgery. While several million dollars annually are allocated for antibiotics at The Cleveland Clinic hospital, this represents only a small fraction of the overall operating budget.

SUPRAINFECTION

Suprainfections are likely to occur by antibiotic-resistant bacteria in patients who have received antibiotic prophylaxis or therapy for other reasons (6). Infectious disease consultants are now seeing a new generation of microbes including methicillin-resistant staphylococci (both *Staphylococcus aureus* and *epidermidis*), aminoglycoside-resistant *Pseudomonas aeruginosa*, and multiple drug-resistant *Serratia marcescens*, in addition to yeasts in patients heavily exposed to antimicrobial agents, particularly those on surgical services. It seems clear that a more prudent use of antibiotics will reduce this problem. Examples are widespread in impoverished areas of the world where unrestricted antibiotic availability has resulted not only in increased resistance of bacteria to antibiotics but an increase in their virulence as well. Such international concerns have caused the World Health Organization to publish a document on the control of antibiotic-resistant bacteria (7). Uncontrolled antibiotic usage in hospitals creates a selective pressure allowing for unique drug resistance problems. By reducing such pressures with strict control, one can reverse some of this, especially in intensive care units where multiple drug-resistant organisms soon replace the patient's normal oral pharyngeal flora after entry to the unit.

ADVERSE DRUG REACTIONS

Toxicity and hypersensitivity may complicate the hospital course of 10 to 20% of patients who receive antibiotics (8). Older patients appear more prone to this problem. For example, people over the age of 50 have an increased frequency of aminoglycoside toxicity. Caldwell and Cluff (9) reported adverse reactions in 3.2% of patients receiving penicillin, 5.2% receiving cephalosporins, and 7% receiving gentamicin. However, since cephalosporins are the most commonly prescribed antibiotics, more adverse reactions occur from them than from both aminoglycosides and penicillins. It is important to note that in Caldwell and Cluff's series, 58% of adverse reactions were severe enough to require a change in therapy, and 45% of reactions extended the hospital stay.

OUTSIDE REGULATORY FORCES

With the rising cost of health care, increasing at least 3 times our inflation rate, the mandate for budget trimming is clear. The most recent approach to encourage cost-saving measures is the diagnosis related groups system (DRG) (10). By this system, the patient's primary and secondary diagnoses, age, sex, discharge diagnoses, and operating procedures define a level of reimbursement accepted by second- and third-party payers. Unfortunately, however, individuals who develop unforeseen complications beyond their DRG will incur expenses beyond what will be reimbursed. Clearly, nosocomial infections with increased morbidity and length of stay will impact on reimbursement. Appropriate use of antibiotics should minimize the likelihood of extended stay. While adverse drug reactions and suprainfections are examples of health care misdirected, appropriate therapy and prophylaxis are needed for optimal

patient care. Recently it was noted that 4 of the top 10 most costly DRGs to a hospital were infection problems, with the greatest single expense being cost of antibiotic therapy (11). After recognizing this, the hospital promoted a cost-effective but therapeutically equivalent formulary. One year later, the pharmacy had turned the tide and actually made money for the hospital! Such a tactic will please administrators and pharmacists, but may be resisted by physicians. They will be closely monitored and held accountable to "certain cost influencing variables within their control." Most physicians need education in both antibiotics and economics. They will need to become more assertive because the DRG system is creating unique financial incentives and competition never before present in our health care system.

In addition to the financial crises, hospitals must also face regularly the Joint Commission on Accreditation of Hospitals (JCAH). In recent years, the highest level of noncompliance with JCAH standards has been the lack of physician peer review on antibiotic usage (12). It is exceptional for a physician or a group of physicians to develop a set of firm rules or guidelines for antibiotic use. It is even rarer for physicians at the other end to accept such dictates. Physicians do not enjoy confronting their colleagues with such issues. JCAH reviews have further noted that little, if any, action occurs after antibiotic usage reviews are completed.

ANTIBIOTIC STANDARDS

One might think the answer to antibiotic abuse is adherence to well established and proven forms of therapy and prophylaxis. Nothing could be further from the truth, for we lack a certain knowledge about treating bacterial infections. There is, perhaps, more known and applied to antibiotic prophylaxis. Therapy guidelines published in textbooks or peer-reviewed journals are often vague or ambiguous. Several years ago the Food and Drug Administration (FDA) asked a selected group of infectious disease experts to consider developing standards based on reliable and adequately controlled information (13). Unfortunately, the golden era of clinical studies comparing sulfa with placebo, penicillin with placebo, or sulfa with penicillin has disappeared. It is unlikely that well controlled clinical trials comparing newer with older antimicrobials will ever take place. Who will fund such studies? Certainly not the pharmaceutical industry which has recently marketed a new antibiotic. Representatives from the FDA stated that the prescribing physician is responsible for judging what antibiotic should be used and openly admitted that the information in the package insert and the *Physicians' Desk Reference* (PDR) is only a general guideline (14). It was further noted that 59% of polled physicians placed a heavy reliance on medical journal advertisements for drug information. After careful review, the panel of experts could not develop guidelines for antibiotic therapy based on existing information. Family practitioners need practical guidelines. Academic physicians may see and interpret problems differently. Recommendations may come after experience with unusual disease problems that a general practitioner is unlikely to encounter.

This problem was illustrated when physicians were asked how they should respond in caring for a 6-month-old infant and a 2-year-old child with acute respiratory disease (15). At least 50% of questionnaires mailed to family physicians, general pediatricians, and infectious disease specialists were returned. The results of the survey were striking. The majority of family practitioners would prescribe antibiotics, whereas the infectious disease specialists were therapeutic nihilists. The general pediatricians fell in between. The problem is, nobody knows who is really right!

The subject of antibiotic prophylaxis also has significant stumbling blocks. A critical evaluation of prophylaxis is nearly impossible because of never ending changes in the practice of medicine and surgery. Even the practice of antibiotic prophylaxis to prevent infective endocarditis is of unproven clinical efficacy, yet such prophylaxis has become a standard practice. Health care providers may suffer litigation if prophylaxis is not given. Dr. William Hewitt (16) has concluded that prophylaxis trials must "undergo the closest scrutiny, but the extent to which valid guidelines can be defined and their application can be proved fruitful and subjected to surveillance deserves close examination in order to prevent wasted research and frustrated compliance." Unfortunately, most prophylaxis studies for surgical procedures have serious problems in their design and implementation. Common flaws in prophylaxis studies have included lack of explanation of patient drop-outs, lack of recording of drug costs and allergic reactions, and lack of assurance that both the technical aspects and duration of the surgical procedures were similar in various study groups (17). Furthermore, most studies have not graded severity of infection. A superficial wound infection is less likely to cause morbidity and

mortality than a deep wound infection. Even well designed trials have failed to show that prophylaxis reduces hospital mortality. Furthermore, there is no evidence that prophylaxis with second or third generation cephalosporins is any better than with the first generation agents (18). Yet, large teaching hospitals have seen the first generation cephalosporins fall by the wayside as newer generation cephalosporins have become available. Credit marketing rather than scientific achievement in accomplishing this goal. Another even greater problem is the misdirected use of antibiotics purely on an empiric basis, where precise microbiologic diagnosis is absent and there are no clinical-laboratory parameters to follow. Cephalosporins with their broad spectrum activity are very appealing for this purpose. They are, however, rarely the drugs of choice for proven bacterial infections.

GENERAL APPROACH TO ANTIBIOTIC SELECTION

The therapeutic needs of any patient must be available at the hospital. Quality of patient care must not be jeopardized by simply reducing expenses. This concept will likely boomerang once DRG standards become established into everyday practice. The responsibility for regulating antibiotic usage in the hospital clearly rests with the physicians. However, most of them are unwilling to accept this responsibility. Directions for antibiotic control are more likely to come from the pharmacy, infection control, and administration. Physicians usually consider antibiotic selection and prescribing a natural right. An essential element to antibiotic control is a strong, capable, and concerned pharmacy and therapeutics com-

Table 15.1. Strategies to Improve Antibiotic Usage in Hospitalized Patients

1. An effective pharmacy and therapeutics committee
2. A "no-frills" hospital formulary
3. Antibiotic prescription forms
4. Reviews of antibiotic usage with feedback to staff
5. Basic in vitro antibiotic susceptibility reporting
6. Education
   a. Informal ("face to face")
   b. Antibiotic therapy and prophylaxis guides
   c. Newsletters
   d. Formal lectures
7. Restriction of select antibiotics
8. Control of pharmaceutical representatives

mittee, chaired by a clinician with a special interest in applied pharmacology (Table 15.1). Any new antibiotic being considered for the formulary must be carefully assessed for efficacy, toxicity, and expense by the committee. Input may come from infectious disease clinicians and any other staff who think a new antibiotic has unique and special properties. Even after acceptance, an antibiotic should not be poured in a concrete formulary. In most instances, the antibiotic should be accepted on a conditional basis for a 6-month trial period. During this time, the pharmacy must monitor the use of the antibiotic. It is critical to assess whether or not the benefit intended of the antibiotic is actually taking place. This information can be gained by the use of a preprinted antibiotic prescription form where specific designation for the antibiotic (prophylaxis, empiric therapy, therapy due to a proven infection) is required, and some relevant clinical information is supplied (Fig. 15.1). Such completed forms are compiled and the data reviewed to provide both the pharmacy and therapeutics committee and the staff feedback on antibiotic prescribing patterns. The form also tends to reduce overprescribing. If prescribing is too easy, the practice will be abused. Some antibiotic forms include automatic stop orders, such as 48 hours for surgical wound prophylaxis and 5 days for therapy, with renewal required for longer duration (19). In this case it

PHYSICIAN'S ORDERS

ANTIBIOTIC ORDER FORM

CORD ALL ALLERGIES AND INTOLERANCES

☐ NO KNOWN ALLERGIES OR INTOLERANCES

IMPRINT

DATE | TIME | USE BALLPOINT PEN ONLY | C | K | R

All systemically absorbed antibiotics must be ordered on this form. Please use this form for each new order, continuation order, or changed order. Include all requested information.

☐ **PROPHYLAXIS (Medical or surgical)**
Operation or condition:
☐ **EMPIRIC THERAPY (For suspected infection)**
Suspected site of infection: Cultures ordered: ☐ Yes ☐ No
☐ **THERAPEUTIC USE (For infection caused by identified pathogen)**
Site of infection/pathogen:
ANTIBIOTIC ORDER (include number of days or doses):

PHYSICIAN SIGNATURE PAGER

☐ **PROPHYLAXIS (Medical or surgical)**
Operation or condition:
☐ **EMPIRIC THERAPY (For suspected infection)**
Suspected site of infection: Cultures ordered: ☐ Yes ☐ No
☐ **THERAPEUTIC USE (For infection caused by identified pathogen)**
Site of infection/pathogen:
ANTIBIOTIC ORDER (include number of days or doses):

PHYSICIAN SIGNATURE PAGER

☐ **PROPHYLAXIS (Medical or surgical)**
Operation or condition:
☐ **EMPIRIC THERAPY (For suspected infection)**
Suspected site of infection: Cultures ordered: ☐ Yes ☐ No
☐ **THERAPEUTIC USE (For infection caused by identified pathogen)**
Site of infection/pathogen:
ANTIBIOTIC ORDER (include number of days or doses):

PHYSICIAN SIGNATURE PAGER

SEND EVERY ORDER COPY TO PHARMACY

F909 ALL ORDERS MUST BE SIGNED BY PHYSICIAN

Figure 15.1. An example of an antibiotic prescription form that asks for specific indication with accompanying clinical and laboratory information.

is important that no time elapse when the clinician wishes the antibiotic to be continued. Close communication between the pharmacy and staff is essential. Success with the form results in substantial cost savings, especially with a reduction in duration of surgical wound prophylaxis.

The clinical microbiology laboratory can also limit antibiotic prescribing by providing selective in vitro antibiotic susceptibility data on microorganisms. A certain amount of clinical judgment is needed to make these decisions; infectious disease consultants should assist in determining what testing is to be reported. In most cases, it is unwise to disclose the results of in vitro testing that is being done with new or nonformulary antibiotics.

Results of antibiotic usage patterns, if reported in a meaningful way, are of considerable benefit to staff as well as to trainees of postgraduate educational programs (20). Selected reporting to departments or individuals may serve a similar purpose to that of reporting surgical wound infection rates to surgeons. If the individual physician sees how he or she stacks up alongside his or her colleagues, some change is more likely to occur. Furthermore, this information plus a concentrated educational program directed at a personal level is more likely to achieve behavioral modification than are erudite and sometimes dry lectures on antibiotics. In addition to these endeavors, the staff should consider distributing pharmacy bulletins or newsletters that contain practical, up-to-date information on antibiotics. Counter-detailing techniques showing that sometimes the older antibiotics remain the drugs of choice for certain infections have been successfully employed by Avorn (21). Infectious disease clinicians can be leaders in their hospital in promoting such basic concepts (never lose the opportunity to use penicillin G!). More formal guidelines can be created, printed, and distributed to staff with updating at regular intervals. Although the initial investment of such a handbook may be costly, in the long run, the guidelines have merit because they address specific problems, perhaps unique to the hospital, and they are authored by respected colleagues. The difficult part about education, however, is the reversal of the learning curve with time. For example, D'Eramo and associates at the University of Texas (22) applied an intense education program for several weeks and noted a significant drop in inappropriate prescribing immediately after their efforts. However, the trend reversed itself within 3 months.

Another recent study from Harvard University examined the value of frequent educational visits by clinical pharmacists to outpatient-based physicians (23). Participating physicians in the study also received information through the mail. The results suggested that direct, personal educational experiences produced the best results. Tighter control on antibiotic prescribing can occur by requiring approval for certain restricted antibiotics before they are released by the pharmacy. In a recent survey, 57% of medical school-affiliated hospitals exercised some form of antibiotic restriction (24). Forty-six percent required authorization by an infectious disease specialist, and 12% required specific written indications before approval. Eighty-five percent of infectious disease specialists agreed with the policy of antibiotic restriction, and 47% of their hospitals had formal education programs. With programs, antibiotic control was easier. These investigators concluded that "Direct, face-to-face, concurrent control methods, are likely to be more effective but also require resourceful and diplomatic controller/educators." This is *not* a place for a bull in a china shop!

SPECIFIC EXAMPLES OF ANTIBIOTIC SELECTION

Although it is impossible to dictate what should or should not be included in a hospital formulary, it is appropriate to review specific antibiotics that are within classes of frequently prescribed parenteral drugs. Such examples will give the reader a flavor of the decision-making process that must take place before an antibiotic is approved for the formulary.

The Antistaphylococcal Penicillins: Methicillin, Oxacillin, and Nafcillin

All three of the antibiotics are similar in in vitro activity against penicillin-resistant staphylococci and in clinical efficacy. Their pharmacokinetics are somewhat different, and related, in part, to differences in serum protein binding and volume distribution (25). After a standard dose is given by intravenous bolus infusion, peak serum concentrations of nafcillin are significantly lower than methicillin or oxacillin. With renal failure, dosage adjustment is usually not necessary with nafcillin or oxacillin. All three antibiotics diffuse into the cerebrospinal fluid in the presence of acute inflammation. Nafcillin spinal fluid concentrations are reported higher. Penicillin-type hypersensitivity reactions can occur, in addition to interstitial nephritis (most frequently reported with methicillin), and hepatitis and neutropenia (most frequently reported with oxacillin). Because of a high reported frequency of cases developing interstitial nephritis after methicillin, hospital formularies usually have only oxacillin or nafcillin. The dosage for all three ranges from 100 to 300 mg/kg/day, with the higher dose for patients with life-threatening infections.

It is obviously essential for an antistaphylococcal penicillin to be on the hospital formulary. Since they are therapeutically equivalent, one must consider other merits, such as toxicity and cost. Competitive bidding may favorably influence the market price. With similar dosing schedules, pharmacy preparation and administration fees should be the same. Finally, the quality of the interaction between the hospital and the individual pharmaceutical firms and local representatives must be considered. Obviously, it is essential that the local representative be knowledgeable, honest, and pleasant in his dealings with the hospital.

After careful consideration, the pharmacy and therapeutics committee approves one antistaphylococcal penicillin for the formulary.

The Antipseudomonas Penicillins: Ticarcillin, Azlocillin, Mezlocillin, and Piperacillin

Carbenicillin, the first antipseudomonas penicillin, came into use in the late 1960s. Over the last several years, it has been largely replaced by newer antipseudomonas penicillins that appear more effective and have less toxicity. Of the four listed above, piperacillin and azlocillin are active against greater numbers of strains of *P. aeruginosa* than ticarcillin or mezlocillin (26). Their pharmacokinetics are similar with comparable peak serum levels after a 2- or 3-g bolus intravenous infusion. Cerebrospinal fluid concentrations are achieved in the presence of inflammation. Although mezlocillin and piperacillin concentrations are reported higher in bile, the clinical significance of this is uncertain. All can cause penicillin hypersensitivity reactions; additional side effects of hypernatremia, hypokalemia, and bleeding are reported with ticarcillin and neutropenia with piperacillin.

Although it might appear that piperacillin or azlocillin would have a slight edge against ticarcillin or mezlocillin because of greater activity against *P. aeruginosa*, this should be corroborated by reviewing the hospital's clinical and laboratory experience. The reported differences in the literature may not represent what is occurring at the local level.

After careful review, one antipseudomonas penicillin should be approved for the formulary.

The Cephalosporins

Cephalothin, the first cephalosporin, became available in 1964. Twenty years later there are now at least 20 different cephalosporins either on the market or currently being investigated. They are the most frequently prescribed group of antibiotics. Strangely, they are not considered the drugs of choice for most infections (27). Their greatest use has been in surgical wound prophylaxis. Another frequently considered indication is for therapy in the patient with a history of penicillin allergy.

First Generation Cephalosporins: Cephalothin and Cefazolin

Both cephalothin and cefazolin have good in vitro activity against gram-positive cocci (excluding enterococci) and against most enteric gram-negative bacilli. Neither is active against *S. marcescens* or *P. aeruginosa*. Cefazolin is more susceptible to inactivation by β-lactamase than cephalothin (28). In vitro activity of cephalothin is slightly better against *S. aureus* and *S. epidermidis*. However, the pharmacokinetic properties of cefazolin are far superior to cephalothin. Peak serum concentrations are at least twice as high with cefazolin and serum half-life is 3 times longer. Cefazolin can be given intramuscularly without causing the pain reported by cephalothin. Adverse drug reactions occur with equal frequency for both.

After comparing activity, pharmacology, and cost, one first generation cephalosporin should be approved for the formulary.

Second Generation Cephalosporins: Cefamandole, Cefoxitin

Cefamandole and cefoxitin have a different spectrum of in vitro antibiotic activity. They cannot be considered therapeutic equivalents (29). Cefamandole is very active against *Enterobacter* species, while cefoxitin is very active against *Bacteroides fragilis*. Although cefamandole is more active against staphylococci than cefoxitin, it is less active than cephalothin. Both cefamandole and cefoxitin have relatively short serum half-lives; frequent dosing is necessary to achieve therapeutic serum concentrations. Toxicity is similar to other cephalosporins; bleeding complications have been reported with cefamandole. Success has been claimed using cefoxitin for prophylaxis during colorectal or gynecologic surgery (30).

After review, the pharmacy and therapeutics committee might conclude that neither agent need be on the formulary, or it might consider approval on a restricted basis. For example, cefoxitin could be approved only for prophylaxis during colorectal or gynecologic surgery or for therapy of *Bacteroides fragilis* infections where alternative agents (for example, metronidazole or clindamycin) are contraindicated.

Third Generation Cephalosporins: Cefotaxime, Moxalactam, and Cefoperazone

All three of the above have broad spectrum in vitro activity against enteric gram-negative bacilli (31). In contrast, none has the same high level of activity against staphylococci as do the first generation cephalosporins. Both cefotaxime and moxalactam are usually more active against *S. marcescens* and *Morganella* species than cefoperazone. However, cefoperazone and moxalactam have modest activity against *P. aeruginosa*. Against *B. fragilis*, moxalactam is clearly the most active of the three. It is obvious here that they cannot be considered therapeutic equivalents. Of the three, cefotaxime has the shortest half-life, with moxalactam longer and cefoperazone the longest. Adverse effects are similar in frequency to other cephalosporins; however, bleeding problems have been reported most frequently with moxalactam (32).

After careful review, the pharmacy and therapeutics committee may conclude that none of these antibiotics needs to be routinely available on the formulary. However, at least one should be available, but restricted for use in meningitis due to enteric gram-negative bacilli or for infection due to antibiotic-restricted bacteria.

Aminoglycosides: Streptomycin, Gentamicin, Tobramycin, Amikacin

Streptomycin, the first aminoglycoside, became available in the 1940s (33). Although its use is now limited because of resistance problems, it remains important with penicillin therapy for infective endocarditis due to streptomycin-sensitive streptococci. In the 1960s with the discovery of gentamicin, and subsequent clinical trials, this aminoglycoside proved effective not only for infections due to most enteric bacilli, but also to *P. aeruginosa*. Ten years later, tobramycin, an aminoglycoside somewhat more active than gen-

tamicin against *P. aeruginosa*, became available. Against *S. marcescens*, however, more strains have remained susceptible to gentamicin. Amikacin, a semisynthetic derivative of kanamycin, came along several years later and has unique activity against most gram-negative bacteria resistant to gentamicin or tobramycin. Unfortunately, for all aminoglycosides, the safety margin between therapeutic efficacy and toxicity is very small. Adverse reactions include nephrotoxicity, ototoxicity, and neuromuscular blockade. Nephrotoxicity, the most common complication, appears to be dose-related and potentiated by hypotension, loop diuretics, old age, and preexisting renal disease (34). Several studies have suggested that tobramycin is less nephrotoxic than gentamicin, but other studies have concluded that toxicity is not significantly different. Toxicity from amikacin occurs with similar frequency. More likely, however, toxicity will occur from any aminoglycoside if the dosing is inappropriate or renal function is not being monitored during therapy.

In summary, the pharmacy and therapeutics committee must decide what aminoglycosides should be on the formulary. Recently, the decision became easier with the loss of patent for gentamicin. This has created healthy competition with considerable cost savings to consumers. At the present time, equivalent generic gentamicin costs one-tenth as much as that of tobramycin or amikacin. If the decision is to accept only gentamicin, the others should be available on a restricted basis for therapy of infections due to gentamicin-resistant bacteria.

This section has briefly reviewed several classes of antibiotics that need to be on the hospital formulary. There are many others that also must be considered: penicillin G, ampicillin, vancomycin, sulfonamide, trimethoprim-sulfamethoxazole, erythromycin, clindamycin, chloramphenicol, tetracycline, metronidazole, and so forth. Detailed information can be found by consulting a current edition of Goodman and Gilman's text, *The Pharmacological Basis of Therapeutics* (35), the *Medical Letter on Drugs and Therapeutics*, as well as critical articles on antibiotics in peer-reviewed medical journals.

THE PHARMACEUTICAL INDUSTRY: A DOUBLE-EDGED SWORD

While the United States pharmaceutical firms have enjoyed considerable financial success over the past several decades, now they are being seriously challenged by the industrial giants of Western Europe and Japan. Funds for research and development have come with reasonable ease from these firms in the past; now the competition is so fierce for the market that monies are being redirected in promotional areas. As a rule, antibiotics must be promoted beyond the goal for which they were originally intended to make a profit. An example of this is the widespread promotion and consequent use of the cephalosporins. An exception to the rule is the growing demand for vancomycin because of the increasing number of infections due to methicillin-resistant staphylococci and to *Clostridium difficile.* Vancomycin is making a sizeable profit without being heavily detailed. Scientific programs on antibiotics are often sponsored by these companies. Unfortunately, sometimes such efforts turn out to be self-serving for marketing needs. Accreditation for some of these programs is questionable, although they may be sanctioned for continuing education credit (36). Even seasoned and gray-haired elder statesmen of high stature in the field of infectious diseases may be caught by a "Seduction in a Grand Hotel" (37). As Dr. Calvin Kunin (38) has recently stated, "The promotional activities of the pharmaceutical industry have infiltrated virtually every aspect of medical education." A major concern of his is how to protect the hospital formulary. He suggests that the pharmacy and therapeutics committee go beyond the activity, pharmacology, toxicity, and cost of an antibiotic for consideration. For example, how much funds are expended by the pharmaceutical company for research and reputable education? What interaction does this pharmaceutical company have with investigators at the hospital? How much money do the investigators receive for research, travel, speaking engagements, and consultation fees? Individuals engaged in such research must adopt a high code of ethics (39). All research projects should be subjected to peer and institutional review before being approved. Every possible effort must be made to avoid conflict of interest; relationships with industry should be disclosed and products should not be endorsed.

EXERCISING RESTRAINTS

Reviewing the prescribing patterns of physicians has certainly paid off for industry. Stolley and Lasagna (40) noted that such data are collected by marketing research firms and sold to drug manufacturers and advertising agencies at premium prices. These data provide inroads for new marketing techniques and allow a company to see where their competition is. Students concerned for more prudent antibiotic prescribing can also learn from these data. While antibiotics are clearly overutilized in outpatient and inpatient settings, restraints from infectious disease colleagues seem almost nonexistent. General practitioners rely more on advertising, mailing, and detailmen than on consultants when choosing antibiotics. Personal factors account for the variability of antibiotic prescribing. Physician leaders, particularly of a scholarly nature, tend to set the stage for changing prescribing habits. However, it is often the persuasive and tenacious detailman who bonds physician to antibiotic. There is a need to restrain the activities of detailmen in the hospital (41). They must schedule their detailing at specific times and make arrangements for educational events, all with the prior approval of the chief-of-staff. They should not be allowed to wander through the hospital, but should confine their detailing to a classroom or similar educational setting. The giving of samples and meals must be discouraged. There is no such thing as a free lunch.

With the DRG system, the clinical microbiology laboratory will need to restrain availability of testing (42). The concept of a cost rather than a profit center will create sweeping changes. Not only will poor quality specimens be rejected, but tests requested on specimens of satisfactory quality if they are not clinically indicated will be also. Low demand tests will either not be done at all or will be farmed out to a regional for-profit laboratory. Nor is it likely that the laboratory will provide 24-hour or weekend service. There is now no greater need for physicians to be properly educated in making microbiologic diagnoses (43). The importance of gram-stained smears needs to be re-emphasized. Specific, rapid diagnostic tests, such as detection of bacterial antigens and direct antibiotic susceptibility testing from blood cultures, should improve selection of appropriate antibiotic therapy. More efficient communication must occur between the microbiology laboratory and clinician. Ackerman and associates (44) have criticized laboratory reports because of "jargon, unfamiliar names of microbes, and ill-defined reporting conventions." They further point out that microbiologists should play a more active role in recommending antibiotic therapy based on their laboratory data. As stated by Edwards (45) more than 10 years ago, "Good clinical judgment in initial ordering of cultures, avoidance of inappropriate use of prophylactic antimicrobial drugs, avoidance of empiric antimicrobial therapy until after necessary cultures are collected from all sites, proper collection and transport techniques, intelligent use of immediate smears from clinical specimens, adherence to standardized laboratory methods, and a consciousness of cost-benefit to the patient are all necessary before effective utilization can be realized."

CONCLUSION

The economics of our times are controlling the destiny of health care as never before. Physicians by their nature are independent and resistant to change and criticism. We have ample evidence that prescribing of antibiotics is grossly abused. Some recent efforts in turning the tide, mainly with antibiotic prophylaxis, have been successful. But more work needs to be done. What knowledge we have must be effectively communicated to our colleagues before it is too late (6). A grassroots education program, directed at staff and residents, is essential. Pharmaceutical detailmen must be restrained, but in a careful and considerate manner. A strong pharmacy and therapeutics committee must control access to the hospital formulary. Antibiotics should be selected on the true needs of the individual hospital. Cost-effective antibiotic programs can be developed without compromising patient care (46).

References

1. Kunin CM: Evaluation of antibiotic usage: a comprehensive look at alternative approaches. *Rev Infect Dis* 3:745–753, 1981.
2. Moss F, McNicol MW, McSwiggan DA, Miller DL: Survey of antibiotic prescribing in a district general hospital. I. Pattern of use. *Lancet* 2:349–352, 1981.
3. Moss FM, McNicol MW, McSwiggan DA, Miller DL: Survey of antibiotic prescribing in a district general hospital. II. Lower respiratory tract infection. *Lancet* 2:407–409, 1981.
4. Moss FM, McNicol MW, McSwiggan DA, Miller DL: Survey of antibiotic prescribing in a district general hospital. III. Urinary tract infection. *Lancet* 2:461–462, 1981.
5. Shapiro M, Townsend TR, Rosner B, Kass EH: Use of antimicrobial drugs in general hospitals: patterns of prophylaxis. *N Engl J Med* 301:351–355, 1979.
6. McGowan JE Jr: Antimicrobial resistance in hospital organisms and its relation to antibiotic use. *Rev Infect Dis* 5:1033–1048, 1983.
7. World Health Organization Scientific Working Group on Antimicrobial Resistance: Control of antibiotic-resistant bacteria: memorandum from a WHO meeting. *Am J Hosp Pharm* 41:1329–1337, 1984.
8. Maki DG, Schuna AA: A study of antimicrobial misuse in a university hospital. *Am J Med Sci* 275:271–282, 1978.
9. Caldwell JR, Cluff LE: Adverse reactions to antimicrobial agents, *JAMA* 230:77–80, 1974.
10. Curtis FR: Pharmacy management strategies for responding to hospital reimbursement changes. *Am J Hosp Pharm* 40:1489–1492, 1983.
11. Rosenthal MH: A timely perspective on DRG's: four years' experience. *Hosp Pharm Cost Containment* 3:1–5, 1984.
12. JCAH cites shortcomings in quality assurance functions. *Hospitals* 58:60–63, 1984.
13. Finland M: Introduction. In McCabe WR, Finland M (eds): *Contemporary Standards for Antimicrobial Usage.* Mount Kisco, NY, Futura, 1977, vol XIII, p ix.
14. Gibson ML: FDA view of standards. In McCabe WR, Finland M (eds): *Contemporary Standards for Antimicrobial Usage.* Mount Kisco, NY, Futura, 1977, vol XIII, p 11.
15. Greenberg RA, Wagner EH, Wolf SH, Cohen SB, Kleinbaum DG, Williams CA, Ibrahim MA: Physician opinions on the use of antibiotics in respiratory infections. *JAMA* 240:650–653, 1978.
16. Hewitt WL: Prophylactic use of antibiotics: considerations of standards in clinical practice. In McCabe WR, Finland M (eds): *Contemporary Standards for Antimicrobial Usage.* Mount Kisco, NY, Futura, 1977, vol XIII, p 157.
17. Hirschmann JV, Inui TS: Antimicrobial prophylaxis: a critique of recent trials. *Rev Infect Dis* 2:1–23, 1980.
18. DiPiro JT, Bowden TA Jr, Hooks VH III: Prophylactic parenteral cephalosporins in surgery: are the newer agents better? *JAMA* 252:3277–3279, 1984.
19. Durbin WA Jr, Lapidas B, Goldmann DA: Improved antibiotic usage following introduction of a novel prescription system. *JAMA* 246:1796–1800, 1981.
20. Echols RM, Kowalsky SF: The use of an antibiotic order form for antibiotic utilization review: influence on physicians' prescribing patterns. *J Infect Dis* 150:803–807, 1984.
21. Avorn J: Reducing inappropriate prescribing. *APUA Newslett* 11:2–3, 1984.
22. D'Eramo JE, DuPont HL, Preston GA, Smolensky MH, Roht LH: The short- and long-term effects of a handbook on antimicrobial prescribing patterns of hospital physicians. *Infect Control* 4:209–214, 1983.
23. Avorn J, Soumerai SB: Improving drug-therapy decisions through educational outreach: a randomized controlled trial of academically based "detailing." *N Engl J Med* 308:1457–1463, 1983.
24. Klapp DL, Ramphal R: Antibiotic restriction in hospitals associated with medical schools. *Am J Hosp Pharm* 40:1957–1960, 1983.
25. Neu HC: Antistaphylococcal penicillins. *Med Clin North Am* 66:51–60, 1982.
26. New HC: Carbenicillin and ticarcillin. *Med Clin North Am* 66:61–77, 1982.
27. Choice of cephalosporins. *Med Lett* 25:57–60, 1983.
28. Quintiliani R, French M, Nightingale CH: First and second generation cephalosporins. *Med Clin North Am* 66:183–197, 1982.
29. Andriole VT, Ryan JL: An approach to formulary

consideration of antimicrobial agents: the cephalosporins. *Hosp Formulary* 16:1149–1163, 1981.

30. Guglielmo BJ, Hohn DC, Koo PJ, Hunt TK, Sweet RL, Conte JE Jr: Antibiotic prophylaxis in surgical procedures: a critical analysis of the literature. *Arch Surg* 118:943–955, 1983.

31. Fass R: Comparative in vitro activities of third-generation cephalosporins. *Arch Intern Med* 143:1743–1745, 1983.

32. Panwalker AP, Rosenfeld J: Hemorrhage, diarrhea, and superinfection associated with the use of moxalactam. *J Infect Dis* 147:171–172, 1983.

33. Andriole VT, Ryan JL: An approach to formulary consideration of antimicrobial agents: the aminoglycosides. *Hosp Formulary* 17:242–247, 1982.

34. Edson RS, Keys TF: The aminoglycosides: streptomycin, kanamycin, gentamicin, tobramycin, amikacin, netilmicin, sisomicin. *Mayo Clin Proc* 58:99–102, 1983.

35. Gilman AG, Goodman LS, Gilman A (eds): *Goodman and Gilman's The Pharmacological Basis of Therapeutics*, ed 6. New York, Macmillan, 1980.

36. Musher DM: Antibiotics: the medium is the message. *Rev Infect Dis* 5:809–812, 1983.

37. Kass EH: Seduction in a grand hotel. *Rev Infect Dis* 5:973–974, 1983.

38. Kunin CM: The relation between clinical investigators and the pharmaceutical industry. *Rev Infect Dis* 6:129–131, 1984.

39. Statement on ethical conduct in research by the Infectious Diseases Society of America. *J Infect Dis* 150:792–793, 1984.

40. Stolley PD, Lasagna L: Prescribing patterns of physicians. *J Chronic Dis* 22:395–405, 1969.

41. Curtiss FR: Pharmacy management strategies for responding to hospital reimbursement changes. *Am J Hosp Pharm* 40:1489–1492, 1983.

42. Winkelman JW, Hill RB: Clinical laboratory responses to reduced funding. *JAMA* 252:2435–2440, 1984.

43. Dans PE, Charache P, Fahey M, Otter SE: Management of pneumonia in the prospective payment era: a need for more clinician and support service interaction. *Arch Intern Med* 144:1392–1397, 1984.

44. Ackerman VP, Pritchard RC, Groot Obbink DJ, Bradbury R, Lee A: Consumer survey on microbiology reports. *Lancet* 1:199–202, 1979.

45. Edwards LD, Levin S, Balagtas R, Lowe P, Landau W, Lepper MH: Ordering patterns and utilization of bacteriologic culture reports. *Arch Intern Med* 132:678–682, 1973.

46. Glackman R, Gantz NM: Cost-effective antibiotic prescribing. *Pharmacotherapy* 3:239–248, 1983.

Chapter 16

Organizing and Managing Product Evaluation

Robert C. Aber, M.D., and William E. O'Brien, B.Sc., R.Ph.

INTRODUCTION

Product evaluation is not new to hospitals or to infection control personnel. Since 1976 the Joint Commission on Accreditation of Hospitals (JCAH) has recommended that the activities of the infection control program include consultation relative to the purchase of all equipment and supplies used for sterilization, disinfection, and decontamination purposes, and to the implementation of any major changes in cleaning products or techniques (1). Until recently, the quality (proven or potential) of an item carried more weight in the decision process to use the product than its cost, since the latter was reimbursable. We have entered an era of transition in the financial support of health care, and the incentives for cost containment and cost reduction are escalating. The cost of health care is viewed as a high priority problem nationally, and infection control programs can expect continued pressure for cost containment. Voluntary efforts at cost containment by the health care industry have been supplanted by recent legislation—most importantly, a system of prospective payment for provision of health care which is not based upon reimbursement for actual costs. We are asked to provide health care of the same quality at reduced cost. As a result, there is increasing concern among health care providers that economic pressures may eventually erode the quality of care provided.

At the same time hospitals are struggling to reduce costs, a highly competitive industry is producing and marketing products at an unprecedented rate and with unprecedented fervor. Most new products are also more expensive, and data which bear on the quality or comparative quality of these products are often inadequate to help hospital committees make valid choices. Administrators have become most attentive to issues of cost containment and cost reduction, whereas health care providers must consider issues of product quality, efficacy, and safety. Furthermore, in most hospitals, the situation is made more complex by the prejudices of health care providers, administrators, and patients with respect to choices of products for use.

Labor and nonlabor hospital costs attributable to materiel management have been estimated to be approximately 40 to 50% of the total hospital budget (2). Hence, it is not surprising that more attention is being given to materiel management programs as a means to contain or to reduce operational costs. Strategies for achieving cost control include the following: (*a*) increased efficiency of materiels use, (*b*) decreased demand for materiels, (*c*) reduction in personnel for managing materiels, and (*d*) control of purchase price through competitive or collaborative purchasing.

Most hospitals have already taken initiatives to control product purchase price through competitive bidding or participation in local, regional, state, or national purchasing pacts.

A balance must be achieved between quality of health care provided and the costs incurred in providing such care; and in order to achieve such a balance, an organized approach to product evaluation and standardization is necessary.

Product standardization is one means to control costs by reducing inventory as well as by bulk purchasing. Its goal is simply to eliminate duplicate products purchased for the same purpose or use; it should be emphasized that it is not to purchase the least expensive product.

Product standardization, in fact, may result in increased costs for some products depending on the quality desired. Besides quality and cost, other factors to be considered before selecting a product as the standard include the availability of the product, the associated service required, and the availability of in-service education to accompany its introduction.

Hence, the problems of product evaluation and

standardization have become increasingly complex for the hospital as well as for the infection control program. It may be prudent and cost effective to integrate product evaluation by the infection control program into a hospital-wide program whenever possible, but this hypothesis has not been rigorously tested.

PRINCIPLES OF PRODUCT EVALUATION AND STANDARDIZATION PROGRAM

We think that there are several basic principles upon which an effective product evaluation and standardization program should be built (3, 4):

1. First and foremost, for a program to be effective, it must have high level administrative and professional support. Such support is usually provided as a written policy which defines the authority, objectives, organizational structure, and responsibilities of the program.
2. An effective program must be able to control *all* products used in the hospital. The only exceptions to the principle include (*a*) one-time use of a product by a physician in the care of a patient (and this should be approved on a case-by-case basis) and (*b*) items purchased and used by only a single department. However, the program should be notified of and approve all such departmental purchases.
3. The program must have broad-based, multidisciplinary participation and support. Organizationally, this is usually accomplished by a committee which includes health care professional groups. Representation from health care consumers may be appropriate as well.
4. There should be prompt evaluation and a prompt decision. The format for the evaluation of a product should be formalized, but the actual evaluation can be tailored to the individual product, and should be based upon clearly specifying the desirable generic or esthetic functions as well as any limiting constraints of the product. Whenever possible, committee members should try to evaluate several brands of a particular product rather than a single brand in order to collect comparative data, including products currently being used in the hospital.
5. There should be effective, rapid communications between program participants, product representatives, and those who will be affected by product evaluations or changes

in a product. There must be ample access and opportunity for all who have an interest in a particular product to participate in the evaluation process and to offer opinions. Hence, the names and types of products being evaluated must be widely disseminated.
6. There should be written documentation of products evaluated and decisions made, at least in the form of committee minutes.
7. There should be in-service education and training linked to the evaluation or introduction of a product. This may be conducted by members of the in-service education department, by representatives from industry, or by other knowledgeable persons.

A PROGRAM MODEL

After sufficient administrative and professional support for such a program has been ascertained, a policy statement should be developed defining the authority, objectives, organizational structure, and responsibilities of the program. An example of such a statement might be as follows:

"It is the policy of this hospital and medical staff that consumable items or products used in the hospital must be approved for such use by the standardization and evaluation committee. Furthermore, all items or products proposed for use are to be evaluated by the committee prior to use. (The only exceptions to this policy are (*a*) one-time use of a product by order of a physician in providing for the care of a patient and (*b*) items used by a single department which are purchased by and unique to that department. For both exceptions to apply, the committee is to be notified promptly of any items or products used. If repeated or continual use is anticipated, committee approval will be necessary.) The product standardization and evaluation committee shall be a multidisciplinary committee of hospital and medical staff charged with the following responsibilities: (*a*) to evaluate promptly all items and products for use in the hospital with respect to quality, efficacy, safety, convenience, suitability, and cost effectiveness; (*b*) to select and standardize such products judged appropriate for use as much as possible and feasible while maintaining the quality of patient care; and (*c*) to introduce products properly for evaluation and use with appropriate education and training.

The objectives of the program include the following: (*a*) to improve patient care by efficient use of effective products, (*b*) to foster fiscal responsibility and cost containment; (*c*) to standardize and centralize the product evaluation efforts within the hospital."

THE COMMITTEE

Much has been written about the composition of a product standardization and evaluation committee based upon job title or description, but it seems that the critical ingredients for selection should be the interest, special knowledge, and influence of its members. Interested and influential members probably enhance the overall effectiveness of the committee proportionately more than knowledgeable but less interested or influential members do. Nevertheless, it is probably important that certain departments and health professional groups be represented to facilitate communications and committee function (Table 16.1).

The chairperson should be selected on the basis of organizational skills and instincts rather than job title or position. He or she should ideally be senior, influential, and trusted throughout the hospital. Committee members should act as liaison between the committee and their respective departments and professional health groups to facilitate communications. They serve also as liaison between this committee and other hospital or medical staff committees. For example, the director of materials management at The Milton S. Hershey Medical Center is in a pivotal position as chairman of the product standardization and evaluation committee as well as chairman of the infection control committee's subcommittee on new products. This liaison is quite efficient and effective for both committees.

THE PROCESS

The format or process for product evaluation and standardization should be formalized and published widely within the institution. Table

Table 16.1. Representation on the Product Standardization and Evaluation Committee

Materiel management
Purchasing
Nursing
Medical staff
Central services
Environmental health
Hospital administration
Infection control program
In-service education
Operating room
Ad hoc members as appropriate

16.2 provides a sample scheme used at The Milton S. Hershey Medical Center. Anyone in the institution may initiate a product evaluation request by completing an appropriate form (Fig. 16.1) and submitting it to the materials management office. The request undergoes a preliminary screen by the director of materials management on behalf of the product standardization and evaluation committee, and may result in an immediate approval to conduct an evaluation, a request for additional information, or discussion by the entire committee at its next scheduled meeting. If evaluation of a product is to be conducted, a product evaluation analysis form (Fig. 16.2) is initiated and tailored to the product. Evaluators are reminded to consider carefully the generic and esthetic functions and qualities as well as any limiting constraints of the product during the evaluation process. Additional information may be sought from experienced users (in-house or elsewhere), purchasing department, product representatives from different companies, and the scientific literature to document quality, convenience, acceptance, suitability, efficacy, safety, and cost of one or more brands of a product. We emphasize the need for valid data published in peer-reviewed journals in the evaluation and selection of products for use. We and others have been disappointed by the scarcity of such for most products.

After all of the data are compiled, tabulated, and summarized, a report is distributed to appropriate departments, committees, and potential users for review. A response (if any) is requested by a specified date. The item is then placed on the agenda for the first committee meeting following the deadline date. Anyone interested in committee deliberations or wishing to offer opinion or testimony is welcome to attend the meeting.

The committee deliberations center around value analysis of the product. The objective is to select a product or brand that provides good value to the user with performance suitable to achieve the desired functions and objectives at the lowest possible cost. The extent to which the maximum value for a product or brand can be obtained depends upon the precision and effectiveness with which the users are able to define the essential generic and esthetic functional characteristics required as well as any limiting constraints.

Five decision options may be exercised by the committee: (*a*) approval for purchase and general use, i.e., the product has become the standard; (*b*) a formal evaluation; (*c*) a limited trial period

Table 16.2.   Scheme for Introducing and Evaluating a Product

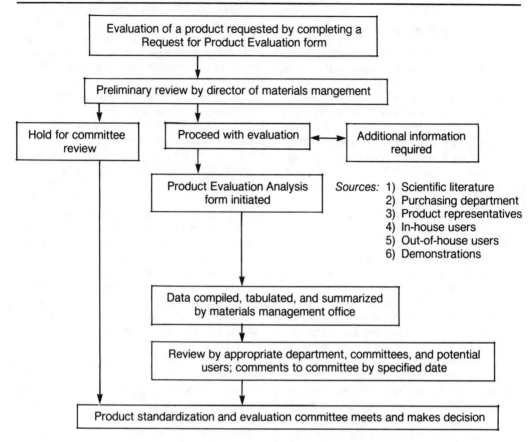

Decision options include: 1) Approve for purchase and general use
2) Initiate an evaluation (for products not yet evaluated)
3) Initiate a limited trial for more extensive evaluation
4) Approve for use by specific or limited groups
5) Do not approve for purchase or use in the hospital

for more extensive evaluation (30 days, 60 days, 90 days, etc); (*d*) approval for use by a specific or limited group of users; or (*e*) not approved for purchase or use in the hospital. Decisions must be promptly disseminated to interested parties and should be accompanied by a brief explanation or justification in the event of disagreement by one or more product advocates.

CAVEATS

We offer the following cautions to the reader based upon personal and published experiences with product standardization and evaluation committees:

1. Be sure that the appropriate high level commitment to the program exists before investing valuable resources.

2. Take time to publicize and describe the goals and objectives of the program to hospital staff, and especially to health care professional groups. Physicians, in particular, are wary of "medicine by committee" and often assume a negative and defensive posture if not convinced of the program's value to them and to their patients. They must understand and believe that the program is intended to improve the quality of care, not just to contain or reduce costs at the expense of that quality. They must also be prepared to make concessions or compromises at times.

3. Be skeptical about "scientific" information provided by sales representatives endorsing their product or brand, but realize that they

Request for Product Evaluation   Request #_____
The Milton S. Hershey Medical Center
The Pennsylvania State University

1. Requesting department:_____ Date_____
   Signature (dept. chairman/director):_____
2. Product: A. Type name:_____
             B. Manufacturer's name:_____
             C. Distributor's name:_____
             D. Approx. cost per unit:_____
3. Is this product an: Addition_____ change_____ to present product used?
4. Does this product replace a current item? Yes_____ No_____
5. If "Yes," what product? (Give name, inventory number, etc.)
6. What is the purpose of this type of product and why do you need it?
   _____
   _____
   _____
7. What are the—Advantages over present: A._____
                                          B._____
                                          C._____
          Disadvantages over present: A._____
                                       B._____
                                       C._____
8. Will this product be used in more than your department or area?
   Explain: (What departments or area will use)
   _____
   _____
9. Will training be necessary for new product?_____ How much?_____
   Will vendor provide training?_____
10. Estimated annual usage/year?_____
11. What is your estimated length of evaluation period needed?_____
12. What quantity of products will be needed for evaluation?_____
13. Will evaluation samples be: Free_____ Purchased_____
14. Additional comments of requestor:_____
    _____
    _____
15. Additional comments and/or questions of standards and evaluation:
    _____
    _____
    _____
    _____
16. Approval to evaluate:_____
    Disapproval to evaluate:_____
    Comments:_____
    _____
    _____
    _____

Signature_____ Date_____
          Chairman, product standards and evaluation committee

Figure 16.1.   Request form for product evaluation.

Product Evaluation Analysis   Request #_____
The Milton S. Hershey Medical Center
The Pennsylvania State University

1. Product: A. Type name:_____
             B. Manufacturer's name:_____
             C. Cost per unit:_____
2. Description and purpose of product:_____
   _____
3. This is an: Addition_____ change_____ to product currently on inventory or used
   in the hospital.
4. What item does this replace, if any?_____
5. Cost comparison per unit: New_____ current_____
6. Evaluation department or area:_____
7. Length of time product evaluated:_____
8. Product—Advantages:
        A._____

        B._____
        Disadvantages:
        A._____

        B._____
9. Is this product useful:
        A. In specific areas of hospital? Yes_____ No_____
            Where?_____
        B. In other areas of hospital? Yes_____ No_____
            Where?_____
10. Is technique improved: Yes_____ No_____
    If "Yes," how?_____
    _____

    _____
11. How does this product compare in quality, effectiveness, and efficiency with product currently
    in use?
    Equal_____ Superior_____ Inferior_____
    Explain:_____

    _____
12. What is reaction of: (good—bad—indifferent)
    Staff using the product:_____
    Patients using the product:_____
13. Does this product: increase_____, decrease_____, same_____ the number of
    items currently being used?
14. Will this product: increase_____, decrease_____, same_____ consumption and/
    or waste?
15. Does this product: increase_____, decrease_____, same_____ labor?
16. How much of present product do we have in stock?_____
17. Will all of existing stock be used before instituting new item?_____
18. Will this product "lock-in" (because of uniqueness) the hospital with a specific supplier?
    Yes_____ No_____
19. What is the experience with this product in other hospitals?
    (Name hospital)_____

    _____
20. Estimate net cost of evaluation:_____
21. Recommend: Further investigation   Yes_____ No_____
                Replace product presently
                  used with new product   Yes_____ No_____
                Reject product   Yes_____ No_____
22. Additional comments:_____

    _____
23. Please return this form to the chairman of the product standards and evaluation committee upon
    completion of evaluation.
24. Signature_____ Date_____
                        (Evaluator)

Figure 16.2. Product evaluation analysis form.

can be a valuable source of information about competitors' products or brands. Make it a practice to request scientific information published in peer-reviewed journals. Such pressure may stimulate industry to fund and promote the necessary scientific documentation of efficacy and safety by independent investigators.

4. Avoid the compulsion to buy the "Cadillac" (top of the line) if the "Chevrolet" will get the job done without sacrificing the quality of care.

5. Be certain to communicate all ongoing evaluations and decisions to all who need or want to know what is going on.

6. Realize ahead of time that you will not please everyone all of the time, but you should please most of them some of the time.

7. In the event the hospital in which you work does not have a hospital-wide standardization and evaluation program, a modified, scaled-down version can be implemented as a subcommittee of the infection control committee. The principles, organization,

and process described herein should still apply.

In summary, the important features of an effective product standardization and evaluation program are as follows: (*a*) high level administrative and professional support and committment; (*b*) control over all products used in the hospital; (*c*) broad-based, multidisciplinary participation; (*d*) an organized system for product evaluation; (*e*) prompt, efficient communication of information and decisions; and (*f*) appropriate in-service training for product introduction.

References

1. Joint Commission on Accreditation of Hospitals: Infection control. In *Accreditation Manual for Hospitals.* Chicago, JCAH, 1984, p 70.
2. Housley CE: The case for materiel management. In *Hospital Materiel Management.* Germantown, MD, Aspen Systems, 1978, p 1.
3. Housley CE: All about the product standardization process. In *Hospital Materiel Management.* Germantown, MD, Aspen Systems, 1978, p 121.
4. Friend PM (ed): Standardization and evaluation of products and equipment. *Hosp Materiel Management Q* 5:1–86, 1983.

Chapter 17

Skin Cleansing

Elaine Larson, Ph.D., F.A.A.N.

For over a century hand washing has been recognized as the primary method to prevent the spread of infectious agents. Like all established traditions, however, hand washing practices have become entrenched with ritual and dogmatism. In this chapter, current understandings about agents and techniques used for patient skin cleansing and surgical scrubbing of the hands and hand washing will be discussed. In the mid-1800s Semmelweis was able to demonstrate, by means of a natural experiment, the importance of disinfection of the skin of the hands in blocking the transmission of infectious agents (Fig. 17.1). Today, there are still many unanswered questions regarding optimal methods and agents for hand washing and skin cleansing, but such questions are now difficult to answer for ethical and practical reasons. It is not ethical, for example, to plan a clinical trial which involves a control group from whom hand washing is withheld. And, as Rotter has recently discussed, thousands of patients would be needed to demonstrate statistically significant differences in infection rates resulting from different hand disinfection regimens (1).

Other problems that make it difficult to plan and interpret hand washing studies include the fact that there is variability within a given individual in bacterial counts on the hands, the fact that an "adequate," clinically significant reduction in bacterial counts on the hands has not been defined, and the fact that results of many studies of hand washing agents or techniques are not comparable because of the wide variety of the study methods and culture techniques used. Problems such as these can result in apparently contradictory findings. Nevertheless, as consistent evidence accumulates, some recommendations can be made with a high degree of certainty.

In 1978, regulations for skin cleansing products were published in the *Federal Register* (2), and seven definitions of products were developed (Table 17.1). Unfortunately, these categories are not particularly helpful in clinical decision making

because they are not mutually exclusive: the same product can fit into several categories.

The Food and Drug Administration (FDA) also recognizes three categories of antimicrobial ingredients for hand washing products: safe and effective for over-the-counter (OTC) use (Category I), not safe or effective for OTC use (Category II), and insufficient data available to permit final classification (Category III). The rigorous testing requirements and monumental expenditures required to accrue sufficient data for classification mean that such agents are often in widespread use well before their safety and efficacy can be unequivocally demonstrated. Examples of this are triclosan and para-chloro-meta-xylenol (PCMX), both contained in many commercially available skin cleansing products and both classified as agents for which insufficient data are available. Even so, when a product for general hand washing is being selected in a health care institution, it is essential that the active ingredients be known so that an informed decision can be made.

PATIENT SKIN CLEANSING
General Skin Care

With the increasing incidence of infections caused by organisms from the patient's own flora, it is surprising that so little attention has been given to keeping the patient's skin as clean as possible. *Staphylococcus epidermidis* and certain coryneforms such as the JK diphtheroid and *Propionibacterium acnes* are examples of bacterial species that reside on the skin and can cause nosocomial infections. In patients hospitalized for more than a few days, gram-negative bacteria and fecal flora are also found with increasing frequency on the skin. It is more than a comfort measure, therefore, to provide the patient with a daily cleansing bath. It is also reasonable to provide patients with means to wash their hands before meals when they are unable to do so.

Though regular, nonmedicated soap is ade-

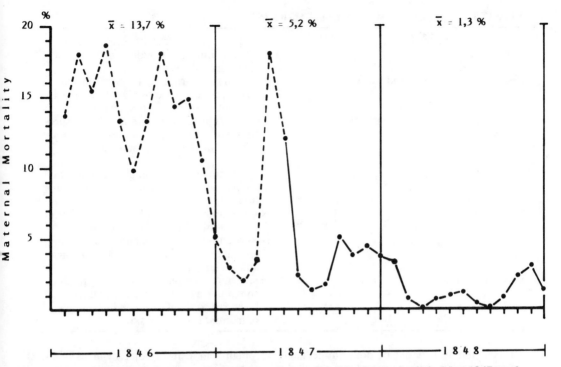

Figure 17.1. Effect of hygienic hand disinfection as introduced by Semmelweis in May 1847 on the maternal mortality at the k.k.l. Obstetric University Clinic in Vienna. - - - = before introduction; — = after introduction. (From Rotter ML: Hygienic hand disinfection. *Infect Control* 5:18–22, 1984.)

quate for most routine bathing, it might be useful for patients at increased risk of infection (those at the extremes of age, with prolonged hospital stays, receiving systemic antimicrobial agents, immunosuppressed, or undergoing major surgery) to use an antibacterial skin cleansing agent for bathing during hospitalization. The substantive effects of such agents might be beneficial in preventing colonization with multiply resistant organisms or organisms endemic in hospital environments. Some investigators have demonstrated dramatic reductions in skin carriage of staphylococci and other flora when total body washes with antibacterial soaps were done (3). Studies of the effect of such washing on subsequent infection rates would determine whether such bathing was of real usefulness.

Whether regular or antibacterial soap is used for bathing, an important aspect of patient skin care is to give special attention to highly sebaceous and/or moist regions (e.g., perineum, anterior nares, axilla, intertriginous spaces) which provide conditions advantageous to microbial proliferation. In addition, patients often have skin areas—such as intravenous insertion sites, wounds, those around monitoring devices and

condom catheters—which are occluded and hence become macerated. Such skin areas are particularly prone to breakdown and infection, and should be routinely cleaned and kept dry.

Skin Preparation for Surgery
Hair Removal

Part of the routine preparation of the patient's operative site has often been a thorough shave to remove all hair, frequently done the day prior to surgery. Mounting evidence suggests, however, that such shaves cause skin damage and increase the risk of bacterial infection (4). In 406 surgical cases, Seropian and Reynolds found a 5.6% wound infection rate after preoperative razor shave, and 0.6% after either a depilatory or after no skin preparation (5). The same findings have been substantiated in other studies (6, 7). Other advantages of a depilatory cream over shaving are that it can be self-administered, is atraumatic, can be used on granulating wounds, and is less expensive (8). Whenever possible, then, hair should not be removed. When it is necessary to remove hair, it should be done with a depilatory or, less desirably, by clipping rather than razor

Table 17.1. Categories of Skin Cleansing Agents (59)

Category	Description
Antimicrobial soap	Soap containing an ingredient active against skin microorganisms.
Health care personnel hand wash	Fast acting, nonirritating preparation containing a broad spectrum antimicrobial ingredient, designed for frequent use.
Patient preoperative skin preparation	Fast acting product containing a broad spectrum antimicrobial agent that significantly reduces numbers of microorganisms on skin.
Skin antiseptic	Nonirritating product containing an antimicrobial agent to prevent overt skin infection.
Skin wound cleanser	Nonirritating product to help remove foreign material from small superficial wounds.
Skin wound protectant	Nonirritating product containing an antimicrobial that provides a protective physical and chemical barrier.
Surgical hand scrub	Fast acting, persistent, nonirritating product containing a broad spectrum antimicrobial, used to significantly reduce numbers of microorganisms on skin.

(9). Hair removal should be done immediately before surgery, since a longer interval between skin preparation and surgery is associated with increased risk of postoperative wound infection (5, 7).

Preoperative Bathing or Showering

Bathing and showering with plain soap result in increased shedding of skin squames containing viable bacteria and subsequent increases in numbers of organisms countable on the surface of the skin. Because of this, preoperative bathing or showering has come into some disfavor. Washing with an antibacterial soap, however, results in decreased shedding of viable bacteria (10). Since there is a relationship between organisms colonizing the skin and those causing subsequent wound infection, it seems reasonable to reduce the skin bacterial reservoirs prior to surgery. Several investigators have recently demonstrated both a reduction in bacterial skin colonization and a reduction in wound infection rates after patients bathed from two to eight times with an antibacterial agent prior to surgery (3, 11–13). In a large trial, 4% chlorhexidine detergent solution used for routine umbilical care in neonates significantly reduced staphylococcal colonization rates over those of controls (14). One Swedish investigator concluded that total body disinfection with such an agent seems to have advantages over local disinfection of the operation field by preventing

contamination from adjacent areas of the skin and delaying recolonization of the skin during the first few postoperative days (13). However, at least one study reported no differences in wound infection rates when patients bathed with nonmedicated bar soap or antimicrobial soap (15). Therefore, evidence is still scanty and the recommendation for such a patient preoperative bathing routine must be made with reservations.

Preparation of Surgical Site

Agents acceptable for skin preparation of patient operative sites are the same as those used for the preoperative scrubs of the hands of the surgical team: agents containing chlorhexidine gluconate or povidone-iodine, and alcohol solutions; 70% (by weight) ethyl and 99% isopropyl alcohol are the most efficient strengths (16). Some investigators feel that chlorhexidine-containing agents have short term advantages over povidone-iodine because of their longer duration of antibacterial activity, the residual effect (17). In an experimental model with artifically contaminated wounds, topically applied chlorhexidine was found to be significantly superior to povidone-iodine in reducing infection rates (18). Povidone-iodine has been reported to cause potential toxic reactions when used in burn patients and when used to irrigate the peritoneal cavity, and to be toxic to phagocytic cells (19, 20). Chlorhexidine, on the other hand, is absorbed very little through skin, and there is no known risk associated with the formulations commercially available (19, 21).

Alcoholic solutions for preoperative skin preparation have fallen into disuse. This is unfortunate, since alcohol is probably still the best skin disinfectant available and its use should be more widespread. In several recent studies, a 1-minute cleansing with alcohol followed by the application of an iodophor-impregnated film to the skin has been found to be equal or superior to the traditional 5-minute scrub with an iodophor for sustaining a mean log reduction in skin bacterial counts for up to 4 hours. The alcohol provides a means to kill bacteria rapidly, and the antimicrobial film may add substantivity. In addition, the alcohol preparation requires about one-third of the time (22, 23). Because "the maximum effect is required on a single application ... alcoholic solutions are always preferred" (24, p 24) for patient preoperative skin preparation. At this time, evidence is insufficient to recommend the use of agents containing PCMX or triclosan for patient presurgical skin cleansing.

HAND WASHING OF HEALTH CARE PERSONNEL
Surgical Scrub

Perhaps no aspect of infection control is more fraught with ritual than is the surgical hand scrub. Some institutions have developed elaborate procedures which can take up to 20 minutes. Available agents and different formulations have proliferated since Semmelweis used a solution of chlorinated lime. Hands of the surgical team are of concern because the majority of gloves become perforated during surgery (16), resulting in considerable wound contamination (25). It is not known, however, what the ideal level of reduction in bacterial populations is (26). Hence, a reasonable goal is that the hands be maximally free of dirt and contaminating organisms and that the colonizing flora be reduced. To meet this goal, an antimicrobial antiseptic should always be part of the regimen for surgical hand scrub.

Agent

Ideally, the choice of scrub agent should be based on studies of differences in wound infection rates. However, such studies have been few, they are often fraught with methodologic problems, and results are equivocal (7, 27). There are three agents which have been evaluated sufficiently to recommend them for use as surgical scrubs: alcoholic solutions (the "gold standard") and agents containing chlorhexidine or povidone-iodine. In general, the latter two result in immediate reductions in bacterial counts of 70 to 80% as compared to 95% reduction with alcohol. Both povidone-iodine and chlorhexidine have increased activity with repeated use, but the substantivity of chlorhexidine has been repeatedly shown to be superior (28–32). In a survey of 623 operating room personnel, chlorhexidine was also shown to be more acceptable, causing fewer skin reactions than povidone-iodine (33). Triclosan has good residual effect, but probably does not result in as high immediate reductions in bacterial counts (24), though some have found it to be quite effective in an alcoholic solution (34, 35).

The alcohol-based hand washes and foams, especially those containing chlorhexidine, have recently been shown to be a highly efficacious, cost- and time-efficient alternative to aqueous solutions for surgical hand scrub and for patient skin disinfection (28–31, 36, 37). In one small study, a "social hand wash" followed by an application of chlorhexidine in methanol was more acceptable to staff, nonirritating to skin, less time consuming, 5 times cheaper, and resulted in no increase in wound infection rates when compared with a standard 5-minute scrub with an aqueous detergent solution containing chlorhexidine (38). Others have found that, contrary to general opinion, the alcoholic preparations available today are not particularly drying to the skin and are quite acceptable to hospital personnel, even after frequent and prolonged use (32, 37, 39). In addition, alcohols have an excellent spectrum of antimicrobial activity and are rapid in their killing effect (40). They seem, therefore, to be the most acceptable products for use as surgical scrubs (41). They are, however, inactivated by proteins and mucus and should, therefore, be applied after dirt is removed by a social hand wash.

Technique

Dineen demonstrated that a 5-minute scrub was as good as a 10-minute scrub in effecting reductions in bacterial counts, regardless of the agent used (42). The 5-minute scrub is now recommended by the Association of Operating Room Nurses (AORN) (43). They also recommend the use of a brush or sponge for scrubbing. The brush or sponge should be single-use or sterilized between uses (40) and should be soft enough to prevent skin trauma. The AORN recommendation to remove rings and watches is reasonable, since rings and watches interfere with effective scrubbing. Probably the most important aspect of a scrub technique is that it be thorough and consistent. The method of application of the disinfectant is as important as the agent itself.

Because it is clear that most long term flora on the hands reside in the nails and the subungual regions, special attention is required for these areas (44). Subungual debris must be carefully removed. A logical procedure for surgical scrub might include a short period of soaking of the hands to loosen subungual debris, a careful cleaning of the nails with a file, a social hand wash with plain or antiseptic soap and drying with a clean towel, followed by application of an alcohol-based antiseptic solution and air drying. There is little evidence that a regimented, longer scrub is of additional benefit.

"Although pre-operative hand disinfection is a rational procedure, it may be that ... a hygienic hand disinfection method (i.e., thorough application of agent for 30 seconds) would be as effective in preventing infection as the usual, more prolonged procedure" (24, p 27).

Hand Washing for General Patient Care

Agents

There is insufficient evidence that soaps containing antibacterial agents are indicated over plain soaps for routine hand washing in health care settings (1, 26). One group of investigators reported a significant reduction in nosocomial infections rates in a medical intensive care unit (ICU), but not the surgical ICU or coronary care unit, when antimicrobial soaps as compared to plain soaps were used for hand washing (45). More such studies are needed. In the meantime, it probably makes sense to use an antimicrobial product such as those mentioned under "Surgical Scrub" during certain high risk situations: before insertion of central catheters or pressure monitoring tubing, and with newborns, the immunosuppressed, and patients with damage to their integumentary system (46). In sites (e.g., home health visits) where adequate hand washing facilities may not be available, antiseptic foams, which can be used without water, are excellent (39).

Though the ecologic balance of the flora of the hand is probably not altered to any great extent by washing with an antiseptic (47), it is most important that agents chosen for hand washing be acceptable to personnel (48, 49). The concern that plain soap can serve as a reservoir to trans-

mission of infection is probably exaggerated (50, 51).

Technique

Of much greater concern than the particular hand washing agent used (since any of those available is probably adequate) is how to motivate personnel to practice acceptable hand washing technique (52–54). Indeed, the observed duration of hand washing of health care personnel in two ICUs was a mean of 8.62 (± 0.29) seconds (55), less than the 10-second minimum time recommended by Centers for Disease Control (40). Others have found that a major observed procedural error of nursing personnel is failure to wash hands (53, 56). It is the author's opinion that the most important way to influence hand washing behavior is by means of role models (57) and by use of other intrinsic and extrinsic motivational techniques (58). In addition, it is essential to continue to study the location of bacteria on the hands. Despite the fact that most of the bacterial flora of the hands resides in the subungual area, the palm and dorsa of the hands receive much more attention during hand washing. In summary, it is suggested that the two most pressing needs in the area of hand washing are (a) the need to improve techniques for motivating staff to wash their hands and (b) the need to identify more specifically the locations of bacteria on the hands and to modify washing techniques to reach these target areas. It should also be pointed out that the relative role of bacteria comprising the nontransient flora on the hands in subsequent nosocomial infection needs further study.

References

1. Rotter ML: Hygienic hand disinfection. *Infect Control* 5:18–22, 1984.
2. Test for health care personnel hand-wash effectiveness. *Federal Register* 43:1210–1249, 1978.
3. Brandberg A, Anderson J: Whole body disinfection by shower-bath with chlorhexidine soap. In Maibach H, Aly R (eds): *Skin Microbiology.* New York, Springer-Verlag, 1981.
4. Hamilton HW, Hamilton KR, Lone FJ: Pre-operative hair removal. *Can J Surg* 20:269–275, 1971.
5. Seropian R, Reynolds BM: Wound infections after preoperative depilatory versus razor preparation. *Am J Surg* 121:251–254, 1971.
6. Count-Brown CM: Pre-operative skin depilation and its effect on post-operative wound infections. *J R Coll Surg Edinb* 26:238–241, 1981.
7. Cruse PJE, Foford R: A five-year prospective study of 23,649 surgical wounds. *Arch Surg* 107:206–210, 1973.
8. Powis SJA, Waterworth TA, Arkell DG: Preoper-

ative skin preparation: clinical evaluation of depilatory cream. *Br Med J* 2:1166–1168, 1976.

9. Alexander JW, Fischer JE, Boyajian M, Palanquist J, Morris MJ: The influence of hair-removal methods on wound infections. *Arch Surg* 118:347–352, 1983.

10. Meers PD, Yeo GA: Shedding of bacteria and skin squames after handwashing. *J Hyg Camb* 81:99–105, 1978.

11. Brandberg A, Holm J, Hanmarsten J, Schersten T: Postoperative wound infections in vascular surgery: effect of preoperative whole body disinfection by shower-bath with chlorhexidine soap. In Maibach H, Aly R (eds): *Skin Microbiology*. New York, Springer-Verlag, 1981.

12. Davies J, Babb JR, Ayliffe GAJ, Wilkins MD: Disinfection of the skin of the abdomen. *Br J Surg* 65:855–858, 1978.

13. Seeberg S, Lindberg A, Bergman BR: Preoperative shower bath with 4% chlorhexidine detergent solution. Reduction of *Staphylococcus aureus* in skin carriers and practical application. In Maibach H, Aly R (eds): *Skin Microbiology*. New York, Springer-Verlag, 1981.

14. Seeberg S, Brinkhoff B: Epidemiology and control of staphylococcal pyoderma among newborn infants. *J Hosp Infect* 5:121–136, 1984.

15. Ayliffe GAJ, Noy MF, Babb JR, et al: A comparison of preoperative bathing with chlorhexidine detergent and non-medicated soap in the prevention of wound infection. *J Hosp Infect* 4:237–244, 1983.

16. Altemeier WA: Surgical antiseptics. In Block SS (ed): *Disinfection, Sterilization and Preservation*, ed 2. Philadelphia, Lea & Febiger, 1977.

17. Goldblum SE, Ulrich JA, Boldman RS, Reed WP, Avasthi PS: Comparison of 4% chlorhexidine gluconate in a detergent base (Hibiclens) and povidone-iodine (Betadine) for the skin preparation of hemodialysis patients and personnel. *Am J Kidney Dis* 2:548–552, 1983.

18. Platt J, Bucknall RA: An experimental evaluation of antiseptic wound irrigation. *J Hosp Infect* 5:181–188, 1984.

19. Kaul AF, Jewett JF: Agents and techniques for disinfection of the skin. *Surg Gynecol Obstet* 152:677–685, 1981.

20. Van den Broek PJ, Buys LFM, Van Furth R: Interaction of povidone iodine compounds, phagocytic cells and microorganisms. *Antimicrob Agents Chemother* 22:593–597, 1982.

21. Rosenberg A, Alatary SD, Peterson AF: Safety and efficacy of the antiseptic chlorhexidine gluconate. *Surg Gynecol Obstet* 143:789–792, 1976.

22. Geelhoed GW, Sharpe K, Simon GL: A comparative study of surgical skin preparation methods. *Surg Gynecol Obstet* 157:265–268, 1983.

23. Ulrich JA, Beck WC: Surgical skin preparation regimens: comparison of antimicrobial efficacy. *Infect Surg* 3:569–572, 1984.

24. Ayliffe GAJ: Surgical scrub and skin disinfection. *Infect Control* 5:23–27, 1984.

25. Cole WR: Preparation of the patient and his operative care. Presented at the First Symposium on Control of Surgical Infections. American College of Surgeons, Fort Lauderdale, FL, 1970.

26. Steere AC, Mallison GF: Handwashing practices for the prevention of nosocomial infections. *Ann Intern Med* 83:683–690, 1975.

27. Davidson AIG, Clarke C, Smith G: Postoperative wound infection: a computer analysis. *Br J Surg* 58:333–337, 1971.

28. Aly R, Maibach HI: Comparative study on the antimicrobial effect of 0.5% chlorhexidine gluconate and 70% isopropyl alcohol on the normal flora of hands. *Appl Environ Microbiol* 37:610–613, 1979.

29. Aly R, Maibach HI: Comparative evaluation of chlorhexidine gluconate (Hibicleus®) and povidone-iodine (E-Z Scrub®) sponge/brushes for presurgical hand scrubbing. *Curr Ther Res* 34:740–745, 1983.

30. LaRocca MAK, LaRocca PT: An evaluation of the antimicrobial effect of a hand sponge-brush impregnated with 4% chlorhexidine gluconate (Hibiclens). In *Developments in Industrial Microbiology*. Arlington, VA, Society for Industrial Microbiology, 1982, vol 23.

31. LaRocca PT, LaRocca MAK: An evaluation of the antimicrobial efficacy of a 0.5% chlorhexidine gluconate-70% isopropyl alcohol solution (Hibitane Tincture) when used for skin antisepsis. In *Developments in Industrial Microbiology*. Arlington, VA, Society for Industrial Microbiology, 1982, vol 23.

32. Ojajarvi J: Effectiveness of handwashing and disinfection methods in removing transient bacteria after patient nursing. *J Hyg Camb* 85:193–203, 1980.

33. Mitchell KG, Rawluk DJR: Skin reactions related to surgical scrub-up: results of a Scottish survey. *Br J Surg* 71:223–224, 1984.

34. Bartzokas CA, Corkill JE, Makin T, Pinder DC: Assessment of the remnent antibacterial effect of a 2% triclosan-detergent preparation on the skin. *J Hyg Camb* 91:521–528, 1983.

35. Bartzoks CA, Gibson MF, Graham R, Pinder DC: A comparison of triclosan and chlorhexidine preparations with 60 per cent isopropyl alcohol for hygienic hand disinfection. *J Hosp Infect* 4:245–255, 1983.

36. Beck WC: Alcohol foam for hand disinfection. *AORN J* 32:1087–1088, 1980.

37. Beck WC: How clean-hands people keep hands clean. *Infect Surg* 1:73–74, 1982.

38. Murie JA, Macpherson SG: Chlorhexidine in methanol for the preoperative cleansing of surgeons' hands: a clinical trial. *Scot Med J* 25:309–311, 1980.

39. Nystrom B: Scandinavian experience differs (letter). *Infect Control* 5:211, 1984.

40. Centers for Disease Control: Antiseptics, handwashing, and handwashing facilities. Guidelines activity, Hospital Infections Branch, Center for Infectious Disease. Atlanta, Department of Health and Human Services, 1981.

41. Rotter M, Koller W, Wewalk G: Povidone-iodine and chlorhexidine gluconate-containing detergents for disinfection of hands. *J Hosp Infect* 1:149–158, 1980.

42. Dineen P: An evaluation of the duration of the surgical scrub. *Surg Gynecol Obstet* 129:1181–1184, 1969.

43. Recommended Practice Subcommittee: Proposed

recommended practices for surgical scrubs. *AORN J* 37:82–85, 1983.

44. Hann JB: The source of the "resident" flora. *Hand* 5:247–252, 1973.
45. Massanari RM, Hierholzer WJ: A crossover comparison of antiseptic soaps on nosocomial infection rates in intensive care units. Presented at Association for Practitioners in Infection Control annual meeting, Washington, DC, 1984.
46. Soule BM (ed): *The APIC Curriculum for Infection Control Practice*. Dubuque, IA, Kendall/Hunt, 1983, vol I, pp 552–560.
47. Larson EL: Persistent carriage of gram-negative bacteria on hands. *Am J Infect Control* 9:112–119, 1981.
48. Ojajarvi J: The importance of soap selection for routine hand hygiene in hospital. *J Hyg Camb* 86:275–277, 1981.
49. Larson E, Killien M: Factors influencing handwashing behavior of patient care personnel. *Am J Infect Control* 10:93–99, 1982.
50. Bannon EA, Judge LF: Bacteriological studies relating to handwashing. I. The inability of soap bars to transmit bacteria. *Am J Public Health* 55:915–922, 1965.
51. Heinze JE: Bar soap and liquid soap (letter). *JAMA* 251:3222–3223, 1984.
52. Albert RF, Condie F: Hand-washing patterns in medical intensive-care units. *N Engl J Med* 304:1465–1466, 1981.
53. Larson EL: Compliance with isolation technique. *Am J Infect Control* 11:221–225, 1983.
54. Taylor LJ: An evaluation of handwashing techniques. *Nurs Times* 74:108–110, 1978.
55. Quraishi ZA, McGuckin M, Blais FX: Duration of handwashing in intensive care units: a descriptive study. *Am J Infect Control* 12:83–87, 1984.
56. McLane C, Chenelly S, Sylvestrak ML, Kirchhoff KT: A nursing practice problem: failure to observe aseptic technique. *Am J Infect Control* 11:178–182, 1983.
57. Larson E, Larson E: Influence of a role model on handwashing behavior (abstract). *Am J Infect Control* 11:146, 1983.
58. Larson E: Current handwashing issue. *Infect Control* 5:15–17, 1984.
59. Eiermann HJ: Antimicrobials: regulatory aspects. In Maibach H, Aly R (eds): *Skin Microbiology*. New York, Springer-Verlag, 1981.

Chapter 18

Disinfection, Sterilization, and Waste Disposal

William A. Rutala, Ph.D., M.P.H.

INTRODUCTION

The necessity for appropriate disinfection, sterilization, and waste disposal procedures has been emphasized by dozens of articles documenting infection after improper decontamination of patient care items and waste disposal practices. Since it is unnecessary to sterilize all patient care items, hospital policies must identify whether cleaning, disinfection, or sterilization is indicated based primarily on an item's intended use but considering other factors, including cost. In this chapter, a pragmatic approach to the judicious selection and proper use of disinfection and sterilization processes is presented, in addition to a discussion of the approved methods for disposal of hazardous waste.

DEFINITION OF TERMS

Sterilization is the complete elimination or destruction of all forms of microbial life and is accomplished in the hospital by physical or chemical processes. Steam under pressure, dry heat, ethylene oxide gas, and liquid chemicals are the principal sterilizing agents used in the hospital. Sterilization is intended to convey an absolute meaning, not a relative one. Unfortunately, some health professionals as well as the technical and commercial literature refer to "disinfection" as "sterilization" and items as "partially sterile." When chemicals are used for the purposes of destroying all forms of microbiologic life, including fungal and bacterial spores, they may be called chemosterilizers. These same germicides used for shorter exposure periods may also be part of the disinfection process.

Disinfection describes a process that eliminates all pathogenic microorganisms on inanimate objects with the exception of the bacterial endospore. The efficacy of disinfection is affected by a number of factors, each of which may nullify or limit the efficacy of the process. Some of the factors that have been shown to affect disinfection efficacy are: the prior cleaning of the object; the organic load present; the type and level of microbial contamination; the concentration of and exposure time to the germicide, the nature of the object (e.g., crevices, hinges, lumens); and the temperature and pH of the disinfection process.

By definition, then, disinfection differs from sterilization by its lack of sporicidal property, but this is obviously an oversimplification. A few disinfectants will kill spores with prolonged exposure times (6 to 10 hours) and are called chemosterilizers. At similar concentrations but with shorter exposure periods (< 30 minutes) these same disinfectants may kill all microorganisms excluding bacterial endospores and are called high level disinfectants. Other disinfectants (low level) may kill the vegetative bacteria, fungi, and lipophilic viruses in a practical period of time (< 10 minutes), whereas others (intermediate level) may be cidal for tubercle bacilli and hydrophilic viruses with longer exposure periods (> 30 minutes). It is apparent that the germicides differ markedly among themselves primarily in their antimicrobial spectrum and rapidity of action. Table 18.1 will be later discussed and consulted in this context.

Cleaning, on the other hand, is the removal of any foreign material (e.g., soil, organic material) from objects, and it is normally accomplished using water with or without detergents. Cleaning must precede disinfection and sterilization procedures. Decontamination is a procedure that removes pathogenic microorganisms from objects so they are safe to handle.

Other terms that deserve discussion because they are found in the literature are words with a "cidal" suffix, such as germicide. A germicide is an agent that destroys microorganisms, particularly pathogenic organisms ("germs"). It is like the word disinfectant with the difference that germicide applies to compounds used on both

Table 18.1. Methods of Sterilization and Disinfection*

			Disinfection	
	Sterilization		High Level	Intermediate to Low Level
Object	*Critical Items:* Will enter tissue or vascular system or blood will flow through		*Semicritical Items:* Will come in contact with mucous membranes but not enter tissue or vascular system	*Noncritical Items:* Will not come in contact with mucous membranes or skin that is not intact
Object	Procedure	Exposure Time (hr)	Procedure (Exposure Time ≥ 10–30 min)†	Procedure (Exposure Time ≤ 10 min)
Smooth, hard surface	A	mfr rec	C	H
	B	mfr rec	D	J
	C	10	E	K
	D	6	F	L
	E	6	G	M
			I	
Rubber tubing and catheters	A	mfr rec	C	
	B	mfr rec	D	
	D	6	E	
	E	6	F	
Polyethylene tubing and catheters‡·§	A	mfr rec	C	
	B	mfr rec	D	
	C	10	E	
	D	6	F	
	E	6	I	
Lensed instruments	B	mfr rec	C	
	C	10	D	
	D	6	E	
	E	6		
Thermometers (oral and rectal)¶	B	mfr rec	I	
	C	10		
	D	6		
	E	6		
Hinged instruments	A	mfr rec	C	
	B	mfr rec	D	
	C	10	E	
	D	6		
	E	6		

* Modified from Simmons BP: CDC guideline for hospital environmental control. *Am J Infect Control* 11:96–115, 1983.

Key:

A Heat sterilization including steam or hot air (see manufacturer's recommendations)

B Ethylene oxide gas (for time, see manufacturer's recommendations).

C Glutaraldehyde-based formulations (2%). A glutaraldehyde-phenate formulation also has been shown to be effective for high level disinfection of respiratory therapy equipment at a glutaraldehyde concentration of 0.13%. Caution should be exercised with all glutaraldehyde formulations when further in-use dilution is anticipated.

D Demand release chloride dioxide (will corrode aluminum, copper, brass, series 400 stainless steel, and chrome with prolonged exposure).

E Six percent stabilized hydrogen peroxide (will corrode copper, zinc, and brass).

F Wet pasteurization at 75°C for 30 minutes after detergent cleaning.

G Sodium hypochlorite (1000 ppm of available chlorine) (will corrode metal instruments)

H Ethyl or isopropyl alcohol (70 to 90%).

I Ethyl alcohol (70 to 90%).

J Sodium hypochlorite (100 ppm of available chlorine).

K Phenolic germicidal detergent solution (follow the product label for use dilution).

L Iodophor germicidal detergent solution (follow the product label for use dilution).

M Quaternary ammonium germicidal detergent solution (follow the product label for use dilution).

† The longer the exposure to a disinfectant, the more likely it is that all bacteria will be eliminated. Ten minutes' exposure may not be adeqeuate to disinfect many objects, especially those that are difficult to clean because they have narrow channels or other areas that can harbor organic material and bacteria. Thirty minutes' exposure may be the minimum time needed to kill *M. tuberculosis* reliably with glutaraldehyde.

‡ Tubing must be completely filled for disinfection.

§ Thermostability should be investigated when indicated.

¶ Do not mix rectal and oral thermometers at any stage of handling or processing.

living tissue and inanimate objects, whereas disinfectants are applied only to inanimate objects. Other words with the suffix "cide" (e.g., virucide, fungicide, bactericide, sporicide, tuberculocide) destroy the microorganism identified by the prefix. For example, a bactericide is an agent that kills bacteria (1–4).

A RATIONAL APPROACH TO DISINFECTION AND STERILIZATION

Nearly 20 years ago a rational approach to disinfection and sterilization of patient care items or equipment was devised by Spaulding (2). This classification scheme is so clear and logical that it has been retained, refined, and successfully used by infection control practitioners and others when planning methods for disinfection or sterilization (1, 3). Spaulding believed that the nature of disinfection could be understood more readily if instruments and items for patient care were divided into three categories based on the degree of risk of infection involved in the use of the items. The three categories of risk of patient care items Spaulding described were critical, semicritical, and noncritical.

Critical Items

Critical items are so called because of the high risk of infection if such an item is contaminated with any microorganism, including bacterial spores. Thus, it is critical that objects which enter sterile tissue or the vascular system be sterile. This category includes surgical instruments, cardiac and urinary catheters, implants, intravenous fluids, and needles. Most of the items in this category should be purchased as sterile or sterilized by autoclaving if possible. If heat-labile, the object may be treated with ethylene oxide or chemosterilizers if other methods are unsuitable. Table 18.1 shows several germicides categorized as chemosterilizers. These include 2% glutaraldehyde-based formulations, 6% stabilized hydrogen peroxide, and demand release chlorine dioxide. The latter procedure can be relied upon to produce sterility only if cleaning precedes treatment and proper guidelines as to organic load, contact time, temperature, and pH are met.

Semicritical Items

It is semicritical that objects which come in contact with mucous membranes or skin that is not intact be free of all microorganisms with the exception of bacterial spores. Intact mucous membranes are generally resistant to infection by common bacterial spores but are susceptible to other organisms, such as tubercle bacilli and viruses. Respiratory therapy and anesthesia equipment, gastrointestinal endoscopes, and thermometers are included in this category. Semicritical items minimally require high level disinfection using wet pasteurization or chemical germicides. Glutaraldehyde, stabilized hydrogen peroxide, ethyl alcohol, and chlorine and chlorine compounds are dependable high level disinfectants provided the factors influencing germicidal procedures are considered (Table 18.1).

It is recommended that these items should be rinsed with sterile water or tap water with at least 10 ppm (milligrams per liter) of chlorine. After rinsing, items must be dried with a method that does not recontaminate the item (e.g., filtered hot air) and are generally packaged prior to use.

Hydrotherapy tanks used for patients with skin that is not intact may be effectively disinfected with high (i.e., chlorine) or intermediate level disinfectants (i.e., phenolic, iodophor).

Noncritical Items

These items come in contact with intact skin but not mucous membranes. Intact skin acts as an effective barrier to most microorganisms, and sterility is "not critical." Examples of noncritical items are bedpans, blood pressure cuffs, crutches, bed rails, linens, some food utensils, bedside tables, and patient furniture. In contrast to critical and some semicritical items, most noncritical reusable items can be cleaned where they are used and do not need to be transported to a central processing area. The low level disinfectants listed for noncritical items in Table 18.1 may be used.

As a guide to the appropriate selection and use of disinfectants, a table was prepared by the Centers for Disease Control (CDC) and is presented in modified form (Table 18.1). This table contains several significant changes from the original guideline. First, formaldehyde-alcohol has been deleted as a chemosterilizer and high level disinfectant because it no longer has a role in disinfection strategies. It is corrosive, irritating, toxic, and not commonly used. Second, a new chemosterilizer, demand release chlorine dioxide, has been added to the table. Third, 3% phenolic and iodophors have been deleted as high level disinfectants because of their unproven efficacy against *Mycobacterium tuberculosis* with an exposure time of ≤ 30 minutes. Lastly, isopropyl alcohol has been excluded as a high level disinfectant because of its inability to inactivate hydrophilic viruses.

PROBLEMS WITH DISINFECTION AND STERILIZATION OF HOSPITAL EQUIPMENT

One problem associated with the aforementioned scheme is oversimplification. For example, it does not consider problems with processing complicated medical equipment (5–7) that is often heat-labile or problems inactivating certain microorganisms. Thus, in some situations it is still difficult to choose a method of decontamination, after considering the categories of risk to patients. This is especially true for medical devices in the semicritical category because, unlike critical and noncritical items which require sterilization and low level disinfection, respectively, there is a controversy about whether to sterilize or high level disinfect semicritical medical devices or patient care equipment. The CDC recommendation is that endoscopes, anesthesia equipment, and respiratory therapy equipment should receive high level disinfection (8). Sterilization would not be a problem if semicritical items could be steam sterilized, but most of these items are heat-labile and sterilization is achieved by using ethylene oxide, which may be too time consuming for routine use between patients. And although the value of sterilization of semicritical items at first seems obvious, evidence that sterilization improves patient care by reducing the infection risk is lacking. In fact, the one study that evaluated the infection benefits of sterilization of semicritical equipment demonstrated that sterile anesthesia breathing circuits did not prevent postoperative pulmonary infections when compared to soap and water-washed reusable breathing circuits (9). Presumably, these reasons account for why the majority of procedures done in most hospitals with semicritical equipment are performed with equipment that has been processed by high level disinfection, not sterilization.

High level disinfection can be expected to destroy all microorganisms, with the exception of bacterial spores. An immersion time from 10 to 30 minutes in the preferred disinfectant, glutaraldehyde, may be required to decontaminate adequately semicritical items such as endoscopes between patient procedures, particularly in view of the disputed tuberculocidal efficacy of the solution. Erring on the side of caution, some have recommended a 30-minute contact time for endoscopes to ensure destruction of microorganisms such as *M. tuberculosis* (6). It must be highlighted that meticulous cleaning must precede any sterilization or disinfection procedures, or outbreaks of infection may occur. Examining

nosocomial infections related only to endoscopes one finds several reports involving numerous microorganisms (e.g., *M. tuberculosis, Pseudomonas aeruginosa, Serratia marcescens, Salmonella* sp) attributable either to inadequate cleaning, improper selection of a disinfecting agent, or a portion of the equipment was not exposed to the disinfectant (10–14). Endoscopic instruments are particularly difficult to disinfect and easy to damage because of their intricate design and delicate materials.

Should we sterilize or high level disinfect semicritical medical devices contaminated with blood from AIDS or hepatitis B virus patients or respiratory secretions from a patient with pulmonary tuberculosis? Again, the CDC recommendation is that these items should receive high level disinfection. The evaluation of chemical disinfectants against hepatitis B virus and the human T lymphotropic virus type III (putative AIDS agent) has been hampered for several reasons, including the inability to culture the hepatitis B virus, but recent experiments have shown that these viruses are not resistant to chemical disinfection (15–17) and the present recommendation of 1:10 household bleach (5.25% sodium hypochlorite) for cleaning blood spills appears adequate (18, 19). Additionally, glutaraldehyde-based products should prove quite sufficient to disinfect medical instruments contaminated with these agents and *M. tuberculosis*.

Another infectious agent that may require unique decontamination recommendations is the virus of Creutzfeldt-Jakob disease. The authors studying this disease recommend autoclaving for 1 hour at a temperature of at least 121°C (15 psi) as the preferred method for the sterilization of contaminated material, but a 1-hour exposure to 1 N sodium hydroxide provides excellent disinfection of inanimate surfaces when autoclaving is impossible (20, 21).

FACTORS AFFECTING THE EFFICACY OF GERMICIDES

The activity of germicides against microorganisms depends on a number of factors, some of which are intrinsic qualities of the organism while others depend on the chemical and external physical environment. An awareness of these factors should lead to a better utilization of disinfection and sterilization processes; thus they will be briefly reviewed. More extensive consideration of these and other factors may be found in the references for this section (1, 2, 22, 23).

Number and Location of Microorganisms

All other conditions remaining constant, the larger the number of microbes present, the longer it takes for a germicide to destroy all of them. This relationship was illustrated by Spaulding when he employed identical test conditions and demonstrated that it took 30 minutes to kill 10 *Bacillus subtilis* spores but 3 hours to kill 100,000 *B. subtilis* spores using 8% formaldehyde-67% isopropanol. This is obviously one reason for scrupulous cleaning of instruments prior to disinfection. By reducing the number of microorganisms present on surfaces which must be inactivated, one correspondingly shortens the exposure time required to kill the entire microbial load.

The location of microorganisms must also be considered when assessing factors affecting the efficacy of germicides. Medical instruments with multiple pieces must be disassembled, and equipment such as endoscopes, which have crevices, joints, and channels, is more difficult to disinfect than a flat surface because problems may arise in the penetration of a disinfectant to all parts of the equipment. Only surfaces in direct contact with the germicide will be disinfected, so there must be no air pockets and the equipment must be completely immersed for the entire exposure period. Manufacturers should be encouraged to produce equipment that is engineered so cleaning and disinfection may be accomplished with facility.

Innate Resistance of Microorganisms

As mentioned throughout this chapter, microorganisms vary greatly in their resistance to chemical germicides. Implicit in all disinfection strategies is the consideration that the most resistant microbial subpopulation controls the sterilization or disinfection time. That is, if one wishes to destroy the most resistant types of microorganisms-bacterial spores, one needs to employ exposure times as well as a concentration of germicides needed to achieve complete destruction. Bacterial endospores possess the most innate resistance to chemical germicides followed by tubercle bacilli, fungal spores, hydrophilic viruses, vegetative fungi, lipophilic viruses, and vegetative bacterial cells. The germicidal resistance exhibited by the gram-positive and gram-negative bacteria is similar with the exception of *P. aeruginosa* which shows greater resistance to some disinfectants (24, 25). These bacteria have also been shown to be significantly more resistant to a variety of disinfectants in their "naturally occurring" state as compared to cells subcultured on laboratory media. Interestingly, antibiotic-resistant hospital strains of common nosocomial pathogens (i.e., *P. aeruginosa*, *Klebsiella pneumoniae*, *Escherichia coli*, *Staphylococcus aureus*, *Staphylococcus epidermidis*, and enterococcus) are equally susceptible to germicides as antibiotic-sensitive strains (25). Unfortunately, rickettsiae, chlamydiae, and mycoplasma cannot be placed in this scale of relative resistance because information on the efficacy of germicides against these agents is lacking. Since these microorganisms contain lipid and are similar in structure and composition to other bacteria, one would suspect that they would be inactivated by the same germicides that destroy lipophilic viruses and vegetative bacterial cells.

Concentration and Potency of Germicides

With other variables constant, and with a few exceptions, the more concentrated the germicide, the greater its efficacy and the shorter the time necessary to achieve microbial kill. Generally not recognized, however, is that all germicides are not similarly affected by concentration adjustments. One can predict how dilution affects the efficiency of a disinfectant via the concentration exponent which is a measure of the effect of changes in concentration to cell death. To illustrate, quaternary ammonium compounds and phenol have concentration exponents of 1 and 6, respectively; thus halving the concentration of a quaternary ammonium compound will only double its disinfecting time, but halving the concentration of a phenol solution will result in a marked increase in its disinfecting time by 2^6 (32 times).

It is also important to consider the length of the disinfection time which is dependent upon the potency of the germicide. This was illustrated by Spaulding, who demonstrated that 70% isopropyl alcohol destroyed 10^4 *M. tuberculosis* using the mucin-loop test in 5 minutes, whereas a simultaneous test with 3% phenolic required 2 to 3 hours to achieve the same level of microbial kill.

Physical and Chemical Factors

Several physical and chemical factors also influence germicidal procedures, including temperature, pH, relative humidity, and water hardness. For example, the activity of most germicides increases as the temperature increases, but there are exceptions (e.g., sodium hydroxide). One must not, however, exceed the point at which the germicide itself degrades, producing a potential health hazard and weakening its germicidal activity.

An increase in pH improves the antimicrobial activity of some germicides (e.g., glutaraldehyde, quaternary ammonium compounds) but decreases the antimicrobial activity of others (e.g., phenols, hypochlorites, iodine). The pH influences the antimicrobial activity by altering the germicidal molecule or the cell surface.

Relative humidity is the single most important factor influencing the activity of gaseous disinfectants such as ethylene oxide or formaldehyde.

Water hardness reduces the rate of kill of certain germicides. This occurs because divalent cations (magnesium and calcium) interact with soap to form insoluble precipitates.

Organic Matter

Organic matter in the form of serum, blood, pus, or fecal material may interfere with the antimicrobial activity of disinfectants in at least two ways. Most commonly the interference occurs by a chemical reaction between the germicide and the organic matter resulting in a complex that is less germicidal or nongermicidal, leaving less of the active germicide available for attacking microorganisms. Chlorine and iodine disinfectants, in particular, are prone to such interaction. Alternatively, organic material may protect microorganisms from attack by acting as a physical barrier. Once again we justify the importance of meticulous cleaning of medical devices before any sterilization or disinfection procedure.

Duration of Exposure

Items must be exposed to the appropriate germicide for certain minimum contact times to be disinfected. The exact times for disinfecting medical items are somewhat elusive because of the complicated interaction of the aforementioned factors on disinfection efficacy. Contact times that have proved reliable for some time are presented in Table 18.1, but one must remember that with exceptions, the longer the germicidal process is allowed to progress the greater is its germicidal effectiveness.

FACTORS AFFECTING THE STERILIZATION PROCEDURES

Most of the factors mentioned above also affect the sterilization process. They include number, type, and location of microorganisms; organic matter; concentration (i.e., ethylene oxide gas); duration of exposure; and some physical factors, such as temperature and relative humidity.

DISINFECTION

A great number of disinfectants are used in the health care setting to include: alcohol; chlorine and chlorine compounds; formaldehyde; glutaraldehyde; hydrogen peroxide; iodophors; phenolics and quaternary ammonium compounds. These germicides are not interchangeable and an overview of the performance characteristics of each is intended to provide the user with sufficient information to select an appropriate disinfectant for any item and to use it in the most efficient way. In addition, it should be recognized that excessive costs may be attributed to incorrect concentrations, inappropriate germicides, and sometimes the selection of name-brand germicides rather than generics.

Chemical Disinfectants

Alcohol

Overview. In the sphere of hospital disinfection the word "alcohol" refers to two water-soluble chemical compounds whose germicidal characteristics are generally underrated; they are ethyl alcohol and isopropyl alcohol (26). These alcohols are rapidly bactericidal rather than bacteriostatic against vegetative forms of bacteria; they are also tuberculocidal, fungicidal, and virucidal, but they do not destroy bacterial spores. Their cidal activity drops sharply when diluted below 50% concentration, and the optimum bactericidal concentration is in the range of 60 to 90% by volume (27). The properties of alcohol are listed in Table 18.2, together with the cost.

Mode of Action. The most feasible explanation for the antimicrobial action is denaturation of proteins. This finds support in the observation that absolute ethyl alcohol, a dehydrating agent, is less bactericidal than mixtures of alcohol and water because proteins are denatured more quickly in the presence of water (28). Protein denaturation is also consistent with the observations by Sykes (29) that alcohol destroys the dehydrogenases of *E. coli* and Dagley and associates (30) that ethyl alcohol increases the lag phase of *Enterobacter aerogenes* and this could be reversed by the addition of certain amino acids. The latter authors concluded that the bacteriostatic action was due to the inhibition of the production of metabolites essential for rapid cell division.

Table 18.2. Some Common Germicides with Their Use Dilutions, Properties, and Cost*†

Germicide	Use Dilution	Level of Disinfection	Inactivates‡						Important Characteristics									Approximate Cost	
			Bacteria	Lipophilic Viruses	Hydrophilic Virus	M. tuberculosis	Mycotic Agents	Bacterial Spores	Shelf life > 1 Week	Corrosive	Residue	Inactivated by Organic Matter	Skin Irritant	Eye Irritant	Respiratory Irritant	Toxic	Easily Obtainable	Purchase ($)/gal	Cost ($)/gal at Use Dilution
Isopropyl alcohol	60–95%	Int	+	+	−	+	+	−	+	−	−	+	−	+	−	+	+	3.75 (70%)	3.75 (70%)
Hydrogen peroxide	3–25%	CS-High	+	+	+	+	+	+	+	+	−	−	+	+	−	+	+	2.37 (3%)	2.37 (3%)
Formaldehyde	3–8%	High-Int	+	+	+	+	+	−	+	−	+	−	+	+	+	+	+	7.94 (37% wt)	0.79 (3.7% wt)
Quaternary ammonium compounds	0.4–1.6% aqueous	Low	+	+	−	−	+	−	+	−	−	+	+	+	+	+	+	8.60–14.40	0.06 (0.4%)– 0.13 (1.6%)
Phenolic	0.4–5% aqueous	Int-Low	+	+	+	−	+	−	+	+	+	−	+	+	−	+	+	8.20–13.90	0.03 (0.4%)– 0.11 (0.8%)
Chlorine	100–1000 ppm free chlorine	High-Int	+	+	+	+	+	−	+	+	+	+	+	+	+	+	+	0.70 (5.25%)	0.07 0.5%
Iodophors	30–50 ppm free iodine	Int	+	+	+	−	+	−	+	+	+	+	+	+	−	+	+	12.80 10%	0.128 0.1%
Glutaraldehyde	2%	CS-High	+	+	+	+	+	+	+	−	−	−	+	+	−	+	+	8.50–11.00	8.50–11.00

* Modified from *Laboratory Biosafety Manual*. Geneva, World Health Organization, 1983.

† Abbreviations: Int, intermediate; CS chemosterilizer; +, yes; −, no.

‡ Inactivates all indicated microorganisms with a contact time of 30 minutes or less, except bacterial spores, which require 6 to 10 hours contact time.

Microbiocidal Activity. Methyl alcohol has the weakest bactericidal action of the alcohols and thus is seldom considered for use as an antibacterial agent (31). It has, however, been found to be sporicidal when freshly prepared and mixed with 2000 ppm of sodium hypochlorite (32) and virucidal (33). The bactericidal activity of ethyl alcohol has been examined by Morton (27) using various concentrations of ethyl alcohol against a variety of microorganisms in exposure periods ranging from 10 seconds to 1 hour. *P. aeruginosa* was killed in 10 seconds by all concentrations of ethanol from 30 to 100% by volume while *S. marcescens, E. coli,* and *Salmonella typhosa* were killed in 10 seconds by all concentrations of ethanol from 40 to 100%. The gram-positive organisms *S. aureus* and *Streptococcus*

pyogenes were slightly more resistant, being killed in 10 seconds by ethyl alcohol concentrations from 60 to 95%. Coulthard and Sykes (34) found isopropyl alcohol (isopropanol) slightly more bactericidal than ethyl alcohol for *E. coli* and *S. aureus.*

Ethyl alcohol is a very potent virucidal agent, inactivating all of the viruses in Table 18.3 within 1 minute. Isopropyl alcohol is nearly inactive against the hydrophilic enteroviruses but is fully active against the lipophilic viruses (35). Recent studies have also demonstrated the ability of ethyl and isopropyl alcohols to inactivate the hepatitis B virus (15, 16) (Table 18.4) and lymphadenopathy-associated virus (17) (Table 18.5), and of ethyl alcohol to inactivate rotavirus and astrovirus (33).

Table 18.3.   Inactivation of Viruses by Germicides*

	Lowest Concentration Inactivating 10^5 to 10^7 Virus in 10 Minutes	
	Lipophilic (Adeno 2, Herpes, Vaccinia, Influenza)	Hydrophilic (Polio 1, Coxsackie B1, ECHO 6)
Sodium hypochlorite	200 ppm	200 ppm
Iodophor	75–150 ppm†	150 ppm
Formalin	2%	2–8%
Glutaraldehyde	0.02%	1–2%
Ethyl alcohol	30–50%	50–70%
Isopropyl alcohol	20–50%	90% (ECHO 6) 95% (neg-polio 1; coxsackie B1)
Phenol	1–5%	5%
O-Phenylphenol	0.12%	12% (neg)
Benzalkonium chloride	1:1,000–1:10,000	10% (neg)

* From Klein M, DeForest A: The chemical inactivation of viruses. *Chem Spec Manuf Assoc Proc* 49:116–118, 1963.
† Variable results dependent on virus. For example, 150 ppm of iodophor are required to inactivate adenovirus 2, but 75 ppm are needed to inactivate herpes, vaccinia, and influenza.

Table 18.4.   Inactivation of Hepatitis B Virus by Disinfectants*

Germicide	Concentration† (10^6 HBV, 10 min, 20°C)	Concentration‡ (5×10^4–10^5 HBV)
Sodium hypochlorite	500 ppm	ND
Glutaraldehyde	2%	0.1% and 1%, 5 min, 24°C
Glutaraldehyde-phenate	0.13% glut– 0.44% phen	ND
Alcohol	70% (isopropyl)	80% (ethyl), 2 min, 11°C
Iodophor	80 ppm	ND
Heat	ND	98°C, 2 min

* HBV, hepatitis B virus; ND, no data.
† Data from Bond et al (15).
‡ Data from Kobayashi et al (16).

Table 18.5.   Inactivation of Human T Lymphotropic Virus Type III/Lymphadenopathy-Associated Virus by Disinfectants*

Germicides	Concentration†	Reduction in RT† (Contact Time)	Concentration‡ (10^5 HTLV III/ LAV ≤10 min, 25°C)
β-Propiolactone	0.25%	100% (1 hr)	ND
	0.025%	none (1 hr)	
Ethyl alcohol	19%	99% (5 min)	50%
Formalin	0.1%	40% (30 min)	ND
Glutaraldehyde	0.01%	95% (1 hr)	ND
	0.0125%	70% (5 min)	ND
Hydrogen peroxide	ND		0.3%
Isopropyl alcohol	ND		35%
Paraformaldehyde	ND		0.5%
Phenolic	ND		0.5%
Sodium hydroxide	30 mmoles/liter	99% (5 min)	
Sodium hypochlorite	0.2%	99% (1 hr)	0.1% (50 ppm)
	0.1%	55% (5 min)	

* Abbreviations: RT, reverse transcriptase; HTLV-III, human T lymphotropic virus type III; LAV, lymphadenopathy-associated virus; ND, no data.

† From Spire B, Montagnier L, Barre-Sinoussi F, Chermann JC: Inactivation of lymphadenopathy- associated virus by chemical disinfectants. *Lancet* 1:899–901, 1984.

‡ From Martin LS, McDougal JS, Loskoski SL: Disinfection and inactivation of the human T lymphotropic virus type III/lymphadenopathy-associated virus. *J Infect Dis* 152:400–403, 1985.

In testing the effect of ethyl alcohol against *M. tuberculosis*, Smith noted that 95% ethanol killed the tubercle bacilli in sputum and water suspensions within 15 seconds (36). In 1964, Spaulding stated that alcohols were the germicide of choice for tuberculocidal activity and they should be the standard by which all other tuberculocides were compared. For example, he compared the tuberculocidal activity of iodophor (450 ppm), a substituted phenol (3%), and isopropanol (70%/volume) using the mucin-loop test (10^6 *M. tuberculosis*/loop) and determined that the contact times needed for complete destruction were 120 to 180 minutes, 45 to 60 minutes, and 5 minutes, respectively. This mucin-loop test is a severe test developed for the purposes of producing long survival times. Thus, these figures should not be extrapolated to the exposure times which are needed when these germicides are being used on medical or surgical material (26).

Seventy percent ethyl alcohol was the most effective concentration for killing the tissue phase of *Cryptococcus neoformans, Blastomyces dermatitidis, Coccidioides immitis,* and *Histoplasma capsulatum* and the culture phases of the latter three organisms aerosolized onto various surfaces. The culture phase was more resistant to the action of ethyl alcohol and required about 20 minutes to disinfect the contaminated surface, compared to < 1 minute for the tissue phase (37, 38).

Uses.   Ethyl alcohol is a high level disinfectant and is used for some types of semi- and noncritical items. Alcohols are not recommended for sterilizing medical and surgical materials principally because of their lack of sporicidal action and their inability to penetrate protein-rich materials. Fatal postoperative wound infections with *Clostridium* have occurred when alcohols were used to sterilize surgical instruments contaminated with bacterial spores (39). Alcohols have been used effectively to disinfect oral and rectal thermometers (40, 41) and to disinfect fiberoptic endoscopes (42, 43). Alcohol towelettes have been used for years to disinfect small surfaces such as rubber stoppers of multiple-dose medication vials or vaccine bottles. Furthermore, alcohol is occasionally used to disinfect external surfaces of equipment (e.g., stethoscopes, ventilators) or medication preparation areas. The documented shortcomings of alcohols on equipment are that they damage the shellac mounting of lensed instruments, tend to swell and harden rubber and certain plastic tubing after prolonged and repeated use, and bleach rubber and plastic tiles (26). They also evaporate rapidly, and this makes extended contact times difficult to achieve unless the items are immersed.

Chlorine and Chlorine Compounds

Overview.   Hypochlorites are the most widely used of the chlorine disinfectants and are available in a liquid (e.g., sodium hypochlorite) or solid (e.g., calcium hypochlorite) form. They have a broad spectrum of antimicrobial activity and are inexpensive and fast acting. Their use in hospitals is limited by their corrosiveness, inactivation by organic matter, and instability. Decomposition of hypochlorite solutions leads to a loss of available chlorine and hence to loss of antimicrobial activity. Decomposition is affected by temperature, concentration, light, and, most importantly, pH value. The microbiocidal activity of chlorine is largely attributed to undissociated hypochlorous acid (HOCl). The dissociation of hypochlorous acid to the less microbiocidal form (hypochlorite ion OCl⁻) is dependent on pH. The disinfecting efficacy of chlorine decreases with an increase in pH which parallels the conversion of undissociated hypochlorous acid to hypochlorite ion (44, 45). A potential hazard is the production of the carcinogen bis-chloromethylether when a hypochlorite solution comes into contact with formaldehyde (46). A mixture of sodium hypochlorite with acid will also affect a rapid evolution of toxic chlorine gas.

Alternative compounds, which release chlorine and are used in the hospital setting, include demand release chlorine dioxide and chloramine T. The advantage of these compounds over the hypochlorites is that they retain chlorine longer and so exert a more prolonged bactericidal effect.

Mode of Action. The exact mechanism by which free chlorine destroys microorganisms has not been elucidated. The postulated mechanism of chlorine disinfection is inhibition of some key enzymatic reactions within the cell, protein denaturation and inactivation of nucleic acid (45).

Microbiocidal Activity. Low concentrations of free chlorine have a biocidal effect on *M. tuberculosis* (50 ppm, 50 to 60°C) and vegetative bacteria (< 1 ppm) in seconds. A concentration of 100 ppm will destroy mycotic agents in < 1 hour (45). Klein and DeForest (47) reported that 25 viruses were inactivated in 10 minutes with 200 ppm of available chlorine. Recent experiments using the Association of Official Analytical Chemists (AOAC) use-dilution method have shown that 100 ppm of free chlorine will kill 10^6 to 10^7 *S. aureus, Salmonella choleraesuis,* and *P. aeruginosa* in < 10 minutes (EC Cole and WA Rutala, unpublished results).

Uses. Inorganic chlorine solution is used for disinfecting tonometer heads (48) and for spot disinfection of countertops and floors. A 1:10 dilution of 5.25% sodium hypochlorite is recommended for cleaning blood spills in rooms of

patients on blood and body fluid precautions (18) and at least 500 ppm of available chlorine for 10 minutes is recommended for decontamination of cardiopulmonary resuscitation training manikins (49). Solutions containing 500 ppm of available chlorine in tap water (pH 9.5) are stable for months when stored at room temperature (23°C) in closed plastic containers (EC Cole, WA Rutala, unpublished data). Chlorine has long been favored as the preferred disinfectant in water treatment. Recently, hyperchlorination of a *Legionella*-contaminated hospital water system resulted in a dramatic decrease (30% to 1%) in the isolation of *L. pneumophila* from water outlets and a cessation of nosocomial Legionnaires' disease in the affected unit (50). Chloramine T (51) and hypochlorites (52) have been evaluated in disinfecting hydrotherapy equipment.

Formaldehyde

Overview. Formaldehyde is used as a disinfectant and sterilant both in the liquid and gaseous states. The liquid form will be considered mainly in this section, and a review of formaldehyde as a gas sterilant may be found elsewhere (53). Formaldehyde is sold and used principally as a water-based solution called formalin, which is 37% formaldehyde by weight. The aqueous solution is a potent bactericide, tuberculocide, fungicide, virucide, and sporicide (46, 54–56). The National Institute for Occupational Safety and Health (NIOSH) indicated that formaldehyde should be handled in the workplace as a potential carcinogen and set an employee exposure standard for formaldehyde that limits an 8-hour time-weighted average exposure to a concentration of ≤ 3 ppm (57). For this reason and others (Table 18.2) employees should have limited direct contact with formaldehyde, and these considerations limit its role in sterilization and disinfection processes.

Mode of Action. Formaldehyde inactivates microorganisms by alkylating the amino and sulfhydral groups of proteins and ring nitrogen atoms of purine bases (1).

Microbiocidal Activity. A wide range of microorganisms is destroyed by varying concentrations of aqueous formaldehyde solutions. Klein and DeForest demonstrated that rapid inactivation (10 minutes) of poliovirus required an 8% concentration of formalin, but all other viruses tested (Table 18.3) were inactivated with 2% formalin. Four percent formaldehyde is a tuberculocidal agent, inactivating 10^4 *M. tuberculosis* in 2 minutes (56), and 2.5% formaldehyde inactivates about 10^7 *Salmonella typhi* in 10 minutes despite the presence of organic matter (55). Rubbo and coworkers demonstrated that the sporicidal action of formaldehyde is slower than that of glutaraldehyde when they performed comparative tests with 4% aqueous formaldehyde and 2% glutaraldehyde against the spores of *Bacillus anthracis* (56). To achieve an inactivation factor of 10^4 the formaldehyde solution required a contact time of 2 hours while glutaraldehyde required only 15 minutes.

Uses. Although formaldehyde-alcohol is a chemosterilizer and formaldehyde is a high level disinfectant, its hospital uses are limited by its irritating fumes and the pungent odor which is apparent at very low levels (< 1 ppm). For these reasons and others, such as evidence of carcinogenicity, this germicide is excluded from Table 18.1. When it is employed there is generally limited direct employee exposure; however, significant exposures to formaldehyde have been documented for employees of renal transplant units (58) and students in a gross anatomy laboratory (59). Formaldehyde is used in the health care setting to prepare viral vaccines (e.g., poliovirus, influenza), as an embalming agent, to preserve anatomic specimens, and in the past for sterilizing surgical instruments, especially when mixed with ethanol. Formaldehyde is also considered the preferred disinfectant for decontaminating equipment associated with hemodialysis systems (24) and is used to disinfect disposable hemodialyzers that are reused. To minimize a potential health hazard to dialysis patients, the dialysis equipment must be thoroughly rinsed and tested for residual formaldehyde before use.

Paraformaldehyde, a solid polymer of formaldehyde, may be vaporized by heat for the gaseous decontamination of laminar flow biological safety cabinets when maintenance work or filter changes require access to the sealed portion of the cabinet.

Hydrogen Peroxide

Overview. The literature contains limited accounts of the properties, germicidal effectiveness, and potential uses for stabilized hydrogen peroxide in the hospital setting. Reports ascribing good germicidal activity to hydrogen peroxide have recently been published and attest to its bactericidal, virucidal, sporicidal, and fungicidal properties (60). The properties of hydrogen peroxide are capsulized in Table 18.2.

Mode of Action. Hydrogen peroxide works by the production of destructive hydroxyl free radicals which can attack membrane lipids, deoxyribonucleic acid (DNA), and other essential cell components. Catalase, produced by aerobic and facultative anaerobes that possess cytochrome systems, may protect cells from metabolically produced hydrogen peroxide by degrading hydrogen peroxide to water and oxygen. This defense is overwhelmed by the concentrations used for disinfection (60).

Microbiocidal Activity. Schaeffer and associates (61) demonstrated the bactericidal effectiveness and stability of hydrogen peroxide in urine against a variety of nosocomial pathogens. They showed that organisms with high cellular catalase activity (*S. aureus*, *S. marcescens*, and *Proteus mirabilis*) required 30 to 60 minutes of exposure to 0.6% hydrogen peroxide for a 10^8 reduction in cell counts, whereas *E. coli*, *Streptococcus* sp, and *Pseudomonas* sp required only 15 minutes exposure (61). Wardle and Renninger investigated 3, 10, and 15% hydrogen peroxide for reducing spacecraft bacterial populations and got a complete kill of 10^6 sporeformers (i.e., *Bacillus* sp) with a 10% concentration and a 60-minutes exposure time. A 3% concentration for 150 minutes killed 10^6 sporeformers in six of seven exposure trials (62). The antiviral activity of hydrogen peroxide against rhinovirus was demonstrated in studies by Mentel and Schmidt (63). The time required for inactivating three serotypes of rhinovirus using a 3% hydrogen peroxide solution was 6 to 8 minutes; this time increased with decreasing concentrations (18 to 20 minutes at 1.5%; 50 to 60 min at 0.75%).

Uses. Commercially available 3% hydrogen peroxide is a stable and effective disinfectant when used on inanimate surfaces. It has been used in concentrations from 3 to 6% for the disinfection of hydrophilic soft contact lenses (60) and ventilators (64). Hydrogen peroxide has also been instilled into urinary drainage bags in an attempt to eliminate the bag as a source of bladder bacteriuria and environmental contamination (65, 66). Concentrations of hydrogen peroxide from 10 to 25% have promise as chemical sterilants but are not yet accepted as comparable to the prime chemosterilizer, glutaraldehyde.

Iodophors

Overview. Iodine solutions or tinctures have long been used by health professionals primarily as antiseptics on skin or tissue and they are discussed in Chapter 17. Iodophors, on the other hand, have enjoyed use as both antiseptics and disinfectants. An iodophor is a combination of iodine and a solubilizing agent or carrier; the resulting complex provides a sustained-release reservoir of iodine and releases small amounts of free iodine in aqueous solution. The best known and most widely used iodophor is povidone-iodine, a compound of polyvinylpyrrolidone with iodine. This product and other iodophors retain the germicidal efficacy of iodine, but unlike iodine are generally nonstaining and are relatively free of toxicity and irritancy (67).

Three recent reports that documented intrinsic microbial contamination of povidone-iodine and poloxamer-iodine (68–70) caused a reappraisal of our concepts concerning the chemistry and use of iodophors (71). Without entering into a discussion over the semantic problems of "free" and "available" iodine, it seems that "free" iodine (I_2) contributes to the bactericidal activity of iodophors, and dilutions of idophors demonstrate more rapid bactericidal action than a full strength povidone-iodine solution. The reason for the observation that dilution increases bactericidal activity is unclear, but it has been suggested that dilution of povidone-iodine results in weakening of the iodine linkage to the carrier polymer with an accompanying increase of free iodine in solution (69).

Mode of Action. Iodine is able to penetrate the cell wall of microorganisms quickly, and it is thought that the lethal effects result from a disruption of protein and nucleic acid structure and synthesis.

Microbiocidal Activity. Published reports on the in vitro antimicrobial efficacy of iodophors are limited (2, 35, 72, 73). These data demonstrate that iodophors are bactericidal and virucidal but may require prolonged contact times to kill *M. tuberculosis* and bacterial spores. Berkelman and associates found that three brands of povidone-iodine solution demonstrated more rapid kill (seconds to minutes) of *S. aureus* and *Mycobacterium cheloni* at a 1:100 and 1:1000 dilution than the stock solution (73). Klein and DeForest demonstrated the virucidal activity of 75 to 150 ppm of available iodine against seven viruses (Table 18.3). Other investigators have questioned the efficacy of iodophors against poliovirus in the presence of organic matter and rotovirus SA-11 in distilled or tap water (74, 75). Manufacturers' data demonstrate that commercial iodophors are not sporicidal but they are tuberculocidal, fungicidal, virucidal and bactericidal at their recommended use dilution.

Uses. Besides their use as antiseptics, iodophors have been used for the disinfection of blood culture bottles and medical equipment, such as hydrotherapy tanks, thermometers, and endoscopes. Antiseptic iodophors are not suitable for use as hard surface disinfectants.

Glutaraldehyde

Overview. Glutaraldehyde is a saturated dialdehyde that has justifiably gained wide acceptance as a high level disinfectant and chemosterilizer. Aqueous solutions of glutaraldehyde are acidic and generally in this state are not sporicidal. Only when the solution is "activated" (made alkaline) by use of alkalinating agents to pH 7.5 to 8.5 does the solution become sporicidal. Once "activated" these solutions have a shelf life of 14 days because of the polymerization of the glutaraldehyde molecules at alkaline pH levels. This polymerization blocks the active sites (aldehyde groups) of the glutaraldehyde molecules that are responsible for its biocidal activity.

Novel glutaraldehyde formulations (e.g., glutaraldehyde-phenate, potentiated acid glutaraldehyde, stabilized alkaline glutaraldehyde) have been produced in the past several years that have overcome the problem of rapid loss of stability while maintaining excellent microbiocidal activity (76–79). Manufacturers' literature for these preparations suggests that the neutral or alkaline glutaraldehydes possess superior microbiocidal and anticorrosion properties when compared to acid glutaraldehydes, and there are a few published reports that substantiate these claims (80–82). The use of glutaraldehyde-based solutions in hospitals is widespread because of their advantages, which include excellent biocidal properties; activity in the presence of organic matter (20% bovine serum); noncorrosive action to endoscopic equipment, thermometers, rubber, or plastic equipment; and does not coagulate proteinaceous material.

Mode of Action. The biocidal activity of glutaraldehyde and its inhibitory effect are a consequence of alkylation with sulfhydral, hydroxyl, carboxy, and amino groups of microorganisms, which alters ribonucleic acid (RNA), DNA, and protein synthesis. For an extensive review of the mechanism of action of glutaraldehydes, the reader is referrerd to Scott and Gorman (83).

Microbiocidal Activity. The in vitro inactivation of microorganisms by glutaraldehydes has been extensively investigated and reviewed (83). Several investigators showed that 2% aqueous solutions of glutaraldehyde, buffered to pH 7.5 to 8.5 with sodium bicarbonate, were effective in killing vegetative bacteria in < 2 minutes; *M. tuberculosis*, fungi, and viruses in < 10 minutes;

and spores of *Bacillus* and *Clostridium* species in 3 hours (84, 85). Collins and Montalbine reported that 2% alkaline glutaraldehyde solution inactivated 10^5 *M. tuberculosis* cells present on the surface of penicylinders within 5 minutes at 18°C (80). A subsequent study conducted by Rubbo and co-workers (56) and more recent investigations (JM Ascenzi, unpublished data) question the mycobacteridal prowess of glutaraldehydes. Rubbo and associates showed that 2% alkaline glutaraldehyde has slow action (> 30 minutes) against *M. tuberculosis* and compares unfavorably with alcohols, formaldehydes, iodine, and phenol. Similarly, a glutaraldehyde manufacturer in collaboration with an independent laboratory tested seven glutaraldehyde-based disinfectants using the AOAC tuberculocidal test and found that none of the disinfectants tested produced total kill of the test population (about 10^5 colony-forming units) (CFU)/ml) of *M. tuberuculosis* var. *bovis* in 10 or 20 minutes at 20°C. These data also identify the actual use of conditions required to assure complete kill of *M. tuberculosis* when 2% glutaraldehyde solution with a 14-day shelf life, 2% glutaraldehyde solution with a 28-day shelf life, and 2.4% glutaraldehyde machine solution are used. They are 70 minutes, 2 hours, and 4 hours at 20°C; and 30 minutes, 30 minutes and 60 minutes at 25°C, respectively (JM Ascenzi, unpublished data).

Uses. Glutaraldehyde is used most commonly as a high level disinfectant for medical equipment, such as endoscopes (42), transducers, anesthesia and respiratory therapy equipment (86), and hemodialysis proportioning and dialysate delivery systems (87).

Phenolics

Overview.   Phenol has occupied a prominent place in the field of hospital disinfection since its initial use as a germicide by Lister in his pioneering work on antiseptic surgery. In the past 20 years, however, work has been concentrated upon the numerous phenol derivatives or phenolics and their antimicrobial properties. Phenol derivatives originate when a functional group (e.g., alkyl, phenyl, benzyl, halogen) replaces one of the hydrogen atoms on the aromatic ring. Two of the phenol derivatives that are found commonly as constituents of hospital disinfectants are *ortho*-phenylphenol and *ortho*-benzyl-*para*-chlorophenol. The antimicrobial properties of these compounds and many other phenol derivatives are much improved over the parent chemical. Phenolics are assimilated by porous materials,

and the residual disinfectant may cause tissue irritation. In 1970, Kahn reported the depigmentation of the skin caused by phenolic germicidal detergents containing paratertiary butyl phenol and paratertiary amylphenol (88).

Mode of Action.   Phenol, in higher concentrations, acts as a gross protoplasmic poison, penetrating and disrupting the cell wall and precipitating the cell proteins. Low concentrations of phenol and higher molecular weight phenol derivatives cause bacterial death by the inactivation of essential enzyme systems and leakage of essential metabolites from the cell wall (89).

Microbiocidal Activity.   Published reports on the antimicrobial efficacy of commonly used phenolic detergents are quite limited (2, 90–93). These data show that three phenolic detergents were bactericidal and tuberculocidal and another phenol (containing 50% Cresol) had little or no virucidal effect against coxsackie B4, echovirus 11, and poliovirus 1. Similarly, Klein and DeForest made the observation that 12% *ortho*-phenylphenol fails to inactivate any of the three hydrophilic viruses after a 10-minute exposure time, although 5% phenol is lethal for these viruses (Table 18.3). Manufacturers' data using the standardized AOAC method demonstrate that commercial phenolic detergents are not sporicidal, but they are tuberculocidal, fungicidal, virucidal, and bactericidal at their recommended use dilution. Generally, these efficacy claims against microorganisms have not been verified by independent laboratories or the Environmental Protection Agency (EPA). Attempts to substantiate the bactericidal label claims of phenolic detergents using the AOAC method have failed (25, 94). Studies are being conducted by the AOAC Use Dilution Method Task Force to determine if these failures are attributed to intrinsic deficiencies of the disinfectants or a methodologic problem.

Uses.   This class of compounds is used for decontamination of the hospital environment, including laboratory surfaces, and for noncritical medical and surgical items. Phenolics are not recommended for semicritical items because of the lack of published efficacy data for many of the available formulations and because the residual disinfectant on porous materials may cause tissue irritation even when thoroughly rinsed.

The use of phenolics in nurseries has been justifiably questioned because of the occurrence of hyperbilirubinemia in infants placed in nurseries that use phenolic detergents (95). In addition, Doan and co-workers demonstrated microbilirubin level increases in phenol-exposed infants compared to nonphenolic-exposed infants when the phenol was prepared according to the manufacturers' recommended dilution (96). If phenolics are used to clean nurseries, they must be diluted according to the recommendation on the product label. It is not recommended that infant bassinettes be cleaned with a phenolic.

Quaternary Ammonium Compounds

Overview. The quaternary ammonium compounds have enjoyed wide usage as disinfectants and until recently as antiseptics. The elimination of such solutions as antiseptics on skin and tissue was recommended by the Centers for Disease Control (3) because of several outbreaks of infections associated with in-use contamination (97–103). There have also been a few reports of nosocomial infections associated with contaminated quaternary ammonium compounds when used to disinfect patient care supplies or equipment such as cytoscopes or cardiac catheters (102, 104, 105). The quaternaries are good cleaning agents but are inactivated by organic materials (e.g., cork, cotton, gauze pads) and, like several other germicides, gram-negative bacteria have been noted to grow in them (106).

Chemically, the quaternaries are organically substituted ammonium compounds in which the nitrogen atom has a valence of 5 and four of the substituent radicals (R1-R4) are alkyl or heterocyclic radicals of a given size or chain length and the fifth (X-) is a halide, sulfate, or similar radical (107).

tion of essential cell proteins, and disruption of the cell membrane. Evidence offered in support of these and other possibilities is provided by Petrocci (108) and Sykes (107).

Microbiocidal Activity. Results from manufacterers' data sheets and from published scientific literature indicate that the quaternaries sold as hospital disinfectants are fungicidal, bactericidal, and virucidal against lipophilic viruses; they are not sporicidal and generally not tuberculocidal or virucidal against hydrophilic viruses (35, 108, 109). Attempts to reproduce the manufacturers' bactericidal claims using the AOAC use dilution method with a limited number of quaternary ammonium compounds have failed (25, 94). Studies are being conducted by the AOAC Use Dilution Method Task Force to determine if these failures are attributed to intrinsic deficiencies of the disinfectants or methodologic problems.

Uses. The quaternaries are recommended for use in ordinary environmental sanitation of noncritical surfaces such as floors, furniture, and walls.

Miscellaneous Inactivating Agents

Other Germicides

There are several compounds that have antimicrobial activity but for various reasons have not been incorporated with our main armamentarium of hospital disinfectants. These include: mercurials, ether, acetone, chloroform, sodium hydroxide, paracetic acid, β-propiolactone, chlor-

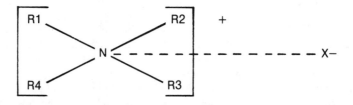

Each compound exhibits its own antimicrobial characteristics, hence the search for finding one compound with outstanding antimicrobial properties. Some of the chemical names of quaternary ammonium compounds that are frequently used in hospitals are alkyldimethylbenzylammonium chloride, alkyldidecyldimethylammonium chloride, and dialkyldimethylammonium chloride.

Mode of Action. The bactericidal action of the quaternaries has been attributed to the inactivation of energy-producing enzymes, denatura-

hexidine gluconate, cetrimide-chlorhexidine, glycols (triethylene and propylene), and the Tego disinfectants. A detailed examination of these agents is presented in two authoritative references (4, 23).

Ultraviolet Radiation (UV)

Microorganisms are inactivated by UV in wavelengths within a range of 240 to 280 nm. The maximum wavelength for microbiocidal activity is 260 nm and modern mercury-vapor lamps emit about 95% of their radiation near (254.7 nm) that level. Inactivation of microorganisms is due to destruction of nucleic acid via induction of thymine dimers. Ultraviolet radiation has several potential applications, but unfortunately its germicidal effectiveness and use are influenced by the following factors: organic matter; wavelength; type of suspension, temperature, type of microorganism; and UV intensity which is affected by distance and dirty tubes (22, 110). The application of UV in the hospital (i.e., operating rooms, isolation rooms, and biologic safety cabinets) is limited to the destruction of airborne organisms or inactivation of microorganisms located on surfaces. The effect of UV radiation used in the operating room on postoperative wound infections has been investigated by means of a double-blind, randomized study in five university medical centers. After following 14,854 patients over a 2-year period, they reported the overall wound infection rate to be unaffected by UV, although there was a significant reduction (3.8 to 2.9%) in postoperative infection in the "refined clean" surgical procedures (111). There are no data that support the use of UV lamps in isolation rooms, and this practice has caused at least one epidemic of ultraviolet-induced skin erythema and keratoconjunctivitis in hospital patients and visitors (112).

Pasteurization

This is not a sterilization process; its purpose is to destroy all pathogenic microorganisms without destroying bacterial spores. The time-temperature relation for hot water pasteurization is generally 77°C (170°F) for 30 minutes. Pasteurization of respiratory therapy (113) and anesthesia equipment (114) is a recognized alternative to chemical disinfection. The efficacy of this process has recently been challenged using an inoculum which the authors believed might simulate contamination by an infected patient. When placing a large inoculum (10^7) of *P. aeruginosa* or *Acinetobacter calcoaceticus* in sets of respiratory tubing before processing, Gurevich and associates demonstrated that machine-assisted chemical processing proved to be a more efficient method than the machine-assisted pasteurization process with a disinfection failure rate of 6% and 83%, respectively (115).

Evaluation and Neutralization of Germicides

Any discussion of germicidal efficacy would be incomplete without a few comments regarding the evaluation of germicides to assure that they meet manufacturers' label claims. Disinfectants in the United States are registered and regulated in interstate commerce by the EPA. For nearly 30 years the EPA also performed intramural pre- and postregistration efficacy testing of chemical disinfectants, but in 1982 this was stopped, presumably for budgetary reasons. Thus, manufacturers presently do not need verification of efficacy claims by the EPA or an independent testing laboratory when registering a disinfectant or chemosterilizer (116). This occurs at a time when the frequency of contaminated germicides and infections secondary to their use have increased (106). Recognizing that the AOAC tests are too complex and expensive for all states or hospitals to commence verification testing, health professionals should demand of chemical manufacturers and their congressman that a verification program be reinstituted either by the EPA or independent laboratories. This program should substantiate the manufacturers' label claim against microorganisms preregistration for chemosterilizers and pre- or postregistration for disinfectants. This would provide assurance that disinfectants and chemosterilizers that meet the test requirements are capable of achieving a known level of antimicrobial activity when used as directed. Unless this and other control measures (106) are instituted, one can confidently predict that reports will continue to emerge in the literature that describe contaminated disinfectants and nosocomial infections secondary to their use.

One of the problems associated with the evaluation of the bactericidal activity of disinfectants is to prevent bacteriostasis due to disinfectant residues that are carried over into the subculture media. Likewise, the presence of small amounts of disinfectants on environmental surfaces may negatively affect accurate enumeration of the bacteria when performing microbiologic sampling of the hospital environment as part of an epidemiologic investigation. One of the ways these problems may be overcome is by employing neutralizers which inactivate residual disinfectants (117, 118). Two commonly used neutralizing media for chemical disinfectants are Letheen Media and D/E Neutralizing Media. The former contains lecithin to neutralize quaternaries and polysorbate 80 (Tween 80) to neutralize phenolics, hexachlorophene, formalin and with lecithin, ethanol. The D/E Neutralizing Media will neutralize a broad spectrum of antiseptic and disinfectant chemicals, including quaternary ammonium compounds, phenols, iodine and chlorine compounds, mercurials, formaldehyde, and glutaraldehyde (119).

STERILIZATION

Sterilization removes or destroys all microorganisms on the surface of an article or in a fluid. Items that enter tissue or the vascular system and equipment (e.g., excorporeal circulator, hemodialysis coil) through which blood or sterile fluids circulate must be sterilized. There are several detailed reviews (23, 120–125) which deal with principles of ethylene oxide and steam sterilization and they have been used as references for this section.

Steam Sterilization

Of all the methods available for sterilization, moist heat in the form of saturated steam under pressure is the most widely used and the most dependable. Steam sterilization is nontoxic, inexpensive, sporicidal, and rapidly heats and penetrates fabrics. For these reasons, steam sterilization should be used whenever possible on all items that are not heat- and moisture-sensitive (e.g., steam sterilizable respiratory therapy and anesthesia equipment), even when not essential to prevent disease transmission. Moist heat destroys microorganisms by the irreversible coagulation and denaturation of enzymes and structural proteins. In support of this opinion, it has been found that the presence of water significantly affects the coagulation temperature of proteins and the temperature at which microorganisms are destroyed.

The basic principle of steam sterilization, as accomplished in an autoclave, is to expose each item to direct steam contact at the required temperature and pressure for the specified time. Thus, there are four parameters of steam sterilization—steam, pressure, temperature, and time. The ideal steam for sterilization is 100% saturated steam, no saturated water in the form of a fine mist. Pressure serves as a means to obtain the high temperatures necessary to kill microorganisms quickly. Specific temperature must be obtained to ensure the microbiocidal activity. The two common steam sterilizing temperatures are 121°C (250°F) and 132°C (270°F). These temperatures must be maintained for a minimum time to kill microorganisms. *Bacillus stearothermophilus* spores are used to monitor the efficacy of steam sterilization. Recognized exposure periods for sterilization of wrapped hospital supplies are 30 minutes at 121°C in a gravity displacement sterilizer and 4 minutes at 132°C in a prevacuum sterilizer. At constant temperatures, sterilization times vary depending on the size and type of item as well as the sterilizer type. The two basic types of steam sterilizers are the gravity displacement autoclave and the high speed prevacuum autoclave. In the former, steam is admitted to the top of the sterilizing chamber and because the steam is lighter than air it forces air out the bottom of the chamber through the drain vent. The gravity displacement autoclaves are primarily used to process laboratory media, water, pharmaceutical products, infectious waste, and nonporous articles whose surfaces have direct steam contact. For gravity displacement sterilizers the penetration time is prolonged by incomplete air elimination. This point is illustrated with the decontamination of microbiologic waste (10 lb) which requires at least 45 minutes at 121°C because the entrapped air remaining in a load of waste greatly retards steam permeation and heating efficiency (126, 127). The high speed prevacuum sterilizers are similar to the gravity displacement sterilizers except they are fitted with a vacuum pump to ensure air removal from the sterilizing chamber and load before the steam is admitted. The advantage of this is that there is nearly instantaneous steam penetration even into porous loads. The Bowie-Dick test using 100% cotton surgical towels (huckaback) is used daily in the first cycle of all vacuum-type autoclaves to evaluate the efficacy of air removal. A new, smaller, disposable test pack has been devised to replace the stack of folded towels for testing the efficacy of the vacuum system in prevacuum sterilizers (128).

Ethylene Oxide

Ethylene oxide (ETO) is used almost exclusively in the United States to sterilize medical products that cannot be steam sterilized. ETO is a colorless gas which is flammable and explosive; however, mixtures of ETO (10 to 12%) with carbon dioxide or the preferred fluoridated hydrocarbons reduce the risk. The effectiveness of ETO sterilization is influenced by four essential elements; gas concentration, temperature, humidity, and exposure time. The operational ranges for each of these four parameters are 450 to 1200 mg/liter, 29 to 65°C, 45 to 85%, and 2 to 5 hours, respectively. Within certain limitations, an increase in gas concentration and temperature may shorten the time necessary for achieving sterilization. ETO inactivates all microorganisms, although the bacterial spores (especially *B. subtilis*) are more resistant than other microorganisms and for this reason *B. subtilis* is the recommended biologic indicator. The microbiocidal activity of ETO is considered to be the result of alkylation of protein, DNA, and RNA. Alkylation, or the replacement of a hydrogen atom with an alkyl group, within cells prevents normal cellular metabolism and replication.

The main disadvantages associated with ETO are the lengthy cycle time, the cost, and its potential hazards to patients and staff; whereas the advantage is that it can sterilize heat- or moisture-sensitive medical equipment without deleterious results. The basic ETO sterilization cycle consist of five stages (i.e., preconditioning and humidification, gassing, exposure, evacuation, and air washes) and takes approximately 2½ hours excluding aeration time. Mechanical aeration for 8 to 12 hours at 50 to 60°C allows desorption of the toxic ETO residual contained in exposed absorbent materials. Ambient room aeration (20°C) will also achieve desorption of toxic ETO but requires 7 days. The direct cost involved in the ETO sterilization process is about 4½ times the cost of steam sterilization ($35 versus $8) for the same size sterilizer (30 ft³).

In recent years, the toxicity of ETO to employees has raised considerable concerns. In June 22, 1984, the Occupational Safety and Health Administration (OSHA) reduced the permissible exposure limit (PEL) for ETO to a time-weighted average (TWA) of 1 ppm, which is a 50-fold reduction from the old standard adopted in 1971. The basis for this action was a determination by the Assistant Secretary of Labor for OSHA that exposure to ETO presents a carcinogenic, mutagenic, genotoxic, reproductive, neurologic, and sensitization hazard to workers. Determination of employee exposure shall be made from breathing zone air samples that are representative of the 8-hour TWA of each employee. For < 0.5 ppm the employer can discontinue the monitoring for affected employees. If > 1 ppm, the employer must establish a regulated area, then must make an effort to comply through work practice alterations and by engineering controls (e.g., extensive ventilation modification, process isolation, and/or effective equipment repair). When these modifications are not sufficient to reduce employee exposure to < 1 ppm, the employer needs to supplement them by use of respiratory protection. Employees who are or may be exposed to ETO at or above the action level of 0.5 ppm for at least 30 days/year are covered by a medical surveillance program. The impact that this regulation will have on hospital sterilization practices is not yet known (129).

Other Sterilization Methods

Dry Heat Sterilizers

This method should be used only for materials (e.g., powders, petroleum products, sharp instruments) that might be damaged by moist heat. The advantages of dry heat are its penetrating power and lack of corrosive properties for metal and sharp instruments; but the slow rate of heat penetration and microbial killing makes this a time-consuming method. The most common time-temperature relationships for sterilization with hot air sterilizers are: 170°C (340°F) for 60 minutes; 160°C (320°F) for 120 minutes; and 150°C (300°F) for 150 minutes. *B. subtilis* spores should be used to monitor the sterilization process for dry heat since they are much more resistant to dry heat than *B. stearothermophilus*. The primary lethal process is considered to be oxidation of cell constituents.

Ionizing Radiation

Sterilization by ionizing radiation, primarily by cobalt 60 gamma rays and electron accelerators, is a low temperature sterilization method which has been used for a host of medical products (e.g., tissue for transplantation, drugs, pharmaceuticals). Because of the high sterilization costs this method is an unfavorable alternative to ethylene oxide sterilization in hospitals but is suitable for large scale sterilization. There are several good reviews dealing with the sources, effects, and application of ionizing radiation (23, 130, 131) that may be referred to for more detail.

Liquid Chemicals

Several EPA-registered liquid chemicals are capable of producing sterile medical and surgical materials after exposure periods of 6 to 10 hours (Table 18.1). Sterilization with liquid chemicals is recommended only for those materials that cannot be sterilized by heat or ethylene oxide.

Filtration

This technology is used to remove bacteria from thermolabile pharmaceutical fluids that cannot be purified by any other means. To remove bacteria, the membrane pore size (e.g., 0.22 μm) must be smaller than the bacteria and uniform throughout (132). Some investigators have questioned whether the removal of microorganisms by filtration really is a sterilization method because there may be slight bacterial and viral passage through filters, and transference of the sterile filtrate into the final container under aseptic conditions entails a risk of contamination (133).

Microwave

Recent reports have shown microwaves to be an effective microbiocide. The microwaves produced by a "home-type" microwave oven (2.45g Hz) have been shown to inactivate bacterial cultures, viruses, and *B. stearothermophilus* spores completely within 60 seconds to 5 minutes depending on the challenge organism (134, 135). Its use in hospitals requires further evaluation.

Sterilizing Practices

Hospitals should perform most cleaning, disinfecting and sterilization of patient care supplies in a central processing department to control quality more easily. Some hospitals are able to promote the same level of efficiency and safety in the preparation of supplies in other areas, like operating room, anesthesia, and respiratory therapy.

Physical Facilities

The central processing area(s) should ideally be divided into at least three areas: decontamination; packaging; and sterilization and storage. Minimally, the decontamination area should be separated by physical barriers from the other sections in order to contain contamination from used items, but ideally all three sections should be separated by physical barriers. In the decontamination area reusable supplies (and possibly disposable items that are reused) are received, sorted, and decontaminated. The packaging area is for assembling and packaging clean but not sterile material. The storage area should be a limited access area with a controlled temperature (65 to 72°C) and relative humidity (35 to 50%). One physical arrangement of processing areas is presented schematically in an acknowledged reference (120).

Cleaning

As repeatedly mentioned, items must be cleaned using water with or without detergents before processing. Precleaning in patient care areas, although not recommended by the CDC (3), may be needed on items that are heavily

soiled with feces, sputum, blood, etc. Items sent to central processing without removing gross soil may be difficult to clean because of dried secretions and excretions.

There are several types of mechanical cleaning machines (e.g., utensil washer-sanitizer, ultrasonic cleaner, washer-sterilizer, dishwasher) that may facilitate cleaning and decontamination of most items. Delicate and intricate objects as well as heat- or moisture-sensitive articles are carefully cleaned by hand. Traditionally, items contaminated or likely to be contaminated with infective material have been contained in an impervious bag before being sent to central processing (3). Such bagging is intended to prevent inadvertent personnel exposure and contamination of the environment. All used items sent to the central processing area, not only known contaminated items, should be considered contaminated and need to be handled with gloves and decontaminated (not necessarily sterilized) by one of the aforementioned methods before or during cleaning to render them safer to handle.

Packaging, Loading, and Storage

Once items are cleaned, dried, and inspected, objects requiring sterilization must be wrapped or packaged. The packaging material must allow penetration of the sterilant and maintain the sterility of the processed item after sterilization. Commonly used packaging material include muslin (140 to 288 thread count/inch), Kraft paper, nonwoven wraps, and paper/plastic peel-down packages.

All items to be sterilized should be arranged so all surfaces will be directly exposed to the sterilizing agent. Packs must not exceed the maximum dimensions, weight, and density of 12 × 12 × 20 inches, 12 lb and 7.2 lb/ft³, respectively.

Safe storage times for sterile packs vary with the porosity of the wrapper and storage conditions (e.g., open versus closed cabinets). Some believe that the practice of outdating packages may itself soon be outdated if hospitals commence wrapping materials in packaging that maintains sterility until time of use and the Joint Commission on the Accreditation of Hospitals modifies their position of dating every sterilized product (136). Until these changes occur, hospitals should continue to assign expiration dates. Heat-sealed, plastic peel-down pouches and wrapped packs sealed in 3-mil (3/1000 inch) polyethylene overwrap have been reported to be sterile for as long as 9 months after sterilization. The 3-mil polyethylene is applied after sterilization to extend the shelf life for infrequently used items (137). Supplies wrapped in double thickness muslin comprising four layers or equivalent remain sterile for at least 30 days. Any item that has been sterilized should not be used after the expiration date has been exceeded or if the sterilized package has been dropped, wet, torn, or punctured.

Monitoring

The sterilization procedure should be monitored routinely by a combination of mechanical, chemical, and biologic parameters. These process parameters evaluate the sterilizing conditions and indirectly the microbiologic status of the processed items. The mechanical techniques for steam sterilization include the daily assessment of cycle time and temperature by examining the temperature record chart as well as an assessment of pressure via the pressure gauge. Unfortunately, two other essential elements for ethylene oxide sterilization (i.e., the gas concentration and humidity) cannot be monitored.

Chemical indicators are affixed on the outside of each pack to show that the package has been processed through a sterilization cycle, but these indicators do not prove that sterilization has been achieved. Preferably, a chemical indicator should also be placed on the inside of each pack to verify steam penetration. Chemical indicators are usually either heat- or chemical-sensitive inks printed on paper which change color when one or more germicidal-related parameters are present.

Biologic indicators are the only process indicators that directly measure sterilization. *B. subtilis* spores (10^6) are used to monitor ethylene oxide and dry heat and *B. stearothermophilus* spores (10^5) are used to monitor steam sterilization. *B. stearothermophilus* is incubated at 55°C and *B. subtilis* is incubated at 35 to 37°C. Steam and ethylene oxide sterilizers should be monitored at least weekly with the appropriate commercial preparation of spores, but each load should be monitored if it contains implantable objects. When feasible, do not use implantable items until results of spore tests are known to be negative. "Flash" steam sterilization, defined as sterilization of an unwrapped object at 132°C for 3 minutes in a gravity displacement autoclave, is not recommended for implantable items because spore tests are not reliable and "flash" sterilization provides no margin of safety.

The procedure to follow in the event of positive spore tests is controversial. The CDC recommendation is that "objects, other than implantable objects, do not need to be recalled for a positive spore test unless the sterilizer or its use is defective." This is in contrast to recommendations from the Association for the Advancement of Medical Instrumentation (AAMI) and the Association of Operating Room Nurses (AORN). The AAMI recommends that materials in the sterilizer with a positive biologic indicator up to the next cycle with a negative biologic indicator must be considered nonsterile and should be retrieved and reprocessed (138). Similarly, AORN states that all items processed in a suspect load are considered nonsterile. The items should be retrieved and, if possible, washed, repackaged, and resterilized in another sterilizer (122). The AORN and AAMI recommendations for a positive spore test should be followed. All positive tests should be gram stained, and if the microscopic evaluation demonstrates gram-positive rods that are representative of *Bacillus*, all items processed in the suspect load(s) should be considered nonsterile and reprocessed. This may be the only defensible position one can assume unless there is strong evidence that the biologic indicator is defective (139) or the growth medium contained a *Bacillus* contaminant (140).

The size and composition of the biologic indicator test pack must be standardized in order to obtain interpretable results. Unfortunately, there is no biologic indicator test pack that has gained acceptance for either steam or gas sterilization. The biologic indicator test pack recommended by the AORN for both types of steam sterilizers consists of 3 muslin surgical gowns, 12 towels, 30 gauze sponges (4 × 4 inches), 5 laparotomy sponges (12 × 12 inches) and 1 muslin drape sheet. The biologic and chemical indicators are placed in the center of the pack but are separated by one towel. The pack should be placed in such a way that the center of the pack is as close to the cold spot as possible. This means that the test pack should be placed on the bottom shelf of a steam sterilizer in the area above the chamber drain (122). The biologic indicator test pack recommended by the AAMI for ethylene oxide sterilizers varies with sterilizer volume but consists of towels, gowns, bedsheets, latex tubing, plastic syringes (with biologic and chemical indicators inside), and a woven or nonwoven overwrap. If only one test pack is placed in the load, it should be in the geometric center of the load (121).

WASTE DISPOSAL

Introduction

Health care facilities that generate infectious, chemical, or radiologic waste have a moral and legal obligation to dispose of these wastes in a manner that poses minimum potential hazard to the environment or public health. The proper disposal of these wastes requires a dynamic waste management plan that conforms to federal, state, and local regulations and provides adequate personnel and financial resources to assure implementation. This section on solid waste disposal will provide an overview of infectious waste management and guidance on chemical and radiologic waste disposal even though only by reference to appropriate regulations.

Infectious Waste

The need for a comprehensive infectious waste management program in hospitals is mandated not only by federal and state regulations but also by a concern about the public image of the hospital as a source of environmental pollution. Considering the critical environmental health problems posed by the improper disposal of hazardous waste, Congress charged the EPA with the responsibility of formulating "cradle-to-grave" regulations over hazardous waste by requiring implementation of Subtitle C of the Resource Conservation and Recovery Act (RCRA) of 1976. Hazardous waste is defined in this Act as "solid waste, or combination of solid wastes, which because of its quantity, concentration or physical, chemical, or infectious characteristics, may a) cause or significantly contribute to an increase in mortality or an increase in serious, irreversible, or incapacitating reversible, illness, or b) pose a substantial present or potential hazard to human health or the environment when improperly treated, stored, transported, or disposed of, or otherwise managed" (141). Thus, by definition infectious waste is considered a subset of hazardous waste. Nonetheless, the EPA has not yet issued regulations to fulfill the Congressional mandate to establish an infectious waste management system. It has, however, prepared a draft manual which is intended to assist hospitals and states so they may establish appropriate programs and/or regulations on infectious waste management. The vast majority of the EPA draft manual is good practice, but as will be discussed, some of its recommendations are highly controversial, and since some states have adopted these guidelines in toto as regulations, it is unfortunate that it was not circulated for review and modified to reflect consensus opinion (142). This section will review some of the problems and principles associated with infectious waste management, but a more detailed description of collection, storage, processing, transporting, and disposal of hospital solid waste may be found elsewhere (143).

A critical step in a waste management program is to determine how much solid waste (materials or objects, biologic or nonbiologic, that are not intended for further use) is produced. Overall, about 13 lb of solid waste/patient/day are generated in acute care hospitals. Using available data one would expect the first five types of infectious waste listed in Table 18.6 to comprise about 5 to 7% of the total hospital waste (143, 144). Thus, a hospital with 100 patients would produce about 1300 lb of solid waste/day and from 65 to 91 lb of infectious waste/day. In contrast, chemical and radiologic waste is generated in much smaller amounts (< 5%) when compared to infectious waste.

Two controversial issues in the management of infectious waste in hospitals are: What are infectious waste and what are the recommended methods for disposal? When one defines infectious waste as a waste capable of producing an infectious disease, this requires a consideration of the factors necessary for induction of disease, which include dose, resistance of host, portal of entry, presence of a pathogen, and virulence. Therefore, for a waste to be infectious, it must contain pathogens with sufficient virulence and quantity so that exposure to the waste by a susceptible host could result in an infectious disease. Infectious waste is unfortunately unlike other hazardous waste because there are no tests that allow infectious waste to be identified objectively. Additionally, there are limited studies that have quantified the microbial load associated with hospital waste, and, if sharps are excluded, there is only one instance of these wastes associated with in-hospital transmission of infection (145). Those studies that have quantified the microbial load associated with different hospital wastes (i.e., operating unit, nursing station, intensive care unit) have found that this waste is no more microbially contaminated than household waste (146). For these reasons, the efforts of responsible agencies to define waste as infectious when it is suspected to contain potentially hazardous levels of microorganisms are imprecise and conflicting. To illustrate, when examining the designation of infectious waste by the CDC and EPA, one recognizes agreement that four and possibly five types of waste are infectious (i.e., microbiologic, blood, pathologic, sharps, and possibly isolation) but disagreement on several other types of hospital

Table 18.6. Types of Solid Waste Designated as Infectious and Recommended Disposal Methods—CDC and EPA*· †

Source/Type of Solid Waste	CDC		EPA	
	Infectious Waste	Disposal Method	Infectious Waste	Disposal Method
Microbiologic	Yes	S, I	Yes	S
Blood and blood products	Yes	S, I, Sew (blood)	Yes	S, I
Communicable disease isolation	Yes/No (?)	HP	Yes	S, I
Pathologic (includes autopsy)	Yes	I	Yes	I, SW, CB
Sharps (e.g., needles)	Yes	S, I	Yes	S
Contaminated lab wastes	No		Yes	S, I
Surgical ("dirty" cases)	No		Yes	S, I
Dialysis unit	No		Yes	S, I
Other (discarded biologicals, animal carcasses and bedding, contaminated equipment and food)	No		Yes	V

* The Joint Commission for the Accreditation of Hospitals requires that there be a system designed to manage hazardous waste safely, and the established system should operate in accordance with federal, state and local regulations (150).

† S, steam sterilization; I, incineration; HP, in accordance with hospital policy; Sew, sanitary sewer; SW, steam sterilization with incineration or grinding; CB, cremation or burial by mortician; V, varied, refer to EPA draft manual.

waste (i.e., "dirty" surgical cases, contaminated lab, dialysis). These contradictory recommendations have resulted in hospitals designating blood, microbiologic, isolation, and pathologic waste as infectious and treating them appropriately, while there is less agreement of the infectious nature of the other types of hospital waste (143). When the recommended methods for disposal of infectious waste from the CDC and the EPA are examined, significant differences are again noted. For example, the EPA recommends steam sterilization for microbiologic waste (i.e., cultures and stock of etiologic agents), whereas the CDC allows steam sterilization or incineration. In addition, the drain is not an acceptable mode of disposal of unautoclaved blood in the EPA guidance manual, while the CDC permits blood to be poured carefully down a drain to the sewer. Fortunately, the EPA is considering modifying these and other differences with the CDC recommendations, but this will not be done until a task force involving these two agencies and several other professional organizations considers these issues (AS Corson, personal communication).

Since differences exist at the present time between the CDC and EPA on what constitutes infectious wastes and how it should be discarded, an important question is: What waste management program should state agencies and hospitals assume to provide protection to human health and the environment? Utilizing available information, this protection can be assured if hospitals considered at least four types of waste as infectious (pathologic, microbiologic, sharps, blood, and possibly isolation) and these wastes are rendered noninfectious by the methods designated by either the EPA or the CDC before final disposal. Other hospital waste should be discarded in a properly sited and operated sanitary landfill since this method is safe and inexpensive (e.g., landfill costs $0.02/lb versus contract incinerator service costs $0.32/lb).

Chemical Waste

Chemical waste generated in health care facilities (relatively small in quantity and chemically varied) must be disposed of in compliance with federal, state, and local regulations. As mentioned, the federal regulation for chemical waste disposal became effective in November 1980 when the EPA promulgated a Hazardous Waste Management System under the RCRA of 1976. A chemical becomes a waste under EPA regulations once a decision is made to discard it. The chemical is a hazardous waste and subject to EPA regulations if it appears on any of the several lists in the regulations or if it meets regulatory characteristics for ignitability, corrosivity, reactivity, or extraction procedure toxicity. For disposal there are several options—landfill, incineration, and sanitary sewer. Landfills and incinerators must have a permit from the EPA or the state to accept hazardous waste, and certain chemicals that undergo violent change are prohibited from landfill disposal. The indiscriminate dumping of chemicals down the drain is not acceptable. There are classes of chemicals that are suitable for drain disposal; however, local regulations must approve the disposal of chemicals into the sanitary sewer system (147, 148).

Until recently the EPA regulations had a provision for exempting modest quantities of chemical waste (1000 kg/month) from regulation. Under the Reauthorization Bill under RCRA this exemption has been reduced substantially to 100 kg/month (i.e., 220 lb/month or 28 gal/month). Thus, many hospitals that were previously exempted and disposed of hazardous chemical waste via municipal sanitary landfills or sanitary sewers will now have to consider other disposal options.

Radioactive Waste

The radioactive waste generated by hospitals is of low specific activity. These low level radioactive materials (e.g., C-14, H-3, Co-57 and 60, I-125 and 131, P-32) are used in the diagnosis or treatment of many diseases. The disposal of these wastes is regulated by the Nuclear Regulatory Commission (NRC), which licenses facilities that produce or use radioactive material. There are also 26 agreement states which have promulgated regulations in conformance with the NRC and are approved as licensing agencies. The NRC (or agreement state) must approve the disposition of these wastes. The approaches that may be approved for final disposal after separated by type are: sanitary sewer within regulatory bounds; storage-for-decay waste with short half-lives; incineration of combustible solid waste, scintillation vials, and carcasses; or transfer to an authorized receiver such as the vendor or approved site (e.g., Barnwell, SC; Richland, WA). Hospitals may choose to store-for-decay only isotopes with half-lives up to 8 days. This includes I-131, which may require 10 weeks' storage. Some hospitals with sufficient storage space have found that isotopes with half-lives of 60 days or less can be stored-for-decay. This includes the commonly used iodine-125, which requires storage for approximately 2 years. In most cases after storage for 10 half-lives these wastes may be disposed of as ordinary waste so long as a sensitive radiologic monitoring device demonstrates no activity. A hospital that cannot implement a storage-for-decay program would have to consider another option, such as transfer to an authorized receiver

such as a licensed waste disposal company (149). Hospitals may also be granted an in vitro clinical laboratory testing general license by the NRC (or agreement state) if their total possession at one time of certain radioisotopes is low (i.e., 200 μCi of I-125, I-131, Fe-54). In this case the laboratory is exempt from the rules governing disposal.

Acknowledgments. The author wishes to thank Kathy Cheek for secretarial assistance, and Mr. Walter W. Bond, Mr. William B. Dennis, LTC Kathleen M. Shafer, Dr. David J. Weber, and Ms. Donna P. Renfrow for reviewing this chapter.

References

1. Favero MS: Chemical disinfection of medical and surgical materials. In Block SS (ed): *Disinfection, Sterilization and Preservation*, ed 3. Philadelphia, Lea & Febiger, 1983, pp 469–492.
2. Spaulding EH: Chemical disinfection of medical and surgical materials. In Lawrence CA, Block SS (eds): *Disinfection, Sterilization and Preservation*. Philadelphia, Lea & Febiger, 1968, pp 517–531.
3. Simmons BP: Guideline for hospital environmental control. *Am J Infect Control* 11:97–115, 1983.
4. Block SS: *Disinfection, Sterilization and Preservation*, ed 3. Philadelphia, Lea & Febiger, 1983.
5. Wenzel RP, Groschel DHM: Sterilization, disinfection and disposal of hospital waste. In Mandell GL, Douglas RG Jr, Bennett JE (eds): *Principles and Practices of Infectious Diseases*, ed 2. New York, John Wiley & Sons, 1984, pp 1609–1612.
6. Bond WW, Favero MS, Mackel DC, Mallison GF: Sterilization or disinfection of flexible fiberoptic endoscopes. *AORN J* 30:350, 352, 1979.
7. Guidelines for cleaning and disinfection of flexible fiberoptic endoscopes (FFE) used in GI endoscopy. *AORN J* 28:907, 910, 1978.
8. Garner JS, Favero MS: *Guideline for Handwashing and Hospital Environmental Control*. Washington DC, US Government Printing Office, 1985, no. 544-436/24441.
9. Feeley TW, Hamilton WK, Xavier B, Moyers J, Eger EI: Sterile anesthesia breathing circuits do not prevent postoperative pulmonary infection. *Anesthesiology* 54:369–372, 1981.
10. Greene WH, Moody M, Hartley R, Effman E, Aisner J, Young VM, Wiernik PH: Esophagoscopy as a source of *Pseudomonas aeruginosa* sepsis in patients with acute leukemia: the need for sterilization of endoscopes. *Gastroenterology* 67:912–919, 1974.
11. Hawkey PM, Davies AJ, Viant AC, Lush CJ, Mortensen NJ: Contamination of endoscopes by *Salmonella* species. *J Hosp Infect* 2:373–376, 1981.
12. Webb SF, Vall-Spinosa A: Outbreak of *Serratia marcescens* associated with the flexible fiberbronchoscope. *Chest* 68:703–708, 1975.
13. Dawson DJ, Armstrong JG, Blacklock ZM: Mycobacterial cross-contamination of bronchoscopy specimens. *Am Rev Respir Dis* 126:1095–1097,

1982.

14. Leers WD. Disinfecting endoscopes: how not to transmit *Mycobacterium tuberculosis* by bronchoscopy. *Can Med Assoc J* 123:275–280, 1980.

15. Bond WW, Favero MS, Petersen NJ, Ebert JW: Inactivation of hepatitis B virus by intermediate-to-high-level disinfectant chemicals. *J Clin Microbiol* 18:535–538, 1983.

16. Kobayashi H, Tsuzuki M, Koshimizu K, Toyama H, Yoshihara N, Shikata T, Abe K, Mizuno K, Otomo N, Oda T: Susceptibility of hepatitis B virus to disinfectants or heat. *J Clin Microbiol* 20:214–216, 1984.

17. Spire B, Montagnier L, Barre-Sinoussi F, Chermann J: Inactivation of lymphadenopathy associated virus by chemical disinfectants. *Lancet* 1:899–901, 1984.

18. Garner JS, Simmons BP: Guideline for isolation precautions in hospitals. *Infect Control* 4:245–325, 1983.

19. Centers for Disease Control: Acquired immune deficiency syndrome (AIDS): precautions for clinical and laboratory staffs. *MMWR* 31:577–580, 1982.

20. Brown P, Gibbs CJ, Amyx HL, Kingsbury DT, Rohwer RG, Sulima MP, Gajdusek DC: Chemical disinfection of Creutzfeldt-Jakob disease virus. *N Engl J Med* 306:1279–1281, 1982.

21. Brown P, Rohwer RG, Gajdusck DC: Sodium hydroxide decontamination of Creutzfeldt-Jakob disease virus. Letter to the editor. *N Engl J Med* 310:727, 1984.

22. Bean HS: Types and characteristics of disinfectants. *J Appl Bacteriol* 30:6–16, 1967.

23. Russell AD, Hugo WB, Ayliffe GAJ: *Principles and Practice of Disinfection, Preservation and Sterilisation*. Oxford, Blackwell, 1982.

24. Favero MS, Petersen NJ, Carson LA, Bond WW, Hindman SH: Gram-negative water bacteria in hemodialysis systems. *Health Lab Sci* 12:321–334, 1975.

25. Rutala WA, Stiegel MM, Sarubbi FA: Ineffectiveness of disinfectants against hospital strains of bacteria. *Abstracts of the Annual Meeting of the American Society for Microbiology*, 1982, Q138, p 233.

26. Spaulding EH: Alcohol as a surgical disinfectant. *AORN J* 2:67–71, 1964.

27. Morton HE: The relationship of concentration and germicidal efficiency of ethyl alcohol. *Ann NY Acad Sci* 53:191–196, 1950.

28. Morton HE: Alcohols. In Block SS (ed): *Disinfection, Sterilization and Preservation*, ed 3. Philadelphia, Lea & Febiger, 1983, pp 225–239.

29. Sykes G: The influence of germicides on the dehydrogenases of *Bact. coli*. Part I. The succinic acid dehydrogenase of *Bact. coli*. *J Hyg Camb* 39:463–469, 1939.

30. Dagley S, Dawes EA, Morrison GA: Inhibition of growth of *Aerobacter aerogenes*: the mode of action of phenols, alcohols, acetone and ethyl acetate. *J Bacteriol* 60:369–378, 1950.

31. Tilley FW, Schaffer JM: Relation between the chemical constitution and germicidal activity of the monohydric alcohols and phenols. *J Bacteriol* 12:303–309, 1926.

32. Coates D, Death JE: Sporicidal activity of mixtures of alcohol and hypochlorite. *J Clin Pathol* 31:148–152, 1978.

33. Kurtz JB, Lee TW, Parsons AJ: The action of alcohols on rotavirus, astrovirus and enterovirus. *J Hosp Infect* 1:321–325, 1980.

34. Coulthard CE, Sykes G: The germicidal effect of alcohol with special reference to its action on bacterial spores. *Pharm J* 137:79–81, 1936.

35. Klein M, DeForest A: The inactivation of viruses by germicides. *Chem Specialists Manuf Assoc Proc* 49;116–118, 1963.

36. Smith CR: Alcohol as a disinfectant against the tubercle bacillus. *Public Health Rep* 62:1285–1295, 1947.

37. Kruse RH, Green TD, Chambers RC, Jones MW: Disinfection of aerosolized pathogenic fungi on laboratory surfaces. 1. Tissue phase. *Appl Microbiol* 11:436–445, 1963.

38. Kruse RH, Green TD, Chambers RC, Jones MW: Disinfection of aerosolized pathogenic fungi on laboratory surfaces. II. Culture phase. *Appl Microbiol* 12:155–160, 1964.

39. Nye RN, Mallory TB: A note on the fallacy of using alcohol for the sterilization of surgical instruments. *Boston Med Surg J* 189:561–563, 1923.

40. Sommermeyer L, Frobisher M: Laboratory studies on disinfection of rectal thermometers. *Nurs Res* 2:85–89, 1953.

41. Frobisher M, Sommermeyer L, Blackwell MJ: Studies on disinfection of clinical thermometers. I. Oral thermometers. *Appl Microbiol* 1:187–194, 1953.

42. Babb JR, Bradley CR, Deverill CEA, Ayliffe GAJ, Melikian V: Recent advances in the cleaning and disinfection of fibrescopes. *J Hosp Infect* 2:329–340, 1981.

43. Garcia de Cabo A, Larriba PLM, Pinilla JC, Sanz FG: A new method of disinfection of the flexible fibrebronchoscope. *Thorax* 33:270–272, 1978.

44. Hoffman PN, Death JE, Coates D: The stability of sodium hypochlorite solutions. In Collins CH, Allwood MC, Bloomfield SF, Fox A (eds): *Disinfectants: Their Use and Evaluation of Effectiveness*. London, Academic Press, 1981, pp 77–83.

45. Dychdala GR: Chlorine and chlorine compounds. In Block SS (ed): *Disinfection, Sterilization and Preservation*, ed 3. Philadelphia, Lea & Febiger, 1983, pp 157–182.

46. Gamble MR: Hazard: formaldehyde and hypochlorites. *Lab Anim* 11:61, 1977.

47. Klein M, DeForest A: The chemical inactivation of viruses. *Fed Proc* 24:319, 1965.

48. Nagington J, Sutehall GM, Whipp P: Tonometer disinfection and viruses. *Br J Ophthalmol* 67:674–676, 1983.

49. Ad Hoc Committee: Recommendations for decontaminating manikins used in cardiopulmonary resuscitation training—1983 update. *Infect Control* 5:399–401, 1984.

50. Helms CM, Massanari RM, Zeitler R, Streed S, Gilchrist MJR, Hall N, Hausler WJ, Sywassink J, Johnson W, Wintermeyer L, Heirholzer WJ: Legionnaires' disease associated with a hospital water system: a cluster of 24 nosocomial cases. *Ann Intern Med* 99:172–178, 1983.

51. Steve L, Goodhart P, Alexander J: Hydrotherapy burn treatment: use of chloramine-T against resistant microorganisms. *Arch Phys Med Rehabil* 60:301–303, 1979.

52. Turner AG, Higgins MM, Craddock JG: Disinfection of immersion tanks (Hubbard) in a hospital burn unit. *Arch Environ Health* 28:101–104, 1974.

53. Tulis JJ: Formaldehyde gas as a sterilant. In Phillips GB, Miller WS (eds): *Industrial Sterilization.* Durham, Duke University Press, 1972, pp 209–238.

54. Emmons CW: Fungicidal action of some common disinfectants on two dermatophytes. *Arch Dermatol Syphil* 28:15–21, 1933.

55. McCulloch EC, Costigan S: A comparison of the efficiency of phenol, liquor cresolis, formaldehyde, sodium hypochlorite and sodium hydroxide against *Eberthella typhi* at various temperatures. *J Infect Dis* 59:281–284, 1936.

56. Rubbo SD, Gardner JF, Webb RL: Biocidal activities of glutaraldehyde and related compounds. *J Appl Bacteriol* 30:78–87, 1967.

57. Formaldehyde: Evidence of carcinogenicity. NIOSH Current Intelligence Bulletin 34. DHEW (NIOSH) Publication No. 81-111, April 15, 1981.

58. NIOSH Report; Formaldehyde exposures in dialysis units. *Dialysis Transplant* 12:43, 1983.

59. Formaldehyde exposures in a gross anatomy laboratory—Colorado. *MMWR* 31:698–700, 1983.

60. Turner FJ: Hydrogen peroxide and other oxidant disinfectants. In Block SS (ed): *Disinfection, Sterilization and Preservation,* ed 3. Philadelphia, Lea & Febiger, 1983, pp 240–250.

61. Schaeffer AJ, Jones JM, Amundsen SK: Bactericidal effect of hydrogen peroxide on urinary tract pathogens. *Appl Environ Microbiol* 40:337–340, 1980.

62. Wardle MD, Renninger GM: Bactericidal effect of hydrogen peroxide on spacecraft isolates. *Appl Microbiol* 30:710–711, 1975.

63. Mentel R, Schmidt J: Investigations on rhinovirus inactivation by hydrogen peroxide. *Acta Virol* 17:351–354, 1973.

64. Judd PA, Tomlin PJ, Whitby JL, Inglis TCM, Robinson JS: Disinfection of ventilators by ultrasonic nebulisation. *Lancet* 2:1019–1020, 1968.

65. Maizels M, Schaeffer AJ: Decreased incidence of bacteriuria associated with periodic instillations of hydrogen peroxide into the urethral catheter drainage bag. *J Urol* 123:841–844, 1980.

66. Thompson RL, Haley CE, Searcy MA, Guenthner SM, Kaiser DL, Groschel DHM, Gillenwater JY, Wenzel RP: Catheter-associated bacteriuria: failure to reduce attack rates using periodic instillations of a disinfectant into urinary drainage systems. *JAMA* 251:747–751, 1984.

67. Gottardi W: Iodine and iodine compounds. In Block SS (ed): *Disinfection, Sterilization and Preservation,* ed 3. Philadelphia, Lea & Febiger, 1983, pp 183–196.

68. Craven DE, Moody B, Connolly MG, Kollisch NR, Stottmeier KD, McCabe WR: Pseudobacteremia caused by povidone-iodine solution contaminated with *Pseudomonas cepacia. N Engl J Med* 305;621–623, 1981.

69. Berkelman RL, Lewin S, Allen JR, Anderson RL, Budnick LD, Shapiro S, Friedman SM, Nicholas P, Holzman RS, Haley RW: Pseudobacteremia attributed to contamination of povidone-iodine with *Pseudomonas cepacia. Ann Intern Med* 95:32–36, 1981.

70. Parrott PL, Terry PM, Whitworth EN, Frawley LW, Coble RS, Wachsmuth IK, McGowan JE Jr: *Pseudomonas aeruginosa* peritonitis associated with contaminated poloxamer-iodine solution. *Lancet* 2:683–685, 1982.

71. Favero MS: Iodine-champagne in a tin cup. *Infect Control* 3:30–32, 1982.

72. Chang SL: Modern concept of disinfection. *J Sanit Eng Div Proc Am Soc Civ Eng,* pp 689–705, 1971.

73. Berkelman RL, Holland BW, Anderson RL: Increased bactericidal activity of dilute preparations of povidone-iodine solutions. *J Clin Microbiol* 15:635–639, 1982.

74. Wallbank AM, Drulak M, Poffenroth L, Barnes C, Kay C, Lebtag I: Wescodyne: Lack of activity against poliovirus in the presence of organic matter. *Health Lab Sci* 15:133–137, 1978.

75. Sattar SA, Raphael RA, Lochnan H, Springthorpe VS: Rotavirus inactivation by chemical disinfectants and antiseptics used in hospitals. *Can J Microbiol* 29:1464–1469, 1983.

76. Boucher RMG: Potentiated acid 1,5 pentanedial solution—a new chemical sterilizing and disinfecting agent. *Am J Hosp Pharm* 31:546–557, 1974.

77. Miner NA, McDowell JW, Willcockson GW, Stark RL, Whitmore EJ: Antimicrobial and other properties of a new stabilized alkaline glutaraldehyde disinfectant/sterilizer. *Am J Hosp Pharm* 34:376–382, 1977.

78. Pepper RE: Comparison of the activities and stabilities of alkaline glutaraldehyde sterilizing solutions. *Infect Control* 1:90–92, 1980.

79. Leach ED: A new synergized glutaraldehyde-phenate sterilizing solution and concentrated disinfectant. *Infect Control* 2:26–30, 1981.

80. Collins FM, Montalbine V: Mycobactericidal activity of glutaraldehyde solutions. *J Clin Microbiol* 4:408–412, 1976.

81. Masferrer R, Marquez R: Comparison of two activated glutaraldehyde solutions: Cidex solution and sonacide. *Respir Care* 22:257–262, 1977.

82. Babb JR, Bradley CR, Ayliffe GAJ: Sporicidal activity of glutaraldehydes and hypochlorites and other factors influencing their selection for the treatment of medical equipment. *J Hosp Infect* 1:63–75, 1980.

83. Scott EM, Gorman SP: Sterilization with glutaraldehyde. In Block SS (ed): *Disinfection, Sterilization and Preservation,* ed 3. Philadelphia, Lea & Febiger, 1983, pp 65–88.

84. Stonehill AA, Krop S, Borick PM: Buffered glutaraldehyde—a new chemical sterilizing solution. *Am J Hosp Pharm* 20:458–465, 1963.

85. Borick PM, Dondershine FH, Chandler VL: Alkalinized glutaraldehyde, a new antimicrobial agent. *J Pharm Sci* 53:1273–1275, 1964.

86. Townsend TR, Wee SB, Koblin B: An efficacy evaluation of a synergized glutaraldehyde-phenate solution in disinfecting respiratory therapy equipment contaminated during patient use. *Infect Control* 3:240–243, 1982.

87. Petersen NJ, Carson LA, Doto IL, Aguero SM, Favero MS: Microbiologic evaluation of a new glutaraldehyde-based disinfectant for hemodialysis systems. *Trans Am Soc Artif Intern Organs* 28:287–290, 1982.

88. Kahn G: Depigmentation caused by phenolic detergent germicides. *Arch Dermatol* 102:177–187, 1970.

89. Prindle RF: Phenolic compounds. In Block SS (ed): *Disinfection, Sterilization, and Preservation*, ed 3. Philadelphia, Lea & Febiger, 1983, pp 197–224.

90. Hegna IK: A comparative investigation of the bactericidal and fungicidal effects of three phenolic disinfectants. *J Appl Bacteriol* 43:177–181, 1977.

91. Hegna IK: An examination of the effect of three phenolic disinfectants on *Mycobacterium tuberculosis*. *J Appl Bacteriol* 43:183–187, 1977.

92. Bergan T, Lystad A: Antitubercular action of disinfectants. *J Appl Bacteriol* 34:751–756, 1971.

93. Narang HK, Codd AA: Action of commonly used disinfectants against enteroviruses. *J Hosp Infect* 4:209–212, 1983.

94. Bavley A: Tests: not all germ killers adequate. *Miami Herald*, December 26, 1982.

95. Wysowski DK, Flynt JW, Goldfield M, Altman R, Davis AT: Epidemic neonatal hyperbilirubinemia and use of a phenolic disinfectant detergent. *Pediatrics* 61:165–170, 1978.

96. Doan HM, Keith L, Shennan AT: Phenol and neonatal jaundice. *Pediatrics* 64:324–325, 1979.

97. Plotkin SA, Austrian R: Bacteremia caused by *Pseudomonas* sp. following the use of materials stored in solutions of a cationic surface-active agent. *Am J Med Sci* 235:621–627, 1958.

98. Malizia WF, Gangarosa EJ, Goley AF: Benzalkonium chloride as a source of infection. *N Engl J Med* 263:800–802, 1960.

99. Lee JC, Fialkow PJ: Benzalkonium chloride—source of hospital infection with gram-negative bacteria. *JAMA* 177:144–146, 1961.

100. Hardy PC, Ederer GM, Matsen JM: Contamination of commercially packaged urinary catheter kits with the pseudomonad EO-1. *N Engl J Med* 282:33–35, 1970.

101. Frank MJ, Schaffner W: Contaminated aqueous benzalkonium chloride. An unnecessary hospital infection hazard. *JAMA* 236:2418–2419, 1976.

102. Dixon RE, Kaslow RA, Mackel DC, Fulkerson CC, Mallison GF: Aqueous quaternary ammonium antiseptics and disinfectants. Use and misuse. *JAMA* 236:2415–2417, 1976.

103. Sautter RL, Mattman LH, Legaspi RC: *Serratia marcescens* meningitis associated with a contaminated benzalkonium chloride solution. *Infect Cont* 5:223–225, 1984.

104. Shickman MD, Guze LB, Pearce ML: Bacteremia following cardiac catheterization. *N Engl J Med* 260:1164–1166, 1959.

105. Ehrenkranz NJ, Bolyard EA, Weiner M, Cleary TJ: Antibiotic-sensitive *Serratia marcescens* infections complicating cardiopulmonary operations: contaminated disinfectant as a reservoir. *Lancet* 2:1289–1292, 1980.

106. Rutala WA, Cole EC: Antiseptics and disinfectants—safe and effective. *Infect Control* 5:215–218, 1984.

107. Sykes G: *Disinfection and Sterilization*, ed 2. London, E & FN Spon, 1965, pp 362–376.

108. Petrocci AN: Surface active agents: quaternary ammonium compounds. In Block SS (ed): *Disinfection, Sterilization, and Preservation*, ed 3. Philadelphia, Lea & Febiger, 1983, pp 309–329.

109. Smith CR, Nishihara H, Golden F, Hoyt A, Guss CO, Kloetzel MC: The bactericidal effect of surface-active agents on tubercle bacilli. *Public Health Rep* 48:1588–1600, 1950.

110. Shechmeister IL: Sterilization by ultraviolet irradiation. In Block SS: *Disinfection, Sterilization and Preservation*, ed 3. Philadelphia, Lea & Febiger, 1983, pp 106–124.

111. National Research Council: Postoperative wound infections—the influence of ultraviolet irradiation of the operating room and of various other factors. *Ann Surg* 160 (suppl 2):1–125, 1964.

112. Sensakovic JW, Smith LG: Nosocomial ultraviolet keratoconjunctivitis. *Infect Control* 3:475–476, 1982.

113. Roberts FJ, Cockcroft WH, Johnson HE: A hot water disinfection method for inhalation therapy equipment. *Can Med Assoc J* 101:30–32, 1969.

114. Craig DB, Cowan SA, Forsyth W, Parker SE: Disinfection of anaesthesia equipment by a mechanized pasteurization method. *Can Anaesth Soc J* 22:219–223, 1975.

115. Gurevich I, Tafuro P, Ristuccia P, Herrmann J, Young AR, Cunha BA: Disinfection of respiratory tubing: a comparison of chemical versus hot water machine-assisted processing. *J Hosp Infect* 4:199–208, 1983.

116. Groschel DHM: Caveat emptor: do your disinfectants work? *Infect Control* 4:144,1983.

117. Russell AD, Ahonkhai I, Rogers DT: Microbiological applications of the inactivation of antibiotics and other antimicrobial agents. *J Appl Bacteriol* 46:207–245, 1979.

118. Russell AD: Neutralization procedures in the evaluation of bactericidal activity. In Collins CH, Allwood MC, Bloomfield SF, Fox A (eds): *Disinfectants: Their Use and Evaluation of Effectiveness*. London, Academic Press, 1981, pp 45–59.

119. Engley FB Jr, Dey BP: A universal neutralizing medium for antimicrobial cleaner. *Chem Spec Manuf Assoc Proc*, pp 100–106, 1970.

120. Perkins JJ: *Principles and Methods of Sterilization in Health Sciences*, ed 2. Springfield, IL, Charles C Thomas, 1969.

121. American Society for Hospital Central Service Personnel: *Ethylene Oxide Use in Hospitals*. Chicago, American Hospital Association, 1982.

122. AORN recommended practices for inhospital sterilization. *Score* 6:12–20, 1981.

123. Joslyn LJ: Sterilization by heat. In Block SS (ed): *Disinfection, Sterilization and Preservation*, ed 3. Philadelphia, Lea & Febiger, 1983, pp 3–46.

124. Caputo RA, Odlaug TE: Sterilization with ethylene oxide and other gases. In Block SS: *Disinfection, Sterilization and Preservation*, ed 3. Philadelphia, Lea & Febiger, 1983, pp 47–64.

125. Mallison GF: Decontamination, disinfection and sterilization. *Nurs Clin North Am* 15:757–767, 1980.

126. Rutala WA, Stiegel MM, Sarubbi FA: Decontam-

ination of laboratory microbiological waste by steam sterilization. *Appl Environ Microbiol* 43:1311–1316, 1982.

127. Lauer JL, Battles DR, Vesley D; Decontaminating infectious laboratory waste by autoclaving. *Appl Environ Microbiol* 44:690–694, 1982.

128. Rhodes P, Zelner L, Laufman H: A new disposable Bowie-Dick type test pack for prevacuum high-temperature sterilizers. *Med Instrum* 16:117–120, 1982.

129. Federal Register. Occupational exposure to ethylene oxide: final standard. Department of Labor, Occupational Safety and Health Administration. 29 CRF Part 1910, June 22, 1984.

130. Silverman GJ: Sterilization by ionizing irradiation. In Block SS: *Disinfection, Sterilization and Preservation*, ed 3. Philadelphia, Lea & Febiger, 1983, pp 89–105.

131. MacClelland DC: Sterilization by ionizing radiation. *AORN J* 26:675–684, 1977.

132. Fifield CW, Leahy TJ: Sterilization filtration. In Block SS (ed): *Disinfection, Sterilization and Preservation*, ed 3. Philadelphia, Lea & Febiger, 1983, pp 125–153.

133. Wallhausser KH: Is the removal of microorganisms by filtration really a sterilization method? *J Parenter Drug Assoc* 33:156–170, 1979.

134. Latimer JM, Matsen JM: Microwave oven irradiation as a method for bacterial decontamination in a clinical microbiology laboratory. *J Clin Microbiol* 6:340–342, 1977.

135. Sanborn MR, Wan SK, Bulard R: Microwave sterilization of plastic tissue culture vessels for reuse. *Appl Environ Microbiol* 44:960–964, 1982.

136. Mayworm D: Sterile shelf life and expiration dating. *J Hosp Supply, Processing Distribution*, Nov–Dec, pp 32–35, 1984.

137. Mallison GF, Standard PG: Safe storage times for sterile packs. *Hospitals* 48:77, 78, 80, 1974.

138. Association for the Advancement of Medical Instrumentation Recommended Practice: Good hospital practice: steam sterilization and sterility assurance. Arlington, VA, AAMI, 1980, p 8.

139. False-positive results of spore tests in ethylene oxide sterilizers—Wisconsin. *MMWR* 30:238–240, 1981.

140. Gurevich I, Holmes JE, Cunha BA: Presumed autoclave failure due to false-positive spore strip tests. *Infect Control* 3:388–392, 1984.

141. Resource Conservation and Recovery Act of 1976 (P.L. 94-580), 42 USC 6091 et seq.

142. *Draft Manual for Infectious Waste Management*. Washington, DC, Environmental Protection Agency, 1982.

143. Rutala WA, Sarubbi FA: Management of infectious waste from hospitals. *Infect Control* 4:198–204, 1983.

144. Rutala WA: Infectious waste. *Infect Control* 5:149–150, 1984.

145. Grieble HG, Bird TJ, Nidea HM, Miller CA: Chute-hydropulping waste disposal system: a reservoir of enteric bacilli and *Pseudomonas* in a modern hospital. *J Infect Dis* 130:602–607, 1974.

146. Kalnowski G, Wiegand H, Ruden H: The microbial contamination of hospital waste. *Zbl Bakt Hyg, I. Abt Orig B* 178:364–379, 1983.

147. National Research Council: *Prudent Practices for Disposal of Chemicals from Laboratories*. Washington, DC, National Academy Press, 1983.

148. Joyce RM: Prudent practices for disposal of chemicals from laboratories. *Science* 224:449–452, 1984.

149. Illinois Commission on Atomic Energy: *Low-Level Radioactive Waste—Near Term Management Options for Illinois*. 1984, pp 30–70.

150. Hazardous waste disposal. In *Accreditation Manual for Hospitals*. Chicago, Joint Commission on Accreditation of Hospitals, 1985, pp 133–134.

Chapter 19

Nosocomial Bloodstream and Intravascular Device-Related Infections

Bruce H. Hamory, M.D.

Bloodstream infections are the most dramatic and life-threatening infections that occur in hospitals. Although the economic consequences of nosocomial bacteremia may be debated, the increased mortality rates associated with it and its clinical significance are unquestioned. The reasons to monitor their occurrence have been cogently summarized by Brenner and Bryan (1) (Table 19.1).

The macroepidemiology of bacteremia has been described in the recent publication of two carefully performed community-based studies (2, 3). Furthermore, the understanding of nosocomial bloodstream infections has been improved by publication of the results of the SENIC study (4), the National Nosocomial Infection Study (NNIS) (5–8), and other published studies (9–25). In addition, a number of well designed, experimental studies have been reported which evaluate many of the available preventative measures proposed for reducing rates of device-related bacteremias.

Recently, the coagulase-negative staphylococci (*Staphylococcus epidermidis* and other species) have been recognized to play an increasingly important role in nosocomial bacteremias. Recognition of the potential importance of slime production by coagulase-negative staphylococci in the pathogenesis of device-related infections has opened new possibilities for preventing some of these infections. This chapter will cover the information published since the exhaustive review of Maki in 1981 (26).

DEFINITIONS

A nosocomial bacteremia is defined as a clinically important blood culture positive for a bacterium or fungus that is obtained more than 48 hours following hospitalization (27). When a culture is unexpectedly positive (in the absence of signs or symptoms) or when only one of *many* cultures is positive for an organism, it can usually be dismissed as a contaminant. Certain organisms, such as *Candida albicans*, are infrequent contaminants, and are difficult to culture, so they should be carefully evaluated before being dismissed as unimportant.

Nosocomial bacteremias have been divided

Table 19.1. Reasons to Perform Bacteremia Surveillance

1. Surveillance of nosocomial infection
    Ongoing surveillance
    Surveillance in high risk patients
    Evaluation of risk factors to nosocomial infection
2. Outbreak investigation
    Outbreaks related to hospital-associated risk factors
    Outbreaks related to extrahospital risk factors
    Interhospital spread of pathogens
3. Microbiology laboratory quality control
    Recognition of pseudoepidemics due to contaminated cultures
    Interpretation of significance of cultures
    Recognition of settings in which blood cultures may be cost ineffective
4. Antibiotic review
    Monitoring of susceptibility trends
    Review of appropriateness of therapy
    Recommendations for empiric initial therapy in defined clinical situations
5. Other
    Data pertaining to the cost of medical care
    Definition of need for research in selected areas because of apparent ineffectiveness of current therapy
    Epidemiology of community-acquired disease, with implications for prevention

into two categories (27). Primary bacteremias occur *without* any recognizable focus of infection with the same organism at another anatomic site (urine, lung, wound). They are considered to be related to intravenous (IV) fluid therapy when an intravenous line is present. A secondary bacteremia is a blood culture positive for the same organism found at another site. If purulent thrombophlebitis exists or if local infection (redness, tenderness, and pus) is present at the site of the IV line, then the bacteremia is considered to be secondary to the intravenous line.

DIAGNOSIS OF BACTEREMIAS AND FUNGEMIAS

Microbiologic culture of blood is the definitive method for diagnosing bacterial invasion of the bloodstream. There are many methods available for shortening the time between sample collection and recognition of a positive sample, each with its advantages and disadvantages (28). The sites used to obtain blood cultures must be carefully chosen and thoroughly cleansed. Techniques for skin preparation have been carefully described (26, 28). Cultures obtained through arterial or venous cannulae should be avoided whenever possible because of the risk of obtaining a contaminated culture (29).

The clinical necessity to identify microorganisms rapidly or to discover a removable focus for the septicemia has resulted in the use of several microscopic techniques. The simplest and most rapid method to discern the presence of microorganisms in peripheral blood is the careful examination of a stained smear of buffy coat from peripheral blood. The techniques used and results obtained have been recently reviewed by Graham (30). In one study (31), a positive test was inversely correlated with survival: 55% of patients with positive blood smears died, and only 18% of patients with positive smears survived. Peripheral blood smears may be particularly helpful when *Staphylococcus aureus* is suspected or for central venous catheters epsis due to fungi (32). Reik and Rubin (33) performed simultaneous buffy coat examinations on 599 blood cultures. Only 3 of 21 positive blood cultures had positive smears. They noted that a positive buffy coat smear required at least 4.0×10^4 colony forming units of bacteria/ml of blood. Four clinical features were suggested which might increase the yield of such smears: (*a*) the presence of serious illness on admission, (*b*) the presence of a debilitating disease, (*c*) infection with gram-positive

organisms, (*d*) bacteremia from pneumonia, cellulitis, or wound infection. However, the long time needed to examine such specimens and the associated high rate of false negatives do not make this a useful technique in the general clinical microbiology laboratory.

Recently, a technique for rapid diagnosis of catheter-related sepsis has been published by Cooper and Hopkins (34). The catheter segments are obtained aseptically and, following semiquantitative culture by the method of Maki et al (35), are rinsed, air dried, and then placed in gentian violet, followed by grams iodine, and counterstained with safranin. When examined under the oil immersion lens of a light microscope for 15 minutes, good correlation between the presence of microorganisms on the surface of the catheter and a positive semiquantitative culture was found. The sensitivity of this technique was 100% with a specificity of 96.9% and a positive predictive value of 83.9%. The authors did not comment on whether the catheters, which were positive by gram stain and by culture, had any associated purulence at the insertion site. This study examined centrally placed catheters, and the findings may not apply to peripheral catheters.

Longfield et al (36) examined the use of membrane filters for the quantitative culture of intravenous fluids and other fluids suspected of being the source of nosocomial bacteremias. In this experimental study, known numbers of microorganisms were inoculated into IV fluids, which were then cultured by each of two methods. When compared to placing 5 ml of IV fluid in an equal amount of enriched infusion broth, the technique of filtering 10 ml of the fluid through a 0.45-μm membrane filter and then incubating it on sheep blood agar was considerably more sensitive and rapid. At very low concentrations of organisms (one organism/ml to one organism/10 ml), all of the membrane filter samples were positive, whereas the maximum number of positives by broth culture was 85% at the one organism/10 ml level. In addition, membrane filter cultures showed evidence of growth by 24 hours, whereas broth cultures required at least 48 hours to achieve their maximal yield. The authors concluded that the membrane filter technique was more sensitive than culture in a broth medium and was suitable for use in hospital laboratories. Anderson et al (37) compared standard pour plate cultures with rapid testing using *Limulus* lysate assay for endotoxin and an ATP procedure. Standard pour plate was the most sensitive method, detecting as few as one organism per milliliter of inoculated IV fluid. However the *Limulus* lysate method was more rapid and sensitive than the ATP procedure, detecting as few as four organisms per milliliter, and becoming positive from 12 to 36 hours before the ATP procedure was positive. They noted that both the Limulus lysate and standard pour plate methods could be used to detect microbial contamination of IV fluids.

EPIDEMIOLOGY OF BACTEREMIA

A community-based study of all bacteremias diagnosed in residents of Charleston County, South Carolina from 1974 through 1976 revealed an incidence rate of 80 cases of bacteremia/ 100,000 population/year, of which 39% were nosocomial (3). The authors excluded all *Staphylococcus epidermidis* isolates as contaminants, and their data probably underestimated the total frequency of nosocomial bacteremia. In the report, only *Klebsiella* and *Pseudomonas* species had significantly higher rates of occurrence in nosocomial infections than among community-acquired infections. Both *Streptococcus pneumoniae* and *Haemophilus influenzae* had much lower rates as nosocomial bacteremias than as community pathogens.

Bryan et al (2) reviewed bacteremia occurring among 300,547 patients discharged from four major acute care hospitals in Columbia, South Carolina between 1977 and 1981. They documented 2,978 episodes of bacteremia, of which 51% were hospital acquired. The rate of hospital-acquired bacteremias ranged from 8.06/1,000 admissions at teaching hospitals to 1.9/1,000 at nonteaching hospitals (Table 19.2). In this hospital-based series, hospital-acquired bacteremias were associated with a 50% higher risk of death than community-acquired bacteremias. This study confirmed previous observations that for both hospital- and community-acquired bacteremias the relative risk of death increases with age, with polymicrobial bacteremia, with the severity of the underlying condition (nonfatal to rapidly fatal and is highest for nosocomial bacteremias). Haley et al (4) reported an incidence rate of 2.7 nosocomial bacteremias/1,000 admissions from the SENIC data of 1975–1976. This rate compares favorably with the rate of 2.95 episodes/ 1,000 patient discharges reported to NNIS during 1975 (6). The rate increased by 20% to 3.55 episodes/1,000 among patients discharged in 1979 (5), representing a small (3.2%) increase over the rates reported in 1978 (38). Primary bacteremias accounted for 47.8% of the total, a

Table 19.2. Rates of Bacteremia

Ref.	Author	Site	Year(s)	Institution	Bacteremia/ 1000 Admissions	Nosocomial Bacteremia/ 1000 Admissions	Nosocomial Bacteremia/ 1000 Days of Care	Mortality Rate/ 1000 Infections
2	Bryan et al	Columbia, SC USA	1977–1981	Teaching Hospital	15.1	8.06		
				Nonteaching Hospital	4.5	1.9		
4	Haley et al	USA	1975–1976	SENIC		2.7	0.34	289.4
39	Duggan et al	Australia	1978–1979	Referral Hospital		2.08		
43	McCormack and Barnes	United Arab Emirates	1980–1982			5.35		
9	Krieger et al	Univ. of Virginia		University Hospital		1.39	2.02	
38	CDC	USA	1978	NNIS		3.44		
5	CDC	USA	1979	NNIS		3.55		
7	CDC	USA	1980–1982	NNIS		2.0		
8	CDC	USA	1983	NNIS		2.4		

proportion unchanged over the preceding several years.

As shown in Table 19.2, the rates of nosocomial bacteremia (both primary and secondary) range from 1.19 to 13.9/1,000 hospital admissions and from 0.3 to 2.02/1,000 days of care. Most rates are in the range of 1 to 3.5/1,000 admissions, with the highest value in the teaching hospitals surveyed by Bryan et al (2). These are rates of *endemic* bacteremia.

Rates of bacteremia in children may represent a special problem. Berkowtiz (40) reported that 5% of all black children admitted to a South African hospital had bacteremia, and that 9/1,000 admissions developed a nosocomial bacteremia. Many of these children were malnourished, and the rate of bacteremia was almost twice as high among the malnourished as among the normally nourished. Nosocomial bacteremias were most frequently caused by *S. pneumoniae*, *Klebsiella pneumoniae*, and *Salmonella* enteriditis. Baker (41) reported rates of nosocomial sepsis and meningitis of 6.5–8.1/1,000 births in a Houston hospital. These rates were reduced to 4.0/1,000 births after institution of an infection control program. However, Bennett et al (46) noted an increase in the rate of neonatal sepsis in a Swedish hospital between 1969–1973 (1.4/1,000 births) and 1979–1983 (2.4/1,000 births). Townsend and Wenzel (42) reported a 4% rate of nosocomial bacteremia among infants admitted to a Newborn intensive care unit. These infections were associated with increased mortality, and were usually secondary to infections at other sites. Although the organisms causing hospital-acquired bacteremia may vary between institutions (46), multiply resistant *S. aureus* and *S. epidermidis* are increasingly recognized as a problem (38, 48). The endemic rates of nosocomial bacteremia vary markedly among areas of the same hospital. Donowitz et al (44) reported a 3-fold increase in the risk of nosocomial infection for intensive care unit (ICU) patients as compared to ward patients (18% versus 6%). Bacteremias were 7.4 times as likely to occur in ICU patients as in ward patients. Daschner (45) reported that bacteremias accounted for 14.2 to 21.8% of all nosocomial infections occurring in ICUs in five hospitals in Germany and Switzerland. The rates of nosocomial bacteremia ranged from 1.13/100 discharges in the heart surgery ICU to 5.45/100 in general surgery, and 44% were secondary to another site of infection. Donowitz and colleagues (44) reported bacteremia rates ranging from 0% in pediatrics to 12% in general surgery,

which allows calculation of rates ranging from 0 bacteremias/1,000 days of care in pediatrics to 19.1/1,000 days of care in the general surgery ICU. The observed rates of bacteremia/1,000 days of care within services were as follows: orthopaedics (0.8/1,000), cardiovascular surgery (6.0/1,000), neurosurgery (7.2/1,000), medicine (18.0/1,000), and urology (16.0/1,000). Organisms causing bacteremias were more likely to be resistant to multiple antibiotics than those from the wards.

Wenzel et al (47) extended these observations using a statewide surveillance system and reported that rates of nosocomial bacteremias ranged from 0.5 to 1.0/100 admissions in ICUs other than burn units. They noted that 8% of all nosocomial bacteremias occurred as a result of an epidemic, and these usually involved small numbers of cases (3 to 19 patients each).

Bacteremia rates in one chronic care facility have been reported to be 0.3 cases/1,000 patient care days (48). Nationally, the predicted number of hospital-acquired bacteremias ranges from 176,000 cases annually (estimated by Bryan et al (2)) to 102,950 episodes annually (projected by SENIC (4)). Bryan et al estimate that these 176,000 hospital-acquired bacteremias directly cause 32,000 deaths and contribute to an additional 38,000 deaths (2). It should be pointed out that about half of these bacteremias are secondary to other foci of infection.

The cost of hospital-acquired bacteremia has been estimated by several methods. Haley et al (49) estimated in 1975–1976 that a primary bacteremia added $931 (±$328) and 7.4 days (± 12.2) to the average hospital stay. A secondary bacteremia added a mean of $1,288 and 8.1 days stay to nosocomial infections for all sites other than lower respiratory tract. If these figures are applied to the estimates of Bryan et al that 176,000 nosocomial bacteremias occur and 50% of these are secondary bacteremias, it can be estimated that approximately 1.4 million extra hospital days and $200 million extra are spent on nosocomial bacteremias for hospitalization alone.

MICROBIAL ETIOLOGY

The species of microorganisms causing nosocomial bloodstream infections at NNIS hospitals (Table 19.3) did not change from 1975 to 1983. However, the proportion of primary bacteremias caused by *S. epidermidis* doubled from 6.5% to 14.2%, and the proportion of candidemias increased from less than 3.5% of all cases to 5.6%. The relative positions of the other organisms were

Table 19.3. Organisms Responsible for Nosocomial Bacteremias

		Primary Bacteremias				
	NNIS				Bryan (2) 1977–1981	
1975 (6)			1983 (8)			
	%			%		%
S. aureus	14.3	Coagulase-negative staphylococci		14.2	S. aureus	15.2
E. coli	14.0	S. aureus		12.8	E. coli	13.6
Klebsiella sp.	9.1	Klebsiella sp.		9.1	S. epidermidis	7.9
S. epidermidis	6.5	Group D streptococci		7.3	Klebsiella sp.	7.3
Bacteroides	6.3	Enterobacter sp.		6.9	Bacteroides sp.	6.6
Group D streptococci	6.0	P. aeruginosa		6.1	Streptococci	5.5
Enterobacter sp.	5.7	Candida sp.		5.6	Proteus mirabilis	5.0
P. aeruginosa	4.5	Bacteroides		3.4	Group D streptococci	4.7
Proteus-Providencia	3.9	Serratia		2.8	P. aeruginosa	4.5
Serratia sp.	3.8	Group D streptococci		2.8	Enterobacter sp.	4.1

		Secondary Bacteremias	
	NNIS		
1975		1983	
	%		%
E. coli	20.2	S. aureus	36.7
S. aureus	18.8	P. aeruginosa	17.8
Klebsiella sp.	11.7	Klebsiella sp.	11.6
P. aeruginosa	8.1	Enterobacter sp.	10.0
Proteus-Providencia	6.2	Coagulase-negative staphylococci	9.5
		Serratia	6.4

maintained. In 1983, *S. aureus* and coagulase-negative staphylococci together accounted for over one-quarter of all nosocomial bacteremias and for almost half of all secondary bacteremias. The study of Bryan et al (2) confirms the NNIS data.

Organisms associated with bacteremias secondary to another focus of infection changed markedly from 1975 to 1983. *Escherichia coli* dropped out of the top six organisms by 1983. The proportions of secondary bacteremias caused by *S. aureus* and *Pseudomonas aeruginosa* both doubled during that interval. *Enterobacter* sp., coagulase-negative staphylococci, and *Serratia* sp. completed the list of the most common agents causing secondary bacteremias. Whether these changes are related to changes in patient populations, new drugs, or biologic variation is not clear.

The sites of origin of secondary nosocomial bacteremias vary with the organism. *S. aureus* bacteremia occurred in association with wound infection, pneumonia, intravenous devices, and hemodialysis fistulae (19–20). The rate of bacteremia following nosocomial urinary tract infections (UTIs) varies with the organism (9), being highest with *Serratia marcescens* (16/100 UTIs) and lowest with *S. epidermidis* (1.8/100 UTIs).

E. coli, the most common cause of UTI, contributed to one-third of the total number of nosocomial bacteremias but infrequently complicated nosocomial *E. coli* UTIs.

Maki (50) has reviewed the difference in the types of microorganisms (Fig. 19.1) causing endemic versus epidemic bacteremias. There is a preponderance of unusual gram-negative rods associated with epidemics reported in the literature. Similarly, epidemics are most commonly identified when they complicate a vascular device or represent pseudobacteremias (Fig. 19.2).

GRAM-NEGATIVE BACTEREMIA

Kreger et al (10) reviewed all episodes of gram-negative bacteremia documented at Boston University Hospital from 1965 through 1974. Bacteremias occurring after the fifth hospital day were considered nosocomial. During the period of their study the incidence of gram-negative bacteremia progressively increased from 7.06/1,000 admissions to 12.75/1,000 admissions. Since 74% of all the bacteremias were nosocomial, the rate of nosocomial gram-negative bacteremia rose from 5.22/1,000 to 9.4/1,000 admissions. Case fatality rates remained constant. The attack rates of bacteremia were highest among individuals

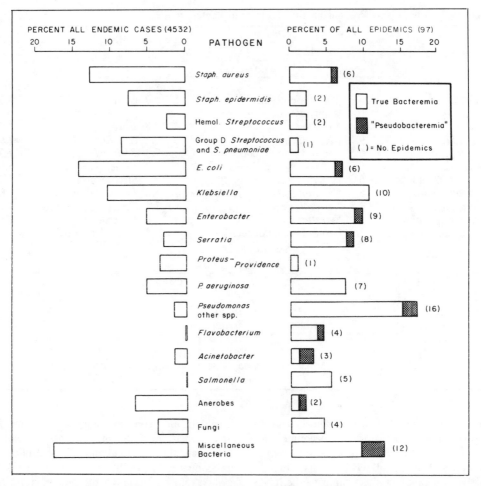

Figure 19.1.   **Microbial pathogens associated with endemic noscomial bacteremias and responsible for 97 epidemics occurring between 1965 and 1978.** Data on 4,532 endemic bacteremias from 83 United States hospitals submitting data on 46,821 nosocomial infections occurring in 1976 to the National Nosocomial Infections Study of the Centers for Disease Control. Data on epidemics were compiled from published reports in the English world literature. Epidemic pathogens in miscellaneous bacteria: *Citrobacter* (four epidemics), *Listeria* (two epidemics), *Bacillus* spp. (two epidemics), *Mycobacterium chelonei* (one epidemic), *Neisseria meningitidis* (one epidemic), *Haemophilus influenzae* (one epidemic), *Moraxella* (one epidemic). (From Maki DG: Epidemic nosocomial bacteremias. In Wenzel RP (ed): *CRC Handbook of Hospital Acquired Infections.* Boca Raton, FL, CRC Press, 1981, pp 371–512.)

over the age of 60 years. Increased rates of gram-negative bacteremia during this period were noted on the general and thoracic surgery services compared to the medicine and urology services, where the rates remained constant. This study confirmed the previous findings of McCabe and Jackson (51) that the case fatality rate for bacteremia was correlated with the severity of underlying disease in the patient. The urinary tract was the source for bacteremia in 34% of instances and the gastrointestinal (GI) tract in 14%. In 30% of

the patients the bacteremia was primary. *Klebsiella pneumoniae* and *Pseudomonas* bacteremias were more often nosocomially acquired than were those due to *E. coli*. There was no significant difference in the case fatality rate in patients with bacteremia due to different bacterial species when the patients were stratified for severity of underlying disease and frequency of appropriate antibiotic therapy. Bryan et al (52) confirmed that mortality rates associated with nosocomial gram-negative bacteremia were elevated by increased

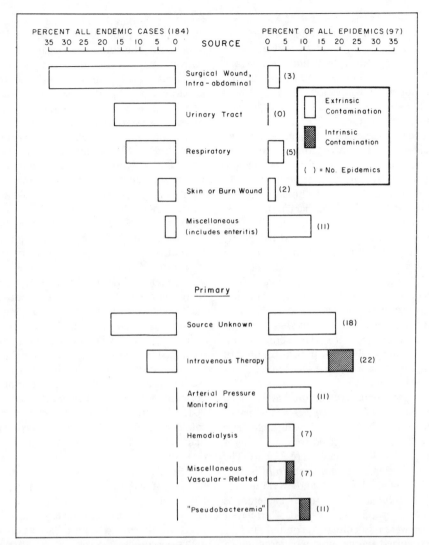

Figure 19.2. Sources of nosocomial bacteremia. Data from the National Study suggest that one-half of endemic nosocomial bacteremias are primary bacteremias, because a culture-proved local infection is not reported. However, prospective studies indicate that the anatomic portal of an individual bacteremia should be identifiable considerably more frequently. To provide a more accurate picture of endemic bacteremia and sharpen the comparison between endemic and epidemic cases with respect to sources, pooled data on 184 endemic bacteremias from prospective studies in three U.S. hospitals, a teaching-community hospital (St. Mary's, Madison, WI), a university hospital (Johns Hopkins, Baltimore, MD), and a municipal hospital (Grady Memorial, Atlanta, GA), are used for comparison with 97 outbreaks reported in the world literature between 1965 and 1978 rather than the otherwise excellent data of the National Study (From Maki DG: Epidemic nosocomial bacteremias. In Wenzel RP (ed): *CRC Handbook of Hospital Acquired Infections.* Boca Raton, FL, CRC Press, 1981, pp 371–512.)

age, and increased severity of underlying disease. Bacteremia secondary to pneumonia, or *Pseudomonas* infection had increased mortality rates in his series.

The continuing importance of *P. aeruginosa* as a nosocomial pathogen has been reaffirmed (11).

P. aeruginosa continues to account for approximately 6% of all primary nosocomial bacteremias and ranks second only to *E. coli* in the number of secondary nosocomial bacteremias. The organism has a predilection for patients suffering from burns, granulocytopenia, immunosuppressed states, or cystic fibrosis. New *Pseudomonas* species are being reported to cause infections in hospitals; for instance, Southern and Kutscher (16) reported a patient with *Pseudomonas paucimonas* bacteremia following vascular surgery, and practitioners are witnessing the emergence of *Pseudomonas maltophilia* and other organisms with distinct antibiograms.

Klebsiella species are also frequent nosocomial bacteremic pathogens. Montgomerie and Ota (12) reported that these bacteremias were secondary to UTI in 27%, GI tract infections in 24%, IV sites in 20%, and lung infections in 15% of cases. Only 10% of *Klebsiella* bacteremias were primary. The crude mortality rate was 37% overall, but it was higher in neonates and the elderly or when the portal of entry was the lung or GI tract. Cryz et al (13) examined the capsular serotypes of 703 bacteremic *Klebsiella* isolates from 13 centers in Europe and North America. Twenty-five serotypes accounted for 70% of all bacteremic isolates, but no individual type accounted for more than 9%. The serotypes involved varied markedly between institutions, but not enough to make a vaccine ineffective, if one could be developed.

Proteus bacteremia (including *Morganella morganii* and *Providencia rettgeri*) was reviewed by Berger (14). In his series, 39% of all bacteremic isolates over an 11-year period were gram-negative bacilli, and 14.4% of these were *Proteus*. The most frequent isolate was *Proteus mirabilis*. In a separate review, McDermott and Mylotte (15) reviewed the *Morganella morganii* bacteremias documented over a 5½-year period. Thirteen of 19 episodes were nosocomially acquired, and 11 of the 13 occurred among surgery patients. Seven nosocomial bacteremias resulted from surgical wound infections, two were secondary to decubitus ulcers and two to other leg lesions, and two were of unknown source. The overall mortality rate was 22%. Polymicrobial bacteremia occurred in 61.5% of instances, presumably because of the nature of the primary infection.

CHANGING EPIDEMIOLOGY OF STAPHYLOCOCCUS AUREUS BACTEREMIA

S. aureus is currently the leading cause of nosocomial bacteremias and has been noted to be an increasing cause of infections in patients with cancer. A report from the National Cancer Institute for the period January 1, 1973 through December 31, 1979 revealed that 32 (23%) of 142 bacteremias among oncology patients were caused by *S. aureus* (17). This rate was significantly higher than the 5% observed in several prior series. The authors reported that a probable primary site was discernible in 39 of 45 total episodes at their institution; skin sources were implicated in 29 and IV sites were specifically implicated in 5. Only 6 of the 45 episodes of bacteremia were associated with granulocytopenia. Shah and Watanakunakorn (19) reviewed the records of 134 patients with *S. aureus* bacteremia. Seventy-three of the 134 patients (54.5%) had nosocomially acquired bacteremia, and 13 additional cases (10%) were associated with chronic hemodialysis. Twenty-two of the 73 nosocomial bacteremias (28.8%) complicated intravenous catheter infections, and four had endocarditis (18%). Overall, 10% of patients with nosocomial *S. aureus* bacteremias had a complicating endocarditis. Bryan et al (20) confirmed these sources of bacteremia, but reported only a 1.7% incidence of endocarditis among nosocomial *S. aureus* bacteremia.

In a separate review, Libman and Arbeit (53) evaluated 39 episodes of *S. aureus* bacteremia occurring during a 1-year period at their Veterans Administration Hospital. Thirty-four of these 39 episodes (87%) were hospital acquired. Of these, 20 (59%) were secondary to infected intravascular catheters, and six (18%) were secondary to a dialysis access site infection (arteriovenous fistula or graft). In one of the remaining six episodes, bacteremia was secondary to a subclavian access which resulted from repeated unsuccessful attempts at subclavian vein catheterization. Of 34 episodes of nosocomial bacteremias, 27 (79%) were directly related to an IV access device or to dialysis access.

The contribution of methicillin-resistant *S. aureus* (MRSA) strains to the level of staphylococcal bacteremias in hospitals has been discussed by Peacock et al (21). During an outbreak at a university hospital, 31 patients were infected over an 8-month period. Of 50 sites from which the organism was isolated, six were bacteremias. Two of the patients with bacteremia died. This outbreak was triggered by the admission of one patient to the hospital with a diffuse dermatitis colonized by methicillin-resistant *S. aureus*. He served as the source for subsequent hand-to-hand spread of the organism to other patients. The virulence of this strain of MRSA was suggested by the high rate of infection following colonization (approximately 50%), and by the 30% rate of bacteremia (six of 19 infections) with a 30% case fatality rate. Craven et al (22) reported an outbreak of nosocomial infections caused by oxacillin and aminoglycoside-resistant *S. aureus* over a period of 16 months. During this time 174 patients were colonized, and 82 patients had 120 nosocomial infections. Twelve (10%) of 120 sites were IV-related infections, and there were 19 episodes of bacteremia (15%). The mortality rate among patients with two or more positive blood cultures (persistent bacteremia, $n = 12$) was 33%. This confirmed the potential of this organism to cause invasive and fatal infection.

Crossley et al (54) reported a 22-month experience with methicillin-resistant *S. aureus* in their large, university-affiliated hospital. During this period, MRSA was isolated from 66 patients on the burn unit and from 42 patients on other services. Among burn patients, 24 of 166 (36%) had infections associated with central venous catheters, and 21 patients (32%) had bacteremias. Of 42 patients in other areas of the hospital, one had an IV-associated infection, and six had bacteremia. In this report, as in others, the length of stay and severity of underlying illness of the patients colonized and infected with MRSA organisms were significantly greater than those in patients colonized by methicillin-sensitive strains.

A report (55) from the Centers for Disease Control suggests that the problem of MRSA predominantly involves tertiary referral centers, which are usually large (> 600 beds) governmental hospitals associated with medical schools. The rate of MRSA bacteremia in these hospitals was not reported. In some instances control of MRSA may be possible with early identification of colonized patients, prompt institution of isolation measures, and careful attention to hand washing practices. Since colonized patients tend to remain colonized, they should be isolated upon readmission to the hospital.

DISTINGUISHING COMPLICATED FROM UNCOMPLICATED STAPHYLOCOCCAL BACTEREMIA

Because of the frequency of nosocomial *S. aureus* bacteremia and its potential for serious metastatic infection, including endocarditis, much attention has been focused on methods for determining an appropriate length of therapy for this infection. Iannini and Crossley (56) observed that patients having a clearly cannula-related *S. aureus* sepsis—defined as (*a*) blood cultures positive for the same *Staphylococcus* as isolated from semiquantitative cultures of the removed cannula and (*b*) absence of any other demonstrable focus

of *Staphylococcus* infection (abscess, pneumonia, wound infection, etc)—could be successfully treated with 2 weeks of parenteral antibiotic therapy following removal or drainage of the focus. Subsequent studies have not always borne out the same observation.

More recently, considerable effort has been devoted to assessing the utility of various serologic tests to distinguish between patients with "uncomplicated bacteremia" from those with "complicated (metastatic?) bacteremia." The tests which have been used include the determination of antibody to teichoic acid (57, 58, 65), and peptidoglycan (59–61). The sensitivity and specificity of these serologic tests for complicated bacteremia are determined by their inherent sensitivity to detect small amounts of antibody to staphylococcal cell well antigens. Ouchterlony gel diffusion is relatively insensitive for those antibodies but more specific for complicated bacteremia, whereas radioimmunoassays appear to be overly sensitive and less specific. When a battery of tests is used for detecting teichoic acid antibody, they are about 80% sensitive in detecting titer rises in individuals with complicated bacteremias as opposed to individuals with simple bacteremias (61). Test batteries that include the use of both teichoic acid antibody and antibody to peptidoglycan increase the sensitivity slightly, but not enough to be clinically applicable. The results of these tests are varied; several authors (62–64) found good separation of complicated from uncomplicated bacteremias by these tests, and others (65, 66) were unable to distinguish them using these tests.

Whether the distinction between "complicated" and "uncomplicated" staphylococcal bacteremias is clinically useful, is open to some question. Bernhardt et al (67) reported the failure of a 2-week course of antibiotics in a patient with IV cannula-associated staphylococcal bacteremia. However, they did not ligate and remove the purulent thrombophlebitic vein. Careful clinical evaluation of each patient is needed to determine the best course of managment (64), although some authorities always treat *S. aureus* sepsis for 4 to 6 weeks with parenteral antibiotics because of the low predictive value for identifying the patient who will develop endocarditis or osteomyelitis.

HOSPITAL-ACQUIRED FUNGEMIA

The incidence of fungemia acquired by hospitalized patients appears to be increasing. Jarvis et al (62) noted that the rate of fungemia due to *Candida* species at NNIS hospitals increased from 0.7/10,0000 discharges in 1980 to 1.5/10,000 discharges in 1984. Horn et al (23) reviewed 200 episodes of fungemia occurring in a large cancer hospital between 1978 and 1982. They observed that the total number of episodes of fungemia increased 30.6% above the earlier figure for the period of 1974 to 1977. Episodes of candidemia in lymphoma or solid tumor patients increased by 73% and 95%, whereas episodes in leukemia patients decreased by about 50%. The most common cause for fungemia in their hospital was *Candida albicans*, which accounted for 44.5% of the total. This was followed by *C. tropicalis* (25.5%), *C. parapsilosis* (11.5%), *Torulopsis glabrata* (11%), and *T. krusei* (3.5%). Most of the episodes were preceded by colonization of some other body site by the same fungal species. Ten of the 23 patients with *C. parapsilosis* infections were found to have infected central venous catheters. Among all patients with fungemia, the prognosis was poor (76% died), and 72% of those on whom autopsies were performed had disseminated fungal infection.

Klein and Watanakunakorn (24) reviewed 85 episodes of hospital-acquired fungemia in 77 patients. No information on the rates of nosocomial fungemia were provided. All patients had intravenous catheters and were receiving multiple antibiotics. Ninety-seven percent also had Foley catheters in place, and a majority had concomitant bacterial infections. Of 56 patients who had more than one positive blood culture, 19 had infected hyperalimentation catheters, and 11 had other infected IV catheters. In 18 of 31 instances, the positive blood culture was preceded by an episode of funguria. In 33 patients (39 episodes) fungemia appeared to resolve simply by removing the IV catheters. In 20 of these 33 episodes there had been only one positive blood culture. However, in four of these patients (five episodes) fungal endophthalmitis subsequently developed. The diagnosis of endophthalmitis was made between 8 and 66 days following the last positive blood culture. Of the 28 patients who received antifungal therapy, six died within 72 hours of beginning antifungal therapy, 12 patients improved but died of an underlying disorder, and 10 patients recovered fully on treatment. Sixteen patients received no antifungal therapy and died of fungal sepsis. In this series *C. albicans* accounted for 51.8%, *C. tropicalis* for 12.9%, and unidentified species for 11.8% of all isolates.

Maksymiuk et al (69) reported a series of 188 episodes of systemic candidiasis occurring over a 4-year period at a large cancer hospital. During this time the overall frequency of systemic infections due to *T. glabrata* was 0.7/100 patients. Patients with acute leukemia had the highest rate of fungemia (10.9 infections/100 patients); the occurrence fell to 1.3% in patients with lymphoma and was very infrequent in patients with solid tumors. Ninety-nine of the 188 episodes had positive blood cultures for yeast. The survival was 29 of 55 instances when only one culture was positive. In 44 instances disseminated infection was documented by the presence of more than one positive blood culture and/or culture of an internal organ. There were only four survivors in this group (9%). Among 55 patients with two positive blood cultures for fungi or disseminated candidemia, all had indwelling intrasvascular catheters. *Candida* was recovered from the catheter tips of 15 of the 55 patients (27%).

Rose (70) reported a prospective study of 69 patients with systemic *Candida* infection seen over 13 years at a veterans hospital. Fifty-five of the 69 episodes (80%) were secondary to venous catheters. Twenty patients (36%) died, and 26 became afebrile following removal of the infected cannula. The remaining nine remained febrile and required amphotericin B therapy, as did four other patients who developed endophthalmitis after the cannula was removed.

Turner et al (71) critically examined the complications of candidemia occurring in pediatric patients in two university hospitals over a 5-year period. Forty-five patients were identified as having candidemia, of whom 18 (40%) were premature infants; 38% had gastrointestinal or hepatic disorders, and 7 (15%) patients had underlying malignancies. In 82% of instances the infection was hospital acquired, and 93% of the instances were associated with IV lines (87% with hyperalimentation). Mortality in this series was very high, and only 49% of patients lived. These series all document the high mortality rate of candida bloodstream infections, especially when multiple cultures are positive.

Suppurative peripheral thrombophlebitis due to *Candida* continues to be a problem. Walsh et al (72) reported seven patients with this infection over a 15-month period. These patients were in the hospital for a longer time (mean 27 days) and were older (median age 64) than other patients. All were on the surgical service. In addition, all patients had received multiple antibiotics for at least 2 weeks prior to the onset of their infection. These authors implicated catheter insertion techniques and the care of the local catheter entry site as possibly being important in the generation of these infections. Torres-Rojas et al (73) reported six cases of *Candida* suppurative thrombophlebitis associated with intravenous cannulae. In all instances persistent candidemia occurred. In two patients the vein was not clinically inflamed but was thrombosed. Surgical excision of the vein and treatment with amphotericin B were curative. Histopathologic examination showed *Candida* invading the vessel wall in all instances (73). New organisms continue to be recognized. Reinhardt et al (74) described a patient with catheter-associated fungemia due to *Candida rugosa*, a previously unrecognized human pathogen.

PSEUDOBACTEREMIAS

Blood cultures that are found to be positive in the laboratory, but that do not truly reflect bacteremia in the patient have been termed "contaminants" and more recently "pseudobacteremia." Kusek (75) and Maki (76) have reviewed the causes of microbiologic results leading to the "recognition" of spurious bacteremia. Since these reviews, several additional outbreaks of pseudobacteremias (77–101) (Table 19.4), and one report of "endemic staphylococcal pseudobacteremia" (102) have appeared.

Because infection control practitioners rely heavily on bacteriologic culture reports to document nosocomial infections (indeed, the only method to document a bacteremia), the number of reported "pseudobacteremia" outbreaks has increased greatly since 1976. These are fairly frequent events as documented by the observation that 11% of 181 nosocomial outbreaks occurring between 1956 and 1975 which were investigated by the CDC were found to be pseudoepidemics of one type or another (103). The potential medical and economic consequences of pseudobacteremias are staggering. Additional cultures, removal or exploration of various catheters or implantable devices, and administration of antibiotics may result. Economically, the cost of pseudobacteremias is quite high when one includes the costs of the additional cultures needed to disprove the false positive, the antibiotics often started before recognizing the problem, and the increased hospital days that may be necessary. John and Bannister (104) have estimated that the cost of pseudobacteremia may exceed $22 million/year in the U.S.

Reported outbreaks have been traced to contamination occurring at any one of several differ-

ent steps in the blood culture process (Table 19.4). The first possibility for contamination is using intrinsically contaminated blood culture media. The second mechanism is the use of contaminated disinfectants either to cleanse the skin prior to venipuncture or to prepare the top of the blood culture bottle prior to inoculation. The third mechanism is contamination caused by collecting blood in nonsterile culture tubes or by contaminating multidraw needles by backflow from nonsterile culture tubes used before collection of blood for culture through the same needle.

The fourth mode is addition of contaminated medication (penicillinase) to blood culture medium. This mechanism has been studied experimentally by McNeil et al (86). They demonstrated contamination of blood cultures in 9.5% of instances when the needle was removed, the hub of the syringe placed inside a contaminated coagulation tube, and then a sterile needle replaced and used to inject the remaining blood into a culture bottle. This rate of contamination was reduced to 4.8% if needles were changed between each step, but increased to 76.2% if the same needle used to inoculate the coagulation tube was subsequently used to inoculate the blood culture bottle. The authors note that drawing blood for multiple tests, including culture, requires strict attention to detail to prevent false positive blood cultures.

The fifth mechanism is contamination of the cultures in the laboratory by a contaminated piece of equipment (such as the tuberculin syringe used to subculture bottles of media onto solid agar), by failure to disinfect the automated needle used in some commercial growth detection systems, or by contamination from the nose or hands of a technologist. The organisms involved in these outbreaks vary. The majority are gram-negative organisms. Staphylococci have been implicated in laboratory contamination from a colonized technician. Spore-forming organisms, such as *Bacillus* and *Clostridium* species, have been isolated from intrinsically contaminated media, as well as from contaminated solutions or soaps used to disinfect the skin or the diaphragm of the blood culture bottle prior to puncture.

Kusek (75) has outlined an approach to the prevention and detection of "pseudo-outbreaks." Given the number of steps involved and the changing skin preparations, techniques, and reagents used to obtain and process blood cultures, it is likely that the problem of "pseudobacteremia" will continue. The well informed infection control practitioner should, with the help of a

Table 19.4.   Methods of Contamination Resulting in "Pseudobacteremia"

Site	Method/Source	Etiologic Agent(s)	Ref	Author
Bedside	*Intrinsic contamination of blood culture medium*	Bacillus sp.	77	Noble and Reeves
	Contaminated skin preparation			
	Benzalkonium chloride	*P. cepacia*	78	Kaslow et al
	Chlorhexidine	*Flavobacterium meningosepticum*	79	Coyle-Gilchrist et al
	Green soap	*P. picketti*	80	Verschraegen et al
	Green soap	*P. stutzeri*	81	Keys et al
	Povidone-iodine	*P. cepacia*	82	Craven et al
		P. cepacia	83	Berkelman et al
	"Touch contamination" of skin			
	Thrombin contamination	*E. cloacae*	84	Graham et al
	Contamination at Collection			
	Backflow from needle holder	*Moraxella nonliquefaciens*	85	Duclos
	Backflow from citrated tubes	*Ewingella americanna*	86	McNeil et al
	Backflow from nonsterile tubes	*S. marcesens*	87	Hoffman
		P. maltophila	88	Semel
	Arterial blood gases on blood before culture	*S. marcesens*	89	Ives et al
	Culture in mist tent	*Acinetobacter calcoaceticus*	90	Snydman
	Contamination after collection			
	Add contaminated penicillinase to bottle	*E. coli*	91	Norden
		Acinetobacter lwoffi	92	Fairs
Laboratory	*Stopper top problems*			
	Inadequate disinfection	*Aerococcus viridans*	93	Spivak
	Contaminated disinfectant			
	Thimerosal	*Cl. sordellii*	94	Lynch et al
	Alcohol pads	*Bacillus* sp.	95	Berger
	Contamination at subculture			
	Lab tech shedder	*S. aureus*	96	Dolan
	Humidified incubator	*Acinetobacter lwoffi*	97	Jones et al
	Radiometric blood culture system	*K. pneumoniae*	98	Greenhood
	Sampling needle not sterile	*S. pyogenes*	99	Griffin
		Streptococcus sp. *S. aureus* *S. epidermidis* *E. coli* *Bacillus* sp.	100	Craven et al
	Dust	*Bacillus* sp.	101	Gurevich et al

capable microbiology laboratory staff, be able to identify such problems before they result in large numbers of patients receiving unnecessary and potentially toxic therapy. Maki (76) has pointed out that one or more of the following strongly suggest pseudobacteremia: (*a*) a cluster of blood cultures positive for a new or unusual pathogen; (*b*) "affected" patients do not consistently show signs or symptoms consistent with bloodstream infection; (*c*) the putative bacteremias are entirely "primary"; (d) most or all blood cultures from an individual are positive.

Of special note is the observation of Stratton (102) that half of all positive blood culture isolates in a university hospital microbiology laboratory were for coagulase-negative staphylococci. This isolation rate was found to be markedly higher in hospitals where cultures were obtained by housestaff than in hospitals where technicians obtained the cultures. Thus, the term "endemic pseudobacteremia" may be appropriate to denote a high rate of contamination during collection of blood cultures by poorly trained personnel.

PRIMARY AND IV DEVICE-RELATED BACTEREMIAS

Most patients admitted to United States hospitals receive intravenous fluids. Patients admitted to intensive care units or those undergoing invasive procedures often have intravascular devices placed to monitor blood pressure or cardiac output, or to permit administration of large volumes of fluid. All of these devices, and the IV fluids they administer, carry a small risk of local site infection or of bacteremia. The degree of risk varies with the device and its use, but risk *increases with time in place* for all of them.

INTRINSIC FLUID CONTAMINATION

Since the nationwide outbreak of intrinsically contaminated IV fluids in the United States in 1971, the problem has not been recognized in this country. A recent report from Greece concerned 63 patients with nosocomial sepsis caused by either *Enterobacter cloacae* or *E. agglomerans* seen in one hospital between April and October of 1981 (105). This epidemic was traced to contamination of the screw caps of bottles containing the intravenous fluids, and it was terminated only when the hospital excluded IV fluids from the incriminated manufacturer. Goldman (106), in an accompanying editorial, pointed out the similarities between this outbreak in Greece and the original description of the *E. agglomerans* sepsis that occurred in the United States in the early 1970s caused by the same mechanism.

At the other end of the spectrum, Daisy et al (107) reported 24 instances of intravenous infusion of IV fluids contaminated with filamentous fungi into patients without notable adverse affects. Arnow (108) has recently reported a single case of *E. coli* sepsis from a contaminated platelet transfusion together with a prospective study of quantitative culture of 500 consecutive units of platelet concentrate. They found an overall rate of contaminated platelet concentrate of 7%, with colony counts ranging from 1 to 1000 organisms/ml.

Unusual microorganisms recovered from catheter-associated IV infections include *Corynebacterium JK* (109, 110), and *Fusarium chlamydosporum* (111).

MULTIDOSE PARENTERAL MEDICATION VIALS

Outbreaks of nosocomial infection have been traced to the contamination of multidose medication vials used for venous admixtures or heparin flushes for arterial or other vascular lines. Highsmith et al (112) artificially contaminated vials of insulin, potassium chloride, heparin, and thiopental using selected microorganisms isolated during the investigation of nosocomial outbreaks. Following inoculation, they incubated the contaminated vials at room temperature and cultured them periodically. Two of the eight medications were lethal to all 13 test organisms within 24 hours. However six medications allowed the survival of some species for as long as 24 hours. Regular insulin allowed survival of *Candida*, enterococci, *Proteus mirabilis*, and *Serratia marcescens* for 48 hours or more at refrigerator temperature. Sheth et al (113) cultured 197 multidose injectable vials recovered from nursing units at their Veterans Administration hospital. In no instance was a bacterium or fungus cultured. They performed several experiments which demonstrated that gross contamination of the needle before entering the vial or of the injection cap was necessary in order to allow introduction of bacteria. Hence, they concluded that multidose vials could be used safely if handling practices were acceptable.

PATHOGENESIS OF CANNULA-RELATED INFECTIONS

The initial step in the pathogenesis of catheter-associated bacteremias has been held to be the establishment of a fibrin sheath around a cannula inserted into the bloodstream. This is followed by the attachment of bacteria to the fibrin. The organisms could migrate from the surface of the skin, be carried by contaminated IV fluids, or be brought by the bloodstream from some distant focus of infection (114) (Fig. 19.3). Once the fibrin sheath is colonized, active bacterial replication occurs, and bacteria are released into the bloodstream and become clinically evident.

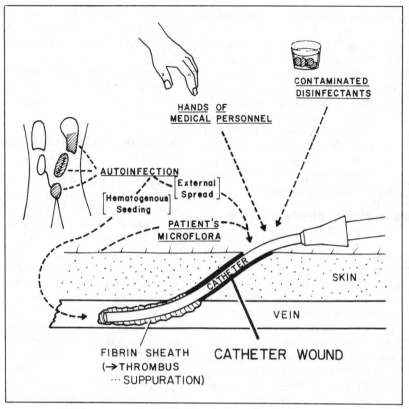

Figure 19.3.   Sources of vascular cannula-related infection. (From Phillips I, Meers PO, D'Arcy PF (eds): *Microbiologic Hazards of Intravenous Therapy*. Lancaster, England, MTP Press, 1977.)

The routes by which bacteria gain access to the catheter may depend most importantly on the type of catheter placed and its specific use. Short plastic catheters placed in peripheral veins seem to be associated with sepsis only when the cannula is colonized, whereas contaminated infusate or infection of a cannula-related clot secondary to another focus of infection is more frequent in centrally placed catheters, such as hyperalimentation catheters, Hickman-Broviac catheters, or central venous lines.

Characteristics of the catheter itself may facilitate colonization and/or infection by certain microorganisms. Bair and Petersen (115) and Locci et al (116) examined plastic cannulae by scanning electron microscopy and found multiple surface irregularities on both the internal and external surfaces. Cannulae used for infusion of IV fluids other than blood all had fibrinous material on the interior surface (115). Peters et al (117) demonstrated the presence of an "amorphous matrix" in which bacterial forms were embedded on the inner surfaces of "infected catheters." Plastic catheters exposed to heavy inocula of coagulase-

negative staphylococci in IV fluids flowing through the catheter for 24 hours regularly showed bacteria deposited at the site of major surface irregularities, especially at the point of sharp-edged cracks or scratches transverse to the direction of flow. With longer perfusion times, the numbers of bacteria at these sites increased, and organisms were also seen in "smooth" regions (117).

Franson et al (118) used scanning electron microscopy to confirm the observations of Locci et al (Fig. 19.4). Both groups found preferential attachment of bacteria to polyvinyl chloride (PVC) cannulae. Sheth et al (119) tried to assess the influence of the catheter material on bacterial colonization by analyzing semiquantitative cultures of 787 catheters consecutively submitted to their microbiology laboratory. No hyperalimentation catheters were examined. Of 77 PVC catheters (used for pulmonary artery pressure monitoring), 19 (24.6%) yielded more than 15 colonies of bacteria, predominantly coagulase-negative staphylococci. Only 48 of 647 Teflon catheters (6.9%) yielded more than 15 colonies per semi-

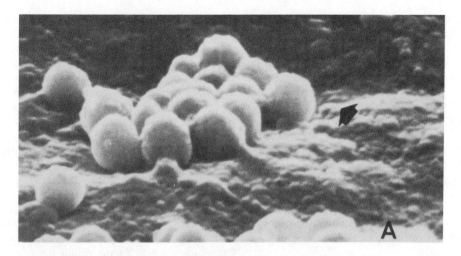

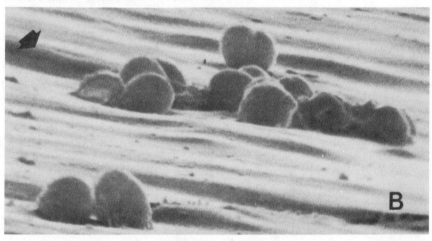

Figure 19.4. Scanning electron micrograph of coagulase-negative staphylococci on the surface of clinically infected (*A*) and in vitro prepared (*B*) PVC catheters: lodgement of organisms in surface irregularities (magnification, ×10,000) (*arrow* indicates ridge-like irregularity on catheter surface). (From Franson TR, Sheth NK, Rose HD, Sohnle PG: Scanning electron microscopy of bacteria adherent to intravascular catheters. *J Clin Microbiol* 20:500–505, 1984.)

quantitative culture (61.9% *S. epidermidis*). They concluded that *S. epidermidis* had an increased affinity for polyvinyl chloride, as opposed to Teflon, cannulae.

The characteristic of microorganisms which are associated with the ability to colonize plastic catheters are also under investigation. Christensen et al (120), using a quantitative microtiter method to assess slime production, found that strains of coagulase-negative staphylococci isolated during an outbreak of intravascular catheter-associated sepsis were significantly more adherent to plastic and produced more slime than were strains isolated from blood culture contaminants or from skin. They also found that the coagulase-negative staphylococcal strains isolated from the spinal

fluid of patients with clinically infected cerebrospinal fluid shunts were more adherent to plastic than were those coagulase-negative isolates from cerebrospinal fluid contaminants. This observation of a possible association of adherence and slime production as features which are associated with the pathogenicity of coagulase-negative staphylococci involved in nosocomial sepsis or nosocomial infection has been confirmed by Ishak et al (121) and by Davenport et al (122). Christensen et al (123) noted that coagulase-negative staphylococci appeared to adhere to smooth plastic surfaces in two separate phases. The first phase was that of adherence, which reached a maximum at approximately 2 hours, and the second was an accumulation phase of increasing numbers of cells and microcolony formation, which reached a maximum at approximately 6 hours.

Ishak et al (121) confirmed a correlation between slime production in *S. epidermidis* and nosocomial bacteremia. However, neither adherence of the organism to Teflon catheters nor phagocytosis and intracellular killing of coagulase-negative staphylococci was influenced by slime production. Davenport et al (122) also verified the association between slime positivity and the invasiveness and pathogenicity of coagulase-negative staphylococci. Furthermore, in their chart review study, antibiotic therapy for infections caused by slime-positive organisms was significantly less effective than that for slime-negative organisms.

Rotrosen et al (124) examined the adherence of various *Candida* species to mucosal cells, fibrin platelet matrixes, vascular endothelial cells, and plastic materials. They noted increased adherence of *Candida* species to polyvinyl chloride catheters as opposed to Teflon catheters and increased adherence of *Candida albicans*, as compared with other *Candida* species, to mucosal cells, fibrin platelet matrixes, and vascular endothelial cells. In contrast, *Candida tropicalis* was more adherent to catheter material than was *C. albicans*. The mannan of *Candida* appears to be important in the initial attachment of these organisms to substrates.

In summary, the attachment of bacteria (*S. epidermis, S. aureus*) and fungi (*C. albicans*) (124) to plastic surfaces appears to be facilitated by the irregularities in the surface of the plastic and, for *S. aureus*, by the presence of fibronectin (125). For *S. epidermidis*, the ability to "eat" into the plastic surface to provide a "pit" which partially covers the organism may facilitate colonization. In addition, coagulase-negative staphylococci and *Pseudomonas aeruginosa* secrete a glycocalyx substrate called "slime" that coats the surface of the organism and the catheter. This may improve their ability to bind to plastic surfaces and impair the host's ability to remove the organism. The establishment of a catheter-associated infection may, therefore, be the net result of the type of cannula placed, the presence of a particle or microorganism on the surface of the cannula, and its rate of growth balanced against the time the cannula is left in place. Whether newer catheter materials can influence the rate of colonizaton/infection remains to be seen.

The role of bacterial colonization of the skin at the entry site of IV cannulae has been subjected to study. Smallman et al (126) randomly assigned patients to peripheral IV catheter insertion with no skin preparation or with a chlorhexidine and ethanol preparation. They observed a 100% phlebitis rate in the no preparation group as opposed to a 34.5% rate in the treated group. Using nonquantitative bacteriology, 86% of the control catheters yielded bacterial growth versus 17.3% of the treated ones.

Snydman et al (127) prospectively evaluated the use of skin cultures taken at the site of entry of total parenteral nutrition catheters in predicting catheter-related infection. They demonstrated that 61% of patients with bacteria present on the skin developed cannula-related infection, whereas more of the patients with negative cultures had such problems within the subsequent week.

PERIPHERAL VENOUS CATHETERS

Peripheral IV catheters may be the most commonly used medical devices in United States hospitals. One recent study reported that IV cannulae were placed in 80.6% of all hospitalized patients (128). They have been intensively studied as a potential source for nosocomial bacteremia, but disagreement still exists over their importance. Tager et al (128) examined the risks of peripheral IV catheters at 10 Rhode Island hospitals. After following 5161 peripheral IV catheters in 3094 patients, they discerned a clinical phlebitis rate of 2.3% and a possible IV catheter-associated bacteremia rate of 0.08%. Since all patients were followed to discharge, these rates presumably are representative of those seen in non-Federal acute care hospitals. Their phlebitis rate is lower than those reported in studies from urban hospitals (129, 130). Examination of day-specific phlebitis rates revealed a highly significant trend toward increased phlebitis rate from 1 day of catheterization to 5 or 6 days of catheterization. Other factors importantly associated were chronologic order of catheter insertion and placement in a patient at high risk for nosocomial infection.

A summary of prospective studies reporting complications of peripheral intravenous cannulae (catheters and steel needles) is presented in Table 19.5. The studies of Tager et al (128) and Tomford et al (129) are observational studies only and do not include any cannula cultures. Combined, these two studies involve more than 6000 cannulae with a phlebitis rate of 15% (range 2.3 to 32%) and a rate of suspected cannula-associated bacteremia of only 0.07%.

Table 19.5. Risks Associated with Peripheral IV Catheters in Prospective Studies

Ref.	Authors	No. of Patients	No. of Cannulae	No. with Phlebitis	No. with Local Infection	Culture-Positive Cannulae	Cannula-Associated Bacteremia
128	Tager et al	3094	5164	118 (2.3[b])		Not Done	4 (0.08%)
129	Tomford et al	445	863	(32)	(2.1)	Not Done	0
			6027	(15)	(0.2)		(0.07%)
132	Maki and Band	381	827			34 (8.9)	6 (0.7%)
131	Righter et al		1696	(35.4)	0	41 (2.4)	0
134	Snydman et al		519	(25.2)	1	26 (5)	1 (0.2)
135	Gantz et al	807	431	(16.7)	2	10 (2.3)	0
133	Ricard et al	?	134	?	0	1 (0.75)	0
136	Wilkins et al	?	50	?	?	13 (20)	0
137	Tully et al	?	468	88 (18.8)	?	7 (1.5)	0
138, 138a	Cheesbrough and Finch	204	209	46 (22)		32 (15.3)	0
139	Hamory et al	805	2258	79 (3.5)	0	44/883 (5)	0
			6592			208 (3.4)	7 (0.11)
			Steel Needles				
137	Tully et al	?	486	43 (8.8)		6 (1.4)	0
140	Band and Maki		148	?	8 (5.4)		3 (2.1)
			634				3 (0.5)
			Heparin Lock				
141	Couchonnal et al	97	120	13		4/39 (10.3)	0
142	Hodder and Stern	89	246			32	0
140	Band and Maki	18					

[a] Semiquantitative culture ($\geq$ 15 colonies/plate).
[b] Percent of total cannulae.

Tomford et al (129) reported a 32% clinical phlebitis rate among patients on the general medicine services of a large city hospital, a rate similar to that observed by Falchuk et al (130) among surgical patients in a large hospital and by Richter et al (131). Both Falchuk and Richter observed their rates with an IV therapy team providing services. Richter confirmed that only 2.7% of cannulae from phlebitic veins were positive on semiquantitative culture.

The next nine studies listed in Table 19.5 are prospective studies of IV cannulae from various patient groups in which cannulae were cultured semiquantitatively. The range of reported clinical phlebitis rates using similar, but not identical, criteria is 3.5 to 35.4%, a 10-fold difference. The rates of positive cannula cultures range from 20% in a neonatal ICU (136) to 0.75% in a mixed adult ICU (133). The average rate (all cannulae positive/all cannulae cultured) is 3.4% culture positive. Among all 208 cannulae which had positive cultures, only 7 were associated with bacteremia for a rate of 3.4%. Of all 6,592 cannulae studies, only 7 or 0.11% were associated with bacteremia. This confirms a very low rate of bacterial infection as a complication of peripheral IV catheterization and a low predictive value of

positive semiquantitative culture for bacteremia. Complication rates for steel needles are similarly low. Though the data reported in the two largest series (137, 140) are incomplete, a bacteremia rate of 3/634 or 0.5% can be estimated from these studies.

Hershey et al (143) followed patients for 48 hours after discontinuation of peripheral IV catheters. They noted that clinical phlebitis appeared 12 hours following removal of the catheter in over half the patients with phlebitis. Furthermore, only 29% of patients who ultimately developed phlebitis had pain, and only 17% had erythema when examined 24 hours before diagnosis or phlebitis. No data are given concerning the rate of positive symptoms that did not progress to phlebitis, but the sensitivity of symptoms and signs 24 hours previously appears to be poor. Patients whose IV cannulae were pulled out at the time of diagnosis had a mean duration of phlebitis of 47 hours compared to a duration of symptoms of 38 hours if the phlebitis developed 12 hours after discontinuation (p = not significant). Both were of much shorter duration than the 77 hours of symptoms if the catheter remained in place at least 12 hours after early signs were detected ($p < 0.0004$). Other features associated with increased duration of phlebitis were diabetes, distant infection, and the use of vancomycin hydrochloride in the infusate.

Evaluations of interventions to reduce the rate of IV-associated bacterial infection have centered on local wound care preparations and on catheter materials. All such studies have used the semiquantitative culture method of Maki et al (35) as the endpoint. Unfortunately, some studies have included several types of cannulae (e.g., central venous lines, arterial cannulae, and peripheral venous cannulae) in the same study (133, 143), thus confounding their results.

Maki and Band (132) evaluated the efficacy of polyantibiotic or povidone-iodine ointment in reducing the rate of cannula-associated sepsis compared to no ointment. Polyantibiotic ointment applied by research nurses significantly reduced the rate of catheter positivity compared to no treatment. Povidone-iodine ointment reduced the rate by 50% compared to control, a difference that was not statistically significant. Of note, three of four *Candida* infections, and the only bacteremia occurred in the polyantibiotic ointment-treated group.

Ricard et al (133) evaluated four methods of protecting the cannula entry wound. They found no significant difference between the four methods studied (Betadine ointment and sterile gauze; Opsite; Opsite spray and film; or Betadine and Opsite film) using a semiquantitative culture method. However, this study illustrates the pitfalls of combining catheter types for analysis. Pulmonary artery catheters accounted for 109 of 708 total catheters, but for 9 of 12 contaminated ones. The authors do not specify the distribution of the catheters, stating only that "each type of catheter was uniformly distributed in the four groups." Richter et al (131) reported cannula culture rates of 2.4% by use of a povidone-iodine skin preparation and transparent dressing only. Most cannulae were removed prior to 72 hours.

As noted, the most widely used method to document cannula-associated sepsis has been the semiquantitative roll plate culture described by Maki et al (35). This generally shows good concordance with bacteremia in patients who are ill, but necessitates removal of the cannula. With the increased use of central and surgically implanted catheters, various approaches have been tried to diagnose catheter-related sepsis without removing the catheter (134, 144, 145). One case reported (144) and a series of 30 episodes of fever in 28 children with Broviac catheters reported complete success in diagnosing catheter-related sepsis by a marked increase in the level of bacteremia (100-fold) seen in cultures obtained through the line compared to peripheral cultures. Snydman et al (134) could not confirm this in a carefully done prospective study. In their hands only 4 of 12 catheter-related infections were detectable by pour plate cultures of blood obtained through the incriminated line.

Cleri et al (146) describe a flush technique for quantitative culture of IV catheters. They found an association of > 1,000 colony forming units of bacteria from the cannula with bacteremia. Furthermore, in all but one instance the intravascular section of the cannula had 1.4 to 1000 times more bacteria than did the intracutaneous segment. *S. epidermidis* was found in nine cannulae without associated bacteremia. The authors suggested that the skin was "the usual portal of entry for the organisms." This observation has not been followed up.

Moyer et al (147) compared several culture methods to document catheter-associated sepsis. Twenty-five of the 82 patients yielding catheters were burn patients, and they accounted for 39% of culture-positive cannulae. These investigators found that semiquantitative cannula cultures and quantitative cannula blood cultures were highly correlated with bacteremia documented by peripheral blood cultures.

Quercia et al (148) studied the contamination rates of IV infusion systems in the intensive care unit. They did not report their data by type of cannula location (peripheral versus central) but did find that 84 of 661 (12%) filter sets yielded bacterial growth, suggesting contamination. In this unit, all admixtures were prepared by unit nursing staff, except for parenteral nutrition. The study conflicts with the report of Gorbea et al (149a), who found contaminated IV burette fluid in only 4% of instances at 48 hours of use. They concluded that 48-hour changes of IV systems containing burettes for drug administration are safe.

Salohemio et al (149) used a laboratory model to demonstrate a higher rate of contamination from venous catheters with a silicone-valved side port than from standard cannulae. The data could not be confirmed in a clinical study (138). Cheesebrough et al (138a) cultured skin, cannula and side port from 51% cannulae removed from patients. In no instance was the same organism isolated from both side port and catheter tip. In half of the instances of positive cannula culture, the local skin was positive for the identical organism, suggesting that the skin was the source for the bacteria cultured from the tip. In contrast, colonization of the side port was usually unrelated to the patient's organism.

EFFECT OF IN-LINE, INTRAVENOUS FILTERS ON REDUCING MICROPARTICULATE-INDUCED PHLEBITIS

A chemically induced or irritative phlebitis in a peripheral vein is the most common complication of IV fluid therapy, occurring in up to 30% of infusions (129–131). Infection accounts for less than 1% of the observed instances of peripheral vein thrombophlebitis (131, 137). Three recent studies (130, 150, 151) have critically examined this issue (Table 19.6). All three studies have reached the same conclusion: a 0.45-μm or 0.22-μm filter placed in the peripheral IV line drastically reduces the rate of chemical or particulate-induced phlebitis. The large study of Falchuck et al (130) was performed using surgical patients with 18 to 20 gauge plastic peripheral IV catheters in place. A reduction in clinical phlebitis rates from 27% among controls to 11% in the filter-treated group was evident by day 3. In none of these studies were quantitative cultures of the peripheral catheter performed, and in none of them is there any comment regarding the occurrence of fever, positive blood cultures, or other evidence of infection. A recent letter concerning a prospective study of adding heparin to peripheral IV lines suggests the possibility of other ways to effect such a reduction (152). Considering the expense of adding catheters to the lines, the need in some instances for such filters to be changed at 24-hour intervals—hence opening the line—and the expense of the manpower needed, a recommendation to routinely use IV filters seems to be premature unless a hospital is observing a substantial rate of phlebitis associated with severe symptoms or complications (153, 154).

EFFECTIVENESS OF A PROFESSIONAL IV THERAPY TEAM

Two prospective studies evaluating the effectiveness of an IV therapy team in reducing the rate of complications associated with peripheral intravenous catheters have been reported (129, 139). Tomford et al (129) used a block design prospectively to monitor the effect of having a professional IV team available during one nursing shift for 5 days a week. Standard techniques for insertion and maintenance of IV therapy catheters were used without in-line filters. Phlebitis was evaluated using standard criteria by two independent and unblinded investigators. No catheters were prospectively cultured. These investigators studied 860 IV cannulae in 445 patients over the course of 2½ months. They demonstrated a significantly higher incidence rate of phlebitis among catheters inserted and maintained by floor staff than among those devices inserted or maintained by the IV therapy team. Overall, nine cases of suppurative phlebitis and one case of cellulitis were observed, only one of which was in a catheter maintained by the IV therapy team. The rate of suppurative phlebitis was therefore 0.2% in the team-inserted catheters versus 1% in the ward staff-inserted groups. For all types of cannulae, the phlebitis rate was 32% among the ward-inserted versus 15% in the team-inserted devices. The authors noted that the difference was not due to insertion technique since many of the catheters maintained by the IV team were inserted by ward housestaff. The rate of 32% phlebitis among ward-inserted catheters is the same as that reported by Falchuck et al (130) among their IV team-inserted catheters without in-line filters.

Table 19.6. Reducing Infusion-Related Phlebitis with In-line IV Filters

Ref.	Author	Patient Population	Filter Size	Cannula Size	Treatment	Group (n)	Phlebitis	p Value
			μm					
150	Rusho and Bair	Orthopaedic surgery	0.45	16 gauge	Control	50	27%	$p < 0.05$
					Filter	50	6%	
151	Allcutt et al	All	0.20	14–18 gauge	Control	93	24%	$p < 0.01$
					Filter	101	9%	
130	Falchuk et al	Surgery	0.22	18–20 gauge	Control	264	57.2%	$p < 0.001$
					Filter	277	25.5%	

Hamory et al (139) reported a prospective, randomized study of all adult patients to the general medical and surgical wards of a university hospital. All patients with IV therapy ordered were randomized to have cannulae inserted and maintained by either a team of professional IV therapy nurses or by standard ward (nurses and housestaff) care. Over a 14-week period, 805 patients with 2258 catheters were entered, randomly allocated, and followed. Catheter care and insertion techniques used were those described by the Centers for Disease Control and were identical in both groups. No in-line filters or differences in types of dressings applied to the site were allowed. Only those catheters *inserted and maintained* by each group were followed. The observers were blinded as to the randomization process and to the group to which the patient had been entered. Catheters were obtained for semiquantitative culture whenever possible at the time catheterization was discontinued. No major complications of IV therapy using peripheral veins were seen. There were no local site complications (such as abscess or purulent thrombophlebitis) and no systemic complications (such as bacteremia). The rate of minimal phlebitis (pain, redness, and induration extending less than 2 cm proximal to the insertion site) was lower in the team-inserted and maintained catheters (25 or 1227 catheters) than in the ward-inserted and maintained devices (54 of 1031, $p < 0.01$). The patient groups were well matched by age, sex, and service. No effect of antibiotic administration or type of fluid was noted. However, substantial differences in the rate of phlebitis according to the cannula size were noted. The IV therapy team preferentially inserted 20 and 22 gauge cannulae, whereas ward staff inserted 16 gauge cannulae in patients going to the operating room; this may account for some of the difference observed. The cost of maintaining a professional IV therapy team to provide service 18 hours a day, 7 days a week, as was done in this study, amounted to approximately $140,000. No effect of savings in usage of catheters or IV tubing was seen, but billing of private patients for IV fluids used was improved.

Both these studies show a benefit to the introduction of IV therapy teams in slightly different settings. The reduction seen in a busy metropolitan general hospital by Tomford et al (129) was greater than that seen at a university hospital with a presumably higher proportion of nursing staff to patients. In the study of Hamory et al (139), an IV team worked on the same floor with nurses who were inserting and maintaining their own

catheters, thus compensating for differences in available patient care personnel time. The effect of adding an IV therapist to a nursing floor may not simply be a reflection of the increased skill of the IV therapist but, rather, of increased total nursing time available to prevent the problem. The study of Hamory et al (139) differed from that of Tomford in that patients were not followed into intensive care areas and were not systematically followed past the point when the IV catheter was discontinued. However, most patients were available for continued observation and repeated cannulae were used on the same patients. Their observations did not reveal major complications—i.e., suppurative phlebitis or bacteremia—in study patients.

In view of published information that reflects an increasing proportion of catheter-associated complications in intensive care units relative to those on general floors, and because the largest number of catheter-associated bacteremias are associated with central catheters, which are not affected by IV therapy insertion and maintenance, the role of an IV therapy team in a general hospital remains ill defined. Although improvements in the rates of phlebitis were found by both Tomford and Hamory and their colleagues, the risk appears to be more related to chemical phlebitis than to bacterial infection. In addition, a recently reported study of the efficacy of the IV filter (130) was from a hospital with a functioning IV therapy team in which the baseline rate of phlebitis was reported to be 30% and was lowered by placement of terminal filters into IV lines. Such studies suggest that, in hospitals with IV therapy teams, the majority of these minor phlebitic episodes are not amenable to intervention by the IV team but rather to a technologic change, such as a filter.

RISK OF BACTEREMIA FOLLOWING CANNULA COLONIZATION

Analysis of the results of semiquantitative cannula cultures from multiple studies (Table 19.7) reveals that the risks of bacteremia following catheter colonization vary markedly between different bacterial species. Organisms in the *Klebsiella-Enterobacter-Serratia* group have the highest rates of bacteremia (25%), followed by *S. aureus* (15%) and *Candida* (10%). *S. epidermidis*, the most common colonizing organism, was only associated with bacteremia in 3% of instances. Certainly all of these cannulae were removed; thus, the true risk may be slightly higher than

Table 19.7. Risk of Bacteremia Secondary to Vascular Catheter Colonization by Organism and Device

Organism	Reference (No. of Devices Sampled[a])											Totals
	137 (465)	141 (39)	140 (148)	132 (827)	131 (1696)	134 (519)	137 (423)	139 (883)	141 (50)	135 (431)	138 (209)	
S. epidermidis	3	4	4 (1)	21 (4)	26	25	4	39	22		28	5/166 (3%)
Other CNS												
S. aureus	3		1 (1)	4	2	1 (1)			2		1	2/13 (15%)
Streptococci				2	13		1				1	0/15
Enterococcus				2 (1)					1			0/3
KES			1	1								1/4 (25%)
E. coli					1			1 (gram-negative rod)				0/2
P. aeruginosa				1								0/1
Acinetobacter sp.					1				1			0/2
Candida sp.				3 (1)	4		1				1	1/10 (10%)
Bacillus sp.				3	5			3			1	0/10
Corynebacterium sp.	1			3	3		1					0/8
Neisseria					4				2			0/6
Micrococcus					3							0/3
Bacteremias/catheter cultured	0/7	0/4	2/8	6/34	0/41	1/26	0/6	0/44	0/23+b		0/10	0/32

[a] A total of 5690 devices was sampled; 0.16% were positive on culture.
[b] Five cultures positive for multiple organisms.

estimated here. On the other hand, several of these studies were done in symptomatic patients, which might have falsely elevated the rate.

PERIPHERAL ARTERIAL PRESSURE MONITORING CATHETERS

Peripheral arterial catheters used for measuring intra-arterial pressure and for monitoring arterial oxygenation are among the most common devices in an intensive care setting. During an 8-month period, Pinilla et al (155) found that 172 arterial catheters were placed in 250 consecutive patients admitted to a surgical intensive care unit. Seven different prospective studies using quantitative culture techniques for catheter colonization of patients have been performed to evaluate radial artery catheters (155–161). The rates of bacterial colonization range from 0.85 to 20% of catheters. The rates of radial artery catheter-associated bacteremia range from 0.56 to 4.6% (Table 19.8).

The observational studies of Singh et al (156) and Russell et al (160) demonstrated an increased rate of catheter colonization (156) or catheter-associated bacteremia (160) among catheters placed in the femoral artery compared to the radial artery. However, the prospective randomized study of Thomas et al (159) failed to show a statistically significant difference in the rate of catheter tip colonization or of catheter-related bacteremia among patients randomly assigned to either radial or femoral arterial pressure monitoring. The only purulent entry site infections seen were in the femoral catheters. In the study the radial artery cannulae were inserted by trained technicians, whereas the femoral artery cannulae were inserted by physicians, and the sample size used was small. Both these factors may account for their failure to detect a difference.

The rate of cannula culture positivity increases with increasing duration of cannulation (157, 160) (Fig. 19.5), especially after the fourth day. Thomas et al (159) and Russell et al (160) performed daily dressing changes of the catheter entry site, whereas Pinella's group (155) changed the dressing at 48 hours. Infusion fluids and tubing were left hanging for 48 hours. No major differences in infection rates due to these differences can be inferred.

ARTERIAL PRESSURE MONITORING SYSTEMS

Outbreaks of nosocomial bacteremia have been traced to contamination of the fluids used for both intra-arterial infusion and for hemodynamic monitoring (26). These outbreaks are often prop-

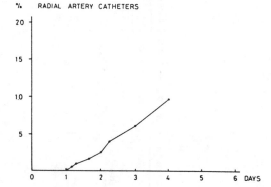

Figure 19.5. The cumulative probability of positive radial artery catheter cultures with time. (From Damen J, Verhoef J, Bolton DT, Middleton NG, Van Der Tweel I, De Jonge K, Wever JEAT, Nijsen-Karelse M: Microbiologic risk of invasive hemodynamic monitoring in patients undergoing open-heart operations. *Crit Care Med* 13:548–555, 1985.)

Table 19.8. Colonization and Infection of Arterial Cannulae

Ref.	Author	No. of Patients	No. of Catheters	Site	Positive Culture	Local Inflammation	Catheter-Associated Bacteremia
156	Singh et al	51	26	Radial	1 (4.0%)		[a]
			26	Femoral	5 (20.0%)		
157	Damen et al	574	584		9 (1.5%)	0	0
158	Samsoondar et al		19		2 (10.5%)	?	0
155	Pinilla et al		172		7 (4.6%)	4% Radial 7% Femoral	0
159	Thomas et al	155	82	Radial	2/68 (2.9%)	0	
			88	Femoral	2/73 (2.7%)	2.3%[b]	
160	Russell et al	231	178	Radial		1.7%	1 (0.56%)
			114	Femoral		0	2 (1.75%)
161	Shinozaki et al	117	117		1 (0.85)	0	0

[a] Twelve of 260 blood cultures through cannula were positive (4.6%).
[b] Pus at site.

agated by failure to sterilize reusable transducers or their domes adequately, or by the presence of small cracks in the transducer membrane that allow bacteria from nonsterile fluid used to transfer pressure to gain access to the sterile fluid path. The published prospective studies of arterial pressure systems are summarized in Table 19.9. Maki and Hassemer (162) prospectively evaluated 102 intra-arterial infusion lines for contamination of the fluid used to flush the monitoring system. They demonstrated that 11.8% of the fluids were contaminated at the site of the chamber dome, and in 7.8% of the total group they were associated with a concordant bacteremia. In each of these instances the transducer chamber dome had been used for more than 2 days. They concluded that 2 days was the maximum length of time during which such a system might be safely maintained.

Shinozaki et al (161) reported the result of a prospective study of 117 patients with arterial pressure monitoring lines. In this system, nondisposable transducers were used and were gas sterilized between patients. The patency of the system was maintained using a catheter flow device that bypassed the transducer dome. Cultures were obtained of the cannula and the stopcock sidearm used for removing arterial blood; quantitative cultures of fluid of the transducer dome were obtained using a loop method. During a 1-year period, 117 arterial lines were studied and "no clinically important vascular complications occurred." The authors reported only one instance where the catheter tip yielded a positive culture (0.85%). This occurred with a *Klebsiella* species that was obtained at autopsy but was not believed to be due to the catheter. There was no instance of transducer fluid contamination. The rates of positive stopcock cultures increased with increasing duration of cannulation, from 6.5% at less than 48 hours to 27.5% for more than 97 hours. The authors attributed their remarkably low rate of contamination to the placement of a continuous flow device distal to the transducer dome such that there was no column of fluid between the sampling port and the transducer dome.

Luskin et al (163) determined the contamination rates of totally disposable pressure transducers used for arterial monitoring. Of 120 courses of arterial monitoring, 62 were in a 2-day change group, and 58 were changed at 4 days or longer (39 every 8 days). Thirty-seven courses involved Swan-Ganz catheters, including 19 in the 2-day group and 18 changed at 4 days or more. The authors concluded that there was no difference in the rate of contamination for transducers changed every 2 days versus those changed every 4 days. The rate did not vary between those devices used for arterial or Swan-Ganz catheters. Among contaminated transducers, gram-negative bacilli were found in 63%. No relationship could be shown between the risk of contaminated transducer fluid and the number of blood specimens drawn through the transducer port. Of interest, five contaminated transducers were sampled periodically. In two instances the bacterial contamination cleared spontaneously. In the remaining three instances the number of gram-negative organisms increased. In one instance the count of *Pseudomonas* rose from 1 colony forming unit (CFU)/ml on the third day of cannulation to 10^4 CFU/ml on day 6. In another patient with a continuous level of *Klebsiella pneumoniae* contamination, a definite transducer-related bacteremia occurred on the first day of recognized contamination of the total group of 569 transducer cultures, 86 contained fewer than 15 CFU of organisms other than enteric gram-negative bacilli or *Pseudomonas*. Of these, 68 were coagulase-negative staphylococci, and 10 were *Acinetobater*. Of 86 catheter tips recovered for cultures, 28.6% had counts of more than 15 CFU/ml. Coagulase-negative staphylococci accounted for 87.5% of these positive cultures and in two instances were associated with bacteremia. The rate of positive catheter tips rose from 23% of those catheters removed by day 4 to 33% of those removed after 5 or more days. Hence, there was a relationship between the duration of cannulation and the number of positive cultures. The authors note that their system has some features in common with that described by Shinozaki et

Table 19.9. Contamination of Arterial Pressure Fluids

Ref.	Author	No. of Patients	No. of Infusions	No. of Contaminants	No. of Bacteremias	Associated Factors
162	Maki and Hassemer	56	102	12	8	Distant focus of infection, > 48-hr use
		31	53	3	0	(All < 48-hr use)
161	Shinozaki	117	0	0	0	
163	Luskin et al	157	569			Disposable transducer

al (161) in that it does not have a standing column of fluid between the transducer and the sampling port. The authors conclude that changing disposable pressure transducers at 48-hour intervals provides acceptably low rates of contamination/bacteremia compared with changing at 24-hour intervals.

CENTRAL VENOUS CATHETERS

Several authors (157, 164–168) have reviewed the complications of central venous catheterization with particular attention to the infectious complications. A comparison of the available information regarding the risks of catheter colonization and/or bacteremia attributable to central venous catheters is presented (Table 19.10). The total number of patients with prospective evaluation including semiquantitative culture of the catheter and peripheral blood cultures for documentation of bacteremia is fairly small ($n =$ 1002). The observed rate of bacteremia ranges from 3.8 to 21% with a mean of 4.3%. Several authors, in evaluating the relationship of sepsis or colonization to risk factors, have implicated infection at a distant focus as a risk for seeding the catheter, contamination of infusion fluid, or bacterial growth at the skin entry site of the organism. Methods for preventing catheter-related sepsis that have been evaluated include daily dressing changes with cleansing of the skin and topical application of a povidone-iodine solution (164), weekly exchange of the catheter over a guidewire with associated disinfection and redressing of the skin (169a) and placement of the catheter in the jugular vein rather than the infraclavicular location (170).

As with other vascular catheters that penetrate the epidermis, duration of catheterization was significantly associated with the increased colonization of the catheter and with bacteremia. Prager and Silver (169) found that 17 of 126 central venous catheters in place for 7 days or less were colonized (13.5%), whereas 23 of 53 catheters in place for more than 8 days (43.4%) became colonized. Only two catheters had associated positive blood cultures in less than 7 days, whereas 13 of 53 had associated bacteremia in the over-7-day group. In Prager's study of peripheral blood cultures obtained before removing the central venous catheters, only three of 15 episodes of documented bacteremia or fungemia were associated with clinically suspected sepsis. The remaining 12 instances were unsuspected. Most of the patients from whom blood cultures were positive had fever. Catheters placed into the internal jugular vein were significantly less apt to be colonized than were subclavian catheters. Of 40 catheters significantly colonized with bacteria, 15 (37.5%) were associated with positive peripheral venous cultures. The rate of both bacteremia and catheter colonization were not influenced by the use of topical povidone-iodine.

Linblad and Wolff (166) evaluated 151 central venous catheterizations during a 1-year period. Insertion of the cannulae was made using sterile gloves and a face mask but without sterile gowns and with dressing changes made every other day. Mural or occlusive thrombosis of the central vein was found in 12%, and autopsy revealed thrombosis in 32% of the 28 patients who came to postmortem examination. Nineteen instances of bacteremia were found; 15 were clearly related to other foci, two were clearly related to central venous catheter tip, and two were possibly related. The high rate of thrombophlebitis in central venous catheterization has also been shown by Curelaru et al (171). In this study of 227 central

Table 19.10.   Central Venous Catheters

Author	Ref.	No. of Catheterized Patients	No. of Catheters Colonized	No. with Bacteremia	Culture		
					Skin	Fluid	Hub
Prager and Silva	169 (Iodine)	84	18 (21%)	7 (8.3%)	Yes	No	No
	(Drsg.)	95	22 (23%)	8 (8.4%)			
Bozzetti	164	140	?	9 (6.4%)	Yes	Yes	No
Lindblad and Wolff	166	151	10 (6.6%)	4/19 (21%)	No	No	No
Michel et al	167	390	47 (12%) Phlebitis	15 (3.8%)	No	No	No
Sketch et al	168	65	3 (4%)	0	No	No	No
Damen et al	157	77	3 (3.9)	0	No		
Total		1002		43 (4.3%)[a]			

[a] Percentage of all catheters.

venous catheters, the majority of episodes of thrombophlebitis occurred within the first 10 days of catheterization. Twenty percent of catheters (44 of 227) in place for 10 days or less were associated with radiographic evidence of thrombophlebitis versus three of 62 in place for more than 10 days. Only one incidence of suppurative thrombophlebitis and catheter sepsis was diagnosed in over 2000 catheterized days. There were no other instances of catheter-related infection. Hence, Curelaru et al demonstrated the alarming frequency of venous thrombosis associated with the placement of a central venous catheter, which may account for the observation of a significant association of bacteremia from a distant focus being associated with catheter colonization with microorganisms.

Michel et al (167) evaluated the risk of microbial colonization of indwelling central venous catheters prospectively. The catheter culture technique was not a semiquantitative one, and hence the precise determination of which organisms represented colonization of the catheter tip is arguable. However, the authors did demonstrate a linear increase in the contamination rate of catheters in patients who had a remote infected focus of infection as well as a significant association statistically between catheter contamination in bacteremia as well as between the catheter contamination and the presence of a tracheostomy. The use of infusion of total parenteral nutrition fluids through the catheter was not associated with an increased risk of catheter colonization. Bacteremia was documented in 33 cases, but the catheter was considered the source in only three episodes. In the other 30 instances a remote infected site was found. These authors recommended the removal of a central venous catheter in any patient with fever and unexplained sepsis.

The necessity for this procedure was examined by Bozetti (164) in an attempt to discern whether cultures of other body sites would permit discrimination between catheter-related sepsis and sepsis secondary to some other source. Catheter tip cultures were performed by a nonquantitative method together with cultures of the skin entry site of the catheter, the infusion fluid, and peripheral blood. Twenty-five of 165 catheter tips had colonization, of which only 13% were with "pathogenic organisms." There were 25 instances of bacteremia, nine of which were associated with the catheter tip culture positive for the same organism. Microorganisms isolated were *S. aureus*, "*S. albis* (*S. epidermidis*)," *Candida*, *Serratia*, and unidentified gram-negative rods. A *Candida* was associated in all instances with a positive tip culture, whereas *S. aureus* was only associated with a 33% positive tip culture. The author demonstrated contamination of infusion fluid in 6.9% of instances using nonquantitative techniques. The risk of contamination of the catheter with the same microorganism was 5.8%. The rate of catheter-related sepsis was 7.6%, and the author estimated that a positive catheter tip culture was associated with "infection" in 25.7% of instances. They found that the predictive value for catheter-related sepsis of cultures of the proximal catheter segment, the infusion fluid, distant fossae of presumed infection, and the point of skin entry of the catheter was quite low, ranging from 3.8 to 7.4%.

Bozetti et al (165) further extended their study to examine the effectiveness of weekly changes of the central venous catheter over a guidewire to prevent sepsis. In a sequel to Bozetti's earlier study, all patients undergoing central venous catheterization had weekly guidewire exchanges performed with cultures of the central venous catheter tip and peripheral blood. The rate of catheter-associated sepsis was 3 of 62 patients (4.8%), and the rate of colonization was 21 of 207 patients (10.1%). The authors claimed that in all instances the catheter contamination (sepsis) resolved with weekly exchanges of the catheter over the guidewire. It is unclear whether antimicrobial agents were given concomittantly. In addition, the authors recognized some risk of pulmonary thromboembolism if subclavian venous thrombosis is present, but they state the probability was 4 to 11.5%. This article occasioned some comments (172) that pointed out that the conclusions were difficult to support because *S. epidermidis* was not considered as a potential pathogen and no quantitative technique was used for culture. An association between central venous catheters and endocarditis has been made. Wheeler and Weesner (173) reported a case of *S. aureus* endocarditis associated with central venous catheterization in an infant. Tsao and Katz (174) presented a case report and literature review documenting 21 previously reported cases of central venous catheter-associated endocarditis. Fourteen of the 21 cases were associated with hyperalimentation. The sepsis rates associated with the use of central venous catheters ranged between 0 and 80%. Few cases of documented endocarditis were reported in papers which collected series of bacteremia associated with central venous catheters.

PULMONARY ARTERY (SWAN-GANZ) CATHETERS

Insertion of ballon-tipped cardiac catheters for monitoring cardiac output and pulmonary artery pressures is quite common in today's intensive care areas. Pinilla et al (155) reported that 37 of 250 consecutively admitted patients in the surgery ICU (14.8%) received such catheters, and Donowitz (175) reported that 1% of all patients admitted to the pediatric ICU at the University of Virginia Hospital had such catheters inserted. These catheters have been associated with various problems, including endocardial lesions and bacterial endocarditis (175–177), as well as sepsis (54, 157, 178–181). These are in addition to the numerous mechanical complications and arrhythmias which also may occur (179, 182).

A review of the published literature (Table 19.11) reveals that among studies in which semiquantitative cultures of Swan-Ganz catheters were performed, the rate of colonization ranged from 2.1 to 33%. Sepsis rates ranged from 0 to 47%.

One of the most complete studies is that of Damen et al (157). It involved cultures of patients undergoing open heart surgery in whom the lines were placed in the operating room and who received antimicrobial cefazolin prophylaxis. The study revealed that of 584 pulmonary artery catheters, 12 (2.1%) had more than 10 colonies recovered from the tip on semiquantitative culture. In all of these series, the majority of organisms isolated were staphylococcal species, predominantly *S. epidermidis*, with a scattering of gramnegative organisms, including *Pseudomonas* and *Acinetobacter*. *Candida* species were recovered from only one patient (181) involved in a prospective study using semiquantitative culture methods. *Candida* species were recovered from the blood of very ill surgical patients with associated bacterial endocarditis who were catheterized for long periods (176). In the study of Michel et al (178), which did not use semiquantitative methodology, two patients had *Candida* recovered from a thioglycollate culture of the catheter tip. One of them had *Candida* recovered from the blood and empyema fluid. The sources for bacteria that colonize or infect the pulmonary artery catheter are still under investigation. In some studies (178, 181–183) the rate of positive blood cultures was explained in more than half of the cases by distant foci that were actively infected with the same organism. Thus, significant rates of catheter colonization were associated with active infected foci at other body sites. Singh et al (156) were unable to confirm this relationship.

Three studies (156, 157, 181) have intensively investigated the risks of contamination of pulmonary artery catheters as measured by semiquantitative culture of the catheter tip, peripheral blood culture, culture of blood obtained through the catheter port, and culture of the skin surrounding the catheter entry site. The rate of catheter tip positivity on semiquantitative culture using the criteria of 10 colonies or more (157), 12 colonies or more (181), and 15 colonies or more (156) were, respectively, 2.1%, 5.8%, and 8.1%. The lowest proportion, that of Damen et al (157), was obtained from cultures of patients undergoing open heart surgery whose catheters were inserted in the operating suite using aspetic technique.

Myers et al (181) and Singh et al (156) demonstrated that skin cultures obtained from the area close to the entry point of the catheter were positive in 12% and 8.1%, respectively, of samples. In both instances, most of these cultures

Table 19.11. Swan-Ganz Catheters

Ref.	Population	No. of Catheters	No. of Colonized Catheters	No. with Sepsis	Mean Duration of Catheterization
					days
183	SICU	33	?		
	SICU (sepsis)	24			
182	ICU	116	5	2 (*S. aureus*)	
178	ICU	190	29/153	0/153	
179	ICU	173	IV catheter patients	1	3.5
156	ICU	37	6 (11.5%)		
180	SICU	211		3 (1.4%)	
181		170	10 (5.8%)		
157		584	12 (2.1%)	0	1.1
158	SICU	12	4 (33%)	0	

were positive for *S. epidermidis*. Blood cultures obtained at the time of fever or other clinical indication by Damen et al were not positive in any instance (157). In their study Myers et al (181) obtained blood cultures every 2 days both through the distal port of the catheter and by peripheral venipuncuture. Of 309 cultures obtained through the distal port of the pulmonary artery catheter, 13.2% were positive in patients with negative semiquantitative catheter cultures. This compared to 8% of peripheral blood cultures obtained from patients with 146 pulmonary artery catheters negative on semiquantitative culture. Of these 67 positive blood cultures obtained from catheter tip-negative patients, 23 (34.3%) yielded *S. epidermidis*, a presumed skin contaminant. Of the nine pulmonary artery catheter tips that were positive on semiquantitative culture, six of 17 blood cultures obtained through the catheter lumen versus eight of 20 obtained through the peripheral blood were positive. Overall, from either peripheral blood or blood through the catheter, 60% of patients with positive catheter tip cultures had a positive blood culture. Noteworthy in this study is the fact that of 10 patients with positive catheter tip cultures, five had remote foci infected with the same organism that was cultured from their catheter tip. Three of these five also had "several blood cultures" that yielded the same organism during the period of catheterization. The authors also noted that 15 of 147 blood cultures taken at the time of insertion of the pulmonary artery catheter were positive. Virtually all of these individuals were receiving systemic cephalosporin antibiotic, and only one of the 15 patients with a positive blood culture at the time of insertion subsequently developed a positive catheter tip culture. The organisms responsible for these 15 cases of bacteremia at the time of catheter insertion are not given. However, since the patients were being catheterized in the surgery ICU for a variety of problems, including systemic and abdominal sepsis, it is unlikely that these were simple contaminants.

Singh et al (156) found that 5% of 119 blood samples obtained either from the right atrial port of the pulmonary artery catheter or from the side port of the cordis introducer were positive. The three pulmonary artery catheters that were positive on semiquantitative culture all yielded micrococcus species. It is not known whether these were *S. epidermidis*. The authors commented that the recovery of microorganisms from skin site swabs of the combined groups of radial artery and pulmonary artery catheters was associated with a marked increase in the rate of catheter positivity. However, they did not provide data that could be analyzed. Of 14 positive skin cultures, five were associated with positive catheter cultures and nine with negative catheter cultures. Conversely, five catheters were positive for both semiquantitative bacteria and skin cultures, and nine of 80 negative catheter tip cultures were positive on skin sampling. Infection at distant foci did not appear to affect the rates of catheter colonization, nor did durations of catheterization influence the rate of colonization. The findings may have been influenced by the addition of peripheral arterial catheters into the group, since Damen et al (157) demonstrated a linear relationship between the length of catheterization with pulmonary artery catheters and the rate of culture positivity; they were unable to show this relationship for either peripheral IV catheters or arterial monitoring catheters.

The contribution of infusate, such as the chilled saline used to perform thermodilution cardiac output measurements, to catheter-related sepsis has not been directly examined under conditions of prolonged in-use circumstances. However, Riedinger et al (184) provided information for a laboratory-based setting, and Yonkman and Hamory (185) provided information based upon observations of nurses performing single injections of chilled injectate using three separate methods. Under laboratory conditions and wearing sterile surgical gowns, gloves, masks, and caps, Riedinger et al filled syringes with sterile D5W and placed the syringes in sterile containers inside an ice bath or at room temperature. The sterile syringes prepared in this manner were then used for routine measurements of thermodilution cardiac output and those not used by the nursing staff were sampled. No contamination was found.

Under conditions of actual use in intensive care areas, Yonkman and Hamory attached Millipore filters to sterile stopcocks inserted at the time of assembly of the Swan-Ganz apparatus. They then sampled the injectate actually delivered to the patient by nursing staff performing these procedures using one of three different methods. The contamination rate of the injectate ranged from 0% with a system in which the injectate was chilled using a blood coil loop and in which a closed system was maintained to almost 30% in a system requiring multiple entries into a liter bag of saline maintained in an ice bath.

Therefore, it seems reasonable to conclude that pulmonary artery catheters that are inserted in an operating room environment in patients undergoing cardiac surgery have lower risks of contamination than those catheters inserted at the bedside in busy ICUs. Additionally, patients who have active bacteremia at the time of catheter insertion have an associated rate of contamination which may be approximately 7%. Contamination of the end of the catheter appears to be related to the presence of a distant focus of infection and to the legnth of time (Fig. 19.6) the catheter is left in place (157). It is not clear how the use of various dressing devices or a permanent introducer that is infused in a side port affects the rate of contamination. Because of the frequency of endocardial and valvular lesions associated with pulmonary artery catheterization, it is recommended that catheters be changed at 72- to 96-hour intervals and that a new site be prepared if they are required for long periods of time.

HICKMAN-BROVIAC INDWELLING CATHETERS

Permanent implantation of intravenous access devices into patients requiring prolonged administration of chemotherapeutic agents, antibiotics, or total parenteral nutrition has become increasingly common. The devices most commonly used are Hickman or Broviac catheters, which are surgically placed central venous catheters tunneled subcutaneously to an exit site on the chest wall at some distance from the entry into the subclavian or external jugular vein. A leading complication of these devices is infection, of which *S. epidermidis* is the primary cause. Begala

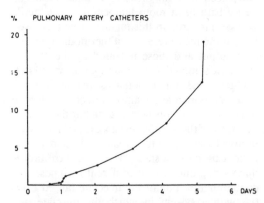

Figure 19.6.   The cumulative probability of positive PA catheter cultures with time. (From Damen J, Verhoef J, Bolton DT, Middleton NG, Van Der Tweel I, De Jonge K, Wever JEAT, Nijsen-Karelse M: Microbiologic risk of invasive hemodynamic monitoring in patients undergoing open-heart operations. *Crit Care Med* 13:548–555, 1985.)

et al (186) prospectively followed 88 patients with 90 central venous catheters inserted over 4 months. The authors demonstrated a 4-fold difference in the rate of catheter infections between Hickman catheters and Broviac catheters. In part this may have been related to the fact that the Broviac catheters were inserted in young patients, whereas the Hickman catheters were inserted in older patients. No association was found between catheter-related infections and age, *disease*, or the administration of blood, medication, or hyperalimentation fluids. The risk of catheter-related infection was approximately 7.5/1000 catheter days, and it remained constant over time. Of the 17 patients with catheter-related infections, seven patients had septicemia with *S. epidermidis* and *S. aureus* in three instances. In 15 of 17 instances in which a catheter-related infection occurred (local site or septicemia), a concurrent focus of infection existed at another body site. In four instances of catheter-related sepsis the organism(s) cultured from blood was also cultured from the other site of infection. These authors concluded that the risk of infection was constant over time and was increased if the patient had another site of active infection. However, they were unable to demonstrate any relationship between the administration of hyperalimentation and/or blood through the catheter and an increased rate of sepsis. The infection rate with the Hickman catheter was greater than that with the Broviac catheter. In this study the Broviac catheter was Teflon coated, whereas the Hickman catheter was not.

Abrahm and Mullen (187) reported on a 3-year prospective study involving 71 silicone catheters, of which 63 were Hickman catheters and eight were Broviac catheters. Rigorous attention was devoted to placement and maintenance of the catheter. There were eight catheter-related infections in the 71 catheters (11%). Three bacteremias occurred (two *S. aureus* and one *S. epidermidis*), and there were five local site infections (one *S. epidermidis*). None of these incidents resulted in death of the patient. Catheters were left in place in 38 patients during systemic infections with various organisms. In only five of the 38 cases was the source of the bacteremia unknown. In the 38 episodes, four catheters were removed, two of which were infected. The rate of all catheter-related infections, including those that were septic and insertion site related, was 1.2 infections/1000 patient days. The authors did not note any relationship between the duration of catheterization and the rate of complication.

Thomas et al (188) reported a rate of catheter-related sepsis in 8 of 6308 catheter days. Jacobs and Yeager (189) provided some information from the Stanford University Hickman experience. In a series of 196 catheters there was an 8% rate of definite catheter-related infections and a 13% rate of possible or probable catheter-related infections. Lowder et al (190) reported 80 immunocompromised patients with 90 catheters in place and 27 episodes of sepsis. They noted an increased proportion of bacteremias in patients with Hickman catheters compared with those who had peripheral lines. Legha et al (191) reported on 65 percutaneously placed silicone elastormer catheters placed in 50 patients. Opsite dressings were used after application of povidone-iodine ointment at the site of insertion with three times weekly dressing changes. All patients had metastatic cancer. Twenty-eight catheters were inserted through the subclavian vein and 37 through a peripheral vein. Sepsis was noted in four patients, cellulitis in one, and phlebitis in one. Both sepsis and phlebitis were more common in the peripherally placed catheters, whereas the only incidence of cellulitis occurred in a patient whose catheter was subclavian. The phlebitis noted occurred within 10 days following insertion with a median of 7 days. There was no evidence of infection in any of these instances. In all four instances of catheter-related sepsis the catheter tip was cultured and was positive for the same organism found in blood. Two of the four infections were caused by *Candida* species, one by *Klebsiella*, and one by *Bacillus cereus*. Many other studies have also been published (187, 190, 192–199).

Svirbely et al (192) have reported infection with *Mycobacterium fortuitum* at the catheter exit site of a Hickman catheter as an unusual complication of such a device. The patient had a large cell histiocytic lymphoma and his catheter was initially inserted for treatment of *Cryptococcus neoformans*. Other complications have included endocarditis (193) and brachial plexus neuritis (194).

Bothe et al (195) report the use of a totally implantable central venous access system that utilizes a small subcutaneous injection port connected to a Silastic catheter. All of it is contained subcutaneously and the catheter accesses a cephalic vein. During a 1-year period, 75 access discs were implanted in 74 patients for treatment of malignancy. All patients were adults, and the access devices were in place for a total of 6762 patient days (1 to 351 days). The duration of

continuous needle placement for infusion was 2207 days with an average of 29 days/patient. Infections were found in seven systems (9%). Six instances involved infections of the subcutaneous pocket, one of which was associated with sepsis. Two had systemic catheter-related infections. Only three infections required removal of the system. No relationship was found between the duration of device implantation and the rate of infection. Neiderhuber et al (200) have also reviewed this topic.

INTRA-AORTIC BALLOON PUMPING

The technique of placing a catheter into the abdominal or thoracic aorta as a blood pressure assistance device has gained wider usage during the last 5 years. Infectious complications of such devices are related primarily to the presence of local wound infection. In one series (203) three of four groin wound infections were caused by *Pseudomonas* infection. An arteritis was documented together with a superficial skin infection. Bacteremia complicated 0.8% of these procedures. The overall rate of local wound infection is 2.4% (201–203).

TOTAL PARENTERAL NUTRITION (TPN)

Prevention of infections associated with TPN catheters has received a great deal of attention, because infection is one of the most common complications, occurring in 6 to 27% of patients (204, 205). These alarming rates have been reduced by strict attention to aseptic insertion practices, care in maintaining a closed system used only for hyperalimentation, and strict attention to techniques of local wound care. However, major complications still occur, including thrombosis of the central vein in up to 71% of catheterized patients.

Recent studies (206–212) have improved the understanding of the routes for bacterial entry into the system. The central catheter and its local skin entry site account for most infections (127, 134, 204). Snydman et al (127) demonstrated that 14 of 21 patients with skin culture yielding bacteria from the site of catheter entry had positive semiquantitative cannula cultures within the next week. Two instances of line-related sepsis were seen in 63 courses of TPN therapy, and both had skin cultures positive for the same organism isolated from blood and the catheter tip. Bjornson et al (204) reported a similar finding, since all five instances of catheter sepsis had semiquantitative cultures of skin at the insertion site positive for $>10^3$ organisms/4 inches^2, and all 15 intravascular catheter segments positive on culture were associated with skin colonization.

Snydman et al (134) prospectively identified the presence of T-connectors (stopcocks) and the occurrence of violations in line management as variables that increase the risk of infection with TPN cannulae. They noted TPN line-related infections within 3 days following such breaks in line protocol as obtaining central venous pressure readings, extracting a clot, and replacing a line under nonsterile conditions.

Sitges-Serra et al (208) have proposed that bacterial colonization of the catheter hub represents an additional route for bacterial entry into the system. This issue requires further study. Additional techniques for precisely identifying coagulase-negative staphylococci are needed in future studies (207, 208).

Techniques that have been evaluated and that do not seem to reduce the rate of infection include the administration of prophylactic vancomycin (210) and "tunneling" a standard subclavian catheter through a 10-cm subcutaneous tract (209). Jarrard et al (213) found that daily dressing changes and skin preparation eliminated their ability to recover bacteria from the skin entry site. However, they did not recommend routine use of this time-consuming and expensive procedure.

UMBILICAL ARTERY CATHETERS

Bacterial infection complicates 1.4 to 2.6% of umbilical artery catheterizations in neonates (214). The subject was reviewed by Thompson et al (215), who noted the lack of good, quality data linking the observed rates of bacteremia to the catheter itself. The authors reported two infants with mycotic aortic aneurysms at the site of the catheter tip and reviewed nine other cases from the literature. The organisms recovered from these cases were similar to those isolated from the umbilical stump of the neonate (coagulase-negative staphylococci, *S. aureus*, and various gram-negative bacilli).

In a prospective study using semiquantitative methodology, Adams et al (214) examined 114 umbilical catheters, 79 of which were arterial. Ten percent of catheter tips were positive on semiquantitative culture, and *S. epidermidis* accounted for 10 of 16 isolates. They found that the rate of catheter positivity increased with increasing duration of catheterization but that cultures of the umbilical stump were not helpful in predicting results of catheter culture.

SUBCLAVIAN VEIN HEMODIALYSIS CATHETERS

Percutaneously inserted catheters used for hemodialysis access have become quite common (216). The rate of infectious complications is time dependent. Local site infections occur at a rate of 1.3 to 37.2 episodes/100 patient months, and catheter-related sepsis occurs at a rate of 0.4 to 20.6 episodes/100 patient months (217). In a retrospective review of their experience, Kozeny et al (216) reported a sepsis rate of 6.8%; the rate was also time dependent. Sherertz et al (217) pointed out that early catheter infections were due to *S. epidermidis*. Concurrent data suggest the need for rigorous attention to local site care to reduce the rate of complications. Raja et al (218) suggested limiting the duration of catheterization to less than 4 weeks to reduce complications.

SUMMARY

Nosocomial bloodstream infections are associated with significantly increased patient mortality. Reducing the rate of nosocomial bacteremia will depend on earlier identification and treatment of the primary sites of nosocomial infection (surgical wound, pneumonias, and UTIs)—responsible for one-half of all bacteremias—in addition to paying closer attention to the use of intravascular devices. Various techniques now exist for reducing the risk of bacteremia that is associated with many types of vascular devices and with infusion therapy. These recommendations have been summarized by Simmons (219).

Future research efforts need to be directed not only toward techniques and devices that may lower the risk of infection or extend the interval that devices may remain in place, but also to methods which encompass effective ways to change the behavior of physicians and nurses.

References

1. Brenner ER, Bryan CS: Nosocomial bacteremia in perspective: a community-wide study. *Infect Control* 2:219–226, 1981.
2. Bryan CS, Hornung CA, Reynolds KL, Brenner ER: Endemic bacteremia in Columbia, South Carolina. *Am J Epidemiol* 123:113–127, 1986.
3. Filice GA, Van Etta LL, Darby CP, Fraser DW: Bacteremia in Charleston County, South Carolina. *Am J Epidemiol* 123:128–136, 1986.
4. Haley RW, Culver DH, White JW, Morgan WM, Emori TG: The nationwide nosocomial infection rate: a new need for vital statistics. *Am J Epidemiol* 121:159–167, 1985.
5. Centers for Disease Control: National nosocomial infections study report: *Annual Summary 1979.*

Issued March 1982.

6. Centers for Disease Control: National nosocomial infections study report: *Annual Summary 1975.* Issued October 1977.

7. Centers for Disease Control: Nosocomial infection surveillance, 1980–82. *CDC Surveillance Summaries.* 32 (no. 4SS):1SS-16SS, 1983.

8. Centers for Disease Control: Nosocomial infection surveillance, 1983. *CDC Surveillance Summaries.* 33 (no. 2SS):955–22SS, 1984.

9. Krieger JN, Kaiser DL, Wenzel RP: Urinary tract etiology of bloodstream infections in hospitalized patients. *J Infect Dis* 148:57–62, 1983.

10. Kreger BE, Craven DE, Carling PC, McCabe WR: Gram-negative bacteremia. III. Reassessment of etiology, epidemiology and ecology in 612 patients. *Am J Med* 68:332–343, 1980.

11. Cross A, Allen JR, Burke J, Ducel G, Harris A, John J, Johnson D, Lew M, MacMillan B, Meers P, Skalova R, Wenzel R, Tenney J: Nosocomial infections due to *Pseudomonas aeruginosa*: review of recent trends. *Rev Infect Dis* 5:S837–S845, 1983.

12. Montgomerie JZ, Ota JK: *Klebsiella* bacteremia. *Arch Intern Med* 140:525–527, 1980.

13. Cryz SJ Jr, Mortimer PM, Mansfield V, Germanier R: Seroepidemiology of *Klebsiella* bacteremic isolates and implications for vaccine development. *J Clin Microbiol* 23:687–690, 1986.

14. Berger SA: *Proteus* bacteraemia in a general hospital 1972–1982. *J Hosp Infect* 6:293–298, 1985.

15. McDermott C, Mylotte JM: *Morganella morganii*: epidemiology of bacteremic disease. *Infect Control* 5:131–137, 1984.

16. Southern PM, Kutscher AE: *Pseudomonas paucimobilis* bacteremia. *J Clin Microbiol* 13:1070–1073, 1981.

17. Carney DN, Fossieck BE Jr, Parker RH, Minna JD: Bacteremia due to *Staphylococcus aureus* in patients with cancer: report on 45 cases in adults and review of the literature. *Rev Infect Dis* 4:1–12, 1982.

18. Munson DP, Thompson TR, Johnson DE, Rhame FS, VanDrunen N, Ferrieri P: Coagulase-negative staphylococcal septicemia: experience in a newborn intensive care unit. *J Pediatr* 101:602–605, 1982.

19. Shah M, Watanakunakorn C: Changing patterns of *Staphylococcus aureus* bacteremia. *Am J Med Sci* 278:115–121, 1979.

20. Bryan CS, Kirkhart B, Brenner ER: Staphylococcal bacteremia: current patterns in nonuniversity hospitals. *South Med J* 77:693–696, 1984.

21. Peacock JE, Marsik FJ, Wenzel RP: Methicillin-resistant *Staphylococcus aureus*: introduction and spread within a hospital. *Ann Intern Med* 93:526–532, 1980.

22. Craven DE, Reed C, Kollisch N, DeMaria A, Lichtenberg D, Shen K, McCabe WR: A large outbreak of infections caused by a strain of *Staphylococcus aureus* resistant to oxacillin and aminoglycosides. *Am J Med* 71:53–58, 1981.

23. Horn R, Wong B, Kiehn TE, Armstrong D: Fungemia in a cancer hospital: changing frequency, earlier onset, and results of therapy. *Rev Infect Dis* 7:646–655, 1985.

24. Klein JJ, Watanakunakorn C. Hospital-acquired fungemia: its natural course and clinical significance. *Am J Med* 67:51–58, 1979.

25. Weinstein MP, Reller LB, Murphy JR, Lichtenstein KA: The clinical significance of positive blood cultures: a comprehensive analysis of 500 episodes of bacteremia and fungemia in adults. I. Laboratory and epidemiologic observations. *Rev Infect Dis* 5:35–53, 1983.

26. Maki DG: Epidemic nosocomial bacteremias. In Wenzel RP (ed): *CRC Handbook of Hospital-Acquired Infections.* Boca Raton, FL, CRC Press, 1981.

27. Center for Disease Control: *Definition Used by the National Nosocomial Infections Study, Quarterly Report, Second Quarter.* 1972, 1973, p 261.

28. Reller LB, Murray PR, Machowry JD: Cumitech 1A: Blood cultures II. Coordinating ed: JA Washington. Washington, DC, American Society for Microbiology, 1982.

29. Vaisanen IT, Michelsen T, Valtonen V, Makelainen A: Comparison of arterial and venous blood samples for the diagnosis of bacteremia in critically ill patients. *Crit Care Med* 13:664–667, 1985.

30. Graham BS: Detection of bacteremia and fungemia: microscopic examination of peripheral blood smears. *Infect Control* 5:448–452, 1984.

31. Smith H: Leukocytes containing bacteria in plain blood films from patients with septicemia. *Aust Ann Med* 15:210–221, 1966.

32. Ascuitto RJ, Gerber MA, Cates KL, Tilton RC: Buffy coat smears of blood drawn through central venous catheters as an aid to rapid diagnosis of systemic fungal infections. *J Pediatr* 106:445–447, 1985.

33. Reik H, Rubin SJ: Evaluation of the buffy-coat smear for rapid detection of bacteremia. *JAMA* 245:357–359, 1981.

34. Cooper GL, Hopkins CC: Rapid diagnosis of intravascular catheter-associated infection by direct gram staining of catheter segments. *N Engl J Med* 312:1142–1147, 1985.

35. Maki DG, Weise CE, Sarafin HW: A semiquantitative culture method for identifying intravenous-catheter-related infection. *N Engl J Med* 296:1305–1309, 1977.

36. Longfield JN, Charache P, Diamond EL, Townsend TR: Comparison of broth and filtration methods for culturing of intravenous fluids. *Infect Control* 3:397–400, 1982.

37. Anderson RL, Highsmith AK, Holland BW: Comparison of the standard pour plate procedure and the ATP and *Limulus* amebocyte lysate procedures for the detection of microbial contamination in intravenous fluids. *J Clin Microbiol* 23:465–468, 1986.

38. Centers for Disease Control: National nosocomial infections study report: *Annual Summary 1978.* Issued March 1981.

39. Duggan JM, Oldfield GS, Ghosh HK: Septicaemia as a hospital hazard. *J Hosp Infect* 6:406–412, 1985.

40. Berkowitz FE: Bacteremia in hospitalized black South African children: A one-year study emphasizing nosocomial bacteremia and bacteremia in severely malnourished children. *Am J Dis Child* 138:551–556, 1984.

41. Baker CJ: Nosocomial septicemia and meningitis

in neonates. *Am J Med* 70;698–701, 1981.

42. Townsend TR, Wenzel RP: Nosocomial blood-stream infections in a newborn intensive care unit: a case-matched control study of morbidity, mortality, and risk. *Am J Epidemiol* 114:73–80, 1981.

43. McCormack JG, Barnes M: Nosocomial infections in a developing Middle East hospital. *Infect Control* 4:391–395, 1983.

44. Donowitz LG, Wenzel RP, Hoyt JW: High risk of hospital-acquired infection in the ICU patient. *Crit Care Med* 10:355–357, 1982.

45. Daschner FD, Frey P, Wolff G, Baumann PC, Suter P: Nosocomial infections in intensive care wards: a multicenter prospective study. *Inten Care Med* 8:5–9, 1982.

46. Bennet R, Eriksson M, Melen B, Zetterstrom R: Changes in the incidence and spectrum of neonatal septicemia during a fifteen-year period. *Acta Paediatr Scand* 74:687–690, 1985.

47. Wenzel RP, Thompson RL, Landry SM, Russell BS, Miller PJ, Ponce de Leon S, Miller GB Jr: Hospital-acquired infections in intensive care unit patients: an overview with emphasis on epidemics. *Infect Control* 4:371–375, 1983.

48. Setia U, Serventi I, Lorenz P: Bacteremia in a long-term care facility: spectrum and mortality. *Arch Intern Med* 144:1633–1635, 1984.

49. Haley RW, Schaberg DR, Von Allmen SD, McGowan JE Jr: Estimating the extra charges and prolongation of hospitalization due to nosocomial infections: a comparison of methods. *J Infect Dis* 141:248–257, 1980.

50. Maki DG: Nosocomial bacteremia: An epidemiologic overview. *Am J Med* 70:719–732, 1981.

51. McCabe WR, Jackson GG: Gram-negative bacteremia. I. Etiology and ecology. *Arch Intern Med* 110:847–855, 1962.

52. Bryan CS, Reynolds KL, Brenner ER: Analysis of 1186 episodes of gram-negative bacteremia in non-university hospitals: the effects of antimicrobial therapy. *Rev Infect Dis* 5:629–638, 1983.

53. Libman H, Arbeit RD: Complications associated with *Staphylococcus aureus* bacteremia. *Arch Intern Med* 144:541–545, 1984.

54. Crossley K, Loesch D, Landesman B, Mead K, Chern M, Strate R: An outbreak of infections caused by strains of *Staphylococcus aureus* resistant to methicillin and aminoglycosides. I. Clinical studies. *J Infect Dis* 139:273–279, 1979.

55. Haley RW, Hightower AW, Khabbaz RF, Thronsberry C, Martone WJ, Allen JR, Hughes JM: The emergence of methicillin-resistant *Staphylococcus aureus* infections in United States hospitals; possible role of the house staff-patient transfer circuit. *Ann Intern Med* 97:297–308, 1982.

56. Iannini PB, Crossley K: Therapy of *Staphylococcus aureus* bacteremia associated with a removable focus of infection. *Ann Intern Med* 84:558–560, 1976.

57. Yamada JK, Inderlied CB, Porschen RK: Detection of antibody to *Staphylococcus aureus* teichoic acid by enzyme-linked immunosorbent assay. *J Clin Microbiol* 17:898–905, 1983.

58. Wheat LJ, Luft FC, Tabbarah Z, Kohler RB, White A: Serologic diagnosis of access device-related staphylococcal bacteremia. *Am J Med* 67:603–607, 1979.

59. Verbrugh HA, Peters R, Rozenberg-Arska M, Peterson PK, Verhoef J: Antibodies to cell wall peptidoglycan of *Staphylococcus aureus* in patients with serious staphylococcal infections. *J Infect Dis* 144:1–9, 1981.

60. Wheat LJ, Wilkinson BJ, Kohler RB, White AC: Antibody response to peptidoglycan during staphylococcal infections. *J Infect Dis* 147:16–22, 1983.

61. Verbrugh HA, Peters R, Goessens WHF, Michel MF: Distinguishing complicated from uncomplicated bacteremia caused by *Staphylococcus aureus*: the value of "new" and "old" serological tests. *J Infect Dis* 153:109–115, 1986.

62. Herzog C, Wood HC, Noel I, Booth JC: Comparison of a new enzyme-linked immunosorbent assay method with counterimmunoelectrophoresis for detection of teichoic acid antibodies in sera from patients with *Staphylococcus aureus* infections. *J Clin Microbiol* 19:511–515, 1984.

63. Bayer AS, Tillman DB, Concepcion N, Guze LB: Clinical value of teichoic acid antibody titers in the diagnosis and management of the staphylococcemias. *West J Med* 132:294–300, 1980.

64. Sheagren JN: Guidelines for the use of the teichoic acid antibody assay. *Arch Intern Med* 144:250–252, 1984.

65. Tenenbaum MJ, Archer GL: Prognostic value of teichoic acid antibodies in *Staphylococcus aureus* bacteremia: a reassessment. *South Med J* 73:140–143, 1980.

66. Kaplan JE, Palmer DL, Tung KSK: Teichoic acid antibody and circulating immune complexes in the management of *Staphylococcus aureus* bacteremia. *Am J Med* 70:769–774, 1981.

67. Bernhardt LL, Antopol SC, Simberkoff MS, Rahal JJ: Association of teichoic acid antibody with metastatic sequelae of catheter-associated *Staphylococcus aureus* bacteremia: a failure of the two-week antibiotic treatment. *Am J Med* 66:355–357, 1979.

68. Drutz DJ, Jarvis WR, de Repentigny L, Rhame FS, Goldmann D: Severe nosocomial yeast infections. *Convers Infect Control* 6(5):1–12, 1985.

69. Maksymiuk AW, Thongprasert S, Hopfer R, Luna M, Fainstein V, Bodey GP: Systemic candidiasis in cancer patients. *Am J Med* 77(4D):20–27, 1984.

70. Rose HD: Venous catheter-associated candidemia. *Am J Med Sci* 275:265–270, 1978.

71. Turner RB, Donowitz LG, Hendley JO: Consequences of candidemia for pediatric patients. *Am J Dis Child* 139:178–180, 1985.

72. Walsh TJ, Bustamente CI, Vlahov D, Standiford HC: Candidal suppurative peripheral thrombophlebitis: recognition, prevention, and management. *Infect Control* 7:16–22, 1986.

73. Torres-Rojas JR, Stratton CW, Sanders CV, Horsman TA, Hawley HB, Dascomb HE, Vial LJ: Candidal suppurative peripheral thrombophlebitis. *Ann Intern Med* 96:431–435, 1982.

74. Reinhardt JF, Ruane PJ, Walker LJ, George WL: Intravenous catheter-associated fungemia due to *Candida rugosa*. *J Clin Microbiol* 22:1056–1057, 1985.

75. Kusek JW: Nosocomial pseudoepidemics and pseudoinfections: an increasing problem. *Am J Infect Control* 9:70–75, 1981.

76. Maki DG: Through a glass darkly: nosocomial

pseudoepidemics and pseudobacteremias. *Arch Intern Med* 140:26–28, 1980.

77. Noble RC, Reeves SA: *Bacillus* species pseudosepsis caused by contaminated commercial blood culture media. *JAMA* 230:1002–1004, 1974.
78. Kaslow RA, Mackel DC, Mallison GF: Nosocomial pseudobacteremia: Positive blood cultures due to contaminated benzalkonium antiseptic. *JAMA* 236:2407–2409, 1976.
79. Coyle-Gilchrist MM, Crewe P, Roberts G: *Flavobacterium meningosepticum* in the hospital environment. *J Clin Pathol* 29:824–826, 1976.
80. Verschraegen G, Claeys G, Meeus G, Delanghe M: *Pseudomonas pickettii* as a cause of pseudobacteremia. 21:278–279, 1985.
81. Keys TF, Melton LJ, Maker MD, Ilstrup DM: A suspected hospital outbreak of pseudobacteremia due to *Pseudomonas stutzeri*. *J Infect Dis* 147:489–493, 1983.
82. Craven DE, Moody B, Connolly MG, Kollisch NR, Stottmeier KD, McCabe WR: Pseudobacteremia caused by povidone-iodine solution contaminated with *Pseudomonas cepacia*. *N Engl J Med* 305:621–623, 1981.
83. Berkelman RL, Lewin S, Allen JR, Anderson RL, Budnick LD, Shapiro S, Friedman SM, Nicholas P, Holzman RS, Haley RW: Pseudobacteremia attributed to contamination of povidone-iodine with *Pseudomonas cepacia*. *Ann Intern Med* 95:32–36, 1981.
84. Graham DR, Wu E, Highsmith AK, Ginsburg ML: An outbreak of pseudobacteremia caused by *Enterobacter cloacae* from a phlebotomist's vial of thrombin. *Ann Intern Med* 95:585–588, 1981.
85. Duclos TW, Hodges GR, Killian JE: Bacterial contamination of blood-drawing equipment; a cause of false-positive blood cultures. *Am J Med Sci* 266:459–463, 1973.
86. McNeil MM, Davis BJ, Anderson RL, Martone WJ, Solomon SL: Mechanism of cross-contamination of blood culture bottles in outbreaks of pseudobacteremia associated with nonsterile blood collection tubes. *J Clin Microbiol* 22:23–25, 1985.
87. Hoffman PC, Arnow PM, Goldman OA, Parrott PL, Stamm WE, McGowan JE Jr: False-positive blood cultures, association with nonsterile blood collection tubes. *JAMA* 236:2073–2073, 1976.
88. Semel JD, Trenholme GM, Harris AA, Jupa JE, Levin S: Pseudomonas maltophilia pseudosepticemia. *Am J Med* 64:403–406, 1978.
89. Ives KN, Evans NAP, Thom BT, Harper EA: *Serratia marcescens* pseudobacteraemia on a special care baby unit. *Lancet* 1:994–995, 1982.
90. Snydman DR, Maloy MF, Broch SM: Pseudobacteremia: false-positive blood cultures from mist tent contamination. *Am J Epidemiol* 106:154–159, 1977.
91. Norden CW: Pseudosepticemia. *Ann Intern Med* 71:789–790, 1969.
92. Fairs HM, Sparling FF: *Micro polymorpha* bacteremia. False-positive cultures due to contaminated penicillinase. *JAMA* 219:76–77, 1972.
93. Spivack ML, Shannon R., Natsios GA, Wood J: Two epidemics of pseudobacteremia due to *Staphylococcus aureus* and *Aerococcus viridans*. *Infect Control* 1:321–323, 1980.

94. Lynch JM, Anderson A, Camacho FR, Winters AK, Hodges GR, Barnes WG: Pseudobacteremia caused by *Clostridium sordellii*. *Arch Intern Med* 140:65–68, 1980.
95. Berger SA: Pseudobacteremia due to contaminated alcohol swabs. *J Clin Microbiol* 18:974–975, 1983.
96. Dolan J, Joachim GR, Khapra A: Pseudobacteremia due to *Staphylococcus aureus*. *Morbid Mort Weekly Rep* 28:82–83, 1978.
97. Jones BC, Stark FR, Reordan R, Lancaster M: Pseudo-positive blood cultures caused by contamination in a humidified incubator. *Am J Infect Control*, pp 109–110.
98. Greenhood GP, Highsmith AK, Allen JR: *Klebsiella pneumoniae* pseudobacteremia due to cross contamination of a radiometric blood culture analyzer. *Infect Control* 2:460–465, 1981.
99. Griffin MR, Miller AD, Davis AC: Blood culture contamination associated with a radiometric analyzer. *J Clin Microbiol* 15:567–570, 1982.
100. Craven DE, Lichtenberg DA, Browne KF, Coffey DM, Treadwell TL, McCabe WR. Pseudobacteremia traced to cross-contamination by an automated blood culture analyzer. *Infect Control* 5:75–78, 1984.
101. Gurevich I, Tafuro P, Krystofiak SP, Kalter RD, Cunha BA: Three clusters of *Bacillus* pseudobacteremia related to a radiometric blood culture analyzer. *Infect Control* 5:71–74, 1984.
102. Stratton CW: Endemic staphylococcal pseudobacteremia. 2:251–252, 1981.
103. Weinstein RA, Stamm WE: Psuedoepidemics in hospital. *Lancet* 1:862–864, 1977.
104. John JF Jr, Bannister ER: Pseudobacteremia. *Infect Control* 5:69–70, 1984.
105. Matsaniotis NS, Syriopoulou VP, Theodoridou MC, Tzanetou KG, Mostrou GI: Enterobacter sepsis in infants and children due to contaminated intravenous fluids. *Infect Control* 5:471–477, 1984.
106. Goldmann D: Intravenous fluid contamination, aegean-style. *Infect Control* 5:469–470, 1984.
107. Daisy JA, Abrutyn EA, MacGregor RR: Inadvertent administration of intravenous fluids contaminated with fungus. *Ann Intern Med* 91:563–565, 1979.
108. Arnow PM, Weiss LM, Weil D, Rosen NR: *Escherichia coli* sepsis from contaminated platelet transfusion. *Arch Intern Med* 146:321–324, 1986.
109. Quinn JP, Arnow PM, Weil D, Rosenbluth J: Outbreak of JK diphtheroid infections associated with environmental contamination. *J Clin Microbiol* 19:668–671, 1984.
110. Riebel W, Frantz N, Adelstein D, Spagnuolo PJ: *Corynebacterium JK*: A cause of nosocomial device-related infection. *Rev Infec Dis* 8:42–49, 1986.
111. Kiehn TE, Nelson PE, Bernard EM, Edwards FF, Koziner B, Armstrong D: Catheter-associated fungemia caused by *Fusarium chlamydosporum* in a patient with lymphocytic lymphoma. *J Clin Microbiol* 21:501–504, 1985.
112. Highsmith AK, Greenhood GP, Allen JR: Growth of nosocomial pathogens in multiple-dose parenteral medication vials. *J Clin Microbiol* 15:1024–1028, 1982.

113. Sheth NK, Post GT, Wisniewski TR, Uttech BV: Multidose vials versus single-dose vials: a study in sterility and cost-effectiveness. *J Clin Microbiol* 17:377–379, 1983.

114. Maki DG, Goldmann DA, Rhame FS: Infection control in intravenous therapy. *Ann Intern Med* 79:867–887, 1973.

115. Bair JN, Petersen RV: Surface characteristics of plastic intravenous catheters. *Am J Hosp Pharm* 36:1707–1711, 1979.

116. Locci R, Peters G, Pulverer G: Microbial colonization of prosthetic devices. I. Microtopographical characteristics of intravenous catheters as detected by scanning electron microscopy. *Zbl Bakt Hyg, I Abt Orig B* 173:285–292, 1981.

117. Peters G, Locci R, Pulverer G: Microbial colonization of prosthetic devices. II. Scanning electron microscopy of naturally infected intravenous catheters. *Zbl Bakt Hyg, I Abt Orig B* 173:293–299, 1981.

118. Franson TR, Sheth NK, Rose HD, Sohnle PG: Scanning electron microscopy of bacteria adherent to intravascular catheters. *J Clin Microbiol* 20:500–505, 1984.

119. Sheth NK, Franson TR, Rose HD, Buckmire FLA, Cooper JA, Sohnle PG: Colonization of bacteria on polyvinyl chloride and Teflon intravascular catheters in hospitalized patients. *J Clin Microbiol* 18:1061–1063, 1983.

120. Christensen GD, Simpson WA, Younger JJ, Baddour LM, Barrett FF, Melton DM, Beachey EH: Adherence of coagulase-negative staphylococci to plastic tissue culture plates: a quantitative model for the adherence of staphylococci to medical devices. *J Clin Microbiol* 22:996–1006, 1985.

121. Ishak MA, Groschel DHM, Mandell GL, Wenzel RP: Association of slime with pathogenicity of coagulase-negative staphylococci causing nosocomial septicemia. *J Clin Microbiol* 22:1025–1029, 1985.

122. Davenport DS, Massanari RM, Pfaller MA, Bale MJ, Streed SA, Hierholzer WJ: Usefulness of a test for slime production as a marker for clinically significant infections with coagulase-negative staphylococci. *J Infect Dis* 153:332–339, 1986.

123. Christiansen GD, Simpson WA, Bachey EH, Bisno AL, Barrett FF: In *Program Abstracts of 22nd Interscience Conference on Antimicrobial Agents and Chemotherapy*, 1982. abstract 649.

124. Rotrosen D, Calderone RA, Edwards JE Jr: Adherence of *Candida* species to host tissues and plastic surfaces. *Rev Infect Dis* 8:73–85, 1986.

125. Vaudaux P, Suzuki R, Waldvogel FA, Morgenthaler JJ, Nydegger UE: Foreign body infection: role of fibronectin as a ligand for the adherence of *Staphylococcus aureus. J Infect Dis* 150:546–553, 1984.

126. Smallman L, Burdon DW, Alexander-Williams J: The effect of skin preparation and care on the incidence of superficial thrombophlebitis. *Br J Surg* 67:861–862, 1980.

127. Snydman DR, Pober BR, Murray SA, Gorbea HF, Majka JA, Perry LK. Predictive value of surveillance skin cultures in total-parenteral-nutrition-related infection. *Lancet.* 2:1385–1388, 1982.

128. Tager IB, Ginsberg MB, Ellis SE, Walsh NE,

Dupont I, Simchen E, Faich GA and The Rhode Island Nosocomial Infection Consortium: An epidemiologic study of the risks associated with peripheral intravenous catheters. *Am J Epidemiol* 118:839–851, 1983.

129. Tomford JW, Hershey CO, McLaren CE, Porter DK, Cohen DI: Intravenous therapy team and peripheral venous catheter-associated complications: a prospective controlled study. *Arch Intern Med* 144:1191–1194, 1984.

130. Falchuk KH, Peterson L, McNeil BJ: Microparticulate-induced phlebitis: its prevention by inline filtration. *N Engl J Med* 312:78–82, 1985.

131. Righter J, Bishop LA, Hill B: Infection and peripheral venous catheterization. *Diagn Microbiol Infect Dis* 1:89–93, 1983.

132. Maki DG, Band JD: A comparative study of polyantibiotic and iodophor ointments in prevention of vascular catheter-related infection. *Am J Med* 70:739–744, 1981.

133. Ricard P, Martin R, Marcoux JA: Protection of indwelling vascular catheters: incidence of bacterial contamination and catheter-related sepsis. *Crit Care Med* 13:541–543, 1985.

134. Snydman DR, Murray SA, Kornfeld SJ, Majka JA, Ellis CA: Total parenteral nutrition-related infections: prospective epidemiologic study using semiquantitative methods. *Am J Med* 73:695–699, 1982.

135. Gantz NM, Presswood GM, Goldberg R, Doern G: Effects of dressing type and change interval on intravenous therapy complication rates. *Diagn Microbiol Infect Dis* 2:325–332, 1984.

136. Wilkins EGL, Manning D, Roberts C, Davidson DC: Quantitative bacteriology of peripheral venous cannulae in neonates. *J Hosp Infect* 6:209–217, 1985.

137. Tully JL, Friedland GH, Baldini IM, Goldmann DA. Complications of intravenous therapy with steel needles and Teflon catheters: a comparative study. *Am J Med* 70:702–706, 1981

138. Cheesbrough JS, Finch RG: Studies on the microbiological safety of the valved side-port of the "Venflon" cannula. *J Hosp Infect* 6:201–208, 1985.

138a. Cheesbrough JS, Finch RG, Macfarlane JT: The complications of intravenous cannulae incorporating a valved injection side port. *J Hyg Camb* 93:497–504, 1984.

139. Hamory BH, Pearson SK, Duffy KR: Efficacy of professional IV therapy team in reducing complications of IV cannulae. In *Annual Meeting of the American Society for Microbiology*, St. Louis, 1984, abstract L2.

140. Band JD, Maki DG: Steel needles used for intravenous therapy: morbidity in patients with hematologic malignancy. *Arch Intern Med* 140:31–34, 1980.

141. Couchonnal GJ, Hodges GR, Barnes WG, Elmets CA, Clark GM: Complications with heparin-lock needles. *JAMA* 242:2098–2100, 1979.

142. Hodder SL, Stern RC: Safety of long duration intravenous heparin-lock needles for administration of antibiotics to cystic fibrosis patients. *J Pediatr* 99:312–314, 1981.

143. Hershey CO, Tomford JW, McLaren CE, Porter DK, Cohen DI: The natural history of intravenous

catheter-associated phlebitis. *Arch Intern Med* 144:1373–1375, 1984.

144. Wing EJ, Norden CW, Shadduck RK, Winkelstein A: Use of quantitative bacteriologic techniques to diagnose catheter-related sepsis. *Arch Intern Med* 139:482–483, 1979.

145. Raucher H, Hyatt AC, Barzilai A, Harris MB, Weiner MA, LeLeiko NS, Hodes DS: Quantitative blood cultures in the evaluation of septicemia in children with brovaic catheters. *J Pediatr* 104:29–33, 1984.

146. Cleri DJ, Corrado ML, Seligman SJ: Quantitative culture of intravenous catheters and other intravascular inserts. *J Infec Dis* 141:781–786, 1980.

147. Moyer MA, Edwards LD, Farley L: Comparative culture methods on 101 intravenous catheters: routine, semiquantitative, and blood cultures. *Arch Intern Med* 143:66–69.

148. Quercia RA, Hills SW, Klimek JJ, McLaughlin JC, Nightingale CH, Drezner AD, Sigman R: Bacteriologic contamination of intravenous infusion delivery systems in an intensive care unit. *Am J Med* 80:364–368, 1986.

149. Salohemio S, Henning C, Hillborgh U: Infection risks from cannulae used to maintain intravenous access. *Acta Anaesthesiol Scand* 28:199–200, 1984.

149a. Gorbea HF, Snydman DR, Delaney A, Stockman J, Martin WJ: Intravenous tubing with burettes can be safely changed at 48-hour intervals. *JAMA* 251:2112–2115, 1984.

150. Rusho WJ, Bair JN: Effect of filtration on complications of postoperative intravenous therapy. *Am J Hosp Pharm* 36:1355–1356, 1979.

151. Allcutt DA, Lort D, McCollum CN: Final inline filtration for intravenous infusions: a prospective hospital study. *Br J Surg* 70:111–113, 1983.

152. Messing B: Infusion-related phlebitis. *N Engl J Med* 312:1452, 1985.

153. Friedland G: Infusion-related phlebitis: is the inline filter the solution? *N Engl J Med* 312:113–115, 1985.

154. Riebel W: Infusion-related phlebitis (Letter). *N Engl J Med* 312:1453–1454, 1985.

155. Pinilla JC, Ross DF, MartinT, Crump H: Study of the incidence of intravascular catheter infection and associated septicemia in critically ill patients. *Crit Care Med* 11:21–25, 1983.

156. Singh S, Nelson N, Acosta I, Check FE, Puri VK: Catheter colonization and bacteremia with pulmonary and arterial catheters. *Crit Care Med* 10:736–739, 1982.

157. Damen J, Verhoef J, Bolton DT, Middleton NG, Van Der Tweel I, De Jonge K, Wever JEAT, Nijsen-Karelse M: Microbiologic risk of invasive hemodynamic monitoring in patients undergoing open-heart operations. *Crit Care Med* 13:548–555, 1985.

158. Samsoondar W, Freeman JB, Coultish I, Oxley C: Colonization of intravascular catheters in the intensive care unit. *Am J Surg* 149:730–732, 1985.

159. Thomas F, Burke JP, Parker J, Orme JF, Gardner RM, Clemmer TP, Hill GA, MacFarlane P: The risk of infection related to radial vs femoral sites for arterial catheterization. *Crit Care Med* 11:807–812, 1983.

160. Russell JA, Joel M, Hudson RJ, Mangano DT,

Schlobohm RM: Prospective evaluation of radial and femoral artery catheterization sites in critically ill adults. *Crit Care Med* 11:936–939, 1983.

161. Shinozaki T, Deane RS, Mazuzan JE Jr, Hamel AJ, Hazelton D: Bacterial contamination of arterial lines: a prospective study. *JAMA* 249:223–225, 1983.

162. Maki DG, Hassemer CA: Endemic rate of fluid contamination and related septicemia in arterial pressure monitoring. *Am J Med* 70:733–738, 1981.

163. Luskin RL, Weinstein RA, Nathan C, Chamberlin WH, Kabino SA: Extended use of disposable pressure transducers: a bacteriologic evaluation. *JAMA* 255:916–920, 1986.

164. Bozzetti F, Terno G, Camerini E, Baticci F, Scarpa D, Pupa A: Pathogenesis and predictability of central venous catheter sepsis. *Surgery* 91:383–389, 1982.

165. Bozzetti F, Terno G, Bonfanti G, Scarpa D, Scotti A, Ammatuna M, Bonalumi MG: Prevention and treatment of central venous catheter sepsis by exchange via a guidewire. *Ann Surg* 198:48–52, 1983.

166. Lindblad B, Wolff T: Infectious complications of percutaneously inserted central venous catheters. *Acta Anaesthesiol Scand* 29:587–589, 1985.

167. Michel L, McMichan JC, Bachy JL: Microbial colonization of indwelling central venous catheters: statistical evaluation of potential contaminating factors. *Am J Surg* 137:745–748, 1979.

168. Sketch MH, Cale M, Mohiuddin SM, Booth RW: Use of percutaneously inserted venous catheters in coronary care units. *Chest* 62:684–689, 1972.

169. Prager RL, Silva J Jr: Colonization of central venous catheters. *South Med J* 77:458–461, 1984.

169a. Malmvall BE, Alestig K, Dottori O, Seeberg S: Septicaemia in patients with central vein catheters. *Acta Chir Scand* 146:155–159, 1980.

170. Eisenhauer ED, Derveloy RJ, Hastings PR: Prospective evaluation of central venous pressure (CVP) catheters in a large city-county hospital. *Ann Surg* 196:560–564, 1982.

171. Curelaru I, Bylock A, Gustavsson B, Hultman E, Linder LE, Stefansson T, Stenqvist O: Dynamics of thrombophlebitis in central venous catheterization via basilic and cephalic veins. *Acta Chir Scand* 150:285–293, 1984.

172. Snydman DR. Letter to the editor. *Ann Surg* 200:101, 1984.

173. Wheeler JG, Weesner KM: *Staphylococcus aureus* endocarditis and pericarditis in an infant with a central venous catheter. *Clin Pediatr* 23:46–47, 1984.

174. Tsao MMP, Katz D. Central venous catheter-induced endocarditis: human correlate of the animal experimental model of endocarditis. *Rev Infect Dis* 6:783–790, 1984.

175. Donowitz LG: High risk of nosocomial infection in the pediatric critical care patient. *Crit Care Med* 14:26–28, 1986.

176. Powell DC, Bivins BA, Bell RM, Sachatello CR, Griffen WO Jr: Bacterial endocarditis in the critically ill surgical patient. *Arch Surg* 116:311–314, 1981.

177. Ford SE, Manley PN: Indwelling cardiac catheters: an autopsy study of associated endocardial

lesions. *Arch Pathol Lab Med* 106:314–317, 1982.

178. Michel L, Marsh HM, McMichan JC, Southorn PA, Brewer NS: Infection of pulmonary artery catheters in critically ill patients. *JAMA* 245:1032–1036, 1981.

179. Darst DJ, Forker AD: Complictions of Swan-Ganz catheterization in a university and Veterans Administration hospital. *Neb Med J* 271–276, 1982.

180. Horst HM, Obeid FN, Vij D, Bivins BA: The risks of pulmonary arterial catheterization. *Surg Gynecol Obstet* 159:229–232, 1984.

181. Myers ML, Austin TW, Sibbald WJ: Pulmonary artery catheter infections: a prospective study. *Ann Surg* 201:237–241, 1985.

182. Elliott CG, Zimmerman GA, Clemmer TP: Complications of pulmonary artery catheterization in the care of critically ill patients: a prospective study. *Chest* 76:647–652, 1979.

183. Applefeld JJ, Caruthers TE, Reno DJ, Civetta JM: Assessment of the sterility of long-term cardiac catheterization using the thermodilution Swan-Ganz catheter. *Chest* 74:377–380, 1978.

184. Riedinger MS, Shellock FG, Shah PK, Weissfeld AS, Ellrodt AG: Sterility of prefilled thermodilution cardiac output syringes maintained at room and ice temperatures. *Heart Lung* 14:8–11, 1985.

185. Yonkman CA, Hamory BH: A comparison of three methods of maintaining a sterile injectate system during cardiac output determinations. *Am J Infect Control* 12:276–281, 1984.

186. Begala JE, Maher K, Cherry JD: Risk of infection associated with the use of Broviac and Hickman catheters. *Assoc Pract Infect Control* 10:17–23, 1981.

187. Abrahm JL, Mullen JL: A prospective study of prolonged central venous access in leukemia. *JAMA* 248:2868–2873, 1982.

188. Thomas JH, MacArthur RI, Pierce GE, et al: Hickman-Broviac catheters: indications and results. *Am J Surg* 140:791–796, 1980.

189. Jacobs MB, Yeager M: Thrombotic and infectious complications of Hickman-Broviac catheters. *Arch Intern Med* 144:1597–1599, 1984.

190. Lowder JN, Larzarus HM, Herzig RH: Bacteremias and fungemias in oncologic patients with central venous catheters: changing spectrum of infection. *Arch Intern Med* 142:1456–1459, 1982.

191. Legha SS, Haq M, Rabinowits M, Lawson M, McCredie K: Evaluation of silicone elastomer catheters for long-term intravenous chemotherapy. *Arch Intern Med* 145:1208–1211, 1985.

192. Svirbely JR, Buesching WJ, Ayers LW, Baker PB, Britton AJ: *Mycobacterium fortuitum* infection of a Hickman catheter site. *Am J Clin Pathol* 80:733–735, 1983.

193. Liepman MK, Jones PG, Kauffman CA: Endocarditis as a complication of indwelling right atrial catheters in leukemic patients. *Cancer* 54:804–807, 1984.

194. Krol TC, O-Keefe P: Brachial plexus neuritis and fatal hemorrhage following *Aspergillus* infection of a Hickman catheter. *Cancer* 50:1214–1217, 1982.

195. Bothe A, Piccione W, Ambrosino JJ, Benotti PN, Lokich JJ: Implantable central venous access system. *Am J Surg* 147:565–569, 1984.

196. Press OW, Ramsey PG, Larson EB, Fefer A, Hickman RO: Hickman catheter-infections in patients with malignancies. *Medicine* 63:189–200, 1984.

197. Martin JK, Beart RW Jr, Mucha P Jr, Hoagland HC: Hickman catheter implantation in the treatment of acute leukemia. *Arch Surg* 118:1224–1226, 1983.

198. Shapiro GD, Wald ER, Nelson KA, Spiegelman KN: Broviac catheter-related bacteremia in oncology patients. *Am J Dis Child* 136:679–681, 1982.

199. Reilly JJ Jr, Steed DL, Ritter PS: Indwelling venous access catheters in patients with acute leukemia. *Cancer* 53:219–223, 1984.

200. Niederhuber JE, Ensminger W, Gyves JW, Liepman M, Doan K, Cozzi E: Totally implanted venous and arterial access system to replace external catheters in cancer treatment. *Surgery* 92:706–711, 1982.

201. Grantham RN, Munnell ER, Kanaly PJ: Femoral artery infection complicating intraaortic balloon pumping. *Am J Surg* 146:811–814, 1983.

202. Harvey JC, Goldstein JE, McCabe JC, Hoover EL, Gay WA Jr, Subramanian VA: Complications of percutaneous intraaortic balloon pumping. *Circulation* 64:114–117, 1981.

203. Pennington DG, Swartz M, Codd JE, Merjavy JP, Kaiser GC: Intraaortic balloon pumping in cardiac surgical patients: a nine-year experience. *Ann Thorac Surg* 36:125–131, 1983.

204. Bjornson HS, Colley R, Bower RH, Duty VP, Schwartz-Fulton JT, Fischer JE: Association between microorganism growth at the catheter insertion site and colonization of the catheter in patients receiving total parenteral nutrition. *Surgery* 92:720–727, 1982.

205. Wistbacka JO, Nuutinen LS: Catheter-related complications of total parenteral nutrition (TPN): a review. *Acta Anaesth Scand* 29:84–88, 1985.

206. Snydman DR: Bacteria in total parenteral nutrition catheters. *Lancet* 940–941, 1983.

207. Sitges-Serra A, Jaurrieta E, Linares J, Perez JL, Garau J: Bacteria in total parenteral nutrition catheters: where do they come from? *Lancet* 1:531, 1983.

208. Sitges-Serra A, Puig P, Linares J, Perez JL, Farrero N, Jaurrieta E, Garau J: Hub colonization as the initial step in an outbreak of catheter-related sepsis due to coagulase negative staphylococci during parenteral nutrition. *J Parent Enteral Nutr* 8:668–672, 1984.

209. von Meyenfeldt MMF, Stapert J, De Jong PCM, Soeters PB, Wesdorp RIC, Greep JM: TPN catheter sepsis: lack of effect of subcutaneous tunnelling of PVC catheters on sepsis rate. *J Parent Enteral Nutr* 4:514–517, 1980.

210. McKee R, Dunsmuir R, Whitby M, Garden OJ: Does antibiotic prophylaxis at the time of catheter insertion reduce the incidence of catheter-related sepsis in intravenous nutrition? *J Hosp Infect* 6:419–425, 1985.

211. Brismar B, Hardstedt C, Malmborg AS: Bacteriology and phlebography in catheterization for parenteral nutrition: a prospective study. *Acta Chir Scand* 146:115–119, 1980.

212. Fonkalsrud EW, Berquist W, Burke M, Ament ME: Long-term hyperalimentation in children

through saphenous central venous catheterization. *Am J Surg* 143:209–211, 1982.

213. Jarrard MM, Olson CM, Freeman JB: Daily dressing change effects on skin flora beneath subclavian catheter dressings during total parenteral nutrition. *J Parent Enteral Nutr* 4:391–392, 1980.

214. Adam RD, Edwards LD, Becker CC, Schrom HM: Semiquantitative cultures and routine tip cultures on umbilical catheters. *J Pediatr* 100:123–126, 1982.

215. Thompson TR, Tilleli J, Johnson DE, Britt W, L'Heureux P, Williams H, Jarvis C, Burke BA: Umbilical artery catheterization complicated by mycotic aortic aneurysm in neonates. In *Mycotic Aortic Aneurysm Complications in UAC.* Chicago, Year Book Medical Publishers, 1980.

216. Kozeny GA, Venezio FR, Bansal VK, Vertuno LL, Hano JE: Incidence of subclavian dialysis catheter-related infections. *Arch Intern Med* 144:1787–1789, 1984.

217. Sherertz RJ, Falk RJ, Huffman KA, Thomann CA, Mattern WD: Infections associated with subclavian Udall catheters. *Arch Intern Med* 143:52–56, 1983.

218. Raja RM, Fernandes M, Kramer MS, Barber K, Rosenbaum JL: Comparison of subclavian vein with femoral vein catheterization for hemodialysis. *Am J Kidney Dis* 2:474–476, 1983.

219. Simmons BP: CDC guidelines for the prevention and control of nosocomial infections: guideline for prevention of intravascular infections. *Am J Infect Control* 11:183–199, 1983.

Chapter 20

Hospital-Acquired Pneumonia

James E. Pennington, M.D.

INTRODUCTION

Terminal bronchopneumonia among hospitalized patients has been recognized from the days of Osler as a relatively common cause of death. Until the late 1950s, pneumococci (and other streptococci), *Haemophilus influenzae*, and occasionally staphylococci were considered to be the most common bacterial etiologies for terminal pneumonia, regardless of whether the infection was community- or hospital-acquired. The "modern era" of hospital-acquired pneumonias began in the late 1950s and early 1960s and has been characterized by the predominance of aerobic gram-negative bacilli as etiologic agents. While the precise reasons for the emergence of gram-negative pathogens as predominant etiologic agents of nosocomial pneumonia are not entirely clear, increased use of broad spectrum antibiotics, the use of prolonged respiratory assistance for victims of poliomyelitis, and newly developed respiratory equipment using mainstream reservoir nebulizers have all been implicated as causative factors in this etiologic evolution (1, 2). In any event, retrospective analyses clearly suggest that a 4-fold increase in the incidence of necrotizing gram-negative pneumonia occurred among hospitalized patients between the late 1950s and early 1960s (3).

Currently, the lung is the third most common site of hospital-acquired infection, accounting for approximately 15% of all nosocomial infections (4, 5). However, in contrast to more frequently involved organs (urinary tract and skin), for which mortalities range from 1 to 4%, the crude mortality rates associated with nosocomial pneumonia range from 20 to 50% (5–8). In fact, it has been estimated that as many as 15% of all deaths occurring in hospitalized patients are directly related to nosocomial pneumonia (9). Thus, hospital-acquired pneumonia is currently the most common fatal nosocomial infection in this country. Based upon one recent epidemiologic analysis, it appears that prevention or better treatment of this infection might result in as many as 40,000 fewer deaths/year in the United States alone (10).

INCIDENCE AND MORTALITY

The incidence of hospital-acquired pneumonia is dependent upon the patient setting. The National Nosocomial Infections Study (NNIS), reporting for the year 1983, recorded an annual incidence of nosocomial lower respiratory infection of approximately 0.55% (5.5 cases/1000 discharges) (4). The incidence was much lower in nonteaching hospitals (0.41%) and small teaching hospitals (0.46%), when compared to larger teaching hospitals (0.75%), however. In a separate study, the incidence of bacteremic nosocomial pneumonia was noted to be 10 times greater in a teaching as compared to a nonteaching hospital (8). The incidence of nosocomial pneumonia ranged widely among various inpatient services in the NNIS report, with highs of 0.5 to 1.0% on medical-surgical services, and lows of 0.03 to 0.3% on obstetrics, gynecology, and pediatrics services. Others have noted an even higher incidence of nosocomial pneumonia in certain settings, such as respiratory intensive care units, 20% (7); postoperative patients, 17.5% (11); and neonatal intensive care units, 7% (12).

It is impossible to estimate the morbidity and excess costs associated with nosocomial pneumonias accurately. However, in patients surviving gram-negative pneumonia, it is not unusual for treatments to require 3 or more weeks (13). The mortality associated with nosocomial pneumonia has been more clearly identified. In one series, including a large number of nonteaching hospital patients, the overall mortality from nosocomial pneumonia was 20% (5). However, crude mortality rates of 50% or greater have been typical for nosocomial pneumonia in teaching hospitals (6, 7). To date, however, no large study has indicated the attributable mortality from hospital-acquired pneumonia. Bacteremia occurs in approximately 2 to 6% of nosocomial pneumonias (4, 5), but is associated with a 3-fold increase in mortality when present (5).

Of particular interest has been the relationship between etiologic agent and mortality from nosocomial pneumonia. The mortality associated with gram-negative bacillary pneumonias is generally about 50% (6, 7), while mortality from gram-positive pneumonias is considerably lower, reported to be 5 to 24% (6, 7). Among gram-negative bacilli, deaths associated with *Pseudomonas aeruginosa* are particularly high, with rates of 70 to 80% reported in several series (7, 8, 13, 14). The 25% mortality reported for nosocomial Legionnaires' disease (15) may be somewhat overstated since a number of fatal cases have been diagnosed retrospectively, without a trial of specific therapy. On the other hand, since nosocomial Legionnaires' disease occurs predominantly in compromised hosts, mortality might be expected to be higher than that reported for sporadic community-acquired Legionnaires' disease. While viral nosocomial pneumonias are usually not fatal, deaths may occur, particularly in children with congenital heart disease (16) or in adults with debilitating diseases (17, 18).

ETIOLOGIES

Over half of all hospital-acquired pneumonias are caused by aerobic gram-negative bacilli. In most cases, single pathogenic isolates have been identified. However, in 10 to 20% of cases, polymicrobial gram-negative pneumonias are reported (4, 8). The NNIS data for 1983 indicate that six of the seven most common etiologic agents causing nosocomial pneumonia are gram-negative rods (Table 20.1). The predominance of gram-negative bacillary pathogens as etiologic agents for nosocomial pneumonia has been noted for community hospitals (5), as well as teaching

Table 20.1.   Most Frequent Etiologic Agents for Hospital-Acquired Pneumonia in the United States, 1980 to 1983*

Pathogen	Frequency (%)
Pseudomonas aeruginosa	15.1
Klebsiella sp.	12.8
Staphylococcus aureus	12.8
Enterobacter sp.	10.0
Escherichia coli	7.1
Proteus sp.	5.8
Serratia marcescens	5.6

* Adapted from Centers for Disease Control: National Nosocomial Infections Study report, annual summary 1983. *MMWR* 33 (no. 255):9SS–21SS, 1985.

centers (7). Among gram-positive bacteria, *Staphylococcus aureus* is by far the most common (4). *Streptococcus pneumoniae*, the most frequent bacterial etiology of community-acquired pneumonia, accounts for less than 3% of nosocomial pneumonias (4). Of some interest has been the observation that specific pathogens occur more commonly on certain hospital services (Table 20.2).

A number of less frequent etiologies exist for nosocomial pneumonia. Several may be more common than is generally acknowledged. This potential for underreporting is due to difficulties with the diagnostic techniques necessary for identifying certain etiologic agents. For example, epidemic viral pneumonia has been recognized in the hospital setting (19–21). However, only with prospective monitoring and careful evaluation of specimens by a diagnostic virology laboratory can the true incidence of endemic viral pneumonias in the hospital setting be determined. In one such survey, it was reported that viral agents accounted for 20% of all nosocomial lower respiratory infections during a 17-month surveillance period in a general hospital (22). The majority of nosocomial viral pneumonia cases in that study occurred on pediatric wards. Others have observed that viral etiologies are, in fact, the most common cause of nosocomial respiratory infections on the pediatric ward (19). Although data are less well established for adults, it appears that nosocomial viral respiratory infections are much less common on adult medical and surgical wards (23).

Attention has recently been directed toward two viral pathogens as important etiologic agents for nosocomial respiratory infection, respiratory syncytial virus (RSV) and influenza A (17, 24, 25). In one study, over 40% of hospitalized infant contacts developed RSV infection during hospitalization (24). In another report (18), seven hospitalized adults with debilitating disease developed nosocomial influenza A pneumonia after exposure to a single index case. Although most studies have emphasized the role of RSV infection among pediatric patients and influenza among adults, it is clear that these viral agents are not limited to such specific settings (26–28). Furthermore, although RSV and influenza appear to be the most common viral agents causing nosocomial pneumonias, occasional outbreaks with such agents as parainfluenza and enterovirus (e.g., neonatal nurseries) have also been reported (19). Since viral cultures are not routinely performed on sputum specimens by most microbi-

Table 20.2. Three Most Frequent Etiologic Agents Causing Hospital-Acquired Pneumonia on Various Services*

Medicine	Surgery	Pediatrics	Newborn Nursery
P. aeruginosa	*P. aeruginosa*	*Klebsiella*	*S. aureus*
S. aureus	*Klebsiella*	*P. aeruginosa*	*P. aeruginosa*
Klebsiella	*Enterobacter*	*S. aureus*	*Coag. neg staph*

* Adapted from Centers for Disease Control: National Nosocomial Infections Study report, annual summary 1983. *MMWR* 33 (no. 255):9SS–21SS, 1985.

ology laboratories, an appreciation that viral agents may cause nosocomial pneumonia is important, particularly during periods of community-wide epidemic viral illness.

It is now evident that *Legionella* sp. account for a certain number of cases of nosocomial pneumonia (15, 29–33). Since the diagnosis of pneumonia caused by *Legionella* sp. requires special serologic and microbiologic techniques, its precise frequency is presently unknown. Estimates of frequency range from 3 to 10% (31, 34, 35). In hospital settings with contamination of potable water by *Legionella* sp., this pathogen may account for up to 30% of all nosocomial pneumonias (30, 36, 37). However, using prospective monitoring, others have documented extremely low frequencies of *Legionella* nosocomial pneumonias (38). Thus, while certain medical centers may encounter a cluster of nosocomial *Legionella* pneumonias due to environmental factors, true estimates of the frequency of sporadic *Legionella* nosocomial pneumonias must await further study.

Other bacterial etiologies for nosocomial pneumonia have been reported under special conditions. For example, *Haemophilus influenzae* is a relatively frequent respiratory isolate among hospitalized patients with chronic lung diseases (39), but is otherwise rarely associated with nosocomial pneumonia (4). Likewise, enterococcal pneumonia has been documented as a superinfection among patients receiving broad spectrum cephalosporin therapy (40). In addition, it should be emphasized that certain hospital centers may experience sporadic outbreaks of nosocomial pneumonia caused by nonfermentative gram-negative bacilli, such as *Acinetobacter* sp. (41), and *Pseudomonas* sp. (42). The outbreaks may be associated with local factors, such as contamination of specific respiratory equipment or fluids, or carriage on skin of individual health care personnel. Finally, while aspiration of upper airway secretions clearly predisposes to nosocomial pneumonia (see below), large volume aspirations leading to anaerobic lung infection appear to be rare in the hospital setting (4).

Nosocomial pneumonia among immunosuppressed patients represents a special problem. The lung remains one of the most common identifiable sites of infection among immunosuppressed patients (43), and nosocomial pneumonia is a potential problem for virtually any immunocompromised host. Neutropenic patients are at particular risk for acquiring aerobic gram-negative bacillary pneumonias, even in the absence of endotracheal instrumentation (44). *Aspergillus* sp. pneumonias have also been associated with neutropenia as well as with corticosteroid usage (45). Construction in or near hospital sites, as well as contaminated fireproofing materials and air conditioning equipment, have all been associated with nosocomial *Aspergillus* pneumonia among compromised hosts (46, 47). Although one report documents a clustering of *Pneumocystis carinii* pneumonia cases within a single medical center (48), there are insufficient epidemiologic data to implicate this protozoal pathogen as a cause of nosocomial pneumonias. Finally, it should be noted that recently published data do not suggest a role for nosocomial transmission of the acquired immunodeficiency syndrome (49).

FACTORS PREDISPOSING TO HOSPITAL-ACQUIRED PNEUMONIA

The most important factor predisposing to nosocomial pneumonia is endotracheal intubation. Both short term intubations for surgery, as well as longer term intubation for respiratory failure, are associated with the highest reported frequencies (17 to 20%) for nosocomial pneumonia (7, 11). In fact, the incidence of nosocomial pneumonia for intubated patients appears to be 4 times higher than that for nonintubated patients, and tracheostomy further increases the risk (50). A number of factors account for the enhanced risk of pneumonia among intubated patients. Apart from the obvious fact that such patients are often the most critically ill, the presence of an endotracheal tube eliminates one of the most effective natural host defense mechanisms of the airway. The usual inertial filtration system of the nose and conducting airways, and the mucociliary clearance system of the airways, are largely bypassed during intubation. Furthermore, mechanical irritation and injury of respiratory mucosa may predispose to local colonization of airways with potential bacterial pathogens (51). Finally, the endotracheal tube and the respiratory equipment utilized for assisted ventilation may serve as a source for bacterial contamination of the lower respiratory tract.

It has been known for many years that respiratory equipment may serve as a source for nosocomial pneumonia (21, 52). It is clear, however, that the major risk of infection was associated with mainstream reservoir nebulizers, designed to deliver aerosols of small particle size suspended in the effluent gas (2, 53, 54). Several epidemics of nosocomial pneumonia were reported shortly after the introduction of nebulization equipment in respiratory care (55–61). A significant correlation between the occurrence of necrotizing gram-negative pneumonia at autopsy and the use of nebulization equipment has, in fact, been documented (3, 62). Virtually any method used to provide microaerosoled material to the lungs may transmit bacteria. These include Venturi jet nebulizers (2, 53, 54), ultrasonic nebulizers (63, 64), and spinning disc nebulizers (65). Of particular interest is a recent report documenting contaminated medication nebulizers as a potential source of nosocomial pneumonia (66). The contamination appeared rapidly (after a single use) and was presumably caused by reflux of contaminated condensate in the ventilator circuit. Based upon these observations, it was suggested that medication nebulizer reservoirs be cleaned or disinfected after each use, rather than after 24-hour periods. Furthermore, the large body of data implicating nebulization equipment with increased risk of gram-negative pneumonia led to the current trends in respiratory therapy to utilize cascade humidifiers. The cascade humidifiers allow gas to bubble through water prior to delivery, but do not generate microaerosols which may become contaminated (67). Subsequently, a marked reduction in respiratory-associated pneumonias was noted (3).

Use of antibiotics in the hospital setting has also been associated with increased risk for nosocomial pneumonia (68–70). These so-called "superinfections" presumably occur as a consequence of selection for more resistant bacterial pathogens during treatment of a primary infection. In one report, 149 patients treated in the hospital with penicillin or erythromycin for community-acquired bacterial pneumonia experienced a 16% incidence of pulmonary superinfections (70). Etiologic agents were either gram-negative bacilli or *S. aureus*. Although a concomitant group of non-antibiotic-treated hospitalized patients was not available in this series for comparison, the incidence is several times that reported in the general hospital population (4).

Surgical procedures appear to be associated with an increased risk for pneumonia (11). One series reported that 50% of all nosocomial pneumonias occurred in postoperative patients (71). Others have reported a 17.5% incidence of nosocomial pneumonia among patients undergoing elective thoracic or abdominal procedures (11). Obesity, advanced age, and severity of underlying disease were all associated with increased risk for nosocomial pneumonia in that study. Considering that intubation and prophylactic antibiotics are commonly used in surgical patients, it is not surprising that nosocomial pneumonias are particularly common on the surgical service.

Several studies suggest that chronic pulmonary diseases are associated with increased risk of nosocomial pneumonia (39, 68). It is noteworthy, however, that these particular patients require assisted ventilation more frequently than others. In one report, mortality rates from nosocomial pneumonia in intubated patients with or without underlying chronic lung disease were not significantly different (7). Other conditions associated with an increased risk for nosocomial pneumonia include advanced age (7, 11) and immunosuppression (see above).

PATHOGENESIS

Hospital-acquired pneumonias may occur as metastatic infections, secondary to bacteremia, or as a primary infection, with pathogens acquired via the respiratory tract. The infrequent association of nosocomial pneumonia with bacteremias suggests that primary respiratory infection is by far the most common route. The majority of nosocomial pneumonias appear to result from aspiration of potential pathogens which have colonized the mucosal surfaces of the upper airways (1, 68). In one study (68), 213 patients admitted to a medical intensive care unit were monitored with frequent cultures of the posterior oropharynx. Ninety-five patients (45%) became colonized with aerobic gram-negative bacilli by the end of 1 week in the hospital. Of these 95 colonized patients, subsequent nosocomial pneumonia developed in 22 (23%). Pneumonia developed in only 4 of 118 noncolonized patients (3.3%). In that same study, the risk of airway colonization increased as a function of time in the hospital. In separate observations, a direct correlation was made between the degree of illness and the risk of airway colonization with gram-negative bacilli (72). Surveillance cultures of oropharyngeal flora revealed aerobic gram-negative bacilli in 0% of psychiatry patients, 16% of moderately ill patients, and 57% of moribund patients. The carriage rate of aerobic gram-negative rods among normal volunteers was 2%. Other factors associated with increased risk of oropharyngeal colonization are use of antibiotics, azotemia, intubation, and underlying pulmonary disease (68, 69, 72).

Since prevention of upper airway colonization with potential bacterial pathogens represents one potential method for decreasing the incidence of nosocomial pneumonia, there is considerable interest in identifying the sources of these colonizing flora. A fecal to oral route of bacterial contamination of airways has long been suspected for bedridden patients. This route could not readily explain the frequency of colonization by organisms such as *P. aeruginosa* or *Acinetobacter*, however, since these organisms are distinctly unusual inhabitants of the human gastrointestinal tract. In a recent study, daily cultures were monitored from rectal, hypopharyngeal, and tracheal sites in 21 patients requiring prolonged intubation (73). Enterobacteriaceae were commonly cultured from the hypopharynx and rectum prior to their appearance in tracheal cultures. In contrast, non-Enterobacteriaceae (e.g., *P. aeruginosa*, *Acinetobacter*) were rarely found in those sites prior to their appearance in the trachea. This suggested that environmental sources existed primarily for non-Enterobacteriaceae, and that colonizing Enterobacteriaceae originated primarily from the patients' endogenous flora. Others have suggested that the most important vector for transmission of environmental flora is the hands of health care personnel (74, 75). While hand washing and other infection control methods may reduce cross-contamination with certain potential pathogens, however, it appears that the patient's endogenous flora will continue to provide a source for upper airway colonization. In addition, the recent popularity for gastric alkalinization to prevent stress ulcers and bleeding in hospitalized patients is producing larger numbers of patients with extensive bacterial overgrowth in the upper gastrointestinal tract. This, in turn, appears to lead to airway colonization secondary to aspiration of gastric microflora (76).

Numerous observations have suggested that the respiratory epithelium in hospitalized patients has increased affinity for the attachment of gram-negative bacilli (77–79). In fact, in vitro bacterial adherence assays using buccal cells from various patient groups appear to be predictive for the risk of subsequent bacterial colonization of airways (77, 78). While most studies have utilized buccal cells for in vitro adherence assays, recent data indicate that tracheal cells may be even more useful for such studies (80). The mechanisms by which aerobic gram-negative bacilli become more adherent to airway mucosa of hospitalized or otherwise debilitated patients have also been the subject of numerous investigations. Bacterial lectins, such as the pili on cell membranes of *P. aeruginosa*, have been identified as important in adherence to airway mucosa (51, 81). Receptors on respiratory epithelial cells may also be important in mediating attachment of gram-negative bacilli. For example, a sialic acid moiety on cell surfaces, or in tracheal mucin, has been implicated as a receptor for *P. aeruginosa* (82). Also, considerable data have been collected suggesting that the mucosal cell surface glycoprotein, fibronectin, plays an integral part in modulating oropharyngeal bacterial ecology. Under normal conditions, buccal cells are coated with fibronectin, which in turn selects for adherence of gram-positive cocci (83). Fibronectin also appears to prevent adherence of *P. aeruginosa* to buccal cells (84). Of particular interest are recent studies documenting increased levels of salivary protease in seriously ill hospitalized patients (85). Increased protease content of saliva was associated with loss of fibronectin from buccal cell surfaces and increased adherence (in vitro) and colonization (in vivo) of airway mucosa with gram-negative bacilli. The implications of the preceding biochemical and biophysical observations are uncertain. Under the best of circumstances, however, the observations might form the basis for new strategies in prevention or reversal of airway bacterial colonization among patient populations at high risk for nosocomial pneumonia.

DIAGNOSIS

The diagnosis of nosocomial pneumonia may be difficult. For example, the clinical significance of respiratory cultures positive for aerobic gram-negative bacilli or *S. aureus* may not be clear. On the one hand, it is known that as many as 75%

of such cultures represent airway colonization rather than invasive infection (68). On the other hand, it is also clear that up to 30% of the time, infection is mistaken for colonization (86). What can account for this diagnostic difficulty? First, patients in the intensive care unit generally have abnormal chest X-rays, whether or not lung infection is present. Similarly, fever and leukocytosis are common in such patients, irrespective of pneumonia, and cough and sputum production have little relevance in the obtunded and intubated patient. Thus, it is not surprising that considerable debate often surrounds the isolation of potential gram-negative (or *S. aureus*) bacillary pathogens from cultures of the airways in such patients. Even when the tracheobronchial secretions are purulent, the differentiation between tracheobronchitis and pneumonia may be difficult.

The presence or absence of infection in patients with adult respiratory distress syndrome is particularly difficult to determine. In one recent report (86), histopathologic and clinical diagnoses were correlated for 30 consecutive adult patients who died in association with adult respiratory distress syndrome. Particular attention was given to whether premortem clinical diagnoses of pneumonia could be verified by autopsy findings. In some cases autopsies revealed unsuspected pneumonia, and in other cases clinically suspected pneumonias were not confirmed by examination of lung tissues. Overall, nosocomial bacterial pneumonia was misdiagnosed in 30% of the patients. Thus, the difficulty in deciphering between bacterial colonization and infection of the lower respiratory tract will inevitably lead to some errors in management. Nevertheless, clinical experience, coupled with careful physical and microbiologic observations should assist the clinician in this difficult setting. The following questions are extremely useful in evaluating these patients: Has there been a change in clinical status, unexplained by other events (e.g., myocardial infarction; pulmonary embolism)? Has there been a sudden increase in lung infiltrate, a drop in arterial pO_2, or a change in fever pattern? Most importantly, has there been an increase in quantity and purulence of respiratory secretions? While such criteria for nosocomial pneumonia may lack both sensitivity and specificity, they may be the only available parameters for the clinician.

Beyond the clinical decision of whether a nosocomial pneumonia exists, is the decision regarding etiology. Microbiologic evaluation of the patient with suspected nosocomial pneumonia may or may not be helpful. Sputum, or respiratory secretions (obtained by endotracheal aspiration), should be examined microscopically using a gram stain. Unfortunately, these specimens are often contaminated with upper airway flora. Likewise, cultures of such specimens may or may not reflect the microbiology of infected lung tissues. In one series, the difficulty in reproducing growth of a single, known bacterial pathogen from multiple respiratory specimens in the hospital setting resulted in a 44% incidence of uncertain etiologies for nosocomial pneumonia (6). Isolation of a single organism from blood cultures may help to decipher between contaminating and infecting bacterial isolates in sputum.

Since microbiologic evaluation of contaminated respiratory specimens may be misleading, a number of invasive methods have been developed in order to obtain noncontaminated specimens for diagnostic evaluation (87). Furthermore, quantitative sputum cultures, "washed" sputum cultures, and microscopic "screening" of sputa for the presence of upper airway cells suggesting contamination have all been evaluated as means for determining the significance of bacterial isolates (88). These methods may be impractical for widespread use, however, and in fact have met with some controversy regarding their actual usefulness. Transtracheal aspiration (not possible in intubated patients), percutaneous thin needle lung aspiration (not advised for patients on positive pressure breathing modes), and shielded-tip bronchoscopic sampling of lower airway secretions have all been suggested as methods to avoid upper airway contamination of respiratory specimens. While these methods may, in fact, increase diagnostic specificity in certain patients, they may not be well tolerated by certain critically ill patients with suspected pneumonia. In addition, several reports have, in fact, illustrated a rather high rate of false positive results for cultures obtained using these procedures (89, 90). To date, almost no information has been available regarding the use of shielded-tip diagnostic bronchoscopy in intubated patients. A recent report, however, compared the accuracy of cultures obtained by shielded-tip bronchoscopy to cultures obtained by lung biopsy in patients with assisted ventilation (91). In each case, specimens were collected from patients immediately after they expired. While excellent microbiologic correlation between lung tissues and bronchoscopic specimens was noted for patients with histologic evidence of pneumonia, there was a high incidence of false positive results among the bronchoscopic specimens obtained from patients without pneumonia. It appears that aspiration of oral flora attendant with invasive diagnostic procedures may result in rather large numbers of false positive microbiologic results during the invasive procedures.

TREATMENT

Treatment of nosocomial pneumonia may be empiric or specific. Furthermore, treatment may be considered conventional or investigational. Empiric treatment is employed for clinically suspected pneumonia in which an identified etiologic agent is not available to guide therapy. If and when the etiology is identified, then specific therapy may be chosen. Intravenous antibiotics remain the conventional form of treatment for nosocomial pneumonia. However, a number of investigational therapies have been proposed, including intrabronchial antibiotics and passive immunization.

When microscopic examination of sputum or tracheal aspirate smears does not provide a presumptive diagnosis, empiric choices of initial antimicrobial therapy must be made for suspected cases of nosocomial pneumonia. Several issues must be considered in selecting appropriate therapy. Patient-related considerations are as follows: Has the patient recently received antibiotics which could select for more resistant organisms? Does the patient have underlying chronic bronchitis, which would increase the risk of *H. influenzae*, or cystic fibrosis, which would increase the risk of *P. aeruginosa* and *S. aureus*? Have recent surveillance cultures of the patient's sputum been consistently positive for a particular organism? Also important is the recent experience with nosocomial pathogens in a given hospital or intensive care unit. For example, has there been a particularly high incidence of pneumonias caused by multiantibiotic-resistant *Acinetobacter* or *Serratia* during recent months? Furthermore, has *Legionella* sp. been noted in the patient's hospital? Relevant to pediatric and psychiatric wards are outbreaks of viral or mycoplasmal respiratory infections in the community. Also important in making an empiric therapeutic decision is a thorough understanding of which pathogens are most likely to cause nosocomial pneumonia (see "Etiologies").

In general, empiric treatment of nosocomial pneumonia should include coverage for aerobic gram-negative bacilli, including highly resistant organisms, such as *P. aeruginosa*, *S. marcescens*, and *Acinetobacter*, and also for *S. aureus*. Based upon these considerations, several regimens have been employed for empiric treatment of nosocomial pneumonia. These include the following: a semisynthetic penicillin plus an aminoglycoside; clindamycin plus an aminoglycoside; or a cephalosporin plus an aminoglycoside. In patients with known chronic lung disease, coverage for *H. influenzae* should also be included. Likewise, in the presence of known large scale aspiration, coverage against anaerobic flora should be maintained. The information in Table 20.3 is meant to serve as a guide for selection of empiric therapy of nosocomial pneumonia, both in general and in specialized situations. In each case, combination therapy has been advocated, and an aminoglycoside has been included in each regimen. While recent reports of single-agent, β-lactam treatment for serious gram-negative infections are encouraging (92), the reliability of β-lactam agents as single drug treatment for *P. aeruginosa* pneumonia has yet to be fully established. Thus, until *P. aeruginosa* can be excluded as a pathogen, most experts would include an aminoglycoside in their empiric regimen (93).

In the event that a specific etiologic agent is identified, other questions regarding proper therapy remain. One issue is whether two potentially synergistic antibiotics might offer therapeutic efficacy superior to that of a single antibiotic with activity against the isolate. Currently available clinical data have not substantiated additional benefits for two active agents in treating *Klebsiella* pneumonia (93). Experimental data do suggest that β-lactam-aminoglycoside combinations may be at least additive in efficacy for treating *P. aeruginosa* pneumonia (94, 95). An additional potential advantage in using two active agents in treating gram-negative pneumonia is the suppression of emerging resistance among microorganisms (96, 97).

Also controversial is the role of aminoglycosides in treating gram-negative pneumonia. While some consider this class of agent to be the cornerstone of therapy for serious gram-negative respiratory infections (93, 98, 99), others have questioned the usefulness of aminoglycosides in treating pneumonia (100, 101). It has been proposed, for example, that the narrow therapeutic ratios for aminoglycosides in serum, and the difficulty in penetration of aminoglycosides from blood into the infected respiratory tissues, may result in local drug concentrations insufficient to treat infecting organisms (102). On the other hand, evidence also exists that aminoglycosides are more

Table 20.3.   Empiric Treatment of Hospital-Acquired Pneumonia

Potential Pathogens	Therapeutic Agents

1. All patients
Staphylococcus aureus
Aerobic gram-negative bacilli
   (including *Pseudomonas aeruginosa*)
 	
Mouth flora (anaerobes)
	Nafcillin plus aminoglycoside
	or
	Cephalosporin plus amino-
	   glycoside
	or
	Clindamycin plus amino-
	   glycoside
	or
	Piperacillin* plus amino-
	   glycoside

2. Patients with chronic lung diseases
Add *Haemophilus influenzae*
	Cefamandole plus aminogly-
	   coside
	or
	Cefotaxime plus aminogly-
	   coside

3. Large aspiration
Maximize anaerobe coverage
	Clindamycin plus aminogly-
	   coside
	or
	Cefoxitin plus aminoglyco-
	   side

4. *Legionella* sp. endemic	Include erythromycin

* For patients with sputum gram stains clearly indicative of gram-negative pathogens.

active than β-lactam antimicrobial agents against certain resistant gram-negative bacilli (such as *P. aeruginosa*) (103, 104). Two separate reports have documented the importance of achieving high peak serum levels of aminoglycosides ($\geq 6 \mu g/ml$ for gentamicin or tobramycin; $\geq 24 \mu g/ml$ for amikacin) in order to treat gram-negative pneumonia successfully with these agents (93, 105). Several other approaches have been utilized to improve delivery of aminoglycosides into infected lung tissues. These include computer-assisted individualized dosing (106), bolus dosing with unconventionally large doses (107), and direct instillation of aminoglycoside into the respiratory tract via an endotracheal or tracheostomy tube (108, 109). In one prospective randomized study (108), groups of patients with nosocomial gram-negative pneumonia were treated with systemic antibiotics plus either 25 mg of sisomicin in saline suspension instilled into the respiratory tract every 8 hours, or saline-placebo instillations. More patients in the group receiving local aminoglycoside treatment experienced improvement, and superinfections with resistant flora were no different between the groups. Despite this encouraging experience, further investigation of lo-

cal aminoglycoside therapy for pneumonia will be necessary before the relative risks and benefits can be defined.

In addition to antibiotics, there exists considerable interest in immunologic methods of treatment of gram-negative pneumonia. A number of passive immune sera, including the J-5 cross-protective antisera (110), and hyperimmune *Pseudomonas* globulin (111), are potentially valuable agents for treatment of gram-negative pneumonias. These sera are currently being evaluated in experimental models of gram-negative pneumonia. However, clinical or experimental data are insufficient to establish a definitive therapeutic role for passive immune sera in nosocomial pneumonia at this time.

PREVENTION

The fundamental objective in preventing nosocomial pneumonia is to reduce the acquisition of potential bacterial pathogens in upper airways, and thus to reduce the potential for aspiration of these organisms into the lower respiratory tract. Three general approaches have been utilized for achieving this objective. These include the following: (*a*) attention to environmental factors (e.g., hand washing, specialized isolation procedures, monitoring of respiratory equipment for bacterial contamination); (*b*) prophylactic antibiotics; and (*c*) immunologic intervention. Great emphasis has been placed upon reducing oropharyngeal bacterial colonization by infection control procedures within the patient's environment. It is clear that careful monitoring, decontamination, and adherence to the usage guidelines of respiratory equipment will decrease the incidence of nosocomial gram-negative pneumonia (3, 52). Additional infection control guidelines for the prevention of nosocomial pneumonia have been published (112). A number of these recommendations are empiric, however, rather than based upon controlled observations. For example, the recommendation that breathing circuit tubing be changed every 24 hours appears to be arbitrary. In one recent report, no significant increase in bacterial contamination of tubing was noted between 24 and 48 hours of use (113). It was estimated in that report that $30 million could be saved annually in the United States if tubing changes were carried out every 48 hours instead of every 24 hours, as recommended in the published guidelines. In another report, the recommendation that nebulizers be changed every 24 hours was shown to be inappropriate, since significant contamination of medication nebulizers occurred after a single use (66). These published guidelines contain many other "common sense" recommendations, such as washing hands between patients, wearing sterile gloves for endotracheal suctioning, and avoiding contact between infected hospital personnel and high risk patients. Remarkably few of the precepts have been carefully studied. However, a recent report documents that hand washing with chlorhexidine may reduce the incidence of nosocomial pneumonias (75).

Several groups have utilized endobronchial prophylactic antibiotics in an attempt to reduce the incidence of nosocomial pneumonia. In one study, aerosolized gentamicin was employed in burn patients with inhalation injury (114). Pulmonary and septic complications were not reduced in the gentamicin group. Furthermore, use of prophylactic gentamicin aerosol was associated with isolation of antibiotic-resistant *Pseudomonas* and *Klebsiella* from sputum. In a separate study, hospitalized patients with tracheostomies were randomized to receive endotracheal instillations of gentamicin (80 mg every 8 hours, suspended in 10 ml of saline) versus saline alone

(115). Prophylactic gentamicin instillations resulted in fewer episodes of purulent sputum, documented chest infiltrates, and positive sputum cultures. However, a slight increase in gentamicin resistance was noted among respiratory isolates from the drug-treated group. In a subsequent study (116), an aminoglycoside-polymyxin B combination was employed in order to reduce resistant flora. Bronchial irritation was noted with that regimen, however. Finally, an extensive analysis of prophylactic polymyxin B aerosol for patients in a respiratory intensive care unit has been described (117–119). Early reports were encouraging, with both reduced colonization of airways (117) and reduced incidence of pneumonia (118) observed in patients receiving polymyxin B. In the final phase of this study, however, emergence of antibiotic-resistant respiratory pathogens and increased pneumonia-related mortalities were both observed (119). Thus, based upon currently available data, routine use of prophylactic endobronchial antibiotics cannot be recommended.

As an alternative to antibiotic prophylaxis, immunization has been proposed as a rational method for prevention of nosocomial pneumonia (5, 120). There are several potential approaches to providing immune enhancement of lung defenses. One method would be to provide organism-specific immunization for pathogens known to be associated with particularly high mortalities. This approach has been evaluated for *P. aeruginosa* pneumonia, using prophylactic immunization with a lipopolysaccharide (LPS) vaccine (121). Although results from that study suggested that immunization reduced the incidence and mortality of *Pseudomonas* pneumonia, the experience was limited to only 34 vaccinated patients. Other concerns for active vaccination with *P. aeruginosa* vaccines include the side effects associated with LPS vaccine, the fact that *P. aeruginosa* accounts for only 10 to 15% of nosocomial pneumonias, and importantly, the insufficient time to develop a full immune response in acutely hospitalized patients. Recent development of a hyperimmune anti-*Pseudomonas* globulin (111) offers the potential for rapid immunization using passive administration of type-specific antibodies. An alternative, and perhaps even more rational, immunologic approach would be to confer protection against the wide range of gram-negative bacillary species which serve as potential pathogens for the human respiratory tract. So-called cross-protective vaccines or antisera, such as the J-5 mutant of *Escherichia coli* 0 111, might be candidate immunogens. While recent clinical studies with J-5 antisera suggest a protective role against gram-negative septicemia (110), the relative degree of pulmonary protection provided by J-5 antisera has not been determined.

Finally, while most attention has been focused upon prevention of aerobic gram-negative pneumonias, effective methods for reducing endemic nosocomial *Legionella* infections have also been reported. These measures have largely employed hyperchlorination of contaminated potable water within the hospital (31, 36). Identification and removal of contaminated air conditioning equipment may also be necessary, however (35). In addition, limited success has been achieved in controlling nosocomial viral respiratory infection. Respiratory syncytial virus (RSV) is spread primarily by direct inoculation of large droplets or by direct contact (i.e., hands, fomites) (122). Thus, secretion precautions have been advocated for known cases. In one study, isolation, cohorting of infected infants, and cohorting of staff to infected infants reduced the spread of RSV among patients but not among hospital personnel (123). Influenza virus, on the other hand, is spread by small particle aerosols. Thus, influenza may be spread more rapidly and is generally even more difficult to control. Prophylactic immunization with influenza vaccines, to include hospital workers, would be the most rational approach to control of nosocomial influenza respiratory infection. Unfortunately, less than 20% of high risk patients are immunized each year (21), and even fewer health care workers receive influenza vaccine (19).

SUMMARY

Hospital-acquired pneumonia continues to be the leading cause of fatal nosocomial infection. The ability to prevent or treat aerobic gram-negative bacillary pneumonias in the critically ill patient has not kept pace with our understanding of the pathogenesis of this infection. As even more is learned regarding the initial phase of oropharyngeal colonization with potential bacterial pathogens, biochemical or immunologic strategies to interrupt this critical initiation step may be developed. In the meanwhile, continued attention to the patients' hospital environment and more judicious use of newer antimicrobial agents will continue to be the cornerstones of prevention and therapy. Recent development of hyperimmune globulins for intravenous use offers the possibility for improved therapies in the near future.

References

1. Lepper MH: Opportunistic gram-negative rod pulmonary infections. *Dis Chest* 44:18–26, 1963.
2. Reinarz JA, Pierce AK, Mays BB, Sanford JP: The potential role of inhalation therapy equipment in nosocomial pulmonary infection. *J Clin Invest* 44:831–839, 1965.
3. Pierce AK, Sanford JP, Thomas GD, Leonard JS: Long-term evaluation of decontamination of inhalation-therapy equipment and the occurrence of necrotizing pneumonia. *N Engl J Med* 282:528–531, 1970.
4. Centers for Disease Control: National Nosocomial Infections Study report, annual summary 1983. *MMWR* 33 (no. 255):9SS–21SS, 1985.
5. Stamm WE, Martin SM, Bennett JV: Epidemiology of nosocomial infections due to gram-negative bacilli: aspects relevant to development and use of vaccines. *J Infect Dis* 136:S151–S160, 1977.
6. Graybill JR, Marshall LW, Charache P, Wallace CK, Melvin VB: Nosocomial pneumonia. *Am Rev Respir Dis* 108:1130–1140, 1973.
7. Stevens RM, Teres D, Skillman JJ, Feingold DS: Pneumonia in an intensive care unit. *Arch Intern Med* 134:106–111, 1974.
8. Bryan CS, Reynolds KL: Bacteremic nosocomial pneumonia. Analysis of 172 episodes from a single metropolitan area. *Am Rev Respir Dis* 129:668–671, 1984.
9. Gross PA, Neu HC, Aswapokee P, Van Antwerpe C, Aswapokee N: Deaths from nosocomial infections: experience in a university hospital and a community hospital. *Am J Med* 68:219–223, 1980.
10. LaForce FM: Hospital-acquired gram-negative rod pneumonias: an overview. *Am J Med* 70:664–669, 1981.
11. Garibaldi RA, Britt MR, Coleman ML, Reading JC, Pace NL: Risk factors for postoperative pneumonia. *Am J Med* 70:677–680, 1981.
12. Hemming VG, Overall JC Jr, Britt MR: Nosocomial infections in a newborn intensive-care unit. *N Engl J Med* 294:1310–1316, 1976.
13. Pennington JE, Reynolds HY, Carbone PP: *Pseudomonas* pneumonia: a retrospective study of 36 cases. *Am J Med* 55:155–160, 1973.
14. Tillotson JR, Lerner AM: Characteristics of nonbacteremic *Pseudomonas* pneumonia. *Ann Intern Med* 68:295–307, 1968.
15. Kirby BD, Snyder KM, Meyer RD, Finegold SM: Legionnaires' disease: report of sixty-five nosocomially acquired cases and review of the literature. *Medicine* 59:188–205, 1980.
16. MacDonald NE, Hall CB, Suffin SC, Alexson C, Harris PJ, Manning JA: Respiratory syncytial viral infection in infants with congenital heart disease. *N Engl J Med* 307:397–400, 1982.
17. Blumenfeld HL, Kilbourne ED, Louria DB, Robers DE: Studies on influenza in the pandemic of 1957–1958. I. An epidemiologic, clinical and serologic investigation of an intrahospital epidemic, with a note on vaccination efficacy. *J Clin Invest*

38:199–212, 1959.
18. Kapila R, Lintz DI, Tecson FT, Ziskin L, Louria DB: A nosocomial outbreak of influenza A. *Chest* 71:576–579, 1977.
19. Hall CB: Nosocomial viral respiratory infections: perennial weeds on pediatric wards. *Am J Med* 70:670–676, 1981.
20. Wenzel RP, Deal EC, Hendley JO: Hospital-acquired viral respiratory illness on a pediatric ward. *Pediatrics* 60:367–371, 1977.
21. Glezen WP: Viral pneumonia as a cause and result of hospitalization. *J Infect Dis* 147:765–770, 1983.
22. Valenti WM, Hall CB, Douglas RG Jr, Menegus MA, Pincus PH: Nosocomial viral infections. 1. Epidemiology and significance. *Infect Control* 1:33–37, 1979.
23. Kimball AM, Foy HM, Cooney MK, Allan ID, Matlock M, Plorde JJ: Isolation of respiratory syncytial and influenza viruses from the sputum of patients hospitalized with pneumonia. *J Infect Dis* 147:181–184, 1983.
24. Hall CB, Douglas RG Jr, Geiman JM, Messner MK: Nosocomial respiratory syncytial virus infections. *N Engl J Med* 293:1343–1346, 1975.
25. Hoffman PC, Dixon RE: Control of influenza in the hospital. *Ann Intern Med* 87:725–728, 1977.
26. Hall CB, Douglas RG Jr: Nosocomial influenza infection as a cause of intercurrent fevers in infants. *Pediatrics* 55:673–677, 1975.
27. Meibalane R, Sedmak GV, Sasidharan P, Garg P, Grausz JP: Outbreak of influenza in a neonatal intensive care unit. *J Pediatr* 91:974–976, 1977.
28. Mathur U, Bentley DW, Hall CB: Concurrent respiratory syncytial virus and influenza A infections in the institutionalized elderly and chronically ill. *Ann Intern Med* 93:49–52, 1980.
29. England AC III, Fraser DW: Sporadic and epidemic nosocomial legionellosis in the United States. *Am J Med* 70:707–711, 1981.
30. Yu VL, Kroboth FJ, Shonnard J, Brown A, McDearman S, Magnussen M: Legionnaires' disease: new clinical perspective from a prospective pneumonia study. *Am J Med* 73:357–361, 1982.
31. Meyer RD, Edelstein PH: *Legionella* pneumonias. In Pennington JE (ed): *Respiratory Infections: Diagnosis and Management*. New York, Raven Press, 1983, pp 283–297.
32. Brown A, Yu VL, Elder EM, Magnussen MH, Kroboth F: Nosocomial outbreak of Legionnaires' disease at the Pittsburgh Veterans Administration Medical Center. *Trans Assoc Am Physicians* 93:52–59, 1980.
33. Gerber JE, Casey CE, Martin P, Winn WC Jr: Legionnaires' disease in Vermont, 1972–1976. *Am J Clin Pathol* 76:816–818, 1981.
34. Balows A, Fraser DW (eds): International symposium on Legionnaires' disease. *Ann Intern Med* 90:481–714, 1979.
35. Dondero TJ Jr, Rendtorff RC, Mallison GF, Weeks RM, Levy JS, Wong EW, Schaffner W: An outbreak of Legionnaires' disease associated with a contaminated air-conditioning cooling tower. *N Engl J Med* 7:365–370, 1980.
36. Cordes LG, Wiesenthal AM, Gorman GW, Phair JP, Sommers HM, Brown A, Yu VL, Magnussen MH, Meyer RD, Wolf JS, Shands KN, Fraser DW: Isolation of *Legionella pneumophila* from hospital shower heads. *Ann Intern Med* 94:195–197, 1981.
37. Stout J, Yu VL, Vickers RM, Zuravleff J, Best M, Brown A, Yee RB, Wadowsky R: Ubiquitousness of *Legionella pneumophila* in the water supply of a hospital with epidemic Legionnaires' disease. *N Engl J Med* 306:466–468, 1982.
38. Girod JC, Reichman RC, Winn WC Jr, Klaucke DN, Vogt RL, Dolin R: Pneumonic and nonpneumonic forms of legionellosis. *Arch Intern Med* 142:545–547, 1982.
39. Simon HB, Southwick FS, Moellering RC, Sherman E: *Haemophilus influenzae* in hospitalized adults: current perspectives. *Am J Med* 69:219–226, 1980.
40. Berk SL, Verghese A, Holtsclaw SA, Smith JK: Enterococcal pneumonia. Occurrence in patients receiving broad-spectrum antibiotic regimens and enteral feeding. *Am J Med* 74:153–154, 1983.
41. Buxton AE, Anderson RL, Werdegar D, Atlas E: Nosocomial respiratory tract infection and colonization with *Acinetobacter calcoaceticus*. Epidemiologic characteristics. *Am J Med* 65:507–513, 1978.
42. Olson B, Weinstein RA, Nathan C, Chamberlin W, Kabins SA: Epidemiology of endemic *Pseudomonas aeruginosa*: why infection control efforts have failed. *J Infect Dis* 150:808–816, 1984.
43. Fanta CH, Pennington JE: Pneumonia in the immunocompromised host. In Pennington JE (ed): *Respiratory Infections: Diagnosis and Management*. New York, Raven Press, 1983, pp 171–185.
44. Valdivieso M, Gil-Extremera B, Zornoza J, Bodey G: Gram-negative bacillary pneumonia in the compromised host. *Medicine* 56:241–254, 1977.
45. Pennington JE: Opportunistic fungal pneumonias: *Aspergillus, Mucor, Candida, Torulopsis*. In Pennington JE (ed): *Respiratory Infections: Diagnosis and Management*. New York, Raven Press, 1983, pp 329–339.
46. Aisner J, Schimpff S, Bennett JE, Young VM, Wiernick PH: *Aspergillus* infections in cancer patients; association with fireproofing in a new hospital. *JAMA* 235:411–412, 1976.
47. Arnow PM, Anderson RL, Mainous PD, Smith EJ: Pulmonary aspergillosis during hospital renovation. *Am Rev Respir Dis* 118:49–53, 1978.
48. Singer C, Armstrong D, Rosen PP, Schottenfeld D: *Pneumocystis carinii* pneumonia: a cluster of eleven cases. *Ann Intern Med* 82:772–777, 1975.
49. Hirsch MS, Wormser GP, Schooley RT, Ho DD, Felsenstein D, Hopkins CC, Joline C, Duncanson F, Sarngadharan MG, Saxinger C, Gallo RC: Risk of nosocomial infection with human T-cell lymphotropic virus III (HTLV-III). *N Engl J Med* 312:1–4, 1985.
50. Cross AS, Roup B: Role of respiratory assistance devices in endemic nosocomial pneumonia. *Am J Med* 70:681–685, 1981.
51. Ramphal R, Sadoff JC, Pyle M, Silipigni JD: Role of pili in the adherence of *Pseudomonas aeruginosa* to injured tracheal epithelium. *Infect Immun* 44:38–40, 1984.
52. Pierce AK, Sanford JP: Aerobic gram-negative

bacillary pneumonias. *Am Rev Respir Dis* 110:647–658, 1974.

53. Edmondson EB, Reinarz JA, Pierce AK, Sanford JP: Nebulization equipment. A potential source of infection in gram-negative pneumonias. *Am J Dis Child* 111:357–360, 1966.

54. Pierce AK, Sanford JP: Bacterial contamination of aerosols. *Arch Intern Med* 131:156–159, 1973.

55. Hoffman MA, Finberg L: *Pseudomonas* infections in infants associated with high-humidity environment. *J Pediatr* 46:626–630, 1955.

56. MacPherson R: Oxygen therapy—an unsuspected source of hospital infections? *JAMA* 167:1083–1086, 1958.

57. Severe JL: Possible role of humidifying equipment in spread of infections from the newborn. *Pediatrics* 24:50–53, 1959.

58. Bishop C, Potts MW, Molloy PJ: A method of sterilization for the Barnet respirator. *Br J Anaesth* 34:121–123, 1962.

59. Bishop C, Roper WAG, Williams SR: The use of an absolute filter to sterilize the inspiratory air during intermittent positive pressure respiration. *Br J Anaesth* 35:32–34, 1963.

60. Bishop C, Robertson DS, Williams SR: The use of ethylene oxide for sterilization of mechanical ventilators. *Br J Anaesth* 36:53–57, 1964.

61. Sykes MK: Sterilizing mechanical ventilators. *Br J Med* 1:561, 1964.

62. Pierce AK, Edmondson EB, McGee G, Ketchersid J, Loudon RG, Sanford JP: An analysis of factors predisposing to gram-negative bacillary necrotizing pneumonia. *Am Rev Respir Dis* 94:309–315, 1966.

63. Moffet HL, Allan D, Williams T: Survival and dissemination of bacteria in nebulizers and incubators. *Am J Dis Child* 114:13–20, 1967.

64. Rhoades ER, Ringrose R, Mohr JA, Brooks L, McKown BA, Felton F: Contamination of ultrasonic nebulization equipment with gram-negative bacteria. *Arch Intern Med* 127:228–232, 1971.

65. Grieble HG, Colton FR, Bird TJ, Toigo A, Griffith LG: Fine-particle humidifiers. Source of *Pseudomonas aeruginosa* infections in a respiratory-disease unit. *N Engl J Med* 282:531–535, 1970.

66. Craven DE, Lichtenberg DA, Goularte TA, Make BJ, McCabe WR: Contaminated medication nebulizers in mechanical ventilator circuits. Source of bacterial aerosols. *Am J Med* 77:834–838, 1984.

67. Shultze T, Edmondson EB, Pierce AK, Sanford JP: Studies of a new humidifying device as a potential source of bacterial aerosols. *Am Rev Respir Dis* 96:517–519, 1967.

68. Johanson WG Jr, Pierce AK, Sanford JP, Thomas GD: Nosocomial respiratory infections with gram-negative bacilli. *Ann Intern Med* 77:701–706, 1972.

69. Louria DB, Kaminski T: The effects of four antimicrobial drug regimens on sputum superinfection in hospitalized patients. *Am Rev Respir Dis* 85:649–665, 1962.

70. Tillotson JR, Finland M: Bacterial colonization and clinical superinfection of the respiratory tract complicating antibiotic treatment of pneumonia. *J Infect Dis* 119:597–624, 1969.

71. Eickhoff JC: Pulmonary infections in surgical patients. *Surg Clin North Am* 60:175–183, 1980.

72. Johanson WG, Pierce AK, Sanford JP: Changing pharyngeal bacterial flora of hospitalized patients. *N Engl J Med* 281:1137–1140, 1969.

73. Schwartz SN, Dowling JN, Benkovic C, De Quittner-Buchanan M, Prostko T, Yee RB: Sources of gram-negative bacilli colonizing the tracheae of intubated patients. *J Infect Dis* 138:227–231, 1978.

74. Maki DG, Alvarado CJ, Hassemer CA, Zilz MA: Relation of the inanimate hospital environment to endemic nosocomial infection. *N Engl J Med* 25:1562–1566, 1982.

75. Maki D, Hecht J: Antiseptic-containing hand-washing agents reduce nosocomial infections—a prospective study. Abstracts of The Twenty-second Interscience Conference on Antimicrobial Agents and Chemotherapy, 1982, no. 699, p 188.

76. Du Moulin GC, Paterson DG, Hedley-Whyte J, Libson A: Aspiration of gastric bacteria in antacid-treated patients: a frequent cause of postoperative colonisation of the airway. *Lancet* 1:242–245, 1982.

77. Johanson WG Jr, Higuchi JG, Chaudhuri TR, Woods DE: Bacterial adherence to epithelial cells in bacillary colonization of the respiratory tract. *Am Rev Respir Dis* 121:55–63, 1980.

78. Johanson WG Jr, Woods DE, Chaudhuri T: Association of respiratory tract colonization with adherence of gram-negative bacilli to epithelial cells. *J Infect Dis* 139:667–673, 1979.

79. Niederman MS, Merrill WM, Ferranti RD, Pagano KM, Palmer LB, Reynolds HY: Nutritional status and bacterial binding in the lower respiratory tract in patients with chronic tracheostomy. *Ann Intern Med* 100:795–800, 1984.

80. Niederman MS, Rafferty TD, Sasaki CT, Merrill WM, Matthay RA, Reynolds HY: Comparison of bacterial adherence to ciliated and squamous epithelial cells obtained from the human respiratory tract. *Am Rev Respir Dis* 127:85–90, 1983.

81. Woods DE, Straus DC, Johanson WG Jr, Berry VK, Bass JA: Role of pili in adherence of *Pseudomonas aeruginosa* to mammalian buccal epithelial cells. *Infect Immun* 29:1146–1151, 1980.

82. Ramphal R, Pyle M: Evidence for mucins and sialic acid as receptors for *Pseudomonas aeruginosa* in the lower respiratory tract. *Infect Immun* 41:339–344, 1983.

83. Abraham SN, Beachey EH, Simpson WA: Adherence of *Streptococcus pyogenes, Escherichia coli,* and *Pseudomonas aeruginosa* to fibronectin-coated and uncoated epithelial cells. *Infect Immun* 41:1261–1268, 1983.

84. Woods DE, Straus DC, Johanson WG Jr, Bass JA: Role of fibronectin in the prevention of adherence of *Pseudomonas aeruginosa* to buccal cells. *J Infect Dis* 143:784–790, 1981.

85. Woods DE, Straus DC, Johanson WG Jr, Bass JA: Role of salivary protease activity in adherence of gram-negative bacilli to mammalian buccal epithelial cells in vivo. *J Clin Invest* 68:1435–1440, 1981.

86. Andrews CP, Coalson JJ, Smith JD, Johanson WG: Diagnosis of nosocomial bacterial pneumonia in acute, diffuse lung injury. *Chest* 80:254–

258, 1981.

87. Bartlett JG: Invasive diagnostic techniques in respiratory infections. In Pennington JE (ed): *Respiratory Infections: Diagnosis and Management*. New York, Raven Press, 1983, pp 55–77.

88. Washington JA II: Noninvasive diagnostic techniques for lower respiratory infections. In Pennington JE (ed): *Respiratory Infections: Diagnosis and Management*. New York, Raven Press, 1983, pp 41–54.

89. Halperin SA, Suratt PM, Gwaltney JM Jr, Gröschel DHM, Hendley JO, Eggleston PA: Bacterial cultures of the lower respiratory tract in normal volunteers with and without experimental rhinovirus infection using a plugged double catheter system. *Am Rev Respir Dis* 125:678–680, 1982.

90. Joshi JH, Wang K-P, De Jongh CA, Newman KA, Wiernik PH, Schimpff SC: A comparative evaluation of two fiberoptic bronchoscopy catheters: the plugged telescoping catheter versus the single sheathed nonplugged catheter. *Am Rev Respir Dis* 126:860–863, 1982.

91. Chastre J, Viau F, Brun P, Pierre J, Dauge M-C, Bouchama A, Akesbi A, Gibert C: Prospective evaluation of the protected specimen brush for the diagnosis of pulmonary infections in ventilated patients. *Am Rev Respir Dis* 130:924–929, 1984.

92. Smith CR, Ambinder R, Lipsky JJ, Petty BG, Israel E, Levitt R, Mellits ED, Rocco L, Longstreth J, Lietman PS: Cefotaxime compared with nafcillin plus tobramycin for serious bacterial infections. A randomized, double-blind trial. *Ann Intern Med* 101:469–477, 1984.

93. Moore RD, Smith CR, Lietman PS: Association of aminoglycoside plasma levels with therapeutic outcome in gram-negative pneumonia. *Am J Med* 77:657–662, 1984.

94. Pennington JE: Use of animal models to evaluate antimicrobial therapy for bacterial pneumonias. In Sande MA, Zak O (eds): *Animal Models in the Evaluation of Chemotherapy of Infectious Diseases*. London, Academic Press, in press.

95. Rusnak MG, Drake TA, Hackbarth CJ, Sande MA: Single versus combination antibiotic therapy for pneumonia due to *Pseudomonas aeruginosa* in neutropenic guinea pigs. *J Infect Dis* 149:980–985, 1984.

96. Eliopoulos GM, Moellering RC Jr: Antibiotic synergism and antimicrobial combinations in clinical infections. *Rev Infect Dis* 4:282–293, 1982.

97. Gerber AU, Vastola AP, Brandel J, Craig WA: Selection of aminoglycoside-resistant variants of *Pseudomonas aeruginosa* in an in vivo model. *J Infect Dis* 146:691–697, 1982.

98. Trenholme GM, McKellar PP, Rivera N, Levin S: Amikacin in the treatment of gram-negative pneumonia. *Am J Med* 62:949–953, 1977.

99. Louria DB, Young L, Armstrong D, Smith JK: Gentamicin in the treatment of pulmonary infections. *J Infect Dis* 119:483–485, 1969.

100. Neu HC: Clinical use of aminoglycosides. In Whelton A, Neu HC (eds): *The Aminoglycosides. Microbiology, Clinical Use and Toxicology*. New York, Marcel Dekker, 1982, pp 611–628.

101. Bodem CR, Lampton LM, Miller DP, Tarka EF,

Everett ED: Endobronchial pH. Relevance to aminoglycoside activity in gram-negative bacillary pneumonia. *Am Rev Respir Dis* 127:39–41, 1983.

102. Pennington JE: Penetration of antibiotics into respiratory secretions. *Rev Infect Dis* 3:67–73, 1981.

103. Bundtzen RW, Gerger AU, Cohn DL, Craig WA: Postantibiotic suppression of bacterial growth. *Rev Infect Dis* 3:28–37, 1981.

104. Corrado ML, Landesman SH, Cherubin CD: Influence of inoculum size on activity of cefoperazone, cefotaxime, moxalactam, piperacillin, and *N*-formimidoyl thienamycin (MK 0787) against *Pseudomonas aeruginosa*. *Antimicrob Agents Chemother* 18:893–896, 1980.

105. Noone P, Pattison JR, Garfield Danies D: The effective use of gentamicin in life-threatening sepsis. *Postgrad Med J* 50 (suppl 7):9–16, 1974.

106. Cipolle RJ, Seifert RD, Zaske DE, Strate RG: Hospital acquired gram-negative pneumonias: response rate and dosage requirements with individualized tobramycin therapy. *Ther Drug Monitoring* 2:359–363, 1980.

107. Martin AJ, Smalley CA, George RH, Healing DE, Anderson CM: Gentamicin and tobramycin compared in the treatment of mucoid *Pseudomonas* lung infections in cystic fibrosis. *Arch Dis Child* 55:604–607, 1980.

108. Klastersky J, Carpentier-Meunier F, Kahan-Coppens L, Thys JP: Endotracheally administered antibiotics for gram-negative bronchopneumonia. *Chest* 75:586–591, 1979.

109. Klastersky J, Geuning C, Mouawad E, Daneau D: Endotracheal gentamicin in bronchial infections in patients with tracheostomy. *Chest* 61:117–120, 1972.

110. Ziegler EJ, McCutchan JA, Fierer J, Glauser MD, Sadoff JC, Herndon D, Braude AI: Treatment of gram-negative bacteremia and shock with human antiserum to a mutant *Escherichia coli*. *N Engl J Med* 307:1225–1230, 1982.

111. Collins MS, Roby RE; Protective activity on an intravenous immune globulin (human) enriched in antibody against lipopolysaccharide antigens of *Pseudomonas aeruginosa*. *Am J Med* 76:168–174, 1984.

112. Simmons BP, Wong ES: Guidelines for prevention of nosocomial pneumonia. *Infect Control* 3:327–333, 1982.

113. Craven DE, Connolly MG Jr, Lichtenberg DA, Primeau PJ, McCabe WR: Contamination of mechanical ventilators with tubing changes every 24 or 48 hours. *N Engl J Med* 306:1505–1509, 1982.

114. Levine BA, Petroff PA, Slade CL, Pruitt BA Jr: Prospective trials of dexamethasone and aerosolized gentamicin in the treatment of inhalation injury in the burned patient. *J Trauma* 18:188–193, 1978.

115. Klastersky J, Huysmans E, Weerts D, Hensgens C, Daneau D: Endotracheally administered gentamicin for the prevention of infections of the respiratory tract in patients with tracheostomy: a double-blind study. *Chest* 65:650–654, 1974.

116. Klastersky J, Hensgens C, Noterman J, Mouawad E, Meunier-Carpentier F: Endotracheal antibiotics for the prevention of tracheobronchial infec-

tions in tracheotomized unconscious patients. A comparative study of gentamicin and aminosidin-polymyxin B combination. *Chest* 68:302–306, 1975.

117. Greenfield S, Teres D, Bushness LS, Hedley-Whyte J, Feingold DS: Prevention of gram-negative bacillary pneumonia using aerosol polymyxin as prophylaxis. *J Clin Invest* 52:2934–2940, 1973.

118. Klick JM, Du Moulin GC, Hedley-Whyte J, Teres D, Bushnell LS, Feingold DS: Prevention of gram-negative bacillary pneumonia using polymyxin aerosol as prophylaxis. II. Effect on the incidence of pneumonia in seriously ill patients. *J Clin Invest* 55:514–519, 1975.

119. Feeley TW, Du Moulin GC, Hedley-Whyte J, Bushnell LS, Gilbert JP, Feingold DS: Aerosol polymyxin and pneumonia in seriously ill patients. *N Engl J Med* 293:471–475, 1975.

120. Pennington JE: Pseudomonas aeruginosa pneumonia: the potential for immune intervention. In Weinstein L, Fields BN (eds): *Seminars in Infectious Diseases*. New York, Thieme-Stratton, 1983, pp 71–80.

121. Polk HC Jr, Borden S, Aldrett JA: Prevention of *Pseudomonas* respiratory infection in a surgical intensive care unit. *Ann Surg* 177:607–615, 1973.

122. Hall CB, Douglas RG Jr: Modes of transmission of respiratory syncytial virus. *J Pediatr* 99:100–103, 1981.

123. Hall CB, Geiman JM, Douglas RG Jr, Meagher MP: Control of nosocomial respiratory syncytial viral infections. *Pediatrics* 62:728–732, 1978.

Chapter 21

Hospital-Acquired Urinary Tract Infections: Epidemiology and Prevention

Richard A. Garibaldi, M.D.

EPIDEMIOLOGY

Recent reports continue to point out the importance of urinary tract infections (UTIs) as a major type of hospital-acquired infections. The urinary tract remains the most common site of nosocomial infection, accounting for as many as 50% of hospital-acquired infections (1, 2). Nonetheless, over recent years, a slight decrease in the incidence of nosocomial UTIs has been noted by some investigators. The National Nosocomial Infections Study (NNIS), conducted by the Centers for Disease Control, has noted a steady decrease in the rate of nosocomial UTIs from 1.47 cases/100 patients discharged in 1975–1976 to 1.41 in 1977 and 1.36 in 1978 (3). This surveillance involves more than 1 million patients in 82 hospitals throughout the United States. A similar trend over time has been noted by Burke et al in a single hospital where the rate of catheter-associated bacteriuria has decreased from an average incidence of 7.0%/day in 1974 to 2.5%/day in 1982 (4, 5). The reasons for this apparent improvement in rates of hospital-acquired UTI are multifactorial; they include changes in the population of catheterized patients, changes in antibiotic prescribing habits, and, hopefully, changes in the utilization, management, and duration of urinary catheterization.

Nonetheless, more than 10% of hospitalized patients continue to be exposed to temporary indwelling urethral catheters, and these catheters continue to represent the most important single risk factor that predisposes patients to infection (2, 6). The most common reasons for catheterization are for management of the surgical patient during the immediate postoperative period and for care of the debilitated, incontinent patient. One-third of patients are catheterized for less than 1 day (4, 6–8); the median duration of catheterization for all patients is 2 days. Approximately 10% of patients undergoing catheterization are bacteriuric at the time of catheter insertion (4, 6–8). Of those patients who are not bacteriuric at the time of catheter insertion and remain catheterized for at least 1 day, approximately 10% will develop bacteriuria during their period of catheterization. From study to study, the rate of occurrence of catheter-associated bacteriuria ranges from 6 to 23% (4, 6–8). Not all patients who become bacteriuric develop clinical symptoms of infection. Approximately 30% of the bacteriuric patients develop symptomatic UTI, and 3% develop secondary bacteremias (6, 9). Stated in another way, symptomatic localized infection and bacteremia complicate 3% and 0.3%, respectively, of episodes of temporary indwelling urethral catheterization (6, 9).

The fact that hospital-acquired UTI is such a common nosocomial infection makes it very important from an infection control point of view. It contributes to the morbidity, mortality, and costs of hospitalization. Cost estimates per case of nosocomial UTI range between $150 and $300 for antibiotic therapy and an added duration of hospital stay of approximately 2 days (1, 10, 11). Although this figure seems relatively unimpressive when compared with the costs per patient of nosocomial infections at other sites, the relatively high frequency of hospital-acquired UTI makes it a very costly infection from a broader, epidemiologic perspective (11). Thus, even a marginal decrease in the overall rate of hospital-acquired UTI would have significant economic implications for hospitals and third-party payers.

During the past few years, there has been a growing awareness of UTI in other groups of institutionalized patients outside of the acute care hospital setting. Patients who reside in extended care facilities or nursing homes are at risk for a number of institutionally acquired infections, including UTIs. They are at increased risk because of their old age, chronic diseases, debilitated status, and exposures to long term indwelling catheters (12). The prevalence of bacteriuria in elderly, noncatheterized nursing home residents ranges between 20 and 50% (13–15). For nursing home residents who require chronic urethral catheterization, the prevalence of asymptomatic bacteriuria approaches 100% (12, 16–18). The rate of symptomatic UTI in nursing home patients is similar to that observed for hospitalized patients, approximately 3% (12, 19, 20). In addition, an increased rate of death has been observed for bacteriuric nursing home residents that apparently is not related to their underlying disease status (21); the reasons for this increased mortality are unclear.

CLINICAL CONSIDERATIONS
Diagnosis of UTI

The clinical and microbiologic criteria for the diagnosis of a hospital-acquired UTI are ambiguous and subject to interpretation. Oftentimes, components of the typical symptom complex of UTI are missing, especially in debilitated, catheterized patients. Thus, the absence of such characteristic signs or symptoms as fever, suprapubic or flank pain, urinary frequency, or dysuria does not rule out the possibility of a clinically significant UTI. On the other hand, in catheterized postsurgical patients or medical patients with grave underlying diseases, the pressure of pyuria, peripheral leukocytosis, and fever may be seen with conditions other than a UTI.

The urine culture remains the most helpful clue to the diagnosis of hospital-acquired UTI. However, new information has made the interpretation of urine culture results even more ambiguous than it formerly had been. It is now almost impossible to distinguish clinically significant from clinically insignificant bacteriuria on the basis of culture results alone. Urine colony counts with $< 10^5$ colony-forming units (CFU)/ml have been shown to be reproducible and have clinical significance for both noncatheterized and catheterized patients. The acute urethral syndrome in dysuric, noncatheterized females is often caused by gram-negative bacteria with colony counts between 10^3 and 10^5 CFU/ml (22). Treatment of these patients with antibiotics brings about a clinical resolution of symptoms

and bacteriologic cure (23). For catheterized patients, bacteriuria with colony counts of $> 10^5$ CFU/ml have the same implication as colony counts of $> 10^5$ CFU/ml. Low level colonization of catheter urine has been shown to progress to high level bacteriuria in more than 95% of patients who are cultured on subsequent days and who do not receive intercurrent suppressive antimicrobial therapy (24). Colony counts as low as 10^2 CFU/ml in urine collected aseptically from catheter tubing have been used by several investigators to diagnose "significant" bacteriuria (4, 5, 25, 26).

In addition to the current rethinking of the significance of bacteriuria with quantitatively low colony counts, there has been a reassessment of the significance of polymicrobial bacteriuria. Previously, urine specimens with more than one bacterial species were considered to be contaminated with skin, vaginal, or periurethral flora. However, contamination from these sources is unlikely in specimens collected from catheter tubing. Polymicrobic bacteriuria is the rule, rather than the exception, in patients with chronic indwelling urinary catheters (12, 16, 17). For these patients, two or three different bacterial species are often recovered from aseptically collected urine specimens, even when no symptoms of UTI are present (12, 16). In symptomatic patients with polymicrobic bacteriuria, it is not possible to tell which organism or combination of organisms is responsible for the clinical infection. In these cases, antibiotic therapy must be guided by the sensitivity test results of all isolates.

Finally, the spectrum of bacteria that are considered to be potential urinary pathogens has been broadened by the inclusion of such organisms as *Chlamydia trachomatis, Mycoplasma hominis, Staphylococcus aureus, Staphylococcus epidermidis, Staphylococcus saprophyticus, Haemophilus influenzae,* and *Candida albicans* (22, 27–31). These bacterial species were formerly considered to be nonpathogens or were not routinely cultured from urine specimens. However, in certain high risk patient populations, such as hospitalized or catheterized patients, virtually any type of microorganism should be considered as a potential uropathogen.

Therefore, the diagnosis of a hospital-acquired UTI requires clinical judgment and must be based on information from the patient's symptoms, physical findings, and clinical microbiology laboratory results. Care must be taken when making cross-comparisons of infection rates from studies or hospitals in which different criteria are used to diagnose patients with UTI (32). Rates of infection may be markedly different in studies in which urine cultures were obtained routinely from all patients regardless of the presence or absence of symptoms, studies in which different criteria for significant colony counts were used, or studies in which the definition of uropathogen was limited to certain species of bacteria.

Consequences of UTI

The majority of patients exposed to short term urethral catheterization remain nonbacteriuric and suffer no clinical consequences of this procedure (6). However, the 10% of patients who become bacteriuric are at increased risk for other complications, including infections at other sites, secondary bacteremia, and death. Surgeons have long recognized that the likelihood of acquiring a postoperative wound infection is increased in patients with active infections at other sites at the time of surgery (2, 33). This association may reflect the debilitated status of the already infected patient and/or the likelihood of endogenous spread of infection from one site to another. Surgery patients with nosocomial bacteriuria are also at increased risk for secondary wound infection with the same organism that was present in the urine (34). Thus, asymptomatic bacteriuria, in addition to symptomatic infection, must be considered as a risk factor for postoperative wound infection.

Even though bacteremia is observed in only 0.3% of episodes of urethral catheterizations, the indwelling urinary catheter and UTI remain the major primary source of hospital-acquired bacteremia. In one study, the urinary tract, particularly the catheterized urinary tract, was identified as the source of infection in 15% of hospital-acquired bacteremias (35). The mortality rate for bacteremias secondary to UTI was 12.5% and was directly associated with the severity of the patient's underlying disease. In addition, a 2- to 3-fold increase in the case/fatality ratios has been observed in both noncatheterized elderly nursing home residents and catheterized hospital patients with asymptomatic bacteriuria (21, 36). This increase in mortality for bacteriuric patients appears not to be related to the underlying debility of the patients nor the development of secondary bacteremia. As yet, no explanations are available to account for these findings. It is possible that previous studies have failed to appreciate the clinical significance of occult, asymptomatic bacteriuria as a risk factor for unexplained deaths. However, two subsequent studies involving nursing home patients and hospitalized patients have failed to confirm a connection between bacteriuria and death (15, 37). Therefore, this association is still subject to question.

PATHOGENESIS

The two major risk factors that predispose to catheter-associated UTI are the presence of potentially pathogenic bacteria in the periurethral area and an indwelling urethral catheter to allow the ingress of bacteria into the urinary bladder. Enhancement of periurethral colonization is the means by which other risk factors act to cause catheter-associated UTI. Thus, catheterized patients who are female, elderly, severely ill, or not receiving antibiotics are more likely to be colonized and more likely to develop infection than their lower risk counterparts (38). In fact, even in the lower risk groups, those patients with positive periurethral cultures have higher rates of bacteriuria than patients with negative cultures. It has now been shown that urethral and/or rectal colonization immediately precedes the development of UTI with identical strains in two-thirds of catheterized women and slightly less than one-third of catheterized men (25). Infections in catheterized women are frequently caused by gastrointestinal flora, such as the Enterobacteriaceae, or enterococci, that migrate across the perineum and colonize the periurethral area prior to infection (39–42). Oftentimes, the bacteria that colonize the gastrointestinal tracts of hospitalized or nursing home patients are highly selected and resistant to commonly prescribed antibiotics (42, 43). Therefore, hospital-acquired UTIs are often caused by antibiotic-resistant bacteria.

Periurethral colonization by potential uropathogens is a major risk factor for the development of UTI in both catheterized and noncatheterized patients (44). It is likely that bacterial virulence is related to the ability of the microorganism to adhere to uroepithelial cells and that host susceptibility is increased in patients whose cell surfaces have an increased affinity for bacterial attachment. The exact stimuli which modulate the reactivity of host cells to permit or resist bacterial adherence are not yet well delineated; however, this is an exciting area for basic and applied research.

In order to cause an infection, bacteria must gain entry into the urinary bladder. In the hospitalized patient, this can be accomplished at the time of catheter insertion, by the retrograde migration of bacteria outside the catheter in the periurethral mucous sheath, and by the reflux of urine and bacteria into the bladder inside the catheter tubing (45). The risk of acquiring bacteriuria after a single in-and-out catheterization is between 0.5 and 8%. However, with severely debilitated, bedridden patients, rates as high as 15 to 30% have been observed. Nonetheless, the major route by which bacteria enter the catheterized bladder is by movement up the urethra in the mucous layer that coats the external surface of the catheter. This route of infection probably accounts for more than 70% of episodes of catheter-associated bacteriuria (4, 8, 46) (Fig. 21.1). The higher frequency of infection in catheterized females is in part due to anatomic differences between the lengths of the female and male urethra and the ease of this route of infection in females. UTI secondary to the intraluminal reflux of bacteria in the catheter tubing occurs much less commonly since the closed, sterile system of catheter drainage has been widely accepted in most U.S. hospitals. Now, contamination of the drainage bag prior to colonization of bladder urine can be identified in from only 7 to 20% of episodes of catheter-associated infection (4, 8, 46).

Symptomatic infection is not an inevitable consequence of all episodes of bacterial colonization of bladder urine. In fact, bladder defense mechanisms, urine acidity and osmolality, complete bladder emptying, and normal urine flow are effective mechanisms to prevent infection (44). However, the presence of an indwelling catheter can impair the protective effect of these defense mechanisms and predispose to colonization or infection. For instance, the catheter can cause damage to the epithelial lining of the bladder wall, induce an inflammatory reaction, and destroy the protective layer of mucopolysaccharide that coats the bladder. This trauma exposes deep bladder mucosal cells to bacteria which are able to adhere avidly to these surfaces (47). In addition, indwelling catheters prevent the complete drainage of bladder urine, allowing residual urine to serve as a culture medium for bacterial growth. Mucous or cellular debris that adheres to the catheter surface may serve as foci for bacterial growth and seed bladder urine. Finally, episodes of temporary obstruction of catheter urine flow due to concretions, kinking, or clamping may produce a situation resembling a closed space infection and set the stage for bacterial invasion of the bladder wall or reflux into the kidney. Episodes of catheter obstruction may be an important predisposing factor to convert asymptomatic bacteriuria into symptomatic infection (16).

Even though the majority of episodes of catheter-associated bacteriuria appear to be secondary

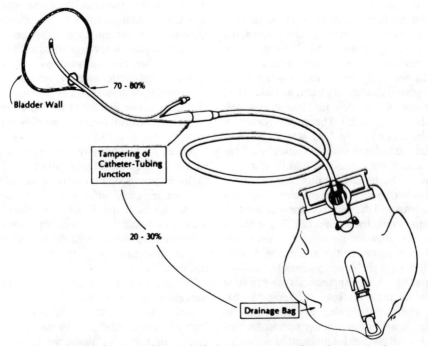

Figure 21.1.   Sources of bacteriuria in short term catheterized patients.

to endogenous colonization of the periurethral area, reports of exogenous contamination of the drainage system from other sources, including other catheterized patients, continue to appear in the literature (42, 48–50). Exogenous contamination is responsible for case clusters and epidemic occurrences of hospital-acquired UTI. One report estimated that as many as 15% of episodes of nosocomial bacteriuria during nonepidemic periods are clustered cases involving two to five patients each (48). Virtually all patients involved in case clusters are catheterized and presumably are infected by cross-contamination of either the external catheter surface or urine collected in the drainage bag. Certain organisms—such as *Serratia marscescens*, *P. aeruginosa*, and *Citrobacter freundii*—are frequently implicated in case clusters, whereas other organisms—such as *Escherichia coli*—are infrequently spread by cross-contamination. Clustered cases are more likely than nonclustered cases to be caused by organisms that are resistant to multiple antibiotics, including gentamicin (48). The nosocomial pathogens involved in clustered cases are selected by their ability to survive in the hospital setting. The epidemiologic characteristics of hospital outbreaks are similar to those described in previous reports of epidemic, hospital-acquired UTI (51). These recent reports stress the importance of clustered patients with indwelling catheters, prior exposure to antimicrobics, circumstances to increase the likelihood of cross-contamination, and infection with bacteria with plasmid-mediated antibiotic resistance as risk factors for the development of epidemic UTI. These reports remind us of the continual need for infection control efforts to limit antibiotic use and to maintain effective barrier precautions to prevent cross-infections among catheterized patients.

PREVENTION AND CONTROL

Beeson's admonition to physicians in his classic editorial in 1958 entitled, "The Case against the Catheter" remains apropros today (52). Catheter use should be restricted to times when it is absolutely necessary. Initiation of catheter drainage should be avoided if possible; indwelling catheters should be removed as soon as they are no longer necessary. A recent report suggests that as many as one-third of catheter days might be unnecessary and that early removal of catheters might prevent as many as 40% of catheter-associated UTIs (9).

In order to avoid the complications of indwelling urethral catheterization, other methods of urinary drainage have been proposed, including intermittent catheterization, suprapubic catheterization, and condom drainage. Intermittent catheterization is an accepted practice for acute spinal cord injury patients (53). It has been suggested that intermittent clean, but not sterile, self-catheterization is an effective and safe method for the long term management of these patients (54). The combination of intermittent catheterization and effective urinary antisepsis with oral methenamine and an intravesicular acidifying agent may make this an even safer procedure in terms of infection prevention (55). Nonetheless, reports of the efficacy and safety of intermittent catheterization have studied only relatively small numbers of patients with neurogenic bladders. As yet, there are no prospective, randomized, controlled clinical trials comparing the use of indwelling urethral catheters with intermittent catheterization in the same patient population. Similarly, no well designed studies are available to demonstrate an advantage of short term or long term suprapubic catheterization over indwelling urethral drainage. Even though there are no comparative studies with condom drainage, the high rates of bacteriuria, urine obstruction, and local penile complications that have been observed with condoms have limited their use (56, 57). In addition, condom catheters have been implicated as a reservoir of *Providencia stuartii* during an epidemic outbreak (58).

Prevention of Endogenous Infection

Most episodes of catheter-associated UTI are caused by intestinal organisms that contaminate the periurethral area and subsequently enter the bladder by migrating up the urethra in the periurethral mucous sheath surrounding the indwelling catheter. Strategies that interrupt this route of infection at any point should prevent infections. The points at which the chain may be broken include (*a*) decreasing intestinal colonization with potential uropathogens, (*b*) preventing attachment of bacteria to uroepithelial cells, (*c*) eradicating organisms that colonize the periurethral area, (*d*) preventing the movement of bacteria up the urethra, and (*e*) removing bacteria that colonize bladder urine before they cause infections.

Several studies have suggested that systemic antibiotics administered during the time of catheterization are effective in decreasing rates of catheter-associated bacteriuria (4, 8, 9). It is well known that systemic antibiotics have a profound effect on intestinal flora and may transiently reduce bacterial numbers. However, systemic antibiotics also allow antibiotic-resistant intestinal or periurethral flora to flourish and predispose patients to urinary infections with these bacteria (41, 42, 59). It has been reported that the prophylactic effect of antibiotics for catheter-associated infections is transient, lasting no more than 4 days (4). After that, patients are at increased risk for colonization with resistant organisms. In a similar vein, studies of bladder irrigations with antibiotic solutions or weak acids have shown some efficacy in preventing bacteriuria. However, these agents also predispose to colonization and infection with resistant organisms (60). Neither systemic antibiotics, chronic urinary suppressants, nor bladder irrigations with urinary antiseptics have been shown to decrease rates of bacteriuria or symptomatic infections in patients with long term indwelling urethral catheters (4, 61–63). On the other hand, these interventions predispose patients to colonization with antibiotic-resistant bacteria.

As yet, no agents are available for clinical use to block the attachment of bacteria to uroepithelial cells. However, other techniques to reduce meatal colonization and to prevent migration of bacteria into the bladder have been evaluated. Randomized, prospective, controlled trials have failed to show any protective efficacy of twice daily meatal cleansing with soap and water or povidone-iodine solution (64). Similarly, twice daily applications of a polyantimicrobic ointment failed to reduce rates of catheter-associated bacteriuria (7). However, more recent data suggest that application of a water-soluble polyantimicrobic cream at the catheter-meatal junction may be effective in preventing infection (65).

When silicone catheters were first introduced, it was thought that they might induce less inflammatory reaction in the urethra than latex catheters and be less likely to allow bacteria to enter the bladder in the periurethral mucous sheath. However, no well designed, prospective, controlled study has been done to evaluate the efficacy of these catheters; and the only data that are available suggest no advantage over latex catheters (9). A recent study suggesting that a specially designed, silver-coated catheter might have dramatic antibacterial properties needs confirmation by a properly designed, prospective clinical trial (66).

The other route by which bacteria gain entry into the catheterized bladder is by external con-

tamination of the downdrain bag or tubing with reflux retrogradely into the bladder. This route of infection was greatly curtailed by the introduction of closed sterile gravity drainage. However, breaks in catheter care technique still occur frequently and are responsible for infections by this route (4, 8, 60). Recently, it has been suggested that retrograde intraluminal spread of bacteria might be further decreased by instilling antiseptic solutions into the drainage bag or by using catheters in which the catheter-tubing junction was presealed. Preliminary uncontrolled reports suggested decreased rates of catheter-associated infection in drainage systems to which povidone-iodine (67), hydrogen peroxide (68, 69), or chlorhexidine solution (70) were added. However, these reports were not confirmed by subsequent prospective clinical trials (46, 71). Given the relative infrequency of infection by this route, the lack of proven efficacy of these techniques, the possibility of toxic side effects, the probable selection of resistant organisms, and the added costs to the patient, these practices have not been recommended for general hospital use (72). On the other hand, presealed catheters have been evaluated and have been shown to lower infection rates in patients not receiving concurrent antibiotics (8). Yet, the added costs, the inconvenience, and the limited impact of this infection control strategy on infection rates (Fig. 21.1) may restrict the general acceptance of these catheters by hospitals.

Another potential strategy to prevent symptomatic catheter-associated infection is to initiate antibiotic treatment for bladder colonization before infection occurs. If antibiotics were restricted to patients with new episodes of bacteriuria who were identified by daily urine cultures, they might prevent symptomatic infections without inducing wide scale resistance. Despite the apparent logic of this infection control strategy, the concept of early treatment has been shown to be ineffective. For most infections, there is no lag time between the onset of asymptomatic bladder colonization and symptomatic infection during which antibiotics could be administered (6). Neither prophylactic antibiotics nor routine monitoring of daily urine cultures from catheterized patients is recommended for the general hospital setting.

Control Measures for Epidemic Hospital-Acquired UTI

The most important step in limiting possible epidemic spread of catheter-associated infection is recognizing case clusters as early as possible.

Epidemic situations sometimes develop insidiously and are easily overlooked. Early identification of epidemics requires ongoing, effective surveillance. This is often accomplished by weekly or monthly reviews of cases of hospital-acquired UTI to identify increased rates, clustered episodes, epidemiologic features, more frequent isolation of specific bacterial species, or unique patterns of antibiotic resistance among different types of bacteria. In some hospitals, this type of intensive surveillance is restricted to certain areas at high risk for epidemic transmission, such as medical or surgical intensive care units, neurosurgical units, genitourinary wards, or rehabilitation centers. In other hospitals, abbreviated surveillance strategies based on microbiology laboratory reports seem comparable to traditional surveillance in monitoring cases of hospital-acquired UTI and in identifying epidemic occurrences (73).

Once case clustering or epidemic spread is identified, active infection control measures must be initiated as soon as possible to limit further transmission. In fact, the identification of even a single isolate of *S. marcescens* or *P. aeruginosa* in a catheterized patient might be sufficient to initiate special precautions. In epidemic situations, specific steps should include an investigation to identify possible common sources of infection and prompt action to eliminate them whenever possible. In cases where catheterized patients are thought to be reservoirs of epidemic bacteria, barrier precautions should be initiated; these include careful hand washing, gloving, and separation of infected patients from other high risk, catheterized patients. Urinary antiseptics instilled in drainage bag reservoirs may be effective in decreasing the likelihood of bag contamination and reducing the possibility of cross-transmission of infection (70, 74). Consideration should also be given to treating colonized patients with urinary suppressants or bladder irrigation. Whenever possible, indwelling catheters should be removed. For patients who must remain catheterized, the techniques of closed sterile catheter care should be re-emphasized.

The Centers for Disease Control developed a practical set of guidelines designed for hospitals, physicians, nurses, and infection control practitioners to prevent catheter-associated UTI (75). These guidelines represent a consensus opinion of investigators and clinicians in the field. The recommendations are ranked according to the degree to which they have been substantiated by scientific data or by their perceived effectiveness

Table 21.1. Recommendations for the Prevention of Catheter-Associated Urinary Tract Infections: Centers for Disease Control, 1980

Category I. Strongly recommended for adoption:
  Educate personnel in correct techniques of catheter insertion and care.
  Catheterize only when necessary.
  Emphasize hand washing.
  Insert catheter using aseptic technique and sterile equipment.
  Secure catheter properly.
  Maintain closed sterile drainage.
  When irrigation is necessary, use intermittent method.
  Obtain urine samples aseptically.
  Maintain unobstructed urine flow.

Category II. Moderately recommended for adoption:
  Periodically re-educate personnel in catheter care.
  Use smallest suitable bore catheter.
  Do not perform continuous irrigation as a routine infection control measure.
  Refrain from daily meatal care with povidone-iodine and polymicrobic ointment.
  Do not change catheters at arbitrary fixed intervals.

Category III. Weakly recommended for adoption:
  Consider alternative techniques of urinary drainage before using an indwelling urethral catheter.
  Replace the collecting system when sterile closed drainage has been violated.
  Spatially separate infected and uninfected patients who have indwelling catheters.
  Avoid routine bacteriologic monitoring.

and practical value (Table 21.1). These guidelines succinctly summarize the state-of-the-art recommendations in 1980 for preventing catheter-associated infections. However, even these guidelines will need updating periodically as new data regarding the epidemiology and pathogenesis of catheter-associated infections become available and new methods for the prevention of infection and control of epidemic spread are developed.

References

1. Krieger JN, Kaiser DL, Wenzel RP: Nosocomial urinary tract infections: secular trends, treatment and economics in a university hospital. *J Urol* 130:102–106, 1983.
2. Haley RW, Hooton TM, Culver DH, Stanley RC, Emori TG, Handison CD, Quade D, Shadtman RH, Schaberg DR, Shah BV, Schaty GD: Nosoco-

mial infections in US hospitals, 1975–1976. Estimated frequency by selected characteristics of patients. *Am J Med* 70:947–959, 1981.

3. Centers for Disease Control: *National Nosocomial Infections Study Report, Annual Summary 1978.* Atlanta, Centers for Disease Control, March 1981, pp 1–14.

4. Garibaldi RA, Burke JP, Dickman ML, Smith CB: Factors predisposing to bacteriuria during indwelling urethral catheterization. *N Engl J Med* 291:215–219, 1974.

5. Burke JP: Status of methods to prevent urinary catheter-associated infections. Presented at a symposium at Harvard Medical School in honor of Dr. Maxwell Finland, Boston, March 13, 1982.

6. Garibaldi RA, Mooney BR, Epstein BJ, Britt MR: An evaluation of daily bacteriologic monitoring to identify preventable episodes of catheter-associated urinary tract infection. *Infect Control* 3:466–470, 1982.

7. Burke JP, Jacobson JA, Garibaldi RA, Conti MT, Alling DW: Evaluation of daily meatal care with polyantibiotic ointment in prevention of urinary catheter-associated bacteriuria. *J Urol* 129:331–334, 1983.

8. Platt R, Polk BF, Murdock B, Rosner B: Reduction of mortality associated with nosocomial urinary tract infection. *Lancet* 1:893–897, 1983.

9. Krieger JN, Kaiser DL, Wenzel RP: Urinary tract etiology of bloodstream infections in hospitalized patients. *J Infect Dis* 148:57–62, 1983.

10. Haley RW, Schaberg DR, Crossley KBV, Von Allman SD. McGowan JE Jr: Extra charges and prolongation of stay attributable to nosocomial infections: a prospective interhospital comparison. *Am J Med* 70:51–58, 1981.

11. Givens CD, Wenzel RP: Catheter-associated urinary tract infections in surgical patients: a controlled study on the excess morbidity and costs. *J Urol* 124:646–648, 1980.

12. Garibaldi RA, Brodine S, Matsumiya S: Infections among patients in nursing homes. Policies, prevalence and problems. *N Engl J Med* 305:731–735, 1981.

13. Kaye D: Urinary tract infections in the elderly. *Bull NY Acad Med* 56:209–220, 1980.

14. Beeman K, Cote J, Graham J, Neuhaus E., Garibaldi R: Pedi bag cultures—a non-invasive technique to collect urine samples from uncooperative female patients (abstract). Presented at the Association of Practitioners in Infection Control meeting, Washington DC, June 1984.

15. Nicolle LE, Bjornson J, Harding GKM, MacDonell JA: Bacteriuria in elderly institutionalized men. *N Engl J Med* 309:1420–1425, 1983.

16. Warren JW, Tenney JH, Hoopes JM, Muncie HL, Anthony WC: A prospective microbiologic study of bacteriuria in patients with chronic indwelling urethral catheters. *J Infect Dis* 146:719–723, 1982.

17. Eddeland A, Hedelin H: Bacterial colonization of the lower urinary tract in women with long-term indwelling urethral catheter. *Scand J Infect Dis* 15:361–365, 1983.

18. Graham J, Beeman K, Cote J, Neuhaus E, Garibaldi R: Prevalence and changing patterns of bacteriuria in nursing home patients (abstract). Presented at the Association of Practitioners in Infection Control meeting, Washington DC, June 1984.

19. Lester M: Looking inside 101 nursing homes. *Am J Med* 64:111–116, 1964.

20. Moody ML, Burke JP: Infections and antibiotic use in a large private hospital, January 1971: comparisons among hospitals serving different populations. *Arch Intern Med* 130:261–266, 1972.

21. Dontas AS, Kasviki-Charvati P, Papanayaotou PC, Marketos SG: Bacteriuria and survival in old age. *N Engl J Med* 304:939–943, 1981.

22. Stamm WE, Wagner KF, Amsel R, Alexander ER, Twok M, Counts GW, Holmes KK: Causes of the acute urethral syndrome in women. *N Engl J Med* 303:409–415, 1980.

23. Stamm WE, Running K, McKevitt M, Counts GW, Twok M, Holmes KK: Treatment of the acute urethral syndrome. *N Engl J Med* 304:956–958, 1981.

24. Stark RP, Maki D: Bacteriuria in the catheterized patient. What quantitative level of bacteriuria is relevant? *N Engl J Med* 311:560–564, 1984.

25. Daifuku R, Stamm WE: Association of rectal and urethral colonization with urinary tract infection in patients with indwelling catheters. *JAMA* 252:2028–2030, 1984.

26. Kevorkian CG, Merritt JL, Ilstrup DM: Methenamine mandelate with acidification: an effective urinary antiseptic in patients with neurogenic bladder. *Mayo Clin Proc* 59:523–529, 1984.

27. Arpi M, Renneberg J: The clinical significance of *Staphylococcus aureus* bacteriuria. *J Urol* 132:697–700, 1984.

28. Bailey RR: Significance of coagulase-negative staphylococcus in urine. *J Infect Dis* 127:179–182, 1973.

29. Hovelius B, Colleen S, March PA: Urinary tract infections in men caused by *Staphylococcus saprophyticus. Scand J Infect Dis* 16:37–41, 1984.

30. Gabre-Kidan T, Lipsky BA, Plorde JJ: *Haemophilus influenzae* as a cause of urinary tract infections in men. *Arch Intern Med* 144:1623–1627, 1984.

31. Hamory BH, Wenzel RP: Hospital-associated candiduria: predisposing factors and review of the literature. *J Urol* 120:444–448, 1978.

32. Maglio S, Hyrb K, Garibaldi R: Postoperative infections in geriatric patients (abstract). Presented at the Association of Practitioners in Infection Control meeting, Washington, DC, June 1984.

33. Postoperative wound infections: the influence of ultraviolet irradiation of the operating room and other factors. *Ann Surg* 160 (Suppl):1–192, 1964.

34. Krieger JN, Kaiser DL, Wenzel RP: Nosocomial urinary tract infections cause wound infections postoperatively in surgical patients. *Surg Gynecol Obstet* 156:313–318, 1983.

35. Bryan CS, Reynolds KL: Hospital-acquired bacteremic urinary tract infection. Epidemiology and outcome. *J Urol* 132:494–498, 1984.

36. Platt R, Polk BF, Murdock B, Rosner B: Mortality associated with nosocomial urinary tract infection. *N Engl J Med* 307:637–641, 1982.

37. Gross PA, Van Antwerpen C: Nosocomial infections and hospital deaths. *Am J Med* 75:658–662, 1983.

38. Garibaldi RA, Burke JP, Britt MR, Miller WA, Smith CB: Meatal colonization and catheter-associated bacteriuria. *N Engl J Med* 303:316–318, 1980.

39. Winterbauer RH, Turck M, Petersdorf RG: Studies

on the epidemiology of *Escherichia coli* infections. V. Factors including acquisition of specific serologic groups. *J Clin Invest* 46:21–29, 1967.
40. Gross PA, Harkavy LM, Barden GE, Flower MF: The epidemiology of nosocomial enterococcal urinary tract infection. *Am J Med Sci* 272:75–81, 1976.
41. Montgomerie JZ, Morrow JW: *Pseudomonas* colonization in patients with spinal cord injury. *Am J Epidemiol* 108:328–336, 1978.
42. Gaynes RP, Weinstein RA, Smith J, Carman M, Kabins SA: Control of aminoglycoside resistance by barrier precautions. *J Infect Control* 4:221–224, 1983.
43. Rose HD, Schreier J: The effect of hospitalization and antibiotic therapy on the gram-negative fecal flora. *Am J Med Sci* 255:228–236, 1968.
44. Sobel JD, Kaye M: Host factors in the pathogenesis of urinary tract infections. *Am J Med* 76:122, 1984.
45. Garibaldi RA: Hospital-acquired urinary tract infections. In Wenzel RP (ed): *Handbook of Hospital-Acquired Infections.* Boca Raton, FL, CRC Press, 1981.
46. Thompson RL, Haley CE, Searcy MA, Guenthner SM, Kaiser DL, Gröschel DHM. Gillenwater JY, Wenzel RP: Catheter-associated bacteriuria. Failure to reduce attack rates using periodic instillation of a disinfectant into urinary drainage systems. *JAMA* 251:747–751, 1984.
47. Vardi Y, Meshulam T, Obedeanu H, Merzbach D, Sobel JD: In vivo adherence of *Pseudomonas aeruginosa* to rat bladder epithelium. *Proc Soc Exp Biol Med* 172:449–456, 1983.
48. Schaberg DR, Haley RW, Highsmith AK, Anderson RL, McGowan JE Jr: Nosocomial bacteriuria: a prospective study of case clustering and antimicrobial resistance. *Ann Intern Med* 93:420–424, 1980.
49. Okuda T, Endo N, Osada Y, Zen-Yoji H: Outbreak of nosocomial urinary tract infections caused by *Serratia marcescens. J Clin Microbiol* 20:691–695, 1984.
50. Echols RM, Palmer DL, King RM, Long GW: Multidrug-resistant *Serratia marcescens* bacteriuria related to urologic instrumentation. *South Med J* 77:173–177, 1984.
51. Schaberg DR, Weinstein RA, Stamm WE: Epidemics of nosocomial urinary tract infection caused by multiple resistant gram-negative bacilli: epidemiology and control. *J Infect Dis* 133:363–366, 1976.
52. Beeson PB: Editorial: the case against the catheter. *Am J Med* 24:1–3, 1958.
53. Guttman L, Frankel H: The value of intermittent catheterization in the management of traumatic paraplegia and tetraplegia. *Paraplegia* 4:63–84, 1966.
54. Lapides J, Diokno AC, Lowe BS, Kalish MD: Follow-up on unsterile intermittent self-catheterization. *J Urol* 111:184–187, 1974.
55. Krebs M, Halvorsen RB, Fishman IJ, Santos-Mendoza N: Prevention of urinary tract infection during intermittent catheterization. *J Urol* 131:82–85, 1984.
56. Johnson ET: The condom catheter: urinary tract infection and other complications. *South J Med* 76:579–582, 1983.
57. Hirsch DD, Fainstein V, Musher DM: Do condom-catheter collecting systems cause urinary tract in-

fections? *JAMA* 242:340–341, 1979.
58. Fierer J, Ekstrom M: An outbreak of *Providencia stuartii* urinary tract infections—patients with condom catheters as a reservoir of the bacteria. *JAMA* 245:1553–1555, 1981.
59. Selden R, Lee S, Wang WLL, Bennett JV, Eickhoff TC: Nosocomial *Klebsiella* infections: intestinal colonization as a reservoir. *Ann Intern Med* 74:657–664, 1971.
60. Warren JW, Platt R, Thomas RJ, Rosner B, Kass EH: Antibiotic irrigation and catheter-associated urinary tract infections. *N Engl J Med* 299:570–573, 1978.
61. Bjork DT, Pelletier LL, Tight RR: Urinary tract infections with antibiotic resistant organisms in catheterized nursing home patients. *Infect Control* 5:173–176, 1984.
62. Warren JW, Anthony WC, Hoopes JM, Muncie HL: Cephalexin for susceptible bacteriuria in afebrile long-term catheterized patients. *JAMA* 248:454–458, 1982.
63. Warren JW, Hoopes JM, Muncie HL, Anthony WC: Ineffectiveness of cephalexin in treatment of cephalexin-resistant bacteriuria in patients with chronic indwelling urethral catheters. *J Urol* 129:71–73, 1983.
64. Burke JP, Garibaldi RA, Britt, MR, Jacobson JA, Conti M: Prevention of catheter-associated urinary tract infections. Efficacy of daily meatal care regimens. *Am J Med* 70:655–658, 1981.
65. Larsen RA, Burke JP: Determinants of the efficacy of urethral care in preventing catheter-associated urinary infection. *Clin Res* 33:100A, 1985.
66. Akiyama H, Okamoto S: Prophylaxis of indwelling urethral catheter infection: clinical experience with a modified Foley catheter and drainage system. *J Urol* 121:40–42, 1979.
67. Evans AT, Cicmenec JF: The role of Betadine microbicides in urine bag sterilization. In *Proceeding of the Second World Congress on Antiseptics 1980.* New York, HP Publishing, 1980, pp 85–86.
68. Maizels M, Schaeffer AJ: Decreased incidence of bacteriuria associated with periodic instillation of hydrogen peroxide into the urethral catheter drainage bag. *J Urol* 123:841–845, 1980.
69. Desautels RE, Chibaro EA, Lang RJ: Maintenance of sterility of urinary drainage bags. *Surg Gynecol Obstet* 154:838–840, 1982.
70. Southampton Infection Control Team: Evaluation of aseptic techniques and chlorhexidine on the rate of catheter-associated urinary tract infection. *Lancet* 1:89–91, 1982.
71. Gillespie WA, Jones JE, Teasdale C, Simpson RA, Nashef L, Speller DCE: Does the additional disinfectant in urine drainage bags prevent infection in catheterized patients? *Lancet* 1:1037–1039, 1983.
72. Kunin CM: Genitourinary infections in the patient at risk: extrinsic risk factors. *Am J Med* 76:131–139, 1984.
73. Costel EE, Mitchell S, Kaiser AB: Abbreviated surveillance of nosocomial urinary tract infections: a new approach. *Infect Control* 6:11–13, 1985.
74. Noy MF, Smith CA, Watterson LL: The use of chlorhexidine in catheter bags. *J Hosp Infect* 3:365–367, 1982.
75. Wong ES, Hooten TM: Guidelines for prevention of catheter-associated urinary tract infections. *Infect Control* 2:126–130, 1981.

Chapter 22

Surgical Infections Including Burns

C. Glen Mayhall, M.D.

INTRODUCTION

More than a century after the contributions of Louis Pasteur, Ignaz Semmelweis, Oliver Wendell Holmes, and Joseph Lister to the understanding of disease transmission and prevention of infection by application of surgical asepsis, it is still necessary to include a chapter on postoperative wound infections in any text on hospital-acquired infections (1). Although great strides have been made in lowering surgical wound infection rates over the last 100 years, it is estimated that 325,000 postoperative wound infections occur each year in the United States, making surgical wound infections the second most frequently encountered hospital-acquired infection (2). Estimates of additional health care costs for postoperative wound infections range between $400 and $2600/wound infection, giving rise to annual costs for surgical wound infections in the United States of between $130 and 845 million/year (3–6). In addition to the morbidity and mortality that result from postoperative wound infections, the additional health care costs due to these infections are substantial and have grown in importance with the increasing concern over rapidly rising health care costs. It is likely that there will be increasing pressure to prevent these types of infectious complications in the future.

Burn wound infections are much more severe and much more difficult to prevent than are postoperative wound infections. The burn wound frequently covers a large area of the body and is an excellent culture medium made up of necrotic tissue and serum. The gastrointestinal tract provides a ready source of bacteria as do the burn wounds of patients in adjacent beds. Data collected from the early 1950s to the early 1960s and in the early 1970s indicated that 80.7% and 73.2% of deaths in burn patients were due to infection (7, 8). More recent data from the National Burn Information Exchange (I Feller, The National Burn Information Exchange, University of Michigan, Ann Arbor, 1978) indicated that infection was the second most common cause of death in burn patients, with 40.1% of fatalities due to infection. Clearly, infection is one of the major causes of death in burn patients. There are no estimates of the excess cost of medical care due to burn wound infections.

POSTOPERATIVE WOUND INFECTIONS

The postoperative wound infection rate for patients admitted to hospitals in the Centers for Disease Control's (CDC) National Nosocomial Infections Study (NNIS) between January, 1980 and December, 1984 was 6.1/1000 patient discharges (Table 22.1). Postoperative wound infection rates for patients in different size hospitals and on different services are shown in Tables 22.1 and 22.2, respectively.

Postoperative (incisional) wound infections may be manifested by local erythema, tenderness, swelling, pain, dehiscence, and discharge of a purulent exudate. Since local signs of inflammation may be difficult to interpret and are not always due to infection, the definition of an incisional wound infection that has been generally accepted is that an infected wound is one that drains purulent exudate. Although all postoperative wounds that drain purulent exudate should be cultured, purulent exudate that is culture positive is not necessary for diagnosis of a postoperative wound infection.

The risk of a postoperative wound's becoming infected is related to the likelihood that the wound will be contaminated by microorganisms. A herniorrhaphy wound is less likely to become infected than is a wound made during an operation on the colon. Even with preoperative antibiotic prophylaxis, there is a risk that bacteria which make up the normal flora of the colon may seed the incisional wound when the colon is

Table 22.1. Surgical Wound Infection Rates by Hospital Category, NNIS,[a] January 1980 to December 1984

Hospital Category	No. of Infections	Rate[b]
NMSA[c]	7,134	4.3
SMSA[d]	9,441	6.1
LMSA[e]	16,624	7.5
Total	33,199	6.1

[a] National Nosocomial Infections Study, Centers for Disease Control.

[b] Number per 1,000 patient discharges.

[c] NMSA, nonmedical school-affiliated hospitals.

[d] SMSA, medical school-affiliated hospital (< 500 beds).

[e] LMSA, medical school-affiliated hospital (≥ 500 beds).

Table 22.2. Surgical Wound Infection Rates by Service, NNIS,[a] January 1980 to December 1984

Service	No. of Infections	Rate[b]
Newborn	207	0.4
Medicine	1,343	0.8
Pediatrics	354	1.1
Obstetrics	5,244	8.4
Gynecology	2,815	9.5
Surgery	23,236	12.6
Total	33,199	6.1

[a] National Nosocomial Infections Study, Centers for Disease Control.

[b] Number per 1,000 patient discharges.

opened during the operation. A widely accepted classification system based on the risk of contamination of the incisional wound at the time of surgery was developed by the National Research Council for the cooperative study on ultraviolet irradiation of operating rooms (9). A modification of this classification scheme is presented below (10, p 28):

Clean Wound

Elective, primarily closed, and undrained
Nontraumatic, uninfected
No inflammation encountered
No break in aseptic technique
Respiratory, alimentary, genitourinary, or oropharyngeal tracts not entered

Clean-Contaminated Wound

Alimentary, respiratory, or genitourinary tracts entered under controlled conditions and without unusual contamination
Appendectomy
Oropharynx entered

Vagina entered
Genitourinary tract entered in absence of culture-positive urine
Biliary tract entered in absence of infected bile
Minor break in technique
Mechanical drainage

Contaminated Wound

Open, fresh traumatic wounds
Gross spillage from gastrointestinal tract
Entrance of genitourinary or biliary tracts in presence of infected urine or bile
Major break in technique
Incisions in which acute nonpurulent inflammation is present

Dirty and Infected Wound

Traumatic wound with retained devitalized tissue, foreign bodies, fecal contamination, or delayed treatment, or from a dirty source
Perforated viscus encountered
Acute bacterial inflammation with pus encountered during operation

Postoperative wound infection rates by class from the National Research Council cooperative study were as follows: (a) refined-clean wounds 3.3%; (b) other clean wounds 7.4%; (c) clean-contaminated wounds 10.8%; (d) contaminated wounds 16.3%; and (e) dirty wounds 28.6%. The distribution of surgical wound infections by class from NNIS is shown in Table 22.3.

Microorganisms That Cause Postoperative Wound Infections

Most incisional wound infections are caused by bacteria. Bacteria most commonly isolated from postoperative wound infections are shown in Table 22.4. Although *Staphylococcus aureus* is the most frequently isolated microorganism, gram-negative bacilli, as a group, are the most common cause of postoperative wound infec-

Table 22.3. Distribution of Surgical Wound Infections by Class, NNIS,[a] January 1980 to December 1984

Surgical Class	No. of Infections	Percentage
Dirty	680	2.1
Contaminated	4,513	13.6
Clean	9,209	27.7
Clean-contaminated	15,181	45.7
Unknown	3,616	10.9
Total	33,199	100.0

[a] National Nosocomial Infections Study, Centers for Disease Control.

Table 22.4.   Distribution of Pathogens Associated with Surgical Wound Infections, NNIS,[a] January 1980 to December 1984

Pathogen	No. of Isolates	Percentage of Isolates
S. aureus	6540	15.7
E. coli	5184	12.5
P. aeruginosa	3160	7.6
S. faecalis	2657	6.4
P. mirabilis	2041	4.9
K. pneumoniae	1643	4.0
E. cloacae	1606	3.9
B. fragilis	1248	3.0

[a] National Nosocomial Infections Study, Centers for Disease Control.

tions. While fungi are much less frequently isolated from postoperative wound infections, they may cause serious infections that are difficult to diagnose and treat. The most commonly isolated fungus is *Candida albicans*. Other fungal causes include *Rhizopus rhizopodiformis* (11–13). In the last decade there have also been several reports of postoperative wound infections caused by atypical mycobacteria (14, 15).

Epidemiology of Postoperative Wound Infections

Almost all postoperative wound infections are acquired at the time of operation. Thus, the epidemiology of postoperative wound infections is closely associated with events in the operating room. Microorganisms are implanted in the operative field from a reservoir or source present at the time of operation, but the reservoir or source is usually not part of the intrinsic operating room environment. Indeed, most microorganisms that enter the wound are transmitted from the operative team or some area of the patient's body immediately adjacent to, or sometimes remote from, the operative wound.

Reservoirs or Sources for Microorganisms That Cause Postoperative Wound Infections

Personnel.   The hands of the members of the operative team are a potential reservoir for microorganisms for wound infection, but the preoperative scrub of the hands combined with use of surgical gloves minimizes the hands as a potential reservoir. Galle and co-workers observed that several scrub techniques using several different antiseptics were very effective in markedly reducing the number of bacteria on the hands by 88.6 to 99.7% (16). The low risk for the hands as a

reservoir was demonstrated by one study that found no postoperative wound infections after 141 operations during which the surgeon's glove was punctured (4). Another study indicated that the gloved hand was more likely to be contaminated from the operative wound than was the wound from the hand when there was a punctured glove (17). Only when dermatitis is present does the gloved hand become an important potential reservoir for microorganisms (17).

Unlike the hands, skin on other areas of the body may be an important reservoir for microorganisms that cause postoperative wound infections. Many materials used in operating room gowns and drapes are not effective barriers for bacteria on the underlying skin and scrub suits (18–20). After penetration of the gown, microorganisms are quickly spread in the operative field (19). One study showed a significant decrease in postoperative wound infection rates after use of more effective barrier materials for gowns and drapes, lending support to the skin of the operative team members as an important reservoir for bacteria (20). Microorganisms penetrate certain barrier materials at a faster rate when these materials become moist (21).

Another possible reservoir for postoperative wound infections is the hair of personnel. Though hair is rarely implicated as a reservoir, two outbreaks due to *S. aureus* carried in the hair of a physician and in the hair of a nurse have been reported (22).

The anus and vagina may be reservoirs for group A β-hemolytic streptococci. Seven outbreaks of postoperative wound infection have been reported due to rectal or vaginal carriage of group A streptococci by physicians and nurses (23–29). None of these carriers had had group A streptococci recovered from cultures of their nasopharynx. Thus, absence of group A streptococci in the upper respiratory tract does not rule out rectal or vaginal carriage.

The upper respiratory tract may be a reservoir for microorganisms that cause wound infections, but it is much less important than the skin surfaces of operating room personnel (18). Most of the bacteria in the operating room air are shed from the skin and not the upper respiratory tract of personnel. The number of microorganisms shed from the upper respiratory tract correlates with the concentration of microorganisms in the saliva (18). The upper respiratory tract is a minor reservoir except in the presence of an acute upper respiratory tract infection.

Patients.   Among the most important reservoirs are various sites in the patient's body. In fact, the majority of surgical wound infections are caused by microorganisms indigenous to the normal flora of the skin and several mucosal surfaces (30). These reservoirs are made up of microorganisms in the normal flora of the skin, gastrointestinal tract, female genital tract, and upper respiratory tract.

Microorganisms may be carried into the wound from the skin if the skin is colonized because of disease or if the skin is not properly prepared with an antiseptic prior to operation. *S. aureus* may be carried in the nose, in the perineum, or in skin lesions of patients. In one study the carrier rate rose from 44.1% on admission to 81.6% after about 2 months in the hospital (31).

In addition to the normal flora of the gastrointestinal, female genital, and upper respiratory tracts, microorganisms that cause infections in the normally sterile urinary tract, lower respiratory tract, and biliary tract may gain entrance to the operative wound when these tracts are opened. Inoculation of the wound with microorganisms contained within a hollow viscus takes place by traumatic perforation of the organ or by surgical operations. Contamination at surgery occurs when a hollow viscus is entered, transected, or resected (30). In addition to the mechanism of direct inoculation, microorganisms may gain access to wounds by lymphogenous or hematogenous seeding of the wound from distant foci of infection.

Environment. The environment of the operating room has rarely been implicated as a reservoir or source of microorganisms that cause postoperative wound infections. Infection due to *Clostridium perfringens* is a rare but devastating complication of surgery. Although these infections appear 24 to 48 hours after surgery, it has not been possible to prove that the reservoir for these microorganisms is in the operating room. In an extensive study of the environment Lowbury and Lilly concluded that *Clostridium welchii* (*perfringens*) was acquired by self-infection from the patient's own gastrointestinal tract at least as often as from the environment (32). Eickhoff reported a small outbreak of *C. perfringens* postoperative wound infections and concluded that the most likely source of *C. perfringens* was contaminated instruments (33). The instruments had apparently been contaminated by a patient with endogenously acquired *C. perfringens* infection who had surgery for small bowel obstruction. It was postulated that the two secondary cases occurred because of failure to sterilize the instruments contaminated by the index case. However, the available data did not allow for firm conclu-

sions with respect to the source of the microorganisms. Fredette investigated a case of gas gangrene in a surgical patient in Montreal and found the operating room heavily contaminated with *C. perfringens* (34). The source of contamination was the air conditioning system. However, he also found *C. perfringens* in the air conditioning systems of three other hospitals where no cases of gas gangrene had been reported. Given the considerable evidence for endogenous infection in many surgical patients with gas gangrene and the difficulty in associating environmental contamination epidemiologically with postoperative infection, it would appear that the operating room is not a significant source of *C. perfringens* implicated in postoperative infections (33).

The usual inanimate reservoirs or sources of microorganisms that gain entrance to surgical wounds are contaminated antiseptics or contaminated dressings. Bassett and co-workers reported an outbreak of postoperative wound infections due to *Pseudomonas multivorans* (35). The reservoir of the microorganism was an antiseptic solution (chlorhexidine 0.05% and cetrimide 0.5%). The antiseptic was probably contaminated with *P. multivorans* from hospital tap water, entering the skin of the incision site where the antiseptic was applied prior to surgery.

The second inanimate source of microorganisms for postoperative wound infections is that of bandages applied to the wound after the operation. In 1978 and 1979 several centers reported postoperative wound infections due to *Rhizopus* sp. (11–13, 36). Investigations at each institution implicated elasticized adhesive tape as the source of the fungus. Infections occurred under the elasticized adhesive tape. The elasticized tape was not marketed as sterile, and one investigation indicated that the tape was contaminated prior to its leaving the manufacturing plant (36). Pearson and co-workers reported an outbreak of postoperative wound infections caused by *C. perfringens*, and an investigation implicated contaminated elastic bandages (37). In four of five cases the infection appeared in an amputation stump to which an elastic bandage had been applied after surgery.

Modes of Transmission for Microorganisms That Cause Postoperative Wound Infections

Contact Transmission. Contact transmission may be subdivided into transmission either by direct or indirect contact. One important potential mode of transmission by direct contact would be with the hands of members of the operative team. Microorganisms could be transmitted from the skin beneath the gloves to the wound through holes in the gloves. There are few data in the literature to indicate that this type of transmission is important. As noted above, there are few bacteria present on the surface of the skin of the gloved hand unless the individual has dermatitis or an infected lesion. Furthermore, glove punctures are not associated with a higher rate of postoperative wound infections.

Although it has long been known that microorganisms rapidly penetrate surgical gowns from skin and garments worn under the gown, it has not been understood how the microorganisms reach the surgical wound. Schwartz and Saunders demonstrated that microorganisms cultured from scrub suits rapidly passed through the gowns of the operative team and could be cultured from the outer surface of the sleeves of the gown (19). Within 5 minutes the microorganism cultured from the sleeve of one surgeon could be recovered from drapes in the operative field and sleeves of other members of the team. Thus, it would appear that direct contact with the surface of the surgical gown may also transfer microorganisms to the wound.

There is also evidence that direct contact of the wound with surgical drapes may transmit microorganisms to the wound. Wiley and Ha'eri showed that human albumin microspheres applied to skin outside the area of the incision could invariably be recovered from the wound at the end of each of 40 operations (38). Human albumin microspheres behave similarly to human skin squames which penetrate materials of which surgical gowns and drapes are made. This study indicates that particles similar to human skin squames may somehow migrate from adjacent areas of skin and penetrate drapes on the margin of the wound.

There are no data on the mode of transmission of the endogenous flora from the various hollow organs to the surgical wound. Such transmission could occur by direct contact with contaminated instruments, sponges, or irrigating solutions, or the hands of the operative team. Ritter and coworkers found that up to 53% of instruments became contaminated during operations in operating rooms with conventional ventilation (39). The study was conducted during clean operations, and the predominant microorganism was the coagulase-negative staphylococcus. This study provided no evidence for transmission of enteric microorganisms.

Wound infections may also occur as a result of direct contact with inanimate sources such as antiseptics and bandages (11–13, 35–37). Microorganisms are transmitted by direct contact when contaminated antiseptics are applied to the incision site just prior to starting the operation. Transmission from bandages to surgical wounds occurs after the operation when dressings are applied to the incision. Microorganisms migrate to the wound from beneath the tape or through the gauze covering the wound, particularly if the gauze becomes moistened by fluids from the wound.

Contamination of the operative wound may occur by indirect contact when droplets of secretions or particles shed from skin or hair fall into the wound. One of the principal concerns for many years has been droplets which may carry bacteria from the nose and mouth to the wound. This led many years ago to the utilization of a mask to cover the nose and mouth. However, there have been published no definitive studies that establish this route as an important mode of transmission when a mask is not worn. Ford and associates noted that microorganisms cultured from the nasopharynges of operating room personnel resembled those recovered from exudates from infected wounds (40). However, they offered no proof that microorganisms were transmitted from the nasopharynx of personnel to the operative wound. Using human albumin microspheres as tracer particles, Ha'eri and Wiley demonstrated that these particles, which range between 10 and 35 μm in diameter, did not pass through the surgical mask but rather fell out from under the lower edge of the mask into the operative wound (41). However, no evidence was provided to indicate that microorganisms were transmitted to the wound in this manner. In another study using tracer particles Letts and Doermer found that the number of human albumin microspheres increased in a simulated wound when subjects talked continuously compared to baseline periods when they spoke two words every 30 seconds (42). The microspheres had been applied to the nostrils and skin on the face covered by the mask. Again, no evidence was presented that microorganisms transmitted from the upper respiratory tract of operating room personnel could cause postoperative wound infections.

The only data suggesting that particles carrying microorganisms may be transmitted from skin to wound by indirect contact has been presented by Wiley and Ha'eri (38). They applied human albumin microspheres to the forehead and temples of the surgeons during 30 operations and demonstrated wound contamination with the microspheres in 100% of cases. It is also entirely possible that microorganisms that penetrate the gown over the upper chest may fall into the operative field and contaminate the wound by indirect contact.

Caps or hoods are worn in the operating room to protect the wound from microbial contamination from the head and facial hair. Although it stands to reason that hair falling into the wound would pose a serious risk of contamination by indirect contact, there are few data to define the risk of contamination from this source. Dineen and Drusin described two outbreaks associated with carriage of *S. aureus* in the hair of a surgeon and a nurse, but did not establish the mode of transmission (22).

Airborne Transmission. Although microorganisms may be transmitted to the surgical wound by way of the air, it has rarely been possible to document airborne transmission from a proven source. It is well known that the sources of microorganisms in the operating room air are people; microorganisms originate either from the patient or operating room staff. Microorganisms are carried on droplet nuclei generated by the upper respiratory tract or on lint or skin squames. However, it has never been proven whether microorganisms in the surgical wound at the end of the operation are deposited by direct or indirect contact or by the airborne route or by both modes of transmission. Thus, it has been difficult to establish the importance of the airborne route in the absence of an exact source for the microorganisms found in the air of the operating room.

The only direct proof of airborne transmission in the operating room has been that provided by several outbreaks of group A β-hemolytic streptococcal infection (23–29). Postoperative wound infections due to group A β-hemolytic streptococci usually appear 24 to 48 hours after surgery and present an acute onset with systemic toxicity and fever. The case-fatality ratio is high for patients who are not treated promptly. There is substantial evidence that these infections are acquired by the airborne route. In six of the seven outbreaks, the same serotype was recovered from the anal or vaginal carrier site and the infected wounds (23, 24, 26–29). In four outbreaks the carriers did not work in the sterile field and therefore had no close contact with the surgical wound (25, 26, 28, 29). Further, the epidemic strain was recovered from the air of the operating room in three of the outbreaks (25, 26, 29). In one outbreak a case occurred in a room that had

been vacated by the carrier just prior to start of the operation (25). Finally, in four of the seven reports investigators uniformly recovered the epidemic strain from settle plates in a room where the carrier exercised (23, 24, 28, 29).

In most instances in which airborne transmission has been implicated in the occurrence of postoperative wound infection, the exact source is never established. Several studies on this type of airborne transmission have been published, but most have failed conclusively to establish transmission by the airborne route. Many of the studies have been carried out during operations for total replacement of joints (43–46). In two studies postoperative wound infection rates in patients operated on in rooms with special ventilation systems to provide ultraclean air were compared with those in patients operated on in rooms with conventional ventilation systems (43, 46). The latter studies have several weaknesses in design. Neither was a randomized study, and neither was blinded as to the type of ventilation in use for each operation. In the first study other variables were changed at the same time as the type of ventilation used. In the second study the infection rate for total knee replacement actually increased for the operations carried out in the room with a clean-air laminar flow system. Other studies are noncomparative or have failed to show a significantly lower infection rate for patients operated on in rooms with ultraclean air (44, 47, 48). Another approach has been to determine the wound contamination rate during surgery in rooms with laminar flow air handling systems and in rooms with conventional ventilation systems (44). Although operative wounds in rooms with ultraclean air are significantly less likely to become contaminated than those in conventionally ventilated rooms, the findings cannot be equated with a significantly lower rate of postoperative wound infections.

The only reports that provide convincing evidence of airborne transmission from unknown sources in the operating room are those of the National Research Council and the multicenter study group in Europe (9, 49). The National Research Council study was a multicenter collaborative effort that examined the effect of ultraviolet irradiation on microbial contamination of operating room air and on postoperative wound infection rates. The study was well designed, prospective, double-blinded, and randomized. Objectives were well defined, definitions were carefully developed, and the study was carefully monitored for quality of data collection throughout the period of data collection. The data indicated that refined clean wounds were significantly less likely to become infected when operations were performed in rooms illuminated with ultraviolet irradiation. Ultraviolet irradiation had no significant effect on the other classes of wounds (other clean, clean-contaminated, contaminated, and dirty) and no effect on the overall postoperative wound infection rate. This lack of effect on infection in other types of wounds was most likely due to the greater risk of contamination with endogenous microorganisms or exogenous contamination by other mechanisms of transmission. Thus, when considering airborne transmission of microorganisms to surgical wounds from unknown sources in the operating room, it can be concluded from the National Research Council study that the airborne route is a mode of transmission of minor importance for postoperative infections of most surgical wounds. It would seem to be of significant importance only for postoperative infections in refined clean wounds.

The multicenter European study was also a well designed, prospective, randomized trial carried out with patients who had total joint replacements. Postoperative wound infection rates for patients operated on in rooms with ultraclean air provided by special ventilation systems or isolators and, in some instances, body-exhaust suits were compared with infection rates for patients operated on in rooms with conventional air handling systems. The only weakness in design was the inability to provide blinding for the type of ventilation system in use for each operation. Nevertheless, the data showed a significantly lower infection rate for operations performed in rooms with ultraclean air. Further evidence for airborne transmission was provided by the observation that the concentration of microorganisms in air of rooms with special ventilation systems or where body-exhaust suits were worn was lower than the concentration in the air of rooms with conventional ventilation. The lower concentrations of microorganisms in the air of rooms with special ventilation systems correlated with the lower number of microorganisms recovered from the wounds of patients operated on in these rooms. A second publication from the multicenter European study provided data on the relationship between the level of air contamination and the joint sepsis rate (50). There was a significant association between the concentration of microorganisms in the air of the operating room and the postoperative infection rate.

The patients in the European study who benefited from operations in rooms with ultraclean air were patients with refined clean wounds. Thus, the National Research Council and European multicenter studies provided strong evidence that when microorganisms are not transmitted to the wound from other sources, airborne transmission may be an important mode of transmission. However, the significance of airborne transmission is lost for other types of wounds in which other sources and modes of transmission produce a heavier contamination of the surgical wound.

Risk Factors for Postoperative Wound Infections

The minimum requirements for development of a postoperative wound infection are a reservoir or source of microorganisms, a mode of transmission for transport of the microorganisms, and a surgical wound into which the microorganisms are deposited. However, whether an infection takes place also depends on the number of microorganisms delivered to the wound (size of the inoculum), the virulence of the microorganism, and the strength of the host's natural defenses.

Certain factors may enhance the risk for infection by increasing the size of the reservoir of the microorganism, by increasing the likelihood that transmission will take place, by increasing the size of the inoculum, or by lowering local and systemic host resistance. Some risk factors may influence more than one of the latter elements at the same time, or they may interact with each other in a complex fashion.

Age. Age has been shown to be a risk factor for postoperative wound infection by the National Research Council study, by Davidson and associates, by Cruse and Foord, and by Simchen and co-workers (9, 51–53). An increase in infection rates with age may be due to the natural waning of host defenses with age.

Sex. Although males were found to have a slightly higher rate of postoperative wound infections than females in the National Research Council study, when adjusted for the larger number of contaminated wounds in males, the rates in males and females were nearly the same (9). In similar fashion Simchen and co-workers were unable to identify sex as a risk factor for postoperative wound infection (53).

Race. The limited data available indicate that race is not a risk factor for postoperative wound infections. Data from the National Research Council study revealed slight differences in the hospital-adjusted race-specific infection rates, but the differences were much smaller than differences in rates related to many other variables (9). In their study of determinants of postoperative wound infections in orthopaedic patients, Simchen and co-workers noted no differences in rates between Jews and Arabs (53).

Month of Operation. The only information available on seasonal postoperative wound infection rates is that from the National Research Council Study (9). There was no association between month of operation and infection rates, even when refined clean wounds were examined separately.

Underlying Diseases. Chronic debilitating diseases may be risk factors for postoperative wound infections by lowering host resistance. For many years diabetes has been considered an important risk factor for postoperative wound infections, but the best data available fail to establish diabetes as a significant factor. Cruse and Foord reported higher rates of surgical wound infection in patients with diabetes (52). However, data from the National Research Council study indicate that when other risk factors, such as age, are controlled for, there is no significant difference in postoperative wound infection rates between diabetics and nondiabetics (9). Likewise, in a study of 3617 clean orthopaedic operations, Lidgren found no significant difference in postoperative wound infection rates between diabetics and nondiabetics (54).

Obesity has been clearly shown to be a risk factor for postoperative wound infection. The infection rate for obese patients in the National Research Council study was 16.5% even after the infection rate had been adjusted for duration of operation (9). Postoperative wound infection rates for obese patients reported by Cruse and Foord and Postlethwait and Johnson ranged between 13.5% and 14.5% (52, 55). Several reasons for the greater susceptibility of obese patients to postoperative wound infections have been postulated. By measuring organ blood flow, circulating blood volume, and blood flow per unit body weight, Alexander and associates inferred that adipose tissue has both a lower blood volume and a lower blood flow per unit weight than lean tissue (56). Such a relative avascularity could make adipose tissue more susceptible to infection. The technical difficulties of handling adipose tissue are associated with longer operations and perhaps more trauma to the abdominal wall. Finally, it may be very difficult to obliterate dead space in the abdominal wall fat (55).

The effect of malnutrition on the postoperative wound infection rate has not been well studied. The infection rate in malnourished patients in the National Research Council study was 22.4% (9). However, much of the effect of malnutrition was confounded by the higher age, longer operations, and a higher rate of contaminated operations in malnourished patients. After correction for hospital distribution and wound classification, rates fell markedly but were still higher than the overall infection rate of 7.4%. Cruse and Foord reported postoperative wound infection rates of 16.6% for malnourished patients (52). None of the studies to date has provided definitive data on the effect of malnutrition on postoperative wound infection.

Steroids. Adrenocorticosteroids are known to have several deleterious effects on host immunity. Unfortunately, there are no definitive data that make it possible to prove or refute the generally held belief that steroid therapy predisposes to surgical wound infection. The data from the National Research Council study were not analyzed to the extent necessary to determine whether steroid therapy is a risk factor for postoperative wound infection (9). As presented, it is not possible to determine what impact the potentially interrelated variables of age, longer duration of surgery, and longer preoperative stay had on the effect of steroid administration. Other studies have also failed to control for interrelated variables. Engquist and co-workers reported increased wound infection rates in patients treated with steroids (57). On the other hand, Cruse and Foord found no effect of steroid therapy on surgical wound infection rates (52). Further studies are needed to determine whether steroids are risk factors for postoperative wound infections.

Remote Infection. Infections in areas of the body other than the surgical wound place the wound at significant risk for postoperative infections. The data from the National Research Council study provided solid evidence that remote infection is a risk factor for postoperative wound infection (9). The infection rate in patients with remote infection was 18.4%. When adjustments were made for other possible differences in the two groups (those with and without remote infection) the infection rate remained the same, indicating that remote infection influenced the infection rate independently. Bruun also found that infection at a remote site was a significant risk factor for postoperative wound infection (31).

Duration of Preoperative Hospitalization. The duration of preoperative hospitalization has been shown to be a risk factor for postoperative wound infections. In the National Research Council study the infection rate associated with a 1-day preoperative stay was 6%, but it rose to 14.7% when the duration of preoperative hospitalization was 21 or more days (9). This association appeared to be at least partially independent of other operative and patient risk factors. Bruun also found a significant association between length of preoperative hospitalization and the rate of postoperative wound infections when multiple factors were examined by multiple regression analysis (31). Cruse and Foord noted a progressive increase in the postoperative wound infection rate with increasing duration of preoperative hospitalization. With a preoperative stay of 1 day, 1 week, and more than 2 weeks, the infection rates were 1.2%, 2.1%, 3.4%, respectively (4). Available data indicate a strong relationship between length of preoperative hospitalization and the postoperative wound infection rate. This may be the result of an increase in the size of the endogenous reservoir of microorganisms due to acquisition of hospital flora or to some adverse effect on host resistance.

Time of Day of Operation. The limited data available on the effect of the time of day when an operation is performed on postoperative wound infection rates are conflicting. When this factor was assessed in the National Research Council study it was found that rates of infection increased through the day from 7:30 a.m. to 12 midnight (9). However, this was due to a disproportionately high number of nonclean and nonelective operations during the evening and night. There was no difference in infection rates for clean wounds between cases done at the beginning of the operative schedule in the morning and those operated on late at night. On the other hand, Cruse and Foord observed an increase in infection rates in clean and clean-contaminated wounds between operations done from 8:00 a.m. to 4:00 p.m. and those performed between midnight and 8:00 a.m. (52). It is not clear whether the differences in rates are significant. Thus, the time of day during which an operation is performed has not been proven or disproven to be a risk factor for postoperative wound infections.

Preoperative Hair Removal. A decade and a half ago Seropian and Reynolds published the results of a prospective randomized study comparing postoperative wound infection rates after hair removal by shaving with a razor with rates after hair removal by a depilatory (58). The rate of infection after shaving with a razor (5.6%) was about 10 times higher than the rate after removal of hair by depilation (0.6%). The difference in

these rates was significant at the 0.02 level. They noted an infection rate of 3.1% when shaving with a razor was done just prior to surgery, 7.1% when the patient was shaved in the 24 hours prior to surgery, and 20% when the patient was shaved more than 24 hours before surgery. About a decade later Cruse and Foord reported the results of their prospective, nonrandomized, 10-year study of 62,939 wounds (4). The postoperative wound infection rate for clean wounds was 2.5% after shaving with a razor, 1.4% after shaving with an electric razor, and 0.9% in patients who had no hair removal. Whether these rates were significantly different was not reported. In 1983 Alexander and associates reported on a prospective, randomized study comparing hair removal by shaving with a razor with hair removal by clipping (59). The overall infection rate after shaving was 4.6% and after clipping it was 2.5% ($p < 0.06$). The infection rate for clean wounds was significantly ($p < 0.01$) lower when the hair was removed by clipping just prior to surgery compared with clipping the night before surgery, shaving just prior to surgery, or shaving the night before surgery. In a smaller, prospective, randomized study Thur de Koos and McComas failed to show a significant difference in postoperative wound infection rates between patients who had hair removal either by shaving or by depilatory cream (60). The infection rate for clean wounds for shaving was 5.6% and for depilatory 5.2%. Two additional smaller prospective randomized studies have also been published. Powis and colleagues found no difference in postoperative wound infection rates in 92 patients randomized to hair removal by either shaving with a razor or application of a depilatory cream (61). Balthazar and co-workers studied 200 patients undergoing inguinal herniorrhaphy who were randomized to either shaving or clipping for preoperative hair removal (62). They observed no difference in postoperative wound infection rates between the two groups.

Data from the best studies now available for the effect of shaving with a razor versus other hair removal techniques indicate that removing hair from the skin at the site of the incision with a razor is a risk factor for postoperative wound infections. This is probably due to release of resident flora deep in the skin from the trauma of shaving and/or a break in the local skin defenses with subsequent colonization and infection by exogenous microorganisms.

Skin Drapes. The type of skin drapes applied to the operative site was noted by Cruse and Foord to affect the postoperative wound infection rate (4). With cotton drapes the infection rate was 1.5% and with adhesive plastic drapes it was 2.3%. The study was not randomized and no statistical analysis was presented. More data are needed to determine whether use of plastic adhesive drapes is a risk factor for postoperative wound infection.

Duration of the Operation. The duration of a surgical operation is a well documented risk factor for postoperative wound infection. Data from the studies of Cruse and Foord and the National Research Council suggested an association between duration of surgery and the postoperative wound infection rate (4, 9). Simchen and co-workers observed a relationship between operations of long duration ($\geq$ 5 hours) and an increase in the postoperative wound infection rate ($p =$ 0.06) in patients undergoing orthopaedic operations (53). The most convincing data for an important effect of duration of operation on infection rates are from the studies of Bruun (31) and Davidson and associates (51). In both studies large numbers of patients were studied and data were tested using multiple regression analysis. Bruun found a significant association at $p < 0.01$, and Davidson and co-workers reported a significant relationship at $p < 0.001$. Although duration of operation is firmly established as a risk factor for postoperative wound infection, it is not clear exactly what effect long duration has on the surgical wound. Several possible adverse effects of a long operative time on the surgical wound have been suggested: (*a*) an increase in number of microorganisms that contaminate the wound; (*b*) increasing damage to tissues from drying, prolonged retraction and manipulation, and increasing amounts of suture and electrocoagulation in the wound; (*c*) greater suppression of systemic host defenses from blood loss, shock, and prolonged anesthesia time; and (*d*) personal fatigue leading to breaks in technique (4, 9, 31, 63).

Operative Technique. Since the days of Kocher and Halsted surgical technique has been thought to be important in the prevention of postoperative wound infections. This has become a basic tenet of surgical practice, and these principles appear logical although they have not been proven effective by scientific studies. Thus, effective hemostasis, maintenance of an adequate blood supply, removal of all devitalized tissue, obliteration of dead space, use of fine nonabsorbed suture material, and wound closure without tension are held as basic to the practice of modern surgery and to the prevention of postoperative wound infection (9).

Use of Electrosurgical Units. There are few data available on use of electrosurgical units as a risk factor for postoperative wound infection. Cruse and Foord noted that use of the electrosurgical unit for cutting and coagulating tissue led to a postoperative wound infection rate twice the rate observed in patients on whom the electrosurgical unit was not used (4). With experience and development of better technique, the rate of infection in patients on whom the unit was used returned to baseline. Further study is needed to determine whether or not and under what circumstances use of an electrosurgical unit significantly contributes to development of postoperative wound infections.

Incidental Appendectomy. The data on the risk of incidental appendectomy are sparse. Cruse and Foord reported that the postoperative wound infection rate for cholecystectomies (1.4%) tripled when an incidental appendectomy was performed at the same time (4). Whether this was a significant difference was not reported. It remains to be proven whether incidental appendectomy is a risk factor for postoperative wound infection.

Drains. The risk inherent in placement of a drain at surgery for subsequent postoperative wound infection has been investigated throughout the 20th century. Most of the studies have not been well designed, and those that are provide conflicting results. One uncontrolled and nonrandomized study suggested that drains are risk factors for postoperative wound infection (52). Two experimental studies in animal models have also suggested that drains are risk factors for infection, and both suggest that the drain provides a portal of entry for microorganisms (64, 65). The National Research Council study identified a high infection rate in drained wounds (11.1%) (9). Although it was not stated whether the difference (11.1% versus 5.0% for undrained wounds) was statistically significant, the difference was great, and the rate remained high even after adjustment for other factors that might have been interrelated with the effects of surgical drains. Lidwell applied multiple regression analysis to retrospectively collected data on postoperative wound infections and identified drains as a risk factor for infection (66).

Five prospective studies have been published that provide statistical analysis of the data. Four studies were nonrandomized and uncontrolled with respect to insertion of drains, but all were analyzed by multiple logistic regression analysis. Bruun found that drains significantly increased the risk of postoperative wound infection (31). Davidson and associates were unable to show a significant association between insertion of a drain and infection (51). Simchen and co-workers prospectively studied patients undergoing colonic surgery, cardiac surgery, and neurosurgery (67). They found no significant association between insertion of drains and postoperative wound infection rates. In another study of postoperative wound infections in orthopaedic patients, Simchen and co-workers observed a significant relationship between open drains and infection but not between closed drains and postoperative wound infection (53). In the only randomized controlled study Maull and co-workers found no significant difference in infection rates between drained and undrained wounds after cholecystectomy (68).

Given the conflicting results of the published studies, it cannot be concluded that drains are risk factors for postoperative wound infections. Furthermore, more data are needed on the risk of the use of drains in specific surgical procedures.

Urgency of Operation. Surgery carried out under emergency conditions has long been considered a risk factor for postoperative wound infections. However, the very limited data available from two prospective studies failed to show a significant relationship between surgical procedures performed under emergency conditions and the rate of postoperative wound infections. In the National Research Council study operations carried out under urgent or emergency conditions had a much higher rate of associated postoperative wound infections, but when adjusted for other factors, particularly the degree of contamination of the wound, there was no difference in infection rates for elective operations and for operations carried out under more urgent circumstances (9). On initial analysis, Davidson and co-workers found a significant association between emergency procedures and the rate of postoperative wound infections, but when the data were subjected to multiple logistic regression analysis, the relationship between emergency operations and the rate of infections became insignificant (51). Emergency surgery does not appear to be a risk factor for postoperative wound infections.

Prevention of Postoperative Wound Infections

A discussion of prevention of postoperative wound infections may be conveniently divided into the following phases: (*a*) prehospitalization measures; (*b*) preoperative measures; (*c*) intraoperative measures; (*d*) postoperative measures; (*e*) preparation of the operative team; (*f*) environmental control; and (*g*) prospective wound surveillance (see "New Aspects of Postoperative Wound Infections," below).

Prehospitalization Measures

Duration of Preoperative Hospitalization. A long duration of hospitalization prior to surgery has been well established as a risk factor for postoperative wound infection. For that reason all correctable conditions that are or may be risk factors for infection should be treated prior to hospitalization. Minimizing the duration of hospitalization prior to operation would appear to be a very important preventive measure.

Underlying Diseases. Underlying conditions should be treated prior to surgery with the goal of eliminating or improving diseases that may increase the risk of postoperative wound infections. Since infection at a remote site is strongly associated with postoperative wound infection, it is very important that such infections be treated, and where possible, eradicated, prior to surgery.

Diabetes and malnutrition have long been implicated as risk factors for infection in the absence of data that provide support for such an association. Although diabetes and malnutrition are not established risk factors for surgical wound infection, diabetes should be well controlled and malnutrition should be treated prior to surgery, because these conditions may have other adverse effects on the surgical patient, such as disturbances in fluids and electrolytes and poor wound healing.

Although obesity is an established risk factor for postoperative wound infection, it may be very difficult to correct this condition prior to surgery. Obese patients should undergo weight reduction prior to surgery, but unfortunately, this probably cannot be carried out successfully in most patients. Indeed, some patients have surgical procedures to treat morbid obesity.

Steroids. Although steroids are known to have a suppressive effect on host immunity, there are no studies that show a significant increase in surgical wound infection rates in patients who are treated with steroids. There is no evidence that adrenocorticosteroids should be withdrawn prior to surgery for the purpose of preventing postoperative wound infections.

Preoperative Measures

Preoperative Showers. Cruse and Foord reported that postoperative infection rates for clean wounds were 2.3% for patients who did not shower, 2.1% for patients who showered with soap, and 1.3% for patients who showered with a preparation containing hexachlorophene (4, 52). Whether these rates were significantly different was not reported. Polk and associates recommended preoperative showers but cited no data on which to base their recommendation (69). It is not known whether preoperative showering or bathing with antiseptic soap is effective in the prevention of postoperative wound infections.

Removal of Hair. Removal of hair by shaving with a razor is a risk factor for postoperative infection in clean wounds, and in the study of Seropian and Reynolds shaving was identified as a risk factor for infection in all classes of wounds (58). Strong consideration should be given to the removal of hair either by clipping with an electric razor or by application of a depilatory. If the method of hair removal used is shaving, the patient should be shaved just prior to operation. When hair is removed by shaving the night prior to surgery or at even longer intervals before operation, the risk of surgical wound infection appears to be higher than when the patient is shaved just prior to operation.

Application of an Antiseptic Solution to the Skin at the Incision Site. Degerming the skin at the site of the surgical incision has been practiced since Lister introduced the application of carbolic acid to the skin for removal of microorganisms prior to operation in 1864. Currently, the most commonly used agents include iodine and iodine compounds, chlorhexidine gluconate, hexachlorophene preparations, ethyl alcohol, and quarternary ammonium compounds (10, p 82). Among these the most frequently used preparations appear to be those containing chlorhexidine, iodophors, and hexachlorophene. Based on the available data, the best compounds seem to be those containing either chlorhexidine or an iodophor. Hexachlorophene is not effective against gram-negative microorganisms and is inactivated by blood and serum proteins. In comparative studies chlorhexidine gluconate causes a greater reduction in skin flora after the first application and after multiple applications than either iodophor preparations or those containing hexachlorophene (70–72). Chlorhexidine has a substantive action after a single application, and it is not inactivated by blood and serum proteins (73). Iodophors do not have a substantive activity and are inactivated by blood and serum protein. However, iodophors exert a bacteriostatic effect as long as they remain on the skin (74).

Chlorhexidine and iodophors have a broad spectrum of antimicrobial activity and rapidly kill microorganisms on the skin. These two types of preparations appear to be the best currently available for degerming the skin in the operative area. These preparations should reduce the skin reservoir of microorganisms to a sufficiently low level to almost eliminate infections due to skin flora.

In addition to the application of antiseptic agents, washing the skin prior to application of these agents continues to be recommended (10, p 82). However, it has never been proven that this is a necessary step in preparation of the skin. Further, two studies have shown that this step may be omitted without any change in the rate of postoperative wound infections (73, 74). In one of the latter studies there was a substantial savings when chlorhexidine gluconate was sprayed on the skin after removal of obvious foreign material with a clean sponge (73).

Drapes. Drapes are used as barriers to prevent microorganisms outside the operative area from entering the wound. It has been shown that microorganisms easily pass through the cotton materials from which drapes and surgical gowns are frequently made (19). This process is accelerated when these materials become moist (21). Materials are available which resist the penetration of microorganisms both in the dry and in the moist state (19, 21). However, there are few data on the effect of permeable versus impermeable materials on the rate of postoperative wound infections. The only study comparing rates of infection for permeable and impermeable materials is that of Moylan and Kennedy (20). They found a significantly lower infection rate ($p = 0.001$) when the gowns and drapes used were made from a spun-bonded olefin material compared with the use of gowns and drapes made of either 140 thread count cotton material or 280 thread count cotton material. This difference was significant for both clean and clean-contaminated wounds. There are too few data available on which to base a firm recommendation with respect to the choice of materials for the manufacture of drapes.

In addition to the drapes used simply to cover the skin, there are drapes made of plastic adhesive that are applied to the skin at the operative site. The incision is made through the drape so that the skin is covered by the adhesive drape right up to the margin of the incision. Theoretically, such a drape should markedly diminish the number of microorganisms from skin that enter the wound. However, Lilly and co-workers found no difference in the number of microorganisms in wounds that had been draped with adhesive drapes versus those to which adhesive drapes had not been applied (75). Wiley and Ha'eri found that adhesive drapes were ineffective in preventing human albumin microspheres applied outside the area of the incision from gaining entrance to the wound (38). In a randomized, prospective, controlled trial, Jackson and associates found no difference in the postoperative wound infection rates between patients draped with adhesive plastic drapes and those operated on without plastic drapes (76). Cruse and Foord found a higher rate of infection when plastic drapes were used than when cotton drapes were used (4). Thus, there are no data to support the routine use of adhesive plastic drapes.

Prophylactic Antibiotics. A comprehensive review of the use of prophylactic antibiotics in surgery is beyond the scope of this chapter. However, antimicrobial prophylaxis may be an important modality for the prevention of certain types of postoperative wound infection. In the two decades after the introduction of antibiotics, they were used empirically for prophylaxis in surgery with no scientific evidence that they prevented postoperative wound infections. Indeed, the National Research Council study carried out in the early 1960s found no benefit from prophylactic use of antibiotics (9). Burke's classic work published in 1961 provided a strong theoretical basis for use of prophylactic antibiotics for certain types of surgery, and this stimulated a number of well designed studies (77).

Antibiotic prophylaxis is justified when there is a high risk of infection or when the risk of infection is not high but when infection is likely to have disastrous consequences, such as infection of a prosthetic implant. Antibiotics for prophylaxis should be chosen based on the antimicrobial susceptibility of the microorganisms most likely to contaminate the wound. The antibiotic should be administered at an appropriate time prior to surgery so that concentrations in tissue are high enough at the time contamination of the wound is likely to take place to suppress the growth of microorganisms that gain entrance to the tissues. Prophylaxis should be given for no longer than 48 hours.

Prophylaxis is indicated for wounds classified as clean-contaminated and contaminated or when a prosthetic device is to be inserted. The 75% of the wounds that are clean do not need prophylaxis, and wounds that are classified as dirty are already infected. Antibiotics adminis-

tered for the latter type of wound are considered therapeutic rather than prophylactic (78).

Antibiotic prophylaxis is indicated for surgery on the stomach and duodenum except for non-obstructing duodenal ulcer (78, 79). Other operations for which prophylaxis is indicated include appendectomy, operations on the colon and rectum, operations on the biliary tract in high risk patients, vaginal hysterectomy, operations on the head and neck, operations for insertion of prosthetic cardiac valves, and orthopaedic operations for placement of prosthetic joints (78–82). Prophylactic antibiotics should not be used in place of other preventive measures, but, rather, their use should complement other modalities of prevention. When used properly, prophylactic antibiotics can be an integral part of an effective prevention program.

Intraoperative Measures

Operative Technique. Good operative technique would appear to be important for the prevention of postoperative wound infections. The application of good surgical technique is the responsibility of the surgeon. The impact of a control program based on postoperative wound surveillance with feedback of infection rates to the surgeon is likely dependent, at least in part, upon changes in operative technique and aseptic technique made by the surgeon when he/she is alerted to a rise in the rate of postoperative wound infections in his/her patients (see below).

Duration of the Operation. Every operation should be performed as quickly as possible within the limits of safety. There is a strong association between duration of operation and postoperative wound infection.

Insertion of Drains. A discussion of the indication for and the proper use of surgical drains is beyond the scope of this chapter. Since there is no conclusive evidence that drains either cause or prevent postoperative wound infections, the decision to drain or not to drain a wound should be based on accepted principles for the use of surgical drains (10, p 131). When drains are inserted, there are two studies that suggest that closed suction drainage is associated with the lowest infection rate (52, 53). However, van der Linden and co-workers found that suction drainage was no better than gravity drainage with respect to postoperative wound infection and that suction drainage impaired rather than enhanced evacuation of intraperitoneal fluid (83). Cruse and Foord reported higher infection rates when drains were brought out through the incisional wound than when they were brought out through a separate stab wound (52). However, in two other studies there was no difference in the rate of postoperative wound infections, whether the drain was brought out through the incision or through a separate stab wound (9, 83). No definitive statement can be made about drains with respect to prevention of postoperative wound infections.

Postoperative Measures

When surgical wounds are not closed at the time of operation, there is a risk of acquiring an infection during postoperative care on the ward. When dressings are changed on open wounds, it is important that aseptic technique be used to prevent cross-infection among patients on the floor. Cruse and Foord stated that postoperative care on the ward was not associated with surgical wound infections (4). However, there is good evidence that wound infections caused by methicillin-resistant S. aureus are acquired on surgical wards by cross-infection (see below).

Preparation of the Operative Team

Surgical Scrub. There are no prospective, randomized, controlled epidemiologic studies that compare rates of postoperative wound infection when different antiseptic detergent hand scrub preparations are used or when hands are scrubbed for different periods of time. The only data available on which to base the selection of antiseptic detergents and to help determine an appropriate duration for the surgical scrub are from microbiologic studies.

Based on microbiologic studies that assessed immediate reduction of skin flora, reduction in bacterial counts after multiple applications, and residual or cumulative antiseptic action on the gloved hand, 4% chlorhexidine gluconate detergent solution is the best antiseptic preparation when compared with antiseptic detergents that contain iodophors or hexachlorophene (70–72). However, there is no evidence that scrubbing with chlorhexidine gluconate detergent is associated with lower infection rates than scrubbing with detergents that contain iodophors or hexachlorophene. There has been a concern that use of hexachlorophene may select out gram-negative bacteria, because it has no antibacterial activity against gram-negative bacilli (84). The available data suggest that detergents containing chlorhexidine and iodophors are the best preparations for the surgical scrub.

There are also no controlled trials that compare postoperative wound infection rates when the duration of the surgical scrub is varied. Although the 10-minute scrub has been used widely and continues to be recommended, two microbiologic studies indicate that a 5-minute surgical scrub duration is as effective in removing skin flora as a 10-minute scrub (16, 85). A longer scrub duration is more likely to cause dermatitis, and this is associated with higher bacterial counts on the skin of the gloved hand (17). Based on the available data, the duration of the surgical scrub need not exceed 5 minutes.

Masks. Although there is a strong theoretical rationale for the use of face masks in surgery, there are no studies that prove that wearing a mask reduces postoperative wound infection rates. All of the data on surgical face masks are from microbiologic or tracer particle studies (40–42, 86, 87). The following conclusions can be drawn from these studies: (*a*) masks varied in their filtering efficiencies; (*b*) all masks filtered large particles (> 3.3 μm diameter) efficiently, but there was variation between masks for small particle (< 3.3 μm diameter) filtration; (*c*) prolonged use and moistening of the more efficient masks did not decrease their ability to filter; (*d*) inefficiency of filtration was probably affected as much by design (stiffness, lack of pleating, and small size) as by the filtration efficiency of the materials from which the mask was constructed; (*e*) cotton fabric masks were as efficient as masks made of synthetic materials when cotton masks were properly designed; (*f*) tracer studies indicated that particles carrying microorganisms probably do not pass through the mask but rather most likely fall out from the lower edge of the mask; (*g*) tracer studies also suggested that reducing the amount of conversation and wearing the face mask beneath an overlapping hood may reduce the number of microorganisms that reach the wound.

The best way to select a surgical mask is to choose the mask associated with the lowest infection rate. Since such data are not available, the selection of a mask should be based on filtration efficiency, maintainence of high efficiency with time and moistening, and cost.

Gowns. There is little evidence for an association between the type of gown that is worn and postoperative wound infection rates. It is clear that microorganisms from the surgical team's scrub clothes and skin readily penetrate the muslin from which surgical gowns are made (19). It is also clear that microbial penetration occurs more quickly when these materials become wet (21). The only study that compared the rates of postoperative wound infections between the use of drapes and gowns made of muslin versus the use of those made of nonpermeable material showed a significantly ($p = 0.001$) higher rate of infections for patients when the gowns and drapes were made of the permeable muslin (20). More studies are needed to determine the relationship between varying degrees of permeability and postoperative wound infection rates. Such studies are needed to provide a scientific basis for selection of appropriate materials for manufacture of surgical gowns.

Caps. Surgical caps are worn routinely in the operating room, and if worn properly, they should prevent hair and skin squames from falling into the wound. Although *S. aureus* and other microorganisms are commonly carried in the hair, there is no evidence that caps prevent transmission of any microorganisms from hair to the surgical wound (88, 89). In the only two outbreaks associated with hair carriers of *S. aureus*, transmission apparently took place while the carriers were wearing caps. Use of caps appears appropriate to prevent loose hair from falling into the operative field, but caps would be effective only if they covered all scalp and facial hair.

Shoe Covers. Use of shoe covers is standard practice in operating rooms, but even in textbooks that recommend their use, no scientific data are cited to justify the practice (10, p 101). Microorganisms on the floor of any room in the hospital have never been associated with nosocomial infections. Indeed, the Medical Research Council of Great Britain and the Centers for Disease Control do not recommend shoe covers, and the American Hospital Association recommends shoe covers only "when laundry facilities permit" (90). The effect of shoe covers on postoperative wound infection rates needs to be studied.

Environmental Control

It has been difficult to establish any environmental reservoir for microorganisms in the operating room that cause postoperative wound infections. Airborne microorganisms may reach the surgical wound, but the reservoir for these microorganisms is either the operative team or the patient. Discussion of all aspects of environmental control—including ventilation systems, ultraviolet irradiation, traffic control, decontamination and sterilization of instruments, wrappers for

sterile materials, shelf life of sterile goods, monitoring autoclaves, use of tacky mats, special precautions for "dirty" cases, and housekeeping practices—is beyond the scope of this chapter. The discussion below will be limited to a few selected areas, including ventilation systems, sterilization of instruments, use of tacky mats, and precautions for "dirty" cases.

Ventilation Systems. There are no studies that relate particular types of ventilation to postoperative wound infection rates except for systems that produce ultraclean air. Recommendations are based on studies that relate the type of ventilation used to the concentration of microorganisms in the air. The minimum requirements set by the Public Health Service are for 25 air changes/hour with 5 units of outside air (10, p 274). It is recommended that air be introduced at the ceiling and exhausted near the floor. Air handling systems that produce ultraclean air would not be expected to result in overall lower postoperative wound infection rates except, perhaps, for insertion of prosthetic joints in orthopaedic surgery (see above). However, even for this type of surgery, rates equal to those achieved in rooms with ultraclean air may be achieved in rooms with standard ventilation systems when good barrier technique and prophylactic antibiotics are used (47, 82, 91). Furthermore, it is possible that postoperative wound infection rates equal to or nearly equal to those attained in rooms with ultraclean air could be realized in rooms with modern standard ventilation systems and exquisite barrier technique. To date, ventilation systems that provide ultraclean air have not been proven to add significantly to control of any type of postoperative wound infection in the United States.

Sterilization of Instruments. Instruments must be thoroughly cleaned before sterilization with removal of all tissue, blood, and secretions. The steam autoclaves in the operating room should be checked and serviced frequently on a regular schedule. Steam autoclaves should be tested at least weekly using commercial preparations of the spores of *Bacillus stearothermophilus* (92).

Tacky Mats. Tacky mats have been placed at the entrance of the operating room suite to remove dirt and microorganisms from the bottom of the shoes of personnel. They are ineffective and expensive (93, 94). There is no evidence that they can reduce postoperative wound infection rates. Also, mats soaked with disinfectant are ineffective in preventing contamination of floors in the operating room (93, 94). Such mats may also be hazardous since the floor becomes slippery after the disinfectant is tracked onto the surface adjacent to the mat.

Dirty Cases. Although 84% of U.S. hospitals still use special procedures for dirty cases, there is no scientific rationale for such special handling of dirty cases (90, 93). Routine housekeeping procedures will effectively decontaminate any operating room after a dirty case or a case in which the patient has a communicable disease.

Summary

There are many recommendations in the literature for measures to prevent postoperative wound infections. However, there are only seven types of intervention that are supported by epidemiologic studies of postoperative wound infection rates. Such preventive measures include: (*a*) minimizing the duration of preoperative hospitalization; (*b*) weight reduction for obese patients; (*c*) eradication of remote infections; (*d*) hair removal by depilatory, clipping with an electric razor, or shaving with a razor just prior to operation; (*e*) minimizing the duration of surgery; (*f*) appropriate use of prophylactic antibiotics; and (*g*) institution of a prospective postoperative wound surveillance program with feedback of postoperative wound infection rates to the surgeons (see below). All other recommendations are based on incomplete data, laboratory studies, theory, or tradition.

New Aspects of Postoperative Wound Infections

Surveillance Program for the Prevention of Postoperative Wound Infections

Although surveillance of postoperative wounds is an integral part of any surveillance program in infection control, a more focused program of postoperative wound surveillance with rapid feedback of infection rates to surgeons has been tested in several medical centers (4, 52, 95, 96). The assumption has been made that, when a surgeon is informed about high or rising postoperative wound infection rates in his/her patients, he or she can make improvements in aseptic and/or operative technique that will result in an improvement in infection rates. An emphasis has been placed on clean wound infection rates for feedback to surgeons, because clean wound infections are usually caused by easily correctable breaks in technique. On the other hand, wound infections related to intrinsic contamination (clean-contaminated, contaminated, and dirty) would not be likely to respond as well as clean wounds to changes in technique since such changes may have little effect on contamination of the wound by microorganisms.

Elements of a Postoperative Wound Surveillance Program. One of the key elements of a postoperative wound surveillance program is a committed infection control practitioner (ICP) who is compulsive in identifying infections and who communicates well with other hospital staff (95). In addition to basic training in infection control, the ICP should be trained by the surgical staff in the identification of postoperative wound infections (95).

Infection rates are reported by wound classifications. Wounds are classified by operating room personnel and verified by the ICP (96). Certain operations, such as dental procedures and transurethral prostatic resections, may be excluded because of difficulty in defining a postoperative wound infection (96). Postoperative wound surveillance is carried out while the patient is in the hospital and for at least 14 days after discharge to identify late onset wound infections (95).

The most important element of the program is frequent feedback of postoperative wound infection rates to surgeons. Clean wound infection rates probably constitute the most important information conveyed to the surgeons. However, it is also appropriate to report infection rates for each wound classification as well as the overall postoperative wound infection rate. Infection reports should be sent to each surgeon and should provide the rates of infection for his patients as well as the average rates and ranges for all surgeons in the division or department. Reports should be kept strictly confidential. Data might also be displayed in the form of a graph in the surgical wards or in the operating room, and infection rates might be discussed at departmental meetings (4, 52).

Objective Evidence for Effectiveness of Postoperative Wound Surveillance Programs. Cruse and Foord were the first to report on the results of a postoperative wound surveillance program (4). Although the study was not randomized or controlled, they observed a decrease in clean wound infection rates from 2.5% to 0.6% over a 10-year period. No results of statistical analysis of the data were reported.

Condon and associates reported a decrease in the clean wound infection rate from 3.5% to less than 1% over 5 years ($p < 0.01$) (95). The changing trend of wound infection rates during the 10 six-month periods of the study was found to be significantly downward ($p < 0.05$) as determined by the Cochrane test for linearity.

In another 5-year prospective study Olson and co-workers noted a decrease in the overall postoperative wound infection rates from 4.2% to 1.9% ($p < 0.05$) (96). The significant decrease in wound infection rates included clean wound and clean-contaminated wounds but not contaminated wounds.

Reporting on the results of the Study on the Efficacy of Nosocomial Infection Control (SENIC), Haley and his colleagues presented data that supported the effectiveness of control programs based on surveillance with feedback of surgical wound infection rates to the hospital's practicing surgeons (97). They identified two important components in such programs: (a) establishment of a strong infection surveillance and control program and feedback of surgical wound infection rates to the hospital's practicing surgeons and (b) presence of an effective hospital epidemiologist. For high risk patients, having both elements of the program resulted in very effective control of surgical wound infections, whereas the presence of one element of the program led to only a moderate reduction in infection rates. When applied to low risk patients, the presence of only the first element of the program resulted in a moderate reduction in infection rates (19%), but when only the second element was present, there was no reduction in infection rates. When both elements were applied to low risk patients, there was a large decrease (41%) in wound infection rates. These observations applied to all hospitals in the sample except for municipal hospitals affiliated with medical schools. None of these hospitals in the sample had very effective control programs utilizing both elements. Moderately effective programs in these institutions had no effect on infection rates in high risk patients but did result in lower infection rates in low risk patients.

A new wound classification system was developed during the SENIC project (98). The new system was derived from stepwise multiple logistic regression analysis of 10 risk factors for surgical wound infections. Four factors were identified that provided most of the predictive power. These included having (a) an operation that involved the abdomen; (b) an operation lasting longer than 2 hours; (c) an operation classified as either contaminated or dirty-infected; and (d)

three or more underlying diagnoses. The regression coefficients were rounded to one, and an index was evolved with wounds being classified from 0 to 4 (low risk to high risk). The authors demonstrated that their index had substantially more predictive power than the traditional wound classification system. They suggested that a similar system be used in postoperative wound surveillance programs. The authors observed that 90% of the infections occurred in a group made up of approximately one-half of the patients with wounds classified 1 to 4. It was recommended that surveillance be limited to this group of patients when a hospital's resources did not permit surveillance of all postoperative wounds.

The wound classification developed during the SENIC project is 10 years old and may no longer be valid for control programs in the 1980s. Haley and his colleagues observed no effect of prophylactic antimicrobial drugs on postoperative wound infection rates (97). Since those data were collected, a number of randomized well controlled studies (see above) on the use of prophylactic antibiotics in surgery have been carried out, and these studies have clearly defined the appropriate use of antibiotic prophylaxis for prevention of postoperative infections. Now that a number of contaminated wounds, particularly in the abdomen, no longer become infected, it is not clear how predictive this wound classification system is in the mid-1980s. Further study of this system is indicated before it is widely adopted.

Other Potential Benefits from Postoperative Wound Surveillance Programs. Both Condon and associates and Olson and co-workers suggested that postoperative wound surveillance provides a mechanism for the early detection of outbreaks (95, 96). Both groups also reported that the surveillance program led to more appropriate use of prophylactic antibiotics. Although only relatively crude estimates of costs were made, Cruse and Foord, Condon and associates, and Olson and co-workers all concluded that postoperative wound surveillance programs were cost effective (4, 95, 96).

Postoperative Wound Infections Caused by Methicillin-Resistant *Staphylococcus aureus*

Methicillin and other semisynthetic penicillins have proven very useful for the treatment of infections due to pencillinase-producing *Staphylococcus aureus*. However, strains resistant to methicillin were recovered from clinical specimens at about the time of its introduction for clinical use (99). During the 1960s, methicillin-resistant *S. aureus* (MRSA) became a clinically significant problem in many countries in Europe. A few cases of infection due to MRSA were reported in the United States in 1967, but the first outbreak in a hospital in this country was reported by Barrett and associates in 1968 (100). Two additional outbreaks occurred in 1968 and 1969, respectively (101, 102). Since the mid-1970s, MRSA has become an increasingly serious problem throughout the country (103).

Infections due to MRSA occur most commonly in surgical patients hospitalized in university-affiliated medical centers (103). This is probably due to the fact that surgical wounds are easily colonized and infected in these high risk patients with severe underlying diseases and injuries who are hospitalized in all too frequently overcrowded intensive care units (103). There are also a number of reported instances of transfer of MRSA between referral centers when colonized or infected patients are transported from one institution to another (104–106; CG Mayhall, unpublished observations).

Microbiology of MRSA. Methicillin resistance in *S. aureus* is not due to penicillinase production and has been termed intrinsic resistance. Another characteristic of this type of resistance is that of heteroresistance; only a small population of cells within each strain of MRSA are resistant to methicillin, and these resistant cells grow more slowly under usual conditions of incubation than do the sensitive cells (107, 108). Since the resistant cells are slow in their growth, routine overnight antimicrobial susceptibility tests may fail to identify methicillin-resistant strains of *S. aureus*. However, there are several techniques that aid in the laboratory detection of MRSA. Addition of 5% sodium chloride to the media or incubation at lower temperatures (either 35° or 30°) increases the rate of growth of the resistant cells (109, 110).

In addition to methicillin, MRSA are generally resistant to all other β-lactam antibiotics and many other antibiotics as well (111–113). Although MRSA may appear susceptible to some cephalosporins, infections due to MRSA usually fail to respond to therapy with cephalosporins (114). The drug of choice for infections due to MRSA is vancomycin (111, 112). There have been no reports of MRSA resistant to vancomycin (112). If therapy with vancomycin fails to eradicate the infection, it may be necessary to add rifampin or an aminoglycoside (112).

Several epidemiologic markers are available for MRSA. In addition to the antibiogram, isolates of MRSA may be typed by phage typing, plasmid pattern, and production of aminoglycoside-inactivating enzymes (113). Archer and Mayhall concluded from their study that plasmid pattern analysis was a better technique for typing MRSA than either phage typing or antibiogram (113).

Epidemiology of MRSA Infections. Most outbreaks of MRSA infections have occurred in surgical patients, and surgical wounds were the most common site from which MRSA was recovered (104–106, 115–121). Other sites from which MRSA have also been cultured include urine, burn wounds, the respiratory tract, blood, stool, bone, chest tubes, intravenous catheter tips, intra-abdominal abscesses, eye, ear, skin and soft tissue, and wounds other than surgical wounds (104–106, 115–121). Except for blood and intra-abdominal abscesses, the above sites may be either colonized or infected. In either case patients are an important reservoir for MRSA during hospital outbreaks. Once colonized or infected, patients may harbor MRSA for many months (122; CG Mayhall, unpublished observations).

A second reservoir for MRSA is found among hospital personnel who carry MRSA in either their nose or on their skin (106, 115, 118–120). The overall importance of this reservoir has not been determined, but it is clear that some patients have been colonized or infected by personnel who are carriers of MRSA. A third potential reservoir is the environment. However, cultures of the environment have usually been negative during MRSA outbreaks (115, 118–120, 123). The only exception to this observation applies to outbreaks in burn units. The environment of burn units has been found to be heavily contaminated (121, 123, 124).

The most important mode of transmission for MRSA is probably contact transmission by the hands of personnel, although the data for this type of transmission are limited. Saroglou and associates, Bock and colleagues, and Boyce and co-workers were unable to recover MRSA from the hands of personnel (104, 105, 118). Peacock and associates cultured the hands of seven nurses who had contact with patients with cultures positive for MRSA, and only one nurse had positive cultures (117). Thompson and co-workers and Crossley and colleagues were able to recover MRSA from hands of personnel immediately after they had handled materials contaminated with MRSA but before they washed their hands

(121, 123). Thus, MRSA may be transferred from one patient to another by direct contact with the contaminated hands of hospital personnel. There is also evidence that MRSA carried in the nares of hospital personnel may be transmitted from this site to patients by hand contact (106,115, 118–120).

There is no evidence for contact transmission by fomites. Except for burn units, air samples in areas of the hospital where MRSA patients are located have been essentially negative (115, 118, 123).

Risk factors for acquisition of MRSA have been identified in several case-control studies (106, 116–118, 120). In four of the five studies, controls were patients from whom methicillin-sensitive S. aureus had been recovered on culture. The most consistent finding of the case-control studies was that prior antibiotic therapy was a risk factor for acquisition of MRSA, particularly with semisynthetic penicillins, cephalosporins, and aminoglycosides. Two other important risk factors included a long duration of hospitalization and the presence of underlying diseases. Only one of the studies identified advanced age and a high number of invasive procedures as risk factors for acquisition of MRSA (120).

Control of Outbreaks of Infection Due to MRSA. Control of outbreaks due to MRSA has been difficult, and routine isolation precautions may not be effective (103). In fact, once introduced, most hospitals have been unable to eradicate MRSA from their patient populations (121). The key to successful control and eradication of MRSA is a continuous assessment of the patient reservoir. Only by continuous and rapid identification of new patients in the reservoir can the spread of MRSA be halted. Since patients may be reservoirs when they are only colonized and not infected, a rapid prospective system to identify new sources is the cornerstone of control. Such a system involves contact tracing. Patients who have been exposed to MRSA cases (infected or colonized) should be cultured at all possible sites using a selective medium. Thus, patients exposed to cases in a given geographic area (perhaps one section of a nursing unit) or exposed to cases by way of a common nursing staff should be cultured once a week until 3 weeks after the last exposure to an MRSA case. Sites for culture would include all wounds, sputum, and nares. Newly identified cases are immediately placed in isolation. An effective selective medium is made by adding 20 μg/ml of methicillin to staphylococ-

cus 110 agar. This rapid identification system should be supplemented with periodic point prevalence culture surveys using the selective medium in high risk areas such as surgical intensive care units or other areas where many cases have occurred. The contact tracing system is further supplemented by screening for MRSA in clinical specimens in the hospital laboratory using appropriate identification techniques for MRSA. All newly identified cases are immediately isolated and all contacts cultured until they are either discharged or are determined to be negative for MRSA, because they have had three negative sets of cultures after their last known contact with an unisolated case. A contact tracing control system is labor intensive, but it may eradicate an outbreak before it becomes widespread in the hospital. At the author's institution, a highly resistant strain of MRSA (including resistance to rifampin) was eradicated from the hospital in 8 months after only eight cases of infection and nine cases of colonization. Culture of patient contacts has been reported in only one publication (120). However, the authors provided no details on the use of this control technique in their hospital.

About 6 months after eradication of MRSA from the author's institution, Thompson and co-workers published the details of their control system for MRSA (121). Two of their three surveillance techniques were similar to two of our three techniques; they carried out periodic point prevalence culture surveys in high risk patients, and they screened clinical specimens for MRSA through the clinical microbiology laboratory. These measures were instituted in response to an increasing prevalence of nosocomial infections due to MRSA. It is possible that the addition of contact tracing to the other surveillance techniques could prevent a large outbreak if applied shortly after introduction of MRSA into a hospital or that a large outbreak could be controlled more rapidly.

Patients who are infected or colonized with MRSA should be isolated. Although the best method of isolation for MRSA cases has not been determined, many authors have used strict isolation in their hospitals (115, 117–120, 123). Since airborne transmission has not been established for MRSA, even in burn units where MRSA may be recovered from the air, strict isolation is probably unnecessary for patients with MRSA in sites other than the lower respiratory tract. However, strict attention must be paid to barrier isolation technique. This would include use of gowns, gloves, strict attention to hand washing, and decontamination of hands with antiseptic agents. Since patients with pneumonia due to methicillin-sensitive *S. aureus* are placed on strict isolation, it would also be appropriate for patients with MRSA pneumonia.

Another control measure that could be employed is that of cohorting. Patients with MRSA infection or colonization could be cared for in one area with hospital personnel assigned to work only with the cohort. This could be combined, where possible, with geographic limitations on transfer of MRSA patients within the hospital.

Since patients and personnel are the most important reservoirs for MRSA, any modality for reducing these reservoirs should contribute to control of outbreaks. Ward and colleagues described an antimicrobial therapy regimen combined with hexachlorophene baths designed to eradicate the MRSA carrier state in patients and personnel (120). They observed that a 5-day course of rifampin, 300 mg orally twice daily, combined with topical application of bacitracin to the nares three times a day was uniformly effective in eradicating MRSA from the anterior nares. To this regimen they added trimethoprim-sulfamethoxazole, one 80/400 mg tablet twice a day, for eradication of MRSA from extranasal carrier sites. The regimen was less successful in clearing MRSA from extranasal sites. Since the authors defined success in eradication by a single negative culture taken at least 2 weeks after completion of antibiotic therapy, the effectiveness of these regimens cannot be considered well established. More studies are needed to confirm the efficacy of these antibiotic combinations.

Locksley and associates reported success in eradication of MRSA from nasal and extranasal sites in eight patients using a combination of intravenous vancomycin and oral rifampin, but three patients relapsed 1 to 3 weeks after completion of therapy (106). Other authors have reported variable results with topical therapy sometimes combined with hexachlorophene baths for hospital personnel who were carriers of MRSA (115, 118, 119). Additional studies are needed to develop effective antimicrobial regimens for the eradication of the MRSA carrier state in patients and personnel.

Another approach to control of MRSA outbreaks might be a form of "protective isolation" for patients at high risk of acquiring MRSA. Thus, patients with severe underlying disease who are treated with antibiotics might be protected by the vigorous application of barrier techniques to decrease their risk of acquiring MRSA. This type of control measure might help in limiting the patient reservoir.

Since patients may carry MRSA for many months after discharge from the hospital, it is important that they be identified immediately on readmission. Such patients should be isolated until it can be determined whether they continue to be infected or colonized with MRSA (121, 122).

Toxic Shock Syndrome Due to Postoperative Wound Infection

In 1978 Todd and associates described a syndrome characterized by high fever, headache, confusion, conjunctival hyperemia, a scarlatiniform rash, subcutaneous edema, vomiting, watery diarrhea, oliguria, acute renal failure, hepatic abnormalities, disseminated intravascular coagulation, and severe prolonged shock (125). The illness occurred in seven children and appeared to be caused by an exotoxin elaborated by *S. aureus*. The latter microorganism was recovered from mucosal sites in four patients and from tissue sites in two patients.

In January, 1980 Andrew G. Dean and Jeffrey P. Davis, state epidemiologists in Minnesota and Wisconsin, reported several cases of toxic shock syndrome (TSS) to the Centers for Disease Control (CDC) (126). It was noted that these cases occurred in women during menstrual periods. It was also observed that many of these women used tampons. After these initial reports, many more cases of TSS were reported to the CDC. Like the earlier cases, most cases were in menstruating women who used tampons.

Clinical Manifestations. The onset of TSS is usually characterized by sudden onset of high fever. This is followed by vomiting, diarrhea, diffuse myalgia, arthralgia, orthostatic dizziness, and a diffuse, blanching macular erythroderma (127). Other manifestations included nonexudative mucous membrane inflammation with pharyngitis, strawberry tongue, conjunctivitis, diffuse vaginal hyperemia, and vulvar edema. The majority of patients were hypotensive, but only a minority had evidence of shock with oliguric renal failure or abnormal peripheral circulation. About half the patients had confusion and agitation. Five to 12 days after the rash had cleared, full thickness desquamation occurred, with the hands and feet most commonly involved. A minority of patients experienced patchy scalp alopecia and loss of fingernails, but these abnormalities were not permanent.

Laboratory Abnormalities. A majority of patients had one or more abnormal laboratory tests, including leukocytosis with an increase in band forms, sterile pyuria, prolonged prothrombin and partial thromboplastin times, hypocalcemia, and low total serum protein and albumin concentrations (127). Most patients also had elevated blood urea nitrogen, alanine transaminase, bilirubin, and creatine kinase levels. Less common laboratory findings included a mild, normochromic, normocytic, nonhemolytic anemia, thrombocytopenia, hypophosphatemia, and elevated serum creatinine.

The overwhelming majority of patients with TSS have cultures positive for *S. aureus* (127–129). The microorganism has been recovered either from sites of infection or from sites of mucosal colonization. Most isolates of *S. aureus* cultured from cases of TSS produce either pyrogenic enterotoxin C or enterotoxin F (127, 129).

Epidemiology. Within 2 years of the first reports of TSS related to menstruation and use of tampons, nonmenstrual cases of TSS were recognized and reported (128–131). The TSS in these cases was related to focal cutaneous and subcutaneous infections, postpartum infections, adenitis, bursitis, deep abscesses, "primary" bacteremia, mastitis, lung abscess, postoperative wound infections, and unknown sites of infection (128, 130, 131). The first case of TSS associated with a postoperative wound infection was reported in 1981 by Silver and Simon (132). The patient had onset of TSS 12 hours after amputation of his left index finger. Since the first report, there have been cases of TSS reported after a wide variety of operations (128, 129, 131, 133–146).

Since there is no laboratory test for the definitive diagnosis of TSS, diagnosis is made by clinical criteria. Most authors have adopted the CDC's case definition of TSS (126). It is important that this case definition be rigorously applied so that cases of TSS can be identified with a high degree of confidence.

The clinical manifestations of TSS are the same for both menstrually and nonmenstrually related cases. However, the demographic characteristics between these two types of TSS are substantially different (128, 130). Patients with nonmenstrual TSS were significantly older than patients with TSS related to menstruation. While 2% of patients with menstrual TSS were nonwhite, 13% of patients with TSS unrelated to menstruation

were nonwhite. Whereas patients with menstruation-associated TSS were obviously all female, the sex distribution for nonpostpartum, nonmenstruation-related cases of TSS was evenly divided among males and females.

More than half of the cases of TSS related to postoperative wound infections had onset of the syndrome within 48 hours of surgery (131). The incubation period in cases related to surgery may be as short as 12 hours and as long as 65 days. However, the overwhelming majority of cases have an onset within 1 week of surgery. The overall case/fatality ratio for nonmenstrual cases of TSS was 1%, but for cases with onset in 1980–1981 it was 6.3% (130). There was no relationship between delay in seeking medical care and a fatal outcome. The cause of death was a combination of irreversible respiratory failure, hypoperfusion, and disseminated intravascular coagulopathy.

One of the striking features of TSS associated with surgical wound infections was the minimal evidence of inflammation of the wound, or in many cases, the absence of signs of infection (128, 130, 131). It would appear that a very small inoculum of *S. aureus* in a surgical wound can cause TSS. Some cases have been associated with a stitch abscess, with only 5 ml of pus aspirated from a normal appearing wound, with failure to recover *S. aureus* from a surgical wound in a male patient, and with recovery of *S. aureus* from hemorrhagic fluid with no evidence of purulent exudate (132, 135, 142, 143). With some cases having onset within 12 hours and with over one-half appearing within 48 hours of surgery, the differential diagnosis of patients appearing with some of the signs and symptoms of TSS may not be limited to but would certainly have to include postoperative infections due to group A β-hemolytic streptococci and *Clostridium perfringens*. However, these latter infections usually have prominent signs of infection at the site of the surgical wound while signs of inflammation are minimal or absent in patients with TSS.

There are very few data on the reservoir or source of *S. aureus* that causes TSS in patients with postoperative wound infections. It is not known whether patients enter the hospital carrying toxigenic strains of *S. aureus* or whether they acquire them after hospitalization. The cases of TSS after nasal surgery suggest that some patients may enter the hospital carrying toxigenic strains of *S. aureus* in their nose (136, 144–146). After nasal surgery, nasal packing is routinely inserted. The combination of packing, blood, and disrupted mucosa is similar to the condition in menstruating women who develop TSS while using tampons. In one report of TSS after nasal surgery a small number of random samples of unopened sterile nasal packing were cultured (136). The cultures were negative.

In only one report was evidence presented of possible transmission in the hospital (131). In this report it was noted that a patient developed TSS within 1 week of another case in an adjacent room. It was not possible to determine whether transmission took place between the patients, because the second patient was not cultured. No other evidence for transmission of toxigenic strains of *S. aureus* in the hospital has been published. No data on risk factors for hospital-acquired TSS have been published.

No hospital outbreaks of TSS related to postoperative wound infections have been reported. There are no data on how to prevent infections with toxigenic strains of *S. aureus*. Of interest is the failure of antibiotic-impregnated nasal packing to prevent TSS after nasal surgery (144, 145).

Median Sternotomy Infections

Since its introduction by Julian and his associates in 1957, the median sternotomy incision has been universally adopted as the incision of choice for cardiac operations (147). Postoperative infections in these wounds may lead to serious morbidity and even to a fatal outcome. Fortunately, the reported incidence of this complication is low. The reported infection rates vary from 0.5% to 7.5%, but the rates from most series are ≤ 2.0% (148–151). Infection rates may also vary between types of procedures; Wells and co-workers observed a median sternotomy infection rate of 2.2% after intracardiac operations but a rate of 7.5% after coronary artery surgery (150).

Clinical Manifestations. Sternal wound infections are usually accompanied by fever and leukocytosis (152). Patients may have spiking fevers and signs of systemic sepsis as well as excessive incisional pain (149). Local signs of infection include erythema, purulent drainage, and sternal dehiscence (149, 152). Median sternotomy infections may be complicated by bacteremia (149). Occasionally sternal wound infections occur without evidence of local purulent exudate or dehiscence (152).

Causative Microorganisms. Most sternal wound infections are caused by bacteria. The most common bacterial causes of median sternotomy infections are staphylococci and gram-

negative bacilli (148, 150–154). Among gram-negative bacilli the most common isolates from sternal wound infections have been *Klebsiella*, *Pseudomonas*, *Escherichia coli*, and *Proteus mirabilis*. There has been only one reported anaerobic infection of a median sternotomy, and this was due to *Bacteroides fragilis* (155). The most common fungal cause of sternal wound infection is *Candida albicans* (149, 152, 156). Although much less common, there have been several outbreaks of sternal wound infections due to a zygomycete (*Rhizopus*) related to elastic bandages contaminated with this fungus (11–13).

The largest outbreak of median sternotomy infections was due to *Mycobacterium fortuitum* (14). In this outbreak 19 patients developed sternal wound infections. Two smaller outbreaks have also been reported (157, 158).

Epidemiology of Median Sternotomy Infections. Little is known about the epidemiology of sternal wound infections. In a few instances reservoirs or sources for the microorganisms that cause sternal wound infections have been documented. In the one reported case of *Pseudomonas cepacia* median sternotomy infection, the reservoir for *P. cepacia* was a contaminated detergent solution used to clean transducers (153). Suction pumps connected to mediastinal tubes were found to be the reservoir for *P. aeruginosa* that caused an outbreak of sternal wound infections in five patients (154). In the only outbreak of *M. fortuitum* infections for which a reservoir was identified, the microorganism was cultured from nonsterile ice used to cool the cardioplegia solution (158). Wells and co-workers provided some circumstantial evidence that bacteria that cause median sternotomy infections after coronary artery bypass surgery are from the patient's leg at the site of the incision made to harvest the saphenous vein (150).

There is also little information on the mode of transmission of microorganisms to the sternal wound. However, two types of transmission have been identified. First, there have been two reports describing contact transmission. In one report *P. aeruginosa* was transmitted by retrograde migration through mediastinal tubes from suction pumps to the mediastinum and sternal wound (154). In the other report there was evidence that ice water containing *M. fortuitum* was dripped into the sterile field (158). In addition to these reports Wells and co-workers suggested that bacteria that colonize the leg were transferred to the sternal wound by saphenous vein grafts (150).

The other mode of transmission is that of hematogenous seeding of the sternum. Weinstein and associates provided evidence that sternal wound infections may occur after bacteria seed the sternal wound during an episode of bacteremia (153).

Many variables have been reported as risk factors for sternal wound infection. However, no prospective epidemiologic studies on risk factors have been published. Breyer and his colleagues carried out a prospective study on sternal wound complications, but, unfortunately, the numbers of complications were small and the majority were noninfectious complications (159). Thus, the variables discussed below that are purported risk factors for median sternotomy infections should be considered possible risk factors for sternal wound infections. Variables that have been reported as risk factors include (a) myocardial revascularization procedures (compared to other types of cardiac surgery); (b) presence of pneumonia prior to surgery; (c) prolonged perfusion time; (d) long duration of the operation; (e) postoperative hemorrhage; (f) re-exploration for control of hemorrhage; (g) postoperative closed chest massage; and (h) depressed cardiac output in the postoperative period. The latter variables should be considered as a starting point for future prospective epidemiologic studies of risk factors for median sternotomy infection. Although use of internal mammary arteries for revascularization has been stated to be a risk factor for sternal wound infection, Nkongho and associates found no relationship between use of the internal mammary artery and infection (148, 149, 151).

In summary the epidemiology of median sternotomy infections involves reservoirs containing moisture where *Pseudomonas* species or atypical mycobacteria may survive and multiply or the skin of the leg colonized by *S. aureus* and gram-negative bacilli. Microorganisms are transmitted by some type of contact and, less commonly, by way of the bloodstream. Possible risk factors emphasize the apparent adverse effects of prolonged duration of extracorporeal circulation, postoperative hemorrhage, reoperation, and depressed cardiac output in the postoperative period.

Prevention of Median Sternotomy Infections. The limited information on the epidemiology of median sternotomy infections provides some basis for preventive measures. Moist reservoirs in the operating room that may provide a risk to patients should be eliminated. Great care should be exercised in harvesting the saphenous vein. The skin of the leg should be properly prepared and draped to prevent transmission of microorganisms from the skin of the leg to the sternum. Wells and co-workers described the technique in detail (150). Infections at other body sites should be eradicated prior to surgery, and all potential sources of bacteremia from use of intravascular devices should be eliminated, such as contaminated transducers. Exquisite attention should be paid to hemostasis during the operation to avoid postoperative hemorrhage and the need for reoperation.

One approach considered for the prevention of postoperative wound infections has been preoperative bathing with antiseptics (see above). Wells and co-workers failed to show a protective effect of preoperative bathing with chlorhexidine for median sternotomies (150). Although cardiac operations are usually considered clean surgery, Fong and associates were able to show a protective effect of methicillin for median sternotomy incisions (160). In a prospective, double-blind, randomized study, 21.3% of the control group developed sternal wound infections while there were no infections among the patients who received methicillin. However, only 105 subjects were studied, and the authors failed to explain satisfactorily the very high rate of infections in the control group. It is not clear at the present time what role prophylactic antibiotics should play in protocols for the prevention of infections in median sternotomies.

BURN WOUND INFECTIONS

The burn wound is made up of avascular necrotic tissue which is a good culture medium. In addition to the surface trauma, thermal injury results in global immunosuppression with a marked impairment in function of neutrophils (161, 162). Thus, the burn wound is very susceptible to infection.

Immediately after the thermal injury has been sustained, few microorganisms colonize the burn wound surface, and those present are usually gram-positive microorganisms (161). However, by the middle of the second postburn week, gram-negative bacteria have become the predominant surface flora of the wound. When microorganisms on the burn wound surface multiply and reach a high density, invasion of the burn eschar may take place. When microorganisms reach the subeschar space, further multiplication may take place (162). Invasion of the viable tissue subjacent to the burn eschar is accompanied by the clinical manifestations of burn wound infection. Penetration of microorganisms into blood vessels and lymphatics in subjacent viable tissue results in septicemia and is associated with a high mortality (163).

Clinical manifestations of burn wound infection (burn wound sepsis) include hypothermia or hyperthermia, altered mental status, ileus, and respiratory distress. In advanced cases of infection oliguria and shock may occur (161). Laboratory manifestations of burn wound infection include hyperglycemia or hypoglycemia, and leukopenia (161).

Burn wound infection is diagnosed by burn wound biopsy. Although microorganisms may be recovered from the surface of the burn wound on culture, such data are not reliable indicators of the presence or absence of burn wound infection. In some instances microorganisms recovered from the surface are different from those invading viable tissue beneath the eschar. The appearance of the burn wound may indicate infection, but again, surface features are not a reliable indicator for the presence or absence of burn wound infection. The definitive technique for diagnosis of burn wound infection is biopsy of the burn wound. A 500-mg sample should be taken from an area of the burn wound that appears infected. The biopsy must contain viable tissue subjacent to the eschar (162). The specimen should be divided into two parts. One portion should be sent to the microbiology laboratory for quantitation and identification of microorganisms, and the other portion should be sent to the pathology laboratory for histopathologic examination. The diagnosis of burn wound infection is made when microorganisms are identified in unburned tissue. Although less definitive, quantitation of microorganisms in the wound may be used for the diagnosis of burn wound infection. The presence of $\geq 10^5$ colony forming units (CFU)/g of burned tissue is suggestive of burn wound infection. Two studies showed a good correlation between burn wound infections and a concentration of 10^5 CFU/g of burned tissue, and one study suggested that institution of antibiotic therapy when concentrations of microorganisms reached 10^4 CFU/g of tissue would prevent burn wound infection (164–166). Woolfrey and associates identified several problems with quantitative burn wound biopsies, including a 25% chance that a microorganism present in the wound will not be detected by a single quantitative eschar culture (167). More recent studies continue to show an association between high concentrations of microorganisms in the burn eschar as determined by quantitative cultures of burn wound biopsies and burn wound infection (168–170). However, from these studies it can only be concluded that counts of 10^8 CFU/g of tissue are associated with burn wound infection and high mortality.

Freshwater and Su state that burn wound biopsies have little value if the residual eschar represents less than 20% of the total body surface area (171). If quantitative burn wound biopsies are used as the only diagnostic modality for burn wound infections, biopsies should be taken from multiple anatomic sites over the period of time that the patient appears to be at risk of burn wound infection (165, 171).

Microorganisms That Cause Burn Wound Infections

Most burn wound infections are caused by bacteria. Bacteria most commonly isolated from burn wound infections are shown in Table 22.5. These data from the CDC's National Nosocomial Infections Study indicate that *S. aureus* is the most frequent cause of burn wound infection. After *S. aureus*, the most frequent causes of burn wound infection are the gram-negative bacilli. As noted (Table 22.5) *Candida albicans* is the eighth most frequently isolated burn wound pathogen, and this reflects the increasing incidence of burn wound infections due to fungi. Spebar and Lindberg reported that 7% of burn patients developed burn wound infections due to fungi between 1973 and 1977 at the U.S. Army Institute of Surgical

Table 22.5. Frequency Distribution of Leading Burn Wound Pathogens, NNIS,[a] 1980 to 1984[b]

Pathogen	No. of Isolates	Percentage of Isolates
S. aureus	202	24.5
P. aeruginosa	159	19.3
Enterococci	97	11.8
E. coli	69	8.4
E. cloacae	64	7.8
S. marcescens	39	4.7
Coagulase-negative staphylococci	29	3.5
C. albicans	23	2.8
K. pneumoniae	20	2.4
P. mirabilis	17	2.1

[a] National Nosocomial Infections Study, Centers for Disease Control.

[b] Through November 13, 1984.

Research (172). Fungi that have been reported as burn wound pathogens include *C. albicans*, zygomycetes, *Asperigillus* species, *Fusarium* species, and *Cephalosporium* species (172–181). In addition to bacteria and fungi, viruses may rarely cause burn wound infections. Foley and associates reported six patients with herpesvirus infections of the burn wound (182).

Epidemiology of Burn Wound Infections

Since infections of the burn wound always develop more than 48 hours after admission, they are, by definition, hospital-acquired infections. It is not surprising that burn wound infections are such an important complication of thermal injury when one considers that these patients have lost at least part of the important mechanical barrier provided by the skin, that the burn eschar provides a rich culture medium, and that the burn wound always becomes colonized with microorganisms.

Reservoirs or Sources for Microorganisms That Cause Burn Wound Infections

Personnel.   There is little evidence that hospital staff are an important reservoir for microorganisms that cause infection of the burn wound. Hands of personnel are considered important vectors for transmission of microorganisms to the burn wound, but since these microorganisms are transient flora of the hands, they are usually easily removed by washing with soap and water. Thus, hands have not been considered a reservoir for these microorganisms. However, there is evidence that some hospital personnel who work in intensive care units and who have frequent contact with gram-negative microorganisms may become hand carriers of gram-negative bacilli (183). Such carriage in burn care personnel could constitute a reservoir for burn wound pathogens.

The nasopharynges of personnel are uncommon reservoirs for microorganisms that infect the burn wound. There have only been two reports in which nasopharyngeal carriers among burn unit staff could be implicated as a source for microorganisms that caused burn wound infection. These reports dealt with outbreaks of infection due to *Streptococcus pyogenes* and *S. aureus* (184, 185). The nasopharynx has not been identified as a reservoir for gram-negative bacilli. The hair has rarely been identified as a reservoir in burn unit staff, and there have been no reports

implicating the rectum as a reservoir for infection (184).

Patients.   The most important reservoir for microorganisms in burn care facilities is the population of the patients. Collectively, the gastrointestinal tracts and burn wounds of patients make up a very large reservoir of diverse types of microorganisms.

Several studies indicate that the gastrointestinal tract may be a reservoir for microorganisms that infect the burn wound. The gastrointestinal tract may be a reservoir for *P. aeruginosa*, Enterobacteriaceae, *Salmonella typhimurium*, *S. aureus*, yeasts, and *Acinetobacter* (186–191). Microorganisms that colonize the burn wound from the gastrointestinal tract may be present on admission (endogenous flora) or they may be acquired after admission. Lowbury and co-workers and Burke and associates have shown that microorganisms from the patient's normal bowel flora may colonize and infect the burn wound (188, 192). On the other hand, microorganisms may colonize the bowel of patients after they have been acquired from other patients, or microorganisms may colonize the gastrointestinal tract after they are ingested in food (190, 193, 194). Kominos and associates were able to recover *P. aeruginosa* from a variety of raw vegetables collected from a hospital kitchen (193). They found that four of the six most common clinical isolates were the same as the four most common types isolated from raw vegetables. In another report Kominos and associates observed that when raw vegetables were removed from the diet of burn patients and other steps were taken to eliminate *P. aeruginosa* from food, the sepsis rate due to *P. aeruginosa* decreased from 32% to 6.25% (194).

The most important patient reservoir for burn wound pathogens is the burn wound itself (186, 195, 196). Collectively, the burn wound surfaces of patients in a burn unit provide a huge reservoir of microorganisms for cross-contamination of other patients.

Environment.   A number of environmental surfaces have been identified as reservoirs or sources for microorganisms that colonize and infect the burn wound, particularly during outbreaks. *P. aeruginosa* has been the microorganism most frequently isolated from environmental surfaces. Shulman and colleagues recovered *P. aeruginosa* from sink faucets, handles, towel racks, and bars of soap during an outbreak in their burn unit (197). MacMillan and co-workers cultured *P. aeruginosa* from counter surfaces and bed rails during a study of endemic infections due to *P. aeruginosa* in a burn intensive care unit (198). Mattresses have been identified as reservoirs for both *P. aeruginosa* and *Acinetobacter calcoaceticus* in burn units (199, 200). Another potential reservoir in burn units is the "blanketrol" unit used for warming and cooling patients (201, p 321). Microorganisms have been cultured from the water that is circulated through these units.

Hydrotherapy equipment has been identified as a reservoir or source for both *Enterobacter cloacae* and *P. aeruginosa* (196–198, 202). It has been stated that sinks are an important reservoir for *P. aeruginosa*. However, data are conflicting, and sinks have never been established as a reservoir for *P. aeruginosa* that colonize and infect burn wounds. Kohn, MacMillan and co-workers, and Holder all suggested that sinks were important reservoirs for *P. aeruginosa* that caused burn wound colonization and infection, but they provided no evidence that *P. aeruginosa* from sinks was transmitted to the burn wounds of patients (186, 198, 203). Wormald and Kominos and associates found no evidence that sinks colonized by *P. aeruginosa* were reservoirs for isolates that colonized the burn wound surfaces of their patients (184, 204).

Modes of Transmission for Microorganisms That Cause Burn Wound Infections

Microorganisms are transferred from the many reservoirs or sources to the burn wound surface of the patient by one or more of several routes. Available epidemiologic data indicate that most, if not all, microorganisms are transmitted to the burn wound by some form of contact.

Feces of Patients. Fecal contamination of the burn wound appears to be a frequent event. That microorganisms from the intestinal reservoir reach the burn wound by way of feces is supported by the distribution of bowel flora on the wound. Microorganisms from the gastrointestinal tract are most commonly found on burn wounds involving groins, buttocks, perineum and inner aspect of the upper part of the thigh (187). Furthermore, a gradient has been found for intestinal flora with a higher frequency of isolation from the perianal area and lower frequencies of isolation for areas more remote from the anus (190). Studies in which burn patients were cared for in isolators also provided evidence that coliform bacteria were transmitted to the burn wound by fecal contamination (188).

Hands of Personnel. The most important mode of transmission for microorganisms that colonize and infect the burn wound is direct contact with contaminated hands of burn unit staff. Most reports that have evaluated hand contamination among personnel have involved studies of endemic or hyperendemic infections or outbreaks of infection due to *P. aeruginosa* (194, 195, 197, 202–204). In these reports up to 38% of personnel cultured had hands contaminated with *P. aeruginosa*. During an outbreak of infections in a burn center due to *E. cloacae*, Mayhall and associates cultured the epidemic strain from 50% of nursing staff who were sampled (196). Wenzel and co-workers found the epidemic strain in 8% of the hand samples taken from personnel during an outbreak caused by *Providencia stuartii* (205).

Although most transmission by contact with the hands of staff probably occurs by direct contact between patients, some contact transmission may be indirect. Thus, hands may be contaminated from environmental surfaces that were previously contaminated by contact with patients or the hands of personnel (195, 197, 203). In addition, microorganisms may be transmitted by hands even when gloves are worn between patients (202; CG Mayhall, unpublished data).

Fomites. There is some evidence that microorganisms may be transmitted to the burn wound by contact with contaminated surfaces of inanimate objects. Articles that have been implicated in the possible transmission of microorganisms in burn units include curtains, toys, books, papers, wash basins, crockery, glassware, clean pillows, urine bottles, bedpans, food trays, a chair, faucets, and the outer surface of a solution bottle (184, 188, 195, 198, 206).

Hydrotherapy equipment could be considered to be in a special category of fomites, since in addition to the potential for contact with contaminated surfaces there is also the possibility of contact with contaminated water. Two outbreaks of infections in burn patients have been related to contaminated hydrotherapy equipment (196, 202). It is not surprising that hydrotherapy equipment may be a vector for transmission of microorganisms between burn patients. Surfaces are moist and some areas of the equipment may not dry between uses. Agitators are very difficult to decontaminate, and water fixtures may become contaminated. Even when agitators are removed and a new disposable liner is used for each patient, cross-contamination of the hydrotherapy water between patients may still occur (196). Such cross-contamination of hydrotherapy water may occur via the hands of personnel. During hydrotherapy treatments, patients' burn wounds may also become colonized by direct contact with the contaminated hands of the staff (202).

Airborne Transmission. The airborne route would appear to be unimportant as a vector for transmission of microorganisms to the burn wound surface. Although it has been possible to demonstrate dispersal of microorganisms into the air from burn wounds, there is no evidence that microorganisms are transferred from the burn wound of one patient to the burn wound of another patient by way of the air. Hambraeus and Laurell and Hambraeus demonstrated dispersal of *S. aureus* into the air from burn wounds with heavier shedding from the larger wounds (185, 207). However, they were unable to show that airborne *S. aureus* was transmitted to the surface of patients' burn wounds. Lowbury and co-workers suggested that *S. aureus* was transmitted by both contact and airborne spread since infection rates were lowered only when patients were nursed in isolators that would block both contact and airborne transmission (188). They did not, however, provide any direct evidence that *S. aureus* was transmitted between patients by the airborne route.

Barclay and Dexter and Lowbury and Fox concluded that *P. aeruginosa* was transmitted between their patients by airborne spread, but they provided no convincing evidence for this route of transmission (187, 195). In their studies Kohn, Lowbury and co-workers, Mayhall and associates, and MacMillan and co-workers found no evidence for airborne transmission of gram-negative bacilli between burn patients (186, 188, 196, 198). Wenzel and co-workers suggested that *P. stuartii* was transmitted between patients by the airborne route during an outbreak in their burn unit (205). However, they recovered *P. stuartii* from the air in very small numbers and could not rule out transmission between patients by contact with the hands of personnel or with fomites.

Most microorganisms are probably transmitted to the burn wound by the contaminated hands of personnel and by feces. Contact with the surface of inanimate objects and water in hydrotherapy tanks is of lesser importance but is probably responsible for colonization of burn wounds in some patients. It would appear unlikely that airborne transmission is of any importance as a

route for transfer of microorganisms between burn patients.

Risk Factors for Colonization of the Burn Wound

The presence of one or more reservoirs and modes of transmission for a given microorganism does not assure that the burn wound surface will be colonized by that microorganism. There are factors which may enhance the risk for colonization of the burn wound. One risk factor may be the virulence of the microorganism, but a discussion of virulence is beyond the scope of this chapter. Other factors of importance include the size of the burn wound and the use of systemic and topical antimicrobial agents.

Size of the Burn Wound. Barclay and Dexter concluded that the distribution of the burn wound on the body was more important than the size of the wound in predicting whether *P. aeruginosa* would contaminate the wound (187). Contrary to this, several authors have reported a relationship between wound size and the likelihood of wound colonization. Wormald found a much higher colonization rate of wounds that covered 30% or more of the body surface than of wounds that covered less than 30% of the surface area (184). Kohn found that 100% of patients with burns $\geq$ 40% of the body surface area became colonized with *P. aeruginosa* (186). He also reported that only 7.1% of patients with less than 10% body surface area burns became colonized, whereas 54.2% of patients with burns $\geq$ 10% surface area had colonization of their burns by *P. aeruginosa.* Lowbury and Fox reported similar findings to those of Wormald and Kohn (195). Twenty-eight of their 30 (93.3%) patients with burns of $\geq$ 21% of the body surface area developed burn wound colonization with *P. aeruginosa* compared with 128 of 301 (42.5%) patients with burns $\leq$ 20% of surface area.

A large burn is a risk factor for colonization with *P. aeruginosa.* There are no published data on the relationship between burn size and other microorganisms that colonize and infect the burn wound. However, burn size should be considered a possible risk factor for colonization with other microorganisms when the epidemiology of burn pathogens other than *P. aeruginosa* is being studied.

Systemic Antibiotics. Although it has been generally accepted that development of antibiotic resistance is related to extensive use of antibiotics and that use of antibiotics to which many microorganisms are resistant will select out resistant strains, there are few data on the use of systemic antibiotics and selection of resistant microorganisms that subsequently colonize the burn wound surface. Lilly and Lowbury observed that withdrawal of erythromycin prophylaxis in a burn unit resulted in a fall in the proportion of *S. aureus* resistant to erythromycin and other antibiotics including methicillin, novobiocin, lincomycin, tetracycline, kanamycin, and cephaloridine (208). Even though the data are sparse, it is likely that systemic administration of antibiotics is a risk factor for colonization of the burn wound with resistant microorganisms.

Topical Antimicrobial Agents. That development of resistance to topical agents is a risk factor for colonization of the burn wound with resistant microorganisms has not been proven. However, it is clear that some burn pathogens develop resistance to the topical agents and that during some outbreaks, the epidemic strain was resistant to the topical agent in use at the time of the outbreak.

There have been several reports of resistance of burn wound pathogens to silver nitrate. Silver nitrate resistance has been reported in *Salmonella typhimurium*, *Klebsiella* sp., *Enterobacter* sp., and *P. aeruginosa* (189, 209–211). Burn wound pathogens may also become resistant to silver sulfadiazine. Wenzel and co-workers observed that the epidemic strain was resistant to silver sulfadiazine during the outbreak in their burn unit due to *P. stuartii* (205). Gayle and associates reported that the strain of *E. cloacae* that caused their outbreak was resistant to silver sulfadiazine with minimal bactericidal concentrations of > 3200 µg/ml (212). In addition to the resistance to silver compounds, microorganisms that colonize the burn wound may become resistant to gentamicin when the latter antibiotic is applied topically to the wound (197, 213). Since gentamicin is a very important drug for treatment of gram-negative sepsis in burn patients, its use topically has largely been discontinued to avoid the marked tendency for selection of resistant microorganisms on the burn surface.

Prevention of Burn Wound Infections

Prevention of burn wound infections involves use of good barrier nursing techniques, prevention of the transfer of microorganisms by fomites and hydrotherapy, elimination of foods that contain potentially pathogenic microorganisms, and use of topical antimicrobial agents to suppress multiplication of microorganisms on the burn wound surface. A much less common approach to prevention of burn wound infections is the use of isolators or special isolation rooms.

Barrier Technique

The most important aspect of barrier technique is the establishment of individual environments for each patient in the unit (201, p 335). All surfaces and objects in each patient's immediate environment are considered contaminated for all of the other patients. In most burn care facilities, burn unit staff wear surgical scrub clothes. Personnel should wear a gown or plastic apron and gloves for contact with each patient. Hands should be washed prior to donning the gloves. After contact with a patient, personnel should consider themselves contaminated for all other patients. While gloved, personnel should not touch surfaces such as cubicle curtains which may later be touched with ungloved hands. After gown or apron and gloves are removed, hands should again be washed. If the surgical scrub suit has been inadvertently soiled, it should be changed prior to contact with the next patient. Contaminated trash and soiled linen should be bagged and removed from the unit as quickly as possible. Surfaces in the environment immediately adjacent to the patient's bed (bedside table, across the bed table, bedrails, etc) should be cleaned with a disinfectant at frequent intervals.

Fomites and Hydrotherapy

Fomites. There is evidence that contact with inanimate surfaces may transmit microorganisms to the burn wound surface (see above). Prevention of this type of transmission involves decontamination of surfaces that can be disinfected, use of disposable devices, and removal of materials, devices, and other articles that cannot be disinfected.

Surfaces of tables, bedrails, and intravenous poles can readily be disinfected. EKG leads would be difficult to disinfect under the usual working conditions and could be replaced with disposable leads. Toys such as stuffed animals that cannot be disinfected should be removed from the burn unit. Each patient should be assigned his own stethoscope and blood pressure cuff so that these items do not have to be shared between patients. Equipment that must be used for the care of all patients must be carefully cleaned and disinfected between patients. Particular attention should be paid to mattresses. After discharge of a patient, the mattress surface should be disinfected. If the mattress cover is perforated or torn, it should be replaced or the mattress should be discarded.

Hydrotherapy. Hydrotherapy equipment must be thoroughly cleaned and disinfected between each patient use. Agitators may be particularly difficult to clean (202). Even when disinfectant is circulated through these devices, all contaminating microorganisms may not be eliminated. This difficulty can be alleviated by removing the agitators and using a disposable plastic liner for each patient. The water is agitated by compressed air forced through channels in the bottom of the liner.

Even when plastic liners are used, cross-contamination of hydrotherapy water may still occur (196). Such cross-contamination may occur by contaminated hands of personnel or by contaminated plumbing. Cross-contamination by personnel may be controlled by using shoulder length disposable gloves and disposable gowns or aprons between patients (196). Contaminated filling hoses should be replaced by plumbing devices that cannot contaminate hydrotherapy water and that can be disinfected (201, p 336).

Another approach to preventing transmission of microorganisms by hydrotherapy water is addition of antiseptic agents to the water. Even when hydrotherapy water is not contaminated prior to contact with the patient, there is some concern that microorganisms from other areas of the body, such as the rectum, may be transferred by the water to the burn wound. Although there are only three studies on addition of antiseptics to hydrotherapy water, there is evidence that the water may be maintained free of microorganisms during treatments. Smith and colleagues found that sodium hypochlorite was very effective in eliminating microorganisms from hydrotherapy water (214). At a concentration of 425 or 850 μg/ml, bacteria were not isolated from the water before, during, or after hydrotherapy. At these concentrations, there was a 1 or 2 log decrease in bacteria/cm^3 of burned sites and normal skin. The authors did not comment on the presence or absence of any untoward reactions. Steve and co-workers tubbed patients in water containing chloramine-T at a concentration of 200 parts per million (215). They observed that cultures of the equipment before and after treatments were negative. They reported that after 5 days of therapy, all gram-negative microorganisms had been eradicated from the burn wounds. The authors observed no side effects in patients or staff. Stone and Kolb added povidone-iodine to hydrotherapy water and found that the rate of residual contamination of hydrotherapy equipment after cleaning decreased from 50% to 12.9% (202). These limited studies indicate that addition of antiseptics to hydrotherapy water may be of value in decreasing the risk of transmission of microorganisms to the burn wound surface. More studies need to be done, and additional antiseptics should be evaluated.

Elimination of Potential Pathogens from the Diet

From the data available, it would appear that raw fruits and vegetables are frequently contaminated with gram-negative bacilli when they arrive at the hospital. There is also evidence that, after ingestion, these microorganisms may pass through the gastrointestinal tract and be transferred from feces to the burn wound (see above). Based on this evidence, burn patients' diets should be made up only of cooked foods. Raw fruits and vegetables should be excluded. It is important to keep in mind that microorganisms may be added to cooked foods inadvertently in the hospital kitchen. Kominos and associates found that cutting boards, knives, a blender, and the hands of some kitchen personnel yielded *P. aeruginosa* on culture (193, 194).

Topical Antimicrobial Agents

Topical antimicrobial agents are applied to the surface of the burn wound to suppress the growth of colonizing microorganisms. Suppression of the surface flora would appear to be important, because multiplication of microorganisms to high concentrations on the wound surface is thought to be necessary for microbial invasion of the burn eschar. Introduction of silver nitrate and mafenide acetate (Sulfamylon) in 1965 appeared to bring about a marked reduction in mortality due to burn wound infection (216). This was followed by the introduction of silver sulfadiazine in 1968 (216). Although these agents are reported to have reduced the incidence of burn wound sepsis and mortality due to burn wound infection, none has been tested in placebo-controlled clinical trials. Topical agents continue to be used, because when compared with historical controls, they appear to have significantly reduced the incidence of burn wound sepsis. Selection of a topical agent should depend on susceptibility tests against the microorganisms most commonly encountered on the burn wounds of patients in a given burn unit as well as the known side effects of each topical preparation.

Resistance of microorganisms to silver nitrate, silver sulfadiazine, and gentamicin has been reported but not to mafenide acetate (189, 197, 205, 209, 211–213, 217). When microorganisms commonly found on the burn wound become resistant to the topical agent in use, a new preparation to which the microorganisms are susceptible should be selected. Preparations such as mafenide acetate and silver sulfadiazine may be alternated every 12 hours with mafenide acetate applied in the morning and silver sulfadiazine in the evening (218).

Protected Environments

Another approach to prevention of burn wound infections is to nurse patients in protected environments such as isolators or isolation rooms with laminar airflow. Personnel don sterile clothing and gloves when caring for patients in these protected environments, but linens and food are not sterilized. Burke and associates compared contamination and infection rates of burn wounds of patients nursed in a protected environment with those nursed in single rooms or in a conventional burn unit (192). They found a significantly higher wound cross-contamination rate in patients nursed in single rooms or a burn unit compared to patients treated in the protected environment. On the other hand, contamination of the wound from the gastrointestinal tract (autocontamination) occurred at about the same rate for all groups of patients. Of most importance was the finding that infection was significantly more likely to occur if the wound was contaminated by a cross-contaminating strain than if it were contaminated by a strain from the gastrointestinal tract.

Demling and colleagues studied the effects of nursing burn patients in a laminar airflow room compared to nursing them in an intensive care unit (219). They noted that cross-contamination did not occur in the laminar airflow room but that it occurred frequently in burn patients nursed in the intensive care unit. Bacterial isolates from patients in the intensive care unit were much more likely to be highly resistant gram-negative bacilli than were those recovered from patients in the laminar airflow room. The mortality rate for patients in the laminar airflow room was 25% compared to a mortality rate of 55% for patients in the intensive care unit.

The limited data available indicate that nursing burn patients in protected environments may be effective in preventing burn wound infections, particularly those due to the more resistant gram-negative bacilli found in the hospital. However, none of the few published studies has been randomized or adequately controlled. Since the airborne route of transmission does not appear to be important for transfer of microorganisms to the burn wound surface (see above), it is doubtful that the laminar airflow is an important part of the protected environment. Indeed, Demling and Maly suggested that protected environments are effective in preventing burn wound infections because sterile and nonsterile areas are well defined and not because of the laminar airflow (220).

Disadvantages of protected environments include substantial psychologic problems for patients and nursing staff and the larger number of staff needed to take care of patients in a protected environment (220). Given the limited data on efficacy and the high capital investment required for establishing protected environments in a hospital, many more studies should be conducted before this modality of prevention is widely accepted for care of burn patients.

New Aspects of Burn Wound Infections

Effect of Systemic Antibiotic Therapy on the Microbial Flora of the Burn Wound

It has been widely stated that systemically administered antimicrobial agents are not very effective in the treatment of burn wound infections, because they penetrate poorly into the vascular burn eschar. However, Polk and co-workers showed that the aminoglycosides gentamicin and tobramycin reach therapeutic concentrations in burn eschar when administered intravenously (221). Therapeutic concentrations of both drugs were attained in both superficial and deep layers of eschar. Mayhall and associates observed that when concentrations of aminoglycoside exceeded the minimal bactericidal concentrations of the microorganisms in the deep layer of the wound, in most instances, the microorganisms were eliminated from the eschar (222). However, of great importance was the additional observation that the burn eschar was often rapidly repopulated by a highly resistant superinfecting gram-negative microorganism. In each case superinfection took place within 4 days of onset of therapy. The microorganism most commonly isolated from the deep layer of the burn wound before systemic antimicrobial therapy was *P. aeruginosa*. The only microorganism isolated from the superinfected wounds was *Serratia marcescens*. Thus, endemic, hyperendemic, and epidemic infections caused by two different microorganisms could occur simultaneously in a burn unit, and the microorganism isolated from the burn wound of a given patient might depend on whether he was on systemic antibiotic therapy. In order to understand the epidemiology of burn wound infections in a given burn unit, frequent burn wound biopsies (see above) need to be done on each patient over the course of his hospitalization. Such information about changes of the microbial flora of wounds is also needed for effective antimicrobial therapy of burn wound sepsis. The interaction between the epidemiology and treatment of burn wound infections is depicted in Figure 22.1.

Burn Wound Infections Due to Methicillin-Resistant *S. aureus*

Outbreaks of burn wound infections due to methicillin-resistant *S. aureus* (MRSA) are par-

ticularly serious because of the large surface area of the body involved and the marked difficulty in controlling such outbreaks. Another important aspect of MRSA infections of burn wounds was the observation by Boyce and colleagues that there was a significant rise of MRSA infections in nonburn patients when new cases of colonization or infection were reported among burn patients (223). Once established, MRSA has seldom been eradicated from a burn unit patient population.

Epidemiology of MRSA Burn Wound Infections. As noted for postoperative wound infections due to MRSA, personnel who are nasal carriers of MRSA may be a reservoir for burn wound infections due to MRSA (106, 118, 123, 223–225). However, the major reservoir for MRSA that causes burn wound infections is made up of the burn wounds of patients who are colonized or infected by MRSA (101, 106, 118, 123, 124, 223, 224). MRSA may be cultured from the rectum of some patients, but the gastrointestinal

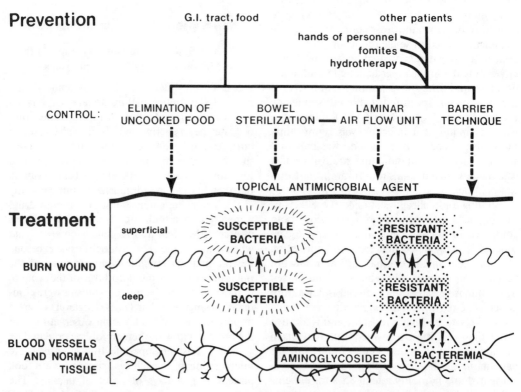

Figure 22.1. Interaction between the epidemiology and treatment of burn wound infection. The burn wound may be rapidly repopulated with resistant microorganisms during systemic antibiotic therapy. (From Mayhall CG, Polk RE, Haynes BW: Infections in burned patients. *Infect Control* 4:454–459, 1983.)

tract does not appear to be a major reservoir for MRSA that infects burn wounds.

Unlike the environment of patients with MRSA postoperative wound infections, the environment of burn patients with MRSA burn wound colonization or infection is frequently contaminated by MRSA (104, 123, 124). Rutala and co-workers carried out a systematic study of environmental contamination by MRSA in a burn unit over a longer period of time than had ordinarily been studied (124). They found that 16%, 31%, and 40% of the bacterial isolates from air, elevated surfaces, and floor surfaces, respectively, were MRSA. The mean counts for air, elevated surfaces, and floor surfaces were 1.9 CFU/cubic foot, 20 CFU/Rodac plate, and 48 CFU/Rodac plate, respectively. Although there is no evidence that MRSA are spread in any patient population by the airborne route, the heavy surface contamination would provide a ready source for contamination of hands of personnel. Another source of MRSA in the environment that has been reported is the silver sulfadiazine ointment used for topical prophylaxis (104). MRSA has also been cultured from hydrotherapy equipment (104, 123, 201, p 323).

As is the case for transmission of other microorganisms to the burn wound surface, the most important mode of transmission for MRSA appears to be by contact with the contaminated hands of personnel (123, 201, p 323). There is no direct evidence for transmission of MRSA by fomites, but the high level of environmental contamination by MRSA in burn units makes this mode of transmission plausible. There are data highly suggestive of transmission by hydrotherapy. First, Saroglou and associates found that the air manifold of a whirlpool bath was contaminated by MRSA (104). Such contamination could lead to inoculation of the hydrotherapy water with MRSA. Second, Crossley and colleagues recovered MRSA from hydrotherapy tubs after disinfection, suggesting that the hydrotherapy water for subsequent patients could become contaminated from the residual contamination of the tanks (123). Third, in one outbreak it appeared that transmission of MRSA to burn patients may have occurred after contamination of the hands of hydrotherapy personnel from hydrotherapy equipment (201, p 323). Although MRSA has been recovered from air samples in burn units, no evidence has been provided that airborne transmission of MRSA occurs (118, 123, 124). When quantitative air samples have been taken, the concentration of MRSA in the air has only

been about 2 CFU/cubic foot of air (124). Airborne transmission does not seem a likely route for spread of MRSA among patients in a burn unit.

Little is known about risk factors for colonization or infection of the burn wound by MRSA. Locksley and colleagues performed a case-control study in an attempt to elucidate risk factors for infection due to MRSA (106). Controls were patients from whom methicillin-sensitive *S. aureus* was isolated. Cases included patients without burns who had other types of infections. They found a significant association between duration of hospitalization before isolation of *S. aureus* and administration of multiple antibiotics and infection due to MRSA. However, since there were many patients with other types of infections among the cases, it is uncertain whether the findings of this case-control study can be applied to patients with burn wound infections.

Prevention of Burn Wound Infection Due to MRSA. Many of the concepts underlying the techniques used to prevent transmission of MRSA among patients with postoperative wounds can also be applied to prevention or control of burn wound infections caused by MRSA (see above). Thus, the patient reservoir must be continuously assessed by contact tracing of the patients who have been exposed to cases of burn wound colonization or infection. Contacts should be cultured weekly using a selective culture medium (see above). All possible sites, including the nares, that could harbor MRSA should be cultured. Multiple burn wound sites should be cultured each time to minimize sampling error since colonization or infection may not involve the entire wound. Contacts are cultured until they become positive for MRSA or until they have had three consecutive negative sets of cultures after their last exposure to a case. Periodic point prevalence culture surveys using the selective medium could be performed in the group of burn patients who are not known to be contacts of cases to identify patients who may have become colonized through unrecognized exposure to a case. The hospital laboratory should monitor all clinical cultures for MRSA.

Patients who have colonization or infection with MRSA should be isolated with rigorous application of barrier techniques (see above). In addition to the barrier techniques described above, patients with positive cultures for MRSA should be moved into private rooms whenever possible. Personnel should be assigned to patients isolated for MRSA colonization or infection, and they should work only with these patients. An attempt should be made to move stable patients with small burns and positive cultures for MRSA out of the unit to a private isolation room. These patients present a lower risk to patients in other areas of the hospital than they do to other patients in the burn unit. On the other hand, nursing personnel who work in other areas of the hospital where there are patients colonized or infected with MRSA should not be pulled to work in the burn unit.

The techniques for prevention of transmission of microorganisms to burn wounds by fomites and hydrotherapy described above also apply to prevention of transmission of MRSA. If patients have colonization or infection due to MRSA at body sites other than the burn wound, an antiseptic might be added to the hydrotherapy water in an attempt to prevent inoculation of the burn wound from the other colonized or infected sites.

An attempt might be made to eradicate MRSA from body sites other than the burn wound using the regimen of Ward and Colleagues (120). The regimen could be used when patients have colonization of nares, sputum, or surgical wounds outside of the burned area. There are no data as to whether this regimen could eradicate colonization of the burn wound. Since topical antimicrobial agents may prevent colonization of the burn wound surface with some microorganisms or at least suppress their multiplication, the antimicrobial susceptibility of MRSA strains to available topical agents should be determined. An agent should be chosen to which the MRSA is susceptible.

Viral Infections in Burn Patients

The first report on viral infections in burn patients was published by Foley and co-workers in 1970 (182). Their report dealt only with viral infections of the burn wound due to *Herpesvirus hominis*. Later that year the same group published a case report of cytomegalovirus infection in a burn patient (226). Since these early reports, little has been published on viral infections in burn patients. Most of the available data have appeared in the literature since 1981. These reports have mostly covered infections caused by the herpesviruses.

Herpes Simplex Virus Infections. Most of the Herpes simplex infections reported have been systemic infections without involvement of the burn wound. However, the first report by Foley and co-workers presented six patients with *Herpesvirus hominis* (herpes simplex) infections of the burn wound (182). Herpetic lesions in the burn wound appeared from 1 week to 1 month postburn. The herpetic infection frequently involved the face, neck, and chest. The lesions were usually found in areas of healing second-degree burns and donor sites. The herpetic infection was frequently complicated by secondary bacterial infection. Secondary bacterial infection was associated with conversion of partial thickness to full thickness skin loss. Two of the six patients developed systemic infection with the herpes simplex virus, and this led to their demise.

Most infections due to herpes simplex virus in burn patients have not been obvious clinically. Linnemann and MacMillan observed that 25% of their patients developed serologic evidence of herpes simplex infection, but only two had clinical evidence of infection; one had fever blisters and one had infection of a perioral burn wound (227). In a prospective study by Kagan and associates, 40% of their burn patients developed infection due to herpes simplex (228). The mean time of infection was 2.2 weeks postburn. Both primary and reactivation infections were observed. Herpes simplex infections were significantly associated with age ≥ 50 years, tracheal intubation, facial burn, smoke inhalation, hospitalization longer than 3 weeks, and full thickness burn. As in the other series, there was an important relationship between facial burns and herpesvirus infection. This relationship is likely a reflection of the fact that the trigeminal ganglion is the site of herpes simplex latency.

Cytomegalovirus Infections. Thirty-three per cent of the burn patients studied prospectively by Linnemann and MacMillan developed infection due to cytomegalovirus (CMV) (227). These authors studied pediatric burn patients who ranged in age from 4 to 14 years. They noted both early and late infections; early infections appeared 7 to 11 days postburn, and late infections appeared 2 to 4 months after the patients had been burned. Patients with early CMV infections were similar to patients who did not develop CMV infections. On the other hand, those with late infections had significantly larger third-degree burns and required significantly more skin grafts and blood transfusions. Patients with late infections also had significantly more febrile days and longer hospitalizations. Kagan and associates also found that 33% of their burn patients developed CMV infections, and infection appeared a mean of 3.8 weeks after burning (228). In a mixed adult and pediatric burn population they found that occurrence of CMV infection was significantly associated only with hospitalization for longer than 3 weeks and having a full thickness burn. They observed both primary and reactivation infections; the onset at a mean of 3.8 weeks may be an average onset when primary and reactivation infections were combined.

The clinical picture of CMV infections in burn patients is one of unexplained fever which lasts for 1 to 4 weeks in a patient whose burn wound is healing well without signs of infection (227, 229). Lymphocytosis occurs in most patients, but hepatitis is seen in a minority of the patients (227, 229). Other common manifestations of CMV, such as myalgias, arthralgias, pneumonia, and retinitis, have not been observed in burn patients (229). The burn wound does not appear to be directly involved by CMV infection. Infections due to CMV in burn patients are not associated with higher mortality (228).

In summary, CMV infections in burn patients may be primary or reactivation infections and usually appear 1 to 4 months postburn. They are observed in patients with the most severe burns who require prolonged hospitalization. They do not involve the burn wound directly but are manifested by prolonged fever and lymphocytosis in patients without signs of burn wound infection. It is important that CMV infections in burn patients be recognized so that the unnecessary administration of toxic antibiotics and the performance of invasive diagnostic procedures can be avoided.

New Topical Antimicrobial Agents

Topical antimicrobial agents appear to suppress the growth of microorganisms on the burn wound surface. Currently, there are only three agents in general use. These include silver nitrate, mafenide acetate (Sulfamylon), and silver sulfadiazine. Unfortunately, resistance has been reported to silver nitrate and silver sulfadiazine (189, 205, 209, 212). Although resistance to mafenide acetate has not been reported, it may cause pain on application, and it may cause acid-base changes (217). Mafenide acetate inhibits carbonic anhydrase, and this may cause a metabolic acidosis. With the development of resistance to two of the most commonly used agents, several investigators have reported on studies of new topical antimicrobial preparations.

Zinc Sulfadiazine. This preparation has been studied only in animals (230). It appeared to be effective against *Pseudomonas aeruginosa* infections in burned mice and rats. There was good uptake of the preparation by the burn wound but negligible absorption into body fluids. Zinc sulfadiazine seemed to have a positive effect on wound healing. This agent may hold some promise as a new topical agent, but it will have to undergo clinical trials before it can be determined whether it is safe and effective in burn patients.

Cerium Nitrate-Silver Sulfadiazine Cream. In a prospective randomized study Munster and co-workers found no difference between cerium nitrate-silver sulfadiazine cream and silver sulfadiazine cream (231). There was no difference in the mortality rate, mortality rate due to sepsis, concentration of microorganisms in the burn wound, or distribution of bacterial isolates by microorganism between the two groups. Cerium nitrate-silver sulfadiazine does not appear to represent a significant advance in topical antimicrobial agents for burn wound prophylaxis.

Phenoxetol-Chlorhexidine Cream. In a controlled clinical trial in which phenoxetol-chlorhexidine cream was compared with a cream containing 0.5% silver nitrate and 0.2% chlorhexidine, Lawrence and colleagues found little difference in the antimicrobial effects of the two preparations (232). The most important differences observed were that phenoxetol-chlorhexidine cream did not cause electrolyte imbalance or stain surfaces with which it came into contact. Since the degree to which phenoxetol is absorbed is unknown, there is some concern about possible systemic toxicity. More clinical trials with determination of phenoxetol serum levels need to be carried out before this new agent can be accepted for general use.

Silver Pefloxacin. In animal studies Modak and co-workers found that the mortality in burned mice due to *P. aeruginosa* dropped from 80% in the group treated with silver sulfadiazine to 10% in groups treated with topical pefloxacin or silver pefloxacin (233). There was little systemic absorption of pefloxacin and no absorption of silver from topical prophylaxis. Furthermore, silver pefloxacin has much more antimicrobial activity in vitro against bacteria and fungi than does silver sulfadiazine. Silver pefloxacin should be tested in clinical studies for safety and efficacy. It may prove to be an important addition to the armamentarium for topical prophylaxis of burn wound infection.

References

1. Doberneck RC, Kleinman R: The surgical garb. *Surgery* 95:694–698, 1984.
2. Dixon RE: Effect of infections on hospital care. *Ann Intern Med* 89 (Part 2):749–753, 1978.

3. Green JW, Wenzel RP: Postoperative wound infection: a controlled study of the increased duration of hospital stay and direct cost of hospitalization. *Ann Surg* 185:264–268, 1977.
4. Cruse PJE, Foord R: The epidemiology of wound infection. A 10-year prospective study of 62,939 wounds. *Surg Clin North Am* 60:27–40, 1980.
5. Haley RW, Schaberg DR, Von Allmen SD, McGowan JE Jr: Estimating the extra charges and prolongation of hospitalization due to nosocomial infections: a comparison of methods. *J Infect Dis* 141:248–257, 1980.
6. Stone HH, Haney BB, Kolb LD, Geheber CE, Hooper CA: Prophylactic and preventive antibiotic therapy. Timing, duration and economics. *Ann Surg* 189:691–699, 1979.
7. Moncrief JA, Teplitz C: Changing concepts in burn sepsis. *J Trauma* 4:233–245, 1964.
8. Alexander JW, MacMillan BG: Infections of burn wounds. In Bennett JV, Brachman PS (eds): *Hospital Infections*. Boston, Little, Brown, and Co, 1979, p 336.
9. National Academy of Sciences-National Research Council: Postoperative wound infections: the influence of ultraviolet irradiation of the operating room and of various other factors. *Ann Surg* 160 (Suppl 2):1–132, 1964.
10. Altemeier WA, Burke JF, Pruitt BA, Sandusky WR (eds): *Manual on Control of Infection in Surgical Patients*, ed 2. Philadelphia, JB Lippincott, 1984.
11. Gartenberg G, Bottone EJ, Keusch GT, Weitzman I: Hospital-acquired mucormycosis (*Rhizopus rhizopodiformis*) of skin and subcutaneous tissue. Epidemiology, mycology and treatment. *N Engl J Med* 299:1115–1118, 1978.
12. Sheldon DL, Johnson WC: Cutaneous mucomycosis. Two documented cases of suspected nosocomial cause. *JAMA* 241:1032–1034, 1979.
13. Everett ED, Pearson S, Rogers W: *Rhizopus* surgical wound infection associated with elasticized adhesive tape dressings. *Arch Surg* 114:738–739, 1979.
14. Robicsek F, Daugherty HK, Cook JW, Selle JG, Masters TN, O'Bar PR, Fernandez CR, Mauney CU, Calhoun DM: *Mycobacterium fortuitum* epidemics after open-heart surgery. *J Thorac Cardiovasc Surg* 75:91–96, 1978.
15. Foz A, Roy C, Jurado J, Arteaga E, Ruiz JM, Moragas A: *Mycobacterium chelonei* iatrogenic infections. *J Clin Microbiol* 7:319–321, 1978.
16. Galle PC, Homesley HD, Rhyne AL: Reassessment of the surgical scrub. *Surg Gynecol Obstet* 147:215–218, 1978.
17. Walter CW, Kundsin RB: The bacteriologic study of surgical gloves from 250 operations. *Surg Gynecol Obstet* 129:949–952, 1969.
18. Hambraeus A, Laurell G: Protection of the patient in the operating suite. *J Hosp Infect* 1:15–30, 1980.
19. Schwartz JT, Saunders DE: Microbial penetration of surgical gown materials. *Surg Gynecol Obstet* 150:507–512, 1980.
20. Moylan JA, Kennedy BV: The importance of gown and drape barriers in the prevention of wound infection. *Surg Gynecol Obstet* 151:465–470, 1980.
21. Laufman H, Eudy WW, Vandernoot AM, Liu D, Harris CA: Strike-through of moist contamination by woven and nonwoven surgical materials. *Ann Surg* 181:857–862, 1975.
22. Dineen P, Drusin L: Epidemics of postoperative wound infections associated with hair carriers. *Lancet* 2:1157–1159, 1973.
23. McKee WM, Di Caprio JM, Roberts CE Jr, Sherris JC: Anal carriage as the probable source of a streptococcal epidemic. *Lancet* 2:1007–1009, 1966.
24. McIntyre DM: An epidemic of Streptococcus pyogenes puerperal and postoperative sepsis with an unusual carrier site—the anus. *Am J Obstet Gynecol* 101:308–314, 1968.
25. Schaffner W, Lefkowitz LB Jr, Goodman JS, Koenig MG: Hospital outbreak of infections with group A streptococci traced to an asymptomatic anal carrier. *N Engl J Med* 280:1224–1225, 1969.
26. Gryska PF, O'Dea AE: Postoperative streptococcal wound infection. The anatomy of an epidemic. *JAMA* 213:1189–1191, 1970.
27. Richman DD, Breton SJ, Goldmann DA: Scarlet fever and group A streptococcal surgical wound infection traced to an anal carrier. *J Pediatr* 90:387–390, 1977.
28. Stamm WE, Feeley JC, Facklam RR: Wound infections due to group A *Streptococcus* traced to a vaginal carrier. *J Infect Dis* 138:287–292, 1978.
29. Berkelman RL, Martin D, Graham DR, Mowry J, Freisem R, Weber JA, Ho JL, Allen JR: Streptococcal wound infections caused by a vaginal carrier. *JAMA* 247:2680–2682, 1982.
30. Altemeier WA, Culbertson WR, Hummel RP: Surgical considerations of endogenous infections—sources, types, and methods of control. *Surg Clin North Am* 48:227–240, 1968.
31. Bruun JN: Post-operative wound infection. Predisposing factors and the effect of a reduction in the dissemination of staphylococci. *Acta Med Scand (Suppl)* 514:1–89, 1970.
32. Lowbury EJL, Lilly HA: The sources of hospital infection of wounds with *Clostridium welchii*. *J Hyg* 56:169–182, 1958.
33. Eickhoff TC: An outbreak of surgical wound infections due to Clostridium perfringens. *Surg Gynecol Obstet* 114:102–108, 1962.
34. Fredette V: The bacteriological efficiency of air-conditioning systems in operating rooms. *Can J Surg* 1:226–229, 1958.
35. Bassett DCJ, Stokes KJ, Thomas WRG: Wound infection with Pseudomonas multivorans. A water-borne contaminant of disinfectant solutions. *Lancet* 1:1188–1191, 1970.
36. Keys TF, Haldorson AM, Rhodes KH, Roberts GD, Fifer EZ: Nosocomial outbreak of *Rhizopus* infections associated with Elastoplast wound dressings—Minnesota. *MMWR* 27:33–34, 1978.
37. Pearson RD, Valenti WM, Steigbigel RT: *Clostridium perfringens* wound infection associated with elastic bandages. *JAMA* 244:1128–1130, 1980.
38. Wiley AM, Ha'eri GB: Routes of infection. A study of using "tracer particles" in the orthopedic operating room. *Clin Orthop* 139:150–155, 1979.
39. Ritter MA, Eitzen HE, French MLV, Hart JB: The effect that time, touch and environment have

upon bacterial contamination of instruments during surgery. *Ann Surg* 184:642–644, 1976.

40. Ford CR, Peterson DE, Mitchell CR: An appraisal of the role of surgical face masks. *Am J Surg* 113:787–790, 1967.

41. Ha'eri GB, Wiley AM: The efficacy of standard surgical face masks: an investigation using "tracer particles." *Clin Orthop* 148:160–162, 1980.

42. Letts RM, Doermer E: Conversation in the operating theater as a cause of airborne bacterial contamination. *J Bone Joint Surg* 65A:357–362, 1983.

43. Charnley J: Postoperative infection after total hip replacement with special reference to air contamination in the operating room. *Clin Orthop* 87:167–187, 1972.

44. Brady LP, Enneking WF, Franco JA: The effect of operating-room environment on the infection rate after Charnley low-friction total hip replacement. *J Bone Joint Surg* 57A:80–83, 1975.

45. Sanderson MC, Bentley G: Assessment of wound contamination during surgery: a preliminary report comparing vertical laminar flow and conventional theatre systems. *Br J Surg* 63:431–432, 1976.

46. Salvati EA, Robinson RP, Zeno SM, Koslin BL, Brause BD, Wilson PD Jr: Infection rates after 3175 total hip and total knee replacements performed with and without a horizontal unidirectional filtered air-flow system. *J Bone Joint Surg* 64A:525–535, 1982.

47. Ha'eri GB, Wiley AM: Total hip replacement in a laminar flow environment with special reference to deep infections. *Clin Orthop* 148:163–168, 1980.

48. Lilly HA, Lowbury EJL, Cason JS: Trial of a laminar air-flow enclosure for the control of infection in a burns operating theatre. *Burns* 10:309–312, 1984.

49. Lidwell OM, Lowbury EJL, Whyte W, Blowers R, Stanley SJ, Lowe D: Effect of ultraclean air in operating rooms on deep sepsis in the joint after total hip or knee replacement: a randomised study. *Br Med J* 285:10–14, 1982.

50. Lidwell OM, Lowbury EJL, Whyte W, Blowers R, Stanley SJ, Lowe D: Airborne contamination of wounds in joint replacement operations: the relationship to sepsis rates. *J Hosp Infect* 4:111–131, 1983.

51. Davidson AIG, Clark C, Smith G: Postoperative wound infection: a computer analysis. *Br J Surg* 58:333–337, 1971.

52. Cruse PJE, Foord R: A five-year prospective study of 23,649 surgical wounds. *Arch Surg* 107:206–210, 1973.

53. Simchen E, Stein H, Sacks TG, Shapiro M, Michel J: Multivariate analysis of determinants of postoperative wound infection in orthopaedic patients. *J Hosp Infect* 5:137–146, 1984.

54. Lidgren L: Postoperative orthopaedic infections in patients with diabetes mellitus. *Acta Orthop Scand* 44:149–151, 1973.

55. Postlethwait RW, Johnson WD: Complications following surgery for duodenal ulcer in obese patients. *Arch Surg* 105:438–440, 1972.

56. Alexander JK, Dennis EW, Smith WG, Amad KH, Duncan WC, Austin RC: Blood volume, cardiac output, and distribution of systemic blood flow in extreme obesity. *Cardiovasc Res Cent Bull* 1:39–44, 1962.

57. Engquist A, Backer OG, Jarnum S: Incidence of postoperative complications in patients subjected to surgery under steroid cover. *Acta Chir Scand* 140:343–346, 1974.

58. Seropian R, Reynolds BM: Wound infections after preoperative depilatory versus razor preparation. *Am J Surg* 121:251–254, 1971.

59. Alexander JW, Fischer JE, Boyajian M, Palmquist J, Morris MJ: The influence of hair-removal methods on wound infections. *Arch Surg* 118:347–352, 1983.

60. Thur de Koos P, McComas B: Shaving versus skin depilatory cream for preoperative skin preparation. A prospective study of wound infection rates. *Am J Surg* 145:377–378, 1983.

61. Powis SJA, Waterworth TA, Arkell DG: Preoperative skin preparation: clinical evaluation of depilatory cream. *Br Med J* 2:1166–1168, 1976.

62. Balthazar ER, Colt JD, Nichols RL: Preoperative hair removal: a random prospective study of shaving versus clipping. *South Med J* 75:799–801, 1982.

63. Koota GM: A study of major postoperative wound sepsis. *Mt Sinai J Med NY* 37:590–602, 1970.

64. Nora PF, Vanecko RM, Bransfield JJ: Prophylactic abdominal drains. *Arch Surg* 105:173–176, 1972.

65. Magee C, Rodeheaver GT, Golden GT, Fox J, Edgerton MT, Edlich RF: Potentiation of wound infection by surgical drains. *Am J Surg* 131:547–549, 1976.

66. Lidwell OM: Sepsis in surgical wounds. Multiple regression analysis applied to records of post-operative hospital sepsis. *J Hyg* 59:259–270, 1961.

67. Simchen E, Shapiro M, Michel J, Sacks T: Multivariate analysis of determinants of postoeprative wound infection: a possible basis for intervention. *Rev Infect Dis* 3:678–682, 1981.

68. Maull KI, Daugherty ME, Shearer GR, Sachatello CR, Ernst CB, Meeker WR, Griffen WO Jr: Cholecystectomy: to drain or not to drain. A randomized prospective study of 200 patients. *J Surg Res* 24:259–263, 1978.

69. Polk HC Jr, Pearlstein L, Jones CE: Operating room-acquired infection: its epidemiology and prevention. In Nyhus LM (ed): *Surgery Annual*. New York, Appleton-Century-Crofts, 1977, p 95.

70. Lowbury EJL, Lilly HA: Use of 4% chlorhexidine detergent solution (Hibiscrub) and other methods of skin disinfection. *Br Med J* 1:510–515, 1973.

71. Smylie HG, Logie JRC, Smith G: From Phisohex to Hibiscrub. *Br Med J* 4:586–589, 1973.

72. Peterson AF, Rosenberg A, Alatary SD: Comparative evaluation of surgical scrub preparations. *Surg Gynecol Obstet* 146:63–65, 1978.

73. Brown TR, Ehrlich CE, Stehman FB, Golichowski AM, Madura JA, Eitzen HE: A clinical evaluation of chlorhexidine gluconate spray as compared with iodophor scrub for preoperative skin preparation. *Surg Gynecol Obstet* 158:363–366, 1984.

74. Ritter MA, French MLV, Eitzen HE, Gioe TJ:

The antimicrobial effectiveness of operative-site preparative agents. *J Bone Joint Surg* 62A:826–828, 1980.

75. Lilly HA, London PS, Lowbury EJL, Porter MF: Effects of adhesive drapes on contamination of operation wounds. *Lancet* 2:431–432, 1970.

76. Jackson DW, Pollock AV, Tindal DS: The value of a plastic adhesive drape in the prevention of wound infection. A controlled trial. *Br J Surg* 58:340–342, 1971.

77. Burke JF: The effective period of preventive antibiotic action in experimental incisions and dermal lesions. *Surgery* 50:161–168, 1961.

78. Gilbert DN: Current status of antibiotic prophylaxis in surgical patients. *Bull NY Acad Med* 60:340–357, 1984.

79. Hurley DL, Howard P Jr, Hahn HH II: Perioperative prophylactic antibiotics in abdominal surgery. A review of recent progress. *Surg Clin North Am* 59:919–933, 1979.

80. Schiessel R, Huk I, Starlinger M, Wunderlich M, Rotter M, Wewalka G, Schemper M: Postoperative infections in colonic surgery after enteral bacitracin-neomycin-clindamycin or parenteral mezlocillin-oxacillin prophylaxis. *J Hosp Infect* 5:289–297, 1984.

81. Kaufman Z, Engelberg M, Eliashiv A, Reiss R: Systemic prophylactic antibiotics in elective biliary surgery. *Arch Surg* 119:1002–1004, 1984.

82. Hill C, Flamant R, Mazas F, Evrard J: Prophylactic cefazolin versus placebo in total hip replacement. *Lancet* 1:795–797, 1981.

83. van der Linden W, Gedda S, Edlund G: Randomized trial of drainage after cholecystectomy. Suction versus static drainage through a main wound versus a stab incision. *Am J Surg* 141:289–294, 1981.

84. Forfar JO, Gould JC, MacCabe AF: Effect of hexachlorophane on incidence of staphylococcal and gram-negative infection in the newborn. *Lancet* 2:177–180, 1968.

85. Dineen P: An evaluation of the duration of the surgical scrub. *Surg Gynecol Obstet* 129:1181–1184, 1969.

86. Dineen P: Microbial filtration by surgical masks. *Surg Gynecol Obstet* 133:812–814, 1971.

87. Quesnel LB: The efficiency of surgical masks of varying design and composition. *Br J Surg* 62:936–940, 1975.

88. Summers MM, Lynch PF, Black T: Hair as a reservoir of staphylococci. *J Clin Pathol* 18:13–15, 1965.

89. Noble WC: *Staphylococcus aureus* on the hair. *J Clin Pathol* 19:570–572, 1966.

90. Garner JS, Emori TG, Haley RW: Operating room practices for the control of infection in US hospitals, October 1976 to July 1977. *Surg Gynecol Obstet* 155:873–880, 1982.

91. Collis DK, Steinhaus K: Total hip replacement without deep infection in a standard operating room. *J Bone Joint Surg* 58A:446–450, 1976.

92. Mallison GF: The inanimate environment. In Bennett JV, Brachman PS (eds): *Hospital Infections*. Boston, Little, Brown, and Co, 1979, p 87.

93. Mallison GF: Housekeeping in operating suites. *AORN J* 21:213–220, 1975.

94. Ayliffe GAJ, Collins BJ, Lowbury EJL, Babb JR,

95. Condon RE, Schulte WJ, Malangoni MA, Anderson-Teschendorf MJ: Effectiveness of a surgical wound surveillance program. *Arch Surg* 118:303–307, 1983.

96. Olson M, O'Connor M, Schwartz ML: Surgical wound infections. A 5-year prospective study of 20,193 wounds at the Minneapolis VA Medical Center. *Ann Surg* 199:253–259, 1984.

97. Haley RW, Culver DH, White JW, Morgan WM, Emori TG, Munn VP, Hooton TM: The efficacy of infection surveillance and control programs in preventing nosocomial infections in U.S. hospitals. *Am J Epidemiol* 121:182–205, 1985.

98. Haley RW, Culver DH, Morgan WM, White JW, Emori TG, Hooton TM: Identifying patients at high risk of surgical wound infection. A simple multivariate index of patient susceptibility and wound contamination. *Am J Epidemiol* 121:206–215, 1985.

99. Jevons MP: "Celbenin"-resistant staphylococci. *Br Med J* 1:124–125, 1961.

100. Barrett FF, McGehee RF Jr, Finland M: Methicillin-resistant *Staphylococcus aureus* at Boston City Hospital. Bacteriologic and epidemiologic observations. *N Engl J Med* 279:441–448, 1968.

101. Everett ED, McNitt TR, Rahm AE Jr, Stevens DL, Peterson HE: Epidemiologic investigation of methicillin resistant *Staphylococcus aureus* in a burn unit. *Milit Med* 143:165–167, 1978.

102. O'Toole RD, Drew WL, Dahlgren BJ, Beaty HN: An outbreak of methicillin-resistant *Staphylococcus aureus* infection. Observations in hospital and nursing home. *JAMA* 213:257–263, 1970.

103. Haley RW, Hightower AW, Khabbaz RF, Thornsberry C, Martone WJ, Allen JR, Hughes JM: The emergence of methicillin-resistant *Staphylococcus aureus* infections in United States hospitals. Possible role of the house staff-patient transfer circuit. *Ann Intern Med* 97:297–308, 1982.

104. Saroglou G, Cromer M, Bisno AL: Methicillin-resistant Staphylococcus aureus: interstate spread of nosocomial infections with emergence of gentamicin-methicillin resistant strains. *Infect Control* 1:81–89, 1980.

105. Bock BV, Pasiecznik K, Meyer RD: Clinical and laboratory studies of nosocomial *Staphylococcus aureus* resistant to methicillin and aminoglycosides. *Infect Control* 3:224–229, 1982.

106. Locksley RM, Cohen ML, Quinn TC, Tompkins LS, Coyle MB, Kirihara JM, Counts GW: Multiply antibiotic-resistant *Staphylococcus aureus*: introduction, transmission, and evolution of nosocomial infection. *Ann Intern Med* 97:317–324, 1982.

107. Sutherland R, Rolinson GN: Characteristics of methicillin-resistant staphylococci. *J Bacteriol* 87:887–899, 1964.

108. Seligman SJ: Methicillin-resistant staphylococci: genetics of the minority population. *J Gen Microbiol* 42:315–322, 1966.

109. Hewitt JH, Coe AW, Parker MT: The detection of methicillin resistance in *Staphylococcus aureus*. *J Med Microbiol* 2:443–456, 1969.

110. Thornsberry C, Caruthers JQ, Baker CN: Effect

of temperature on the in vitro susceptibility of *Staphylococcus aureus* to penicillinase-resistant penicillins. *Antimicrobiol Agents Chemother* 4:263–269, 1973.

111. Sorrell TC, Packham DR, Shanker S, Foldes M, Munro R: Vancomycin therapy for methicillin-resistant *Staphylococcus aureus. Ann Intern Med* 97:344–350, 1982.

112. Watanakunakorn C: Treatment of infections due to methicillin-resistant *Staphylococcus aureus. Ann Intern Med* 97:376–378, 1982.

113. Archer GL, Mayhall CG: Comparison of epidemiological markers used in the investigation of an outbreak of methicillin-resistant *Staphylococcus aureus* infections. *J Clin Microbiol* 18:395–399, 1983.

114. Acar JF, Courvalin P, Chabbert YA: Methicillin-resistant staphylococcemia: bacteriological failure of treatment with cephalosporins. *Antimicrob Agents Chemother*, pp 280–285, 1971.

115. Klimek JJ, Marsik FJ, Bartlett RC, Weir B, Shea P, Quintiliani R: Clinical, epidemiologic and bacteriologic observations of an outbreak of methicillin-resistant Staphylococcus aureus at a large community hospital. *Am J Med* 61:340–345, 1976.

116. Crossley K, Loesch D, Landesman B, Mead K, Chern M, Strate R: An outbreak of infections caused by strains of *Staphylococcus aureus* resistant to methicillin and aminoglycosides. I. Clinical studies. *J Infect Dis* 139:273–279, 1979.

117. Peacock JE Jr, Marsik FJ, Wenzel RP: Methicillin-resistant *Staphylococcus aureus*: introduction and spread within a hospital. *Ann Intern Med* 93:526–532, 1980.

118. Boyce JM, Landry M, Deetz TR, DuPont HL: Epidemiologic studies of an outbreak of nosocomial methicillin-resistant *Staphylococcus aureus* infections. *Infect Control* 2:110–116, 1981.

119. Craven DE, Reed C, Kollisch N, DeMaria A, Lichtenberg D, Shen K, McCabe WR: A large outbreak of infections caused by a strain of Staphylococcus aureus resistant to oxacillin and aminoglycosides. *Am J Med* 71:53–58, 1981.

120. Ward TT, Winn RE, Hartstein AI, Sewell DL: Observations relating to an inter-hospital outbreak of methicillin-resistant *Staphylococcus aureus*: role of antimicrobial therapy in infection control. *Infect Control* 2:453–459, 1981.

121. Thompson RL, Cabezudo I, Wenzel RP: Epidemiology of nosocomial infections caused by methicillin-resistant *Staphylococcus aureus. Ann Intern Med* 97:309–317, 1982.

122. McNeil JJ, Proudfoot AD, Tosolini FA, Morris P, Booth JM, Doyle AE, Louis WJ: Methicillin-resistant *Staphylococcus aureus* in an Australian teaching hospital. *J Hosp Infect* 5:18–28, 1984.

123. Crossley K, Landesman B, Zaske D: An outbreak of infections caused by strains of *Staphylococcus aureus* resistant to methicillin and aminoglycosides. II. Epidemiologic studies. *J Infect Dis* 139:280–287, 1979.

124. Rutala WA, Katz EBS, Sherertz RJ, Sarubbi FA Jr: Environmental study of a methicillin-resistant *Staphylococcus aureus* epidemic in a burn unit. *J Clin Microbiol* 18:683–688, 1983.

125. Todd J, Fishaut M, Kapral F, Welch T: Toxic-shock syndrome associated with phage-group-1 staphylococci. *Lancet* 2:1116–1118, 1978.

126. Shands KN, Schmid GP, Dan BB, Blum D, Guidotti RJ, Hargrett NT, Anderson RL, Hill DL, Broome CV, Band JD, Fraser DW: Toxic-shock syndrome in menstruating women. Association with tampon use and *Staphylococcus aureus* and clinical features in 52 cases. *N Engl J Med* 303:1436–1442, 1980.

127. Tofte RW, Williams DN: Clinical and laboratory manifestations of toxic shock syndrome. *Ann Intern Med* 96 (Part 2):843–847, 1982.

128. Reingold AL, Hargrett NT, Dan BB, Shands KN, Strickland BY, Broome CV: Nonmenstrual toxic shock syndrome. A review of 130 cases. *Ann Intern Med* 96 (Part 2):871–874, 1982.

129. Chow AW, Wong CK, MacFarlane AMG, Bartlett KH: Toxic shock syndrome: clinical and laboratory findings in 30 patients. *Can Med Assoc J* 130:425–430, 1984.

130. Reingold AL, Dan BB, Shands KN, Broome CV: Toxic-shock syndrome not associated with menstruation. A review of 54 cases. *Lancet* 1:1–4, 1982.

131. Bartlett P, Reingold AL, Graham DR, Dan BB, Selinger DS, Tank GW, Wichterman KA: Toxic shock syndrome associated with surgical wound infections. *JAMA* 247:1448–1450, 1982.

132. Silver MA, Simon GL: Toxic shock syndrome in a male postoperative patient. *J Trauma* 21:650–651, 1981.

133. Dornan KJ, Thompson DM, Conn AR, Wittmann BK, Stiver HG, Chow AW: Toxic shock syndrome in the postoperative patient. *Surg Gynecol Obstet* 154:65–68, 1982.

134. Moore PG, James OF: Toxic-shock syndrome complicating recovery from elective cholecystectomy. *Anaesth Intens Care* 10:56–59, 1982.

135. Portnoy D, Hinchey EJ, Marcus-Jones OW, Richards GK: Postoperative toxic shock syndrome in a man. *Can Med Assoc J* 126:815, 817, 1982.

136. Thomas SW, Baird IM, Frazier RD: Toxic shock syndrome following submucous resection and rhinoplasty. *JAMA* 247:2402–2403, 1982.

137. Bach MC: Topical agents in postoperative toxic shock syndrome. *JAMA* 247:3083, 1982.

138. Dunn SR, Capp CD, Ferguson DW: Toxic shock syndrome following ureterolithotomy. *J Urol* 128:1305–1306, 1982.

139. Aganaba T, Evans RP, O'Neill P: Toxic shock syndrome after orchidectomy. *Br Med J* 286:685, 1983.

140. Brier AM: Toxic shock syndrome presenting as postoperative diarrhea in a postmenopausal woman. *J Clin Gastroenterol* 5:77–80, 1983.

141. Barnett A, Lavey E, Pearl RM, Vistnes LM: Toxic shock syndrome from an infected breast prosthesis. *Ann Plast Surg* 10:408–410, 1983.

142. Morrison VA, Oldfield EC III: Postoperative toxic shock syndrome. *Arch Surg* 118:791–794, 1983.

143. Henny CP, Knot EAR, Ten Cate JW, Peters M, Ten Veen JH, Roos J: An acquired antithrombin III deficiency in the course of toxic shock syndrome after elective orthopaedic surgery. *Neth J Med* 26:133–137, 1983.

144. Hull HF, Mann JM, Sands CJ, Gregg SH, Kaufman PW: Toxic shock syndrome related to nasal packing. *Arch Otolaryngol* 109:624–626, 1983.

145. Toback J, Fayerman JW: Toxic shock syndrome following septorhinoplasty. Implications for the head and neck surgeon. *Arch Otolaryngol* 109:627–629, 1983.

146. Barbour SD, Shlaes DM, Guertin SR: Toxic-shock syndrome associated with nasal packing: analogy to tampon-associated illness. *Pediatrics* 73:163–165, 1984.

147. Julian OC, Lopez-Belio M, Dye WS, Javid H, Grove WJ: The median sternal incision in intra-cardiac surgery with extracorporeal circulation: a general evaluation of its use in heart surgery. *Surgery* 42:753–761, 1957.

148. Grmoljez PF, Barner HH, Willman VL, Kaiser GC: Major complications of median sternotomy. *Am J Surg* 130:679–681, 1975.

149. Culliford AT, Cunningham JN Jr, Zeff RH, Isom OW, Teiko P, Spencer FC: Sternal and costochondral infections following open-heart surgery. A review of 2,594 cases. *J Thorac Cardiovasc Surg* 72:714–726, 1976.

150. Wells FC, Newsom SWB, Rowlands C: Wound infection in cardiothoracic surgery. *Lancet* 1:1209–1210, 1983.

151. Nkongho A, Luber JM, Bell-Thomson J, Green GE: Sternotomy infection after harvesting of the internal mammary artery. *J Thorac Cardiovasc Surg* 88:788–789, 1984.

152. Engelman RM, Williams CD, Gouge TH, Chase RM Jr, Falk EA, Boyd AD, Reed GE: Mediastinitis following open-heart surgery. Review of two years' experience. *Arch Surg* 107:772–778, 1973.

153. Weinstein RA, Jones EL, Schwarzmann SW, Hatcher CR Jr: Sternal osteomyelitis and mediastinitis after open-heart operation: pathogenesis and prevention. *Ann Thorac Surg* 21:442–444, 1976.

154. Stiver HG, Clark J, Kennedy J, Cohen M: *Pseudomonas* sternotomy wound infection and sternal osteomyelitis. Complications after open heart surgery. *JAMA* 241:1034–1036, 1979.

155. Cerat GA, McHenry MC, Loop FD: Median sternotomy wound infection and anterior mediastinitis caused by *Bacteroides fragilis*. *Chest* 69:231–232, 1976.

156. Thomas FE Jr, Martin CE, Fisher RD, Alford RH: Candida albicans infection of sternum and costal cartilages: combined operative treatment and drug drug therapy with 5-fluorocytosine. *Ann Thorac Surg* 23:163–166, 1977.

157. Hoffman PC, Fraser DW, Robicsek F, O'Bar PR, Mauney CU: Two outbreaks of sternal wound infections due to organisms of the *Mycobacterium fortuitum* complex. *J Infect Dis* 143:533–542, 1981.

158. Kuritsky JN, Bullen MG, Broome CV, Silcox VA, Good RC, Wallace RJ Jr: Sternal wound infections and endocarditis due to organisms of the *Mycobacterium fortuitum* complex. *Ann Intern Med* 98:938–939, 1983.

159. Breyer RH, Mills SA, Hudspeth AS, Johnston FR, Cordell AR: A prospective study of sternal wound complications. *Ann Thorac Surg* 37:412–416, 1984.

160. Fong IW, Baker CB, McKee DC: The value of prophylactic antibiotics in aorto-coronary bypass

operations. A double-blind randomized trial. *J Thorac Cardiovasc Surg* 78:908–913, 1979.

161. Pruitt BA Jr, Lindberg RB, McManus WF, Mason AD Jr: Current approach to prevention and treatment of *Pseudomonas aeruginosa* infections in burned patients. *Rev Infect Dis* 5 (Suppl 5): S889–S897, 1983.

162. Pruitt BA Jr: The diagnosis and treatment of infection in the burn patient. *Burns* 11:79–91, 1984.

163. McManus WF, Goodwin CW, Mason AD Jr, Pruitt BA Jr: Burn wound infection. *J Trauma* 21:753–756, 1981.

164. Pruitt BA Jr, Foley FD: The use of biopsies in burn patient care. *Surgery* 73:887–897, 1973.

165. Volenec FJ, Clark GM, Mani MM, Humphrey LJ: Burn wound biopsy bacterial quantitation: a statistical analysis. *Am J Surg* 138:695–697, 1979.

166. Loebl EC, Marvin JA, Heck EL, Curreri PW, Baxter CR: The method of quantitative burn-wound biopsy cultures and its routine use in the care of the burned patient. *Am J Clin Pathol* 61:20–24, 1974.

167. Woolfrey BF, Fox JM, Quall CO: An evaluation of burn wound quantitative microbiology. I. Quantitative eschar cultures. *Am J Clin Pathol* 75:532–537, 1981.

168. Bharadwaj R, Phadke SA, Joshi BN: Bacteriology of burn wound using the quantitative full thickness biopsy technique. *Indian J Med Res* 78:337–342, 1983.

169. Bharadwaj R, Joshi BN, Phadke SA: Assessment of burn wound sepsis by swab, full thickness biopsy culture and blood culture—a comparative study. *Burns* 10:124–126, 1983.

170. Tahlan RN, Keswani RK, Saini S, Miglani OP: Correlation of quantitative burn wound biopsy culture and surface swab culture to burn wound sepsis. *Burns* 10:217–224, 1984.

171. Freshwater MF, Su CT: Potential pitfalls of quantitative burn wound biopsy cultures. *Ann Plast Surg* 4:216–218, 1980.

172. Spebar MJ, Lindberg RB: Fungal infection of the burn wound. *Am J Surg* 138:879–882, 1979.

173. Nash G, Foley FD, Pruitt BA Jr: *Candida* burn-wound invasion. A cause of systemic candidiasis. *Arch Pathol* 90:75–78, 1970.

174. MacMillan BG, Law EJ, Holder IA: Experience with *Candida* infections in the burn patient. *Arch Surg* 104:509–514, 1972.

175. Rabin ER, Lundberg GD, Mitchell ET: Mucormycosis in severely burned patients. Report of two cases with extensive destruction of the face and nasal cavity. *N Engl J Med* 264:1286–1289, 1961.

176. Foley FD, Shuck JM: Burn-wound infection with Phycomycetes requiring amputation of hand. *JAMA* 203:154, 1968.

177. Nash G, Foley FD, Goodwin MN Jr, Bruck HM, Greenwald KA, Pruitt BA Jr: Fungal burn wound infection. *JAMA* 215:1664–1666, 1971.

178. Bruck HM, Nash G, Foley FD, Pruitt BA Jr: Opportunistic fungal infection of the burn wound with Phycomycetes and *Aspergillus*. *Arch Surg* 102:476–482, 1971.

179. Bruck HM, Nash G, Stein JM, Lindberg RB:

Studies on the occurrence and significance of yeasts and fungi in the burn wound. *Ann Surg* 176:108–110, 1972.

180. Majeski JA, MacMillan BG: Fatal systemic mycotic infections in the burned child. *J Trauma* 17:320–322, 1977.

181. Wheeler MS, McGinnis MR, Schell WA, Walker DH: Fusarium infection in burned patients. *Am J Clin Pathol* 75:304–311, 1981.

182. Foley FD, Greenwald KA, Nash G, Pruitt BA Jr: Herpesvirus infection in burned patients. *N Engl J Med* 282:652–656, 1970.

183. Knittle MA, Eitzman DV, Baer H: Role of hand contamination of personnel in the epidemiology of gram-negative nosocomial infections. *J Pediatr* 86:433–437, 1975.

184. Wormald PJ: The effect of a changed environment on bacterial colonization rates in an established burns centre. *J Hyg* 68:633–645, 1970.

185. Hambraeus A, Laurell G: Infections in a burns unit. An attempt to study the airborne transfer of bacteria. In *Staphylococci and Staphylococcal Infections*. Warsaw, Polish Medical Publishers, 1973, p 467.

186. Kohn J: A study of Ps. pyocyanea cross infection in a burns unit. Preliminary report. In Wallace AB, Wilkinson AW (eds): *Research in Burns*. Edinburgh, E and S Livingstone, 1966, p 493.

187. Barclay TL, Dexter F: Infection and cross-infection in a new burns centre. *Br J Surg* 55:197–202, 1968.

188. Lowbury EJL, Babb JR, Ford PM: Protective isolation in a burns unit: the use of plastic isolators and air curtains. *J Hyg* 69:529–546, 1971.

189. McHugh GL, Moellering RC, Hopkins CC, Swartz MN: Salmonella typhimurium resistant to silver nitrate, chloramphenicol, and ampicillin. A new threat in burn units? *Lancet* 1:235–240, 1975.

190. van Saene HKF, Nicolai JPA: The prevention of wound infections in burn patients. *Scand J Plast Reconstr Surg* 13:63–67, 1979.

191. Hendriks WDH, Cech M, Kooy P: Isolation efficiency and its clinical importance in patients with burns. *Antonie van Leeuwenhoek* 47:247–254, 1981.

192. Burke JF, Quinby WC, Bondoc CC, Sheehy EM, Moreno HC: The contribution of a bacterially isolated environment to the prevention of infection in seriously burned patients. *Ann Surg* 186:377–387, 1977.

193. Kominos SD, Copeland CE, Grosiak B, Postic B: Introduction of *Pseudomonas aeruginosa* into a hospital via vegetables. *Appl Microbiol* 24:567–570, 1972.

194. Kominos SD, Copeland CE, Delenko CA: *Pseudomonas aeruginosa* from vegetables, salads, and other foods served to patients with burns. In Young VM (ed): *Pseudomonas aeruginosa: Ecological Aspects and Patient Colonization*. New York, Raven Press, 1977, p 70.

195. Lowbury EJL, Fox J: The epidemiology of infection with *Pseudomonas pyocyanea* in a burns unit. *J Hyg* 52:403–416, 1954.

196. Mayhall CG, Lamb VA, Gayle WE Jr, Haynes BW Jr: *Enterobacter cloacae* septicemia in a burn center: epidemiology and control of an outbreak. *J Infect Dis* 139:166–171, 1979.

197. Shulman JA, Terry PM, Hough CE: Colonization with gentamicin-resistant *Pseudomonas aeruginosa*, pyocine type 5, in a burn unit. *J Infect Dis* 124 (Suppl):S18–S23, 1971.

198. MacMillan BG, Edmonds P, Hummel RP, Maley MP: Epidemiology of *Pseudomonas* in a burn intensive care unit. *J Trauma* 13:627–638, 1973.

199. Fujita K, Lilly HA, Kidson A, Ayliffe GAJ: Gentamicin-resistant Pseudomonas aeruginosa infection from mattresses in a burns unit. *Br Med J* 283:219–220, 1981.

200. Sherertz RJ, Sullivan ML: An outbreak of infections with *Acinetobacter calcoaceticus* in burn patients: contamination of patients' mattresses. *J Infect Dis* 151:252–258, 1985.

201. Mayhall CG: Infections in burn patients. In Wenzel RP (ed): *Handbook of Hospital Acquired Infections*. Boca Raton, FL, CRC Press, 1981, p 321.

202. Stone HH, Kolb LD: The evolution and spread of gentamicin-resistant pseudomonads. *J Trauma* 11:586–589, 1971.

203. Holder IA: Epidemiology of *Pseudomonas aeruginosa* in a burns hospital. In Young VM (ed): *Pseudomonas aeruginosa: Ecological Aspects and Patient Colonization*. New York, Raven Press, 1977, p 86.

204. Kominos SD, Copeland CE, Grosiak B: Mode of transmission of *Pseudomonas aeruginosa* in a burn unit and an intensive care unit in a general hospital. *Appl Microbiol* 23:309–312, 1972.

205. Wenzel RP, Hunting KJ, Osterman CA, Sande MA: *Providencia stuartii*, a hospital pathogen: potential factors for its emergence and transmission. *Am J Epidemiol* 104:170–180, 1976.

206. Edmonds P, Suskind RR, MacMillan BG, Holder IA: Epidemiology of *Pseudomonas aeruginosa* in a burns hospital: surveillance by a combined typing system. *Appl Microbiol* 24:219–225, 1972.

207. Hambraeus A: Dispersal and transfer of *Staphylococcus aureus* in an isolation ward for burned patients. *J Hyg* 71:787–797, 1973.

208. Lilly HA, Lowbury EJL: Antibiotic resistance of *Staphylococcus aureus* in a burns unit after stopping routine prophylaxis with erythromycin. *J Antimicrob Chemother* 4:545–550, 1978.

209. Cason JS, Jackson DM, Lowbury EJL, Ricketts CR: Antiseptic and aseptic prophylaxis for burns: use of silver nitrate and of isolators. *Br Med J* 2:1288–1294, 1966.

210. Lowbury EJL: Advances in the control of infection in burns. *Br J Plast Surg* 20:211–217, 1967.

211. Bridges K, Kidson A, Lowbury EJL, Wilkins MD: Gentamicin- and silver-resistant Pseudomonas in a burns unit. *Br Med J* 1:446–449, 1979.

212. Gayle WE Jr, Mayhall CG, Lamb VA, Apollo E, Haynes BW Jr: Resistant *Enterobacter cloacae* in a burn center: the ineffectiveness of silver sulfadiazine. *J Trauma* 18:317–323, 1978.

213. Snelling CFT, Ronald AR, Waters WR, Yaworski DS, Drulak K, Sunderland M: Comparison of silver sulfadiazine and gentamicin for topical prophylaxis against burn wound sepsis. *Can Med Assoc J* 119:466–470, 1978.

214. Smith RF, Blasi D, Dayton SL, Chipps DD: Effects of sodium hypochlorite on the microbial

flora of burns and normal skin. *J Trauma* 14:938–944, 1974.

215. Steve L, Goodhart P, Alexander J: Hydrotherapy burn treatment: use of chloramine-T against resistant microorganisms. *Arch Phys Med Rehabil* 60:301–303, 1979.

216. Lindberg RB, Pruitt BA Jr, Mason AD Jr: Topical chemotherapy and prophylaxis in thermal injury. In Williams JD, Geddes AM (eds): *Chemotherapy.* New York, Plenum, 1976, vol 3, p 352.

217. Lindberg RB, Pruitt BA Jr, Mason AD Jr: Topical chemotherapy and prophylaxis in thermal injury. In Williams JD, Geddes AM (eds): *Chemotherapy.* New York, Plenum, 1976, vol 3, p 353.

218. Pruitt BA Jr, Goodwin CW Jr: Current treatment of the extensively burned patient. *Surg Ann* 15:331–364, 1983.

219. Demling RH, Perea A, Maly J, Moylan JA, Jarrett F, Balish E: The use of a laminar airflow isolation system for the treatment of major burns. *Am J Surg* 136:375–378, 1978.

220. Demling RH, Maly J: The treatment of burn patients in a laminar airflow environment. *Ann NY Acad Sci* 353:294–299, 1980.

221. Polk RE, Mayhall CG, Smith J, Hall G, Kline BJ, Swensson E, Haynes BW: Gentamicin and tobramycin penetration into burn eschar. Pharmacokinetics and microbiological effects. *Arch Surg* 118:295–302, 1983.

222. Mayhall CG, Polk RE, Haynes BW: Infections in burned patients. *Infect Control* 4:454–459, 1983.

223. Boyce JM, White RL, Causey WA, Lockwood WR: Burn units as a source of methicilln-resistant *Staphylococcus aureus* infections. *JAMA* 249:2803–2807, 1983.

224. Linnemann CC Jr, Mason M, Moore P, Korfhagen TR, Staneck JL: Methicillin-resistant *Staphylococcus aureus*: experience in a general hospital over four years. *Am J Epidemiol* 115:941–950, 1982.

225. Espersen F, Nielsen PB, Lund K, Sylvest B, Jensen K: Hospital-acquired infections in a burns unit caused by an imported strain of *Staphylococcus aureus* with unusual multi-resistance. *J Hyg* 88:535–541, 1982.

226. Nash G, Asch MJ, Foley FD, Pruitt BA Jr: Disseminated cytomegalic inclusion disease in a burned adult. *JAMA* 214:587–589, 1970.

227. Linnemann CC Jr, MacMillan BG: Viral infections in pediatric burn patients. *Am J Dis Child* 135:750–753, 1981.

228. Kagan RJ, Naraqi S, Matsuda T, Jonasson OM: Herpes simplex virus and cytomegalovirus infections in burned patients. *J Trauma* 25:40–45, 1985.

229. Deepe GS Jr, MacMillan BG, Linnemann CC Jr: Unexplained fever in burn patients due to cytomegalovirus infection. *JAMA* 248:2299–2301, 1982.

230. Fox CL Jr, Modak SM, Stanford JW: Zinc sulfadiazine for topical therapy of Pseudomonas infection in burns. *Surg Gynecol Obstet* 142:553–559, 1976.

231. Munster AM, Helvig E, Rowland S: Cerium nitrate-silver sulfadiazine cream in the treatment of burns: a prospective evaluation. *Surgery* 88:658–660, 1980.

232. Lawrence JC, Cason JS, Kidson A: Evaluation of phenoxetol-chlorhexidine cream as a prophylactic antibacterial agent in burns. *Lancet* 1:1037–1040, 1982.

233. Modak S, Stanford J, Friedlaender J, Fox P, Foxjun CL: Control of burn wound infections by pefloxacin and its silver derivative. *Burns* 10:170–178, 1984.

Chapter 23

Infections in Implantable Prosthetic Devices

Louis D. Saravolatz, M.D.

INTRODUCTION

In the last two decades medicine and biomedical technology have made significant advances in prolonging the lives of patients by the implantation of prosthetic devices. These implants include joints, heart valves, dialysis access sites, and central nervous system shunts. Although this list is not exhaustive, it contains the most frequently inserted prosthetic devices. Despite their advantages, all prostheses run the risk of causing infection at the time of insertion or even later by hematogenous spread. Also common to all prostheses are the predominance of pathogens from skin flora and the lack of response to medical therapy until the prosthesis is removed. This chapter includes discussions of the major prosthetic devices with special emphasis on the pathogenesis and preventive aspects of infection.

INFECTION IN IMPLANTABLE JOINTS

The development of joint prostheses is a remarkable advance in biomedical technology. When implanted, they significantly reduce discomfort and improve the patient's mobility. Joint replacement is a now commonly performed operative procedure, and an estimated 80,000 to 100,000 hip replacements and 40,000 knee arthroplasties are performed each year in the United States (1, 2). However, this advance has not been achieved without some morbidity—that is, the secondary occurrence of infection of the prosthesis and, less significantly, of the wound. Although less frequent than mechanical failures, infectious causes of failure of a joint prosthesis are more serious.

Epidemiology

Between 1969 and 1972 the incidence of deep wound infection in England and the United States was reported at 8.9% to 9.0% (3, 4), but this figure has been significantly reduced by new developments aimed at preventing joint replacement infections (see below). In seven studies in which the number of patients ranged between 1013 and 5800 per study, the infection rate ranged between 0.6% and 2.0% for total hip replacements (5–11). In another study of 3215 total hip replacements in which follow-ups ranged from 2 to 5 years, the infection rate was 1.3% (12). These data more closely reflect an acceptable incidence of infection for hip replacement based on the operating room and technical expertise currently available.

A patient's risk of developing infection after joint replacement depends upon several factors; these include rheumatoid arthritis, diabetes mellitus, old age, infection remote to the site of joint replacement, and previous infection in the joint replacement (1, 13, 14). Other risk factors for surgical wound infection that may contribute but have not been unequivocally confirmed for joint replacements include obesity, immunosuppressive therapy, malnutrition, duration of the operative procedure, and prolonged hospitalization before surgery. Moreover, certain groups of patients, such as the elderly, are at a higher risk of developing infection (15).

Types of Joint Prostheses

The rate of infection also varies with the joint involved, as well as with the material used to make the prosthesis (Table 23.1). In hip surgery, a prosthesis such as the McKee-Farrar prosthesis may be used. However, this prosthesis has a greater tendency to loosen, as do all metal-on-metal-bearing prostheses (16). The rate of infection as well as other complications from these prostheses is reportedly higher than for the low friction, metal-to-polyethylene arthroplasty developed by Charnley (17). Other hip prostheses that have been developed include ceramic-to-

Table 23.1.   Deep Infection Rates of Joint Replacements

Author	Year	Joint	Operations	Infections	%
Poss et al (1)	1984	Hip	2012	18	0.89
Moggio et al (59)	1979	Hip: UV light	1322	13	0.98
The Hip Society (55)	1984	Hip: clean air, no antibiotics	6800	85	1.25
The Hip Society (55)	1984	Hip: clean air, plus antibiotics	3875	35	0.90
The Hip Society (55)	1984	Hip: antibiotics without clean air	5173	56	1.08
Poss et al (1)	1984	Knee: metal-on-plastic	1957	11	0.57
Insall et al (19)	1979	Knee: nonhinged	220	3	1.36
Vahvanen and Vainio (20)	1979	Knee	91	4	4.4
Poss et al (1)	1984	Knee: hinged	156	17	10.9
Jones (21)	1979	Knee: hinged			15.0
Neer et al (22)	1982	Shoulder	273	1	0.37
Cofield (23)	1982	Shoulder	204	3	1.4
Engelbrecht et al (24)	1980	Shoulder	101	2	2.0
Poss et al (1)	1984	Elbow	115	7	6.0
Morrey and Bryan (26)	1983	Elbow	156	14	9.0
Brumfield et al (27)	1981	Elbow	30	1	3.3
Volz (23)	1984	Wrist	111	2	2.0
Beckenbaugh (23)	1982	Wrist	150	4	2.6

polyethylene and ceramic-to-ceramic components, although experience with these joints is insufficient to evaluate their clinical usefulness.

The infection rates for knee prostheses have also been significantly reduced (18–20). In this case, the type of prosthesis seems more clearly related to the rate of infection. Metal-on-metal joints clearly caused more problems, with a high incidence of loosening and resultant synovitis from the metal and cement debris (1). Although associated with a high infection rate, the GUEPAR (hinged) prosthesis produced better functional results and was used in the worst knees in some series (1, 18, 21). Thus, the infection rate is only one factor to be evaluated in judging the benefit of a joint prosthesis.

Replacement of the shoulder joint can be critical to maintain the axis of motion for the mobility needed for the upper extremity. Fortunately, infection rates are generally less than 2%, which is an acceptably low rate (22–24). In wrist replacement, the risk of infection does not differ much from the rates for shoulder infection. Reported rates vary from 2.0% to 2.67% (23, 25).

By contrast, replacement of the elbow has an appreciably higher infection rate, possibly the highest among all prosthetic joints. Rates range from 3.3% to 9.0%, which is considerably higher than the currently accepted rates of less than 2% for both hip and knee replacements (1, 26, 27). Several features may accont for the higher rate of infection. Among 156 elbow replacement proce-

dures, 112 were for patients with rheumatoid arthritis and 40 were for traumatic arthritis (26). Both conditions are associated with a higher risk of infection in joint replacements. Also, 32% of the rheumatoid patients received steroid therapy, and 31.4% (49/156) of the elbow replacement patients had had previous surgery, two other features known to increase the risk of subsequent infection.

Pathogenesis

The source of microorganisms may be exogenous, in which bacteria are implanted in the operative wound during surgery, or it may be endogenous.

Exogenous bacterial pathogens in prosthetic joint infections come from several sources. Exogenous sources of *Staphylococcus aureus* from carriers who are shedders are significant factors in wound and subsequent prosthetic contamination and infection. Airborne spread of infection has also been implicated (see "Prevention," below).

Endogenous sources of infection also have several mechanisms. The most common is implantation of the patient's own microbial flora into a joint replacement at the time of the operation. A second mechanism may arise from hematogenous spread from a distant focus of infection, such as a urinary tract, pulmonary, dental, skin, or gastrointestinal source. The third source of endogenous infections may be an earlier infection at the site of the joint, since a quiescent pyogenic or tuberculous osteomyelitis may be reactivated.

Evidence for an endogenous source from the patient's own microflora comes from the increased risk of infection that patients experience with prolonged preoperative hospitalization; this suggests that alteration of the patient's own flora and debilitated state requiring preoperative hospitalization may enhance the risk of surgical wound infection. In addition, *S. aureus*, the most common pathogen in joint replacement infections, is seldom found in cultures of air samples from operating rooms, thus supporting the view that endogenous sources are most important. Lidwell et al evaluated patients, surgeons, and other operating room staff for colonization with *S. aureus* and phage-typed isolates from both infected prostheses and carriers (28). In 2 of 14 prosthetic joint infections, patients were carriers of the same phage type, and in 10, the surgeon or other staff were identified as carriers. In the remaining 2 patients, no carrier was identified. Thus, while endogenous sources of *S. aureus* are important, they are identifiable in only a few cases where primary operative seeding is suspected, in contrast to the cases of hematogenous infection in which endogenous sources of *S. aureus* account for most cases.

Hematogenous infections have been responsible for a minority of infections in joint prostheses; for example, Ahlberg et al reported an incidence of only 0.29% (5 of 1,716) (29). In view of established prosthetic joint infection rates, hematogenous sources probably account for no more than one-fourth of all postoperative hip replacement infections. However, it is important to recognize a primary focus of infection in the patient undergoing a prosthetic joint replacement so that it can be appropriately treated preoperatively. These infections occur most frequently with *S. aureus* (46%), streptococci (23%), *Staphylococcus epidermidis* (8%), and gram-negative aerobic enteric pathogens (18%) (30). Sites of origin include the respiratory tract (18%), skin (16%), urinary tract (14.8%), dental (11.4%), and gastrointestinal tract (6.6%). In 23% (14 of 61) of infections presumed to be hematogenous, the primary focus was not identified. In addition, even in cases in which a dental focus was implicated as the primary focus, viridans streptococci were found in only one case, whereas organisms not usually responsible for dental infections, such as *S. aureus* and *S. epidermidis*, were implicated in several cases in which an odontogenic primary focus was suspected.

If a primary infection occurs during childhood or adolescence, the infection is more likely to resolve completely than if it occurs in adults and older patients. However, a quiescent infection may be reactivated, especially in adults, after joint replacement (2). In all patients who have an earlier history of osteomyelitis, careful microbiologic and histologic examination of the involved bone must be performed at the time of joint replacement. In cases of tuberculosis, irrespective of the patient's age, acid-fast bacilli are often identified when a tuberculous hip is replaced. Thus, antituberculous treatment should be carefully considered for such patients, and it may be initiated pending results of prolonged incubation (6 weeks) of bone appropriately cultured for *Mycobacterium tuberculosis* (31).

Microbiology

Gram-positive organisms are the predominant organisms in prosthetic joint infection, and *S. aureus* and *S. epidermidis* are the two most commonly isolated pathogens in most series (Table 23.2) (1, 17, 32–38). While the role of anaerobes has been minimized, presumably because attempts to recover them have been unsuccessful or because laboratory support is inadequate, 5.3% of cases in the collected series disclosed an anaerobic pathogen.

Bacteria less frequently implicated in joint infections include *Salmonella, Haemophilus influenzae, Enterobacter aerogenes, Enterobacter cloacae, Klebsiella pneumoniae, Pseudomonas* sp, *Serratia marcescens, Acinetobacter* sp, *Pasteurella multocida, Bacteroides fragilis*, and *Pepto-*

Table 23.2. Microbial Etiology of Prosthetic Joint Infections*

	No. of Isolates	%
Gram-positive	275	68.9
S. epidermidis	86	21.6
S. aureus	129	32.3
Micrococcus	13	3.3
Diphtheroid	4	1.0
Other	43	10.8
Gram-negative	86	21.6
E. coli	31	7.7
Proteus	21	5.3
Other	34	8.5
Anaerobes	21	5.3
Mixed	17	4.3
Total	399	100.0

*Compilation of nine series of arthroplasty infections from 1972 to 1984 (1, 17, 32–38).

streptococcus sp. In addition, both *Mycobacterium fortuitum* and *M. tuberculosis* have been reported as causes of prosthetic joint infection, with the latter secondary to reactivation of a latent infection (31, 39). Fungal pathogens, including *Candida albicans*, *Candida glabrata*, and *Candida parapsilosis*, have also been reported to cause joint replacement infections (40, 41). Although other fungi, such as *Aspergillus* sp., have been implicated in the genesis of prosthetic heart valve infection, it is surprising that these organisms have rarely, if at all, been implicated in prosthetic joint replacements. Possibly better environmental control is exercised in orthopaedic operating rooms than in thoracic surgery theaters. Nonetheless, airborne fungi may be implanted in the joint when the prosthesis is inserted, and their occurrence may suggest a need to review operating room air control systems.

Mixed infection in joint replacements occurred in 4.3% of 399 cases. Other etiologic factors that have not yet been identified include viruses, *Chlamydia*, and L-form bacteria.

Diagnosis

Diagnosis of deep infection after surgery may be difficult for even the most capable clinician. The differential diagnosis includes superficial infection, mechanical loosening, hematoma, and heterotopic ossification. The cardinal sign of deep infection is pain. If infection occurs in the early period (Table 23.3), the patient usually appears to be toxic, and there is evidence of local inflammation with erythema and induration. Patients have fever with leukocytosis and an elevated erythrocyte sedimentation rate. In Carlson's follow-up study of the erythrocyte sedimentation rate in 75 uncomplicated total hip replacements, the sedimentation rate returned to the preoperative level in 3 to 6 months (42). However, the sedimentation rate for infected joints was significantly higher at 1 month and never returned to normal preoperative levels. The clinician must determine whether there is actual joint tenderness that would indicate a deep wound infection rather than a superficial wound infection. Also, deep wound infections will have more drainage and induration than superficial infections, and drainage also will persist longer for a deep infection.

In differentiating mechanical loosening from deep infection, the patient's clinical course may be helpful. Deep infections are usually associated with a history of poor wound healing, which is not found with mechanical loosening. Additionally, deep infections frequently cause trouble from the time of surgery onward, whereas loos-

Table 23.3.   Clinical Categories of Prosthetic Joint Infections

	Early	Delayed	Hematogenous
ONSET	Before or immediately after discharge (< 3 months)	> 3 months	Any time (3–66 months after surgery)
PATHOGENESIS	Direct implantation in the operating room	Airborne	Primary source of bacteremia; suspected or identified in 77%
PATHOGENS	*S. aureus* *S. epidermidis*	*S. epidermidis* *Propionibacterium acnes* *Peptococcus*	*S. aureus* Group B streptococcus *S. pneumoniae*
CLINICAL ILLNESS	Drainage and wound dehiscence, fever, ↑WBC, ↑ESR*	"Subacute" presentation; minimal to no fever; ESR ~35–40, near normal WBC; painful joint (never becomes pain-free after surgery)	Pain-free interval between surgery and joint infection; fever, rigors
SERIOUSNESS	Moderate to serious illness	Milder illness; nontoxic clinical illness	Life-threatening
OUTCOME	Loss of joint	Loss of joint	Loss of joint

* WBC, white blood cell count; ESR, erythrocyte sedimentation rate.

ening has a symptom-free period between the joint replacement and the loosening. Also, the pain caused by infection is present constantly and may be relieved by antibiotics, whereas the pain associated with loosening is aggravated during the day with activity but alleviated in the evening with rest. Moreover, temperature, white blood count, and erythrocyte sedimentation rate should all be normal if loosening is the problem, in contrast to the abnormalities seen in these areas if infection is the cause.

Differentiating deep infection from hematoma is occasionally difficult. The acute onset of pain following activity accompanied by a drop in hemoglobin would suggest hematoma. Patients may have fever along with leukocystosis and appear to be septic.

When infection is suspected, aspiration or open biopsy will confirm the diagnosis, although aspiration does not always establish the etiology. In a series by Fitzgerald from the Mayo Clinic, the etiology could be established in only 11 of 15 cases (12). While aspiration can easily be performed in the elbow and knee, it is technically much more difficult for the hip because image intensification and, in some cases general anesthesia are required. In addition, aspiration of the joint space may be inadequate since the infection may reside between the prosthesis and the native bone in the cement interface. Thus, it may be necessary to perform a biopsy or aspiration of the cement bone juncture as part of an open procedure to improve the bacterial yield for establishing an etiology. The arthrogram has also been suggested as an adjunct in the diagnosis to ensure needle placement or to confirm sinus tract formation deep in the joint. Although some concern has been expressed about performing arthrograms in the face of substantial evidence of infection, possibly because of the risk of precipitating septicemia or extending the infectious process, little in the literature supports such concerns. Arthrograms have had variable results in assessing postoperative pain and are probably of limited value in helping to establish the etiologic diagnosis of pain after total hip replacement (43).

Radiologic evaluation of the prosthesis should be performed first with plane radiography. For the hip, loosening of the femoral component can readily be detected in approximately 92% of cases but in only 63% of the acetabular components (44). Once loosening is established, radionuclide bone imaging should be performed to differentiate mechanical from infectious causes of loosening. At least two authors have reported that the increased radionuclide uptake activity observed after total joint hip replacement should return to normal levels in 6 months (45, 46). The distribution of uptake was helpful in differentiating infection from loosening, as infection revealed a diffuse pattern around both components of the hip prosthesis, while loosening revealed focal and discrete activity. Other scans, such as gallium 67 and In-111 tagged leukocytes, have been suggested as specific and sensitive studies to be used as adjunct tests to the technetium scan (47, 48).

Treatment

Medical treatment of infected prostheses should be based on the etiologic agent and on susceptibility testing. However, lack of agreement exists on several questions about the management of infected joint protheses. How long should antibiotic therapy be administered? At what point is medical therapy judged to be inadequate, and should the prosthesis be removed? How long should antibiotics be administered after the prosthesis has been removed? Is oral therapy appropriate in the medical management? When, if ever, can a new prosthesis be implanted? These issues have no clear-cut answers, although several authors have expressed opinions. Reported duration of therapy ranges from 4 weeks to 12 months. Most authors utilized 4 to 8 weeks of parenteral therapy, and some used oral antibiotics in follow-up therapy.

The surgical approach for an infected prosthesis varies. Burton and Schurman managed eight deep infections without removing the prosthesis surgically in all but two cases (49). His surgical approach was radical debridement of all necrotic debris and removal of the prosthesis when it was loose or when infection involved the bone. However, this study was limited by its inadequate follow-up period of between 11 and 20 months.

Another surgical approach is a girdlestone arthroplasty, which involves removing the femoral head, removing the prosthesis, and curretting both the femoral and acetabular cavities in order to remove infected cement. The disadvantage of this surgical procedure is the patient's functional disability. Although Bourne et al reported satisfactory relief of pain in 91% of 33 patients undergoing a girdlestone arthroplasty and control of infection in 97% (50), the leg discrepancy and Trendelenburg gait made walking difficult. Only 42% of the patients were satisfied with their functional ability.

The outcome of the infected prosthesis is poor at best. In a nationwide survey in Canada, Hunter and Dandy found that only 18 of 135 patients were able to retain their prosthesis after infection. Infection usually, but not always, implies the need to remove the prosthesis (51).

Prevention

Operating Room

To prevent prosthetic joint infections, one should first consider environmental control efforts and patient-related maneuvers.

Control of the air within the operating room is an important but controversial issue from several standpoints. First, air control systems can be extremely costly. In 1984 in England, the cost for capital acquisition of an air control system was £15,000 ($22,650), and the annual operational cost was £700 ($1,057) (52). Second, if such a system can be justified for prosthetic joint replacements, should it not also be used to prevent infection in other clean surgical cases? Certainly, infection after ophthalmic, cardiac, neurosurgical, or vascular surgery cases can have equally catastrophic consequences.

In 1972, Charnley emphasized the need to reduce airborne bacterial contamination in the operating room and established that a reduction in infection rates correlated with reduction in quantitative counts of bacteria in operating room air samples (5). Over a 6-year period, he reported a reduction in the infection rate from 8.9% to 1.3%. However, Laufmann criticized, crediting the reduced infection rates to a clean airflow system alone and suggested that several factors were implemented that might have improved infection rates. These innovations included double-glove techniques, unidirectional airflow, and personnel isolator systems (53, 54).

Laminar airflow clean room systems operate by unidirectional airflow from a blower through high efficiency particulate air (HEPA) filters on entry into the operating room and then through vents to air in the outside environment. These filters remove particles $\geq 0.5 \ \mu m$ with a 99.7% efficiency. This system can provide an air turnover rate of 500 times/hour, as compared to 25 to 40 times/hour in conventional operating rooms. Of the two types of airflow systems, the vertical and the horizontal, the former has a greater effect on reducing airborne bacteria in the operating room.

Air control is clearly important in reducing airborne bacterial contamination at or near the wound as well as reducing wound contamination rates. Since implantation of bacteria into the wound during surgery is the major cause of prosthetic joint infections, efforts to eliminate this event should be beneficial. Since shedding of bacteria by humans can occur in very large numbers (> 5,000/minute) (55), the ability of air control systems to reduce these bacterial contaminants would be expected to reduce infection. Nelson summarized the data on 15,843 total hip replacements as reported by 20 authors (55). In clean rooms with air control systems, the infection rate was 0.7% (18 of 2,730), whereas in regular operating rooms, the infection rate was 5.8% (109 of 1,880). Antibiotics were not used for prophylaxis in either setting. Such comparisons can be criticized because technical expertise and surgical ability vary; however, as the numbers become larger and more centers are included in studies of both settings, one might expect that variations in technical aspects will be a less significant factor in accounting for the difference in infection rates.

In another study, Salvati reviewed infection rates with clean air versus standard operating room air. Total hip replacement infection rates were reduced from 1.4% to 0.9%, whereas total knee replacement rates were significantly increased from 1.4% to 3.9% (56). No reason other than the operating room environment could be found in a multifactorial analysis to explain the increased incidence of knee infections. Salvati postulated that the operating team's position in relation to the directional airflow accounted for the increased rate of knee infections because bacteria were blown down wind into the wound in the knee surgeries but not during the hip surgeries. Since the operating room staff did not wear special isolator systems, one could argue that inadequate barriers existed between operating room personnel and the patient.

Finally, a recent prospective and randomized study demonstrated a 50% reduction (from 0.85% to 0.42%) when clean rooms were used as compared to conventional rooms (57). This multicenter study is, to date, the best designed study that supports the benefits of laminar airflow systems in reducing infection rates.

Personnel isolator systems have also been used to reduce exogenous sources of bacterial contamination. Such a system includes garments of low porosity material that impede transfer of bacteria shed from the body and a helmet that fully encloses the head. Nelson showed that airborne bacterial contamination was reduced when personnel isolator systems were used. When this system was used in conjunction with a clean air system, Lidwell et al showed an additional 25% reduction in infection rates (57). However, to date, no other prospective, well designed studies corroborate Lidwell's findings of a reduction not only in airborne bacteria but also in infection rates. In addition, the body exhaust suits in personnel isolator systems may cost $6,000 each plus operational costs. Moreover, in spite of the Lidwell study, several centers have reported low infection rates of about 1% when neither airflow control nor personnel isolator systems were used (58).

Ultraviolet light is an economical alternative to expensive clean air control systems to reduce infection in prosthetic joints. Both Duke University and Peter Bent Brigham hospitals employed ultraviolet (UV) systems and reported infection rates of about 1% (59, 60). These systems are rapidly bactericidal; for example, Hart demonstrated that UV irradiation killed *S. aureus* within 1 to 3 minutes (61). In addition, UV systems are inexpensive and easy to install. However, the limitation of ultraviolet light is that UV radiation may be hazardous to both patient and personnel. Conjunctivitis, skin erythema, and corneal burns have all been reported, although these can be avoided by wearing protective glasses with side shields, hoods, and gowns. Not only would these protective measures protect personnel from UV burn, but they may also reduce the spread of airborne bacteria from personnel who are shedders. Patients may also need a sun screen to protect exposed areas. Damage to the patient's skin may reduce healing potential, although this risk has not been a problem at institutions where UV radiation has been used.

Traditional methods of reducing airborne bacterial contamination of the operating room should also be implemented in all clean surgeries. These include reducing personnel movement, minimizing the number of personnel in the operating theaters, excluding personnel with infections, and maintaining air pressure in the operating room above that of the adjacent rooms, hallways, and scrubrooms.

Antibiotic Prophylaxis

The same principles of prophylaxis with antibiotics apply for prosthetic joint surgery as for other surgical cases. Antimicrobial agents should be given if evidence clearly shows their benefit or if the consequences of an infection at the surgical site are catastrophic. Antimicrobial agents may be administered systemically or mixed with the bone cement to reduce the risk of infection. However the effect of antimicrobial prophylaxis cannot be evaluated by studies that use retrospective controls because technical advances in operating room modifications, such as air control systems and personnel isolator systems, that have been added at various centers and at different times would skew the results of such studies.

While antimicrobial prophylaxis is probably beneficial in prosthetic joint surgery, its benefits are not without equivocation. Nelson showed that administration of antimicrobial prophylaxis reduced the infection rate from 5.8% (109 of 1880) to 1.3% (90 of 6791) when all surgeries were performed in regular operating rooms (55). However, when the surgery was performed in operating rooms with air control systems, the rate of infection was 0.6% (17 of 2754) when antimicrobial agents were administered as compared to 0.7% (18 of 2730) when no antimicrobial agents were given. Thus, it would appear that antimicrobial agents may not significantly reduce infection rates if reduction of airborne bacteria can be achieved by air control systems.

An additional study by Hill and associates also demonstrated in 2,137 patients that infection rates after total hip replacement were reduced with the administration 5 days of cefazolin as compared to a placebo (0.9% versus 3.3%, respectively) (62). However, these authors also noted that the benefits of antimicrobial prophylaxis were limited to patients who had operations in conventional theaters, whereas there was no significant benefit for those patients in centers with air control systems. Additional prospective, randomized, double-blind studies also support the use of prophylactic antimicrobial agents for total hip replacement (63, 64).

The same principles for selecting an antimicrobial agent apply to total hip replacement surgery as to other surgical cases. An agent should be effective against the predominant pathogens, be parenteral, penetrate the target tissue, be present at the surgical site at the time of surgery, and be given for a short time. In the past, the ability of antibiotics to penetrate the bone in sufficient amounts to inhibit bacterial growth has been questioned, although several studies showed that antibiotics rapidly penetrate bone in sufficient concentrations to inhibit bacterial growth (65, 66). Thus, antibiotics can be started just before the surgical incision is made. Antibiotic administration should not last a long time, less than 48 hours. Nelson showed that infection rates did not differ significantly whether antibiotics were given for 1 day or for 7 (67). When Muller evaluated

1-day antibiotic prophylaxis for hip replacement, he found no deep infections among 238 patients after at least 1 year of follow-up (68).

Cephalosporins are the agents most often selected because of their spectrum of activity against *S. aureus* and *S. epidermidis* as well as against *E. coli*, *K. pneumoniae*, and *P. mirabilis*. Any of the first generation cephalosporins may be used—cefazolin, cephalothin, cephradine, or cephapirin. Cefazolin has the advantage of a longer half-life and can be given every 8 hours. Some of the newer cephalosporins such as ceftriaxone and cefonicid have an even longer half-life and need be given only once a day. However, the patient who has had an IgE-mediated allergic reaction to penicillin should not be given a cephalosporin or it should be administered only after extreme precautionary measures, including skin testing and desensitization. An alternate prophylactic agent is vancomycin. Semisynthetic penicillins, such as nafcillin, methicillin, or oxacillin, may also be selected but are less active against *S. epidermidis* and have no gram-negative activity. Since up to 40% of *S. epidermidis* at our institution is resistant to semisynthetic penicillins, these agents are not appropriate for prophylaxis. In addition, since most *S. aureus* the leading microbial agents in prosthetic joint infection, are β-lactamase producers, penicillin, ampicillin, and ureidopenicillins are not appropriate agents for prophylaxis.

Antibiotic irrigation is another consideration, although no conclusive evidence supports its practice. In fact, irrigating solutions of certain antibiotics, such as neomycin, have been associated with serious side effects. Neomycin may readily be absorbed, and in some cases when large doses were used for irrigation, deafness resulted (69). If neomycin is used for irrigation, the dose should not exceed 15 mg/kg/day or 1.0 g/day for longer than 3 days (70).

Although many studies support the use of systemic antibiotics in prosthetic joint insertion, few well designed studies support the usefulness of local instillation of antibiotics. The rationale for topical instillation or antibiotic-impregnated cement is that, because of the risk of deep tissue necrosis and hematoma formation, higher antibiotic concentrations provide an additional margin of safety over the systemic antibiotic. Gentamicin has been the main antibiotic impregnated into cements, although others have also been used, such as tobramycin, erythromycin, colistin, carbenicillin, chloraphenicol, and cephalothin. In one prospective, randomized, placebo-controlled study that evaluated gentamicin-impregnated cement in 476 total hip replacements, the rate of infection was 1.1% (3 of 274) in the group receiving the gentamicin cement compared to 5.9% (12 of 202) in the placebo group (71).

In another prospective, randomized, multicenter study, 1633 patients undergoing total hip replacements who received either gentamicin-impregnated bone cement or systemic antibiotics were followed for 1 to 2 years. The differences in deep infection rates between the two groups were statistically significant ($p = 0.01$): 1.6% (13 of 812) for the systemic antibiotic group versus 0.37% (3 of 820) for the gentamicin-impregnated bone cement group (72).

Some of the concerns about using antibiotic-impregnated cement include the effect on the mechanical properties of the cement, allergic reactions, and selection for resistant organisms. Since aqueous forms of an antibiotic adversely affect the mechanical properties of the cement, only a powder form of the agent should be used. The danger of an allergic reaction to the antibiotic impregnated in the cement has raised some concern among orthopaedic surgeons, since it would not be easy to remove the offending allergen, as can be done when antibiotics are administered systemically. Fortunately, allergic reactions have not been a problem, although gentamicin-impregnated cement has been used in over 1500 reported cases (73). Finally, concern has been raised in a few cases that persistent antibiotic concentrations in the bone may result in the selection of resistant organisms if a subsequent infection occurs. This problem may emerge after longer follow-up, more widespread use, or alteration in hospital flora because of gentamicin-resistant organisms.

What should be recommended to prevent infection in total joint replacement? Based on the Lidwell study, one would assume that clean air control, systemic and local antibiotics, and personnel isolator systems should all be employed (57). However, other factors play a role in the final infection rate reported in total hip replacements. When Eftekar conducted a retrospective study of members of the "Hip Society" at centers where more than 1000 hip operations had been performed, he found that the lowest infection rates were at centers where air control systems were not used (58). Infection rates were 0.36% and 0.69% in two centers performing 1000 and 5000 total hip replacements, respectively, whereas the infection rate was 0.4% to 1.46% when clean air was employed. When data from all 17 centers were reviewed (Table 23.1), the lowest rates occurred in areas where clean air and antibiotics were used. Although the difference seems small, it was significant ($\chi^2 = 5.86$, $p < 0.05$) when rates of 1.25% (85 of 6800) for clean air without antibiotics were compared to rates of 0.90% (35 of 3875) for clean air with antibiotics. The survey did not show a significant difference between institutions which used antibiotics with or without clean air systems. Consequently, while the Lidwell study has shown that control measures such as clean air systems and personnel isolators systems are beneficial, centers that do not employ these standards may still have acceptably low infection rates.

INFECTION IN PROSTHETIC HEART VALVES

The replacement of native heart valves with mechanical or bioprosthetic valves has favorably improved the prognosis for patients who have hemodynamic problems secondary to valvular dysfunction. Insertion of a prosthetic heart valve has become a common procedure both at university hospitals and in many community hospitals. Because of the frequency of valve replacement surgery, prosthetic valve endocarditis (PVE) has also become an important disorder. It is essential to recognize PVE as soon as possible so that appropriate medical and surgical therapy may reduce the high mortality from this entity.

Epidemiology

In a review of 11,873 operations from 21 centers, Watanakunakorn found that the incidence of PVE varied from 0% to 9.52%, with an overall incidence of 2.34% (74). Early endocarditis, occurring within 60 days of the prosthetic valve replacement, had the same frequency rate as late endocarditis (> 60 days): 1.14% versus 1.20%, respectively. However, the incidence rates for early and for late PVE differed over time. In early PVE, the incidence rate had dropped from 2.53% for series published before 1969 to 0.75% for series published between 1969 and 1976, whereas, for the same period, the incidence rate of late PVE has not changed significantly, dropping from 1.43% to 1.13%. Factors responsible for the reduction in early PVE include prophylactic antibiotics, improved surgical techniques and preoperative medical care, and earlier surgical intervention to prevent patients from becoming severely debilitated at the time of surgery (75). The

role of each of these factors is difficult to define since they have evolved in recent years.

Types of Heart Valve Prostheses

Heart valves may be replaced either with a mechanical valve made from plastic or metal or with a bioprosthetic valve made of cloth-covered struts and homologous or heterologous tissue. Initially, the bioprosthesis was believed to have several advantages. While the mechanical valve has more problems with thromboembolic phenomena and requires continuous anticoagulation, the bioprosthesis does not. Originally, it was also suggested that the porcine bioprosthetic valve had lower infection rates. However, Rossiter et al found no difference in infection rates between mechanical and bioprosthetic valves which were implanted at the same institution (Stanford) (76). Magilligan et al's and Clarkson and Barratt Boyes' reports of an incidence between 2.4% and 2.6%, respectively, are similar to Rossiter et al's report of a 2.6% infection rate for the Starr-Edwards mechanical valves (77, 78).

The site of valve insertion appears to be important for the development of infection, although the reason is unclear. Aortic valve infections outnumbered mitral valve prosthetic infections almost 2:1 in a review of 398 reported cases of PVE (79). The incidence of infection after insertion of an aortic prosthesis was 2.6%, as compared to 1.7% for a mitral prosthesis. In contrast to the predilection of prosthetic valve endocarditis to involve the aortic rather than the mitral valve, native valve endocarditis involves the mitral more often than the aortic valve.

Pathogenesis

The division of PVE into early and late relates to its pathogenesis. Early PVE, which results from bacterial implantation during surgery, becomes clinically apparent during the first 2 months postoperatively, whereas late PVE occurs after the first 2 postoperative months. Bacteria may come from endogenous or exogenous sources. Endogenous sources may arise from native valve infection, shedding of the patient's own skin flora into the operative site, or hematogenous seeding from a distant infection.

In patients with active endocarditis who are having a valve replaced, the native valve may be a source of bacterial contamination, but this complication occurs in less than 2% of such cases (80, 81). In a review of 31 cases of surgery for endocarditis, Rathod et al found no cases that became reinfected with the same organism if surgery was performed during therapy for the acute episode, although 42% (13/31) had culture-positive valves at the time the valve was removed (82). Others, however, have reported that as many as 15% of PVE replacements acquired recurrent PVE from the initial organism (83).

A second mechanism for endogenous spread is the shedding of organisms from the patient's own flora into the wound. When Kluge and associates evaluated the intraoperative contamination of the operative site in open heart surgery, they found that the most commonly contaminated site was the repaired area of the heart (64.1%) or the prosthesis (51.6%) (84). The most common organisms were diphtheroids and *S. epidermidis*, which accounted for 93.8% (45 of 48) of all organisms recovered. Not only do these organisms represent normal skin flora and common air contaminants in operating rooms, but they are also common causes of endocarditis (85). Interestingly, no endocarditis occurred in the follow-up of patients in Kluge's study.

It is not clear whether these organisms are endogenous, from the patient's own flora, or exogenous, from operating room shedders, although some indirect evidence suggests that endogenous sources may be more likely. A colonization survey of the staff, air, and inanimate environment of a cardiac surgery operating room produced very few methicillin-resistant staphylococci, yet 79% of 70 isolates in a series of *S. epidermidis* cultured from PVE cases were methicillin-resistant (86, 87). In addition, while only 6% of cardiac surgery patients were colonized preoperatively with methicillin-resistant *S. epidermidis*, 68% became colonized with such strains within 7 days of surgery after they received antimicrobial prophylaxis (88). Other studies have shown that the *S. epidermidis* from both skin flora and documented cases of PVE infection have similar plasmid band profiles and antibiograms (89). Against the likelihood of exogenous sources is Archer's finding that plasmid profiles did not match *S. epidermidis* isolates from colonizing patients and from hospital staff (86). Thus, the only definite conclusion is that cardiac surgery patients under the intense selective pressure of antimicrobial agents become colonized and infected with *S. epidermidis*. Whether the source of the infection is their own flora or is selected from the hospital environment is not clear at this point.

The third possible mechanism from an endogenous source is hematogenous spread from a septic complication of the valvular surgery. In a review of 19 cases of early PVE, Dismukes et al found 9 patients who had sites of infection that yielded the same organism subsequently identified as the cause of PVE (90). The sources included a contaminated intravenous catheter, postoperative pneumonia, postoperative wound infection, urinary tract infection, and dental caries. In the Dismukes series, late PVE also had extracardiac sources of infection; operative wound infection and pneumonia were less common, but dental manipulation and skin infection were more common in predisposing to late PVE.

Exogenous sources of PVE include insertion of a contaminated prosthesis, airborne sources, such as operating room staff shedding their flora into the operative site, a contaminated ventilation system, or contamination of the bypass pump.

Contamination from a xenograft prosthesis, specifically the Hancock porcine aortic valve, was reported by Laskowski and associates. They noted that *Mycobacterium chelonei* were recovered from six prosthetic valves and persisted in glutaraldehyde packing solution at 0.2% with a pH = 7.4, which is not mycobactericidal (91).

The airborne route is generally considered of minor importance. However, outbreaks of *Aspergillus* infection, including prosthetic valve infection, have been related to defects in ventilation systems and associated air contamination with *Aspergillus* (92, 93). Correcting these defects generally eliminated the pathogen from PVE. However, a recent article reported that wound infection increased after surgery if a contaminated case was performed within 48 hours before the cardiac surgery case (94). This study also suggests that the airborne route may need to be considered as a potential source during outbreak situations.

The other major exogenous source of bacterial contamination is the extracorporeal circulation from the cardiopulmonary bypass equipment, which may expose the whole blood volume to environmental air contamination drawn through suction lines. Blakemore et al found that the extracorporeal unit was contaminated in 75% of 32 patients who were undergoing a cardiopulmonary bypass procedure (85). Despite this high rate of contamination, in only two cases were organisms of the same species recovered from the blood in the pump as well as from sites of clinically significant infection.

Microbiology

Organisms responsible for early and late PVE are listed in Table 23.4. Isolation of a particular organism by itself does not warrant the distinction between early and late PVE. Staphylococci, both *epidermidis* and *aureus*, are common infecting agents in both forms, whereas streptococci, especially *viridans*, are more apt to occur late in the pathogenesis of PVE. Moreover, while Table 23.4 lists the most frequently found organisms, a variety of rare and unusual organisms has been found in many cases reported.

Clinical Diagnosis

In general, cases of prosthetic valve endocarditis are indistinguishable from native valve endocarditis caused by the same organism. Fever, changing murmur, and systemic embolization are the major clinical clues; however, any one, or all three, may be absent and endocarditis may still be present. Likewise, the clinician must aggressively pursue the slightest clue to this diagnosis to prevent the illness from progressing to mechanical disruption of the valve and catastrophic congestive heart failure. If a new anemia, leukocytosis, hematuria, or petechiae develop, blood cultures should be obtained in order to exclude PVE even if the patient has no fever.

The presence of bacteremia in the diagnosis of PVE is extremely important. Generally, the bacteremia is continuous and results in multiple, positive blood cultures in over 90% of patients. Although two to three separate blood cultures are usually collected within a 24-hour interval, in a patient with PVE, recent antimicrobial therapy or concerns over a fastidious organism would justify an additional two to three blood cultures during the 24- to 48-hour period after the original three sets (95). In addition, the clinician should alert the microbiology laboratory to incubate the blood culture for 2 weeks rather than for the customary 7 days since many fastidious organisms require longer incubation periods.

Table 23.4. Pathogens Responsible for Prosthetic Valve Endocarditis*

	Early PVE	Late PVE	Total
	%	%	%
S. epidermidis	30	23	27
S. aureus	19	10	14
Streptococci	11	39	26
Gram-negative bacilli	18	11	14
Diphtheroids	10	5	7
Candida	9	4	6
Aspergillus	3	1	2
Other or culture-negative	0	7	4

* Based on 576 pathogens isolated from 546 patients (79).

The clinician must be equally cautious about overdiagnosing PVE if a blood culture from a patient with a prosthetic heart valve is positive. Sande et al identified an extracardiac source for the bacteremia in 12 of 13 patients with prosthetic valves who developed bacteremia (96). Thus, more substantial clinical evidence than merely the presence of bacteremia should support the diagnosis of PVE.

Certain fastidious organisms, such as *Aspergillus* and *Histoplasmosis*, are almost uniformly associated with negative blood cultures. Additionally, the yield of *Candida* will be significantly reduced if the vacuum bottles are unvented (97).

Echocardiograhy has also been proposed as a useful adjunct in the diagnosis of infective endocarditis. Bioprosthetic valves are easier to assess by echocardiography than mechanical valves, although the prosthesis may generate sufficient echoes that small vegetations will be obscured. However, in a review in which patients with dysfunction due to primary tissue failure were compared to patients with infective endocarditis, echocardiography was not considered helpful (98).

Therapy

Therapy for PVE is more complicated than the management of native valve endocarditis, although the principles are similar, that is, parenteral therapy with a bactericidal agent that can readily achieve serum levels in excess of 8 times the minimal inhibitory concentration. In addition, the therapy must be well tolerated for 6 weeks. Initially, antibiotic selection should be empiric to ensure that an agent active against the most common isolate is selected. Since most *S. epidermidis* are methicillin-resistant, vancomycin should be part of the initial empiric regimen either alone or combined with other antimicrobial agents. Even when organisms were susceptible to β-lactams, vancomycin was more effective (87).

The three most effective antibiotics against methicillin-resistant *S. epidermidis* are vancomycin, rifampin, and gentamicin. However, other agents, such as teichoplanin, quinolones, and fusidic acid, may also be active against isolates of *S. epidermidis* and may prove to be useful alternate agents in the future.

The other specific therapy for PVE involves carefully performed in vitro susceptibility testing, as well as synergy testing and serum antibiotic measurements. These tests should be performed by laboratories familiar with their intricacies.

Another critical but not well defined issue is the timing of surgical intervention. In a series of 396 patients, the mortality rate for medical therapy was 55.4%, as compared to 50.7% for combined medical-surgical therapy (79). The indications for surgical intervention are similar to those for native valve endocarditis, i.e., major emboli, hemodynamic alteration, and uncontrolled infection. While opinions differ about the number of major emboli that necessitate surgical intervention, emboli to major vessels, including the central nervous system, or to extremities are sufficient to prompt valve and vegetation excision. Also, hemodynamic problems, specifically, moderate to severe heart failure, warrant prompt surgical intervention, as does prosthetic instability, which may portend dehiscence or valve obstruction from vegetations. The third nebulous indication is uncontrolled sepsis. Generally, fungal endocarditis requires excision for cure. In addition, some authors have recommended that the presence of bacteremia for more than 1 week warrants surgical intervention. By itself, however, prolonged bacteremia may be present in native valve endocarditis; and without emboli or hemodynamic defects, it is a questionable indication for surgery if the patient otherwise appears to be well. In such instances, the selection of antimicrobial agents should be carefully evaluated.

Prevention

Operating Room

Factors implicated in the development of PVE have been reviewed in the section on pathogenesis. The general principles of operating room asepsis, preoperative skin decontamination, good surgical techniques, the reduction of traffic flow, and operating room design that conforms to current standards are all essential to minimize the hazard of infection after cardiac surgery. However, several areas deserve special mention. Since distant foci of infection have clearly been implicated in PVE, they need to be effectively treated before surgery (96). Once the valve is inserted, a patient must be protected when undergoing certain procedures recognized as associated with bacteremia (Table 23.5). While producing a prosthesis free of contamination is the manufacturer's responsibility, contamination of such a prosthesis, preoperatively, has resulted in clusters of *Mycobacterium chelonei* infection (91). Some surgeons have considered swabbing cardiac valve prostheses before they are inserted, but this precaution is not routinely performed.

Air control of the operating room during cardiac surgery should conform to the standards of the Joint Commission on Accreditation of Hospitals and the requirements of the Public Health Service. An operating room in the United States should have a properly installed and maintained vertical flow, unidirectional air system that delivers a minimum of 25 changes/hour of high efficiency particulate air filtered into an operating room. The air should be exhausted low on the walls by an active exhaust system to maintain unidirectional air flow. Although air sampling is not routinely recommended, clear air has been defined, microbiologically, by the Committee on Operating Room Environment (CORE) (99).

Although the above-mentioned standards of clean air should be maintained in all modern operating rooms, cardiac bypass surgery deserves some special consideration. In most operating rooms, suction lines aspirate blood from wounds and discard the effluent, but in cardiac surgery, the blood is returned to the heart-lung machine to be recirculated into the patient. When blood is not being suctioned, room air is drawn into the heart-lung machine. In 1 hour on the bypass machine, the patient will be exposed to a minimum of 900 CFU in most operating rooms (99).

Table 23.5.   Indications and Regimens for Prophylaxis of Infective Endocarditis in Patients with Prosthetic Heart Valves

Procedure	Regimen	Penicillin-Allergic Patient
All dental (including cleaning), tonsillectomy and adenoidectomy, surgery of the respiratory mucosa (including bronchoscopy)	Penicillin plus streptomycin	Vancomycin
Surgery or instrumentation of gastrointestinal tract, gallbladder, and genitourinary tract	Penicillin or ampicillin and Gentamicin or streptomycin	Vancomycin and Streptomycin

Thus, the longer the time required for the operation, the greater will be the degree of bacterial contamination of the prosthetic valve. If environmental factors are addressed, special measures should be considered, such as turning the suction off when it is not being used or developing a check valve that will prevent the machine from suctioning air into the heart.

Contamination of air systems may arise either from air delivered to the room or from personnel in the room. The latter problem may be partly addressed by prohibiting an employee who has an acute, active bacterial infection from working in the operating room. However, transmission of pathogenic organisms from a shedder is impossible to identify until after a cluster of operating room-associated infections has occurred. Prompt, effective measures are required, including eradication of carriage and removal of the carrier from the operating room.

Antimicrobial Prophylaxis

Antimicrobial prophylaxis has become widely accepted among thoracic surgeons to prevent bacterial endocarditis in prosthetic heart valves. This practice is supported by the early experience of Geraci and associates who reported a 10% incidence of staphylococcal prosthetic valve endocarditis when patients did not receive antimicrobial prophylaxis (100). The prophylactic regimen should be active against staphylococci and streptococci, and a cephalosporin is usually selected. Prophylaxis should last 24 hours or less, as there is no evidence that longer administration is beneficial. Patients who have long operations may require an intraoperative dose. For this reason, cephalosporins, such as cefazolin, ceforanide, or cefonicid, that can be given at 8-, 12-, and 24-hour dosing schedules, respectively, may be better than cephalosporins with a shorter half-life. If the patient is allergic to penicillin, vancomycin is an acceptable alternative. However, although antimicrobial prophylaxis has significantly reduced early PVE, it has had little or no beneficial effect on late PVE.

INFECTIONS IN IMPLANTABLE DIALYSIS ACCESS SITES

Over 55,000 patients in the United States who have end-stage renal disease need chronic dialysis (101). About 90% are maintained on hemodialysis and the rest on peritoneal dialysis (102), but both forms of dialysis carry the risk of infection.

Hemodialysis

Infection in a patient on hemodialysis can be especially serious because of bacteremia and its attendant complications.

Epidemiology

Since patients with end-stage renal failure can all be considered immunocompromised, they are at increased risk for infection. Infection rates for local infection vary from 6 to 20%, and for bacteremia they vary from 1.7 to 12%, depending on the type of vascular access. As one would expect, distant foci of infection with associated bacteremia constitute an important risk factor (103), as is site of graft insertion. The rate of infection nearly doubles if a femoral graft is selected over a brachial graft (12.4% versus 7.6%, respectively)(103).

Types of Implantable Devices

Several types of angioaccess are available for hemodialysis, and they differ in terms of their lifespan (patency), infection rates, and other complications. The arteriovenous cannulas, including the Scribner and Thomas shunts, have been extensively used, but these devices have a short lifespan (usually less than 1 year) because they have a high rate of infection and thrombosis. In general, they have been replaced by arteriovenous fistulas (AVF), grafts, or prosthetic devices. An AVF has a good lifespan; in one study, more than 90% of 163 dialysis patients needed only one AVF over a 6-year period (104). However, because 30% of patients have an inadequate caliber for an anastomosis, an AVF cannot be used for their initial access, and other grafts must be used as secondary approaches for dialysis access (105). These include saphenous homografts, bovine heterografts, and synthetic grafts of polytetrafluoroethylene and knitted Dacron velour. While the bovine heterograft probably has the highest incidence of both local as well as bacteremic infection, it has remained patent for up to 12 months in 75% of patients who have had a previous access failure (105). Synthetic grafts have a lower incidence of infection, as reported by some centers (105), although this rate may vary with surgical expertise. In some centers, infection rates as high as 25% have been reported (106), a rate higher than reported for bovine heterografts.

Pathogenesis

Graft infection may occur early or late in onset. Early onset infection (< 3 months) may develop from grafts implanted at the time of surgery, but it also may occur from wound breakdown, which leads to subsequent colonization and then infection with pathogenic flora. Invariably, these grafts must be removed. Late onset infection (> 3 months) may arise from slow growth of a surgically implanted pathogen, insertion of a needle, or hematogenous seeding after endothelial disruption. The presence of local hematoma or devitalized tissue and fistula phlebitis all may increase the risk of infection at the site of dialysis access. In addition, frequent breaks in the integument not only increase the rate of skin colonization from pathogenic organisms such as *S. aureus*, but they may also lead to the formation of microabscesses in the integument which may, via contiguous spread, infect the vascular access site (107).

Microbiology

The microbiology of hemodialysis-associated infection is given in Table 23.6. As would be expected from pathogenic mechanisms, the gram-positive cocci, *S. aureus*, *S. epidermidis*, and streptococci are responsible for most bacteremias associated with local infection at a vascular access site. Anaerobic bacteria and fungi seldom are seen.

Clinical Manifestations

Clinical infections include perigraft infection with cellulitis, infected hematoma, or an infected pseudoaneurysm. If the infection becomes dis-

seminated with bacteremic-associated complications, such as septic pulmonary emboli, endocarditis, or osteomyelitis, the seeding of the vital structures may occur. Unfortunately, the clinical signs that point to an access site source of infection may be absent in over 30% of patients who have a vascular access-related bacteremia (109). Thus, the clinician should aspirate for gram stain and culture the access site directly, especially if there is no overt evidence of inflammation in the dialysis patient who has an unexplained fever.

Prevention

A major effort has been made to tabulate infection rates related to access sites, as illustrated by the many publications in this area. Still, further information needs to be compiled on the newest bioprostheses for vascular access. Certainly, meticulous surgical and aseptic techniques must be followed when the access device is inserted.

After the graft has been inserted, prophylactic antibiotics appear to help prevent infection. One study showed that a 5-day course of a semisynthetic penicillin combined with a single injection of gentamicin reduced the infection rate from 33% (6 of 18) in a group that received no antimicrobial agents to 12.5% (2 of 16) in the group that received the agents. Although the p value was statistically insignificant ($p = 0.05$ to 0.1), the data suggested a trend toward a significant difference (110). Although further work needs to

Table 23.6. Pathogens in Dialysis Patients

	Hemodialysis Patients: Blood Isolates Associated with Local Infection (108)		Chronic Peritoneal Dialysis Patients: Peritoneal Isolates (105)	
	No.	%	No.	%
Gram-positive	58	79.5	274	66.5
S. epidermidis	20	27.4	144	35.0
S. aureus	35	47.9	88	21.4
Streptococci	3	4.1	42	10.2
Gram-negative	15	20.5	105	25.5
Klebsiella, Enterobacter	4	5.5		
E. coli	4	5.5		
P. aeruginosa	1	1.4		
S. marcescens	4	5.5		
Proteus	1	1.4		
Others	1	1.4		
Fungi	0	0	33	8.0
C. albicans			25	6.1
Others			8	1.9

be performed in this area, it seems reasonable to use short course prophylaxis when a graft is inserted or manipulated.

Moreover, since some dialysis patients have a higher rate of colonization with *S. aureus*, eradicating the carrier state might be considered (107). However, this area has not been sufficiently studied to determine either the risk/benefit ratio or the preferred agent to use.

Treatment

Treatment of the access site combines medical (antimicrobial) therapy with surgical drainage or excision of the access site. However, the optimal surgical approach has not been clearly defined. The selection of antimicrobial therapy should be dictated not only by culture and sensitivity of the recovered pathogen, but also by knowledge of the pharmacokinetics and problems of antimicrobial therapy associated with renal failure.

Infections Associated with Chronic Peritoneal Dialysis

Chronic ambulatory peritoneal dialysis (CAPD) offers significant benefit as an alternative to hemodialysis for patients with chronic renal failure. Nevertheless, these advantages, including the benefit of outpatient therapy at home, have been tempered by a high infection rate. The average incidence of infection is 2.1 episodes/patient year (105). Since infection probably arises from the indwelling peritoneal catheter or its tunnel in the abdominal wall (111, 112), the responsible organisms are skin flora or flora from the perineum (Table 23.6).

Clinical manifestations are either local inflammation surrounding the catheter or peritonitis, as manifested by abdominal pain, fever, and a cloudy dialysate. The white blood count is usually ≥ 100 cells/mm³. A gram stain and culture and sensitivity of the peritoneal fluid should be performed to give specific direction in selecting an appropriate antimicrobial agent.

For CAPD patients, prevention measures play a crucial role in reducing infections. Patients must be well trained in the need to adhere to aseptic techniques in order to minimize their infection risks. Some patients who have repeated episodes of peritonitis while on CAPD may not be following good aseptic technique.

At the same time, improvements have been made in the delivery systems. For example, the use of plastic bags instead of glass bottles has significantly reduced the incidence of peritonitis

(102). Also, since a major source of contamination is the number of connections and disconnections used in the delivery systems, they should be designed to reduce the number needed (114). In addition, one study evaluated the role of povidone-iodine by aspirating it into the dialysis line during the bag exchange (115). Although this procedure reduced the incidence of peritonitis to 0.33 episodes/patient year, this was not a controlled study. While no evidence of iodinism occurred, and the procedure seemed safe, it must be evaluated further before it can be routinely adopted.

Finally, do prophylactic antibiotics help prevent CAPD-associated peritonitis? One controlled study evaluated oral cephalexin (500 mg, twice daily) in 50 patients over a 6-month period. The incidence of peritonitis was 1.05 episodes/patient year for the placebo group and 1.23 episodes/patient year for the cephalexin group (116). In addition, the incidence of cephalexin-resistant organisms in the treatment group was twice that of the placebo group. Thus, at this time, prophylactic oral antibiotics have no proven advantage in preventing peritonitis in CAPD patients, while the potential for selecting resistant organisms may be increased.

INFECTIONS IN IMPLANTABLE CENTRAL NERVOUS SYSTEM DEVICES

Central nervous system (CNS) devices may be implanted for several reasons: to permit the intraventricular instillation of chemotherapeutic or diagnostic agents, to permit unidirectional shunting of cerebrospinal fluid (CSF), and to monitor CSF pressure. As with the insertion of any implantable device, infection in these patients is a major concern, as are morbidity and mortality.

Epidemiology

The incidence of shunt infections ranges from 2 to 27%, and for ventriculostomies it ranges from 0 to 27% (117, 118). The infection rate from shunts is higher in children under 1 year of age than in older children (13% versus 8%, respectively) (117). Factors such as underlying disease, type of hydrocephalus, earlier meningitis, and diagnostic entry into the central nervous system do not seem to increase the risk of subsequent shunt infection (119). However, in one study, infection was more often found in patients with meningomyelocele than in noninfected patients (117).

A detailed epidemiologic study of ventriculostomies evaluated risk factors for ventriculostomy-related infection (118); these included duration of ventricular catheterization (more than 5 days), intracerebral hemorrhage with intraventricular hemorrhage, intracranial pressure greater than 20 mm Hg, neurosurgical operation, and irrigation of the ventriculostomy drainage system. Other factors that did not appear to increase the risk of infection included underlying disease, ventriculostomy performed in the intensive care unit, leak of the catheter, or previous ventriculostomy.

Types of Implantable Devices

A variety of devices can be implanted into the central nervous system to serve different functional needs. Some reservoirs are implanted without shunting capabilities and are used mainly for drug injection. Infection hazards in these instances are less than for other CNS devices because their use for chemotherapy is of limited duration.

The most commonly used CNS devices are shunting devices, which vary in complexity with the number of valves, dome elements, pumping ability, and reservoirs. Some shunts permit only unidirectional flow to the atrium or peritoneum, while others are bidirectional and permit access to both the ventricle and distal lines. Although understanding the biomechanical intricacies of a shunt is important for managing shunt obstruction, surgical insertion techniques and distal catheter location are more important considerations for managing infection (120). Currently, most CSF shunts are ventriculoperitoneal shunts, which have an infection rate similar to that of ventricular-atrial shunts (119). A ventriculostomy is essentially a small plastic catheter attached by tubing to a transducer with ports for sampling and monitoring and a drainage bag. These devices may be sewn to the scalp to prevent them from being dislodged.

Pathogenesis

Infections from implantable CNS devices arise from one of three routes. First, acute or early onset infections are caused by organisms implanted surgically from skin flora that contaminate either the device or the wound. These endogenous infections, primarily *S. epidermidis* and *S. aureus*, develop during the first 2 to 4 weeks after surgery.

The second method of acquisition is caused primarily by gram-negative bacilli colonizing the distal end of the catheter as a result of either bowel perforation or contamination of the abdominal wound by enteric flora (117, 121). Since this colonization occurs after implantation, most of these infections, called delayed onset infections, begin after the first 2 weeks of surgery. When bowel perforation occurs and retrograde infection results, a polymicrobic ventriculitis may result from enteric gram-negative bacilli, enterococci, and anaerobes.

A third source for ventriculitis from an implantable device is hematogenous seeding from a distal focus. This mechanism may explain the viridans streptococci from dental origins as well as the association of some enteric pathogens with urinary tract infections. Not only can atrial catheters become colonized and serve as portals for spread of ventriculitis, but other catheters may be seeded even if they are not located in the vascular system. Urinary tract infections may cause ventriculitis by spread of bacteria from the bladder into a cannulated ureter of a ventriculoureteral shunt or by hematogenous spread in other shunts.

Recently, scanning electon microscopic studies have provided additional information on the pathogenesis of shunt infections (122, 123). Ventricular catheters may have structural abnormalities that encourage staphylococci to adhere to their surface. As a result, catheter components may break down, and a slime layer is produced over the bacterial colonies that increases adherence and sequesters the organisms from antimicrobial therapy (124).

Microbiology

The two most commonly isolated bacteria from shunt and ventriculostomy infections are *S. epidermidis* and *S. aureus* (Table 23.7). In 10 to 15% of cases (117, 119), shunt infection may be polymicrobial; however, anaerobes are very rarely isolated in shunt infections.

Clinical Manifestatins

Ventriculitis is usually manifested by fever, change in the sensorium, irritability, shunt malfunction, nausea, and vomiting; however, in no more than 10% of cases does a shunt catheter drained into the abdomen show signs of peritonitis (117). Unfortunately, the clinical manifestations of ventriculitis for both shunt and ventriculostomy infections tend to be nonspecific, and meningeal signs are present in only one-quarter of the patients (117, 119). If the patient has fever or the shunt malfunctions, the CSF should be

Table 23.7. Bacteria Isolated from the Cerebrospinal Fluid from Patients with CSF Shunt- or Ventriculostomy-Related Infections

Pathogen	CSF Shunt (117, 119)		Ventriculostomy (118)	
	No.	%	No.	%
Gram-positive	136	74.7	9	47
S. epidermidis	77	42.3	6	32
S. aureus	42	23.1	1	5
Enterococcus	6	3.3	1	5
S. viridans	6	3.3	1	5
β streptococcus	2	1.1		
S. pneumoniae	2	1.1		
Diphtheroid	1	0.5		
Gram-negative	25	13.7	10	53
Others	21	11.5		

evaluated and bacteriologic cultures should be taken. The presence of an elevated leukocyte count with a predominance of segmented cells, elevated CSF protein, and hypoglycorrhachia all suggest infection. In addition, blood cultures should be obtained, since 25% of patients may be bacteremic (117).

Therapy

Therapy for shunts has long challenged the skill of the clinician. One major concern is CSF penetration of systemically administered antimicrobial agents, since agents commonly used for ventriculitis, such as vancomycin, have variable CSF penetration. The clinician must carefully monitor CSF penetration of the antimicrobial agent as well as the bacteriologic response in the CSF. Another concern is whether the shunt should be removed and, if so, when a new shunt should be implanted. Although patients may be cured without shunt removal, the cure rates are much higher when the shunt is removed (89 to 100%) than when it is not (30 to 62%) (117, 125). Thus, surgical removal and replacement may be the preferred mode of therapy, since the relapse rate after medical therapy and the malfunction rates are high. Whether a shunt is replaced immediately or later does not seem to affect the cure rate; a prospective study in which patients were randomized to immediate or delayed shunt replacements showed no difference in cure rates (125).

Prevention

Among published series on shunts and ventriculostomies, few preventive measures have been clearly identified. For a ventriculostomy, sug-

gested ways to reduce infection rates include minimizing the duration, avoiding irrigation, and using meticulous techniques to maintain the system (118). For shunts, meticulous insertion techniques should be observed to avoid bacterial implantation during insertion of the device.

Although prophylactic antimicrobial agents have been used by some neurosurgeons, this practice is not supported by convincing data; most such studies include historical controls but do not control for other variables. Further studies are needed to evaluate implantable CNS devices and the role of antimicrobial prophylaxis, as well as other measures that may reduce the hazard of infection.

References

1. Poss R, Thornhill TS, Ewald FC, Thomas WH, Batte NJ, Sledge CB: Factors influencing the incidence and outcome of infection following total joint arthroplasty. *Clin Orthop* 182:117–126, 1984.
2. Eftekhar NS: The natural history of infection in joint replacement surgery. In Eftekhar NS (ed): *Infection in Joint Replacement Surgery.* St Louis, CV Mosby, 1984, pp 26–96.
3. Charnley J, Eftekhar N: Postoperative infection in total prosthetic replacement arthroplasty of the hip-joint with special reference to the bacterial content of the air in the operating room. *Br J Surg* 56:1461–649, 1969.
4. Wilson PD Jr: Total hip replacement with fixation by acrylic cement: a preliminary study of 100 consecutive McKee-Farrar prosthetic replacements. *J Bone Joint Surg* 54A:207, 1972.
5. Charnley J: Postoperative infection after total hip replacement with special reference to air contamination in operating rooms. *Clin Orthop* 87:167, 1972.
6. Aventry MB: 2012 total hip arthroplasties: a study of postoperative course and early complications. *J Bone Joint Surg* 56A:273, 1974.
7. Ring PA: Problems of uncemented total hip replacement. *J Bone Joint Surg* 55B:209, 1973.
8. Nicholson OR: Total hip replacement. *Clin Orthop* 95:217, 1973.
9. Smith RE, Turner RJ: Total hip replacement using methylmethacrylate cement. *Clin Orthop* 95:231, 1973.
10. Buccholz HW, Novack G: Results of the total hip prosthesis design: "St. George." *Clin Orthop* 95:201, 1973.
11. Dandy DJ, Theodorou BC: The management of local complications of total hip replacement by the McKee-Farrar technique. *J Bone Joint Surg* 57B:30, 1975.
12. Fitzgerald RH Jr, Nolan DR, Lestrup DM, Van Scoy RE, Washington JA, Coventry MB: Deep wound sepsis following total hip arthroplasty. *J Bone Joint Surg* 59:847–855, 1977.
13. Poss R, Maloney JP, Ewald FC, Thomas WH, Battes NJ, Hartness C, Sledge CB: Six to 11 year results of total hip arthroplasty in rheumatoid

arthritis. *Clin Orthop* 182:109–116, 1974.

14. Fitzgerald RH, Kelly PJ: Total joint arthroplasty. *Mayo Clin Proc* 54:590–596, 1979.

15. Sheppeard H, Cleak DK, Ward DJ, O'Connor BT: A review of early mortality and morbidity in elderly patients following Charnley total hip replacement. *Arch Orthop Trauma Surg* 97:243–248, 1980.

16. Dunn AW: Replacement and resurfacing of joints. *Postgrad Med* 67:225–237, 1980.

17. Charnley J: The long-term results of low-friction arthroplasty of the hip performed as a primary intervention. *J Bone Joint Surg* 54B:61–76, 1972.

18. Insall JN, Ranawat CS, Aglietti P: A comparison of four models of total knee replacement prostheses. *J Bone Joint Surg* 58A:754–765, 1976.

19. Insall JN, Scott N, Ranawat CS: The total Condylar knee prosthesis. *J Bone Joint Surg* 61A:173–180, 1979.

20. Vahvanen V, Vainio U: Arthroplasty of the knee joint. *Scand J Rheumatol* 8:17–26, 1979.

21. Jones EC: GUEPAR knee arthroplasty results and late complications. *Clin Orthop* 140:145, 1979.

22. Neer C, Watson K, Stanton FJ: Recent experiences in total shoulder replacement. *J Bone Joint Surg* 64A:319, 1982.

23. Volz RG: Upper extremity joint replacement infection; diagnosis and management. In Eftekhar NS (ed); *Infection in Joint Replacement Surgery*. St Louis, CV Mosby, 1984, p 377.

24. Engelbrecht E, et al: Erfahrungen mit der Anwendung von Schultergelenksendoprothesen. *Chirurg* 51:794, 1980.

25. Volz RG: Total wrist arthroplasty: a clinical and biomechanical analysis. In *American Academy of Orthopaedic Surgeons: Symposium on Total Joint Replacement of the Upper Extremity*. St Louis, CV Mosby, 1982.

26. Morrey BF, Bryan RS: Infection after total elbow arthroplasty. *J Bone Joint Surg* 65A:330–338, 1983.

27. Brumfield RH, Volz RG, Green JF: Total elbow arthroplasty. *Clin Orthop* 158:137, 1981.

28. Lidwell OM, Lowbury EJL, Whyte W, Blowers R, Stanley SJ, Lowe D: Bacteria isolated from deep joint sepsis after operation for total hip or knee replacement and the sources of the infection with *Staphylococcus aureus*. *J Hosp Infect* 4:19–29, 1983.

29. Ahlberg A, Carlsson A, Lindberg L: Hematogenous infection in total joint replacement. *Clin Orthop* 137:69–75, 1978.

30. Blomgren G: Hematogenous infection of total joint replacement. *Acta Orthop Scand* 187:7–55, 1981.

31. Hecht RH, Meyer MH, Thornhill JM, Montgomerie JZ: Reactivation of tuberculous infection following total joint replacement. *J Bone Joint Surg* 65:1015–1016, 1983.

32. Salvati EA: Infection complicating total hip replacement. In *The Hip Society: The Hip Proceedings of the Fourth Open Scientific Meeting of The Hip Society*. St Louis, CV Mosby, 1976.

33. Fitzgerald RH: Contamination of the surgical wound in the operating room. *J Bone Joint Surg* 56A:849, 1974.

34. Hunter G, Dandy D: The natural history of pa-

tients with an infected total hip replacement. Presented at the Annual Meeting of the American Academy of Orthopedic Surgeons, New Orleans, 1976.

35. Murray WR: Results in patients with total hip replacement arthroplasty. *Clin Orthop* 95:80–90, 1973.

36. Patterson FP, Brown CS: The McKee-Farrar total hip replacement: preliminary results and complications of 368 operations performed in five general hospitals. *J Bone Joint Surg* 54A:257, 1972.

37. Benson MKD, Hughes SPF: Infection following total hip replacement: general hospital without special orthopedic facilities. *Acta Orthop Scand* 46:968, 1975.

38. Nelson JP: Operating room, clean rooms and personnel isolator systems. In *American Academy of Orthopaedic Surgeons: Instructional Course Lectures*. St Louis, CV Mosby, 1977, vol 26.

39. Horadam VW, Smilack JD, Smith EF: *Mycobacterium fortuitum* infection after total hip replacement. *South Med J* 75:244–246, 1982.

40. Younkins S, Evarts CM, Steigbigel RT: *Candida parapsilosis* infection of a total hip-joint replacement. *J Bone Joint Surg* 66:142–143, 1984.

41. Goodman JS, Seibert DG, Reahl GE, Geckler RW: Fungal infection of prosthetic joints. *J Rheumatol* 10:494–495, 1983.

42. Carlsson AS: Erythrocyte sedimentation rate in infected and noninfected total hip arthroplasties. *Acta Orthop Scand* 49:287–290, 1978.

43. Murray WR, Rodrigo JJ: Arthrography for the assessment of pain after total hip replacement: a comparison of arthrographic findings in patients with and without pain. *J Bone Joint Surg* 57:1060–1065, 1975.

44. O'Neill DA, Harris WH: Failed total hip replacement: assessment by plane radiographs, arthrograms, and aspiration of the hip joint. *J Bone Joint Surg* 66:540–546, 1984.

45. Williamson BR, McLaughlin RE, Wang GW, Miller CA, Teates CD, Bray ST: Radionuclide bone imaging as a means of differentiating loosening and infection in patients with a painful total hip prosthesis. *Radiology* 133:723–725, 1979.

46. Williams ED, Tregonning RJ, Hurley PJ: 99 Tcm-diphosphonate scanning as an aid to diagnosis of infection in total hip-joint replacements. *Br J Radiol* 50:562–566, 1977.

47. Williams F, McCall IW, Park WM, O'Connor BT, Morris V: Gallium-67 scanning in the painful total hip replacement. *Clin Radiol* 32:431–439, 1981.

48. Mulumba L, Ferrant A, Leners N, de Neyes P, Rombauts JJ, Vincent A: Indium III leukocyte scanning in the evaluation of painful hip arthroplasty. *Acta Orthop Scand* 54:695–697, 1983.

49. Burton DS, Schurman DJ: Salvage of infected total joint replacements. *Arch Surg* 112:574–578, 1977.

50. Bourne RB, Hunter GA, Rorabeck CH, Macnab JJ: A six-year follow-up of infected total hip replacements managed by Girdlestone's arthroplasty. *J Bone Joint Surg* 66:340–343, 1984.

51. Hunter G, Dandy D: The natural history of the patient with an infected total hip replacement. *J Bone Joint Surg* 59:293–297, 1977.

52. Lidwell OM: The cost implications of clean air

systems and antibiotic prophylaxis in operations for total joint replacement. *Infect Control* 5:36–37, 1984.

53. Laufmann H: Surgical hazard control: effect of architecture and engineering. *Arch Surg* 107:552, 1973.
54. Laufmann M: Current status of special air handling systems in operating rooms. *Med Instrum* 7:7, 1973.
55. Nelson JP: Operating room environment: clean room and personnel isolator systems. In Eftekhar NS (ed): *Infection in Joint Replacement Surgery.* St Louis, CV Mosby, 1984, pp 166–177.
56. Salvati EA: Infection rates after 3175 total hip and total knee replacements performed with and without a horizontal unidirectional filtered airflow system. *J Bone Joint Surg* 64A:525, 1982.
57. Lidwell OM, Lowbury EJL, Whyte W: Effect of ultraclean air in operating rooms on deep sepsis in the joint after total hip or knee replacement: a randomized study. *Br Med J* 285:10–14, 1982.
58. Eftekhar NS: Combined use of chemoprophylaxis and ultraclean-air technology in preventing infection. In Eftekhar NS (ed): *Infection in Joint Replacement Surgery.* St Louis, CV Mosby, 1984, pp 250–266.
59. Moggio M, Goldner JL, McCollum DE, Beissinger SF: Wound infection in patients undergoing total hip arthroplasty. *Arch Surg* 114:815–823, 1979.
60. Lowell JD, Kundsin RB: The operating room and the ultraviolet environment. *Med Instrum* 12:181–184, 1978.
61. Hart D: Bactericidal ultraviolet radiation in the operating room. *JAMA* 172:1019–1028, 1960.
62. Hill C, Flamant R, Mazus F, Evrard J: Prophylactic cefazolin versus placebo in total hip replacement. *Lancet* 1:795–796, 1981.
63. Boyd RJ, Burke JF, Colton T: A double-blind clinical trial of prophylactic antibiotics in hip fractures. *J Bone Joint Surg* 55A:1251, 1973.
64. Pavel A: Prophylactic antibiotics in clean orthopedic surgery. *J Bone Joint Surg* 56A:777, 1974.
65. Schurman DJ: Cefazolin concentration in bone and synovial fluid. *J Bone Joint Surg* 60A:359, 1978.
66. Schurman DJ: Cephalothin and cefamandole bone, joint fluid, and hematoma penetration in joint replacement surgery. *J Bone Joint Surg* 62A:981, 1980.
67. Nelson CL, Green TG, Porter RA, Warren RD: One day versus seven days of preventive antibiotic therapy in orthopedic surgery. *Clin Orthop* 176:258, 1983.
68. Muller JC, Cheng N, Van Tornout B, Vandepette J, Debruyne H: The effect of the combined use of a clean air system and one day prophylactic administration of cefamandole in total hip replacement. *Arch Orthop Trauma Surg* 98:29–33, 1981.
69. Weinstein AJ, McHenry MC, Garan TL: Systemic absorption of neomycin irrigating solution. *JAMA* 238:152–153, 1977.
70. Kucers A, McK Bennett N: Neomycin, framycetin, and paromomycin. In Kucers A, McK Bennett N (eds): *The Use of Antibiotics.* London,

Heinemann, 1979, p 410.
71. Wannske M, Tscherne H: Ergebresse prophylacktischer anwerdung von refobasin palacos bei der implantation von endoprosthesen der muftgelenkes in hannoven. In Burri C, Ruter A (eds). *Actual Problems in Surgery and Orthopedic Surgery.* Berne, 1979, vol 12.
72. Josefsson G: Gentamicin-impregnated bone cement in total hip replacement: prevention and treatment of deep infection. Dissertation, Westfred and Soner. Boktryckeri AB, Gavle, 1980.
73. Nelson CI, Bergman BR: Antibiotic-impregnated acrylic composites. In Eftekhar NS (ed): *Infection in Joint Replacement Surgery.* St Louis, CV Mosby, 1984, p 274.
74. Watanakunakorn C: Prosthetic valve infective endocarditis. *Prog Cardiovasc Dis* 22:181–192, 1979.
75. Wilson WR, Danielson GK, Giuliani ER, Geraci JE: Prosthetic valve endocarditis. *Mayo Clin Proc* 57:155–161, 1982.
76. Rossiter SJ, Stinson EB, Oyer PE: Prosthetic valve endocarditis: comparison of heterograft tissue valves and mechanical valves. *J Thorac Cardiovasc Surg* 76:795–803, 1978.
77. Magilligan DJ, Quinn EL, Davila JC: Bacteremia, endocarditis, and the Hancock valve. *Ann Thorac Surg* 24:508–518, 1977.
78. Clarkson PM, Barratt-Boyes BG: Bacterial endocarditis following homograft replacement of the aortic valve. *Circulation* 42:987–991, 1970.
79. Gnann JW, Cobbs CG: Infection of prosthetic valves and intravascular devices. In Mandell GL, Douglass RG, Bennett JE (eds): *Principles and Practice of Infectious Diseases.* New York, John Wiley & Sons, 1984, p 530.
80. Wilson WR, Danielson GK, Giuliani ER: Valve replacement in patients with active infective endocarditis. *Circulation* 58:585–588, 1978.
81. Karchmer AW, Stinson EB: The role of surgery in infective endocarditis. In Swartz M, Remington J (eds): *Current Clinical Topics in Infectious Diseases.* New York, McGraw-Hill, 1980, p 124.
82. Rathod M, Quinn E, Saravolatz L, Magilligan D, del Busto R, Pohlod D, Lewis J: Quantitative cultures of cardiac valves from patients with infective endocarditis (IE). *23rd Interscience Conference on Antimicrobial Agents and Chemotherapy,* no. 863, October 1983.
83. Baumgartner WA, Miller DC, Reitz BA: Surgical treatment of prosthetic valve endocarditis. *Ann Thorac Surg* 35:87, 1974.
84. Kluge RM, Calia FM, McLaughlin JS, Hornick RB: Sources of contamination in open heart surgery. *JAMA* 23:1415–1418, 1974.
85. Blakemore WS, McGarrity GJ, Thorer RJ: Infection by airborne bacteria with cardiopulmonary bypass. *Surgery* 70:830–838, 1971.
86. Archer GL: *Staphylococcus epidermidis*: the organism, its diseases and treatment. In Swartz M, Remington J (eds): *Current Clinical Topics in Infectious Diseases.* New York, McGraw-Hill, 1985, p 25.
87. Karchmer AW: *Staphylococcus epidermidis* prosthetic valve endocarditis: microbiological and clinical observations as guides to therapy. *Ann Intern Med* 98:447, 1983.

88. Archer GL, Armstrong BC: Alteration of staphy-lococcal flora in cardiac surgery patients receiving antibiotic prophylaxis. *J Infect Dis* 147;642, 1983.

89. Archer GL: Plasmid pattern analysis of *Staphylococcus epidermidis* isolates with prosthetic valve endocarditis. *Infect Immun* 35:627, 1982.

90. Dismukes WE, Karchner AW, Buckley MJ, Austin GW, Swartz MN: Prosthetic valve endocarditis. *Circulation* 48:365–377, 1973.

91. Laskowski LF, Marr JJ, Spoernoga JF, Frank NJ, Barner HB, Kaiser G, Tyras DH: Fastidious mycobacteria grown from porcine-heart-valve cultures. *N Engl J Med* 297:101–102, 1977.

92. Gage AA, Dean DC, Schimert G, Minsley N: *Aspergillus* infection after cardiac surgery. *Arch Surg* 101:384–387, 1970.

93. Petheram IS, Seal RM: *Aspergillus* prosthetic valve endocarditis. *Thorax* 31:380–390, 1976.

94. deSilva MI, Rissing JP: Postoperative wound infections following cardiac surgery: significance of contaminated cases performed in the preceding 48 hours. *Infect Control* 5:371–377, 1984.

95. Washington JA: The role of the microbiology laboratory in the diagnosis and antimicrobial treatment of infective endocarditis. *Mayo Clin Proc* 57:22–32, 1982.

96. Sande MA, Johnson WD, Hook EW, Kaye D: Sustained bacteremia in patients with prosthetic cardiac valves. *N Engl J Med* 286:1067, 1972.

97. Gantz NM, Mederios AA, Swain JL, O'Brien TF: Vacuum blood-culture bottles inhibiting growth of *Candida* and fostering growth of *Bacteroides*. *Lancet* 2:1174–1176, 1974.

98. Effron MK, Popp RL: Two-dimensional echocardiographic assessment of bioprosthetic valve dysfunction and infective endocarditis. *J Am Coll Cardiol* 2:4:597–606, 1982.

99. Altemeier WA, Burke JA, Pruitt BA, Sandusky WR: Preparation and maintenance of a safe operating room environment. In *Manual on Control of Infection in Surgical Patients*. Philadelphia, JB Lippincott, 1984, p 111.

100. Geraci JE, Dale AJD, McGoon DC: Bacterial endocarditis and endarteritis following cardiac operations. *Wisc Med J* 62:302–317, 1963.

101. Salvatierri O: Analysis of costs and outcomes of renal transplants at one center: its implications. *JAMA* 241:1469, 1974.

102. Levey AS, Harrington JT: Continuous peritoneal dialysis for chronic renal failure. *Medicine* 61:330, 1982.

103. Nghiem DD, Schulak JA, Corry RJ: Management of the infected hemodialysis access grafts. *Trans Am Soc Artif Intern Organs* 29:360–362, 1983.

104. Zerbino VR: A six-year clinical experience with arteriovenous fistula and bypasses for hemodialysis. *Surgery* 76:1018, 1974.

105. Steigbigel RT, Cross AS: Infection associated with hemodialysis and chronic peritoneal dialysis. In Swartz M, Remington J (eds): *Current Clinical Topics in infectious Diseases*. New York, McGraw-Hill, 1984, vol 5, pp 124–144.

106. Munda R, First R, Alexander JW, Linnemann CC, Fidler JP, Kitter D: Polytetrafluoroethylene graft survival in hemodialysis. *JAMA* 249:219–222, 1983.

107. Kirmani N, Tuazon CU, Murrary HW: *Staphy-lococcus aureus* carriage rate of patients receiving long-term hemodialysis. *Arch Intern Med* 138:1657–1659, 1978.

108. Keane WF, Shapiro FJ, Raij L: Incidence and type of infection occurring in 445 chronic hemodialysis patients. *Trans Am Soc Artif Intern Organ* 23:41–47, 1977.

109. Dobkin JF: Septicemia in patients on chronic hemodialysis. *Ann Intern Med* 88:28, 1978.

110. Oduring A, Slapak M: The use of Goretex (P.T.E.E.) for angio-access for chronic haemodialysis: the place of peri-operative antibiotics. *Br J Clin Pract* 134–137, 1984.

111. Fenton SS, Wu G, Cattran D, Wadigymer A, Allen AF: Clinical aspects of peritonitis in patients on CAPD. *Peritoneal Dial Bull* 1:54–56, 1981.

112. Williams C, Cattran D, Fenton SS, Khanne K, Manuel R, Saiphao C, Oreopoulous DG, Roscoe J: Peritonitis in CAPD: three years' exposure in Toronto. *Peritoneal Dial Bull* 1:57–58, 1981.

113. Rubin J: Peritonitis during continuous ambulatory peritoneal dialysis. *Ann Intern Med* 92:7, 1980.

114. Oreopoulous DG: A simple and safe technique for continous ambulatory peritoneal dialysis (CAPD). *Trans Am Soc Artif Intern Organ* 24:484, 1978.

115. Yee E: Use of povidone iodine in continuous ambulatory peritoneal dialysis (CAPD): a technique to reduce the incidence of infectious peritonitis. *Trans Am Soc Artif Intern Organ* 26:223, 1980.

116. Low DE: Prophylactic cephalexin ineffective in chronic ambulatory peritoneal dialysis. *Lancet* ii:753, 1980.

117. Odio C, McCracken GH, Nelson JD: CSF shunt infections in pediatrics. *Am J Dis Child* 138:1103–1108, 1984.

118. Mayhall CG, Archer NH, Lamb V, Spadora AC, Baggett JW, Ward JD, Narayan RK: Ventriculostomy-related infections. *N Engl J Med* 310:553–559, 1984.

119. Schoenbaum SC, Gardner P, Shilleto J: Infections of cerebrospinal fluid shunts: epidemiology, clinical manifestations, and therapy. *J Infect Dis* 131:543–552, 1975.

120. Sells CJ, Shortleff DB: Cerebrospinal fluid shunts. *West J Med* 127:93–98, 1977.

121. Brook I, Johnson N, Overturf: Mixed bacterial meningitis: a complication of ventriculo- and lumboperitoneal shunts: report of two cases. *J Neurosurg* 47:961–964, 1977.

122. Baystin R, Penny SR: Excessive production of mucoid substances in *Staphylococcus* S11A: a possible factor in colonization of Holter shunts. *Dev Med Child Neurol* 14:25–28, 1972.

123. Guevara JA, LaTorre J, Denoya C: Microscopic studies in shunts for hydrocephalus. *Child's Brain* 8:284–293, 1981.

124. Peters G, Locci R, Pulverer G: Adherence and growth of coagulase-negative staphylococci on surfaces of intravenous catheters. *J Infect Dis* 146:479–482, 1982.

125. James HE, Walsh JW, Wilson HD, Connor JD, Bean JR, Tibbs PA: Prospective randomized study of therapy in cerebrospinal fluid shunt infection. *Neurosurgery* 7:459–463, 1980.

Chapter 24

Nosocomial Gastrointestinal Infections

James M. Hughes, M.D., and William R. Jarvis, M.D.

INTRODUCTION

Nosocomial gastroenteritis may be defined as an acute infectious gastrointestinal illness acquired by a hospitalized patient. More specifically, this entity has been defined as a positive culture for a pathogen or unexplained diarrhea lasting 2 or more days (1) or as onset of infectious diarrhea in the hospital (2). The usual incubation period for an agent is important to consider in determining whether a given infection is nosocomial. Definitions of diarrhea itself vary considerably but generally include some consideration of stool consistency (e.g., liquid or watery) and frequency (e.g., ≥ three/24 hours or more frequent than normal for the individual). No single definition of diarrhea may be adequate for use in all areas of the hospital; for example, the normal frequency and consistency of the stools of neonates need to be considered in defining a case of diarrhea in a neonatal unit.

The definition of a case of nosocomial gastroenteritis requires exclusion of patients who have illnesses with noninfectious etiologies. In addition to underlying diseases that have diarrhea as a manifestation, a number of substances to which hospitalized patients are frequently exposed may cause diarrhea (e.g., antacids, laxatives, cathartics, cytotoxic drugs, enteral hyperalimentation fluids, and lactulose).

In cases of presumed nosocomial gastroenteritis, it is not always possible to identify an etiologic agent. Although identification of some enteric pathogens (e.g., *Salmonella*, *Campylobacter*, and *Shigella*) is well within the capability of clinical microbiology laboratories, identification of other agents (e.g., enterotoxigenic *Escherichia coli* and Norwalk agent) requires techniques usually available only in reference or research laboratories.

The purpose of this chapter is to review the magnitude of the problem of nosocomial gastroenteritis, the risk factors, and the modes of

transmission. Selected gastroenteritis syndromes will be described, and infectious agents capable of causing nosocomial gastroenteritis will be discussed. The problems of gastroenteritis in patients in extended care facilities in developed countries and gastroenteritis in hospitalized patients in developing nations will also be addressed. Finally, priority areas for future research will be identified.

MAGNITUDE OF THE PROBLEM

Data on the magnitude of the problem of nosocomial gastroenteritis are limited. Information reported by hospitals participating in the Centers for Disease Control's (CDC) National Nosocomial Infections Study (NNIS) during 1980 to 1984 indicate that the nosocomial gastroenteritis infection rate was 1.3/10,000 discharges. The infection rate varied by service, with the highest rates in patients on the pediatric (4.2/10,000 discharges) and newborn (3.3/10,000 discharges) services (Table 24.1), and by hospital category, with the highest rates in patients in the large medical school-affiliated hospitals (1.8/10,000 discharges) (Table 24.2). Forty-one percent of all infections occurred in infants (Table 24.3). An etiologic agent was identified in 57% of the cases, and bacteria accounted for 78% of the reported etiologic agents. *Clostridium difficile* was the most common nosocomial pathogen identified and accounted for 45% of infections of known etiology. *Salmonella* spp. ranked second, accounting for 12% of infections. However, since most NNIS hospitals lack diagnostic virology laboratories, the relative importance of viruses in the etiology of nosocomial gastroenteritis is certainly underestimated by these data.

In a 1-year prospective study conducted in a children's hospital, the gastrointestinal tract was the second most common site of nosocomial infection; in this study, 65 (56%) of 117 gastrointestinal tract infections were of known etiology,

Table 24.1. Nosocomial Gastroenteritis Infection Rates by Service, NNIS Hospitals, 1980 to 1984

Service	No. of Infections	Rate*
Pediatrics	133	4.2
Newborn	175	3.3
Medicine	188	1.1
Surgery	178	1.0
Gynecology	15	0.5
Obstetrics	15	0.2

* Per 10,000 discharges.

Table 24.2. Nosocomial Gastroenteritis Infection Rates by Hospital Category, NNIS Hospitals, 1980 to 1984

Hospital Category*	No. of Infections	Rate†
NMSA	88	0.5
SMSA	224	1.5
LMSA	393	1.8

* NMSA, non-medical school-affiliated; SMSA, small (≤ 500 beds) medical school-affiliated; LMSA, large (> 500 beds) medical school-affiliated.
† Per 10,000 discharges.

Table 24.3. Distribution of Nosocomial Gastroenteritis Cases by Age Group, NNIS Hospitals, 1980 to 1984

Age Group	No. of Infections	% of Total
< 1 month	179	25.5
1–11 months	109	15.5
1–2 years	35	5.0
3–19 years	38	5.4
20–59 years	151	21.5
≥ 60 years	190	27.1

and all were viral (3). In a 17-month prospective study of patients in a medical school-affiliated hospital caring for both adults and children, nosocomial viral infections were encountered most frequently on the pediatric service, and most nosocomial gastrointestinal tract infections had a viral etiology (4).

In a review of nosocomial outbreaks investigated by epidemiologists from the Centers for Disease Control (CDC) between 1956 and 1979, 21% of the 223 epidemics involved infections of the gastrointestinal tract (5). From 1971 to 1979, nosocomial gastroenteritis epidemics accounted for 17% of all epidemic investigations conducted by CDC epidemiologists. In contrast, nosocomial gastroenteritis accounted for fewer than 1% of

endemic nosocomial infections reported by hospitals participating in NNIS (5). The gastrointestinal tract may also be involved in nosocomial pseudoepidemics. In a review of 20 pseudoepidemics investigated by CDC epidemiologists from 1956 to 1975, 4 (20%) involved the gastrointestinal tract (6).

No studies have clearly estimated attributable morbidity or mortality from nosocomial gastroenteritis. Furthermore, the direct economic burden of such infections is unknown.

RISK FACTORS

Patients at highest risk for nosocomial gastroenteritis include neonates, the elderly, and patients with achlorhydria. Risk factors for nosocomial gastroenteritis can be divided into two groups: extrinsic and intrinsic factors. Intrinsic risk factors involve impairment of specific or nonspecific immunity, gastric acidity, or intestinal motility and alteration of the normal enteric flora. Specific and nonspecific immunity, provided by the humoral and cell-mediated immune systems, play a major role in resistance to gastrointestinal infection. Patients in whom immune function is abnormal, such as bone marrow transplant patients and those with severe immunodeficiency syndromes, are at an increased risk of developing nosocomial gastroenteritis (7, 8). Yolken et al showed that 40% of bone marrow transplant patients developed nosocomial gastroenteritis, which had a 55% crude mortality rate (7). Specific immunity, such as antirotaviral antibody, either may protect against infection or, if infection occurs, may ameliorate disease. Nonspecific immune components, such as phagocytes, appear to be important in preventing invasive infections with *Candida* spp. Gastric acidity acts as a barrier preventing pathogens from reaching the small and large bowel. Patients with reduced gastric acidity, such as those receiving antacids or those who have undergone gastrectomies, are at increased risk for nosocomial gastroenteritis and may develop more severe disease if infection occurs (9, 10). Intestinal motility is also important in eliminating invasive pathogens; in patients in whom motility is reduced, severity of diseases may be increased (11, 12). Alteration of the normal enteric flora (e.g., by antimicrobials) may also place the patient at increased risk for nosocomial gastroenteritis (13).

Extrinsic risk factors are those outside of the host. Although all hospitalized patients are at risk of acquiring nosocomial gastroenteritis, those in intensive care units appear at greatest risk. In one study, 41% of patients admitted to an intensive care unit during 1 year developed nosocomial gastroenteritis (9). These patients were significantly more likely to have had a nasogastric feeding tube and to have received cimetidine than were those who did not develop gastroenteritis. Thus, factors that bypass or alter host resistance mechanisms or increase the likelihood of colonization increase the risk of nosocomial gastroenteritis.

MODES OF TRANSMISSION

Infectious agents causing gastroenteritis are transmitted by the fecal-oral route. Transmission of nosocomial gastroenteritis typically involves either contact spread from person to person, which may be direct or indirect, or common-vehicle spread (Table 24.4). Airborne and vector-borne spread play little if any role in transmission of nosocomial gastroenteritis. Although common-vehicle transmission has been documented in outbreaks of nosocomial gastroenteritis, the majority of endemic cases result from contact spread. The large number of organisms excreted in the feces, many of which can survive for prolonged periods in the inanimate and animate environment, serve as a major potential reservoir for transmission (14). Inadequate hand washing by medical personnel and inadequate sterilization or disinfection of patient care equipment increase

Table 24.4. Relative Importance of Different Routes of Transmission and Fomites in the Spread of Selected Agents Causing Epidemic Nosocomial Gastroenteritis*

Agent	Contact			Common Vehicle	Fomites
	Direct	In-direct	Droplet		
Salmonella	++	+	±	++	±
Shigella	++	−	−	−	−
Y. enterocolitica	++	?	−	−	−
E. coli	++	?	−	+	−
C. difficile	?	?	−	−	?
Rotavirus	++	?	?	−	?
Norwalk agent	++	?	?	?	?
Adenovirus	+	?	?	?	?
Cryptosporidium	+	?	−	−	?

* Key: ++, Common
+, Occasional
±, Rare
−, Little or no evidence
?, Unknown.

the likelihood of patient colonization and the risk of developing nosocomial gastroenteritis.

SYNDROMES

Necrotizing Enterocolitis (NEC)

A syndrome of segmental intestinal gangrene was described as early as 1891 by Genersich (15). Subsequently, a similar syndrome known as enteritis necroticans was described in Germany following World War II and one known as pigbel was described in New Guinea in association with pork feasts (16, 17). Clinically the patients all had abdominal distension and vomiting and abdominal radiographs which demonstrated small amounts of gas in the intestinal wall, peritoneal cavity, and occasionally in the portal venous tract. In recent years the most common setting for NEC has been in newborn infants, primarily in those who are premature or of low birth weight. In these patients, the syndrome consists of abdominal distension, feeding intolerance, vomiting, bloody stools, and radiographic evidence of pneumatosis intestinalis, with or without portal or peritoneal air (18).

Prior to 1970 most cases of NEC were sporadic. However, since that time, many outbreaks of NEC have been reported. Risk factors for NEC that have been described include low Apgar scores or asphyxia, presence of a patent ductus arteriosus, maternal anesthesia, antimicrobial exposure of the mother or infant, exposure to hyperalimentation or dextrose solutions, gavage feedings, premature rupture of membranes, respiratory distress syndrome, umbilical arterial or venous catheterization, polycythemia or hyperviscosity, apnea, exchange transfusions, and hypertonic feedings. However, it must be recognized that most of these risk factors have been identified by either retrospective or observational studies. In 1980, Ryder et al reported the results of a prospective collaborative study conducted at 12 medical centers (19). Cases included all patients with NEC, and controls were patients selected from the same institutions matched for weight and duration of hospitalizaton. This study showed that low Apgar scores or asphyxia, the presence of a patent ductus arteriosis, maternal anesthesia, antimicrobial exposure, exposure to solutions containing 10% dextrose, and premature rupture of membranes were associated with cases of NEC. However, a subsequent study by Kliegman et al, conducted in a similar fashion, failed to confirm Ryder et al's findings and found only vaginal delivery as a risk factor for NEC (20). Since many of the studies of risk factors for NEC failed to examine similarly defined parameters, comparison of results is difficult.

Several observations suggest that an infectious agent is responsible for NEC. These include the finding that the gas present in the pneumatosis of NEC is hydrogen of probable microbial origin, the frequent finding of positive blood and peritoneal fluid cultures in cases of NEC, the clinical similarity of NEC to cases of infectious gastroenteritis, and the frequent clustering of cases of NEC in nurseries. Numerous bacterial and viral agents have been identified as the putative "etiologic agent" of NEC (Table 24.5). However, in the majority of these studies, the microbiologic testing was either inadequate to identify other potential organisms or the authors failed to examine a control population for the presence of similar organisms. In these studies, a wide variety of bacterial and viral pathogens has been identified: enterotoxigenic and nonenterotoxigenic *E. coli*, *Klebsiella pneumoniae* serotype 26, various *Clostridium* spp., coxsackie B2, *Enterobacter cloacae*, coronavirus, rotavirus, and toxigenic and nontoxigenic strains of *C. difficile*. Some case-control studies have implicated rotavirus, *C. difficile*, and a heat-labile enterotoxin-producing *E. coli* strain (22, 25, 41). However, in other case-control studies, Ryder et al found a lack of association of NEC with heat-stable enterotoxigenic *E. coli* (42), and Lishman et al and Sherertz and Sarubbi found no association between *C. difficile* or its toxin and NEC (43, 44). Thus, no single agent has yet emerged as the etiologic agent of NEC.

The exact pathophysiologic mechanism involved in NEC is unknown. Evidence suggests that the hypoxemia or hypotension that results in ischemic injury to the bowel almost always precedes the onset of NEC. Susceptibility to such injury appears to be related to gastrointestinal maturity. In such a setting either bacteria or their enterotoxins or viruses may result in NEC.

Successful management of NEC depends on a high index of suspicion and early recognition. Oral feedings should be discontinued and supportive parenteral therapy instituted. Patients with sporadic cases should be placed on enteric precautions. When clusters of cases occur, ill infants should be placed on enteric precautions, and personnel and ill and exposed infants should be cohorted.

Table 24.5. Agents Associated with Necrotizing Enterocolitis

Organism	Country	Year	No. of Cases	Reference
Anaerobic Bacteria				
Clostridium sp.	U.S.	1979	1	21
Clostridium sp.	U.S.	1981	8	22
C. butyricum	England	1977	9	23
C. butyricum	U.S.	1980	1	24
C. difficile	Canada	1983	13	25
C. perfringens	U.S.	1979	7	26
C. perfringens	U.S.	1984	2	27
Aerobic Bacteria				
E. coli NE*	U.S.	1976	7	28
E. coli LT†	U.S.	1983	7	29
E. cloacae	Canada	1980	12	30
E. coli/K. pneumoniae	U.S.	1979	UK‡	31
K. pneumoniae	U.S.	1975	38	32
K. pneumoniae	U.S.	1979	6	33
Salmonella sp.	England	1972	6	34
Salmonella Group C	U.S.	1984	UK	35
Viruses				
Coronavirus	France	1982	23	36
Coronavirus	U.S.	1983	5	37
Coronavirus	France	1984	9	38
Coxsackie B2	U.S.	1977	1	39
Rotavirus	Israel	1983	2	40
Rotavirus	U.S.	1983	11	41

* NE, nonenterotoxigenic.
† LT, heat-labile enterotoxin producing.
‡ UK, unknown.

Antibiotic-Associated Diarrhea/ Pseudomembranous Colitis

After several year of reports of colitis following exposure to clindamycin and other antimicrobials, *C. difficile* was identified in 1977 as the etiologic agent of antibiotic-associated pseudomembranous colitis (PMC) (45–47). The *C. difficile* isolates recovered from patients with PMC were shown to produce a toxin in vitro similar to that found in feces from patients with PMC and were found to induce a fatal enterocolitis when orally administered to hamsters pretreated with vancomycin (45–49). Between 89 and 96% of PMC patients have either *C. difficile* or its toxin in fecal specimens (50–52).

The toxin in stools from PMC patients produces actinomorphic changes in cells in tissue culture, which could be neutralized by antisera to *Clostridium sordellii*. In animals the toxin produces pathologic changes similar to those seen in patients with PMC; the changes appear as white plaques, consisting of lymphoid aggregates in the submucosa and lamina propria. Underlying these plaques, or pseudomembranes, are dilated crypts filled with mucus, fibrin, leukocytes, and cellular debris (53). Subsequently, studies have shown that *C. difficile* strains actually produce two toxins, toxins A and B, which can be detected by enzyme-linked immunosorbent assay (ELISA) and that produce different effects in tissue culture (54, 55). Whether toxin A or B or both are responsible for producing colitis is not clear. Both toxins are cytotoxic and lethal in animals. Toxin A is an enterotoxin and causes interstitial fluid accumulation and mucosal necrosis, and toxin B is a cytotoxin and produces the cytopathic effect in tissue culture by causing disorganization of actin-containing myofilament bundles (56–58). In serosurveys approximately 64% of those older than 2 years have antibody to toxin A and 66% of those older than 6 months have antibody to toxin B, suggesting that exposure to toxins occurs early in life (59). Furthermore, elevations in IgM antibody titers to toxins A and B are found in patients with *C. difficile* colitis (59). Whether these antitoxins play any protective role is presently unknown.

Initially PMC was thought to result from toxin production by endogenous *C. difficile* in the gastrointestinal tract when patients were exposed to antimicrobial therapy. However, initial reports of clusters of PMC raised the possibility that PMC might result from nosocomial transmission (60). Subsequently there have been several reports of nosocomial outbreaks of PMC (Table 24.6). No common source was found in any of the outbreaks; however, inanimate objects, including floors, walls, and bedpans, have been culture-positive, and in some instances *C. difficile* has been recovered from the hands or stools of medical personnel. In most instances, person-to-person transmission was suspected but was not definitively demonstrated. In two outbreaks, attempts were made to type the recovered *C. difficile* strains. In one outbreak, polyacrylamide gel electrophoresis followed by electroblot analysis showed that 9 of 10 strains were similar (68).

Table 24.6. Summary of Reported Clusters of Antibiotic-Associated Pseudomembranous Colitis

Country	Year	Ward	No. of Cases	Duration	Typing Methods Employed	Evaluation of Risk Factors	Reference
U.S.	1975	Multiple	10	2 months	None	No	61
England	1981	Transplant	10	8 months	None	Yes*	62
England	1981	Medical	8	11 days	None	No	63
New Zealand	1982	Medical	4	NS†	Antimicrobial susceptibility	No	64
Switzerland	1982	Surgical	15	8 months	Agarose gel electrophoresis, Protein profiles, Bacteriophage typing	No	65
Australia	1982	Intensive care unit	3	NS	Antimicrobial susceptibility	No	66
U.S.	1982	Multiple	10	2 months	Antimicrobial susceptibility	Yes‡	60
U.S.	1983	NS	2	19 days	None	No	67

* Gut decontamination implicated.

† NS, not specified.

‡ Gastrointestinal tract manipulation (e.g., nasogastric tubes, enemas) implicated.

Other investigators have used the analysis of radiolabeled sulfur-methionated proteins to show similarity of strains (69). These data strongly suggest that *C. difficile* can be transmitted within the hospital setting. However, definitive studies are needed to identify the mode of transmission from patient to patient. Since several studies have documented that areas where PMC patients are hospitalized have been contaminated, that *C. difficile* can survive on environmental surfaces for up to 5 months, and that medical personnel are more commonly colonized if they take care of PMC patients, the potential for nosocomial transmission exists (70–73).

Following the diagnosis of PMC, treatment includes withdrawal of the implicated drug, institution of oral vancomycin, and supportive therapy. Patients with diarrhea should be placed on enteric precautions. Small series suggest that using metronidazole, bacitracin, or rifampin may be an alternative to vancomycin therapy, but larger studies are necessary to document their efficacy (74–76). Approximately 14 to 24% of PMC patients relapse following discontinuation of vancomycin therapy (75, 77, 78), and a second course of vancomycin may be successful in eradicating the organism.

Since the discovery of an association between *C. difficile* and PMC, additional studies have demonstrated an association between *C. difficile* and antibiotic-associated diarrhea in adults and in children (52, 79, 80). Whereas *C. difficile* is seldom recovered from the stools of healthy adults, it is recovered from between 29 and 56% of adults with antibiotic-associated diarrhea. The presenting signs and symptoms of *C. difficile*-associated diarrhea are highly variable; the least severe form of disease may consist only of mild diarrhea, while patients with severe disease may present with high fever, leukocytosis, severe abdominal cramping, marked abdominal tenderness, and profuse diarrhea. Both PMC and antibiotic-associated gastroenteritis have followed exposure to a wide variety of antimicrobial agents.

The role that *C. difficile* plays in antibiotic-associated diarrhea in infants and young children has been more difficult to establish, because *C. difficile* is commonly recovered from the stools of infants and preschool children. Between 2 and 30% of healthy newborns and up to 35% of neonates admitted to intensive care nurseries have toxigenic *C. difficile* recovered from their stools (81–83). Data suggest that infants are exposed to *C. difficile* early in life and that carriage

decreases with age, beginning in early childhood (84). In some instances intestinal colonization may be acquired during hospitalization (43, 81, 85). In one nursery, 65 (71%) of 92 infants became colonized with *C. difficile* (85). Stool cultures of the mothers of these infants were negative for *C. difficile*, suggesting that the infants became colonized in the nursery after delivery. Further support for this hypothesis was the finding that the infants were all negative for *C. difficile* on admission but became colonized from 6 to 35 days after admission to the nursery. This high colonization rate in asymptomatic infants has made it difficult to determine the role of *C. difficile* in antibiotic-associated diarrhea in this population. In studies that have controlled for this factor, no association has been found between *C. difficile* and antibiotic-associated diarrhea in infants (86). Further carefully designed studies will be needed to clarify this issue.

Patients with hematologic malignancy appear to be at increased risk of colonization with *C. difficile* and of development of PMC. Several authors have reported episodes of PMC in hematologic malignancy patients following therapy with antineoplastic drugs (71, 87, 88). However, a prospective study of hematologic malignancy patients found that *C. difficile* colonization present on admission to the hospital was associated with prior antimicrobial therapy. However, there was no association between antineoplastic therapy and either *C. difficile* colonization or PMC (89).

The diagnosis of *C. difficile*-associated PMC or antibiotic-associated diarrhea depends on the presence of *C. difficile* in stool culture or the demonstration of the cytotoxic effect of the stool or culture filtrate in tissue culture assays. Rapid assays for detecting *C. difficile* toxin have been developed, but to date, none is sensitive or specific enough to replace the stool culture and tissue culture toxin assay tests. Although several authors have found the countercurrent immunoelectrophoresis (CIE) assay to be sensitive and specific (90–92), others have found the tests to lack sensitivity or specificity and to have a poor predictive value (93–96).

Food Poisoning

The syndrome of food poisoning can be caused by a wide variety of organisms, including bacteria, viruses, and protozoa, as well as by various chemical toxins. Clues to the etiology of a common-source foodborne outbreak are provided by the symptoms and incubation period (97, 98). Considerations for symptoms include whether most ill patients have upper gastrointestinal symptoms (e.g., nausea and vomiting), lower gastrointestinal symptoms (abdominal cramps, diarrhea, tenesmus), or neurologic symptoms (motor, sensory). In addition, examination of fresh stool specimens for the presence of polymorphonuclear leukocytes may provide a useful diagnostic clue to the presence of an invasive pathogen (e.g., *Campylobacter*, *Shigella*). Foodborne diseases which may be transmitted by food whose primary manifestations are outside the gastrointestinal tract (e.g., hepatitis A, trichinosis) will not be considered in this chapter.

The true incidence of foodborne disease outbreaks in hospitals and extended care facilities is not known. However, surveillance data from the United States (99) and Great Britain (100–102) indicate that such outbreaks are not uncommon. Review of foodborne disease outbreak surveillance data in the United States indicates that the majority of all reported outbreaks in these settings are caused by bacterial foodborne pathogens (99). *Salmonella*, *Staphylococcus aureus*, and *Clostridium perfringens* are the most commonly identified etiologic agents. The most common food handling error contributing to outbreaks caused by bacteria in this setting is storage of food at inappropriate temperatures (99, 103).

Because hospitalized patients are at increased risk for illness when exposed to potential foodborne pathogens and because of the continuous operation of hospital food services with the need to provide a wide variety of dietary items, it is critically important that appropriate food handling practices be maintained. Not only are patients who ingest contaminated food at risk for illness, but also other patients and hospital personnel are at risk for secondary transmission if a foodborne outbreak does occur (104). Several large foodborne outbreaks in hospitals have resulted in staffing problems because personnel have been too ill to work (105, 106).

Confirmation of the diagnosis of a foodborne disease outbreak due to certain etiologic agents (e.g., *Salmonella* and *Campylobacter*) is well within the capability of the clinical microbiology laboratory. However, certain etiologic agents (e.g., enterotoxigenic *E. coli* and Norwalk agent) will require a specialized laboratory for identification.

Because a small proportion of all foodborne outbreaks is related to contaminated commercial products and because such outbreaks have occasionally occurred in a hospital setting (107, 108), it is essential to notify appropriate public health authorities when such an outbreak is recognized.

Diarrhea in the Compromised Host

Compromised hosts are at increased risk not only for developing nosocomial gastroenteritis but also for systemic complications, including bacteremia, should such infections occur. These individuals are at risk for infection by all of the enteric pathogens discussed in this chapter, including *Cryptosporidium* (109). In addition, recent reports suggest that these patients are also at increased risk for gastroenteritis caused by more unusual pathogens. Furthermore, such patients are at increased risk for diarrhea resulting from the pharmacologic agents they receive.

Limited data are available on the incidence of such infections. Bone marrow transplant recipients are one group of immuncompromised patients that appears to be at increased risk for nosocomial gastroenteritis, which may be mistaken for a manifestation of acute graft-versus-host disease (110). An outbreak of nosocomial gastroenteritis due to coxsackievirus A1 in one bone marrow transplant unit was associated with an increased mortality rate in infected patients (110). Neither the source nor the mode of transmission was identified. In a prospective study lasting 9 months in the same unit, 31 (40%) of 78 patients had evidence of viral or *C. difficile* infection of the gastrointestinal tract. Twenty-two (28%) had viral infections; agents identified included adenovirus in 12, rotavirus in 9, and coxsackievirus in 4. The mortality rate was significantly higher in infected patients (55% versus 13%) (7). No other bacterial pathogens were identified. Imunocompromised patients also appear to be at increased risk for PMC, even if they are not receiving antimicrobial therapy.

AGENTS

Many individual agents are recognized as definite or potential causes of nosocomial gastroenteritis. Selected clinical, epidemiologic, and laboratory features of illness caused by many of the specific agents discussed in this chapter are summarized in Table 24.7.

Salmonella

Three biochemically distinct species of *Salmonella* exist: *S. typhi*, *S. cholerae-suis*, and *S.*

Table 24.7. Summary of Clinical, Epidemiologic, and Laboratory Features of Selected Agents Capable of Causing Nosocomial Gastroenteritis*

Agent	Frequency	Symptoms			Incubation Period	Pathogenesis	Fecal PMNs	Fecal Blood	Place of Diagnosis	Type of Test	Typing	Rapid Test
		Fever	UGI	LGI								
Salmonella	Common	+	±	+	16–72 hr	Penetration, ± ET	+	±	CL	C	A, ST, P, PH	No
Shigella	Uncommon	+	±	+	16–72 hr	Invasion	+	+	CL	C	A, ST, P	No
C. jejuni	Rare	+	±	+	1–7 d	Invasion, ± ET	+	+	CL	C	A, ST, BT, P	No
Y. enterocolitica	Uncommon	+	±	+	16–48 hr	Invasion, ET	+	−	CL†	C	A, ST	No
E. coli												
ETEC	Uncommon	−	−	+	16–72 hr	ET	−	−	RL	T	A, ST, P	No
EIEC	Rare	+	−	+	6–48 hr	Invasion	+	+	RL	S	A, ST, P	No
EPEC	Uncommon	±	−	+	6–24 hr	Adherence, CT, ±ET	±	±	RL	ST	A, ST, P	No
EHEC	?	−	±	+	72–120 hr	?CT	−	+	RL	ST	A, P	No
C. difficile	Common	+	±	+	?	Invasion, ET, CT	+	+	CL†	C, T	PH, OMP	Yes
Aeromonas	?	+	±	+	?	?ET, ?CT	±	±	CL†	C	A	No
Plesiomonas	?	+	±	+	18–24 hr	?	?	−	CL†	C	A	No
Rotavirus	Common	+	+	+	48–72 hr	Infection of villus tips	−	−	CL	EM, E	ST, EL	Yes
Norwalk agent	Common	+	+	+	24–48 hr	Infection of villus tips	−	−	RL	IEM, SER	IEM, RIA	No
Adenovirus	?	±	±	+	?	?	−	−	RL	EM, C, SER	IEM, EL	No
Giardia	Rare	±	−	+	7–14 d	?	−	−	CL	M	−	Yes
Cryptosporidium	?	−	−	+	3–10 d	?	−	−	CL†	M, SER	−	Yes

* Key: +, Frequently present
±, Occasionally present
−, Rarely present
ET, Enterotoxin
CT, Cytotoxin
CL, Clinical laboratory
RL, Research laboratory
C, Stool culture
† If laboratory alerted to seek organism.

S, Sereny test
ST, Serotyping
T, Enterotoxin testing
EM, Electron microscopy
E, ELISA
IEM, Immune electron microscopy
SER, Serology
M, Miscroscopic examination

A, Antibiogram
P, Plasmid profile
PH, Phage typing
BT, Biotyping
OMP, Outer membrane protein
EL, Electropherotyping
RIA, Radioimmunoassay.

enteritidis. Within *S. enteritidis,* over 2000 serotypes have been identified. *S. typhimurium* remains the most common serotype, accounting for 34% of all isolates reported to the CDC in 1983 (111). *Salmonella* may cause enteric fever, bacteremia with or without subsequent focal infection, and gastroenteritis. These organisms cause disease as a result of tissue penetration; some strains have also been reported to produce enterotoxins.

Salmonella is frequently reported as causing nosocomial gastroenteritis outbreaks. *Salmonella* is also among the most frequently identified causes of endemic nosocomial gastroenteritis.

Even though the dose of several serotypes shown to infect 50% of healthy adult volunteers (ID_{50}) is relatively high, in outbreaks where the infectious dose has been known or estimated, it has actually often been quite low (112). In 6 of 11 outbreaks caused by *Salmonella* species in which the ingested dose could be calculated, it was less than 10^3 organisms (112).

Outbreaks in nurseries are most frequently a result of contact transmission (113). Those occurring on pediatric and adult wards are most often related to a contaminated common vehicle. Examples of common vehicles reported to cause nosocomial salmonellosis include numerous foods, medications such as pancreatic enzyme and thyroid hormone preparations, and diagnostic reagents. These organisms survive for prolonged periods in the environment, and fomites and environmental reservoirs have occasionally been implicated during outbreak investigations (113). Recently reported nosocomial salmonellosis outbreaks (Table 24.8) illustrate the potential for such outbreaks to involve patients or personnel and infants or adults, the importance of both contact and common vehicle transmission, the potential for transmission from patients to personnel and vice versa, the potential role of the inanimate environment (specifically, inadequately disinfected endoscopes, duodenal tubes, and suction tubing), and the ability of multiply resistant organisms to spread in the hospital setting.

Antimicrobial resistance occurs in both community-acquired and nosocomial *Salmonella* isolates and is increasing in the United States (122). The case-fatality rate is significantly higher in outbreaks caused by resistant strains (123). In a recent study of endemic infections, risk factors for infection with resistant organisms included infection with *Salmonella heidelberg,* Hispanic

origin of the patient, and exposure of the patient to a penicillin compound during the 4 weeks prior to the positive stool culture (124).

The relationship of antimicrobial resistance in humans to the use of antimicrobials in animal feeds is a topic that generates considerable debate (125, 126). In two reported outbreaks, a link has been established between antimicrobial-resistant *Salmonella* in animals and nosocomial infections in humans. In one outbreak, three infants in a newborn nursery and the mother of the index infant were infected with an *S. heidelberg* strain resistant to chloramphenicol, tetracycline, and sulfamethoxazole (127). The mother appeared to have acquired the infection on her father's farm shortly before delivery. In the second outbreak, which involved 17 community-acquired infections due to *Salmonella newport* resistant to ampicillin, carbenicillin, and tetracycline, one additional case resulted from nosocomial transmission. This case occurred in a 69-year-old man with a history of abdominal trauma and splenectomy, who appeared to have acquired his infection during sigmoidoscopy with a scope that may have been inadequately disinfected following a procedure performed on one of the community-acquired cases. This patient died of septicemia 20 days after the procedure (128).

Salmonella typhimurium has recently been reported as a cause of gastroenteritis and bacteremia in patients with acquired immunodeficiency syndrome (AIDS) (129–131). Although these infections have appeared to be community-acquired, frequent recurrences are common, sometimes while the patient is hospitalized.

Routine clinical microbiology laboratories are capable of identifying these organisms. Serotyping can be performed by state public health laboratories. Phage typing and plasmid profile analyses, which are superior to antimicrobial susceptibility testing in detecting epidemiologically related isolates of *Salmonella* (132, 133), are available from specialized laboratories.

Shigella

Four species of *Shigella* exist: *S. dysenteriae, S. flexneri, S. boydii,* and *S. sonnei.* Multiple serotypes of each of the first three species also exist. These organisms cause disease as a result of tissue invasion (134).

S. sonnei is the most common cause of shigellosis in the United States and is followed by *S. flexneri* (135). *S. dysenteriae* and *S. boydii* serotypes are rare causes of shigellosis in the United

Table 24.8. Features of Selected Nosocomial Salmonellosis Outbreaks Reported from 1979 to 1984

| Location | Population Affected | | Organism | Risk Factors | Comments | Reference |
	Patients	Personnel				
U.S.	4 adults	1 nurse	*S. typhimurium*	Nasogastric tube	Indirect contact transmission between patients related to contaminated plastic suction tubing attached to intermittent suction machine; direct contact transmission from ill patient to nurse in intensive care unit; original source not identified.	114
U.S.	3 adults	46 personnel	*S. chester* *S. tennessee* *S. habana*	Consumption of pre-cooked roast beef and cold cuts	Common-vehicle (food-borne) transmission to personnel by commercially distributed precooked roast beef and cross-contaminated cold cuts; direct contact transmission from ill nurse to patients.	108
U.S.	7 adults	None	*S. typhimurium*	Upper gastrointestinal endoscopy	Indirect contact transmission by inadequately disinfected endoscope over 3 1/2-month period; suction tubing and collection bottle also contaminated; original source not identified.	115
England	20 adults	1 nurse	*S. kedougou*	Upper gastrointestinal endoscopy	Indirect contact transmission by inadequately disinfected endoscope over 6-month period; original source not identified.	116

England	4 adults	None	*S. typhi*	Duodenal intubation	Indirect contact transmission by inadequately disinfected, reused polyvinyl tube; original source a chronic carrier; transmission within 2 to 3 days of use on infected person.	117
England	2 infants 1 adult	None	*S. typhi*	None	Vertical transmission from acute case to infant before or during delivery with subsequent transmission in maternity ward and nursery, presumably by direct contact.	118
England	15 infants 13 children	2 personnel	*S. muenchen*	None	Presumably direct contact transmission of multiply resistant strain; outbreak controlled only after hospital closed to new admissions for 5 days.	119
U.S.	10 infants	None	*S. nienstedten*	None	Presumably direct contact transmission; prolonged incubation period (median 10 days) delayed recognition of outbreak; original source not identified.	120
U.S.	5 infants	None	*S. typhimurium*	None	Presumably direct contact transmission of strain resistant to ampicillin, chloramphenicol and trimethoprim-sulfamethoxazole; index case acquired strain in Southeast Asia.	121

States. *Shigella* are rarely reported to cause either endemic or epidemic nosocomial gastroenteritis. Vertical transmission has been reported (136), and on occasion, limited nosocomial transmission has occurred in nurseries (137). The group at highest risk for community-acquired shigellosis consists of children in the 1- to 5-year-old age group (135).

Since the infectious dose of *Shigella* is low and since the organisms are an important cause of acute diarrheal disease in day care centers (138) and custodial institutions (139), it would be reasonable to expect that they would be important causes of nosocomial gastroenteritis. Although the reasons why they are not are unclear, possible explanations are that asymptomatic excretion of *Shigella* is rare and that hospitalized patients with shigellosis may be likely to be identified and placed on enteric precautions at the time of admission.

In the reported instances of transmission in nurseries, person-to-person spread by direct contact as a result of transient contamination of hands of hospital personnel has been suspected. In one reported outbreak in an acute care setting in a chronic care institution, person-to-person transmission appeared to be mediated by transient hand contamination of a health care worker (140).

Shigella can be identified by routine clinical microbiology laboratories if fresh specimens are available for culture. Serogrouping can also be done by these laboratories, and more definitive serotyping is available from state health department laboratories. In *Shigella* outbreaks, plasmid profiling may be an additional useful epidemiologic tool (141, 142).

Campylobacter jejuni

During the past 10 years, *C. jejuni* has been recognized as a common cause of community-acquired acute diarrheal disease. The relative importance of two recently identified, closely related species (*Campylobacter coli* and *Campylobacter laridis*) in the etiology of acute diarrheal disease requires definition. *C. jejuni* has a worldwide distribution. Although its exact mechanism of pathogenesis has not been fully elucidated, tissue invasion is involved, and some strains have been reported to produce a heat-labile enterotoxin (143).

As a cause of community-acquired diarrheal disease, *C. jejuni* is at least as common as *Salmonella* and *Shigella*, and in some areas it is the most frequently identified enteric bacterial pathogen (144). Vertical transmission has been reported, but nosocomial outbreaks have not been reported (145). Thorough investigation of a recently reported cluster of four cases occurring in a nursery during a 5-day period in term infants indicated that the cases were unrelated and that each resulted from vertical transmission (146).

Infants, children, and young adults appear to be at highest risk for community-acquired infection (147, 148). Several community-acquired outbreaks caused by *C. jejuni* have been reported. The lack of occurrence of nosocomial outbreaks due to this organism may in part be due to the fact that asymptomatic infection is uncommon in developed countries (149) and the fact that individuals with diarrhea due to this organism may be sufficiently ill when hospitalized that the need for enteric precautions is usually promptly appreciated.

Vehicles which are frequently identified during the investigation of community-acquired *C. jejuni* outbreaks include raw milk (150–152), inadequately cooked chicken (153), and inadequately treated water (154–156). Person-to-person transmission following common vehicle outbreaks appears to be uncommon but has been reported among members of extended families (157). Investigation of sporadic cases of community-acquired infection have identified drinking raw water and raw milk, eating undercooked chicken, living in a household with a cat, and close contact with infected puppies as risk factors (158–161).

As a result of recent developments of selected media for the isolation of *C. jejuni*, diagnosis of this organism is now well within the capability of the routine clinical microbiology laboratory. In addition to antimicrobial susceptibility results, serotyping, biotyping, and plasmid analysis may provide useful information during epidemic investigations.

Yersinia enterocolitica

Y. enterocolitica causes mesenteric adenitis which may be mistaken for acute appendicitis or acute diarrheal disease as a result of tissue invasion. Many strains also produce a heat-stable enterotoxin similar to STa produced by enterotoxigenic *E. coli* strains (162).

The organism is a rare cause of nosocomial gastroenteritis. Two outbreaks in which transmission appeared to have occurred from person to person by direct contact have been reported. In one, transmission occurred from a 9-year-old girl who had abdominal pain and diarrhea to 6 hospital personnel on the two wards where she was hospitalized (163). In the other, transmission occurred by direct contact from one asymptomatic and one symptomatic patient with community-acquired infections to four and two patients, respectively, on 2 hospital wards (164).

Although the nosocomial epidemic potential appears to be somewhat limited, several community-acquired common-source outbreaks have been reported. Vehicles have included pasteurized milk (165, 166) and tofu (167). Person-to-person transmission in these outbreaks has been infrequently reported.

Identification of these organisms is well within the capability of the routine clinical microbiology laboratory. Recovery of these strains can be enhanced by the use of cold enrichment techniques.

Escherichia coli

E. coli strains that cause acute diarrheal disease may be classified into four groups: enterotoxigenic, enteroinvasive, enteropathogenic, and enterohemorrhagic (168). Diarrheal disease caused by enterotoxigenic E. coli (ETEC) is mediated by heat-labile or heat-stable enterotoxins (LT and ST, respectively). LT is antigenically similar to cholera toxin; its mechanism of action is also similar, that is, LT activates adenylate cyclase (169). Two STs have been described: STa activates guanylate cyclase, resulting in increased levels of cyclic guanosine monophosphate (170–172), and the mechanism of action of STb is unknown (173). STa causes disease in humans, while the importance of STb in diarrhea in humans is unknown. Enteroinvasive E. coli strains cause disease as a result of tissue invasion. Although a few strains of enteropathogenic E. coli (EPEC) have been reported to produce an enterotoxin (174), recent evidence indicates that some strains of EPEC produce shiga toxin-like material (175) and produce a plasmid-mediated pathognomonic intestinal lesion visible by electron microscopy as a result of adherence to enterocytes (168, 176–179). The recently described enterohemorrhagic E. coli (180–182) of serotype 0157 produces a cytotoxin for Vero cells (183) which is similar to shiga toxin produced by S. dysenteriae type 1 (182, 184).

The reported incidence of nosocomial gastroenteritis caused by these four groups of E. coli is low. However, since identification of these organisms is generally beyond the capability of

routine clinical microbiology laboratories, the true incidence may be higher. ETEC are common causes of diarrheal disease in developing countries and in travelers to these areas. Enteroinvasive E. coli are relatively rare in developing countries and are also rarely reported to cause outbreaks of community-acquired gastroenteritis in developed countries. EPEC strains were first implicated as causing nosocomial gastroenteritis outbreaks during the 1940s (168). Outbreaks were reported with considerable frequency during the 1950s and 1960s but have been less frequently reported during the past 15 years (168). To date, enterohemorrhagic E. coli have been reported to cause community-acquired epidemic (180, 185) and endemic (181, 186) diarrheal disease, with the exception of one outbreak in a Canadian institution for elderly patients (183, 187), and to be associated with some cases of the hemolytic uremic syndrome (181, 186, 188, 189).

An outbreak of nosocomial gastroenteritis caused by an STa-producing E. coli strain has been reported in infants in a special care nursery in one hospital (190). Neonates appear not only to be at increased risk for infection but also to have more severe disease.

The rarity with which outbreaks caused by these four groups of E. coli are reported probably reflects the facts that enterotoxigenic and enteroinvasive organisms are only infrequently found in this country, that the infectious dose, at least for healthy adults, is relatively high for ETEC and EPEC (168), and that the diagnosis is unlikely to be made in routine microbiology laboratories, where enterotoxin testing and serotyping capability are not generally available.

Reported outbreaks have generally been due to contaminated food or water. In the nursery outbreak caused by STa-producing E. coli, exposure to extrinsically contaminated infant formula was associated with illness (190). Because the infectious dose of these organisms is high, person-to-person transmission is unlikely to be important outside the nursery setting.

Aeromonas and Plesiomonas Infections

Aeromonas and Plesiomonas species have recently received attention as possible enteric pathogens. These organisms are gram-negative oxidase-positive, polarly flagellated, facultative anaerobes frequently found in soil and natural aquatic environments (191). Their survival in the environment depends on the presence of moisture and organic material.

The role of these organisms in human gastrointestinal disorders remains unresolved. *Aeromonas* and *Plesiomonas* species are rarely found in stool specimens of asymptomatic individuals (192); several studies show that between 0 and 3.2% of persons without evidence of gastrointestinal disease are culture-positive (192–194).

As early as 1937, studies showed that *Aeromonas* spp. could be isolated from human stool specimens (195). Since that time, others have reported sporadic cases or small outbreaks of gastroenteritis associated with *Aeromonas* spp. In the majority of these reports, the patients have had acute onset of a mild, watery, nonmucoid, nonbloody diarrhea. The incubation period is unknown. The illness is usually self-limited, lasting 1 to 7 days in healthy individuals, although symptoms may be protracted in immunocompromised or pediatric patients. In at least two instances, *Aeromonas* spp. have been associated with a cholera-like illness (196, 197). Recently, Pitarangsi, et al assessed the role of *Aeromonas* by comparing the frequency of recovery of *Aeromonas* from people with and without diarrhea (198). Among American travelers, *Aeromonas* spp. were isolated significantly more frequently from those with travelers' diarrhea than from those without diarrhea. The majority of strains isolated from individuals with and without diarrhea produced a cytotoxin, hemolyzed rabbit erythrocytes, and caused distension of mouse intestines using either whole culture or culture filtrates. In addition, cytotoxin-producing strains of *Aeromonas* spp. were found to cause blunting of villi and degeneration of enterocytes. Debate continues as to whether the virulence mechanism is mediated by a cytotonic or cytotoxic enterotoxin (199). These and other data suggest that only enterotoxigenic strains of *Aeromonas* cause gastroenteritis.

Two recent studies add to the evidence that toxigenic strains of *Aeromonas* species can cause gastroenteritis in children. Janda et al described 12 patients between 2 months and 17 years of age (mean 2 years) who presented with bloody diarrhea, fever, vomiting, and abdominal pain (200). In two patients, symptoms were severe enough to necessitate hospitalization for supportive care. In all patients, *Aeromonas* strains were isolated in the absence of other known enteropathogens. All 12 strains were cytotoxic to HeLa cells, and both strains tested hemolyzed rabbit erythrocytes.

Burke et al studied nearly 1000 children with diarrhea and controls without diarrhea matched for age and sex (201). Enterotoxigenic *Aeromonas* species, identified by the suckling mouse test, were found in fecal specimens of 10.8% of patients with diarrhea but in only 0.7% of those without diarrhea. When patients with other known enteropathogens were excluded, enterotoxigenic *Aeromonas* strains were still significantly more frequent in children with diarrhea than in those without diarrhea (8% versus 0.7%). All but two of the enterotoxigenic strains produced hemolysins. The frequency of recovery of enterotoxin-negative strains of *Aeromonas* spp. was similar in patients with and without diarrhea. Overall, *Aeromonas* spp. were recovered more frequently from children with diarrhea than were *Salmonella, Shigella, Campylobacter*, or enterotoxigenic *E. coli* and were second in frequency only to rotavirus (12.7% versus 10.8%).

In all studies to date, there has been a striking seasonality in the isolation of *Aeronomas*; peak isolation rates from patients and water sources occur during the summer and early fall. The findings that *Aeromonas* can sometimes be isolated from tap water and from hospital water sources and that the frequency of isolating *Aeromonas* from patients parallels that of their isolation from environmental sources suggest that nosocomial infections due to this organism may occur. In many cases, routine laboratory procedures for culturing stool specimens would not permit isolation of *Aeromonas*; for instance, if all lactose-positive colonies are disregarded, isolates of *Aeronomas* would be overlooked. Thus, an increased awareness of these organisms by laboratory personnel is needed if the link between these organisms and disease is to be appreciated. To date, nosocomial gastroenteritis due to *Aeromonas* species has not been reported, but improvements in isolation techniques and the development of typing systems may allow it to be documented in the future.

Less is known about the role of *Plesiomonas* spp. in gastrointestinal disease. This organism has been reported to cause a mild, self-limited, nonmucoid, nonbloody diarrhea with acute onset. Additional studies also suggest that *Plesiomonas* is associated with gastroenteritis; in a study in Thailand, *Plesiomonas* strains were isolated twice as frequently from patients with diarrhea as from age- and sex-matched controls (15% versus 6%) (198). Furthermore, in two large outbreaks of gastroenteritis involving over 1000 ill persons in Japan, *Plesiomonas* was the predominant organism isolated. *Plesiomonas* spp. have been reported to cause food poisoning (202), and in addition, this genus has been reported to cause cholera-like diarrhea in some patients (203).

The mechanism by which *Plesiomonas* spp. causes gastroenteritis is unknown. Isolates obtained from patients with gastroenteritis have not been found to be enteropathogenic in the laboratory; these organisms have no effect in ligated rabbit ileal loops, Y1 mouse adrenal cells, the suckling mouse assay, or the rabbit skin test. Thus, *Plesiomonas* strains do not produce an enterotoxin detectable by current methods. In the two studies where an incubation period could be determined, the onset of illness occurred 20 to 24 hours after exposure (199). To date, nosocomial transmission of *Plesiomonas* gastroenteritis has not been documented.

Vibrio

Vibrio cholerae serogroup 01 (the etiologic agent of cholera) and *Vibrio cholerae* non-01 strains have long been recognized as important causes of acute, often severe, diarrheal disease in developing countries. During the past few years, these organisms have also been reported to cause sporadic cases and, in the case of *V. cholerae* 01, epidemics of acute diarrheal disease in the United States (204). *Vibrio parahaemolyticus* has been recognized as a cause of acute diarrheal disease in this country for approximately 15 years. During the past few years, a number of additional *Vibrio* species have been identified and associated with gastroenteritis; examples include *V. mimicus*, *V. fluvialis*, *V. furnissii*, and *V. hollisae* (205). The infectious dose of *V. cholerae* is high in healthy adult volunteers, though it is lower when organisms are ingested with food or buffer. To date, nosocomial infections caused by these organisms have not been reported in developed countries. Isolation of these organisms is within the capability of the routine clinical microbiology laboratory if appropriate selective media are used.

Other Enterotoxigenic Bacteria

Members of the family Enterobacteriaceae other than *E. coli* have been reported on occasion to produce enterotoxins (206, 207). Specific examples include *K. pneumoniae* and *Citrobacter* spp. One outbreak in a neonatal nursery in which several such strains were implicated has been reported (208). In this outbreak, transmission appeared to occur from person to person by direct contact due to transient hand contamination of nursery personnel. Although recognition of such enterotoxigenic organisms is beyond the capability of most routine clinical microbiology laboratories, such organisms appear to be an infrequent cause of epidemic nosocomial gastroenteritis.

Methicillin-Resistant *Staphylococcus aureus*

During the past 10 years, the reported frequency of outbreaks caused by methicillin-resistant *S. aureus* (MRSA) and the reported incidence of nosocomial MRSA endemic infections in the United States have increased (209, 210). These infections occur primarily in surgical intensive care units, trauma units, and burn units in large medical school-affiliated hospitals. Recent reports from Australia (211) and Italy (212) suggest that MRSA may cause occasional cases of antibiotic-associated diarrhea.

Rotavirus

In 1973, Bishop et al, utilizing electron microscopy, reported the association of rotaviruses with diarrheal disease (213). Since that time, rotaviruses have been recognized as the single most common cause of childhood gastroenteritis in developed countries. Rotaviruses are spherical, 70 nm in diameter, with a double capsid layer, and a double-stranded RNA genome in 11 segments; they are included in the family Reoviridae. The human rotaviruses resist heating up to 56°C, and a pH of 3. Rotaviruses are worldwide in distribution. The human rotaviruses account for approximately half of the hospitalized cases of childhood diarrhea each year; in the summer from 0 to 20% of gastroenteritis is associated with rotavirus, whereas during the winter 70 to 80% of gastroenteritis is associated with rotavirus. During the first year of life the annual rate of rotavirus diarrhea ranges from 0.82 to 1.05 episodes/child (214, 215).

There is an increased incidence of dehydration and hospitalization associated with rotaviruses that is only surpassed by infections caused by *V. cholerae*. It is estimated that approximately 3.7 of 1000 infants < 1 year of age and 2.2 of 1000 infants 12 to 24 months of age require hospitalization for rotavirus gastroenteritis annually (216). Rotavirus infection is one of the leading causes of mortality in infants and children in the world, and approximately 1 million deaths/year have been estimated to occur as a result of rotavirus gastroenteritis (217).

The incubation period following exposure to rotavirus typically ranges from 48 to 72 hours (216). Characteristically, there is an abrupt onset of vomiting and diarrhea. Upper respiratory symptoms have been reported in from 20 to 75% of patients with rotavirus infections. In studies by Rodriguez et al, vomiting was present in nearly all infected patients (218). In many cases, the onset of vomiting preceded the onset of diarrhea; 60 to 100% of patients with rotavirus infections developed fever. In most cases of rotavirus gastroenteritis, the fever and vomiting resolve within the first 2 days, and the diarrhea resolves wtihin 8 days. Excretion of rotavirus in the stools usually occurs from the third to the eighth day of illness. Laboratory studies show that rotavirus can persist for prolonged periods on environmental surfaces. Household studies reveal that rotavirus infection is highly contagious for both children and adults. In four studies approximately 40% of parents seroconverted to rotavirus following exposure to children with rotavirus gastroenteritis (219–222). In all age groups, infection with rotavirus may be asymptomatic.

The site of multiplication of rotavirus is the mucosa of the small intestine. Biopsies of proximal intestine show shortening of the villi and mononuclear cell infiltration of the lamina propria. Animal studies have demonstrated abnormalities of glucose-coupled sodium transport and increased thymidine kinase activity, while adenylate and guanylate cyclase are not activated. Infected feces contain high titers of virus, as high as 10^{10} viral particles/g. Infection of humans with rotavirus typically follows contact with infected individuals. Rotaviruses are stable in stool and are relatively resistant to commonly used disinfectants. Prolonged environmental survival of rotavirus as well as recent evidence of asymptomatic carriage of rotavirus by infants, children, and adults complicate the control of spread of rotavirus within the hospital.

Rotaviruses are a common cause of nosocomial infection. Such infections have been reported from well-baby and intensive care nurseries, pediatric wards, pediatric chronic care facilities, and among adults who have had contact with pediatric patients, or who have been admitted to long term care facilities for the elderly.

In the late 1970s and 1980s, several outbreaks of rotavirus infections in neonates were reported from England and Australia (Table 24.9). In England and Australia, small outbreaks of diarrhea in nurseries were associated with rotavirus (223, 225, 228). During these outbreaks nearly all the infants in the nursery were infected, and most developed diarrhea (225). Following the out-

breaks, rotavirus became endemic in some of the hospitals leading to large numbers of colonized infants. Subsequent prevalence studies at these and other hospitals showed that between 8 and 50% of the infants admitted during periods without outbreaks became infected with rotavirus and that 8 to 30% of the infected infants became symptomatic; thus, most infected neonates remained asymptomatic and would not normally have been detected. These studies also showed that transmission did not usually occur from mother to infant but rather resulted from spread from infant to infant by direct contact involving medical personnel.

Although rotavirus infections in England and Australia were common findings in the late 1970s and early 1980s, prevalence studies in the United States failed to identify rotavirus as a common infection in well-baby nurseries (Table 24.9). In studies by Dean et al and by Santosham et al, less than 1% of over 1200 infants studied were found to be infected with rotavirus (230, 233). However, in the early 1980s several reports of rotavirus infections in well-baby and intensive care nurseries in the United States appeared.

In 1982 Rodriguez et al reported two outbreaks of human rotavirus infections in their special care nurseries (234). In the first outbreak, 10 infants in three of the six nursery rooms were infected. After the patients were isolated, the involved rooms were closed to further admissions, and the infants and staff were cohorted, no further cases were identified. No source or index case was identified. In the second outbreak, 12 infants were affected following the admission of patients with failure to thrive and poor feeding, who were later found to be excreting rotavirus. During the two outbreak periods, rotavirus was detected in 39 of 101 stool specimens from 22 patients. Rotavirus was found in 15 (25%) of 61 stools designated as either loose, mucoid, or watery, and in 24 (11%) of 214 normal stools. These data suggest that once a nursery outbreak is recognized all nursery patients should be screened for rotavirus, infected patients and contacts should be cohorted, and personnel should be cohorted.

In another study of neonates admitted to intensive care nurseries, Krause et al found that 34 (52%) of 66 neonates were asymptomatically excreting rotavirus (231). Neonates were found to excrete rotavirus in their stool as early as the third day after admission. Four premature neonates were found to excrete rotavirus in their stools for 24 to 101 days. Thus, in some nurseries, a high

Table 24.9.   Rotavirus Infections in Nurseries

Country	Year	No. (%) Infected	No. (%) Symptomatic	Study Period	References
England	1975	29/64 (45)	6 (21)	1 month	223
Australia	1975	14/55 (26)	?	PPS*	224
Australia	1976	11/32 (34)	8 (73)	PPS	225
England	1976	76/174 (44)	7 (8)	2 months	226
Australia	1977	304/628 (49)	84 (28)	9 and 11 months	227
England	1978	343/1056 (33)	27 (8)	12 months	228
Australia†	1980	40/81 (50)	?	?	229
		11/133 (8)	?	?	
United States	1980	0/100 (0)	0	4 months	230
United States	1981	34/66 (52)	0 (0)	4 months	231
England	1982	35/109 (33)	24 (69)	12 months	232
United States	1982	13/1025 (1)	0 (0)	12 months	233
United States	1982	22/102 (22)	15 (68)	7 months	234
England	1983	76/196 (39)	32 (42)	12 months	235
United States	1984	61/1688 (4)	0 (0)	11 months	236

* PPS, Point-prevalence survey.
† Two hospitals studied.

incidence of infection, as well as chronic excretion of rotavirus by patients, can complicate infection control efforts. Additional reports of outbreaks of rotavirus infection in well-baby and intensive care nurseries have recently appeared (236, 237).

Rotavirus was first recognized as an important cause of nosocomial infections on pediatric wards. The incidence of nosocomial rotavirus infections was found to parallel that of community-acquired infections. Both sporadic and epidemic infections have been reported. In 1974, Flewett et al described two outbreaks of acute diarrhea among children in an orthopaedic hospital (238). Patients ranged in age from 3 months to 3 years. During a 6-week period, 6 (23%) of 26 infants on the ward developed an acute diarrheal illness. The incubation period was estimated to be as short as 2 days. Rotavirus was excreted in the feces for between 9 and 23 days after the onset of symptoms. Rotavirus was not detected in the stools of any of the asymptomatic children on the ward.

Ryder et al conducted a prospective study of nosocomial rotavirus infections on infant and toddler wards during a community outbreak of rotavirus gastroenteritis (239). All patients with stools positive for rotavirus on admission or those hospitalized for less than 72 hours were excluded from the study. Of the remaining 60 children at risk for acquiring nosocomial gastroenteritis, twelve (20%) developed diarrhea more than 72 hours after admission to the hospital. Ten of these 12 had rotavirus detected in their stool specimens.

Nine of the 10 infections occurred on the infant ward. The spectrum of disease in the infants with community-acquired and nosocomial infections was similar. The development of nosocomial rotavirus gastroenteritis added significantly to the duration of hospitalization and was estimated to have a mean direct cost of $836/nosocomial infection for diagnostic and therapeutic measures.

During a 12-month period, Middleton et al examined the stools of 669 patients with symptoms of diarrhea, vomiting, and fever (240). Rotavirus was detected in 385 (58%) of the 669 specimens. Seventy-five (19%) of the 385 rotavirus infections detected developed after 7 days of hospitalization and were classified as nosocomial. Although no epidemiologic investigation was conducted, the mode of transmission for the nosocomial rotavirus infections was thought to be person-to-person transmission. Since asymptomatic infection is relatively uncommon in children other than neonates, infection control measures should concentrate on identifying patients with gastroenteritis and instituting enteric precautions.

Rotavirus can also cause chronic gastrointestinal infections in patients with immunodeficiency disorders. Saulsbury et al described one immunodeficient patient with X-linked agammaglobulinemia and one patient with severe combined immunodeficiency who had chronic, symptomatic rotavirus infections (241). In both cases, rotavirus was excreted in the stool for more than 6 weeks. Jarvis et al described three patients with severe combined immunodeficiency who developed rotavirus gastroenteritis. The duration of shedding of rotavirus ranged from < 7 days to > 215 days in the immunodeficient children (8). These studies show that patients with immunodeficiency disorders are at risk for the development of nosocomial rotavirus infections and that when such infections occur the duration of excretion of the virus can be prolonged.

In a 1-year prospective study of hospitalized children under 2 years of age, Champsaur et al found that 82 (29%) of 283 children who were admitted to the general pediatric ward at a hospital in Paris were excreting rotavirus in their stools (242). Rotavirus was found in 43 (36%) of 119 children with diarrhea and in 40 (24%) of 164 children without diarrhea; thus, 40 (48%) of 83 children shedding rotavirus were asymptomatic. Shedding rotavirus was not associated with diarrhea in 71% of neonates, in 50% of 1- to 6-month-old children, and in 26% of 7- to 24-month-old children. The only symptom complex associated with rotavirus shedding was diarrhea with fever and vomiting.

In an attempt to differentiate carriage from asymptomatic infection, these authors evaluated the serologic response to rotavirus and virus shedding in 179 children between 1 week and 24 months of age (243). A stool specimen and paired serum samples were available from 179 hospitalized children. Thirty-six (20%) of the 179 children had rotavirus infections demonstrated by excretion of the virus and a serologic response, 41 (23%) of the children were diagnosed as carriers (those shedding the virus but having no serologic response), and 101 (56%) of the children were neither shedding the virus nor had a serologic response. The frequency of rotavirus infection or disease in these infants and young children increased with age, but the frequency of virus carriage decreased with age. These findings suggest that intestinal maturity may play a role in the development of disease. Data from this study as well as others (225) show that passively or actively acquired immunity does not prevent virus replication; thus, reinfection may occur frequently. The data of Champsaur et al show that the recovery of rotavirus does not necessarily indicate true infection (242, 243). In future studies, the demonstration of a rise in antibody titer should be included in studies to confirm rotaviral infection. This demonstration of rotavirus carriers has important infection control implications, as these patients may act as reservoirs of the virus and can represent a source for dissemi-

nation of rotavirus in the hospital if good patient care practices are not maintained.

Several studies have documented that adults can acquire rotavirus infections following contact with infected children, and also that infected adults may transmit the virus to susceptible children. Most such illnesses are mild and self-limited. However, there have been occasional reports of severe infections leading to death. There have also been several reports of outbreaks of rotavirus gastroenteritis in geriatric patients (244, 245). The majority of patients have been ill with diarrhea and/or vomiting. However, in at least one study, 40% of the asymptomatic patients on whom serologic studies were performed had elevations in their complement fixation antibody titers suggesting asymptomatic infection (244).

Understanding of the epidemiology of rotavirus gastroenteritis has been limited by inability to characterize infecting strains fully. Recently, the use of electropherotyping, the biochemical characterization of rotaviruses by analyzing the mobility of virion RNA segments following polyacrylamide gel electrophoresis, has been evaluated as an epidemiologic tool. The human rotaviruses, when subjected to electrophoretic separation, show extensive diversity in their segmented genomic patterns or electropherotypes. Although it was initially thought that electropherotype and serotype corresponded (246), subsequent work has raised questions about this correlation. Differences in electropherotypic patterns do not necessarily indicate differences in either antigenic or biologic properties. Furthermore, strains with identical electropherotypes may not have identical RNAs. Rodriguez et al and Spencer et al have reported identifying isolates with 12 genome segments, suggesting the possibility of an infection by two or more rotavirus strains of differing electropherotypes (247, 248). With such mixed infections, reassortment between different viruses may occur, resulting in a large number of electropherotypes.

Although these problems hamper the use of electropherotyping for classifying rotaviruses, this technique appears to be an excellent tool for the epidemiologic study of the spread of viruses during discrete outbreaks. In 1983 Rodriguez et al used this molecular epidemiologic tool in the study of 2 nosocomial outbreaks in an intensive care nursery (247). Twenty-two (22%) of 102 infants in the neonatal intensive care unit were infected with rotavirus. Initial epidemiologic studies suggested infant-to-infant spread of the rotavirus during each outbreak. By the use of electrophoresis of RNA from the infecting rotavirus strains, the authors were able to demonstrate nosocomial transmission from infant to infant and to identify at least 10 different rotavirus strains within a 2-month period. In addition, they showed that multiple strains could spread independently and in parallel to different infants during a single outbreak. In a similar study during two epidemics of rotavirus infections in hospitalized patients in Japan, Konno et al demonstrated the existence of a predominant rotaviral electropherotype during the first 2 to 3 months of each outbreak (249). Great variation in the genomic RNA segmented patterns of the rotavirus strains was encountered subsequently. These data suggest that mobility changes in the rotavirus RNA segments may occur during the course of an outbreak, possibly related either to multiple infections or to antigenic drift and reassortment. The use of antibody testing and genome analysis should improve our understanding of the epidemiology of rotavirus infection in the hospital setting and facilitate the development of more efficacious control strategies.

Norwalk and Related Agents

These viruses, of which the Norwalk agent virus is the prototype, are a common cause of epidemic acute nonbacterial gastroenteritis. Numerous community-acquired outbreaks have been reported (250–253). Vehicles associated with gastroenteritis outbreaks caused by the Norwalk or Norwalk-like agents include contaminated drinking water, green salad, raw oysters, and other shellfish, such as cockles (250, 251, 253–256).

In the majority of patients infected with these viruses, there is an abrupt onset of acute gastroenteritis of short duration. The incubation period is typically 24 to 48 hours and the median duration of illness is 24 hours. The majority of patients have diarrhea, nausea, and vomiting. Crampy abdominal pain occasionally occurs, and low grade fever occurs in approximately 20% of cases.

Although these viruses, which are 25 to 32 nm in diameter, can be visualized in the stools of patients with acute gastroenteritis using immune electron microscopy, attempts to cultivate these viruses in tissue culture have been unsuccessful. Until recently, antigen and antibody detection methods were unavailable. Greenberg et al have developed a solid phase radioimmunoassay for detecting Norwalk virus antigen and antibody that appears to be sensitive and specific (257).

Studies suggest that several serologically distinct viruses exist; these include the Norwalk, Hawaii, Ditchling, and Marin agents (255, 258–260).

Evidence suggests that these viruses are associated with nosocomial gastroenteritis. In a study of viruses associated with gastroenteritis in young children, Middleton et al found that 75 (11%) of 669 infants with gastroenteritis had 27-nm viruses visualized by electron microscopy of their stools (240). Evidence for nosocomial acquisition was found in 38 (51%) of the 75 cases. These viruses have also been associated with an outbreak of acute nonbacterial gastroenteritis in an extended care facility (260). During a 3-month period, 95 (51%) of 187 convalescent home residents and 22 (12%) of 180 personnel developed acute infectious nonbacterial gastroenteritis. A 27-nm virus was detected by immune electron microscopy in the stools of 4 of 32 patients examined. In addition, a serologic response to the 27-nm virus was detected by immune electron microscopy in 6 of 18 patients. All patients developed mild diarrhea of approximately 3 days' duration. Nausea and vomiting were uncommon, and fever occurred in less than 15%. Upon further study, the 27-nm virus isolated was designated the Marin agent when it was found to be morphologically similar but serologically unrelated to the Norwalk and Hawaii agents. The further development and use of sensitive and specific diagnostic tests for these viruses should simplify the identification of nosocomial outbreaks associated with these agents and improve our understanding of the epidemiology of these viruses.

Adenovirus

Adenoviruses are icosahedral, nonenveloped, double-stranded DNA viruses that have been associated with a wide range of infections in humans. Adenoviruses 40 and 41, which are also referred to as fastidious enteric adenoviruses, have recently been recognized as a cause of gastroenteritis in infants and children. These viruses are referred to as fastidious and noncultivable because they can be readily detected by direct electron microscopic examination of stool specimens from patients with gastroenteritis, but they do not grow in conventional cell cultures used for cultivation of adenoviruses, in particular, KB', HEP-2, HeLa, and human amnion and embryonic kidney cells (261).

In 1977 Middleton et al found that 86 (31%) of 669 patients with acute gastroenteritis had adenoviruses detectable by electron microscopy of their stools (240). In a subsequent study by Brandt et al, adenoviruses were found to be second only to rotaviruses in their frequency of detection by electron microscopy of stool specimens from patients with acute gastroenteritis (262).

In the majority of patients in whom gastroenteritis has been associated with adenovirus, symptoms have been mild and self-limiting. Although in many instances the gastroenteritis was community-acquired, several reports of hospital-acquired adenovirus gastroenteritis have been documented. In 1975, Flewett et al reported the acute onset of diarrhea in 6 of 19 children on their pediatric wards (238). In all of the affected infants, the duration of symptoms was 24 to 48 hours. None of the children vomited, and only one child had low grade fever. Symptoms also developed at the same time in a nurse on the ward where these children were hospitalized. Adenovirus-like particles were visualized by direct electron microscopy in stools from four of the six infants and the nurse; no adenovirus-like particles were visualized in stools from any of the other 13 children on the ward. Numerous attempts to cultivate these adenoviruses failed.

In 1982 Yolken et al evaluated the role of enteric adenoviruses in gastroenteritis in hospitalized infants (263). During a 12-week period, 14 of 27 (52%) infants with diarrhea had adenoviruses detected in their stools; similar adenoviruses were detected in only 1 of 72 children without diarrhea. The mean duration of adenovirus gastroenteritis in the infected children was 8 days. Thirteen (93%) of the 14 children with adenovirus gastroenteritis had respiratory symptoms.

In 1983 Chiba et al reported that seven children in an orphanage in Sapporo, Japan developed diarrhea during an 11-day period (264). Symptoms were mild in all patients and lasted from 3 to 8 days. Respiratory symptoms were not observed in any of the patients. The authors were able to detect an antibody response using immune electron microscopy in all seven patients with gastroenteritis and in all four contacts present in the same room, suggesting that subclinical infection had occurred. These data suggest that enteric adenoviruses can cause gastroenteritis, that asymptomatic infection can occur, and that the virus can spread in the hospital (265).

Inability to cultivate the enteric adenovirus has severely hampered investigations of the epidemiology of enteric adenoviruses. Recently, Gary et al and Johansson et al have shown that the enteric adenoviruses associated with acute gastroenteritis in infants and children are distinct adenoviruses as determined by antigenic structure and restriction endonuclease banding techniques (266, 267). Takiff et al have demonstrated that adenoviruses isolated from children with gastroenteritis, which could not be cultivated in tissue culture used to isolate respiratory viruses, could be grown in 293 cells, a cell line transformed by infections with adenovirus type 5 (268). In 1981, Kidd and Madeley demonstrated that the enteric adenovirus could also be cultivated in Chang's conjunctival cells (269). Using these tissue culture techniques, Jong et al have shown that about 200 antigenically related adenoviruses isolated from infants with gastroenteritis had no relationship to the 39 known human adenovirus species by either neutralization tests or by hemagglutination inhibition tests (261). Neutralization tests have also shown that these enteric adenoviruses have at least two distinctive variants, which are often referred to as adenoviruses 40 and 41. Although these adenoviruses appear identical by hemagglutination inhibition tests, DNA restriction enzyme analysis shows that these two viruses have considerably different genomes. These and other advances in our understanding of the antigenic and genomic character of the enteric adenoviruses should facilitate the study of the epidemiology of enteric adenoviruses to determine the importance of enteric adenoviruses as a cause of nosocomial gastroenteritis.

Other Viruses

Although rotaviruses account for most cases of nosocomial viral gastroenteritis, other viruses can cause gastroenteritis and may be transmitted within the hospital. Echoviruses have been implicated in two outbreaks of gastroenteritis in the hospital setting (270, 271). In one outbreak, echovirus 11 was recovered from three laboratory workers; in the other, echovirus 18 was found in the stools of 15 (88%) of 17 infants developing gastroenteritis in a nursery and in 0 of 19 infants without gastroenteritis. Minirotavirus or minireovirus, a distinct 32-nm particle, has been reported to be associated with nosocomial gastroenteritis in infants in two hospitals (240, 272). Caliciviruses, 28-nm particles, have been associated with infantile gastroenteritis and appear to spread in the hospital (272). Astroviruses have been associated with sporadic gastroenteritis, but little is known of their epidemiology (273, 274).

Giardia lamblia

G. lamblia is a protozoan parasite that causes acute and chronic diarrhea (275). The prevalence of Giardia infections appears to be highest in infants and toddlers (276, 277). The most consistent feature of Giardia gastroenteritis is the finding that diarrhea persists for more than 5 days. This is commonly accompanied by abdominal cramps, bloating, anorexia, and/or weight loss. Clinical illness varies from mild and self-limiting to severe. Malabsorption and chronic diarrhea have been reported in untreated cases of giardiasis. In such untreated patients, the organisms may be passed in the patient's stool for several months. Among infants and children, asymptomatic infection has been reported to occur in 20 to 50% of those examined in outbreak settings.

Giardia trophozoites are the motile forms of the parasite that attach to and invade the bowel wall; these forms are responsible for symptoms. Once the trophozoite re-enters the intestinal lumen it becomes round, develops an exterior membrane, and is passed as a cyst. Cysts are the infectious form of the organism.

Several studies have recently shown that day care-associated giardiasis is a frequent occurrence (278). Black et al showed that the prevalence of Giardia ranged from 29 to 54% in children between the ages of 6 months and 3 years who attended three day care centers in Atlanta (277). The prevalence of Giardia in age- and neighborhood-matched controls who did not attend day care centers was only 2%. In a similar study in day care centers in Tucson, Arizona, approximately half of 21 infants with gastroenteritis and 70% of asymptomatic children in a day care center who had a past history of diarrhea had Giardia (278). Infants and children with symptomatic or asymptomatic Giardia infections may infect day care center workers and family members. In 14 families of infected day care center children investigated in Atlanta, 25% of family members were found to have Giardia infections (277). Since cysts may survive for a prolonged period in the environment, both direct and indirect contact may play an important role in the transmission of Giardia. Furthermore, infants, children, and staff who have asymptomatic infections may serve as an important reservoir for giardiasis. Although contaminated water has been a frequent vehicle in community-acquired outbreaks of giardiasis, children in day care centers most likely become infected following either direct contact with an infected individual or by indirect contact with fecally contaminated environmental sources. Although nosocomial outbreaks of giardiasis have not been reported, conditions similar to those seen in day care centers exist within hospitals, and nosocomial outbreaks of giardiasis could occur.

Cryptosporidium

Cryptosporidium, an intestinal protozoan parasite, was first reported to be a cause of gastroenteritis in humans in 1976 (279). Prior to that time, Cryptosporidium had for many years been recognized as a cause of diarrhea in animals. Recently, reports of cryptosporidial enteritis in humans have increased dramatically (279).

Immunologic status has been a major determinant of disease severity; asymptomatic or self-limited infection occurs in individuals with an intact immune system, while chronic diarrhea occurs in those with immune abnormalities. Recently, outbreaks of Cryptosporidium gastroenteritis have been reported from day care centers in five states (280). In all outbreaks, illness has been characterized by an afebrile gastroenteritis without nausea or vomiting. In one outbreak, 11 (65%) of 17 symptomatic children and 3 (11%) of 28 asymptomatic children had Cryptosporidium detectable in stool specimens. Characteristically, cryptosporidial enteritis presents as profuse, watery diarrhea, often accompanied by mild abdominal cramping pain, nausea, and vomiting. The incubation period appears to be approximately 3 to 10 days. The duration of symptoms ranges from 5 to 6 days in patients with normal immune function to 2 to 18 months in those with abnormal immune function; asymptomatic fecal carriage of Cryptosporidium has been reported in both healthy and immunodeficient patients (281). In AIDS patients, Cryptosporidium has been associated with asymptomatic carriage as well as severe prolonged diarrhea (282, 283).

One reason for the increased reporting of cryptosporidial enteritis in humans may be the development of improved diagnostic methods. Prior to 1978, Cryptosporidium was identified by light or electron microscopic examination of intestinal biopsies. Recently developed methods allow Cryptosporidium to be identified in stool specimens (284, 285). Cryptosporidium may be missed if a routine "ova and parasite" examination of the stool is performed, as the oocysts are small and can be overlooked or mistaken for yeasts. A sensitive and specific serologic method for diagnosing cryptosporidiosis has recently been developed (286).

Recently, transmission of *Cryptosporidium* has been reported in day care centers and hospital settings (280, 287). In the day care center outbreaks, up to 50% of infants have had diarrhea and up to 65% of symptomatic infants have had *Cryptosporidium* detected in their stools (280). In one report of transmission within a hospital, a nurse, working on a ward where a 13-month-old child with cryptosporidial enteritis was hospitalized, developed abdominal cramps and watery diarrhea; cryptosporidial oocysts were detected in her feces (287). Current laboratory methods are insufficient to identify epidemiologically related strains; until further typing methods are developed, proof of nosocomial transmission will depend on epidemiologic evidence. Another recent report documents the potential for spread from an infected patient to hospital personnel (288). Eight (31%) of 25 personnel exposed to an ill patient had positive *Cryptosporidium* antibody titers, and 2 had diarrhea. The frequency of positivity was higher in nurses, house officers, and medical students than in attending physicians and respiratory therapists.

In patients with cryptosporidial enteritis, fecal shedding of oocysts appears to be irregular and prolonged; in patients with normal immune function, fecal shedding of oocysts has been reported to last for 12 to 21 days. The principal mode of transmission of *Cryptosporidium* appears to be from person to person by direct or indirect contact. At present, rapid identification of patients with cryptosporidial enteritis and institution of enteric precautions is the best form of prevention, as no effective treatment has yet been identified.

Entamoeba histolytica

E. histolytica, like *G. lamblia*, can cause both acute and chronic gastroenteritis. Although nosocomial transmission of *E. histolytica* has not been reported, one recent report suggests that nosocomial transmission could occur. During a 30-month period, Istre et al reported 36 cases of amebiasis occurring in patients who had colonic irrigation therapy in the office of a chiropractor (289). An epidemiologic investigation implicated the colonic irrigation machine, and testing showed that after routine cleaning this machine was heavily contaminated with *E. histolytica*. Patients at greatest risk for the development of amebiasis were those who underwent colonic irrigation immediately following a person with

bloody diarrhea. This report suggests that transmission could occur if endoscopic equipment is not adequately disinfected or sterilized following use in a patient with amebiasis.

Infection control personnel should also be aware that pseudoepidemics of intestinal amebiasis may occur. During a 3-month period in 1983, 38 cases of intestinal amebiasis were reported to the Los Angeles County Department of Health Service (290). When 71 slides from the 38 reported patients were examined by other laboratories, only 4 slides from 2 (5.3%) of the patients were found to have *E. histolytica*. Slides from 34 of 36 patients found not to have *E. histolytica* contained polymorphonuclear neutrophils and/or macrophages. *E. histolytica* can be confused with other intestinal protozoa and, more commonly, with leukocytes or macrophages in stool specimens.

Candida

Candida spp. have been associated with gastroenteritis in two settings: noninvasive enteritis in healthy persons and invasive enteritis in patients with underlying diseases. *Candida* is a normal saprophyte in humans and is present in approximately 60% of stool specimens (291). Thus, the presence of *Candida* spp. in feces has been considered a normal finding, and the etiologic role of *Candida* spp. in enteritis has been uncertain. In neonates *Candida* spp., often acquired from exposure during birth, can lead to watery diarrhea when this organism overgrows in the intestine (292). A similar picture of watery diarrhea with abdominal cramping has been reported in adults (293). In most patients gastroenteritis associated with *Candida* spp. is characterized by intermittent, watery, explosive diarrhea which is not bloody and is rarely accompanied by fever, nausea, anorexia, or vomiting. Stool cultures are seldom helpful as *Candida* spp. grow poorly on most media used for routine stool cultures and certain intestinal organisms, in particular Enterobacteriaceae, inhibit their growth. However, when stool specimens are stained with iodine and examined under high power light microscopy, large numbers of yeast cells may be visualized. *Candida* spp. diarrhea can have a protracted course, lasting as long as 3 months. Although the factors that lead to the transformation of *Candida* spp. from a saprophytic organism to a pathogen are ill defined, risk factors associated with disease include recent exposure to antimicrobials, use of oral contraceptives, and travel to areas where sanitation is poor (294). Healthy patients who develop *Candida* spp. gastroenteritis do not develop candidemia and usually respond to either nystatin or clotrimazole within 72 hours (293).

Candida spp., in particular *Candida albicans*, can also invade the gastrointestinal tract of patients with immunodeficiency diseases such as those with hematologic malignancies. In such patients, agranulocytosis and antimicrobial therapy predispose to disease (295). In this setting *Candida* spp. diarrhea often goes unrecognized until tissue invasion by the yeast occurs and disseminated candidiasis develops. In most cases, *Candida* spp. cause multiple scattered ulcerations of the small bowel with necrotic tissue at the base of the ulceration and masses of yeast cells invading blood vessels of the bowel wall. This occasionally results in perforation and hemorrhage with massive bleeding, and the diagnosis is often not made prior to postmortem examination.

Current typing systems for *Candida* species do not permit differentiation of endogenous from exogenous infections. Thus, although nosocomial *Candida* spp. gastroenteritis has been reported, improvements in laboratory methods for typing will be necessary before nosocomial transmission can be definitively demonstrated.

Candidate Agents

Intestinal spirochetes, which cause acute gastrointestinal disease in animals, have been suspected as a possible cause of gastroenteritis in humans (296). To date, no cases of nosocomial gastroenteritis due to these organisms have been identified, but recognition of this group of potential etiologic agents is beyond the capability of most clinical microbiology laboratories.

CONTROL

Since all enteric pathogens can be transmitted from person to person by the fecal-oral route, careful attention to appropriate hand washing practices is the single most important measure in the control of nosocomial transmission of enteric pathogens. Because such pathogens can also be transmitted by contaminated foods, careful attention to maintenance of appropriate food handling practices in hospitals is essential. Because contaminated breast milk has been implicated as a source of infection for neonates, careful maintenance of aseptic practices in collection and storage of this material is also critical (297).

Patients with acute diarrheal disease for which an infectious etiology is suspected should be placed on isolation precautions (298). For hospitals using the category-specific approach to isolation, the enteric precautions category is appropriate. For hospitals using a disease-specific approach to isolation, a private room is indicated if patient hygiene is poor, gowns should be worn if soiling of clothes is likely, and gloves should be worn if infective material is likely to be touched. The recommended duration of maintenance of the precautions varies for different agents (298).

Personnel with acute diarrheal disease for which an infectious etiology is suspected should be promptly evaluated by a physician and removed from patient care activities pending the results (299). Data suggest that the risk of transmission of nontyphi *Salmonella* spp. from infected health care personnel to patients is greater than that of transmission of other enteric bacteria or protozoa. Although personnel infected with other pathogens can generally return to patient care activities when they are clinically well (provided they are instructed about the need to observe scrupulous personnel hygiene practices), it appears prudent to require at least two negative stool cultures collected at least 24 hours apart before permitting personnel with *Salmonella* infections to return to patient care activities. Over 50% of such individuals can be expected to be culture-negative within 5 weeks and 90% within 9 weeks (300).

GASTROENTERITIS IN EXTENDED CARE FACILITIES

Elderly patients in extended care facilities are at increased risk for the development of gastroenteritis because of the increased incidence of achlorhydria and the frequent use of antacids in this patient population. In addition, such patients are at increased risk for mortality should such infections occur.

The incidence of institutionally acquired gastroenteritis in patients in extended care facilities appears to be higher than in acute care institutions. In a prevalence survey conducted in seven skilled care nursing homes, gastroenteritis was the sixth most common infection, occurring in 1.3% of all patients. A cluster of five cases was identified in one facility (301). *Salmonella* and *Shigella* spp. have been implicated in outbreaks in this setting (302–304). Foodborne outbreaks in this setting appear to be particularly likely to be caused by *C. perfringens* and *Salmonella* (99, 302). Viral gastroenteritis outbreaks caused by

Table 24.10 Characteristics of Selected Nosocomial Gastroenteritis Outbreaks in Developing Areas

Country	Year	Unit	Hospital	Organism	Multiply Resistant	No. of Cases	No. of Deaths	Bacteremia	Source	Transmission	Reference
India	1980	Neonatal	Children's	S. oranienburg	Yes	11	4	Yes	CA* infection	Vertical/direct contact	307
India	1978–1981	Neonatal/pediatric	General	S. typhimurium	Yes	295	?	?	CA infection	Direct contact	308
India	1980	Pediatric/adult	General	S. oranienburg	Yes	7	0	Yes	CA infection	?	309
India	1979	Neonatal/pediatric	Children's	S. bareilly	Yes	11	2	?	CA infection	Direct contact	310
India	1972	Pediatric/adult	General	S. weltevreden	Yes	84†	1	Yes	CA infection	Direct contact	311
India	1979	Neonatal	General	C. freundii	Yes	7	1	Yes	?	? Direct contact	312
India	1977–1978	Neonatal	General	? EPEC	Yes	18	0	No	?	? Indirect contact	313
India	?	Neonatal	General	K. pneumoniae/ETEC	Yes	25	0	Yes	?	?	314
Hong Kong	1974	Pediatric	General	S. johannesburg	Yes	12	0	No	?	? Direct contact	315
Tanzania	1977–1983	Pediatric	General	V. cholerae 01	Yes	216	?	No	CA infection	? Direct contact	316
Puerto Rico	1971–1972	Pediatric	General	S. heidelberg	Yes	55	8	Yes	CA infection	Direct contact	317
Republic of China	1984	Neonatal	General	S. cerro	?	109	0	Yes	?	Direct contact	318

* CA, community-acquired.
† Includes both patients and personnel

Norwalk-like viruses and rotavirus due to person-to-person transmission are being recognized with increasing frequency in these institutions (245, 305, 306). Secondary transmission occurs frequently following common vehicle outbreaks caused by *Salmonella* or viruses.

NOSOCOMIAL GASTROENTERITIS IN DEVELOPING COUNTRIES

Outbreaks of nosocomial gastroenteritis are being reported with increasing frequency from developing parts of the world (Table 24.10). As there is no established mechanism for reporting such outbreaks routinely, many more outbreaks have certainly occurred. The fact that the majority of the outbreaks summarized in Table 24.10 occurred in India undoubtedly reflects not only their frequency of occurrence, but also the local level of interest in investigating such outbreaks and in reporting the results in the scientific literature.

Because of the high incidence of community-acquired diarrheal disease, the existence of crowded facilities, and the frequent lack of attention to careful hand washing, nosocomial gastroenteritis appears to be more of a problem in these settings than in developed countries. Patients hospitalized in developing countries are at risk for development of nosocomial gastroenteritis due to any of the agents causing diarrhea in that locale. Malnourished children are at particular risk for *Salmonella* bacteremia complicating gastroenteritis (319).

Salmonella spp. are the most common cause of nosocomial gastroenteritis outbreaks reported from developing countries (Table 24.10); reported outbreaks typically occur in nurseries and pediatric units and are often caused by strains resistant to multiple antibiotics. Infections acquired in the community are the usual source of the pathogens. Person-to-person transmission by direct contact commonly occurs. The precise mode of nosocomial transmission of cholera in Tanzania is uncertain, but observations suggest that some person-to-person transmission may occur on pediatric wards under extremely crowded conditions (316). In some situations, nosocomial transmission has accounted for a substantial proportion of all cases occurring in nationwide outbreaks (315, 316). Interhospital spread has been reported to result from admission of a patient who acquired the infection during a prior admission at another hospital (317). In addition, a recent case-control study in Brazil has identified

hospitals as a likely source of infection of children with multiply resistant *Salmonella* in Brazil (320).

PRIORITIES FOR THE FUTURE

Future research efforts in the area of nosocomial gastroenteritis need to address a number of important issues. Better data on the incidence of and risk factors for nosocomial gastroenteritis are needed. The relative importance of certain enteric pathogens such as enterohemorrhagic *E. coli*, *Aeromonas hydrophila*, *Plesiomonas shigelloides*, adenoviruses, and a number of candidate viral agents needs to be determined. Investigations of epidemic and endemic infections are needed to identify new vehicles of transmission (e.g., enteral nutrition). Improved diagnostic techniques are needed to facilitate diagnosis of pathogenic *E. coli*, other enterotoxigenic bacteria, and viruses. Effective strategies to improve hand washing behavior need to be identified. Research is needed in extended care facilities to better define the incidence of, risk factors for, and etiologic agents of gastroenteritis. Effective means of interrupting person-to-person transmission in this setting need to be identified. In developing countries data are needed on the magnitude of the problem of nosocomial gastroenteritis in different patient populations in different types of hospitals. In this setting, research should also focus on definition of modes of transmission and on the evaluation of alternative control strategies.

References

1. Wenzel RP, Osterman CA, Hunting KJ, Gwaltney JM Jr: Hospital-acquired infections. I. Surveillance in a university hospital. *Am J Epidemiol* 103:251–260, 1976.
2. Centers for Disease Control: National Nosocomial Infections Study. Instruction manual for completion of "line listing of nosocomial infections" and "monthly discharges by service" forms. Atlanta, Revised December, 1982.
3. Welliver RC, McLaughlin S: Unique epidemiology of nosocomial infection in a children's hospital. *Am J Dis Child* 138:131–135, 1984.
4. Valenti WM, Hall CB, Douglas RG, Menegus MA, Pincus PH: Nosocomial viral infections. I. Epidemiology and significance. *Infect Control* 1:33–37, 1980.
5. Stamm WE, Weinstein RA, Dixon RE: Comparison of endemic and epidemic nosocomial infections. *Am J Med* 70:393–397, 1981.
6. Weinstein RA, Stamm WE: Pseudoepidemics in hospital. *Lancet* 2:862–864, 1977.
7. Yolken RH, Bishop CA, Townsend TR, Bolyard EA, Bartlett J, Santos GW, Saral R: Infectious gastroenteritis in bone-marrow-transplant recipients. *N Engl J Med* 306:1010–1012, 1982.
8. Jarvis WR, Middleton PJ, Gelfand EW: Signifi-

cance of viral infections in severe combined immunodeficiency disease. *Pediatr Infect Dis* 2:187–192, 1984.

9. Kelly TW, Patrick MR, Hillman KM: Study of diarrhea in critically ill patients. *Crit Care Med* 11:7–9, 1983.

10. Gitelson S: Gastrectomy, achlorhydria, and cholera. *Isr J Med Sci* 7:663–666, 1971.

11. Sprinz H: Pathogenesis of intestinal infections. *Arch Pathol* 87:556–561, 1969.

12. DuPont HL, Hornick RB: Adverse effect of Lomotil therapy in shigellosis. *JAMA* 226:1525–1528, 1973.

13. Bohnhoff M, Miller CP, Martin WR: Resistance of the mouse's intestinal tract to experimental *Salmonella* infection. II. Factors responsible for its loss following streptomycin treatment. *J Exp Med* 120:817–828, 1964.

14. Holzman RS, Florman AL, Podrid PJ, Simberkoff MS, Toharsky B: Drug-associated diarrhoea as a potential reservoir for hospital infections. *Lancet* 1:1195–1196, 1974.

15. Genersich A: Bauchfellentzundung beim neugeborenen in folge von perforation des ileums. *Arch Pathol Anat* 126:485–492, 1891.

16. Murrell TGC, Roth L: Necrotizing jejunitis: a newly discovered disease in the highlands of New Guinea. *Med J Aust* 1:61–68, 1963.

17. Zeissler J, Rassfeld-Sternberg L: Enteritis necroticans due to *Clostridium welchii* type F. *Br Med J* 1:267–272, 1936.

18. Kliegman RM, Pittard WB, Fanaroff AA: Necrotizing enterocolitis in neonates fed human milk. *J Pediatr* 95:450–453, 1979.

19. Ryder RW, Shelton JD, Guinan ME: Necrotizing enterocolitis: a prospective multicenter investigation. *Am J Epidemiol* 112:113–123, 1980.

20. Kliegman RM, Hack M, Jones P, Fanaroff AA: Epidemiologic study of necrotizing enterocolitis among low-birthweight infants: absence of identifiable risk factors. *J Pediatr* 100:440–444, 1982.

21. Edmund BJ: Clostridia species and necrotizing enterocolitis. *Am J Dis Child* 133:971, 1979.

22. Cashore WJ, Peter G, Lauermann M, Stonestreet BS, Oh W: Clostridia colonization and clostridial toxin in neonatal necrotizing enterocolitis. *J Pediatr* 98:308–311, 1981.

23. Howard FM, Bradley JM, Flynn DM: Outbreak of necrotizing enterocolitis caused by *Clostridium butyricum*. *Lancet* 2:1099–1102, 1977.

24. Sturm R, Staneck JL, Stauffer LR, Neblett WW: Neonatal necrotizing enterocolitis associated with penicillin-resistant, toxigenic *Clostridium butyricum*. *Pediatrics* 66:928–931, 1980.

25. Han VKM, Sayed H, Chance GW, Brabyn DG, Shahred WA: Outbreak of *Clostridium difficile* necrotizing enterocolitis: a case for oral vancomycin therapy? *Pediatrics* 71:935–941, 1983.

26. Kliegman RM, Fanaroff AA, Izant R, Speck WT: Clostridia as pathogens in neonatal necrotizing enterocolitis. *J Pediatr* 95:287–289, 1979.

27. Warren S, Schreiber JR, Epstein MF: Necrotizing enterocolitis and hemolysis associated with *Clostridium perfringens*. *Am J Dis Child* 138:686–688, 1984.

28. Speer ME, Taber LH, Yow MD: Fulminant neonatal sepsis and necrotizing enterocolitis associated with a "nonenteropathogenic" strain of *Escherichia coli*. *J Pediatr* 89:91–95, 1976.

29. Cushing AH: Necrotizing enterocolitis with *Escherichia coli* heat-labile enterotoxin. *Pediatrics* 71:626–630, 1983.

30. Powell J, Bureau MA, Pare C, Gaildry ML, Cabana D: Necrotizing enterocolitis. Epidemic following an outbreak of *Enterobacter cloacae* type 3305573 in a neonatal intensive care unit. *Am J Dis Child* 134:1152–1154, 1980.

31. Bell MJ, Feigin RD, Ternberg JL, Brotherton T: Evaluation of gastrointestinal microflora in necrotizing enterocolitis. *J Pediatr* 92:589–592, 1978.

32. Frantz ID, L'heureux P, Engel RR, Hunt CE: Necrotizing enterocolitis. *J Pediatr* 86:259–263, 1975.

33. Hill HR, Hunt CE, Matsen JM: Nosocomial colonization with *Klebsiella* type 26 in a neonatal intensive-care unit associated with an outbreak of sepsis, meningitis, and necrotizing enterocolitis. *J Pediatr* 85:415–419, 1974.

34. Stein H, Bek J, Solomon A, Schmaman A: Gastroenteritis with necrotising enterocolitis in premature babies. *Br Med J* 2:616–619, 1972.

35. Richardson RJ, Chan TK, McKenzie R, Yapp S: Necrotizing enterocolitis and *Salmonella* group C. *Ann Trop Paediatr* 4:55, 1984.

36. Chaney C, Moscovici O, Lebon P, Rousset S: Association of coronavirus infection with neonatal necrotizing enterocolitis. *Pediatrics* 69:209–214, 1982.

37. Siegel JD, Luby JP, Laptook AR, Butler S: Identification of coronavirus in a premature nursery during an outbreak of necrotizing enterocolitis and diarrhea. *Pediatr Res* 17:181A, 1983.

38. Rofusset S, Moscovici O, Lebon P, Barbet JP, Helardot P, Mac'e B, Bargy F, Le Tan Vinh, Chany C: Intestinal lesions containing coronavirus-like particles in neonatal necrotizing enterocolitis: an ultrastructural analysis. *Pediatrics* 73:218–224, 1984.

39. Johnson FE, Crnic DM, Simmons MA, Lilly JR: Association of fatal coxsackie B2 viral infection and necrotizing enterocolitis. *Arch Dis Child* 52:802–804, 1977.

40. Mogilner BM, Bar-Yochai A, Miskin A, Shif I, Aboudi Y: Necrotizing enterocolitis associated with rotavirus infection. *Isr J Med Sci* 19:894–896, 1983.

41. Rotbart HA, Levin MJ, Yolken RH, Manchester DK, Jantzen J: An outbreak of rotavirus-associated neonatal necrotizing enterocolitis. *J Pediatr* 103:454–459, 1983.

42. Ryder RW, Buxton AE, Wachsmuth IK, Mason E, Barrett FF: Heat-stable enterotoxigenic *Escherichia coli* and necrotizing enterocolitis: lack of an association. *J Pediatr* 91:302–303, 1977.

43. Lishman AH, Al Jumaili IJ, Elshibly E, Hay E, Record CO: *Clostridium difficile* isolation in neonates in a special care unit: lack of correlation with necrotizing enterocolitis. *Scand J Gastroenterol* 19:441–444, 1984.

44. Sherertz RJ, Sarubbi FA: The prevalence of *Clostridium difficile* and toxin in a nursery population. A comparison between patients with necrotizing

enterocolitis and an asymptomatic group. *J Pediatr* 100:435–439, 1982.

45. Larson HE, Parry JV, Price AB, Davies DK, Dolby J, Tyrell DA: Undescribed toxin in pseudomembranous colitis. *Br Med J* 1:1246–1248, 1977.
46. Larson HE, Price AB, Honour P, Borriello SP: *Clostridium difficile* and the aetiology of pseudomembranous colitis. *Lancet* 1:1063–1066, 1978.
47. Bartlett JG, Chang TW, Gurwith M, Gorbach SL, Onderdonk AB: Antibiotic-associated pseudomembraneous colitis due to toxin-producing Clostridia. *N Engl J Med* 298:531, 1978.
48. Rifkin GD, Fekety FR, Silva J Jr, Sack RB: Antibiotic-induced colitis: implication of a toxin neutralized by *Clostridium sordelli* antitoxin. *Lancet* 2:1103–1106, 1977.
49. Bartlett JG, Onderdonk AB, Cisneros RL, Kasper DL: Clindamycin-associated colitis due to a toxin-producing species of *Clostridium* in hamsters. *J Infect Dis* 136:701–705, 1977.
50. George WL, Rolfe RD, Harding GKM, Klein R, Putnam CW, Finegold SM: *Clostridium difficile* and cytotoxin in feces of patients with antimicrobial agent-associated pseudomembranous colitis. *Infection* 10:205–208, 1982.
51. George WL, Rolfe RD, Finegold SM: *Clostridium difficile* and its cytotoxin in feces of patients with antimicrobial agent-associated diarrhea and miscellaneous conditions. *J Clin Microbiol* 15:1049–1053, 1982.
52. Viscidi R, Willey S, Bartlett JG: Isolation rates and toxigenic potential of *Clostridium difficile* isolates from various patient populations. *Gastroenterology* 81:5–9, 1981.
53. Pesce CM, Colacino R, Gallelli FT, Giampalmo A: Histopathology of pseudomembranous colitis. *Zentralbl Allg Pathol* 129:101–104, 1984.
54. Laughon BE, Viscidi RP, Gdovin SL, Yolken RH, Bartlett JG: Enzyme immunoassays for detection of *Clostridium difficile* toxins A and B in fecal specimens. *J Infect Dis* 149:781–788, 1984.
55. Rothman SW, Brown JE, Diecidue A, Foret DA: Differential cytotoxic effects of toxins A and B isolated from *Clostridium difficile*. *Infect Immun* 46:324–331, 1984.
56. Libby JM, Donta ST, Wilkins TD: *Clostridium difficile* toxin A in infants. *J Infect Dis* 148:606, 1983.
57. Wedel N, Toselli P, Pothoulakis C, Faris B, Oliver P, Franzblau C, LaMont T: Ultrastructural effects of *Clostridium difficile* toxin B on smooth muscle cells and fibroblasts. *Exp Cell Res* 148:413–422, 1983.
58. Lyerly DM, Saum KE, MacDonald DK, Wilkins TD: Effects of *Clostridium difficile* toxins given intragastrically to animals. *Infect Immun* 47:349–352, 1985.
59. Viscidi R, Laughon BE, Yolken R, Bo-Linn P, Moench T, Ryder RW, Bartlett JC: Serum antibody response to toxins A and B of *Clostridium difficile*. *J Infect Dis* 148:93–100, 1983.
60. Pierce PF Jr, Wilson R, Silva J Jr, Garagusi VF, Rifkin GD, Fekety R, Nunez-Montiel O, Dowell VR Jr, Hughes JM: Antibiotic-associated pseudomembranous colitis: an epidemiologic investigation of a cluster of cases. *J Infect Dis* 145:269–274, 1982.
61. Kabins SA, Spira TJ: Outbreak of clindamycin-associated colitis. *Ann Intern Med* 83:830–831, 1975.
62. Rogers TR, Petrou M, Lucas C, Chung JTM, Barrett AJ, Borriello SP, Honour P: Spread of *Clostridium difficile* among patients receiving non-absorbable antibiotics for gut decontamination. *Br Med J* 283:408–409, 1981.
63. Greenfield C, Burroughs A, Szawathowski M, Bass N, Noone P, Pounder R: Is pseudomembraneous colitis infectious? *Lancet* 1:371–372, 1981.
64. Bruce D, Ritchie C, Jennings LC, Lynn KL, Bailey RR, Cook HB: *Clostridium difficile*-associated colitis: cross infection in predisposed patients with renal failure. *NZ Med J* 95:265–267, 1982.
65. Wust J, Sullivan NM, Hardegger U, Wilkins TD: Investigation of an outbreak of antibiotic-associated colitis by various typing methods. *J Clin Microbiol* 16:1096–1101, 1982.
66. Walters BAJ, Stafford R, Roberts RK, Seneviratne E: Contamination and crossinfection with *Clostridium difficile* in an intensive care unit. *Aust NZ J Med* 12:255–258, 1982.
67. Savage AM, Alford RH: Nosocomial spread of *Clostridium difficile*. *Infect Control* 4:31–33, 1983.
68. Poxton IR, Aronsson B, Mollby R, Nord CE, Collee JG: Immunochemical fingerprinting of *Clostridium difficile* strains isolated from an outbreak of antibiotic-associated colitis and diarrhoea. *J Med Microbiol* 17:317–324, 1984.
69. Tabaqchali S, O'Farrell S, Holland D, Silman R: Typing scheme for *Clostridium difficile*: its application in clinical and epidemiological studies. *Lancet* 1:935–938, 1984.
70. Malamou-Ludas H, O'Farrell S, Nash JQ, Tabaqchali S: Isolation of *Clostridium difficile* from patients and the environment of hospital wards. *J Clin Pathol* 36:88–92, 1983.
71. Cudmore MA, Silva J Jr, Fekety R, Liepman MK, Kim KH: *Clostridium difficile* colitis associated with cancer chemotherapy. *Arch Intern Med* 142:333–335, 1982.
72. Mulligan ME, George WL, Rolfe RD, Finegold SM: Epidemiological aspects of *Clostridium difficile*-induced diarrhea and colitis. *Am J Clin Nutr* 33:2533–2538, 1980.
73. Kim KH, Fekety R, Batts DH, Brown D, Cudmore M, Silva J Jr, Waters D: Isolation of *Clostridium difficile* from the environment and contacts of patients with antibiotic-associated colitis. *J Infect Dis* 143:42–50, 1981.
74. Tedesco FJ: Bacitracin therapy in antibiotic-associated pseudomembranous colitis. *Dig Dis Sci* 25:783–784, 1980.
75. Bartlett JG: Treatment of antibiotic-associated pseudomembranous colitis. *Rev Infect Dis* 6:S235–S241, 1984.
76. Teasley DG, Gerding DN, Olson MM, Peterson LR, Gebhard RL, Schwartz MJ, Lee JT Jr: Prospective randomised trial of metronidazole versus vancomycin for *Clostridium difficile*-associated diarrhoea and colitis. *Lancet* 2:1043–1046, 1983.
77. Bartlett JG, Tedesco FJ, Shull S, Lowe B, Chang T: Symptomatic relapse after oral vancomycin

therapy of antibiotic-associated pseudomembranous colitis. *Gastroenterology* 78:431–434, 1980.

78. George WL, Rolfe RD, Finegold SM: Treatment and prevention of antimicrobial agent-induced colitis and diarrhea. *Gastroenterology* 79:366–372, 1980.

79. Falsen E, Kaijser B, Nehls L, Nygren B, Svedhem A: *Clostridium difficile* in relations to enteric bacterial pathogens. *J Clin Microbiol* 12:297–300, 1980.

80. Gilligan PH, McCrathy LR, Genta VM: Relative frequency of *Clostridium difficile* in patients with diarrheal disease. *J Clin Microbiol* 14:26–31, 1981.

81. Donta ST, Myers MG: *Clostridium difficile* toxin in asymptomatic neonates. *J Pediatr* 100:431–434, 1982.

82. Jarvis WR, Feldman R: *Clostridium difficile* and gastroenteritis: how strong is the association in children? *Pediatr Infect Dis* 3:4–6, 1984.

83. Larson HE, Barclay FE, Honour P, Hill ID: Epidemiology of *Clostridium difficile* in infants. *J Infect Dis* 146:727–733, 1982.

84. Stark PL, Lee A, Parsonage BD: Colonization of the large bowel by *Clostridium difficile* in healthy infants: quantitative study. *Infect Immun* 35:895–899, 1982.

85. Al-Jumaili IJ, Shibley M, Lishman AH, Record CO: Incidence and origin of *Clostridium difficile* in neonates. *J Clin Microbiol* 19:77–78, 1984.

86. Elstner CL, Lindsay AN, Book LS, Matsen JM: Lack of relationship of *Clostridium difficile* to antibiotic-associated diarrhea in children. *Pediatr Infect Dis* 2:364–366, 1983.

87. Fainstein V, Bodey GP, Fekety R: Relapsing pseudomembranous colitis associated with cancer chemotherapy. *J Infect Dis* 143:865, 1981.

88. Miller SD, Koornhof HJ: *Clostridium difficile* colitis associated with the use of antineoplastic agents. *Eur J Clin Microbiol* 3:10–13, 1984.

89. Morris JG, Jarvis WR, Nunez-Montiel OL, Towns ML, Thompson FS, Dowell VR, Hill EO, Vogler WR, Winton EF, Hughes JM: *Clostridium difficile*: colonization and toxin production in a cohort of patients with malignant hematologic disorders. *Arch Intern Med* 144:967–969, 1984.

90. Ryan RW, Kwasnik I, Tilton RC: Improved immunologic detection of *Clostridium difficile* antigen by counter immunoelectrophoresis. *Diagn Microbiol Infect Dis* 1:59–63, 1983.

91. Welch DF, Menge SK, Matsen JM. Identification of toxigenic *Clostridium difficile* by counterimmunoelectrophoresis. *J Clin Microbiol* 11:470–473, 1980.

92. Rennie RP, Elliott JM, Nardini MA, Thornley JH: Criteria for detection of *Clostridium difficile* toxin production by counterimmunoelectrophoresis. *J Clin Microbiol* 20:923–926, 1984.

93. Sands M, Yungbluth M, Sommers HM: The nonvalue of counterimmunoelectrophoresis for the direct rapid detection of *Clostridium difficile* toxin in stool filtrates. *Am J Clin Pathol* 79:375–377, 1983.

94. Kurzynski TA, Cembrowski GS, Kimball JL: The use of CIE for the detection of *Clostridium difficile* toxin in stool filtrates: laboratory and clinical correlation. *Am J Clin Pathol* 79:370–374, 1983.

95. Wu TC, Fung JC: Evaluation of the usefulness of counterimmunoelectrophoresis for diagnosis of *Clostridium difficile*-associated colitis in clinical specimen. *J Clin Microbiol* 17:610–613, 1983.

96. Jarvis WR, Nunez-Montiel O, Thompson F, Dowell V, Towns M, Morris G, Hill E: Comparison of bacterial isolation, cytotoxicity assay, and counterimmunoelectrophoresis for the detection of *Clostridium difficile* and its toxin. *J Infect Dis* 147:778, 1983.

97. Horwitz MA: Specific diagnosis of foodborne disease. *Gastroenterology* 73:375–381, 1977.

98. Hughes JM: Food poisoning. In Mandell GL, Douglas RG Jr, Bennett JE (eds): *Principles and Practice of Infectious Diseases*, ed 2. New York, John Wiley & Sons, 1985, pp. 680–691.

99. Hughes JM, Gangarosa EJ: Hospital food Services: role in prevention of nosocomial foodborne disease. In Bennett JV, Brachman PS (eds): *Hospital Infections*, ed 2. Boston, Little, Brown, and Co, in press.

100. Editorial: food poisoning in hospitals. *Lancet* 1:576–577, 1980.

101. Sharp JCM, Collier PW, Gilbert RJ: Food poisoning in hospitals in Scotland. *J Hyg (Camb)* 83:231–236, 1979.

102. Palmer SR, Rowe B: Investigation of outbreaks of *Salmonella* in hospitals. *Br Med J* 287:891–893, 1983.

103. Thomas M, Noah MD, Male GE, Stringer MF, Kendall M, Gilbert RJ, Jones PH, Phillips KD: Hospital outbreak of *Clostridium perfringens* food-poisoning. *Lancet* 1:1046–1048, 1977.

104. Steere AC, Craven PJ, Hall WJ III, Leotsakis N, Wells JG, Farmer JJ III, Gangarosa EJ: Person-to-person spread of *Salmonella typhimurium* after a hospital common-source outbreak. *Lancet* 1:319–321, 1975.

105. Centers for Disease Control: Shigellosis in a children's hospital—Pennsylvania. *MMWR* 28:498–499, 1979.

106. Centers for Disease Control: Hospital-associated outbreak of *Shigella dysenteriae* type 2—Maryland. *MMWR* 32:250–257, 1983.

107. Centers for Disease Control: Multistate outbreak of salmonellosis caused by precooked roast beef. *MMWR* 30:391–392, 1981.

108. Spitalny KC, Okowitz EN, Vogt RL: Salmonellosis outbreak at a Vermont hospital. *South Med J* 77:168–172, 1984.

109. Collier AC, Miller RA, Meyers JD: Cryptosporidiosis after marrow transplantation: person-to-person transmission and treatment with spiramycin. *Ann Intern Med* 101:205–206, 1984.

110. Townsend TR, Bolyard EA, Yolken RH, Beschorner WE, Bishop CA, Burns WH, Santos GW, Saral R: Outbreak of coxsackie Al gastroenteritis: a complication of bone-marrow transplantation. *Lancet* 1:820–823, 1982.

111. Centers for Disease Control: Human *Salmonella* isolates—United States, 1983. *MMWR* 33:693–695, 1984.

112. Blaser MJ, Newman LS: A review of human salmonellosis. I. Infective dose. *Rev Infect Dis* 4:1096–1106, 1982.

113. Baine WB, Gangarosa EJ, Bennett JV, Barker WH Jr: Institutional salmonellosis. *J Infect Dis* 128:357–360, 1973.

114. Aber RC, Banks WV: An outbreak of nosocomial *Salmonella typhimurium* infection linked to environmental reservoir. *Infect Control* 1:386–390, 1980.

115. Beecham HJ III, Cohen ML, Parkin WE: *Salmonella typhimurium*: transmission by fiberoptic upper gastrointestinal endoscopy. *JAMA* 241:1013–1015, 1979.

116. O'Connor BH, Bennett JR, Alexander JG, Sutton DR, Leighton I, Mawer SL, Dunlop JM: Salmonellosis infection transmitted by fibreoptic endoscopes. *Lancet* 2:864–866, 1982.

117. Maudgal DP, Shafi MS, Northfield TC: Duodenal intubation as a source of typhoid fever. *Dig Dis Sci* 27:549–552, 1982.

118. Ayliffe GAJ, Geddes AM, Pearson JE, Williams TC: Spread of *Salmonella typhi* in a maternity hospital. *J Hyg (Camb)* 82:353–359, 1979.

119. Kumarasinghe G, Hamilton WJ, Gould JDM, Palmer SR, Dudgeon JA, Marshall WC: An outbreak of *Salmonella muenchen* infection in a specialist paediatric hospital. *J Hosp Infect* 3:341–344, 1982.

120. Seals JE, Parrott PL, McGowan JE Jr, Feldman RA: Nursery salmonellosis: delayed recognition due to unusually long incubation period. *Infect Control* 4:205–208, 1983.

121. Lamb VA, Mayhall CG, Spadora AC, Markowitz SM, Farmer JJ III, Dalton HP: Outbreak of *Salmonella typhimurium* gastroenteritis due to an imported strain resistant to ampicillin, chloramphenicol, and trimethoprim-sulfamethoxazole in a nursery. *J Clin Microbiol* 20:1076–1079, 1984.

122. Ryder RW, Blake PA, Murlin AC, Carter GP, Pollard RA, Merson MH, Allen SD, Brenner DJ: Increase in antibiotic resistance among isolates of *Salmonella* in the United States, 1967–1975: *J Infect Dis* 142:485–491, 1980.

123. Holmberg SD, Wells JG, Cohen ML: Animal-to-man transmission of antimicrobial-resistant *Salmonella*: investigations of U.S. outbreaks, 1971–1983. *Science* 225:833–835, 1984.

124. Riley LW, Cohen ML, Seals JE, Blaser MJ, Birkness KA, Hargrett NT, Martin SM, Feldman RA: Importance of host factors in human salmonellosis caused by multiresistant strains of *Salmonella*. *J Infect Dis* 149:878–883, 1984.

125. Levy SB: Playing antibiotic pool: time to tally the score. *N Engl J Med* 311:663–664, 1984.

126. Brunton J: Drug-resistant *Salmonella* from animals fed antimicrobials. *N Engl J Med* 311:1698–1699, 1984.

127. Lyons RW, Samples CL, DeSilva HN, Ross KA, Julian EM, Checko PJ: An epidemic of resistant *Salmonella* in a nursery: animal-to-human spread. *JAMA* 243:546–547, 1980.

128. Holmberg SD, Osterholm MT, Senger KA, Cohen ML: Drug-resistant *Salmonella* from animals fed antimicrobials. *N Engl J Med* 311:617–622, 1984.

129. Glaser JB, Morton-Kute L, Berger SR, Weber J, Siegal FP, Lopez C, Robbins W, Landesman SH: Recurrent *Salmonella typhimurium* bacteremia associated with the acquired immunodeficiency syndrome. *Ann Intern Med* 102:189–193, 1985.

130. Jacobs JL, Gold JWM, Murray HW, Roberts RB, Armstrong D: *Salmonella* infections in patients with the acquired immunodeficiency syndrome. *Ann Intern Med* 102:186–188, 1985.

131. Smith PD, Macher AM, Bookman MA, Boccia RV, Steis RG, Gill V, Manischewitz J, Gelmann EP: *Salmonella typhimurium* enteritis and bacteremia in the acquired immunodeficiency syndrome. *Ann Intern Med* 102:207–209, 1985.

132. Holmberg SD, Wachsmuth IK, Hickmann-Brenner FW, Cohen ML: Comparison of plasmid profile analysis, phage typing, and antimicrobial susceptibility testing in characterizing *Salmonella typhimurium* isolates from outbreaks. *J Clin Microbiol* 19:100–104, 1984.

133. Riley LW, Diferdinando GT Jr, DeMelfi TM, Cohen ML: Evaluation of isolated cases of salmonellosis by plasmid analysis: introduction and transmission of a bacterial clone by precooked roast beef. *J Infect Dis* 148:12–17, 1983.

134. Speelman P, Kabir I, Islam M: Distribution and spread of colonic lesions in shigellosis: a colonoscopic study. *J Infect Dis* 150:899–903, 1984.

135. Blaser MJ, Pollard RA, Feldman RA: *Shigella* infections in the United States, 1974–1980. *J Infect Dis* 147:771–775, 1983.

136. Haltalin KC: Neonatal shigellosis. *Am J Dis Child* 114:603–611, 1967.

137. Salzman TC, Scher CD, Moss R: Shigellae with transferable drug resistance: outbreak in a nursery for premature infants. *J Pediatr* 71:21–26, 1967.

138. Weissman JB, Gangarosa EJ, Schmerler A, Marier RL, Lewis JN: Shigellosis in day-care centres. *Lancet* 1:88–90, 1975.

139. Levine MM, Gangarosa EJ, Barrow WB, Weiss CF: Shigellosis in custodial institutions. V. Effect of intervention with streptomycin-dependent *Shigella sonnei* vaccine in an institution with endemic disease. *Am J Epidemiol* 104:88–92, 1976.

140. Weissman JB, Hutcheson RH: Shigellosis transmitted by nurses. *South Med J* 69:1341–1346, 1976.

141. Tacket CO, Cohen ML: Shigellosis in day care centers: use of plasmid analysis to assess control measures. *Pediatr Infect Dis* 2:127–130, 1983.

142. Tacket CO, Shahid N, Huq MI, Alim ARMA, Cohen ML: Usefulness of plasmid profiles for differentiation of *Shigella* isolates in Bangladesh. *J Clin Microbiol* 20:300–301, 1984.

143. Ruiz-Palacios GM, Torres J, Torres NI, Escamilla E, Ruiz-Palacios BR, Tamayo J: Cholera-like enterotoxin produced by *Campylobacter jejuni*: characterisation and clinical significance. *Lancet* 2:250–252, 1983.

144. Blaser MJ, Wells JG, Feldman RA, Pollard RA, Allen JR, Collaborative Diarrheal Disease Study Group: *Campylobacter* enteritis in the United States: a multicenter study. *Ann Intern Med* 98:360–365, 1983.

145. Mawer SL, Smith BAM: *Campylobacter* infection of premature baby. *Lancet* 1:1041, 1979.

146. Karmali MA, Norrish B, Lior H, Heyes B, Monteath A, Montgomery H: *Campylobacter* enterocolitis in a neonatal nursery. *J Infect Dis* 149:874–877, 1984.

147. Blaser MJ, Taylor DN, Feldman RA: Epidemiology of *Campylobacter jejuni* infections. *Epidemiol Rev* 5:157–176, 1983.
148. Finch MJ, Riley LW: *Campylobacter* Infections in the United States: results of an 11-state surveillance. *Arch Intern Med* 144:1610–1612, 1984.
149. Blaser MJ, Reller LB: *Campylobacter* enteritis. *N Engl J Med* 305:1444–1452, 1981.
150. Taylor PR, Weinstein WM, Bryner JM: *Campylobacter* fetus infection in human subjects: association with raw milk. *Am J Med* 66:779–783, 1979.
151. Blaser MJ, Cravens J, Powers BW, Laforce FM, Wang W-LL: *Campylobacter* enteritis associated with unpasteurized milk. *Am J Med* 67:715–718, 1979.
152. Robinson DA, Jones DM: Milk-borne *Campylobacter* infection. *Br Med J* 282:1374–1376, 1981.
153. Istre GR, Blaser MJ, Shillam P, Hopkins RS: *Campylobacter* enteritis associated with undercooked barbecued chicken. *Am J Public Health* 74:1265–1267, 1984.
154. Vogt RL, Sours HE, Barrett T, Feldman RA, Dickinson RJ, Witherell L, Investigation team: *Campylobacter* enteritis associated with contaminated water. *Ann Intern Med* 96:292–296, 1982.
155. Mentzing LO: Waterborne outbreaks of *Campylobacter* enteritis in central Sweden. *Lancet* 2:352–354, 1981.
156. Palmer SR, Gully PR, White JM, Pearson AD, Suckling WG, Jones DM, Rawes JCL, Penner JL: Water-borne outbreak of *Campylobacter* gastroenteritis. *Lancet* 1:287–290, 1983.
157. Blaser MJ, Waldman RJ, Barrett T, Erlandson AL: Outbreaks of *Campylobacter* enteritis in two extended families: evidence for person-to-person transmission. *J Pediatr* 98:254–257, 1981.
158. Hopkins RS, Olmstead R, Istre GR: Endemic *Campylobacter jejuni* infection in Colorado: identified risk factors. *Am J Public Health* 74:249–250, 1984.
159. Taylor DM, McDermott KT, Little JR, Wells JG, Balser MJ: *Campylobacter* enteritis from untreated water in the Rocky Mountains. *Ann Intern Med* 99:38–40, 1983.
160. Blaser MJ, Weiss SH, Barrett TJ: *Campylobacter* enteritis associated with a healthy cat. *JAMA* 247:816, 1982.
161. Blaser M, Cravens J, Powers BW, Wang WL: *Campylobacter* enteritis associated with canine infection. *Lancet* 2:979–981, 1978.
162. Boyce JM, Evans DJ Jr, Evans DG, Dupont HL: Production of heat-stable, methanol-soluble enterotoxin by *Yersinia enterocolitica. Infect Immun* 25:532–537, 1979.
163. Toivanen P, Toivanen A, Olkkonen L, Aantaa S: Hospital outbreak of *Yersinia enterocolitica* infection. *Lancet* 1:801–803, 1973.
164. Ratnam S, Mercer E, Picco B, Parsons S, Butler R: A nosocomial outbreak of diarrheal disease due to *Yersinia enterocolitica* serotype 0:5, biotype 1. *J Infect Dis* 145:242–247, 1982.
165. Black RE, Jackson RJ, Tsai T, Medvesky M, Shayegani M, Felley JC, Macleod KIE, Wakelee AM: Epidemic *Yersinia enterocolitica* infection due to contaminated chocolate milk. *N Engl J Med* 298:76–79, 1978.
166. Tacket CO, Narain JP, Sattin R, Lofgren JP, Konigsberg C, Rendtorff RC, Rausa A, Davis BR, Cohen ML: A multistate outbreak of infections caused by *Yersinia enterocolitica* transmitted by pasteurized milk. *JAMA* 251:483–486, 1984.
167. Centers for Disease Control: Outbreak of *Yersinia enterocolitica*—Washington state. *MMWR* 31:562–564, 1982.
168. Levine MM, Edelman R: Enteropathogenic *Escherichia coli* of classic serotypes associated with infant diarrhea: epidemiology and pathogenesis. *Epidemiol Rev* 6:31–51, 1984.
169. Evans DJ Jr, Chen LC, Curlin GT, Evans DG: Stimulation of adenyl cyclase by *Escherichia coli* enterotoxin. *Nature New Biol* 236:137–138, 1972.
170. Field M, Graf LH Jr, Laird WJ, Smith PL: Heat-stable enterotoxin of *Escherichia coli*: in vitro effects on guanylate cyclase activity, cyclic GMP concentration, and ion transport in small intestine. *Proc Natl Acad Sci USA* 75:2800–2804, 1978.
171. Hughes JM, Murad F, Chang B, Guerrant RL: Role of cyclic GMP in the action of heat-stable enterotoxin of *Escherichia coli. Nature* 271:755–756, 1978.
172. Guerrant RL, Hughes JM, Chang B, Robertson DC, Murad F: Activation of intestinal guanylate cyclase by heat-stable enterotoxin of *Escherichia coli*: studies of tissue specificity, potential receptors, and intermediates. *J Infect Dis* 142:220–228, 1980.
173. Kennedy DJ, Greenberg RN, Dunn JA, Abernathy R, Ryerse JS, Guerrant RL: Effects of *Escherichia coli* heat-stable enterotoxin ST_b on intestines of mice, rats, rabbits, and piglets. *Infect Immun* 46:639–643, 1984.
174. Ryder RW, Kaslow RA, Wells JG: Evidence for enterotoxin production by a classic enteropathogenic serotype of *Escherichia coli. J Infect Dis* 140:626–628, 1979.
175. O'Brien AD, LaVeck GD, Thompson MR, Formal SB: Production of *Shigella dysenteriae* type 1-like cytotoxin by *Escherichia coli. J Infect Dis* 146:763–769, 1982.
176. Ulshen MH, Rollo JL: Pathogenesis of *Escherichia coli* gastroenteritis in man: another mechanism. *N Engl J Med* 302:99–101, 1980.
177. Clausen CR, Christie DL: Chronic diarrhea in infants caused by adherent enteropathogenic *Escherichia coli. J Pediatr* 100:358–361, 1982.
178. Moon HW, Whipp SC, Argenzio RA, Levine MM, Giannella RA: Attaching and effacing activities of rabbit and human enteropathogenic *Escherichia coli* in pig and rabbit intestines. *Infect Immun* 41:1340–1351, 1983.
179. Rothbaum R, McAdams AJ, Giannella R, Partin JC: A clinicopathologic study of enterocyte-adherent *Escherichia coli*: a cause of protracted diarrhea in infants. *Gastroenterology* 83:441–454, 1982.
180. Riley LW, Remis RS, Helgerson SD, McGee HB, Wells JG, Davis BR, Herbert RJ, Olcott ES, Johnson LM, Hargrett NT, Blake PA, Cohen ML: Hemorrhagic colitis associated with a rare *Escherichia coli* serotype. *N Engl J Med* 308:681–685,

1983.

181. Remis RS, MacDonald KL, Riley LW, Puhr ND, Wells JG, Davis BR, Blake PA, Cohen ML: Sporadic cases of hemorrhagic colitis associated with *Escherichia coli* 0157:H7. *Ann Intern Med* 101:624–626, 1984.

182. O'Brien AD, Lively TA, Chen ME, Rothman SW, Formal SB: *Escherichia coli* 0157:H7 strains associated with haemorrhagic colitis in the United States produce a *Shigella dysenteriae* 1 (shiga) like cytotoxin. *Lancet* 1:702, 1983.

183. Johnson WM, Lior H, Bezanson GS: Cytotoxic *Escherichia coli* 0157:H7 associated with haemorrhagic colitis in Canada. *Lancet* 1:76, 1983.

184. O'Brien AD, Lively TA, Chang TW, Gorbach SL: Purification of *Shigella dysenteriae* 1 (shiga)-like toxin from *Escherichia coli* 0157:H7 strain associated with hemorrhagic colitis. *Lancet* 2:573, 1983.

185. Centers for Disease Control: Isolation of *E. coli* 0157:H7 from sporadic cases of hemorrhagic colitis—United States. *MMWR* 31:580–585, 1982.

186. Pai CH, Gordon R, Sims HV, Bryan LE: Sporadic cases of hemorrhagic colitis associated with *Escherichia coli* 0157:H7: clinical, epidemiologic, and bacteriologic features. *Ann Intern Med* 101:738–742, 1984.

187. Centers for Disease Control: Outbreak of hemorrhagic colitis—Ottawa, Canada. *MMWR* 32:133–134, 1983.

188. Karmali MA, Steele BT, Petric M, Lim C: Sporadic cases of haemolytic-uraemic syndrome associated with faecal cytotoxin and cytotoxin-producing *Escherichia coli* in stools. *Lancet* 1:619–620, 1983.

189. Centers for Disease Control: Hemolytic-uremic syndrome associated with *Escherichia coli* 0157:H7 enteric infections—United States, 1984. *MMWR* 34:20–21, 1985.

190. Ryder RW, Wachsmuth IK, Buxton AE, Evans DG, Dupont HL, Mason E, Barrett FF: Infantile diarrhea produced by heat stable enterotoxigenic *Escherichia coli. N Engl J Med* 295:849–853, 1976.

191. Hazen TC, Fliermans CB, Hirsch RP, Esch GW: Prevalence and distribution of *Aeromonas hydrophila* in the United States. *Appl Environ Microbiol* 36:731–738, 1978.

192. von Graevenitz A, Zinterhofer L: The detention of *Aeronomas hydrophila* in stool specimens. *Health Lab Sci* 7:124–127, 1970.

193. Slotnick IJ: *Aeromonas* species isolates: *Ann NY Acad Sci* 174:503–510, 1970.

194. Lautrop H: *Aeromonas hydrophila* isolated from human feces and its possible pathological significance. *Acta Pathol Microbiol Scand* 51 (Suppl 144):299–301, 1961.

195. Miles AA, Halnan ET: A new species of microorganism (*Proteus melanovogenes*) causing black rot in eggs. *J Hyg (Camb)* 37:79–97, 1937.

196. Chatterjee BD, Neogy KN: Studies of *Aeromonas* and *Plesiomonas* species isolated from cases of choleraic diarrhoea. *Indian J Med Res* 60:520–524, 1972.

197. Millership SE, Curnow SR, Chattopadhyay B: Faecal carriage rate of *Aeromonas hydrophila. J*

Clin Pathol 36:920–923, 1983.

198. Pitarangsi C, Echeverria P, Whitmire R, Tirapat C, Formal S, Dammin GJ, Tingtalapong M: Enteropathogenicity of *Aeromonas hydrophila* and *Plesiomonas shigelloides*: prevalence among individuals with and without diarrhea in Thailand. *Infect Immun* 35:666–673, 1982.

199. Holmberg SD, Farmer JJ III: *Aeromonas hydrophila* and *Plesiomonas shigelloides* as causes of intestinal infections. *Rev Infect Dis* 6:633–639, 1984.

200. Janda JM, Bottone EJ, Skinner CV, Calcaterra D: Phenotypic markers associated with gastrointestinal *Aeromonas hydrophila* isolates from symptomatic children. *J Clin Microbiol* 17:588–591, 1983.

201. Burke V, Gracey J, Robinson J, Peck D, Beaman J, Bundell C: The microbiology of childhood gastroenteritis: *Aeromonas* species and other infective agents. *J Infect Dis* 148:68–74, 1983.

202. Ueda S, Yamasaki S, Horik M: The isolation of paracolon C27 and halophilic organisms from an outbreak of food poisoning. *Jpn J Public Health* 10:67–70, 1963.

203. Chatterjee BD, Neogy KN: Studies on *Aeromonas* and *Plesiomonas* species isolated from cases of choleraic diarrhea. *Indian J Med Res* 60:520–524, 1972.

204. Shandera WX, Hafkin B, Martin DL, Taylor JP, Maserang DL, Wells JG, Kelly M, Ghandi K, Kaper JB, Lee JV, Blake PA: Persistence of cholera in the United States. *Am J Trop Med Hyg* 32:812–817, 1983.

205. Morris JG Jr, Black RE: Cholera and other vibrioses in the United States. *N Engl J Med* 312:343–350, 1985.

206. Klipstein FA, Horowitz IR, Engert RF, Schenk EA: Effect of *Klebsiella pneumoniae* enterotoxin on intestinal transport in the rat. *J Clin Invest* 56:799–807, 1975.

207. Cushing AH, Smart J: Gastrointestinal carriage of toxigenic bacteria: relation to diarrhea and to serum response. *J Infect Dis* 151:114–123, 1985.

208. Guerrant RL, Dickens MD, Wenzel RP, Kapikian AZ: Toxigenic bacterial diarrhea: nursery outbreak involving multiple bacterial strains. *J Pediatr* 89:885–891, 1976.

209. Haley RW, Hightower AW, Khabbaz RF, Thornsberry C, Martone WJ, Allen JR, Hughes JM: The emergence of methicillin-resistant *Staphylococcus aureus* infections in United States hospitals. *Ann Intern Med* 97:297–308, 1982.

210. Wenzel RP: The emergence of methicillin-resistant *Staphylococcus aureus. Ann Intern Med* 97:440–442, 1982.

211. McDonald M, Ward P, Harvey K: Antibiotic-associated diarrhoea and methicillin-resistant *Staphylococcus aureus. Med J Aust* 1:462–464, 1982.

212. Scopetti F, Orefici G, Biondi F, Benini F: *Staphylococcus aureus* resistant to methicillin and gentamicin as a cause of outbreak of epidemic enteritis in a hospital. *Boll Ist Sieroter Milan* 62:406–411, 1983.

213. Bishop RF, Davidson GP, Holmes IH, Rusk RJ: Virus particles in epithelial cells of duodenal mu-

cosa from children with acute gastroenteritis. *Lancet* 2:1281–1284, 1973.

214. Koopman JS, Turkish VJ, Monto AS, Gouvea V, Srivastava S, Isaacson RE: Patterns and etiology of diarrhea in three clinical settings. *Am J Epidemiol* 119:114–123, 1981.

215. Gurwith M, Wenman W, Hinde D, Feltham S, Greenberg H: A prospective study of rotavirus infection in infants and young children. *J Infect Dis* 144:218–224, 1981.

216. Kapikian AZ, Greenberg HB, Wyatt RG, Kalica AR, Kim HW, Brandt CD, Rodriguez WJ, Parrott RH, Chanock RM: Viral gastroenteritis. In Evans AJ (ed): *Viral Infections of Humans: Epidemiology and Control*, ed 2. New York, Plenum, 1983.

217. Vesikari T, Isolauri E, Delem A, D'Hondt E, Andre' FE, Zissis G: Immunogenicity and safety of live oral attenuated bovine rotavirus vaccine strain RIT 4237 in adults and young children. *Lancet* 2:807–811, 1983.

218. Rodriguez WJ, Kim HW, Arrobio JO, Brandt CD, Chanock RM, Kapikian AZ, Wyatt RG, Parrott RH: Clinical feature of acute gastroenteritis associated with human reovirus-like agent in infants and young children. *J Pediatr* 91:188–193, 1977.

219. Tufvesson B, Johnsson T, Persson B: Family infections by reo-like virus. *Scand J Infect Dis* 9:257–261, 1977.

220. Haug KW, Orstavik I, Kvelstad G: Rotavirus infections in families. *Scand J Infect Dis* 10:265–269, 1978.

221. Kim HW, Brandt CD, Kapikian AZ, Wyatt RG, Arrobio JO, Rodriguez WJ, Chanock RM, Parrott RH: Human reo-like virus infection. *JAMA* 237:404–406, 1977.

222. Tallett S, MacKenzie C, Middleton P, Kerzner B, Hamilton R: Clinical, laboratory and epidemiologic features of a viral gastroenteritis in infants and children. *Pediatrics* 60:217–222, 1977.

223. Chrystie IL, Totterdell B, Baker MJ, Scopes JW, Banatvala JE: Rotavirus infections in a maternity unit. *Lancet* 2:79, 1975.

224. Murphy AM, Albrey MB, Hay PJ: Rotavirus infections in neonates. *Lancet* 2:452–453, 1975.

225. Bishop RF, Hewstone AS, Davidson GP, Townley RRW, Holmes IH, Ruck BJ: An epidemic of diarrhoea in human neonates involving a reovirus-like agent and "enteropathogenic" serotypes of *Escherichia coli. J Clin Pathol* 29:46–49, 1976.

226. Totterdell BM, Chyrstie IL, Banatvala JE: Rotavirus infections in a maternity unit. *Arch Dis Child* 51:924–928, 1976.

227. Murphy AM, Albrey MB, Crewe EB: Rotavirus infections of neonates. *Lancet* 2:1149–1150, 1977.

228. Chrystie IL, Totterdell BM, Banatvala JE: Asymptomatic endemic rotavirus infections in the newborn. *Lancet* 2:1176–1178, 1978.

229. Crewe E, Murphy AM: Further studies on neonatal rotavirus infections. *Med J Aust* 1:61–63, 1980.

230. Dean AG, Bowden DK, Easa D, Waxman SH, Courtney P, Poon KA: Rotavirus in newborn nurseries: negative results from Honolulu and the New Hebrides. *Hawaii Med J* 39:170–171, 1980.

231. Krause PJ, Hyams JS, Ballow M, Klemas BW: Nosocomial rotavirus infection in a neonatal intensive care unit. Twenty-first Interscience Conference on Antimicrobial Agents and Chemotherapy, 1981, Chicago, abstract 704.

232. Bryden AS, Thouless ME, Hall CJ, Flewett TH, Wharton BA, Mathew PM, Craig I: Rotavirus infections in a special-care baby unit. *J Infect Dis* 4:43–48, 1982.

233. Santosham M, Pathak A, Kottapalli S, Vergara J, Wong S, Frochlick J, Sack RB: Neonatal rotavirus infection. *Lancet* 1:1070–1071, 1982.

234. Rodriguez WJ, Kim HW, Brandt CD, Fletcher AB, Parrott RH: Rotavirus: a cause of nosocomial infection in the nursery. *J Pediatr* 101:274–277, 1982.

235. Dearlove J, Latham P, Dearlove B, Pearl K, Thomson A, Lewis IG: Clinical range of neonatal rotavirus gastroenteritis. *Br Med J* 286:1473–1475, 1983.

236. Srinivasan G, Azarcon E, Muldoon MRL, Jenkins G, Polavarapu S, Kallick CA, Pildes RS: Rotavirus infection in normal nursery: epidemic and surviellance. *Infect Control* 10:478–481, 1984.

237. Harris JS, Kundin WD, Lenahan MF, Bischone A: Outbreaks of rotavirus diarrhea in a fullterm nursery. 23rd Interscience Conference on Antimicrobial Agents and Chemotherapy, Las Vegas, 1983, abstract 417.

238. Flewett TH, Bryden AS, Davies H: Epidemic viral enteritis in a long-stay children's ward. *Lancet* 1:4–5, 1975.

239. Ryder RW, McGowan JE, Hatch MH, Palmer EL: Reovirus-like agent as a cause of nosocomial diarrhea in infants. *J Pediatr* 90:698–702, 1977.

240. Middleton PJ, Szymanski MT, Petric M: Viruses associated with acute gastroenteritis in young children. *Am J Dis Child* 131:733–737, 1977.

241. Saulsbury FT, Winkelstein JA, Yolken RH: Chronic rotavirus infection in immunodeficiency. *J Pediatr* 97:61–65, 1980.

242. Champsaur H, Questiaux E, Prevot J, Henry-Amar M, Goldszmidt D, Bourjouane M, Bach C: Rotavirus carriage, asymptomatic infection, and disease in the first two years of life. I. Virus shedding. *J Infect Dis* 149:667–674, 1984.

243. Champsaur H, Henry-Amar M, Goldszmidt D, Prevot J, Bourjouane M, Questiaux E, Bach C: Rotavirus carriage, asymptomatic infection, and disease in the first two years of life. II. Serological response. *J Infect Dis* 149:675–682, 1984.

244. Marrie TJ, Spencer SHL, Faulkner RS, Ethier J, Young CH: Rotavirus infection in a geriatric population. *Arch Intern Med* 142:313–316, 1982.

245. Cubitt WD, Holzel H: An outbreak of rotavirus infection in a long-stay ward of a geriatric hospital. *J Clin Pathol* 33:306–308, 1980.

246. Kalica AR, Greenberg HB, Espejo RT, Flores J, Wyatt RG, Kapikian AZ, Chanock RM: Distinctive ribonucleic acid patterns of human rotavirus subgroups 1 and 2. *Infect Immun* 33:958–961, 1981.

247. Rodriguez WJ, Kim HW, Brandt CD, Gardner MK, Parrott RH: Use of electrophoresis of RNA from human rotavirus to establish the identity of strains involved in outbreaks in a tertiary care nursery. *J Infect Dis* 148:34–40, 1983.

248. Spencer E, Avendano F, Araya M: Characteristics

and analysis of electropherotypes of human rotavirus isolated in Chile. *J Infect Dis* 148:41–48, 1983.

249. Konno T, Sato T, Suzuki H, Kitaoka S, Katsushima N, Sakamoto M, Yazaki N, Tshida N: Changing RNA patterns in rotavirus of human origin: demonstration of a single dominant pattern at the start of an epidemic and various patterns thereafter. *J Infect Dis* 149:683–687, 1984.

250. Taylor JW, Gary GW, Jr., Greenberg HB: Norwalk-related viral gastroenteritis due to contaminated drinking water. *Am J Epidemiol* 114:584–592, 1981.

251. Griffin MR, Surowiec JJ, McCloskey DI, Capuano B, Pierzynski B, Quinn M, Wojnarski R, Parkin WE, Greenberg H, Gary GW: Foodborne Norwalk virus. *Am J Epidemiol* 115:178–184, 1982.

252. Greenberg HB, Valdesuso J, Yolken RH, Gangarosa E, Gary W, Wyatt RG, Konno T, Suzuki H, Chanock RM, Kapikian AZ: Role of Norwalk virus in outbreaks of nonbacterial gastroenteritis. *J Infect Dis* 139:564–568, 1979.

253. Gunn RA, Janowski HT, Lieb S, Prather EC, Greenberg HB: Norwalk virus gastroenteritis following raw oyster consumption. *Am J Epidemiol* 115:348–351, 1982.

254. Morens DM, Zweighaft RM, Vernon TM, Gary GW, Eslien JJ, Wood BT, Holman RC, Dolin R: A waterborne outbreak of gastroenteritis with secondary person-to-person spread: association with a viral agent. *Lancet* 1:964–966, 1979.

255. Appleton H, Periera M: A possible virus aetiology in outbreaks of food-poisoning from cockles. *Lancet* 2:780–781, 1977.

256. Murphy AM, Grohmann GS, Christopher PJ, Lopez WA, Davey GR, Millsom RH: An Australia-wide outbreak of gastroenteritis from oysters caused by Norwalk virus. *Med J Aust* 2:329–333, 1979.

257. Greenberg HB, Wyatt RG, Valdesuso J, Kalica AR, London WT, Chanock RM, Kapikian AZ: Solid-phase microtiter radioimmunoassay for detection of the Norwalk strain of acute nonbacterial, epidemic gastroenteritis virus and its antibodies. *J Med Virol* 2:97–108, 1978.

258. Kapikian AZ, Wyatt RG, Dolin R: Visualization by immune electron microscopy of a 27-nm particle associated with acute infectious nonbacterial gastroenteritis. *J Virol* 10:1075–1081, 1972.

259. Wyatt RG, Dolin R, Blackow MR, DuPont HL, Buscho RF, Thornhill TYS, Kapikian AZ, Chanock RM: Comparison of three agents of acute infectious nonbacterial gastroenteritis by cross-challenge in volunteers. *J Infect Dis* 129:709–714, 1974.

260. Oshiro LS, Haley CE, Roberto RR, Riggs JL, Croughan M, Greenberg H, Kapikian A: A 27-nm virus isolated during an outbreak of acute infectious nonbacterial gastroenteritis in a convalescent hospital: a possible new serotype. *J Infect Dis* 143:791–795, 1981.

261. de Jong JC, Wigand R, Kidd AH, Wadell G, Kapsenberg JG, Muzerie CJ, Wermenbol AG, Firtzlaff RG: Candidate adenovirus 40 and 41: fastidious adenovirus from human infant stool. *J Med Virol* 11:215–231, 1983.

262. Brandt CD, Kim HW, Rodriguez WJ, Thomas L, Yolken RH, Arrobio JO, Kapikian AZ, Parrott RH, Chanock RM: Comparison and direct electron microscopy, immune electron microscopy, and rotavirus enzyme-linked immunosorbent assay for detection of gastroenteritis viruses in children. *J Clin Microbiol* 13:976–981, 1981.

263. Yolken RH, Lawrence F, Leister BA, Takiff HE, Strauss SE: Gastroenteritis associated with enteric type adenovirus in hospitalized infants. *Pediatrics* 101:21–26, 1982.

264. Chiba S, Nakamura I, Urasawa S, Nakata S, Taniguchi K, Fujinaga K, Nakao T: Outbreak of infantile gastroenteritis due to type 40 adenovirus. *Lancet* 1:954–957, 1983.

265. Brandt CD, Kim HW, Rodriguez WJ, Arrobio JO, Jeffries BC, Stallings EP, Lewis C, Miles AJ, Gardner MK, Parrott RH: Adenoviruses and pediatric gastroenteritis. *J Infect Dis* 151:437–443, 1985.

266. Gary GW, Hierholzer JC, Black RE: Characteristic of noncultivable adenoviruses associated with diarrhea in infants: a new subgroup of human adenoviruses. *J Clin Microbiol* 10:96–103, 1979.

267. Johansson ME, Uhnoo I, Kidd AH, Madeley CR, Wadell G: Direct identification of enteric adenovirus, a candidate new serotype, associated with infantile gastroenteritis. *J Clin Microbiol* 12:95–100, 1980.

268. Takiff HE, Straus SE, Garon CF: Propagation and in vitro studies of previously noncultivable enteral adenoviruses in 293 cells. *Lancet* 2:832–834, 1981.

269. Kidd AH, Madeley CR: In vitro growth of some fastidious adenoviruses from stool specimens. *J Clin Pathol* 34:213–216, 1981.

270. Klein JO, Lerner AM, Finland M: Acute gastroenteritis associated with echovirus, type 11. *Am J Med Sci* 240:749–753, 1960.

271. Eichenwald HF, Ababio A, Arky AM, Hartman AP: Epidemic diarrhea in premature and older infants caused by echovirus type 18. *JAMA* 166:1563–1566, 1958.

272. Spratt HC, Marks MI, Gomersal M, Gill P, Pai CH: Nosocomial infantile gastroenteritis associated with minirotavirus and calicivirus. *J Paediatr* 93:922–926, 1978.

273. Madeley CR, Cosgrove BP: Viruses in infantile gastroenteritis. *Lancet* 2:124, 1975.

274. Madeley CR, Cosgrove BP: 28 nm particles in faeces in infantile gastroenteritis. *Lancet* 2:451–452, 1975.

275. Meyer EA, Jarroll EL: Giardiasis. *Am J Epidemiol* 111:1–12, 1980.

276. Gehlbach SH, MacCormack JN, Drake BM: Spread of disease by fecal-oral route in day nurseries. *Health Care Rep* 88:320–321, 1973.

277. Black RE, Dykes AC, Sinclair MS: Giardiasis in day-care centers: evidence of person-to-person transmission. *Pediatrics* 60:486–491, 1977.

278. Child Day Care Infectious Disease Study Group: Public health considerations of infectious diseases in child day care centers. *J Pediatr* 105:683–701, 1984.

279. Navin TR, Juranek DD: Cryptosporidiosis: clini-

cal, epidemiologic, and parasitologic review. *Rev Infect Dis* 6:313–326, 1984.

280. Centers for Disease Control: Cryptosporidiosis among children attending day-care centers—Georgia, Pennsylvania, Michigan, California, New Mexico. *MMWR* 33:599–601, 1984.

281. Current WL, Reese NC, Ernst JV, Bailey WS, Heyman MB, Weinstein WM: Human cryptosporidiosis in immunocompetent and immunodeficient persons: studies of an outbreak and experimental transmission. *N Engl J Med* 308:1252–1257, 1983.

282. Soave R, Danner RL, Honig CL, Ma P, Hart CC, Nash T, Roberts RB: Crytposporidiosis in homosexual men. *Ann Intern Med* 100:504–511, 1984.

283. Zar F, Geisler J, Brown VA: Asymptomatic carriage of *Cryptosporidium* in the stool of a patient with acquired immunodeficiency syndrome. *J Infect Dis* 151:195, 1985.

284. Ma P, Soave R: Three step stool examination for cryptosporidiosis in 10 homosexual mean with protracted watery diarrhea. *J Infect Dis* 147:824–828, 1982.

285. Garcia LS, Bruckner DA, Brewer TC, Shimizu RY: Techniques for the recovery and identification of *Cryptosporidium* oocysts from stool specimens. *J Clin Microbiol* 18:185–190, 1983.

286. Campbell PN, Current WL: Demonstration of serum antibodies to *Cryptosporidium* sp. in normal and immunodeficient humans with confirmed infections. *J Clin Microbiol* 18:165–169, 1983.

287. Baxby D, Hart CA, Taylor C: Human cryptosporidiosis: a possible case of hospital cross infection. *Br Med J* 287:1760–1761, 1983.

288. Koch KL, Phillips DJ, Aber RC, Current WL: Cryptosporidiosis in hospital personnel: evidence for person-to-person transmission. *Ann Intern Med* 102:593–596, 1985.

289. Istre GR, Kreiss K, Hopkins RS, Healy GR, Benziger M, Canfield TM, Dickinson P, Englert TR, Compton RC, Mathews HM, Simmons RA: An outbreak of amebiasis spread by colonic irrigation at a chiropractic clinic. *N Engl J Med* 307:339–341, 1982.

290. Centers for Disease Control. Pseudo-outbreak of intestinal amebiasis—California. *MMWR* 34:125–126, 1985.

291. Cohen R, Roth FJ, Delgado E, Ahearn DC, Kalser MH: Fungal flora of the normal human small and large intestine. *N Engl J Med* 280:638–641, 1969.

292. Kozinn PJ, Taschdjian CL: Enteric candidiasis. *Pediatrics* 30:71–85, 1962.

293. Brabander JOW, Blank F, Butas CA: Intestinal moniliasis in adults. *Can Med Assoc J* 77:478–480, 1957.

294. Chretien JH, Garagusi VF: Current management of fungal enteritis. *Med Clin North Am* 66:675–687, 1982.

295. Krick JA, Remington JS: Opportunistic invasive fungal infections in patients with leukemia and lymphoma. *Clin Haematol* 5:249–310, 1976.

296. Editorial: intestinal spirochaetes. *Lancet* 1:720, 1984.

297. Ryder RW, Crosby-Ritchie A, McDonough B, Hall WJ III: Human milk contaminated with

Salmonella kottbus: a cause of nosocomial illness in infants. *JAMA* 238:1533–1534, 1977.

298. Garner JS, Simmons BP: CDC guideline for isolation precautions in hospitals. *Infect Control* 4:245–325, 1983.

299. Williams WW: CDC guideline for infection control in hospital personnel. *Infect Control* 4:326–349, 1983.

300. Buchwald DS, Blaser MJ: A review of human salmonellosis. II. Duration of excretion following infection with nontyphi *Salmonella*. *Rev Infect Dis* 6:345–355, 1984.

301. Garibaldi RA, Brodine S, Matsumiya S: Infections among patients in nursing homes: policies, prevalence, and problems. *N Engl J Med* 305:731–735, 1981.

302. Anand CM, Finlayson MC, Garson JZ, Larson ML: An institutional outbreak of salmonellosis due to a lactose-fermenting *Salmonella newport*. *Am J Clin Pathol* 74:657–660, 1980.

303. Bachrach SJ: Successful treatment of an institutional outbreak of shigellosis. *Clin Pediatr* 20:127–131, 1981.

304. Horan MA, Gulati RS, Fox RA, Glew E, Ganguli L, Kaeney M: Outbreak of *Shigella sonnei* dysentery on a geriatric assessment ward. *J Hosp Infect* 5:210–212, 1984.

305. Kaplan JE, Schonberger LB, Varano G, Jackman N, Bied J, Gary GW: An outbreak of acute nonbacterial gastroenteritis in a nursing home: demonstration of person-to-person transmission by temporal clustering of cases. *Am J Epidemiol* 116:940–948, 1982.

306. Kaplan JE, Gary GW, Baron RC, Singh N, Schonberger LB, Feldman R, Greenberg HB: Epidemiology of Norwalk gastroenteritis and the role of Norwalk virus in outbreaks of acute nonbacterial gastroenteritis. *Ann Intern Med* 96:756–761, 1982.

307. Mehta G, Prakash K, Sharma KB: *Salmonella oranienburg* infection in a neonatal unit in New Delhi. *Indian J Med Res* 75:480–484, 1982.

308. Bhat P, Macaden R: Outbreak of gastroenteritis due to multidrug resistant *Salmonella typhimurium* phage type 66/122 UT in Bangalore. *Indian J Med Res* 78:454–458, 1983.

309. Rangnekar VM, Banker DD, Jhala HI: R-plasmids in *Salmonella oranienburg* isolated from hospital outbreak. *Indian J Med Res* 76:353–357, 1982.

310. Aggarwal P, Sarkar R, Singh M, Grover BD, Anand BR, Chowdhuri ANR: *Salmonella bareilly* infection in a paediatric hospital of New Delhi. *Indian J Med Res* 78:22–25, 1983.

311. Chitkara YK, Gill MK: Outbreak of gastroenteritis due to *Salmonella weltevreden* in a hospital. *Indian J Med Res* 64:1280–1287, 1976.

312. Parida SN, Verma IC, Deb M, Bhujwala RA: An outbreak of diarrhea due to *Citrobacter freundii* in a neonatal special care nursery. *Indian J Pediatr* 47:81–84, 1980.

313. Pawa RR, Hobbs BC: Control of infection in a neonatal nursery. *Indian J Pediatr* 47:375–380, 1980.

314. Deb M, Bhujwala RA, Singh S, Singh M: *Klebsiella pneumoniae* as the possible cause of an outbreak of diarrhoea in a neonatal special care unit.

Indian J Med Res 71:359–362, 1980.
315. Teoh-Chan CH, Chau PY, Tse D, Sin WK, Ip HMH, Lan R: Hospital *Salmonella johannesburg* infection and its possible role in the community spread of the infection in Hong Kong. *J Hyg (Camb)* 78:113–119, 1977.
316. Mhalu FS, Mtango FDE, Msengi AE: Hospital outbreaks of cholera transmitted through close person-to-person contact. *Lancet* 2:82–84, 1984.
317. Rice PA, Craven PC, Wells JG: *Salmonella heidelberg* enteritis and bacteremia: an epidemic on two pediatric wards. *Am J Med* 60:509–516, 1976.
318. Bureau of Disease Control, Department of Health, Republic of China: Nursery epidemic of *Salmonella cerro* in a Taipei hospital. *Epidemiol Bull* 1:9–11, 1985.
319. Berkowitz FE: Bacteremia in hospitalized black South African children: a one-year study emphasizing nosocomial bacteremia and bacteremia in severely malnourished children. *Am J Dis Child* 138:551–556, 1984.
320. Riley LW, Ceballos BSO, Trabulsi LR, Fernandes de Toledo MR, Blake PA: The significance of hospitals as reservoirs for endemic multiresistant *Salmonella typhimurium* causing infection in urban Brazilian children. *J Infect Dis* 150:236–241, 1984.

Chapter 25

Uncommon Infections: Eye and Central Nervous System

James E. Peacock, Jr., M.D.

Within the category of "other nosocomial infections," comprising less than 4% of the total (1), are those involving the eye and central nervous system. Although relatively insignificant in terms of absolute numbers, these infections are of major clinical importance because of the involvement of one of the specialized sensory organs, their often devastating impact upon integrated function of the central nervous system, and their potential for significant long term patient morbidity and disability. Nevertheless, despite their apparent clinical and economic significance, they are mentioned briefly if at all in many recent texts dealing with nosocomial infections (2–4). As a result, there exists a relative dearth of information about the infections, including concise data on incidence, risk factors for acquisition, associated morbidity and mortality, and recommended preventive measures. In this chapter, a practical classification of these infections will be proposed, diagnostic criteria presented, existing data on incidence examined, and major causative pathogens explored. In addition, the epidemiology of these infections will be critically examined, risk factors for acquisition identified wherever possible, and prudent measures for prevention and control reviewed.

NOSOCOMIAL EYE INFECTIONS

Hospital-acquired infections of the eye are estimated to occur at an approximate rate of 3.6 to 4.7 infections/10,000 discharges and as such represent less than 1% of all nosocomial infections (5; W Jarvis, Centers for Disease Control (CDC), personal communication). The incidence of nosocomial eye infections varies considerably with hospital service, with the highest incidence seen in the nursery (20.2 to 22.1/10,000 discharges) and on pediatrics (3.8 to 6.3/10,000 discharges) (5; W Jarvis, CDC, personal communication). The predominant pathogens are coagulase-nega-

tive staphylococci (22% of all isolates), *Staphylococcus aureus* (19% of all isolates), and *Pseudomonas aeruginosa* (9% of all isolates) (W Jarvis, CDC, personal communication). Given the general lack of emphasis placed upon these infections and the often poor documentation of their occurrence in the patient record, available figures undoubtedly underestimate the true incidence of disease.

Classification of Infections

Nosocomial eye infections can be broadly classified into those which are postsurgical and those which are nonsurgically related.

Postsurgical Eye Infections. The three major categories of postsurgical eye infections are shown in Table 25.1. Conspicuously absent from this list are wound infections and superficial infections such as keratoconjunctivitis, both of which are exceedingly rare as postoperative infectious complications. The rarity of these types of infections is probably a reflection of the routine use of topical and/or systemic antibiotics in the perioperative period for most forms of ophthalmic surgery. It should be noted that the recognition and diagnosis of postsurgical nosocomial eye infections will be largely confined to the practicing ophthalmologist.

Nonsurgically Related Eye Infections. Four major categories of nonsurgically related nosocomial eye infections can be readily delineated (Table 25.1). These infections may involve ancillary structures such as the eyelids (blepharitis), superficial surfaces (keratitis, conjunctivitis), or intraocular cavities (endophthalmitis) (Fig. 25.1). Panophthalmitis, viewed as an extension of endophthalmitis with involvement of Tenon's capsule or the soft tissues of the orbit, will not be classified as a separate entity. Infections of the uveal tract, retina, and optic nerve, although oc-

Table 25.1. Nosocomial Eye Infections

Type of Infection	Clinical Criteria for Diagnosis	Major Causative Agents
Postsurgical		
Dacryocystitis	Acute—pain, redness and swelling of the lacrimal sac and overlying skin	*S. pneumoniae*, staphylococci, *P. aeruginosa*, *H. influenzae*
	Chronic—tearing on the affected side with purulent secretions	*S. pneumoniae*, staphylococci, *P. aeruginosa*, *Candida* sp., atypical mycobacteria
Episcleritis	Ocular pain, discharge, conjunctival injection, subconjunctival hemorrhage, bloody tears, and/or fistula formation in conjunction with loss of prominence of the internal buckle or protrusion or exposure of the implant	*S. epidermidis*, enteric gram-negative bacilli
Endophthalmitis	Ocular pain, swelling and redness of the upper lid, chemosis, corneal edema, hypopyon, loss of the red reflex, and/or decrease in light perception and visual acuity	Staphylococci, enteric gram-negative bacilli, fungi
Nonsurgically related		
Blepharitis	Burning, itching, tearing, local irritation, crust formation, edema of the lid, necrotic lesions	Staphylococci, streptococci, *P. aeruginosa*
Conjunctivitis	Eye irritation with redness, edema, and hyperemia; mucopurulent secretions; photophobia; sensation of foreign body; pseudomembrane formation	Staphylococci, streptococci, *Haemophilus* sp., *Neisseria* sp., *Chlamydia*, viruses
Keratitis	Corneal/periorbital pain, sensation of foreign body, tearing, perilimbic redness with chemosis, abundant secretions, reduced vision, corneal opacities, inflammatory reaction in anterior chamber	Staphylococci, streptococci, enteric gram-negative bacilli, fungi, viruses
Endophthalmitis	As above	As above

casionally nosocomial in origin, are sufficiently rare so as to justify their exclusion from consideration. It should be noted that nosocomial eye infections which are not related to prior surgery generally occur on inpatient services other than ophthalmology and as such are initially encountered by physicians frequently unfamiliar with eye diseases and their manifestations. This factor contributes greatly to their underrecognition and underdiagnosis and perhaps accounts for the rather limited data available on these infections.

Diagnostic Criteria

In general, the clinical manifestations of the ocular infections under consideration are sufficiently distinct to provide an adequate basis for definitive diagnosis, even in the absence of supportive microbiologic data. As such, the diagnos-

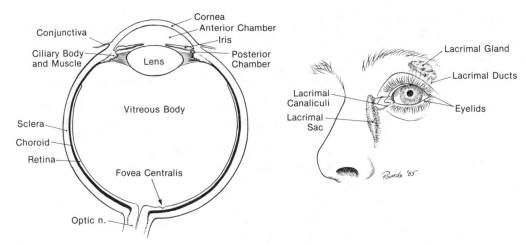

Figure 25.1. Anatomy of the eye. *Left,* cross-sectional schematic diagram of the eye. *Right,* the external eye and associated structures.

tic criteria used for case identification and reporting are largely clinical, although specialized ophthalmologic examination may be necessary in selected instances to confirm clinical impressions definitively. Although determination of a microbiologic etiology for the process under consideration is not an absolute requirement of the case definition, it is obviously desirable whenever possible since certain of the clinical entities may on occasion be noninfectious in origin (e.g., conjunctivitis, endophthalmitis).

By convention, a *postsurgical eye infection* is defined as any clinical infection arising in the postoperative period which can reasonably be related to the preceding surgical procedure. In general, the "postoperative period" encompasses not only the time within the hospital but also the 10- to 14-day period after discharge. However, it should be remembered that the incubation period for postsurgical infection is often uncertain and highly variable and can be greatly influenced by such factors as use of perioperative antibiotics, virulence of the pathogen, inoculum size and site, tissue health, and innate host resistance. The variability in incubation period is especially true for infections related to prosthetic eye devices or implants. Not infrequently, prosthetic device infections, originating in the hospital, may be so indolent in their course that clinical expression may not appear until weeks or months after discharge. Accordingly, good clinical judgment and a careful evaluation of the epidemiologic circumstances may be necessary to classify the site of acquisition of these infections properly.

Nonsurgically related nosocomial eye infections

are those which are not present or incubating at the time of hospital entry and only become manifest beyond 48 to 72 hours after admission. Eye infections appearing within 10 to 14 days of discharge should also be considered to be nosocomial unless available epidemiologic data indicate otherwise.

The clinical criteria for the diagnosis of the various types of nosocomial eye infections are presented in Table 25.1 (6). Since many of the anatomically involved structures are contiguous in location, infections are occasionally mixed in type (i.e., blepharoconjunctivitis, keratoconjunctivitis).

Clinical Aspects/Incidence/Causative Pathogens

Postsurgical Infections

Dacryocystitis. Infection of the lacrimal sac occurs primarily as a complication of dacryocystorhinostomy (DCR), especially when DCR is coupled with implantation of prosthetic silicone tubing for drainage (7). Dacryocystitis occurring postoperatively is usually indolent in onset and chronic in type. The major clinical manifestation is increased tearing on the affected side, often accompanied by mucopurulent secretions emanating from the conjunctival orifice (6). Its true incidence is unknown but, based on published reports, appears to be infrequent. Major causative pathogens include *Streptococcus pneumoniae,* staphylococci, and enteric gram-negative bacilli (6). Although less frequent, opportunistic organisms such as *Candida* species and rapid growing atypical mycobacteria also appear capable of producing this infection (6, 8). In fact, a recent outbreak of dacryocystitis occurring post-DCR in four patients was traced to *Mycobacterium chelonei* (8). Because of the potential contribution of various fungi and atypical mycobacteria to this syndrome, appropriate stains and cultures for these organisms should be obtained during the diagnostic evaluation if routine cultures fail to identify potential pathogens.

Episcleritis. Episcleral infection, characterized clinically by ocular pain, conjunctival injection/discharge, subconjunctival hemorrhage, bloody tears, and/or fistula formation (9), is primarily a complication of retinal detachment surgery utilizing a scleral buckling procedure (10). In this procedure, restoration of chorioretinal contact is accomplished by producing scleral indentation via placement of episcleral silicone implants after which chorioretinal adhesion around the break is induced by cryopexy or diathermy (11). Infectious complications of the procedure can be either intraocular (endophthalmitis) or extraocular (episcleritis), with the former being rarely if ever encountered (12, 13). External postoperative infections (episcleritis) are usually related to the silicone implants and can become manifest as early as a few weeks after the buckling procedure. In addition to the clinical findings noted above, careful ophthalmologic examination may reveal loss of prominence of the internal buckle, granuloma formation, and/or protrusion or exposure of the implant (9).

The incidence of infectious episcleritis following retinal detachment surgery has varied from 0.24 to 4% in four recently published series (9, 13–15). Since perioperative antibiotics and/or antibiotic-impregnated implants were routinely used in all of these series, the true incidence of infection in the absence of antibiotic prophylaxis cannot be readily ascertained.

The predominant pathogen in most cases of infectious episcleritis appears to be *Staphylococcus epidermidis* (9, 15), with *S. aureus* and various enteric gram-negative bacilli also causing a significant proportion of cases as well.

Endophthalmitis. The most devastating infectious complication of ocular surgery continues to be postoperative endophthalmitis (10, 16). Presenting symptoms and signs are variable, but they usually appear within 24 to 72 hours of surgery (10, 16). Ocular pain, especially if it recurs after a pain-free period, is often one of the initial findings in developing endophthalmitis (10, 16).

Soon thereafter, additional signs—including decreasing visual acuity, progressive loss of light perception, swelling and redness of the upper lid, marked chemosis with hyperemia, anterior chamber hypopyon, vitreous haze, and loss of the red reflex—may rapidly appear (10, 16). Alteration, or delay in presentation, of these classic symptoms and signs may occur in special situations, most commonly in mycotic infections or in infections with less virulent organisms (10, 16). Patients who receive perioperative subconjunctival antibiotics, those who receive topical corticosteroids after surgery, and those with conjunctival filtering blebs may also manifest subacute or delayed endophthalmitis as well (16).

Once initiated, the course of infection is usually relentlessly progressive. If vision in the affected eye is to be preserved, swift and definitive diagnostic and therapeutic interventions are mandated. Therefore, in any case of suspected endophthalmitis, anterior chamber paracentesis or vitreous aspiration is usually indicated in an attempt to establish a specific microbiologic etiology (10, 16). Definitive therapy can then be dictated by the results of smears, stains, and cultures.

Recent reviews suggest that the overall incidence of infectious endophthalmitis following intraocular surgery ranges from 0.05 to 0.5% or approximately 1 to 2 cases/1000 operative procedures (10, 16, 17). The current incidence contrasts with a rate of 1% or greater in the decade prior to 1950 (16, 17). Although endophthalmitis occurs most often following cataract operations (18), any form of ophthalmic surgery may be complicated by this infection. The incidence of postoperative endophthalmitis following various types of ophthalmic surgical procedures is summarized in Table 25.2 (17, 18–28). It should be noted that endophthalmitis following filtering surgery for glaucoma is often a late complication which may or may not be nosocomial in origin (10); the fistulous communication established between the anterior chamber and the subconjunctival space predisposes the intraocular cavities to exogenous infection arising from conjunctival flora which may have been acquired either in the hospital or in the community.

The causes of postsurgical endophthalmitis are protean (Table 25.2), although staphylococci, *Proteus* species, and *P. aeruginosa* tend to predominate (16, 18, 29). Various fungi have occasionally been implicated (10, 16, 17, 29) and rarely may cause explosive and clinically devastating outbreaks of disease (30, 31).

Table 25.2. Postsurgical Endophthalmitis

Type of Procedure	No. of Infections/ No. of Procedures	(%)	Causative Organisms	References
Cataract extraction	417/118,755	(0.35)	Staphylococci Enteric gram-negative bacilli Fungi	17, 19–22
Intraocular lens implantation	13/4,397	(0.3)	As above	23, 24
Pars plana vitrectomy	3/1,500	(0.2)	Staphylococci Streptococci	25
Penetrating keratoplasty	4/1,876	(0.2)	Streptococci Staphylococci Gram-negative bacilli	26
Filtering procedures for glaucoma	18/497	(3.6)	Staphylococci Diphtheroids Gram-negative bacilli	27, 28

Nonsurgically Related Infections

Blepharitis. Infection of the eyelids may arise secondary to local factors (e.g., local irritation or trauma, obstruction of eyelid sebaceous glands) or may occur as a metastatic complication of disseminated blood-borne infection (6, 32). Clinical manifestations include edema and hyperemia of the lid margins accompanied by crust formation in the cilia and nasal angle. The eyelashes are often matted together by yellowish exudate and are easily shed from the lid. Accompanying symptoms may include burning, intense pruritus, chronic tearing, local irritation, and mild photophobia (6). Most nosocomially acquired cases are metastatic in origin and present in an acute to subacute fashion. Given the metastatic nature of the lesion, the ocular symptoms and signs are frequently overshadowed by the concurrent systemic manifestations of infection. Nevertheless, local infection, especially if due to virulent pathogens such as *Pseudomonas* (32–34), may progress in a malignant fashion which can culminate in total lid necrosis and panophthalmitis if unrecognized and untreated. Underlying host immunocompromise may predispose to the more severe manifestations of metastatic blepharitis (33, 34).

The incidence of hospital-acquired blepharitis cannot be estimated on the basis of available data. Isolated case reports in the literature suggest that, although unusual, blepharitis is by no means rare. Major etiologic agents include the staphylococci and various gram-negative bacilli such as *P. aeruginosa* (6). Sporadic cases may be due to certain of the herpesviruses, especially herpes simplex virus and varicella-zoster virus (6).

Conjunctivitis. Perhaps the most commonly encountered nonsurgically related nosocomial eye infection is conjunctivitis (35). Most episodes of infectious conjunctivitis appear to be local in pathogenesis, arising when local eye defenses (tearing, lysozyme, IgA antibody, phagocytic cells) are overwhelmed by inoculum size, virulence of the putative pathogen, or enhancing coexistent factors (foreign bodies, trauma, underlying diseases). Infection is typically unilateral but may spread to involve the contralateral eye. Because the surface epithelium of the eyelids and cornea is contiguous with that of the conjunctivae, conjunctivitis is often associated with blepharitis and/or keratitis (6). The cardinal manifestation of acute conjunctivitis is an intensely red eye (6, 35). Other prominent clinical signs include chemosis, eyelid swelling, and variable amounts of discharge which may be serous or purulent (6, 35). Accompanying symptoms include a scratchy (foreign body) sensation, moderate photophobia, and blurring of vision secondary to the exudate (6, 35).

Among the various types of nosocomial conjunctivitis, ophthalmia neonatorum is probably the most frequent in occurrence (18). Although it may be diagnosed any time during the first 28 days of life (6), most cases become apparent within 14 days of birth (18) and as such are properly classified as nosocomial infections.

Occasional outbreaks of nosocomial conjunctivitis have been described (36–38) and deserve special mention because of their occurrence during the provision of routine eye care. Most such outbreaks are viral in etiology and occur in conjunction with community epidemics of disease which spread to the hospital (37).

The overall incidence of nosocomial conjunctivitis is difficult to estimate. Data from the CDC's National Nosocomial Infections Study (NNIS) suggest that nosocomial superficial infections of the eye, most of which presumably are conjunctivitis, occur at a rate of 3.6/10,000 discharges (5). The incidence ranges from 22.1 in the nursery to 0.1 on gynecology, with rates of 3.8 and 2.4 on pediatric and medical services, respectively (5). It is reasonable to assume that the majority of the superficial eye infections in the nursery represent ophthalmia neonatorum, giving an estimated rate of 2/1,000 discharges for that entity. Other studies have found similar though slightly higher attack rates of neonatal conjunctivitis, 3.0/1,000 live births at a public hospital in New York City and 8.6/1,000 live births at a county hospital in Atlanta (39, 40). Other types of nosocomial conjunctivitis are sporadic in occurrence, and no accurate estimate of their incidence can be made. However, secondary attack rates of 10% have been recorded during epidemics of viral conjunctivitis (41).

The microbiologic causes of nosocomial conjunctivitis are varied and include viruses, *Chlamydia*, staphylococci, *N. gonorrheae*, and other assorted bacteria, such as *S. pneumoniae*, *Streptococcus pyogenes* and *Haemophilus influenzae* (6, 18). The latter three bacteria and staphylococci are said to account for the vast majority of cases of acute conjunctivitis (6, 18). *Chlamydia trachomatis* has recently emerged as the predominant pathogen of ophthalmia neonatorum, accounting for 25 to 40% of all culture-proven cases (39, 40). In contrast, *N. gonorrheae* can currently be implicated in only 3 to 15% of cases (39, 40). In industrialized nations, adjusted attack rates for these two pathogens are 0.4/1000 deliveries for *N. gonorrheae* and 1.1 to 1.4/1000 deliveries for *C. trachomatis* (5, 42, 43). Among viral causes of nosocomial conjunctivitis, adenoviruses, especially types 3 and 8, account for most epidemic outbreaks (6, 37), whereas sporadic cases are often due to herpes simplex virus or varicella-zoster virus, usually in the setting of reactivation infection (6).

Keratitis. Infections of the cornea may occur as an isolated event or in association with concurrent infections of the eyelids or conjunctivae. The clinical types of infection are varied, though ulcerative lesions and stromal infiltrates are perhaps most common (6). Most infections are local in their pathogenesis, arising secondary to direct inoculation of pathogens or from reactivation of latent viruses in the trigeminal ganglion. Clinical manifestations are protean and are somewhat dependent upon the type of clinical infection and its anatomic locations. Pain is the most common symptom and is often exacerbated by movement of the eyelids over the cornea; other frequently encountered symptoms include a variable decrease in vision, reflex tearing, photophobia, and blepharospasm (44). Unlike conjunctivitis, discharge is relatively uncommon unless purulent corneal ulcerations are present. The first, albeit subtle, sign of keratitis is a loss of corneal transparency often accompanied by a ciliary flush (44). Localized epithelial defects may develop early and progress rapidly to ulcer formation followed by perforation if untreated. Associated intraocular inflammation is common, and occasional patients may develop a hypopyon (44). As documented in several recent reports, nosocomial keratitis frequently occurs in critically ill patients, many of whom are obtunded (45, 46).

The exact incidence of nosocomial corneal infection is indeterminant. In a recent investigation of nosocomial eye infections in intensive care units (46), the overall incidence of eye infections, most of which were keratitis, was 1.3%. The incidence increased to 3% in intubated patients and to 14% in intubated patients with respiratory infections.

Bacteria account for approximately 65 to 90% of all cases of infectious keratitis, with the most common pathogens being *S. aureus, S. pneumoniae, P. aeruginosa*, and *Moraxella* (6, 44). In the 12 obtunded patients in intensive care settings cited above who developed keratitis (45, 46), *Pseudomonas* was the etiologic agent in six. Viral causes of keratitis include herpes simplex, varicella-zoster, and adenoviruses (44). Fungi are implicated in 20 to 35% of cases, with *Fusarium solani* the most common offending agent (44). *Aspergillus* and *Candida* are also occasionally etiologic, especially in immunosuppressed patients (47, 48).

Endophthalmitis. Intraocular infection unassociated with prior ocular surgery may arise via contiguous spread from extraocular infection (e.g., keratitis) or may reach the eye by bloodborne spread from a distant site of infection (49). In fact, the sudden onset of endophthalmitis in an unoperated nontraumatized eye should immediately raise the specter of hematogenous spread from a distant focus of infection (49, 50). In general, the clinical picture is similar to that seen in postsurgical endophthalmitis except that the posterior segment of the eye is usually involved and the patients are frequently severely ill and often immunocompromised (49).

A special category of hematogenous (endogenous) endophthalmitis is that due to fungi, especially *Candida* (49, 51). In most patients with endogenous fungal endophthalmitis, the ocular involvement may be the first or only manifestation of disseminated fungal disease (49). Typically, the initial symptom is a decrease in visual acuity. Examination usually reveals a preretinal vitreous haze which progresses rapidly over the next several days to fluffy white exudates in the vitreous just anterior to the retina (49, 51). In such cases, prompt therapeutic intervention is necessary to preserve vision.

Another variant of endogenous endophthalmitis occurring in hospitalized, usually immunocompromised, patients is cytomegalovirus retinitis (49, 52). This process is most frequently seen in severely immunosuppressed hosts such as organ transplant recipients or patients with the acquired immunodeficiency syndrome (53, 54). Initial symptoms consist of blurring of vision and scotomas without pain (49). Funduscopic examination typically reveals retinal edema, scattered retinal hemorrhages, yellow-white exudates, and vessel attenuation and sheathing, an appearance which is virtually diagnostic (49, 52, 53).

The incidence of nonsurgically related (endogenous) endophthalmitis is difficult to ascertain. Cases of bacterial disease tend to occur sporadically as an unpredictable complication of bacteremia. The most frequent settings in which hematogenous bacterial endophthalmitis occurs appear to be in association with acute bacterial endocarditis, abdominal infection, or central nervous system infection (50, 55). In a recent review of 28 heroin addicts with acute endocarditis (56), 3 cases of metastatic endophthalmitis developed for an overall attack rate of 11%. Likewise, endogenous fungal endophthalmitis tends to occur in a sporadic fashion, though cases tend to be restricted to certain categories of patients—those receiving broad spectrum antibiotics, those receiving parenteral hyperalimentation, and those who are severely immunocompromised (49). A recent prospective study of 131 seriously ill patients receiving parenteral hyperalimentation indicated that *Candida* endophthalmitis developed in 13 or approximately 10% (57). As noted above, viral retinitis tends to occur almost exclusively in severely immunosuppressed patients. A prospective survey of 39 patients who

had received allogenic renal transplants found a 5% incidence of acute cytomegalovirus retinitis post-transplantation (58).

The major causative pathogens of endogenous nosocomial endophthalmitis have been alluded to above. Staphylococci, other gram-positive cocci, and gram-negative bacilli, especially *Proteus* species and *P. aeruginosa*, comprise the major bacterial etiologies (6, 18, 49, 50). The predominant fungal pathogen in this setting is *Candida* though *Aspergillus* species are also a well documented cause of disease (49, 59). Among viral causes, cytomegalovirus is most common with herpes simplex, varicella-zoster, and measles occasionally implicated as well (49).

Epidemiology of Infection

Postsurgical Infections

As summarized by O'Day (10) and Jaffe (17), four *potential sources of infection* can be readily identified in patients undergoing ocular surgery: (*a*) airborne contaminants, (*b*) contaminated tissue, (*c*) contaminated fluids, and (*d*) contaminated instruments and implants. Although airborne spread of organisms in the operating room is a theoretical risk (60), available data do not support its having a major role in the pathogenesis of postoperative ocular infections (17, 20). In contrast, the presence of potentially pathogenic bacteria along the lid margins and in the conjunctival secretions poses an obvious threat of postoperative infection (61). The role of these "contaminated tissues" (ie., lid margins and conjunctivae) in the pathogenesis of postsurgical ocular infections has now been well established in a number of studies (19, 62) which have shown that preoperative reduction in colony counts or elimination of potential pathogens from the conjunctival sac results in a reduction in postoperative infection rates (62). Contaminated fluids (e.g., optic solutions, medications, and irrigants; tissue disinfectants) are also well documented sources for postsurgical eye infections (61, 63) and are especially important considerations when clusters of infections occur (17). Last, the role of contaminated instruments and surgical materials in postoperative eye infections has been dramatically illustrated by several recent outbreaks of endophthalmitis traced to implantation of contaminated intraocular lens (30, 31, 64). Cadaveric corneal buttons stored in contaminated media have also led to endophthalmitis (65).

Predisposing *risk factors* for the development

of postsurgical eye infections have been tentatively identified for a number of ophthalmic procedures, but, in general, the supporting observations are uncontrolled and noncomparative. A summary of various ophthalmic surgical procedures, their complicating infections, and possible predisposing risk factors for infection are shown in Table 25.3. In addition to the factors identified in Table 25.3, various postoperative complications—such as wound leaks, unplanned filtering blebs, vitreous wick syndromes, deep sutures, epithelial ingrowth, and retained lens material—may also predispose to bacterial endophthalmitis (49).

Nonsurgically Related Infections

The *sources of infection* for nosocomial eye infections not related to surgery include exogenous organisms introduced to the eye via direct contact spread or endogenous organisms normally present in the eye or transmitted to the eye from other sites via contact or droplet spread or by hematogenous dissemination. Direct contact spread of exogenous organisms to the eye usually occurs via the hands of health care workers, but contact with contaminated mucous membranes (as with ophthalmia neonatorum) or contaminated devices or solutions may also contribute in selected instances. Endogenous organisms normally present along the lids and in the conjunctival secretions may develop a pathogenic potential if trauma or drying of the cornea is superimposed. Pathogenic organisms present in secretions at other body sites may be inadvertently introduced into the eye either by direct spread or droplet spread; the physical proximity of the nose and oropharynx invite transfer of organisms from the oropharyngeal or respiratory secretions to the eye, especially in the patient with a depressed level of consciousness. Last, pathogens causing infection at other body sites which gain access to

Table 25.3. Predisposing Risk Factors for the Development of Postsurgical Eye Infections

Type of Ophthalmic Procedure	Nature of Complicating Infection	Predisposing Risk Factors	References
Dacryocystorhinostomy	Dacryocystitis Keratitis Conjunctivitis	?Concurrent implantation of Silastic drainage tubing	8
Retinal detachment surgery (scleral buckling)	Episcleritis	Positive preoperative conjunctival culture for pathogenic bacteria Use of solid silicone implants Use of multiple versus single sponges Reoperations	9, 15
Cataract extraction	Endophthalmitis	Positive preoperative conjunctival culture for pathogenic bacteria Extracapsular extraction Secondary needling ? Vitreous loss	17, 19–21
Intraocular lens implantation	Endophthalmitis	None identified	23, 24
Vitrectomy	Endophthalmitis	None identified	25
Keratoplasty	Endophthalmitis	Positive cultures from donor rim	26
Glaucoma surgery (filtering procedures)	Endophthalmitis	Anterior dissection of the superficial scleral flap Trephination procedures	27, 28

the bloodstream can seed the eye hematogenously and produce metastatic ocular infection.

Risk factors for infection have been identified for selected types of nonsurgically related ocular infections. The occurrence of nosocomial blepharitis appears to be largely confined to the immunocompromised host, with infection usually representing a metastatic, hematogenously disseminated focus (32–34). Studies on neonatal conjunctivitis have shown that race may be a predisposing factor in the acquisition of chlamydial conjunctivitis, with rates in blacks significantly exceeding those in whites (40); the development of gonococcal conjunctivitis was correlated only with prolonged rupture of fetal membranes (40). No definite risk factors for acquisition of nosocomial viral conjunctivitis have been identified beyond contact exposure to the various infecting agents (37, 38). Recently published studies on patients with hospital-acquired corneal ulcers have suggested that critically ill, obtunded patients in intensive care settings are at major risk for acquisition of this infection (45, 46). Predisposing factors would include a depressed level of consciousness which impairs voluntary protection of the eye, impaired or absent corneal reflexes, tracheostomy or intubation, copious respiratory secretions harboring pathogenic organisms, and respiratory care with tracheal suctioning (45, 46). Hilton and colleagues nicely demonstrated that bacterial dispersal during tracheal suctioning was significantly greater in patients with copious secretions than in those whose secretions were scant (46). In explaining the observed selective involvement of the left eye of most affected patients, these investigators found that right-handed health care workers tended to withdraw suction catheters diagonally across the patient's face, thus allowing direct inoculation of bacteria into the often open and uncovered left eye (46). Studies on endogenous endophthalmitis have been concentrated primarily on those cases due to *Candida*. In patients with *Candida* endophthalmitis, common clinical features include a history of gastrointestinal or biliary tract disease, recent surgery, prolonged use of intravenous catheters, recent bacterial sepsis, and intensive treatment with broad spectrum antimicrobics (51). In the prospective study by Henderson and colleagues (57), gastrointestinal hemorrhage was the only underlying illness statistically associated with the development of candidal endophthalmitis. Other predisposing risk factors identified by the investigators included the use of central

venous or Swan-Ganz catheters, the presence of mucocutaneous candidal infection, and documented candidemia (57). Opportunistic viral retinitis has been clearly shown to occur almost exclusively in severely immunocompromised patients with predominant deficits in cell-mediated immune function (52, 53); primary infection appears to carry an enhanced risk of disseminated disease with a greater likelihood of retinal involvement.

Prevention and Control

Postsurgical Infections

As with most surgically related infections, the cornerstones of prevention are good asepsis (16, 61) and elimination of potential sources of infection (17). The necessary procedures for achieving good surgical asepsis are now well established and have been extensively reviewed by Allen (61). The approach to elimination of potential sources of postoperative infection can be conveniently divided into the control of environmental sources and control of tissue sources (66).

Control of environmental sources of infection is directed toward airborne contaminants, surgical objects and materials, and ophthalmic solutions and medications (66). In general, acceptable reduction of airborne contaminants can be achieved by air filtration (capable of removing ≥ 90% of particles 3 μm in diameter or larger) and frequent air exchanges (no fewer than 12 exchanges/hour) (66). Although some authors advocate micropore filtration of operating room air (17), filtration to this degree is probably not warranted. Elimination of microbes from surgical objects and materials is achieved via routine sterilization using accepted techniques (61). Ophthalmic solutions and medications can be eliminated as sources of infection by strict adherence to the manufacturer's recommendations for usage and by minimizing the use of multiple dose dispensers. To insure the sterility of ophthalmic solutions further, some authors would recommend terminal micropore filtration prior to use in order to remove both contaminating microorganisms and particulate debris (17).

The control and elimination of tissue sources of infection constitute a difficult and often prohibitive task for the eye surgeon (66). As noted by Allen (66), "human tissues are at once the most common, the most prolific, and the most intimate sources of contaminants of surgical wounds." Since many forms of intraocular surgery are elective, a careful preoperative evaluation to identify and correct active infections in the periocular tissues is indicated (17). In the absence of clinical evidence of active infection, the role of routine preoperative smears and cultures to detect potential pathogens is controversial. Although some authors advocate the use of such cultures and further recommend employing specific preoperative antibiotic therapy to eliminate selected pathogens if they are recovered (19, 62), others do not (17, 67). However, whether or not preoperative cultures are obtained, most authors agree that preoperative prophylactic antibiotics, administered either topically or subconjunctivally, are warranted in most ophthalmic procedures to achieve relative control of the local flora of the lid margins and conjunctival secretions and thus reduce the risk of postoperative infection (19, 20, 62, 66). Despite the widespread acceptance of the need for preoperative antibiotic prophylaxis, the evidence for a reduction in incidence of postoperative infection, especially endophthalmitis, is inconclusive (17, 21). Although accumulated series reveal a higher incidence of endophthalmitis in studies in which no antibiotics are used than in those when topical or subconjunctival antibiotics are used, the studies are nonrandomized, noncomparative trials, and the controls are historical (17). In addition to the inconclusive evidence suggesting clinical benefit, other factors arguing against the routine use of preoperative topical antibiotics include the fact that they rarely sterilize the external eye, they do not provide significant intraocular drug concentrations during surgery, and they are expensive, inconvenient, and possibly toxic (17). Since subconjunctivally administered antibiotics achieve good concentrations in the aqueous humor and persist for several hours postinjection, their use in perioperative prophylaxis is perhaps more rational (17). Situations in which subconjunctival antibiotics appear to be useful include unplanned extracapsular lens extraction, operative loss of vitreous, and excessive surgical manipulation, all situations in which the risk of complicating endophthalmitis is enhanced (17).

Nonsurgically Related Infections

Since many of the nonsurgically related nosocomial eye infections arise endogenously, with metastatic seeding of the eye as a secondary event, their prevention is largely predicated upon the control and eradication of the primary focus of infection. However, for selected infections in which the pathogenesis involves exogenous inoculation of pathogens, additional specific preventive measures are warranted. The prevention and control of ophthalmia neonatorum are markedly enhanced by the routine use of topical ocular antimicrobial therapy in the newborn (18, 35). The standard method of prophylaxis for *N. gonorrheae* has traditionally been the administration of 1% silver nitrate drops (5, 18, 35). Although still somewhat controversial, more recent recommendations are the use of topical erythromycin to provide prophylaxis both for gonococcal and chlamydial conjunctivitis (35). As a further preventive measure, all infants born to mothers with proved or suspected gonococcal or chlamydial infection should be appropriately cultured and placed under secretion precautions until effective therapy has been administered for 24 hours (5). Since available epidemiologic evidence strongly suggests that epidemic nosocomial viral conjunctivitis may be propagated by health care workers and/or ophthalmic devices and solutions (35, 37), stringent protocols for strict hand washing, rigorous cleaning of equipment (e.g., tonometers), and elimination of potentially contaminated solutions should be enforced during outbreak periods. The prevention of bacterial corneal ulcers largely depends upon the provision of routine eye care to critically ill and/or obtunded patients which will minimize the occurrence of exposure keratopathy (46). In addition, respiratory care and tracheal suctioning should be performed only if eyes are covered and protected, in order to prevent inadvertent inoculation of the eye via droplet dispersal of organisms (46). The role, if any, for routine prophylactic topical ocular antibiotics in comatose patients is undefined. The prevention of endogenous fungal and viral endophthalmitis/retinitis is difficult. Henderson and colleagues made no recommendations regarding prevention of *Candida* endophthalmitis, though the association of mucocutaneous candidiasis with subsequent *Candida* endophthalmitis suggests that intensive efforts to provide prophylaxis against mucosal disease in high risk patients might decrease the incidence of metastatic eye disease (57). Since retinitis due to cytomegalovirus (CMV) and other opportunistic viruses appears to be closely linked to primary infection and severe immunosuppression, attempts to provide "protective matching" of donor and recipient pairs to reduce the risk of primary infection are theoretically attractive but probably of limited practical value (68). Likewise, prophylactic antiviral therapy in high risk patients is under investigation but not currently available as a preventive option (68). Last, the use of active immunization (e.g., CMV vaccine) in high risk patients prior to the onset of immunosuppression is an appealing possibility. In fact, preliminary vaccine trials with a CMV vaccine have already been conducted, and, although humoral and cell-mediated immunity can be induced, absolute protection does not appear to be conferred (68). Further work is obviously necessary.

Overall Clinical Impact

Clinical Outcomes.   Limited data are available on the overall outcome of nosocomial eye infections. Nosocomial conjunctivitis, especially ophthalmia neonatorum, appears to respond promptly to appropriate therapy with few if any long term sequelae (40). Adverse outcomes appear to be more frequent with hospital-acquired keratitis (corneal ulcers). Seven of the 12 patients reported by Hutton and Sexton (45) and Hilton and colleagues (46) experienced complications; of those seven, four ultimately lost useful vision in the affected eye. Among patients who contract infectious episcleritis after retinal detachment surgery, removal of implants is almost universally necessary (9, 15). In the series reported by Ulrich and Burton (9), 13 of the 37 (35%) postoperative infections were associated with surgical failure and were subsequently deemed inoperable. Furthermore, among those patients having implants removed, 13 to 33% will develop recurrent detachment, only approximately 50% of which can be surgically repaired (9, 15). The outcome with endophthalmitis is very guarded. Although Bohigian suggests that useful vision can be preserved in up to 50% of postoperative cases (16), other authors are more pessimistic (17, 18, 22, 69). In several early series reported by Allen and Mangiaracine (20, 70), final visual acuity in the affected eye was light perception only or blindness in 77% of cases. The results of more contemporary series are only minimally more encouraging in that final vision of 20/400 or better is reported in only about 25 to 44% of culture-proven cases (29, 71). The recent experience of Diamond is noteworthy in that 73% of patients with culture-proven endophthalmitis, most of which were postsurgical in origin, had preservation of useful vision in the affected eye post-therapy (72). As summarized by Barza (69), the outcome of endophthalmitis is dependent on the rapidity with which treatment is initiated and on the nature of the infecting pathogen. Culture-negative disease and infections due to *S. epidermidis* do well, whereas infection with *S. aureus* and gram-negative bacilli has a much poorer prognosis.

Economic Consequences.   No accurate estimates are available on the prolongation of hospital stay and additional economic costs of nosocomial eye infections. Uncomplicated infections such as conjunctivitis probably contribute little if any to prolongation of stay, whereas complicated infections such as episcleritis and endophthalmitis undoubtedly add a significant increment to the costs of care since repeat surgery and prolonged antibiotic use are often necessary.

NOSOCOMIAL CENTRAL NERVOUS SYSTEM INFECTIONS

Hospital-acquired infections of the central nervous system (CNS) are relatively infrequent but often clinically devastating. Although initial data accumulated from NNIS for the years 1971 to 1974 suggested a rate of 1 nosocomial CNS infection/10,000 discharges (1), subsequent data from the period 1975 to 1982 estimated the rate to be 8.4/10,000 discharges (73). Based on the earlier figures, nosocomial CNS infections would comprise only about 0.3% of all nosocomial infections (1, 74), whereas the more recent data suggest that perhaps 2 to 2.5% of all nosocomial infections involve the CNS (73). The overall incidence of nosocomial CNS infections is highest on newborn services (15/10,000 discharges), followed by surgery (14.1/10,000 discharges), pediatrics (10.3/10,000 discharges), and medicine (3.9/10,000 discharges) (73). The rate of nosocomial CNS infections in the nursery, where these infections account for about 4% of all infections (75), is significantly higher than on all other services combined (73). Overall, the majority of nosocomial CNS infections are caused by coagulase-negative staphylococci (25%), *S. aureus* (18%), and gram-negative bacilli (15%) (W Jarvis, CDC, personal communication).

Classification of Infections

In general, nosocomial CNS infections can be classified into those which are related to surgical procedures or devices and those which are non-surgically related.

Postsurgical CNS Infections.   The three major categories of postsurgical CNS infections are shown in Table 25.4. The category of meningitis/ventriculitis is broadly representative of those infections which diffusely involve the subarach-

Table 25.4.   Nosocomial CNS Infections*

Classification	Categories of Infection	Associated Procedures or Clinical Settings

Postsurgical	Meningitis/ventriculi-tis
	Focal suppuration
	  Brain abscess
	  Subdural empyema
	  Epidural abscess
	Meningoencephalitis
		Ventriculostomy
		Subarachnoid bolt
		CSF shunt
		CNS reservoir
		Craniotomy
		Corneal transplantation

Nonsurgically related	Meningitis Brain abscess	Contiguous paramenin-geal infection S/P head trauma S/P neuroinvasive pro-cedures Sepsis The neonatal period Host immunocom-promise

* CNS, central nervous system; CSF, cerebrospinal fluid; S/P, status post.

noid and ventricular spaces. Focal suppurative infections include processes such as brain abscess, subdural empyema, and epidural abscess, infections which are localized to the brain parenchyma or epidural or subdural spaces. Meningoencephalitis, a relatively uncommon entity, refers to an infectious process which diffusely involves the meningeal and cortical surfaces. The vast majority of postsurgical CNS infections occur following neurosurgical procedures. By definition, postneurosurgical CNS infections are related etiologically to a preceding neurosurgical intervention which may be simple craniotomy alone, intracranial placement of a neurosurgical device (ventriculostomy, subarachnoid bolt, cerebrospinal fluid (CSF) shunt, CNS reservoir), or some combination of the two. Rarely, nosocomial CNS infections arise following other types of surgical procedures (e.g., corneal transplantation).

Nonsurgically Related CNS Infections. The major category of nonsurgically related CNS infection is hospital-acquired meningitis (Table 25.4). Although a small percentage of these infections will have an encephalitic component, and perhaps should more properly be classified as meningoencephalitis, all such infections will be referred to as "meningitis" for the sake of simplicity. Nosocomial meningitis typically occurs in six defined clinical settings: (*a*) contiguous parameningeal infection, (*b*) status/post (S/P) head trauma, with or without overt skull fracture, (*c*) S/P neuroinvasive procedures (lumbar puncture, myelography, spinal anesthesia), (*d*) sepsis, (*e*)

the neonatal period, and (*f*) host immunocompromise. A less common but nonetheless important category of nonsurgically related CNS infection is that of brain abscess. Brain abscesses may be single or multiple in number and "macro" or "micro" in size. Most arise as a consequence of bloodborne dissemination of infection, usually in the immunocompromised host.

Diagnostic Criteria

The definitions of postsurgical and nonsurgically related nosocomial infection, as applied to CNS infections, are in principle the same as were utilized for eye infections. For neurosurgical device-related infections, a very liberal designation of infection as nosocomial in origin is appropriate since most of these infections are thought to arise from intraoperative or perioperative contamination (76). Despite the often indolent and delayed clinical presentations of these infections, most become clinically apparent within 2 to 8 weeks of surgery (76).

Nosocomial meningitis, whether postsurgical or not, can be defined as infectious inflammation of the meninges manifested clinically as fever, headache, nausea, vomiting, altered mentation, and/or stiff neck; focal neurologic signs including seizures may or may not be present (74). Since the findings are not specific for infection and can sometimes occur even in the absence of meningeal inflammation, CSF analysis is a prerequisite for diagnosis. The CSF findings in nosocomial infectious meningitis are varied but generally will fall into one of three profiles (77). Of the CSF profiles, the one most typically encountered in nosocomial meningitis, most cases of which are bacterial in etiology, is the purulent or neutrophilic profile characterized by an increased number of neutrophilic leukocytes and hypoglycorrhachia (77); the protein concentration is usually but not invariably elevated as well. Since many neurosurgical operative and diagnostic procedures may induce CSF inflammatory changes which mimic those seen with infection (CSF pleocytosis, increased protein concentrations), the diagnosis of postneurosurgical meningitis is frequently difficult. In such cases, the presence of hypoglycorrhachia is probably the most sensitive indicator of infection since decreased glucose concentrations, especially those less than 10 mg/dl, rarely occur as a sequelae of the diagnostic or operative procedure itself (74). Another clinical clue suggesting the presence of complicating infection is the occurrence of a neutrophilic rather than a lymphocytic pleocytosis, the latter being more common with noninfectious inflammation. Whatever the setting, a definitive diagnosis of nosocomial infectious meningitis can only be established by the demonstration of organisms in the CSF (74). Acceptable methods of demonstration of organisms would include positive smears or stains, positive immunodiagnostic tests for microbial antigens (rarely useful with nosocomial meningitis) or positive cultures (74). Occasionally, a presumptive diagnosis of infectious nosocomial meningitis can be made in the absence of microbiologic confirmation if the clinical suspicion of meningitis is strong and the CSF findings are typical (74). This situation is most frequently encountered in the setting of prior antimicrobial therapy, a particularly common occurrence in critically ill hospitalized patients. Thus, a definitive diagnosis of nosocomial infectious meningitis is entertained in the patient with clinical features of meningitis which manifest themselves greater than 48 hours after admission, compatible CSF findings, and isolation of a pathogen from the spinal fluid (74, 75, 78). A presumptive case exhibits compatible clinical findings and CSF abnormalities but lacks microbiologic confirmation of the diagnosis. As always, a physician's diagnosis of meningitis, with or without positive CSF cultures, should be tabulated as a "case" for surveillance purposes (74).

A *focal suppurative infection* can be defined as localized infectious inflammation confined to a restricted anatomic site. The most usual sites of focal CNS suppuration occurring in hospitalized patients would include the brain parenchyma (brain abscess), the subdural space (subdural empyema or abscess), and the epidural space (epidural abscess). Clinical manifestations are diverse but will usually include some combination of fever, altered mentation, and focal neurologic findings. Given the focal nature of these processes, CSF analysis is usually not advisable but, if performed, reveals CSF pleocytosis, predominantly lymphocytic in type, and elevated protein concentrations, findings consistent with a parameningeal process (77). The CSF glucose concentration may or may not be depressed (77). Diagnosis of these processes is usually based upon compatible clinical findings and demonstration of a focal process with inflammatory characteristics by one of a number of neurodiagnostic studies (radionuclide brain scan, computerized axial tomography, magnetic resonance imaging, myelography) (77, 79). Clinical confirmation of the diagnosis is accomplished via operative intervention which demonstrates focal collections of pus. The microbiologic etiology of the process will hopefully be established by culture or histopathologic examination of operative specimens, but it is not invariably so. Thus, diagnostic criteria for case surveillance purposes include compatible clinical findings and demonstration of a focal inflammatory process by neurodiagnostic studies; confirmation surgically and microbiologically is desirable but not essential for case reporting.

Meningoencephalitis can be defined as diffuse inflammation which involves the meningeal and cortical surfaces. Affected patients may exhibit protean clinical manifestations, but prominent signs include fever, a depressed level of consciousness, and impaired higher cortical function. Focal neurologic signs may or may not be present. The results of CSF analysis are highly dependent upon the type of infecting agent. Pleocytosis is an invariable finding but may be either neutrophilic or lymphocytic in type; absolute cell counts tend to be somewhat lower than in "pure" meningitis, but there is considerable overlap (77). Protein concentrations are usually elevated, but the presence of hypoglycorrhachia is highly pathogen-specific. Neurodiagnostic studies may or may not reveal abnormalities; the most usual finding would be diffuse meningeal enhancement on CT scan (79). Given the often unusual or fastidious nature of the causative agents, microbiologic confirmation of etiology is often difficult and is frequently supplanted by serodiagnostic techniques. Diagnostic criteria therefore include a compatible clinical syndrome and CSF abnormalities consistent with the diagnosis; definitive microbiologic information is not a necessary prerequisite. The major features differentiating meningitis from meningoencephalitis therefore are the more common occurrence of positive CSF cultures in the former and the more pronounced depression in level of consciousness and impairment of higher integrative function in the latter.

A summary of the diagnostic criteria for the various types of nosocomial CNS infections is shown in Table 25.5.

Clinical Aspects/Incidence/Causative Pathogens

Postsurgical Infections

Meningitis/ventriculitis. Meningitis/ventriculitis may occur as a complication of craniotomy

Table 25.5. Nosocomial CNS Infections: Diagnostic Criteria*

Type of Infection	Clinical Criteria for Diagnosis
Meningitis	Compatible clinical features (fever, headache, altered mentation, stiff neck) Supportive CSF findings Positive CSF culture†
Focal suppuration (brain abscess, subdural empyema, epidural abscess)	Compatible clinical features (fever, altered sensorium, focal neurologic findings) Positive neurodiagnostic study Surgical confirmation†
Meningoencephalitis	Compatible clinical features (fever, depressed level of consciousness, impaired higher integrative function) Supportive CSF findings

* CNS, central nervous system; CSF, cerebrospinal fluid.

† Requirement not absolute if clinical findings are otherwise typical.

or after placement of various intracranial neurosurgical devices (74). As such, these infections are largely local in their pathogenesis, arising from microbial contamination of the surgical wound or intracranial devices intraoperatively or perioperatively. In patients with neurosurgical devices, the presence of an intracranial foreign body undoubtedly serves to enhance the pathogenic potential of organisms normally considered to be of low virulence. The clinical presentation of the infections is extremely varied. Since most of the affected patients have underlying neurologic disease, it may be difficult to ascertain the presence or absence of typical clinical symptoms and signs such as headache, altered sensorium, depressed level of consciousness, and meningismus. The findings, even if present, may merely be secondary to the surgical procedure itself rather than to superimposed infection. The persistence of the signs beyond 72 hours after the procedure and the presence of significant fever which is otherwise unexplained are two clues which should suggest the possibility of complicating infection (74). Nevertheless, the average time between onset of symptoms and confirmation of the diagnosis in one series was 4.8 days (78). Once suspected, the diagnosis should be pursued by analysis of CSF. As noted above, the CSF findings are extremely variable and are influenced by the surgical procedure itself, the infecting pathogen, and the frequent use of perioperative antibiotic prophylaxis. The presence of either a neutrophilic pleocytosis or hypoglycorrhachia should lead to a presumptive diagnosis of infectious meningitis. The microbial etiology of infection can be identified in 75% or more of cases, notwithstanding the use of antibiotic prophylaxis (75, 78).

Meningitis/ventriculitis associated with intracranial neurosurgical devices may exhibit a number of rather unique features which should heighten clinical suspicion of complicating infection. In patients with ventriculoperitoneal shunts, inflammation along the subcutaneous tract of the shunt or development of peritoneal signs should raise the possibility of shunt infection (76, 80, 81). Likewise, the presence of unremitting fever, multiple positive blood cultures, splenomegaly, and/or hypocomplementemic glomerulonephritis should suggest ventriculoatrial shunt infection (80). In patients with subcutaneous CSF reservoirs, malfunction of the reservoir should raise the possibility of infection as the precipitating event (82).

The true incidence of meningitis/ventriculitis

following neurosurgical operative procedures is difficult to ascertain. Carey, after reviewing nine published series on craniotomy and associated complications, concluded that the overall risk of postoperative infection was 3 to 6% (83). However, the types of postoperative infections and the relative occurrences of each were not delineated. Likewise, Green and colleagues, in reviewing the experience in their neurosurgical unit over a 2-year period, found a postoperative infection rate of 2.6% for clean cranial procedures, excluding shunting operations (84). Again, the proportion of cases attributable to meningitis/ventriculitis was not identified. When attempting to define the incidence of postneurosurgical meningitis/ventriculitis accurately, one should analyze rates associated with individual procedures in order to be most practical and revealing. Accordingly, the incidence of meningitis/ventriculitis as a complication of five separate neurosurgical operative procedures is shown in Table 25.6. As noted, the incidence figures given are those for infections per operative procedure; incidence figures based on infections per patient will accordingly be higher, in many cases strikingly so, since single patients often undergo multiple procedures. The disparity between infection rates for patients versus infection rates based on total number of procedures is perhaps best exemplified by the incidence of meningitis/ventriculitis following CSF shunting procedures. If the percentage of patients developing ventriculitis following CSF shunt procedures is calculated for the series cited in Table 25.6 (80, 99–102), an incidence of 12.1% would be found, a rate approximately twice that of the rate for infections per procedure. This latter figure is consistent with the patient infected rates for ventriculitis cited by Stamm in his review of infections related to medical devices (105). As noted by others (106), the true incidence of meningitis/ventriculitis after many neurosurgical procedures is difficult to establish, partly because of the tendency of writers to group all infections into a general category without delineating types of infections and partly because of the differences in case definition. Nevertheless, the incidence figures shown in Table 25.6 should be representative estimates.

Representative pathogens causing most cases of postneurosurgical meningitis/ventriculitis are shown in Table 25.6. Overall, staphylococcal species, both S. aureus and S. epidermidis, and gram-negative bacilli account for the majority of infections (1, 74, 78). However, a very diverse number of pathogens are capable of causing sporadic cases

of postneurosurgical meningitis (74). The role of S. epidermidis is particularly important in infections of intracranially implanted neurosurgical devices such as shunts and reservoirs, whereas S. aureus and gram-negative bacilli are more prominent pathogens following craniotomy or ventriculostomy.

Focal Suppurative Infection. Focal suppurative infections of the types noted (Table 25.4), although relatively infrequent, may occur in association with any neurosurgical procedure. The majority of the infections arise via local spread of microbes from contaminated wounds or neurosurgical devices. Most are accompanied by nonspecific clinical manifestations such as fever and headache. The anatomic site of the suppurative process, the total area of involvement, and the rapidity of accumulation will determine the nature of the focal neurologic signs which are seen in about 50% of cases (77). The presence of focal neurologic signs is the main clinical feature which distinguishes this group of infections from meningitis/ventriculitis and should prompt the clinician to forego CSF analysis in favor of other neurodiagnostic tests. The diagnosis can readily be confirmed in most cases by cranial CT scan, though other studies such as angiography or radionuclide brain scanning may occasionally be necessary (77, 79).

The clinical presentation of focal CNS suppuration may be acute, subacute, or chronic, with a subacute onset perhaps most common (77). As such, these infections may not become apparent until weeks after surgery which may obscure their relationship to the preceding surgical procedure. Nevertheless, most arise from organisms introduced intraoperatively or perioperatively and are therefore procedure-related.

The incidence of focal suppurative infections as a postneurosurgical complication is admittedly low. The estimated incidence of these infections, considered as a whole, for the various neurosurgical procedures is shown in Table 25.6. Again, rates are expressed as numbers of infections per procedure rather than infections per patient.

The spectrum of pathogens producing postneurosurgical focal suppurative infections is largely the same as for meningitis/ventriculitis. However, S. aureus and gram-negative bacilli tend to supercede S. epidermidis in importance.

Meningoencephalitis. Meningoencephalitis is an unusual postsurgical CNS infection in that it arises almost exclusively from non-neurosurgical procedures. This extremely rare postsurgical infectious complication has been documented only

Table 25.6. Incidence of Nosocomial CNS Infections after Selected Neurosurgical Procedures*

Neurosurgical Procedure	Meningitis/Ventriculitis			Focal Suppurative Infection			References
	No. of Infections/ No. of Procedures	(%)	Causative Organisms	No. of Infections/ No. of Procedures	(%)	Causative Organisms	
Craniotomy† (clean)	82/12,068	(0.7)	*S. aureus* *S. epidermidis* GNRs	7/12,068	(0.06)	Staphylococci GNRs	85–90
Ventriculostomy	80/1,428	(5.6)	GNRs *S. epidermidis* *S. aureus*	0/1,428	(0)		91–95
Subarachnoid pressure monitors	2/295	(0.7)	*S. aureus* *E. coli*	2/295	(0.7)	*S. aureus*	96–98
CSF shunts	200/3,277	(6.1)	*S. epidermidis* *S. aureus* GNRs Diphtheroids	3/3,277	(0.09)	Staphylococci	80, 99–102
CSF reservoirs	15/191	(7.8)	*S. epidermidis* Diphtheroids GNRs	0/191	(0)		82, 103, 104

* CNS, central nervous system; CSF, cerebrospinal fluid; GNRs, gram-negative rods.
† Includes small but indeterminant number of clean spinal procedures.

in association with corneal transplantation, resulting from the dissemination of neurotropic viruses (rabies, the slow virus of Creutzfeld-Jakob disease) which were unrecognized contaminants of the transplant (107, 108). Incubation periods post-transplantation were 18 months and 4.5 weeks for Creutzfeld-Jakob disease and rabies, respectively. The affected patients exhibited very typical clinical manifestations of their respective infections and both expired.

Nonsurgically Related Infections

Meningitis. Nosocomial meningitis which is not associated with neurosurgical procedures tends to occur in a number of well defined clinical settings (Table 25.4). The pathogenesis may be via local spread of contiguous organisms or infection, introduction of potential pathogens via fractures (apparent or inapparent) or procedures (lumbar puncture), or bloodborne dissemination with seeding of the meninges. The onset of infection may be acute or subacute depending on such variables as the etiologic agent, the inoculum size, concurrent antibiotic use, and the integrity of host defenses. Clinical manifestations may be typical or atypical (77, 78, 88) and generally include some combination of fever, headache, altered mentation, and nuchal rigidity. Superimposed illness or preceding procedures may modify or render uninterpretable many of these findings (74, 78). As previously noted, confirmation of the diagnosis is obtained by CSF analysis with cultural identification of the etiologic pathogen.

The most typical parameningeal infections leading to meningitis include acute sinusitis, acute or chronic ear infections, chronic vertebral osteomyelitis, and chronic sacral decubitus ulcers (74, 77, 78). Since sinus and ear infections are rarely indications for hospitalization, the latter group of chronic bone and skin infections may be more important in contributing to nosocomial meningitis via contiguous spread. In patients who develop "meningeal symptoms and signs" with known foci of infection contiguous to the CNS, the possibility of meningeal extension of infection should be strongly entertained and pursued.

Patients with facial and head trauma, whether or not skull fractures or penetrating injuries are present, are at enhanced risk of developing meningitis (74, 88, 109–112). The development of CNS infection is often obscured by the clinical manifestations of the primary injury. Findings which should suggest the presence of complicating meningitis would include persistent unex-

plained fever or the new onset, or persistence beyond a week, of a CSF leak (112).

Meningitis may occasionally arise when organisms are introduced directly into the subarachnoid space via spinal anesthesia or during diagnostic or therapeutic lumbar puncture (74, 78, 113–115). The source of the causative organisms may be the patient's skin, contaminated skin disinfectants (116), contaminated needles or instruments (113, 114), or contaminated solutions administered intrathecally (117). An infectious complication of the procedure should be suspected if new meningeal symptoms develop afterward and persist beyond 48 hours (74).

Meningitis arising as a complication of sepsis, either primary in type or secondary to a distant focus of infection, is a well recognized clinical event (74, 78). Although a potential possibility in any patient with documented bloodborne infection, hematogenous seeding of the meninges is a particularly common event in neonatal populations (74, 118). The possibility of metastatic CNS infection should accordingly be considered in any patient with suspected or proven sepsis who develops signs suggestive of meningitis.

A special subset of nosocomial meningitis is that which occurs in neonates. Although often associated with sepsis (118), neonatal meningitis may arise in the absence of documented bacteremia (119, 120). Nasopharyngeal colonization with virulent pathogens followed by direct mucosal invasion and spread to the CNS by venous and lymphatic channels is the postulated pathogenesis of the infections. Also within the category of neonatal nosocomial meningitis are cases of viral meningoencephalitis due to herpes simplex virus (121) or the enteroviruses (122) which presumably represent CNS involvement during the course of systemic infection.

The last clinical setting in which nosocomial meningitis is frequently encountered is in immunocompromised host populations (123–125). These patients, because of underlying defects in host defense, are peculiarly susceptible to infection by a diverse group of opportunistic pathogens. Infection is often widely disseminated, with certain opportunistic agents exhibiting a propensity for invasion of the CNS (124, 125). Because of the patient's underlying disease or concurrent immunosuppressive therapy, the clinical manifestations of CNS infection are often atypical and muted.

The overall incidence of nonsurgically related nosocomial meningitis is difficult to estimate. Hodges and Perkins found only 18 cases of nosocomial meningitis over a 25-year period (78); of these, 9 or 50% were nonsurgically related. An exact case rate cannot be determined since discharge data for the study period were not provided but the "rough" rate would be 1 case every 2 to 3 years. Overall, 2.6% of all cases of bacterial meningitis seen during the study period would have been classified as nonsurgically related hospital-acquired meningitis. Further information on the incidence of nonsurgically related nosocomial meningitis in each of the clinical settings noted in Table 25.4 can be delineated from selected published reports. Analysis of the data reported by Hodges and Perkins provides insight into the occurrence of meningitis secondary to spread from contiguous infection. They found that three of their nonsurgically related cases were secondary to contiguous spread of infection (78), a sporadic and relatively rare event. Although head trauma as a predisposing cause of nosocomial meningitis is felt to be especially important (74), Hodges and Perkins identified no cases arising from head trauma alone (78). Similarly, Buckwold and colleagues (88), in reviewing their experience with hospital-acquired bacterial meningitis, found only 6 cases of meningitis in 1100 patients admitted with skull fracture and/or CSF leak. Of the 6 cases, 5 had undergone craniotomy which introduced a second predisposing factor and obscured the true occurrence due to head trauma alone. Among their cases of gram-negative bacillary meningitis encountered over an 8-year period, Mombelli and co-workers (111) noted that 19 of 34 (56%) were related to head injuries. Although 5 of these 19 patients also underwent craniotomy, the remaining 14 had no predisposing factor except their head injury. Unfortunately, no data were provided on total numbers of patients with head injury admitted during the study period so the incidence of meningitis in this population cannot be calculated. Hodges and Perkins further noted that 2 of their 9 cases of nosocomial meningitis arose following myelography (78). Although the overall frequency of post-lumbar puncture meningitis cannot be accurately determined, estimates suggest that meningitis occurs as a complication of spinal anesthesia once in every 20,000 to 30,000 cases (74). The overall occurrence of meningitis in association with sepsis is indeterminant. Studies in neonates, the highest risk population, suggest an attack rate of 4.0 to 10 cases/1000 live births (75, 118). The case rate for neonatal bacterial meningitis not associated with sepsis cannot be readily established. Recent data suggest that the inci-

dence of neonatal herpes simplex infection approximates 0.26 case/1000 deliveries (126). Since approximately 50% of cases develop CNS infection, the overall occurrence of herpetic meningoencephalitis would be 0.13 case/1000 deliveries. Among the infectious complications of immunocompromise, meningitis accounts for a minority of the total infections. Nevertheless, it is estimated that 5 to 10% of renal transplant recipients and lymphoma patients develop CNS infections (124), many of which become manifest during periods of hospitalization. Chernik and colleagues identified 146 CNS infections in their oncology population over a 16-year period, with an overall incidence of 0.2 to 0.3% of all hospital admissions (123). Of these 146 infections, 104 (71%) represented meningitis. More recently, Hooper and co-workers analyzed 55 CNS infections in chronically immunosuppressed patients occurring over 10 years, approximately 80% of which were meningitis or meningoencephalitis (124). Based upon the findings of the two series, 4.6 to 6.5 cases of meningitis in compromised hosts may be encountered each year, with perhaps one-third to one-half of these becoming manifest in the hospital.

The pathogens causing nosocomial meningitis not related to prior neurosurgery are extremely varied. Overall, enteric gram-negative bacilli and staphylococci predominate (74, 78). However, the relative importance of the various pathogens depends upon the clinical setting in which disease occurs. For example, meningitis occurring early after head trauma (i.e., $\leq$ 3 days) is primarily due to *S. pneumoniae*, whereas late disease is more typically caused by gram-negative bacilli (109, 127). Prominent pathogens causing post-lumbar puncture meningitis include *S. aureus* and *Pseudomonas* (74). Neonatal meningitis is caused predominantly by gram-negative bacilli (especially *E. coli*), *Listeria*, and group B streptococci (118). Meningitis in the compromised host is predominantly due to *Cryptococcus neoformans*, *Listeria monocytogenes*, and gram-negative bacilli (123, 124).

Brain Abscess. Compared to meningitis, brain abscess is a relatively uncommon nosocomial CNS infection, especially in the absence of a prior neurosurgical procedure. The pathogenesis of most such infections is thought to be direct inoculation of pathogens into the CNS (head trauma) or hematogenous seeding from a distant focus, though occasional cases may arise from contiguous spread (sinusitis). In general, these infections present in an indolent fashion. The clinical manifestations and approach to diagnosis are as outlined above.

Development of brain abscess following head trauma may occur when bone fragments from a skull fracture penetrate the brain and are not debrided or when bone or missile fragments are not removed from the brain following gunshot wounds (112). The incidence of this complication is unknown. Causative pathogens in this setting include gram-negative bacilli and staphylococci (112).

Micro- or macroabscesses of the brain may also arise from hematogenous seeding of the brain parenchyma during the course of disseminated systemic infection. Such lesions occur not uncommonly during the course of infectious endocarditis, especially in acute presentations with virulent pathogens such as *S. aureus*, fastidious gram-negative bacilli, or fungi (128), but are much less common with sepsis not arising from an endovascular focus. Among patients with infective endocarditis who manifest neurologic findings, 4% will have antemortem or postmortem evidence of brain abscess, with most exhibiting multiple microfoci of infection (128). Brain abscess is also a complication of disseminated infection in immunocompromised hosts (123–125). Chernik and colleagues (123) found that brain abscesses accounted for 39 of 146 documented CNS infections (27%) in their cancer patients. The majority of these abscesses occurred in patients with leukemia and arose within the hospital during periods of neutropenia. Almost 50% of these abscesses were due to gram-negative bacilli with fungi accounting for approximately one-third of cases (123). Recent reviews would suggest that the occurrence of candidal CNS infection in this setting has been markedly underestimated (125). Data from Lipton and colleagues suggest that approximately 50% of patients with systemic candidiasis develop CNS involvement, with the predominant pathologic lesion being brain abscess (125).

Epidemiology of Infection

Postsurgical Infections

The *origin of infecting pathogens* producing postneurosurgical CNS infection can be from either environmental sources or tissue sources. Potential environmental sources would include airborne contaminants, contaminated surgical solutions, and contaminated instruments and devices. At present, there is very little evidence to suggest that any of these sources contributes significantly to postneurosurgical infection (83). Of these potential environmental sources, the one of greatest concern is perhaps airborne contamination of surgical wounds in the operating room (83). As summarized by Carey (83), studies by Velghe showed a 25% contamination rate of neurosurgical wounds presumably from airborne contaminants, a rate which increased with the duration of surgery and was reduced by utilizing more frequent air exchanges. However, despite documentation of operative wound contamination, no correlation could be made between these results and subsequent postoperative infection. Given the absence of convincing data which support environmental sources of infection, most authors now accept the principle that the patient's skin and tissues are the most important reservoir for microbes producing postoperative CNS infections (80, 83). Current thoughts on pathogenesis conclude that most pathogens are introduced into the wound or onto neurosurgical devices, presumably from the skin, during the perioperative period (76, 80). Growth and replication of a nidus of organisms in the postoperative period would then account for most observed postsurgical infections. This hypothesis is supported by outbreaks of disease which can be traced to skin contamination in the perioperative period (129). Patient-to-patient spread of pathogenic organisms in the postoperative period is also a documented source of infection in this patient population (130). In this circumstance, infected or colonized patients are themselves the reservoirs for the pathogenic organisms, with hand-to-hand spread from staff to patients the usual mode of transmission.

Risk factors implicated as predisposing to postneurosurgical CNS infection are protean. In many instances, observations are uncontrolled or anecdotal. Factors most commonly cited as being important in the pathogenesis of postoperative infection have included duration of surgery, use of postoperative drains, and wound re-explorations (131), but such factors vary from series to series (132). An overall summary of putative risk factors for acquisition of postoperative infection following various neurosurgical procedures is shown in Table 25.7. Several points are worthy of note. As regards ventriculostomy-associated infections, the recent report by Mayhall and colleagues (95), because of its prospective design and exhaustively complete analysis, is probably the most informative. The published experience with subarachnoid pressure monitors is rather limited compared to other neurosurgical procedures, so conclusions regarding risk factors for infection (97) must be viewed as tentative. Last, although a number of authors suggest that ventriculoatrial shunts are associated with higher infection rates than ventriculoperitoneal shunts (99, 135), other authors dispute this conclusion (80, 102). Thus, the risk factors shown in Table 25.7 must be regarded as representing a compendium of views based on available data which may be modified or evolve further with time.

Nonsurgically Related Infections

The *origin of infecting pathogens* producing the majority of nosocomial CNS infections not related to prior surgery is the patient's own indigenous flora. The causative organisms may be endogenous (present on admission) or exogenous (acquired from the hospital environment after admission). In patients who develop CNS infec-

tion secondary to a contiguous focus, the organisms producing the CNS process are the same as those causing the parameningeal infection, whether those organisms were endogenous in origin or exogenously acquired. Patients manifesting meningitis or brain abscess following head trauma generally exhibit two distinct groups of pathogens, differentiated clinically by the time of onset of infection postinjury and the presence or absence of penetrating injuries (74). Meningitis occurring early after the injury or in the absence of penetrating injuries is usually due to *S. pneumoniae*, an endogenous organism present in the paranasal sinuses, whereas late infections or those accompanying penetrating trauma are most often secondary to *S. aureus* or gram-negative bacilli, organisms acquired exogenously from the hospital environment which then colonize mucous membranes or wounds (109, 112, 127). The or-

Table 25.7. Potential Risk Factors for the Development of Postneurosurgical CNS Infections*

Type of Neurosurgical Procedure	Nature of Complicating Infection	Potential Risk Factors	References
Craniotomy	Meningitis/ventriculitis Focal suppurative infections	Length of operation External drainage Re-exploration Operations through sinuses	86, 131
Ventriculostomy	Meningitis/ventriculitis	Other neurosurgical operations Prolonged duration of drainage (>5 days) Air-vented system Large dural opening ICP > 20 Irrigation	92–95
Subarachnoid pressure monitors	Meningitis Focal suppurative infections	Age of patient Duration of monitoring Concurrent use of corticosteroids	97
CSF shunts	Meningitis/ventriculitis Focal suppurative infections	Length of operation Thrombus formation (VA shunts) Externally communicating wound Age of patient Increasing numbers of operations Inexperience of the surgeon Type shunt (VA > VP)	99, 102, 133–135
CSF reservoirs	Meningitis/ventriculitis	Repetitive puncture	82

* CNS, central nervous system; ICP, intracranial pressure; CSF, cerebrospinal fluid; VA, ventriculoatrial; VP, ventriculoperitoneal.

ganisms producing post-lumbar puncture meningitis are somewhat of an exception in that many arise from environmental sources such as contaminated needles, solutions, or medications (74, 113, 114, 116, 118); organisms acquired in this fashion are usually resistant gram-negative bacilli which are directly inoculated into the CNS. Organisms which enter the CNS via hematogenous seeding may arise either endogenously or exogenously but are almost always associated with an intermediate stage of colonization at some body site or infection at a focus outside the CNS. Neonatal CNS infections are somewhat unique in that many of the causative organisms are acquired from the mother during the birth process as the neonate traverses the birth canal (74, 118). Nevertheless, a small percentage of etiologic agents appears to be acquired exogenously after birth from the hospital environment (hands of personnel, contaminated solutions/equipment). Studies from Baker (118) suggest that approximately 10% of cases of neonatal meningitis fall into this latter category. Likewise, nosocomial meningoencephalitis in neonates appears to arise in a similar fashion, with the majority of cases originating from the mother (122, 126) but a small percentage arising from other environmental reservoirs (136). The sources of pathogens producing nosocomial CNS infections in immunocompromised hosts are complex; most appear to arise from the patient's own flora, whether endogenous or exogenous in origin. In patients with predominant deficits in cell-mediated immune function, most complicating infections, including those involving the CNS, tend to arise from endogenous (latent) pathogens (124). In contrast, patients with quantitative deficits in phagocytic cells tend to manifest CNS infections due to exogenously acquired organisms (124), with CNS infection due to *Aspergillus* a prototype example of this phenomenon (137).

Risk factors for the acquisition of nonsurgically related CNS infection are primarily defined by the clinical settings in which these infections occur (Table 25.4). Thus, most factors relate to the host and any coexistent illnesses, immune deficits, injuries, or neuroinvasive interventions. However, in several of these settings, a few additional risk factors have been defined as well. For example, in patients with head trauma complicated by CSF leak, the risk of meningitis is markedly enhanced if the leak does not spontaneously resolve within 7 days (112). In one series, only 11% of patients whose leaks stopped within 7 days developed meningitis, whereas 88% of the

patients with persistent fistulae developed meningitis (138). Similarly, the risk of neonatal meningitis has been shown to be enhanced by a number of factors, including prematurity, prior exposure to antibiotics, prolonged hospitalization, contaminated life support equipment, and conditions which foster infant contact with multiple antibiotic-resistant gram-negative enteric bacteria (crowding, high nurse-to-infant ratios, poor hand washing practices) (118). Last, in the immunosuppressed host, the nature, severity, and duration of immune deficits are all factors contributing to risk.

Prevention and Control
Postsurgical Infections

Since the prevailing thought on the origin of postneurosurgical CNS infections is that most of these infections arise from the patient's own skin flora (80, 83), the primary preventive techniques should logically be directed toward optimizing surgical asepsis. Thus, emphasis upon traditional surgical principles of infection prevention (thorough skin preparation, isolation of the skin by sterile plastic drapes, prevention of contact between skin and surgical devices during insertion, meticulous surgical care, brief operations) (83) is both proper and mandatory.

Nevertheless, even when meticulous application of the above techniques is unfailingly accomplished, it is recognized that the surgical field will never be sterile. Accordingly, many authors have chosen to utilize perioperative antibiotics in an attempt to eradicate persisting organisms on the skin and in the wound and thus to prevent or reduce the incidence of postneurosurgical infection. At present, the use of perioperative antibiotic prophylaxis for many if not all neurosurgical procedures is well established. However, it should be noted that studies on the effectiveness of prophylactic antibiotics in neurosurgery are limited in number and that few if any are randomized, controlled, prospective trials (83). Other factors contributing to the difficulty which arises in interpreting these studies include widely differing methodologies, noncomparable antibiotic regimens, diverse study populations, and major differences in durations of surgery (83). The lack of uniformity in study design perhaps accounts for the often contradictory conclusions reached by the different investigators. For example, Wright (131), Quadery et al (132), and Llewellyn et al (139) concluded that prophylactic antibiotics, as employed in their studies during routine craniotomies, did not alter postoperative infection rates, whereas Malis (89) and Quartey and Polyzoidis (90) felt strongly that antibiotic prophylaxis was extremely efficacious and strongly warranted. In fact, Malis achieved the "ideal" with the use of parenteral gentamicin and vancomycin and topical streptomycin of no postoperative infections in 1732 major clean cases (89). Similarly conflicting conclusions can be found when analyzing the results obtained using prophylactic antibiotics in procedures involving placement of intracranial devices. In reviewing their experience with ventriculostomy-associated infections, Wyler and Kelly (93) found a reduction in infection rates in those patients who received "prophylactic" antibiotics, a finding not confirmed in the more recent study by Mayhall and colleagues (95). Similar results have been reported with shunt-related infections. Selected studies have demonstrated an advantage of antibiotic prophylaxis (140, 141), whereas others have not (80, 102). The ultimate conclusion to be derived from these studies is that the role of prophylactic antibiotics in clean neurosurgical cases is undefined at present and requires further investigation.

Infection prevention guidelines not related to surgical technique and the use of prophylactic antibiotics are limited in number. In their recent review of ventriculostomy-related infections, Mayhall and co-workers found that these infections may be prevented by maintenance of a closed drainage system and by timely removal of the ventricular catheter (95). They further concluded that if monitoring was required for more than 5 days, removal of the catheter and reinsertion at a different site were indicated.

Nonsurgically Related Infections

Since many nosocomial CNS infections not related to surgery arise secondary to spread of infection from contiguous or remote foci, a significant proportion may be inevitable and cannot be readily prevented (74). The only potentially useful preventive interventions are primary prevention of extra-CNS nosocomial infections by strict adherence to sound principles of patient care and infection control and prompt recognition and treatment of extra-CNS infections in order to prevent local spread or dissemination.

Utilization of proper aseptic technique and sterile solutions should minimize the risk of postlumbar puncture meningitis.

The use of prophylactic antibiotics in the prevention of nonsurgically related CNS infections is controversial (74) but is occasionally practiced in two settings. In patients with significant head trauma, with or without CSF leak, prophylactic antibiotics are frequently utilized to minimize the risk of complicating meningitis (74, 83). As with neurosurgical antibiotic prophylaxis, the data supporting or refuting antibiotic prophylaxis in patients with head trauma are conflicting. Several studies suggest a beneficial effect of prophylactic antibiotics upon the incidence of meningitis following basal skull fracture and CSF leakage (138, 142) whereas others fail to support the use of antibiotic prophylaxis in this setting (143–145). Ignelzi and VanderArk further demonstrated that prophylactic antibiotics encouraged the growth of gram-negative bacilli in the nasopharynx and thus might predispose to gram-negative meningitis (143). Based upon his review of pertinent literature, Carey concluded that the weight of the available evidence was against the use of prophylactic antibiotics in this setting (83).

The second clinical setting in which antibiotic prophylaxis is sometimes used is in the prevention of selected forms of neonatal meningitis, especially group B streptococcal disease. Although theoretically appealing, the use of penicillin or ampicillin chemoprophylaxis in women during pregnancy, parturients at the time of delivery, or neonates at birth has not gained widespread acceptance (146). Accordingly, alternative and perhaps more effective prevention measures such as immunoprophylaxis are now being explored (146).

Last, the prevention of neonatal meningoencephalitis due to herpes simplex (HSV) is contingent upon recognition of women who are at increased risk of active genital HSV infection during the third trimester of pregnancy (147). Although controversial, cesarean section is believed to be warranted whenever active maternal genital HSV infection is present at term, provided that the fetal membranes are intact or have been ruptured for no more than 4 hours (147).

Overall Clinical Impact

Clinical Outcomes. Nosocomial CNS infections are frequently devastating illnesses with significant accompanying morbidity and mortality. Data accumulated through NNIS for the years 1975 through 1982 revealed that 315 of 2146 (15%) patients with nosocomial CNS infections expired (73). Of these total deaths, 125 (40%) were judged to be directly attributable to the CNS infection (73). Preliminary NNIS data for 1983 reveal a slight reduction in overall mortality, with 8% (15 of 192) of all patients expiring but only 13% of these deaths directly attributable to the CNS infection (W Jarvis, CDC, personal communication). An earlier report from Hodges and Perkins (78) noted that 12 of 18 (67%) patients with nosocomial meningitis expired, all ostensibly from their infection. In their summary of the NNIS data, Jarvis and colleagues (73) reported that the proportion of nosocomial CNS infections causing death was highest on newborn (12%), pediatric (10%), and medicine (8%) services. Infections caused by aminoglycoside-resistant gram-negative bacilli were also associated with a higher risk of death than were susceptible strains.

Data on procedure-specific case-fatality ratios are rather limited. As shown in Table 25.6, 89 CNS infections developed following clean craniotomy in 12,068 cases for a case-infection ratio of 0.7% (85–90). Of the 89 infected patients with either meningitis/ventriculitis or focal suppurative infection, 23 (26%) subsequently expired, though the relationship of their death to the CNS infection could not always be ascertained. Therefore, the maximal case-fatality ratio for clean craniotomy which is attributable to infection would be approximately 0.2%. A comparable case-fatality ratio for ventriculostomy-related infection cannot be calculated due to the absence of information on deaths in the reported series (91–95). Stamm reported that the case-fatality ratio for ventriculitis associated with CSF shunts was 30 to 35% (105), a figure somewhat greater than the 1.7 to 8.7% range for case-fatality ratios reported by Horwitz and Rizzoli (106).

Economic Consequences. The economic consequences of CNS infection are potentially great given the often chronic nature of these illnesses, the need for frequent and repetitive operative intervention, the frequent use of prolonged courses of parenteral antibiotics, and the often severe residual disability in survivors which necessitates long term nursing home or institutional care. However, data on this aspect of infection are largely unavailable. Balch, in his review of postneurosurgical infections (86), noted that these infections can be "financially catastrophic." He reported that the duration of hospital stay for patients who developed postsurgical infection was 48 days versus an average stay of 15.3 days for the uncomplicated case (86). Similarly, Green and colleagues found that patients with postcraniotomy infections were hospitalized an average of 41 days compared to the average length of stay

of 14 days for neurosurgical patients in general (84). For the 41 neurosurgical nosocomial infections occurring during the 2-year period of his review, he estimated that these infections resulted in 981 extra days of hospitalization at a total cost of $100,000, excluding costs due to antibiotics, consultants, procedures, and loss of income (84).

References

1. Bennett JV: Incidence and nature of endemic and epidemic nosocomial infections. In Bennett JV, Brachman PS (eds): *Hospital Infections.* Boston, Little, Brown, and Co, 1979, pp 233–238.
2. Wenzel RP: *Handbook of Hospital Acquired Infections.* Boca Raton, FL, CRC Press, 1981.
3. Castle M: *Hospital Infection Control. Principles and Practice.* New York, John Wiley & Sons, 1980.
4. Lowbury EJL, Ayliffe GAJ, Geddes AM, Williams JD: *Control of Hospital Infection. A Practical Handbook.* London, Chapman and Hall, 1981.
5. Stamm WE, Steere AC, Dixon RE: Selected infections of the skin and eye. In Bennett JV, Brachman PS (eds): *Hospital Infections.* Boston, Little, Brown, and Co, 1979, pp 355–380.
6. Michaud R, Rousseau A: Eye infections. In Pechere J-C, Acar J, Armengaud M, Grenier B, Moellering R Jr, Sande M, Waldvogel F, Zinner S (eds): *Infections: Recognition, Understanding, Treatment.* Philadelphia, Lea & Febiger, 1984, pp 501–528.
7. Milder B: Complications in lacrimal surgery. In Waltman SR, Krupin T (eds): *Complications in Ophthalmic Surgery.* Philadelphia, JB Lippincott, 1980, pp 233–251.
8. Centers for Disease Control: *Mycobacterium chelonei* infections following eye surgery—Texas. *MMWR* 32:591–598, 1983.
9. Ulrich RA, Burton TC: Infections following scleral buckling procedures. *Arch Ophthalmol* 92:213–215, 1974.
10. O'Day DM: Intraocular infections. In Spaeth GL (ed): *Ophthalmic Surgery. Principles and Practice.* Philadelphia, WB Saunders, 1982, pp 103–117.
11. Escoffery RF: Complications of retinal detachment surgery. I. Operative complications. In Waltman SR, Krupin T (eds): *Complications in Ophthalmic Surgery.* Philadelphia, JB Lippincott, 1980, pp 266–279.
12. Arribas N: Complications of retinal detachment surgery. II. Postoperative complications. In Waltman SR, Krupin T (eds): *Complications in Ophthalmic Surgery.* Philadelphia, JB Lippincott, 1980, pp 279–291.
13. McMeel JW, Naegele DF, Pollalis S, Badrinath SS, Murphy PL: Acute and subacute infections following scleral buckling operations. *Ophthalmology* 85:341–349, 1978.
14. Lean JS, Chignell AH: Infection following retinal detachment surgery. *Br J Ophthalmol* 61:593–594, 1977.
15. Hahn YS, Lincoff A, Lincoff H, Kreissig I: Infection after sponge implantation for scleral buckling. *Am J Ophthalmol* 87:180–185, 1979.
16. Bohigian GM: Postoperative infection: en-

dophthalmitis. In Waltman SR, Krupin T (eds): *Complications in Ophthalmic Surgery.* Philadelphia, JB Lippincott, 1980, pp 28–45.

17. Jaffe NS: *Cataract Surgery and Its Complications.* St Louis, CV Mosby, 1984, pp 497–529.

18. Baum JL: Current concepts in ophthalmology. Ocular infections. *N Engl J Med* 299:28–31, 1978.

19. Locatcher-Khorazo D, Gutierrez E: Eye infections following cataract extraction. With special reference to the role of *Staphylococcus aureus. Am J Ophthalmol* 41:981–987, 1956.

20. Allen HF, Mangiaracine AB: Bacterial endophthalmitis after cataract extraction. A study of 22 infections in 20,000 operations. *Arch Ophthalmol* 72:454–462, 1964.

21. Christy NE, Lall P: Postoperative endophthalmitis following cataract surgery. Effects of subconjunctival antibiotics and other factors. *Arch Ophthalmol* 90:361–366, 1973.

22. Allen HF: Symposium: postoperative endophthalmitis. Introduction: incidence and etiology. *Ophthalmology* 85:317–319, 1978.

23. Drews RC: Symposium: complications of modern surgical procedures. Inflammatory response, endophthalmitis, corneal dystrophy, glaucoma, retinal detachment, dislocation, refractive error, lens removal, and enucleation. *Ophthalmology* 85:164–175, 1978.

24. Kraff MC, Sanders DR: Symposium: intraocular lenses. The Medallion suture lens. Management of complications. *Ophthalmology* 86:643–654, 1979.

25. Blankenship GW: Endophthalmitis after pars plana vitrectomy. *Am J Ophthalmol* 84:815–817, 1977.

26. Leveille AS, McMullan FD, Cavanagh HD: Endophthalmitis following penetrating keratoplasty. *Ophthalmology* 90:38–39, 1983.

27. Tabbara KF: Late infections following filtering procedures. *Ann Ophthalmol* 8:1228–1231, 1976.

28. Freedman J, Gupta M, Bunke A: Endophthalmitis after trabeculectomy. *Arch Ophthalmol* 96:1017–1018, 1978.

29. Forster RZ, Zachary IG, Cottingham AJ Jr, Norton EWD: Further observations on the diagnosis, cause and treatment of endophthalmitis. *Am J Ophthalmol* 81:52–56, 1976.

30. Centers for Disease Control: Eye infections after plastic lens implantation. *MMWR* 24:437–438, 1975.

31. O'Day DM: Fungal endophthalmitis caused by *Paecilomyces lilacinus* after intraocular lens implantation. *Am J Ophthalmol* 83:130–131, 1977.

32. Treister G, Frankl O, Cohen S, Stein R: Metastatic gangrene of the lid in *Pseudomonas* septicemia. *Ann Ophthalmol* 7:639–641, 1975.

33. Bodey GP, Bolivar R, Fainstein V, Jadeja L: Infections caused by *Pseudomonas aeruginosa. Rev Infect Dis* 5:279–313, 1983.

34. Rosenoff SH, Wolf ML, Chabner BA: *Pseudomonas* blepharoconjunctivitis. A complication of combination chemotherapy. *Arch Ophthalmol* 91:490–491, 1974.

35. Hirst LW, Thomas JV, Green WR: Conjunctivitis. In Mandell GL, Douglas RG Jr, Bennett JE (eds): *Principles and Practice of Infectious Diseases,* ed 2. New York, John Wiley & Sons, 1985, pp 749–754.

36. Leopold IH: Characteristics of hospital epidemics of epidemic keratoconjunctivitis. *Am J Ophthalmol* 43:93–97, 1957.

37. Laibson PR, Ortolan G, Dupre-Strachan S: Community and hospital outbreak of epidemic keratoconjunctivitis. *Arch Ophthalmol* 80:467–473, 1968.

38. Levandowski RA, Rubenis M: Nosocomial conjunctivitis caused by adenovirus type 4. *J Infect Dis* 143:28–31, 1981.

39. Stenson S, Newman R, Fedukowicz H: Conjunctivitis in the newborn: observations on incidence, cause, and prophylaxis. *Ann Ophthalmol* 13:329–334, 1981.

40. Armstrong JH, Zacarias F, Rein MF: Ophthalmia neonatorum: a chart review. *Pediatrics* 57:884–892, 1976.

41. Guyer B, O'Day DM, Hierholzer JC, Schaffner W: Epidemic keratoconjunctivitis: a community outbreak of mixed adenovirus type 8 and type 19 infection. *J Infect Dis* 132:142–150, 1975.

42. Rothenberg R: Ophthalmia neonatorum due to *Neisseria gonorrhoeae:* prevention and treatment. *Sex Transm Dis* 6:187–191, 1979.

43. Schachter J: Chlamydial infections. *N Engl J Med* 298:428–435, 490–495, 540–549, 1978.

44. Hirst LW, Thomas JV, Green WR: Keratitis. In Mandell GL, Douglas RG Jr, Bennett JE (eds): *Principles and Practice of Infectious Diseases,* ed 2. New York, John Wiley & Sons, 1985, pp 754–760.

45. Hutton WL, Sexton RR: Atypical *Pseudomonas* corneal ulcers in semicomatose patients. *Am J Ophthalmol* 73:37–39, 1972.

46. Hilton E, Uliss A, Samuels S, Adams AA, Lesser ML, Lowry FD: Nosocomial bacterial eye infections in intensive-care units. *Lancet* 1:1318–1320, 1983.

47. Searl SS, Udell IJ, Sadun A, Hyslop NE Jr, Albert DM, Kenyon KR: *Aspergillus* keratitis with intraocular invasion. *Ophthalmology* 88:1244–1250, 1981.

48. Polack FM, Kaufman HE, Newmark E: Keratomycosis: medical and surgical treatment. *Arch Ophthalmol* 85:410–416, 1971.

49. Hirst LW, Thomas JV, Green WR: Endophthalmitis. In Mandell GL, Douglas RG Jr, Bennett JE (eds): *Principles and Practice of Infectious Diseases,* ed 2. New York, John Wiley & Sons, 1985, pp 760–767.

50. Gamel JW, Allansmith MR: Metastatic staphylococcal endophthalmitis presenting as chronic iridocyclitis. *Am J Ophthalmol* 77:454–458, 1974.

51. Griffin JR, Pettit TH, Fishman LS, Foos RY: Blood-borne *Candida* endophthalmitis. *Arch Ophthalmol* 89:450–456, 1973.

52. Murray HW, Knox DL, Green WR, Susel RM: Cytomegalovirus retinitis in adults: a manifestation of disseminated viral infection. *Am J Med* 63:574–584, 1977.

53. Egbert PR, Pollard RB, Gallagher JG, Merigan TC: Cytomegalovirus retinitis in immunosuppressed hosts. II. Ocular manifestations. *Ann Intern Med* 93:664–670, 1980.

54. Holland GN, Gottlieb MS, Yee RD, Schanker HM, Pettit TH: Ocular disorders associated with

a new severe acquired cellular immunodeficiency syndrome. *Am J Ophthalmol* 93:393–402, 1982.

55. Farber BP, Weinbaum DL, Dummer JS: Metastatic bacterial endophthalmitis. *Arch Intern Med* 145:62–64, 1985.

56. Dreyer NP, Fields BN: Heroin-associated infective endocarditis. A report of 28 cases. *Ann Intern Med* 78:699–702, 1973.

57. Henderson DK, Edwards JE Jr, Montgomerie JZ: Hematogenous *Candida* endophthalmitis in patients receiving parenteral hyperalimentation fluids. *J Infect Dis* 143:655–661, 1981.

58. Porter R, Crombie AL, Gardner PS, Uldall RP: Incidence of ocular complications in patients undergoing renal transplantation. *Br Med J* 3:133–136, 1972.

59. Clarkson JG, Green WR: Endogenous fungal endophthalmitis. In Duane TD (ed): *Clinical Ophthalmology.* Hagerstown, MD, Harper & Row, 1976, vol 4, chap 11.

60. Walter CW, Kundsin RB, Brubaker MM: The incidence of airborne wound infections during operation. *JAMA* 186:908–913, 1963.

61. Allen HF: Aseptic technique in ophthalmology. In Locatcher-Khorazo D, Seegal BC (eds): *Microbiology of the Eye.* St Louis, CV Mosby, 1972, pp 86–118.

62. Locatcher-Khorazo D, Seegal BC, Gutierrez EH: Postoperative infections of the eye. In Locatcher-Khorazo D, Seegal BC (eds): *Microbiology of the Eye.* St Louis, CV Mosby, 1972, pp 77–85.

63. Ayliffe GAJ, Barry DR, Lowbury EJL, Roper-Hall MJ, Walker WM: Postoperative infection with *Pseudomonas aeruginosa* in an eye hospital. *Lancet* 1:1113–1117, 1966.

64. Gerding DN, Poley BJ, Hall WH, LeWin DP, Clark MD: Treatment of *Pseudomonas* endophthalmitis associated with prosthetic intraocular lens implantation. *Am J Ophthalmol* 88:902–908, 1979.

65. Shaw EL, Aquavella JV: Pneumococcal endophthalmitis following grafting of corneal tissue from a (cadaver) kidney donor. *Ann Ophthalmol* 9:435–440, 1977.

66. Allen HF: Prevention of postoperative endophthalmitis. *Ophthalmology* 85:386–389, 1978.

67. Starr MB: Prophylactic antibiotics for ophthalmic surgery. *Surv Ophthalmol* 27:353–373, 1983.

68. Hirsch MS: Herpes group virus infections in the compromised host. In Rubin RH, Young LS (eds): *Clinical Approach to Infection in the Compromised Host.* New York, Plenum, 1981, pp 402–406.

69. Barza M: Treatment of bacterial infections of the eye. In Remington JS, Swartz MN (eds): *Current Clinical Topics in Infectious Diseases.* New York, McGraw-Hill, 1980, vol 1, pp 158–194.

70. Allen HF, Mangiaracine AB: Bacterial endophthalmitis after cataract extraction. II. Incidence in 36,000 consecutive operations with special reference to preoperative topical antibiotics. *Arch Ophthalmol* 91:3–7, 1974.

71. Peyman GA: Antibiotic administration in the treatment of bacterial endophthalmitis. II. Intravitreal injections. *Surv Ophthalmol* 21:332–346, 1977.

72. Diamond JG: Intraocular management of endophthalmitis. A systematic approach. *Arch Ophthalmol* 99:96–99, 1981.

73. Jarvis W, Hughes J, Munn V, Culver D, Haley R: Epidemiology of nosocomial central nervous system infections in the United States, 1975–1982 (abstract). Proceedings of the 23rd Interscience Conference on Antimicrobial Agents and Chemotherapy, Las Vegas, 1983, abstract 796.

74. Beaty HN: The central nervous system: meningitis. In Bennett JV, Brachman PS (eds): *Hospital Infections.* Boston, Little, Brown, and Co, 1979, pp 409–418.

75. Hemming VG, Overall JC Jr, Britt MR: Nosocomial infections in a newborn intensive-care unit. Results of forty-one months of surveillance. *N Engl J Med* 294:1310–1316, 1976.

76. Weinstein RA, Young LS: Other procedure-related infections. In Bennett JV, Brachman PS (eds): *Hospital Infections.* Boston, Little, Brown, and Co, 1979, pp 498–499.

77. Swartz MN: Neurology—VIII Infections. In Rubenstein E, Federman DD (eds): *Scientific American Medicine.* New York, Scientific American, 1982, pp 11 VIII-1–11 VIII-27.

78. Hodges GR, Perkins RL: Hospital-associated bacterial meningitis. *Am J Med Sci* 271:335–341, 1976.

79. New PFJ, Davis KR: The role of CT scanning in diagnosis of infections of the central nervous system. In Remington JS, Swartz MN (eds): *Current Clinical Topics in Infectious Diseases.* New York, McGraw-Hill, 1980, vol 1, pp 1–33.

80. Schoenbaum SC, Gardner P, Shillito J: Infections of cerebrospinal fluid shunts: epidemiology, clinical manifestations, and therapy. *J Infect Dis* 131:543–552, 1975.

81. Tomaszek DE, Jones FD: Treatment of infected intracranial shunts and reservoirs. *Infect Surg* (July):489–492, 1984.

82. Ratcheson RA, Ommaya AK: Experience with the subcutaneous cerebrospinal-fluid reservoir. Preliminary report of 60 cases. *N Engl J Med* 279:1025–1031, 1968.

83. Carey ME: Infectious diseases. In Rosenberg RN (ed): *The Clinical Neurosciences.* New York, Churchill Livingstone, 1983, pp II:1211–II:1256.

84. Green JR, Kanshepolsky J, Turkian B: Incidence and significance of central nervous system infections in neurosurgical patients. *Adv Neurol* 6:223–228, 1974.

85. Sklutety FM, Nishioka H: Report on the Cooperative Study on Intracranial Aneurysms and Subarachnoid Hemorrhage. Section VIII, part 2. The results of intracranial surgery in the treatment of aneurysms. *J Neurosurg* 25:683–704, 1966.

86. Balch RE: Wound infections complicating neurosurgical procedures. *J Neurosurg* 26:41–45, 1967.

87. Savitz MH, Malis LI, Meyers BR: Prophylactic antibiotics in neurosurgery. *Surg Neurol* 2:95–100, 1974.

88. Buckwold FJ, Hand R, Hansebout RR: Hospital-acquired bacterial meningitis in neurosurgical patients. *J Neurosurg* 46:494–500, 1977.

89. Malis LI: Prevention of neurosurgical infection by

intraoperative antibiotics. *Neurosurgery* 5:339–343, 1979.

90. Quartey GRC, Polyzoidis K: Intraoperative antibiotic prophylaxis in neurosurgery: a clinical study. *Neurosurgery* 8:669–671, 1981.

91. White RJ, Dakters G, Yashon D, Albin MS: Temporary control of cerebrospinal fluid volume and pressure by means of an externalized valve-drainage system. *J Neurosurg* 30:264–269, 1969.

92. Sundbarg G, Kjallquist A, Lundberg N, Ponten U: Complications due to prolonged ventricular fluid pressure recording in clinical practice. In Brock M, Dietz H (eds): *Intracranial Pressure. Experimental and Clinical Aspects.* Berlin, Springer-Verlag, 1972, pp 348–352.

93. Wyler AR, Kelly WA: Use of antibiotics with external ventriculostomies. *J Neurosurg* 37:185–187, 1972.

94. Smith RW, Alksne JF: Infections complicating the use of external ventriculostomy. *J Neurosurg* 44:567–570, 1976.

95. Mayhall CG, Archer NH, Lamb VA, Spadora AC, Baggett JW, Ward JD, Narayan RK: Ventriculostomy-related infections. A prospective epidemiologic study. *N Engl J Med* 310:553–559, 1984.

96. Vries JK, Becker DP, Young HF: A subarachnoid screw for monitoring intracranial pressure. Technical note. *J Neurosurg* 39:416–419, 1973.

97. Rosner MJ, Becker DP: ICP monitoring: complications and associated factors. *Clin Neurosurg* 23:494–519, 1976.

98. Winn HR, Dacey RG, Jane JA: Intracranial subarachnoid pressure recording: experience with 650 patients. *Surg Neurol* 8:41–47, 1977.

99. Little JR, Rhoton AL Jr, Mellinger JF: Comparison of ventriculoperitoneal and ventriculoatrial shunts for hydrocephalus in children. *Mayo Clin Proc* 47:396–401, 1972.

100. Venes JL: Control of shunt infection. Report of 150 consecutive cases. *J Neurosurg* 45:311–314, 1976.

101. Sayers MP: Shunt complications. *Clin Neurosurg* 23:393–400, 1976.

102. George R, Leibrock L, Epstein M: Long-term analysis of cerebrospinal fluid shunt infections. A 25-year experience. *J Neurosurg* 51:804–811, 1979.

103. Diamond RD, Bennett JE: A subcutaneous reservoir for intrathecal therapy of fungal meningitis. *N Engl J Med* 288:186–188, 1973.

104. Borzone M, Capuzzo T, Rivano C, Silvestro C: Utilization of one hundred subcutaneous reservoirs in neurosurgery. *J Neurosurg Sci* 24:21–25, 1980.

105. Stamm WE: Infections related to medical devices. *Ann Intern Med* 89 (part 2):764–769, 1978.

106. Horwitz NH, Rizzoli HV: *Postoperative Complications of Intracranial Neurological Surgery.* Baltimore, Williams & Wilkins, 1982, pp 389–395.

107. Duffey P, Wolf J, Collins G, DeVoe AG, Streeten B, Cowen D: Possible person-to-person transmission of Creutzfeldt-Jakob disease. *N Engl J Med* 290:692–693, 1974.

108. Houff SA, Burton RC, Wilson RW, Henson TE, London WT, Baer GM, Anderson LJ, Winkler WG, Madden DL, Sever JL: Human-to-human transmission of rabies virus by corneal transplant. *N Engl J Med* 300:603–604, 1979.

109. Jones SR, Luby JP, Sanford JP: Bacterial meningitis complicating cranial-spinal trauma. *J Trauma* 13:895–900, 1973.

110. Romig DA, Voth DW, Liu C, Brackett CE: Bacterial flora and infection in patients with brain injury. *J Neurosurg* 38:710–716, 1973.

111. Mombelli G, Klastersky J, Coppens L, Daneau D, Nubourgh Y: Gram-negative bacillary meningitis in neurosurgical patients. *J Neurosurg* 58:634–641, 1983.

112. Katz PM, Cooper PR: Infectious complications of neurosurgical trauma. *Infect Surg* (Jan):22–32, 1985.

113. Kremer M: Meningitis after spinal analgesia. *Br Med J* 2:309–313, 1945.

114. Cutler M, Cutler P: Iatrogenic meningitis. *J Med Soc NJ* 50:510–514, 1953.

115. Kilpatrick ME, Girgis NI: Meningitis—a complication of spinal anesthesia. *Anesth Analg* 62:513–515, 1983.

116. Sautter RL, Mattman LH, Legaspi RC: *Serratia marcescens* meningitis associated with a contaminated benzalkonium chloride solution. *Infect Control* 5:223–225, 1984.

117. Sarubbi FA Jr, Wilson MB, Lee M, Brokopp C: Nosocomial meningitis and bacteremia due to contaminated amphotericin B. *JAMA* 239:416–418, 1978.

118. Baker CJ: Nosocomial septicemia and meningitis in neonates. *Am J Med* 70:698–701, 1981.

119. Graham DR, Anderson RL, Ariel FE, Ehrenkranz NJ, Rowe B, Boer HR, Dixon RE: Epidemic nosocomial meningitis due to *Citrobacter diversus* in neonates. *J Infect Dis* 144:203–209, 1981.

120. Morgan MEI, Hart CA: *Acinetobacter* meningitis: acquired infection in a neonatal intensive care unit. *Arch Dis Child* 57:557–559, 1982.

121. Whitley RJ, Nahmias AJ, Soong S-J, Galasso GG, Fleming CL, Alford CA: Vidarabine therapy of neonatal herpes simplex infection. *Pediatrics* 66:495–501, 1980.

122. Rantakallio P, Lapinleimu K, Mantyjarvi R: Coxsackie B5 outbreak in a newborn nursery with 17 cases of serous meningitis. *Scand J Infect Dis* 2:17–23, 1970.

123. Chernik NL, Armstrong D, Posner JB: Central nervous system infections in patients with cancer. *Medicine* 52:563–581, 1973.

124. Hooper DC, Pruitt AA, Rubin RH: Central nervous system infection in the chronically immunosuppressed. *Medicine* 61:166–188, 1982.

125. Lipton SA, Hickey WF, Morris JH, Loscalzo J: Candidal infection in the central nervous system. *Am J Med* 76:101–108, 1984.

126. Nahmias AJ, Keyserling HL: Neonatal herpes simplex in context of the TORCH complex. In Holmes KK, Mardh P-A, Sparling FP, Wiesner PJ (eds): *Sexually Transmitted Diseases.* New York, McGraw-Hill, 1984, pp 816–826.

127. Hand WL, Sandford JP: Posttraumatic bacterial meningitis. *Ann Intern Med* 72:869–874, 1970.

128. Pruitt AA, Rubin RH, Karchmer AW, Duncan GW: Neurologic complications of bacterial endocarditis. *Medicine* 57:329–343, 1978.

129. Ayliffe G, Lowbury E, Hamilton J, Small J, Asheshov E, Parker M: Hospital infection with *Pseudomonas aeruginosa* in neurosurgery. *Lancet* 2:365–368, 1965.

130. Price DJE, Sleigh JD: Control of infection due to *Klebsiella aerogenes* in a neurosurgical unit by withdrawal of all antibiotics. *Lancet* 2:1213–1215, 1970.

131. Wright RL: A survey of possible etiologic agents in postoperative craniotomy infections. *J Neurosurg* 25:125–132, 1966.

132. Quadery LA, Medlery AV, Miles J: Factors affecting the incidence of wound infection in neurosurgery. *Acta Neurochir (Wien)* 39:133–141, 1977.

133. Forrest DM, Cooper DGW: Complications of ventriculo-atrial shunts. A review of 455 cases. *J Neurosurg* 29:506–512, 1968.

134. Shurtleff DB, Christie D, Foltz EL: Ventriculoauriculostomy-associated infection. A 12-year study. *J Neurosurg* 35:686–694, 1971.

135. Keucher TR, Mealey J Jr: Long-term results after ventriculoatrial and ventriculoperitoneal shunting for infantile hydrocephalus. *J Neurosurg* 50:179–186, 1979.

136. Linnemann CC Jr, Light IJ, Buchman TG, Ballard JL, Roizman B: Transmission of herpes-simplex virus type 1 in a nursery for the newborn. Identification of viral isolates by DNA "fingerprinting." *Lancet* 1:964–966, 1978.

137. Aisner J, Schimpff SC, Bennett JE, Young VM, Weirnik PH: *Aspergillus* infections in cancer patients. Association with fireproofing materials in a new hospital. *JAMA* 235:411–412, 1976.

138. Raaf J: Posttraumatic cerebrospinal fluid leaks. *Arch Surg* 95:648–651, 1967.

139. Llewellyn RC, Jarrott DM, Meriwether RP: Intraoperative prophylactic antibiotic therapy. A prospective study of the effectiveness, cost and complications. Presented at the annual meeting of the American Academy of Neurological Surgery, Munich, Germany, 1978.

140. McCullough DC, Kane JG, Presper JH, Wells M: Antibiotic prophylaxis in ventricular shunt surgery. I. Reduction of operative infection rates with methicillin. *Child's Brain* 7:182–189, 1980.

141. Epstein MH, Kumor K, Hughes W, Lietman P: The use of prophylactic antibiotics in pediatric shunting operations—a double blind prospective randomized study. Presented at the American Association of Neurological Surgeons Meeting, Honolulu, 1982.

142. Brawley BW, Kelly WA: Treatment of basal skull fractures with and without cerebrospinal fluid fistulae. *J Neurosurg* 26:57–61, 1967.

143. Ignelzi RJ, VanderArk GD: Analysis of the treatment of basilar skull fractures with and without antibiotics. *J Neurosurg* 43:721–726, 1975.

144. Hoff JT, Brewin A, U HS: Antibiotics for basilar skull fracture. *J Neurosurg* 44:649, 1976.

145. Klastersky J, Sadeghi M, Brihaye J: Antimicrobial prophylaxis in patients with rhinorrhea or otorrhea: a double blind study. *Surg Neurol* 6:111–114, 1976.

146. Edwards MS, Baker CJ: *Streptococcus agalactiae* (group B streptococcus). In Mandell GL, Douglas RG Jr, Bennett JE. (eds): *Principles and Practice of Infectious Diseases*, ed 2. New York, John Wiley & Sons, 1985, pp 1155–1161.

147. Oxman MN, Richman DD, Spector SA: Management at delivery of mother and infant when herpes simplex, varicella-zoster, hepatitis or tuberculosis have occurred during pregnancy. In Remington JS, Swartz MN (eds): *Current Clinical Topics in Infectious Diseases.* New York, McGraw-Hill, 1983, vol 4, pp 224–280.

Chapter 26

Prevention of Postcesarean Febrile Morbidity

Margaret Lynn Yonekura, M.D.

In 1984, there were 3.7 million live births in the United States; of these, approximately 20% were cesarean births. During recent decades, the cesarean birth rate in the United States increased 3-fold from 5.5% in 1970 to 15.27% in 1978 (1–5). Eighty percent of the overall increase in the cesarean section rate has been related to the following four indications: dystocia, previous cesarean section, breech presentation, and fetal distress (4–10). However, regardless of the indication cited, the increased frequency of cesarean birth has been accompanied by an absolute decrease in perinatal mortality. A similar dramatic increase in the cesarean birth rate is evident internationally. In Canada, the rate doubled in the 1970s, from 6 to 13.9% (11, 12); likewise, in Sweden, it rose from 5.5% in 1973 to 11.9% in 1979 (13–15).

Any dramatic increase in the frequency of a major operative procedure is inevitably shrouded in controversy. Currently, there is a growing consensus that the cesarean rate has probably exceeded that which can be justified purely on the grounds of improving perinatal mortality (16–19). Presently, more attention is being focused on maternal morbidity and mortality related to cesarean birth (13, 20, 21).

In light of the rapidly increasing cesarean birth rate, it is important to know the mortality risk for women who undergo cesarean section compared with the risk for women who deliver vaginally. Overall, in the United States, maternal mortality per 100,000 deliveries decreased from 25.7 in 1970 to 14.3 in 1978. Mortality in patients delivered by cesarean section has also dropped dramatically, but, nevertheless, remains at least 2 to 4 times higher than that following vaginal delivery (22). Petitti et al reported that in the United States the maternal mortality rate in 1978 was 40.9/100,000 cesarean sections compared with a maternal mortality rate of 9.8/100,000

vaginal deliveries (22). However, wide variations in current estimates of relative safety exist; maternal mortality associated with cesarean section has been reported to be 0 to 26 times greater than that for vaginal delivery (8, 16, 22–27). Currently, the major causes of cesarean section-related deaths include: pulmonary embolism (26, 27), anesthesia-related complications (21, 26, 27), and sepsis (8, 24, 28).

While maternal mortality is low, maternal morbidity is more frequent and likely to be more severe following cesarean section than after vaginal delivery (7, 8, 13, 16, 20, 21). Patients who undergo cesarean section are at least 10 times more likely to experience postpartum morbidity than patients who deliver vaginally (16). Moreover, patients undergoing primary cesarean sections are at an even greater risk for morbidity compared to those undergoing elective, repeat cesarean sections. The most common causes of postcesarean morbidity are infection, hemorrhage, and, less often, injury to the urinary tract (13, 16, 20, 29–31). In this chapter postcesarean infectious morbidity will be reviewed and an attempt made to define rational prevention strategies as well as optimal treatment regimens.

POSTCESAREAN ENDOMYOMETRITIS

Cesarean section is the most important factor predisposing to both the frequency and severity of postpartum endometritis (32–37). Endometritis occurs 7 to 30 times more frequently after cesarean section than after vaginal delivery (37). Bacteremia occurs in 8 to 20% of patients with postcesarean endometritis (38–42), but in only 5% of infected patients who deliver vaginally (43). Moreover, pelvic abscess or septic pelvic thrombophlebitis complicates the course of 4 to 9% of postcesarean endometritis patients (38, 39, 44) and only 1.9% of vaginally delivered endometritis patients (43).

Currently, postcesarean endomyometritis is the most common nosocomial infection treated by obstetrician/gynecologists. It complicates 5 to 6% of elective cesarean sections performed prior to the onset of labor or membrane rupture (7, 13) and 22 to 85% of nonelective cesarean sections (7, 13, 45–47). Moreover, approximately 4% of parturients who develop postcesarean endomyometritis suffer potentially life-threatening complications including septic pelvic thrombophlebitis and pelvic abscess (38, 39, 44). Postcesarean endomyometritis is costly not only in terms of febrile morbidity and infection-related morbidity, but also in terms of direct patient care costs (prolonged hospital stay, antibiotic therapy, secondary operative procedures, etc). Postcesarean endomyometritis prolongs the postpartum hospital stay an average of 3 days (13, 48) and significantly increases the cost of hospitalization (48, 49).

One important prevention strategy is the use of perioperative antibiotic prophylaxis for parturients at "high risk" for developing postcesarean endomyometritis. However, the identification of these "high risk" patients remains problematic. Numerous clinical risk factors have been identified in the literature and are reviewed in detail elsewhere (35, 37, 46, 50). Important intrinsic risk factors include indigent socioeconomic status (33, 34, 51–53), anemia (13, 45, 53, 54), and preterm gestational age at the time of cesarean section (55–59). The three most consistently identified extrinsic risk factors include labor prior to cesarean section (13, 35, 45, 54, 60, 61), duration of ruptured chorioamniotic membranes (13, 45, 47, 54, 60–62), and the number of preoperative vaginal examinations (45, 60, 62, 63) (Table 26.1). Even in the absence of these risk factors, various intraoperative findings or complications may identify the parturient as being at "high risk" for postcesarean endomyometritis. For example, emergency cesarean sections performed for antepartum hemorrhage or fetal distress are associated with a significantly higher postoperative infection

rate (13, 45, 64, 65); a number of confounding variables contribute to their increased infectious morbidity including inadequate operative field prep, breaks in sterile technique, use of general anesthesia, and, perhaps, the tracking of a large inoculum of cervicovaginal flora into the lower uterine segment by the assistant, elevating the fetal presenting part off a prolapsed umbilical cord. Total operating times greater than 60 minutes (20, 60), intraoperative hypotension (13, 45, 53), or meconium-stained amniotic fluid (66, 67) are also useful risk factors for postcesarean endomyometritis that should prompt the obstetrician to initiate antibiotic prophylaxis.

The debate over the use of antibiotic prophylaxis was succinctly reviewed by Mead (68). While recognizing the demonstrated efficacy of prophylactic antibiotics for cesarean section, he cited five problem areas: (a) potential increase in nosocomial infections with resistant organisms and alteration of microflora in treated patients; (b) antimicrobial toxicity; (c) cost; (d) failure to prevent serious pelvic infections (i.e., pelvic abscess or septic pelvic thrombophlebitis); and (e) pediatric considerations. To elaborate on this latter point, he expressed concern about exposing the fetus to such antibiotics if the first dose was given "on call" to the operating room, as was the standard procedure for gynecologic surgery. Since most antibiotics used for prophylaxis readily cross the placenta, pediatricians expressed concern about the potential for hidden or delayed neonatal infections, altered neonatal flora, emergence of resistant pathogens, or the development of superinfections. Some felt compelled to treat these neonates, many of whom were at high risk for neonatal sepsis, with a full course of antibiotic therapy since neonatal cultures obtained after delivery might be falsely negative (69, 70). Several studies have now documented that antibiotic prophylaxis begun immediately after umbilical cord clamping is as effective as that begun preoperatively in terms of decreasing the incidence of postcesarean infectious morbidity (70–73).

Table 26.1. Extrinsic Risk Factors for Postcesarean Endomyometritis*

Risk Factor	Gibbs et al (62)	Hawrylyshyn et al (45)	Green and Sarubbi (54)
Labor	4.1	1.0	1.8
Ruptured membranes	2.6	2.2	NS
Number of vaginal exams	2.2	1.5	NS
Internal fetal monitoring	1.0	NS	NS

* Numbers represent the relative risk found in study, i.e., the increased risk of infection developing when a given risk factor is present compared to the risk without that risk factor. Without risk factor, relative risk = 1. NS, not significant (37, 45).

Another concern voiced against routine use of antibiotic prophylaxis at cesarean section was that severe infectious complications such as septic pelvic thrombophletibis or pelvic abscess were not prevented (68). However, if one successfully decreases the overall incidence of postcesarean endomyometritis, one will necessarily decrease the incidence of these serious complications as well; moreover, a better understanding as to the optimal treatment of postcesarean endomyometritis has simultaneously resulted in a decrease in these complications (44).

There is now general agreement that perioperative antibiotic prophylaxis should begin immediately after cord clamping, or at least within 2 hours after making the skin incision (74), in patients deemed at "high risk" for postcesarean endomyometritis (46, 75). However, there is no concensus about the routine use of antibiotic prophylaxis for "low risk" cesarean sections (45, 60, 71, 76–82). Many suggest that, in the case of the latter, the risk:benefit ratio is > 1 and the cost of preventing every infected case is too great to warrant the routine use of antibiotic prophylaxis (75).

Selection of the ideal antibiotic for prophylaxis is also a controversial subject. Overall, various antibiotics used alone or in combinations have succeeded in reducing the incidence of postcesarean infectious morbidity by 50% compared to a placebo control (46, 68, 75). However, the spectrum of activity of such antibiotics or antibiotic combinations has varied widely, suggesting that the optimal spectrum of activity is not known. To address this issue, we studied the microbiology of amniotic membrane cultures obtained from 452 consecutive afebrile parturients undergoing cesarean section; cultures were obtained after umbilical cord clamping and prior to the initiation of antibiotic prophylaxis (83). Table 26.2 summarizes the distribution of organisms recovered. In light of these data and the expand-

Table 26.2. Distribution of Amniotic Membrane Culture Isolates from 452 Afebrile Parturients Undergoing Cesarean Section (83)

Bacterial Isolates	Number
No growth	55
Low virulence isolates	462 (59%)
Aerobic gram-positive	141 (18%)
Aerobic gram-negative	33 (4%)
Anaerobic gram-positive	72 (9%)
Anaerobic gram-negative	78 (10%)
Total isolates	786

ing body of literature documenting the problems of antibiotic resistance, particularly with respect to certain aerobic gram-negative bacteria exposed to second and third generation cephalosporins (68, 84–87), it may be preferable to use antibiotics which provide more selected coverage for cesarean section prophylaxis, rather than to continue the present "shotgun" approach. The enhanced gram-negative spectra offered by second and third generation cephalosporins may not be necessary since facultative gram-negative bacilli resistant to first generation cephalosporins are rarely recovered from amniotic fluid or amniotic membrane cultures obtained at cesarean section. Moreover, the decreased aerobic gram-positive coverage provided by these newer cephalosporins may decrease their efficacy in preventing postcesarean infectious morbidity. Thus, their excessive cost seems unwarranted since they offer no particular advantage over less expensive first generation cephalosporins (88–90).

The next issue to consider is the optimal route of delivery for antibiotic prophylaxis—intravenous, intramuscular, or intrauterine and intraperitoneal lavage? In 1980, Long et al (91) published their experience irrigating the uterus, abdominal gutters, and abdominal incision with a solution containing 2 g of cefamandole in 800 ml of saline. They documented a significant decrease in the incidence of postcesarean endomyometritis in the cefamandole lavage group compared to those irrigated with saline alone or not irrigated at all. Follow-up studies by the same authors reinforced the efficacy of this method of prophylaxis (92, 93). In their opinion, this technique provided high concentrations of antibiotic to the site of bacterial contamination without producing significant serum levels of antibiotic. This technique quickly became quite popular among obstetricians. Other antibiotics delivered by the lavage technique were also studied (94–97). Duff et al (97) documented antibiotic pharmacokinetics resulting from intraoperative irrigation at the time of cesarean section. They concluded that although the primary effect of intraoperative irrigation may be to provide a high concentration of antibiotic directly to injured and heavily contaminated tissue, at least part of the effect is due to systemic absorption of the drug with subsequent redistribution to the surgical site. This technique of prophylaxis is, therefore, not devoid of risk for antibiotic-induced allergic reactions or for other potential antibiotic-related complications (antibiotic-associated colitis, shifts in puerperal cervicovaginal flora, etc). Moreover, low serum concentrations of broad spectrum antibiotics delivered by this technique may create selective pressures for the emergence of drug-resistant microorganisms. In addition, there is a potential detrimental effect if the lavage procedure is not done as originally outlined (91)—that is, if the lavage fluid is not completely suctioned out. As Dunn et al (98) have recently demonstrated, large volumes of irrigation fluid left in the peritoneal cavity may prove detrimental by diluting out opsonins, as well as by hindering phagocytosis. Therefore, the irrigation technique offers no advantages over the intravenous administration of the prophylactic antibiotic, is time consuming for the surgeon, and has been shown in one study to be less effective than the intravenous administration of the same antibiotic (96).

The optimal duration of antibiotic prophylaxis for cesarean section has progressively decreased from 5 days to 1 day (46, 68, 72, 75, 81, 99–102). Currently, there is growing support for single-dose antibiotic prophylaxis at cesarean section (96, 101, 102); such protocols offer advantages both to the hospital (decreased number of intravenous piggybacks, decreased nursing time, decreased antibiotic costs) and the parturient (less exposure to drug-induced side effects, shorter need for intravenous line, and, therefore, better ability to bond with neonate, shower, ambulate, etc).

In summary, a single intravenous dose of a first generation cephalosporin with a long half-life given immediately after clamping of the umbilical cord would seem the ideal method of preventing a significant percentage of postcesarean infectious morbidity. Care must be taken to use the proper dose of such an antibiotic in light of the higher glomerular filtration rate typical of pregnancy since subinhibitory doses of antibiotics may impose unique selection pressures for the proliferation of antibiotic-resistant microorganisms (103, 104).

As important as a rational prevention strategy for postcesarean infectious morbidity is the prompt identification of prophylaxis failures and their proper treatment. Any postcesarean patient who has an oral temperature ≥ 101°F during the first 24 hours or ≥ 100.4°F on two occasions at least 4 hours apart on any day thereafter should be carefully evaluated. During the first 24 hours postoperative atelectasis and dehydration are common causes of fever. Infections that usually present in the first 48 hours include postcesarean endomyometritis, urinary tract infections, and respiratory infections. The work-up of patients who become febrile after receiving antibiotic prophylaxis must include a thorough physical examination including a complete pelvic examination; the cervical os must be well dilated to allow egress of lochia and no placental fragments or other foreign bodies should remain in the uterus. At the time of bimanual examination, the size and consistency of the uterus as well as the degree of uterine tenderness can be assessed; the presence of an adnexal mass or pelvic abscess can also be ascertained. A complete blood count, urinalysis, and blood, urine, and endometrial cultures should be obtained (37). The endometrial culture should be obtained preferably using a sheathed technique to avoid contamination of the specimen with cervicovaginal flora (105–107). Endometrial cultures for aerobic and anaerobic bacteria as well as for *Chlamydia trachomatis* should be submitted. Since many patients with postcesarean endomyometritis have evidence of peritonitis, as a result of direct intraperitoneal contamination with intra-amniotic bacteria at the time of delivery, culdocentesis has also been recommended as a useful technique of obtaining a culture specimen (37).

There are important pitfalls to avoid in treating a patient who fails antibiotic prophylaxis and develops post cesarean endomyometritis. First, appropriate pretreatment cultures must be obtained because the antibiotic used for prophylaxis may have selected out unusual pathogens or microorganisms with unusual antibiograms (102, 108–110); such culture results might be crucial, particularly if the patient fails to respond to initial antibiotic therapy. Second, the antibiotic used for prophylaxis should not be used for therapy (109); for example, if a patient received cefoxitin for perioperative prophylaxis, the same agent should not be continued for a longer course of "prophylaxis" if the patient becomes febrile, nor should it be restarted to treat that patient's endomyometritis. Such thoughtless behavior delays the initiation of proper therapy and may thereby prolong the patient's hospital stay and increase the likelihood of serious complications such as septic pelvic thrombophlebitis (SPT) or pelvic abscess formation.

Our improved understanding of the microbiology of postcesarean endomyometritis has dramatically changed our approach to its antibiotic therapy (37, 40, 44). Previously, initial therapy consisted of penicillin plus an aminoglycoside; gram-negative anaerobic coverage was only provided for those who failed to defervesce after 48 to 72 hours (38, 39). However, diZerega et al (40,

44) documented a superior response if initial antibiotic therapy included broad spectrum anaerobic as well as aerobic coverage; in their studies the initial combination of clindamycin plus gentamicin proved superior to the traditional combination of penicillin and gentamicin in terms of decreased febrile morbidity, shorter postoperative hospital stays, and a decrease in serious complications (SPT, pelvic abscess) (Table 26.3). Others have confirmed their findings (111, 112), and currently the combination of clindamycin-aminoglycoside is the gold standard against which all new single agents or combinations for the treatment of postcesarean endomyometritis are compared (42, 113, 114). Iams and Chawla (49) emphasized that therapeutic efficacy of initial antibiotic therapy, frequency of drug administration, and need for ancillary services for each treatment regimen significantly affect the patient's costs.

Penicillin is added when a patient fails to defervesce 48 to 72 hours after the initiation of clindamycin plus gentamicin (40, 44); the rationale is to provide better synergistic coverage for the enterococcus. Patients who remain febrile on triple therapy are re-evaluated completely; a new set of cultures is obtained and a repeat pelvic examination is performed. At this point, the differential diagnosis includes the following: endomyometritis involving organisms resistant to the current therapeutic regimen, SPT, pelvic abscess, wound infection, and mastitis. Another commonly overlooked factor is anemia; in this author's experience the combination of intraoperative and postoperative blood loss coupled with sepsis-related hemolysis may result in hematocrits

Table 26.3. Postcesarean Endomyometritis Treatment Regimens

Author	Treatment Regimen	No.	Cured with Initial Therapy	Additional Antibiotics	Pelvic Abscess	SPT	Wound Infection
diZerega et al (44)	Clindamycin/gentamicin	100	86	5 (5%)	0	0	8
	Penicillin/gentamicin	100	64	29 (29%)	1	2	16
Gibbs et al (38)	Penicillin/kanamycin	160	125	35 (22%)	4	3	11
Cunningham et al (39)	Penicillin/tetracycline	61	52	9 (15%)	4	NS*	8
	Penicillin/tobramycin	45	32	13 (29%)	6	NS	4
Sen et al (111)	Clindamycin/gentamicin	54	54	0	0	0	0
	Cefazolin/gentamicin	51	43	8 (16%)	0	0	0
Duff et al (155)	Penicillin/gentamicin	18	11	7 (39%)	0	1	2
	Cefoxitin	14	7	7 (50%)	1	2	0
Monif and Hempling (112)	Clindamycin/ampicillin	50	40	10 (20%)	0	0	1
	Clindamycin/ampicillin	50	38	12 (24%)	0	0	0
	Penicillin/kanamycin	50	39	11 (22%)	1	4	3
Gibbs et al (113)	Clindamycin/gentamicin	106	93	6 (6%)	0	0	11
	Cefamandole	92	76	13 (14%)	0	0	18
Gibbs et al (42)	Clindamycin/gentamicin	57	51	2 (4%)	0	0	3
	Moxalactam	56	51	4 (7%)	0	0	7
Blanco et al (114)	Clindamycin/tobramycin	35	30	5 (14%)	0	0	2
	Ceftazidime	34	30	4 (12%)	0	0	4
Hemsell et al (156)	Clindamycin/gentamicin	39	37	2 (5%)	1	NS	1
	Cefotaxime	81	79	2 (2.5%)	1	NS	1

* NS, not stated in paper.

in the low twenties. Such patients are sometimes slow to respond to antibiotic therapy and only do so after transfusion to a hematocrit of at least 30%, preferably ~35%; perhaps improved oxygen-carrying capacity is responsible for this observed response.

SPT is a diagnosis of exclusion that complicates the clinical course of 2% of patients with postcesarean endomyometritis (38, 44, 115). This subject has recently been reviewed in detail by Duff and Gibbs (116). Typically, the patient clinically improves after being started on broad spectrum antibiotic therapy; however, she has persistent spiking temperatures and associated tachycardia. The patient does not appear critically ill and positive physical findings are usually absent. Rarely, on pelvic examination, one can feel extremely tender, worm-like indurated pelvic sidewall veins in the lateral fornices. There are no helpful diagnostic radiographic studies; instead, one begins a trial of heparin therapy while continuing broad spectrum antibiotic therapy (117, 118). Heparin therapy must prolong the partial thromboplastin time 2 to 2½ times control; minidose heparin, sometimes used to prevent deep vein thrombophlebitis, is not adequate for the treatment of SPT. If the patient defervesces within 24 to 48 hours, the diagnosis of SPT is confirmed; the combination of heparin plus antibiotics is continued for a minimum of 7 to 10 days, thus allowing the intima of the pelvic vessels to heal and the infected clots to be sterilized. Long term anticoagulation with oral agents does not appear to be necessary unless the patient develops septic pulmonary emboli. The prompt treatment of SPT is important in order to avoid this latter complication; as many as 30 to 40% of patients who develop SPT embolize. Such emboli may involve lungs, liver, or kidneys and may, in turn, result in secondary abscess formation (119).

Approximately 1% of patients with postcesarean endomyometritis develop a pelvic abscess. This may be manifested clinically as an indistinct fullness or as a palpable, fluctuant mass posterior to the uterus in the cul-de-sac which sometimes dissects into the lower portion of the rectal-vaginal septum. Various diagnostic technques have been recommended in the past; however, currently, pelvic ultrasound and CT scans are the most popular diagnostic modalities (120, 121). When a pelvic abscess is appreciated, the patient's antibiotic therapy must be re-evaluated since not all antibiotics are equally efficacious in penetrating and sterilizing abscesses (122). SPT is a common concurrent problem in these patients; there-

fore, heparin therapy may also be required. If the patient defervesces with medical management alone, the size of the abscess can be followed after the patient's discharge home. However, if the patient remains febrile, surgical drainage of the abscess may be necessary. If the abscess is fluctuant and dissects the rectal-vaginal septum to the level of the cervix, it may be amenable to colpotomy drainage (123, 124). On the other hand, an exploratory laparotomy may be necessary, and, in these cases, a total abdominal hysterectomy and bilateral salpingo-oophorectomy are often required to remove all of the infected tissue. At the time of laparotomy, a thorough exploration for secondary abscesses must also be carried out.

Table 26.4 outlines suggested guidelines for the operative management of patients with a postcesarean pelvic abscess.

POSTCESAREAN WOUND INFECTIONS

An infection of the abdominal incision complicates 1.6 to 18% of cesarean sections and is perhaps a more serious infectious complication than endomyometritis (125). Wound infections double the average duration of the patient's postoperative hospital stay, a factor made even more important by today's Diagnosis-Related Groups (126, 127), and significantly increase the cost of hospitalization (126).

Patients at high risk for wound infection include those also at high risk for postcesarean

Table 26.4. Surgical Management of Postcesarean Pelvic Abscess

1. Preoperative intravenous fluid resuscitation
    Optimal preoperative hematocrit > 35%
2. Parenteral broad spectrum antibiotics
    Achieve therapeutic levels preoperatively
3. Foley catheter
4. Intraoperative central monitoring
5. Position of patient on operating room table: not Trendelenburg
6. Anesthesia: general not regional
7. Intraoperative placement of Cantor or Miller-Abbot tube
8. Removal of all infected tissue and drainage of all pus
9. Careful exploration for secondary abscesses: subdiaphragmatic, between loops of bowel
10. Copious intraperitoneal irrigation with normal saline
11. Smead-Jones closure of peritoneum and fascia with monofilament nylon or wire
12. Delayed primary closure of abdominal incision

endomyometritis (127), those with intra-amniotic infection (128, 129), those who become hypotensive during surgery, obese patients, diabetics, patients on steroid therapy, and those who had prolonged preoperative hospital stays or prolonged operating times (130–132). High wound infection rates occur among women with bacteria present in amniotic fluid at the time of cesarean section (47). Eschenbach recovered virtually the same organism from the abdominal wound as from the uterus following cesarean delivery of the infant (37). These data suggest that the abdominal wound becomes contaminated following cesarean section in a manner analogous to contaminated cases during intestinal surgery.

One prevention strategy includes the use of perioperative antibiotic prophylaxis for all afebrile "high risk" patients; as suggested by Burke (74), in order to be effective in the prevention of wound infections, such antibiotic prophylaxis must begin within 2 hours of making the skin incision. The wound infection rate in 18 controlled studies of women undergoing cesarean section was 3% among 1064 who received prophylactic antibiotics and 7.6% among 838 who did not (46). However, in only 3 of the 18 studies was a statistically significant decrease observed among patients who received perioperative antibiotic prophylaxis. Delayed primary wound closure has also been suggested as a safe, simple, and effective means of reducing the incidence of wound infection, particularly for patients with clinical intra-amniotic infection at the time of cesarean section (133). The rate of wound infection was 4% in patients with delayed closure, but 26% in patients with immediate wound closure when infection existed prior to cesarean section. Delay of wound closure actually enhances wound strength through greater metabolism and collagen synthesis; increased angiogenesis increases blood flow and tissue Po_2. Increased oxygen delivery to tissue, in turn, has been shown to decrease the infection rate (134).

In light of the data promulgated by Cruse (130), patients are not routinely shaved for cesarean section, the skin incision is made with a knife rather than an electrocautery device, the wound is irrigated with saline after the fascia is closed and then blotted dry, no sutures or drains are placed in the subcutaneous layer, and, when possible, the skin is closed with a subcuticular technique (135, 136). Attention is paid to the construction of the wound dressing; the first layer consists of a hydrophilic petroleum gauze (Vaseline or Xeroform), the middle layer is an absorbent layer (Intersorb gauze), and the other wrap (Sta-tite) provides stability for the rest of the dressing and enough pressure to obliterate dead space (137). The purpose of the surgical dressing is to prevent wound contamination. Therefore, the wound is kept dressed in this fashion for a variable duration of time depending on the closure technique: for tape or subcuticular closures, 12 to 24 hours; for mattress sutures, 48 hours; for clips, 72 hours (138). Daily care of the suture line, which is particularly important for wounds closed by clips, involves removing any congealed serum and debris with a Q-tip soaked in dilute H_2O_2 and then putting Polysporin ointment along the suture line before redressing the wound. Because ascorbic acid is an essential vitamin for collagen synthesis, all postoperative patients also receive ascorbic acid, 500 mg twice daily.

With the exception of wound infections caused by group A β-hemolytic streptococci, wound infections usually do not become manifest until 5 to 7 days after surgery. The wound is inspected daily for evidence of erythema and induration. If present, warm, moist packs are applied to the incision, often causing the abscess to point and drain spontaneously. If significant quantities of serum, pus, or blood are observed oozing from the wound, it may be necessary to open the wound. Typically, in such cases, removal of the skin sutures or clips and gentle probing of the wound with a sterile Q-tip are all that is necessary to open it completely. Under adequate analgesia, the wound is opened over its entire extent. The wound discharge is gram-stained immediately and submitted for aerobic and anaerobic culture. Wound debridement is the most important part of managing an infected wound; it removes tissue heavily contaminated with bacteria, protecting the patient from invasive infection, and it removes devitalized tissues which impair the wound's ability to resist infection. If major debridement is necessary, it should be performed in the operating room under adequate anesthesia. Minimal amounts of debridement can be accomplished by using soft, highly porous sponges, preferably surfactant-soaked (138). The wound is thoroughly irrigated with dilute Dakin's solution and packed with Dakin's soaked gauze; wet-to-wet dressings are changed at least every 8 hours. Within 24 hours, the wound should be stabilized; i.e., infected, poorly perfused tissue should have been excised and there should be no undrained dead space. Beyond that, wound care consists of waiting for healthy granulation tissue to close the wound secondarily or to close the wound by tertiary intention. Care must be taken not to "poison" the wound with H_2O_2, betadine, or iodoform gauze nor to damage the fragile granulation tissue with abrasives or dry wound packing materials (139). After adopting the above protocol for infected wounds, our average spontaneous closure time decreased dramatically.

There are three serious complications of abdominal wound infections: necrotizing fasciitis, synergistic bacterial gangrene, and wound dehiscence. Although necrotizing fasciitis and synergistic bacterial gangrene are rare complications, the inordinately high mortality rate associated with these complications (20 to 50%) necessitates their prompt diagnosis and aggressive treatment (140). Several points in their differential diagnosis will be briefly mentioned. Necrotizing fasciitis is often, but not exclusively, due to infection by group A, β-hemolytic streptococci (141); it becomes manifest early in the postoperative period, progresses rapidly, and is marked by high spiking fevers and severe systemic signs (142). A pathognomonic sign of necrotizing fasciitis is a dusky discoloration of the skin and small purplish patches with ill defined borders. Synergistic bacterial gangrene, on the other hand, is a slower, more indolent disease process which is initially indistinguishable from other wound infections (143); however, by the tenth day, an erythematous zone surrounding the wound sharply delineates the circumferentially expanding gangrenous zone. Another important differential sign is that in necrotizing fasciitis, there is skin anesthesia at the site of necrosis because underlying cutaneous nerves have been destroyed; in synergistic bacterial gangrene, on the other hand, the lesions are persistently painful. Treatment of both entities consists of early, wide surgical excision and systemic antibiotics.

Wound dehiscence occurred in 12.5% of postcesarean patients with wound infections, and 38% required surgical repair (127). Helmkamp found that dehiscence usually occurred on postoperative day 7 (range: 3 to 5), primarily in midline abdominal incisions closed with catgut (144). Important predisposing factors include (a) wound infection; (b) mechanical factors that place increased tension on the incision line; and (c) metabolic factors that interfere with normal wound healing.

POSTCESAREAN PNEUMONIA

In general, pneumonia is a relatively rare cause of postcesarean febrile morbidity complicating the postpartum course of 0.5 to 3.4% of patients (6, 13) and ranking as the fourth most common nosocomial infection in postcesarean patients. Risk factors predisposing to postoperative pneumonia include the following: obesity ($\geq$ 250 lb), history of chronic pulmonary disease or smoking, American Society of Anesthesiologists classification $\geq$ 2, preoperative hospitalization $\geq$ 2 days, and prolonged operating times (145). In the postoperative period, additional factors such as incisional pain, abdominal muscle dysfunction, narcotics, abdominal distension, and restrictive dressings contribute to altered breathing patterns, thus promoting hypoventilation, progressive microatelectasis, and pulmonary dysfunction.

One prevention strategy is the identification of patients at high risk for postoperative pneumonia who are likely to be delivered by cesarean section; such patients should have a thorough preoperative evaluation of pulmonary function and prompt initiation of any necessary treatment (antibiotics, bronchodilators, or expectorants). The choice of anesthesia must be carefully considered for these high risk patients and the operating time minimized. Another useful approach is preoperative patient education for patients being scheduled for elective cesarean sections or for patients at increased risk for being delivered nonelectively by cesarean section (breech presentation, multiple gestation, previous cesarean section, diabetes mellitus, etc). Patients are taught what they can do both before and after surgery to avoid pulmonary complications. Postoperative pain and pain relief are described, and ways to splint the incision during coughing and deep breathing are demonstrated. Most importantly, the patients are taught how to use the incentive spirometer; preoperative training is then reinforced by the nursing staff during the early postoperative period. Nonelective surgical patients receive instructions on the use of the spirometer within the first 2 hours postoperatively. The incentive spirometer the author prefers (Spirocare) has selectable volume ranges, provides immediate positive reinforcement to encourage the patient to perform sustained maximum inspiratory maneuvers, and also tallies the number of times this goal is achieved. At least one hundred sustained maximal inhalations each day are required to achieve a successful outcome with incentive spirometric therapy (146).

In addition to the use of the incentive spirometer, patients are encouraged to get out of bed and ambulate as soon as practical postoperatively. If this is not possible, the time-honored method of frequent turning, coughing, and deep breathing is utilized to prevent atelectasis and clear tracheobronchial secretions. Morphine is given in small titrated doses to provide adequate postoperative pain relief without depressing the respiratory center.

The clinical manifestations of atelectasis usually become apparent within the first 48 to 72 hours postoperatively. Tachycardia and tachypnea may be the first signs of atelectasis; however, the fever that occurs with atelectasis is not evidence of early pneumonia and does not necessitate antibiotic therapy. Nevertheless, if not aggressively treated, atelectasis will progress to pneumonia. The chapter on nosocomial pneumonia will provide a more complete discussion of this topic.

Aspiration pneumonia is a much feared pulmonary complication resulting in high maternal morbidity and mortality even today (147). At term, the normal pinch-cock mechanisms of the gastroesophageal junction does not prevent gastroesophageal reflux. Moreover, gastric emptying time is prolonged during late pregnancy and especially during labor. Therefore, parturients are at particularly high risk for regurgitation of gastric contents. The rapid induction technique for general anesthesia used for cesarean section also increases the risk of regurgitation and aspiration. Various prevention strategies are utilized to avoid this complication. Patients are instructed not to eat or drink once labor commences. For pain relief in labor, epidural anesthesia is preferred over repetitive doses of narcotics or sedative-tranquilizers, all of which prolong gastric emptying time. Clear antacids are given to all laboring patients every 3 to 4 hours and again just prior to cesarean section (148). When possible, general anesthesia is avoided in favor of regional anesthesia; however, when necessary, endotracheal intubation is carried out after the induction of anesthesia and before delivery of the infant.

POSTCESAREAN URINARY TRACT INFECTIONS

Urinary tract infections (UTIs) are the etiology of febrile morbidity in 2 to 16% of postcesarean patients (7, 13). Some authors report an even higher incidence of UTIs (6), emphasizing the difficulty in interpreting the significance of bacteriuria in a febrile postpartum patient. Such patients may have a lower urinary tract infection, pyelonephritis, endometritis with incidental asymptomatic bacteriuria, or concomitant endometritis and urinary tract infection (37).

Two to 12% of pregnant patients have asymptomatic bacteriuria; the prevalence is higher among multiparous, indigent patients, those with sickle cell trait, and those with a history of clinically apparent UTIs (149). It is well documented that 20 to 40% of pregnant patients with asymptomatic bacteriuria (ASB) will develop an acute symptomatic UTI during pregnancy or the puerperium if ASB is not treated. Intrapartum bladder catheterization causes subsequent bacteriuria in 15% of women who had no prior UTI (150), and patients who have multiple intermittent catheterizations or an indwelling catheter are at higher risk than those who have a single intermittent catheterization. Fortunately, 75% of cases of bacteriuria documented immediately postpartum will spontaneously resolve by the third postpartum day (151).

The prevention of postcesarean UTIs logically begins with the prenatal identification and treatment of patients with ASB. Patients with recurrent UTIs, pyelonephritis during pregnancy, a history of renal stones, or documented urinary tract anomalies are maintained on antibiotic prophylaxis, such as Macrodantin (nitrofurantoin), 100 mg every night, to prevent the development of ASB during pregnancy. Instrumentation of the urinary tract is avoided whenever possible; however, when laboring patients require two or more catheterizations, an indwelling catheter is placed. Moreover, when an indwelling catheter is used, it is kept in place a minimum duration of time; the catheter is generally inserted just prior to surgery and, preferably, removed as soon as the patient is fully recovered from anesthesia. When the patient is being transported with an indwelling catheter, the collecting bag is never raised above the level of the patient's bladder, thus avoiding retrograde spread of bacteria from collecting bag to bladder. Additionally, a closed drainage system must be meticulously maintained.

Occasionally lower uterine segment lacerations occurring at cesarean section come dangerously close to the ureters (20, 31). In such cases, it may be wise to open the dome of the bladder to check the patency of the ureters (indigo-carmine test) and/or to place ureteral stints so that the ureters are not inadvertently ligated during the repair procedure. The bladder is then closed in two layers and, preferably, drained with a suprapubic catheter for ~10 days (31).

Nosocomial UTIs are discussed in more detail in Chapter 21; however, a few general statements will be made here. The empiric treatment of postcesarean urinary tract infections should be based on the typical antibiogram of community-acquired *Escherichia coli* at one's institution since this organism is responsible for 80 to 90% of UTIs. However, the need for obtaining a pretreatment culture cannot be overly stressed, particularly in light of the selection pressures often imposed by perioperative antibiotic prophylaxis. For example, a significant increase in the incidence of postcesarean enterococcal urinary tract infections has been documented after the use of various second and third generation cephalosporins. Moreover, patients who develop puerperal pyelonephronephritis should have a thorough urologic work-up including an intravenous pyelogram 2 to 3 months postpartum; many of these patients have urinary tract abnormalities predisposing to UTI (152, 153).

SUMMARY

In conclusion, the current high cesarean birth rate necessitates a two-pronged approach to the successful prevention of postcesarean section febrile morbidity. First, we must lower the cesarean birth rate by reevaluating the growing list of indications for cesarean section and identifying patients who might be safely delivered vaginally. Second, the various prevention strategies discussed in this chapter must be integrated into obstetrical practice. Moreover, we must not forget the simple, inexpensive, yet effective measures that can significantly decrease puerperal infectious morbidity (49, 154); rigorous application of aseptic techniques is still the key to preventing nosocomial infections.

References

1. Placek PJ, Taffel SM: Trends in cesarean section rates in the United States, 1970–78. *Public Health Rep* 95:540, 1980.
2. Petitti D, Olson RO, Williams RL: Cesarean section in California—1960 through 1975. *Am J Obstet Gynecol* 133:391–397, 1979.
3. Bottoms SF, Rosen MG, Sokol RJ: The increase in cesarean birth rate. *N Engl J Med* 302:559–563, 1980.
4. NIH Consensus Development Task Force: Statement on cesarean childbirth. *Am J Obstet Gynecol* 139:902–909, 1977.
5. *Cesarean Childbirth: Report of the NICHD Task Force on Cesarean Childbirth.* Bethesda, National Institutes of Health, 1981.
6. Haddad H, Lundy LE: Changing indications for cesarean section. A 38 year experience at a community hospital. *Obstet Gynecol* 51:133–137, 1978.
7. Farrel SJ, Anderson HF, Work BA: Cesarean section: indications and post-operative morbidity. *Obstet Gynecol* 56:696–700, 1980.
8. Amirika H, Zarewych B, Evans TN: Cesarean section: a 15-year review of changing incidence, indications, and risks. *Am J Obstet Gynecol* 140:81–86, 1981.
9. Sokol RJ, Rosen MG, Bottoms SF, Chik L: Risks preceding increased primary cesarean birth rates. *Obstet Gynecol* 59:340–346, 1982.
10. Gilstrap LC, Hauth JC, Toussaint S: Cesarean section: changing incidence and indications. *Obstet Gynecol* 63:205–208, 1984.
11. Anderson GM, Lomas J: Determinants of the increasing cesarean birth rate. Ontario data 1979 to 1982. *N Engl J Med* 311:887–892, 1984.
12. Baskett TK, McMillen RM: Cesarean section: trends and morbidity. *Can Med Assoc J* 125:723–726, 1981.
13. Nielsen TF, Hokegard K-H: Postoperative cesarean section morbidity: a prospective study. *Am J Obstet Gynecol* 146:911–916, 1983.
14. Johnell HE, Osteberg H, Wahlstrand T: Increasing caesarean section rate. *Acta Obstet Gynaecol Scand* 55:95–100, 1978.
15. Patek E, Larsson B: Cesarean section, a clinical study with special reference to the increasing section rate. *Acta Obstet Gynaecol Scand* 57:245–248, 1978.
16. Minkoff HL, Schwarz RH: The rising cesarean section rate: can it safely be reversed? *Obstet Gynecol* 56:135–143, 1980.
17. Sachs BP, McCarthy BJ, Rubin G, Burton A, Terry J, Tyler CW: Cesarean section: risk and benefits for mother and fetus. *JAMA* 250:2157–2159, 1983.
18. O'Driscoll K, Foley M: Correlation of decrease in perinatal mortality and increase in cesarean section rates. *Obstet Gynecol* 61:1–5, 1983.
19. Pearson JW: Cesarean section and perinatal mortality. A nine-year experience in a city/county hospital. *Am J Obstet Gynecol* 148:155–159, 1984.
20. Nielsen TF, Hokegard K-H: Cesarean section and intraoperative surgical complications. *Acta Obstet Gynaecol Scand* 63:103–108, 1984.
21. Jones OH: Cesarean section in present-day obstetrics. *Am J Obstet Gynecol* 126:521–530, 1976.
22. Petitti DB, Cefalo RC, Shapiro S, Whalley P: In-hospital maternal mortality in the United States: time trends and relation to method of delivery. *Obstet Gynecol* 59:6–12, 1982.
23. Benaron HB, Tucker BE: The effect of obstetric management and factors beyond clinical control on maternal mortality rates at the Chicago Maternity Center from 1959 to 1963. *Am J Obstet Gynecol* 110:1113–1118, 1971.
24. Evrard JR, Gold EM: Cesarean section and maternal mortality in Rhode Island. Incidence and risk factors, 1965–1975. *Obstet Gynecol* 50:594–597, 1977.
25. Frigoletto FD, Ryan KJ, Phillippe M: Maternal mortality rate associated with cesarean section: an appraisal. *Am J Obstet Gynecol* 136:969–970, 1980.
26. Rubin GL, Peterson HB, Rochat RW, McCarthy BJ, Terry JS: Maternal death after cesarean section in Georgia. *Am J Obstet Gynecol* 139:681–685, 1981.
27. Moldin P, Hokegard K-H, Nielsen TF: Cesarean section and maternal mortality in Sweden 1973–1979. *Acta Obstet Gynaecol Scand* 63:7–11, 1984.

28. Stevenson CS, Behney CA, Miller NF: Maternal death from puerperal sepsis following cesarean section. A 16-year study in Michigan. *Obstet Gynecol* 29:181–191, 1967.

29. Evrard JR, Gold EM, Cahill TF: Cesarean section: a contemporary assessment. *J Reprod Med* 24:147–152, 1980.

30. Buckspan MB, Simha S, Klotz PG: Vesicouterine fistula: a rare complication of cesarean section. *Obstet Gynecol* 62:64S–66S, 1983.

31. Eisenkop SM, Richman R, Platt LD, Paul RH: Urinary tract injury during cesarean section. *Obstet Gynecol* 60:591–596, 1982.

32. Goplerud CP, White CA: Postpartum infection. A comparative study for the period 1926 through 1961. *Obstet Gynecol* 25:227–231, 1965.

33. Sweet RL, Ledger WJ: Puerperal infectious morbidity. A two-year review. *Am J Obstet Gynecol* 117:1093–1100, 1973.

34. Gibbs RS, Weinstein AJ: Puerperal infection in the antibiotic era. *Am J Obstet Gynecol* 124:769–787, 1976.

35. Gibbs RS: Clinical risk factors for puerperal infection. *Obstet Gynecol* 55:178S–183S, 1980.

36. Filker R, Monif G: The significance of temperature during the first 24 hours postpartum. *Obstet Gynecol* 53:358–361, 1979.

37. Eschenbach DA: The diagnosis of fever occurring in a postpartum patient. In Remington J, Swartz M (eds): *Current Clinical Topics in Infectious Diseases.* New York, McGraw-Hill, 1983, vol 4, pp 186–223.

38. Gibbs RS, Jones PM, Wilder C: Antibiotic therapy of endometritis following cesarean section: treatment successes and failures. *Obstet Gynecol* 52:31–37, 1978.

39. Cunningham FG, Hauth JC, Strong JD, Kappus SS: Infectious morbidity following cesarean section. Comparison of two treatment regimens. *Obstet Gynecol* 52:656–661, 1978.

40. diZerega GS, Yonekura ML, Keegan K, Roy S, Nakamura R, Ledger W: Bacteremia in post-cesarean section endomyometritis: differential response to therapy. *Obstet Gynecol* 55:587–590, 1980.

41. Gibbs RS, Huff RW: Cefamandole therapy of endomyometritis following cesarean section. *Am J Obstet Gynecol* 136:32–37, 1980.

42. Gibbs RS, Blanco JD, Duff P, Castaneda Y, St Clair PJ: A double-blind, randomized comparison of moxalactam versus clindamycin-gentamicin in treatment of endomyometritis after cesarean section delivery. *Am J Obstet Gynecol* 146:769–772, 1983.

43. Gibbs RS, Rodgers PJ, Castaneda YS, Ramzy I: Endometritis following vaginal delivery. *Obstet Gynecol* 56:555–558, 1980.

44. diZerega GS, Yonekura ML, Roy S, Nakamura R, Ledger WJ: The treatment of post-cesarean section endomyometritis. *Am J Obstet Gynecol* 134:238–242, 1979.

45. Hawrylyshyn PA, Bernstein P, Papsin FR: Risk factors associated with infection following cesarean section. *Am J Obstet Gynecol* 139:294–298, 1981.

46. Swartz WH, Grolle K: The use of prophylactic antibiotics in cesarean section. A review of the literature. *J Reprod Med* 26:595–609, 1981.

47. Gilstrap LC, Cunningham FG: The bacterial pathogenesis of infection following cesarean section. *Obstet Gynecol* 53:545–549, 1979.

48. Donowitz LG, Wenzel RP: Endometritis following cesarean section. A controlled study of the increased duration of hospital stay and direct cost of hospitalization. *Am J Obstet Gynecol* 137:467–469, 1980.

49. Iams JD, Chawla A: Patient costs in the prevention and treatment of post-cesarean section infection. *Am J Obstet Gynecol* 149:363–366, 1984.

50. Yonekura ML: Risk factors for post-cesarean endomyometritis. *Am J Med* 78:177–187, 1985.

51. Harger JH, English DH: Selection of patients for antibiotic prophylaxis in cesarean sections. *Am J Obstet Gynecol* 141:752–758, 1981.

52. Gall SA: The efficacy of prophylactic antibiotics in cesarean section. *Am J Obstet Gynecol* 134:506–511, 1979.

53. Ott WJ: Primary cesarean section: factors related to postpartum infection. *Obstet Gynecol* 57:171–176, 1981.

54. Green SL, Sarubbi FA: Risk factors associated with post cesarean section febrile morbidity. *Obstet Gynecol* 49:686–690, 1977.

55. Larsen B, Galask RP: Host resistance to intraamniotic infection. *Obstet Gynecol Surv* 30:675–691, 1975.

56. Schlievert P, Johnson W, Galask RP: Amniotic fluid antibacterial mechanisms. Newer concepts. *Semin Perinatal* 1:59–70, 1977.

57. Schlievert P, Larsen B, Johnson W, Galask RP: Bacterial growth inhibition by amniotic fluid. III. Demonstration of the variability of bacterial growth inhibition by amniotic fluid with a new plate-count technique. *Am J Obstet Gynecol* 122:809–813, 1975.

58. Daikoku NH, Kaltreider DF, Khouzami VA, Spence M, Johnson JWC: Premature rupture of membranes and spontaneous preterm labor: maternal endometritis risks. *Obstet Gynecol* 59:13–20, 1982.

59. Minkoff HL, Henry V, DeCresce R, Schwarz RH: The relationship of amniotic fluid phosphate-to-zinc ratios to post-cesarean section infection. *Am J Obstet Gynecol* 14:988–991, 1982.

60. Rehu M, Nilsson CG: Risk factors for febrile morbidity associated with cesarean section. *Obstet Gynecol* 56:269–273, 1980.

61. Duff P, Gibbs RS, St Clair PJ, Weinberg LC: Correlation of laboratory and clinical criteria in the prediction of post cesarean endomyometritis. *Obstet Gynecol* 63:781–786, 1984.

62. Gibbs RS, Jones PM, Wilder C: Internal fetal monitoring and maternal infection following cesarean section. *Obstet Gynecol* 52:193–197, 1978.

63. D'Angelo LJ, Sokol RJ: Time-related peripartum determinants of postpartum morbidity. *Obstet Gynecol* 55:319–323, 1980.

64. Hagglund L, Christensen KK, Christensen P, Kamme C: Risk factors in cesarean section infection. *Obstet Gynecol* 62:145–150, 1983.

65. Wallace RL, Yonekura ML: The use of prophylactic antibiotics in patients undergoing emergency primary cesarean section. *Am J Obstet Gynecol* 147:533–536, 1983.

66. Florman AL, Teubner D: Enhancement of bacterial growth in amniotic fluid by meconium. *J Pediatr* 74:111–114, 1969.

67. Bryan C: Enhancement of bacterial infection by meconium. *Johns Hopkins Med J* 121:9, 1967.

68. Mead PB: Prophylactic antibiotics and antibiotic resistance. *Semin Perinatal* 1:101–111, 1977.

69. Siegel JD, McCracken GH: Sepsis neonatorum. *N Engl J Med* 304:642–647, 1979.

70. Cunningham FG, Leveno KJ, DePalma RT, Roark M, Rosenfeld CR: Perioperative antimicrobials for cesarean delivery: before or after cord clamping? *Obstet Gynecol* 62:151–154, 1983.

71. Gordon HR, Phelps D, Blanchard K: Prophylactic cesarean section antibiotics: maternal and neonatal morbidity before or after cord clamping. *Obstet Gynecol* 53:151–156, 1979.

72. Padilla SL, Spence MR, Beauchamp PJ: Single-dose ampicillin for cesarean section prophylaxis. *Obstet Gynecol* 61:463–466, 1983.

73. Wong R, Gee CL, Ledger WJ: Prophylactic use of cefazolin in monitored obstetric patients undergoing cesarean section. *Obstet Gynecol* 51:407–411, 1978.

74. Burke JF: The effective period of preventative antibiotic action in experimental incisions and dermal lesions. *Surgery* 50:161–168, 1961.

75. Cartwright PS, Pittaway DE, Jones HW, Entman SS: The use of prophylactic antibiotics in obstetrics and gynecology. A review. *Obstet Gynecol Surv* 39:537–554, 1984.

76. Kreutner AK, DelBene V, Delamar D, Huguley V, Harmon P, Mitchell K: Perioperative antibiotic prophylaxis in cesarean section. *Obstet Gynecol* 52:279–284, 1978.

77. Tully JL, Klapholz H, Baldini LM, Friedland GH: Perioperative use of cefoxitin in primary cesarean section. *J Reprod Med* 28:827–832, 1983.

78. Phelan JP, Pruyn SC: Prophylactic antibiotics in cesarean section. A double-blind study of cefazolin. *Am J Obstet Gynecol* 133:474–478, 1979.

79. Gibbs R, DeCherney A, Schwarz R: Prophylactic antibiotics in cesarean section. A double-blind study. *Am J Obstet Gynecol* 114:1048–1053, 1972.

80. Itskovitz J, Paldi E, Katz M: The effect of prophylactic antibiotics on febrile morbidity following cesarean section. *Obstet Gynecol* 53:162–165, 1979.

81. Apuzzio JJ, Reyelt C, Pelosi M, Sen P, Louria D: Prophylactic antibiotics for cesarean section: comparison of high- and low-risk patients for endomyometritis. *Obstet Gynecol* 59:693–698, 1982.

82. Duff P, Smith P, Keiser JF: Antibiotic prophylaxis in low-risk cesarean section. *J Reprod Med* 27:133–138, 1982.

83. Yonekura ML, Boucher M, Appleman M: Amniotic membrane cultures: bacteriologic correlates of clinical risk factors predisposing to post-cesarean endometritis. Presented at the Annual Meeting of the Infectious Disease Society for Obstetrics and Gynecology, Grand Bahamas Island, July 1983.

84. Gootz TD, Sanders CC, Goering RV: Resistance to cefamandole: derepression of β-lactamases by cefoxitin and mutation in *Enterobacter cloacae*. *J Infect Dis* 146:34–42, 1982.

85. Sanders CC: Novel resistance selected by the new expanded-spectrum cephalosporins: a concern. *J Infect Dis* 147:585–589, 1983.

86. Sanders CC, Moellering RC, Martin RR, Perkins RL, Strike DG, Gootz TD, Sanders WE: Resistance to cefamandole: a collaborative study of emerging clinical problems. *J Infect Dis* 145:118–125, 1982.

87. Sanders CC, Sanders WE: Microbial resistance to newer generation β-lactam antibiotics: clinical and laboratory implications. *J Infect Dis* 151:399–406, 1985.

88. Kreutner AK, DelBene VE, Delamar D, Bodden J, Loadholt C: Perioperative cephalosporin prophylaxis in cesarean section: effect on endometritis in the high-risk patient. *Am J Obstet Gynecol* 134:925–933, 1979.

89. Stiver H, Forward K, Livingstone R, Fugere P, Lemay M, Verschelder G, Hunter J, Carson G, Beresford P, Tyrrell D: Multicenter comparison of cefoxitin versus cefazolin for prevention of infectious morbidity after nonelective cesarean section. *Am J Obstet Gynecol* 145:158–163, 1983.

90. Rayburn W, Varner M, Galask R, Petzold C, Piehl E: Comparison of moxalactam and cefazolin as prophylactic antibiotics during cesarean section. *Antimicrob Agents Chemother* 27:337–339, 1985.

91. Long WN, Rudd E, Dillon M: Intrauterine irrigation with cefamandole nafate solution at cesarean section: a preliminary report. *Am J Obstet Gynecol* 138:755–758, 1980.

92. Rudd E, Long W, Dillon M: Febrile morbidity following cefamandole nafate intrauterine irrigation during cesarean section. *Am J Obstet Gynecol* 141:12–16, 1981.

93. Rudd E, Cobey E, Long W, Dillon M, Matthews M: Prevention of endomyometritis using antibiotic irrigation during cesarean section. *Obstet Gynecol* 60:413–416, 1982.

94. Levin D, Gorchels C, Andersen R: Reduction of postcesarean section infectious morbidity by means of antibiotic irrigation. *Am J Obstet Gynecol* 147:273–277, 1983.

95. Flaherty J, Boswell G, Winkel C, Elliott J: Pharmacokinetics of cefoxitin in patients at term: lavage versus intravenous administration. *Am J Obstet Gynecol* 146:760–766, 1983.

96. Conover W, Moore T: Comparison of irrigation and intravenous antibiotic prophylaxis at cesarean section. *Obstet Gynecol* 63:787–791, 1984.

97. Duff P, Gibbs R, Jorgensen J, Alexander G: The pharmacokinetics of prophylactic antibiotics administered by intraoperative irrigation at the time of cesarean section. *Obstet Gynecol* 60:409–412, 1982.

98. Dunn DL, Barke RA, Ahrenholz DH, Humphrey EW, Simmons RL: The adjuvant effect of peritoneal fluid in experimental peritonitis. Mechanisms and clinical implications. *Ann Surg* 199:37–43, 1984.

99. D'Angelo L, Sokol R: Short- versus long-course prophylactic antibiotic treatment in cesarean section patients. *Obstet Gynecol* 55:583–586, 1980.

100. DePalma R, Cunningham FG, Leveno K, Roark M: Continuing investigation of women at high risk for infection following cesarean delivery. 3-dose perioperative antimicrobial therapy. *Obstet Gynecol* 60:53–59, 1982.

101. Hawrylyshyn P, Bernstein P, Papsin F: Short-term antibiotic prophylaxis in high-risk patients following cesarean section. *Am J Obstet Gynecol* 145:285–289, 1983.

102. Gonik B: Single- versus three-dose cefotaxime prophylaxis for cesarean section. *Obstet Gynecol* 65:189–192, 1985.

103. Washington JA: The effects and significance of subminimal inhibitory concentrations of antibiotics. *Rev Infect Dis* 1:781–786, 1979.

104. Shibl A: Effect of antibiotics on production of enzymes and toxins by microorganisms. *Rev Infect Dis* 5:865–875, 1983.

105. Pezzlo MT, Hesser J, Morgan T: Improved laboratory efficiency and diagnostic accuracy with new double-lumen-protected swab for endometrial specimens. *J Clin Microbiol* 9:56, 1979.

106. Knuppel RA, Scerbo J, Dzink J, Mitchell G, Cetrulo C, Bartlett J: Quantitative transcervical uterine cultures with a new device. *Obstet Gynecol* 57:243–248, 1981.

107. Duff P, Gibbs R, Blanco J, St Clair P: Endometrial culture techniques in puerperal patients. *Obstet Gynecol* 61:217–222, 1983.

108. Gibbs R, Weinstein A: Bacteriologic effects of prophylactic antibiotics in cesarean section. *Am J Obstet Gynecol* 126:226–229, 1976.

109. Gibbs R, St Clair R, Castillo M, Castaneda Y: Bacteriologic effects of antibiotic prophylaxis in high-risk cesarean section. *Obstet Gynecol* 57:277–282, 1981.

110. Stiver H, Forward K, Tyrrell D, Krip G, Livingstone R, Fugere P, Lemay M, Verschelden G, Hunter J, Carson G, Beresford P: Comparative cervical microflora shifts after cefoxitin or cefazolin prophylaxis against infection following cesarean section. *Am J Obstet Gynecol* 149:718–721, 1984.

111. Sen P, Apuzzio J, Reyelt C, Kaminski T, Levy F, Kapila R, Middleton J, Louria D: Prospective evaluation of combinations of antimicrobial agents for endometritis after cesarean section. *Surg Gynecol Obstet* 151:89–92, 1980.

112. Monif G, Hempling R: Antibiotic therapy for the Bacteriodaceae in post-cesarean section infections. *Obstet Gynecol* 57:177–181, 1981.

113. Gibbs R, Blanco J, Castaneda Y, St Clair P: A double-blind, randomized comparison of clindamycin-gentamicin versus cefamandole for treatment of post-cesarean endomyometritis. *Am J Obstet Gynecol* 144:261–267, 1982.

114. Blanco J, Gibbs R, Duff P, Castaneda Y, St Clair P: Randomized comparison of ceftazidime versus clindamycin-tobramycin in the treatment of obstetrical and gynecological infections. *Antimicrob Agents Chemother* 24:500–504, 1983.

115. Cohen M, Pernoll M, Gevirtz C, Kerstein M: Septic pelvic thrombophlebitis: an update. *Obstet Gynecol* 62:83–89, 1983.

116. Duff P, Gibbs R: Pelvic vein thrombophlebitis: diagnostic dilemma and therapeutic challenge. *Obstet Gynecol Surv* 38:365–373, 1983.

117. Josey W, Cook C: Septic pelvic thrombophlebitis. Report of 17 patients treated with heparin. *Obstet Gynecol* 35:891–897, 1970.

118. Josey W, Staggers S: Heparin therapy in septic pelvic thrombophlebitis: a study of 46 cases. *Am J Obstet Gynecol* 120:228–233, 1974.

119. Griffith G, Maul K, Sachatello C: Septic pulmonary embolization. *Surg Gynecol Obstet* 144:105–108, 1977.

120. Maklad N, Doust B, Baum J: Ultrasound diagnosis of postoperative intraabdominal abscess. *Radiology* 113:417–422, 1974.

121. Norton L, Eule J, Burdick D: Accuracy of tests to detect intraperitoneal abscesses. *Surgery* 84:370, 1978.

122. Bartlet J: Recent developments in the management of anaerobic infections. *Rev Infect Dis* 5:235–245, 1983.

123. Rubenstein P, Mishell DR, Jr, Ledger W: Colpotomy drainage of pelvic abscess. *Obstet Gynecol* 48:142–145, 1976.

124. Rivlin M: Clinical outcome following vaginal drainage of pelvic abscess. *Obstet Gynecol* 61:169–173, 1983.

125. Gibbs R, Hunt J, Schwarz R: A follow-up study on prophylactic antibiotics in cesarean section. *Am J Obstet Gynecol* 117:419–422, 1973.

126. Green J, Wenzel R: Postoperative wound infection: a controlled study of the increased duration of hospital stay and direct cost of hospitalization. *Ann Surg* 185:264–268, 1977.

127. Gibbs R, Blanco J, St Clair P: A case-control study of wound abscess after cesarean delivery. *Obstet Gynecol* 62:498–501, 1983.

128. Koh K, Chan F, Monfared A, Ledger W, Paul RH: The changing perinatal and maternal outcome in chorioamnionitis. *Obstet Gynecol* 53:730–734, 1979.

129. Gibbs R, Castillo M, Rodgers P: Management of acute chorioamnionitis. *Am J Obstet Gynecol* 136:709–713, 1980.

130. Cruse PJ, Foord R: A five year prospective study of 23,649 surgical wounds. *Arch Surg* 107:206–209, 1973.

131. Dineen P: A critical study of 100 consecutive wound infections. *Surg Gynecol Obstet* 113:91–96, 1961.

132. Cruse PJ, Foord R: The epidemiology of wound infection. A 10-year prospective study of 62,939 wounds. *Surg Clin North Am* 60:27–40, 1980.

133. Brown S, Allen H, Robins R: The use of delayed primary wound closure in preventing wound infections. *Am J Obstet Gynecol* 127:713–717, 1977.

134. Gottrup F, Fogdestam I, Hunt TK: Delayed primary closure: an experimental and clinical review. *J Clin Surg* 1:113–124, 1982.

135. Galle PC, Homesley H: Ineffectiveness of povidone-iodine irrigation of abdominal incisions. *Obstet Gynecol* 55:744–746, 1980.

136. Alexander J, Kaplan J, Altemeier W: Role of suture materials in the development of wound infections. *Ann Surg* 165:192–199, 1967.

137. Noe J, Lamb D: The function of a dressing: wound healing, a dynamic approach. *Hosp Care* 5:5–13, 1974.

138. Edlich R, Rodeheaver G, Thacker J, Edgerton M: Technical factors in wound management. In Hunt TK, Dunphy JE (eds): *Fundamentals of Wound Management.* New York, Appleton-Century-Crofts, 1979, pp 364–454.

139. Hunt TK, VanWinkle W: Normal repair. In Hunt TK, Dunphy JE (eds): *Fundamentals of Wound*

Management. New York, Appleton-Century-Crofts, 1979, pp 2–67.

140. Borkowf H, Mattingly R: Bacterial gangrenous infection. In Schaefer G, Graber E (eds): *Complications in Obstetric and Gynecologic Surgery*. Hagerstown, MD, Harper and Row, 1981, pp 140–156.

141. Meleny FL: Hemolytic streptococcal gangrene. *Arch Surg* 9:317, 1924.

142. Golde S, Ledger W: Necrotizing fasciitis in postpartum patients. *Obstet Gynecol* 50:670–673, 1977.

143. Meleny FL: A differential diagnosis between certain types of infectious gangrene of the skin. *Surg Gynecol Obstet* 56:847, 1933.

144. Helmkamp BF: Abdominal wound dehiscence. *Am J Obstet Gynecol* 128:803–807, 1977.

145. Garibaldi R, Britt M, Coleman M, Reading J, Pace N: Risk factors for postoperative pneumonia. *Am J Med* 70:677–680, 1981.

146. Craven J, Evans G, Davenport R, Williams B: The evaluation of the incentive spirometer in the management of post-operative pulmonary complications. *Br J Surg* 61:793–797, 1974.

147. Mendelson C: The aspiration of stomach contents into the lungs during obstetrical anesthesia. *Am J Obstet Gynecol* 52:191–205, 1946.

148. Roberts R, Shirley M: Reducing the risk of acid aspiration during cesarean section. *Anesth Analg* 53:859–868, 1974.

149. Whalley P: Bacteriuria in pregnancy. *Am J Obstet Gynecol* 97:723–738, 1967.

150. Warren JW, Platt R, Thomas K: Antibiotic irrigation and catheter associated urinary tract infection. *N Engl J Med* 299:570–573, 1980.

151. Marraro R, Harris R: Incidence of spontaneous resolution of postpartum bacteruria. *Am J Obstet Gynecol* 128:722–723, 1977.

152. Zinner S, Kass E: Long-term (10–14 years) follow-up of bacteriuria in pregnancy. *N Engl J Med* 285:820–823, 1971.

153. Kincaid-Smith P, Bullen M: Bacteriuria in pregnancy. *Lancet* 2:395–399, 1965.

154. Iffy L, Kaninetzky H, Maidman J, Lindsey J, Arrata W: Control of perinatal infection by traditional preventive measures. *Obstet Gynecol* 54:403–410, 1979.

155. Duff P, Keiser J, Strong S: A comparative study of two antibiotic regimens for the treatment of operative site infections. *Am J Obstet Gynecol* 142:996–1003, 1982.

156. Hemsell D, Cunningham F, DePalma R, Nobles B, Heard M, Hemsell P: Cefotaxime sodium therapy for endomyometritis following cesarean section: dose-findings and comparative studies. *Obstet Gynecol* 62:489–497, 1983.

Chapter 27

Infection in the Newborn

Leigh G. Donowitz, M.D.

INTRODUCTION

The topic of neonatal infection includes neonatal immunity, the changing epidemiology of infectious diseases in this population, sources of infection, diagnosis, therapy, and prevention.

The incidence of infection in the fetus and newborn is significant. One to 2% of babies are infected in utero and as many as 10% of neonates are infected prior to 2 months of age (1, 2). Fetal infection results in fetal demise with abortion, stillbirth or fetal resorption, congenital malformations, prematurity, growth retardation and numerous complications of chronic postnatal infection. Perinatal infection may result in severe systemic disease with death, persistent infection, or long term chronic sequelae.

IMMUNE DEFICIENCIES OF THE NEWBORN

The fetus and neonate are immunocompromised with an increased susceptibility to infection when compared to the older child or adult. If one looks at the major categories of the human immune system, deficiencies have been documented in each of the main components of this anatomic system.

Mechanical Barrier to Infection

The skin and mucous membranes of newborns have been shown to be more permeable to exogenous antigen then those in older patients. There is poor development of the stratum corneum before 26 weeks of gestation. This usual barrier to exogenous antigen is only a few cells thick and is poorly keratinized. Harpin and Rutter (3) studied 70 newborns from 25 to 41 weeks of gestation and showed that the application of phenylephrine, a powerful α-agonist, to the skin caused no skin blanching and no water loss in babies with gestational ages greater than 37 weeks. However, there was marked skin blanching and water loss at the site of phenylephrine application in premature newborns less than 32 weeks of gestation. After 2 weeks of age, regardless of gestational age, the skin matures, and the stratum corneum develops. This immature barrier to infection is a very real source of bacterial entry into the newborn and, specifically, the premature newborn.

Phagocyte Function

Migration of polymorphonuclear leucocytes (PMNs) toward a site of exogenous antigen, ingestion of the foreign substance, and successful completion of bactericidal mechanisms of ingested microorganisms constitute a complex biologic phenomenon. Current information suggests that the neonatal granulocyte demonstrates abnormalities in migration and ingestion but has fairly reliable intracellular bacterial killing.

Miller showed that neonatal PMNs were significantly less effective than adult PMNs in migrating toward any of the usual chemotactic stimuli (4). Similarly, Pahwa et al demonstrated that cord blood PMNs were significantly less effective in movement than adult PMNs (5). Furthermore, Klein et al looked at PMN and monocyte migration under agarose gel technique and showed that newborn PMNs migrated at levels less than 50% of normal adult chemotaxis, and monocytes migrated at approximately 25% of adult values (6). Numerous other studies have documented the decreased phagocytic cell movement, decreased deformability of the cell membranes, decreased lectin-induced aggregation (7) and decreased capping of PMNs when exposed to concanavalin A (8). The significance of the latter finding is that PMN receptors do not orient normally, or cap as they would in the adult or older child. These findings all suggest a functional and developmental membrane defect in the neonatal PMN.

Ingestion of phagocytosis by neonatal PMNs has been studied, and the data reliably show that neonatal PMNs in the presence of adult sera have normal phagocytic properties (9–11). At adult serum concentrations of less than 3%, neonatal PMNs did not phagocytize as well as adult PMNs (12). Thus, there appears to be a serum factor in neonates responsible for defective phagocytosis.

Bacterial intracellular killing of ingested microorganisms has been shown in many studies to be normal by PMNs obtained from normal term and preterm infants (10, 13, 14). Mills et al (15) showed decreased chemoluminescence of newborn PMNs and concluded that neonates have decreased oxidative metabolic responsiveness and lowered bactericidal activity. Other authors have found variations in premature bactericidal activity of PMNs and abnormalities in PMN bactericidal activity in sick infants. These data suggest that intracellular PMN killing is reliable and at adult levels against most microorganisms in the well newborn.

Immunoglobulins

IgM is the first immunoglobulin synthesized by the fetus at 30 weeks of age or greater gestation, but normal IgM production occurs as a result of stimulation from gastrointestinal colonization. IgM is the major antibody that is synthesized during the first few months of extrauterine life, and levels are at approximately 80% of adult values by 1 year of age. The identification of a newborn with elevated IgM levels suggests that there has been increased fetal antigenic stimulation and is suggestive of intrauterine infection (16).

Maternal IgG is transferred to the fetus in only negligible quantities until the second trimester of pregnancy. By term, the levels of IgG measured in the fetus generally exceed the maternal levels because an active transport of IgG takes place during the third trimester of pregnancy (17). Significant synthesis of IgG commences at 6 months of extrauterine life and reaches only 60% of adult levels by 1 year. With rapid disappearance of maternal IgG the newborn is essentially hypogammaglobulinemic from 3 to 6 months of age.

The infant born to a mother with high circulating levels of antibody against a specific antigen, such as measles or rubella, is protected. If the immune mother's antibody levels are low and her own immunity is based on a brisk anamnestic response, such as prior immunization against tetanus or diphtheria, the infant will have only partial or poor immunity. Mothers who have had diseases which primarily result in the production of IgM antibodies for protection (e.g., *Salmonella, Escherichia coli*) confer no immunity to their newborns because IgM is not transplacentally transferred.

Complement

Complement studies have shown a decrease in classic pathway activity in the neonate, but the most pronounced deficiencies are those of the alternate pathway. The most important deficiency in the complement system is markedly decreased opsonic activity when compared to adult values (18). Fibronectin, a large opsonic glycoprotein which promotes reticuloendothelial clearance of bacteria, has been studied by Gerdes et al (19) and has been shown to be present at approximately 50% of normal adult values in the term infant. The fibronectin serum level reaches adult values at 2 months of age.

The reticuloendothelial system and specifically the spleen in newborns has been shown to be deficient in removing exogenous antigen from the circulating blood. Holyrode et al (20) looked at red blood cell (RBC) pocking as a measure of asplenia or functional asplenia. They demonstrated that 2.6% of RBCs are pocked in the normal adult, 24% of RBCs are pocked in the term infant, and 47.2% are pocked in the preterm infant. These latter values compare to the prevalence of pocked RBCs seen in traumatically splenectomized or autosplenectomized adult patients.

SOURCES OF INFECTION IN THE NEWBORN
Fetal Infection

Multiple factors affect the infection risk of the developing fetus. Maternal immunity and her exposure to and subsequent development of infection are the major issues. The major infections during pregnancy are self-limited viral infections of the gastrointestinal tract or the upper airway which have no known untoward effects on the fetus. However, transplacental spread of more disseminated maternal infection (e.g., rubella, syphilis, toxoplasmosis, cytomegalovirus, varicella, tuberculosis, or bacterial infection) can cause significant fetal disease resulting in fetal death, prematurity, significant perinatal morbidity, and/or the severe congenital sequelae associated with these infections.

As fetal diagnostic and therapeutic technology advances, so do the infectious complications of the newer procedures. Amniocentesis is associated with amnionitis and fetal infection with significant associated morbidity and mortality (21–23). Intrauterine transfusions for severe fetal hydrops have resulted in infection of the fetus. In one case a fetus developed cytomegalovirus infection from a contaminated intrauterine blood transfusion (24), and a second baby developed *Acinetobacter calcoaceticus* bacteremia from blood transfused in utero that was later shown to be contaminated with that organism (25). There have been mutiple reports (26–37) of scalp abscesses, cellulitis, skull osteomyelitis, and septicemia caused by fetal blood sampling from the scalp or from infection at the site of internal fetal monitor electrode placement.

The diagnosis of congenital infection is a difficult one because infants with disseminated infection of bacterial, protozoan, or viral etiology have many of the same clinical signs and symptoms on presentations. Infants born with purpura, jaundice, hepatosplenomegaly, meningoencephalitis, or pneumonia have a large differential diagnosis which includes bacterial septicemia or toxoplasmosis, rubella, cytomegalic inclusion disease, herpes simplex disease, and syphilis. The distinguishing charateristics of each syndrome coupled with culture, biopsy, and serologic information usually confirm the etiology.

Prevention is the hallmark of successful medical intervention of fetal infections because the significant morbidity, mortality, and devastating sequelae are very poorly affected at the time of postnatal diagnosis. The major effects of this group of illnesses are on central nervous system, ocular, cardiac, and skeletal embryogenesis and development. Table 27.1 describes the more common fetal pathogens, the reservoir and mode of

transmission of maternal infection, and the most effective methods available for preventing these infections in the pregnant mother.

Cytomegalovirus (CMV) infection is an example of this group of pathogens, and because of its widespread prevalence in normal healthy children, it is not currently possible to reliably interrupt transmission of this organism to pregnant women. Forty-two percent of pregnant women in one study (38) of 10,847 patients were seronegative and thus at risk of acquiring their primary infection during pregnancy. The incidence of CMV infection during pregnancy was less than 1%. This virus is found in high prevalence in normal healthy children, in transplant and dialysis patients, in immunosuppressed oncology patients, and in hospitalized neonates and infants. Blood product (39–44) and human milk (45–50) are common sources of viral transmission to neonates, but the organism can be found in most body secretions and is most reliably cultured from the urine of infected patients. Many studies of hospital employees working in low and high incidence settings for CMV infection have been performed in an attempt to determine whether pregnant women working in such settings are at geater risk of infection and delivering congenitally

Table 27.1. Sources, Transmission, and Prevention of Fetal Infection

Microorganism	Common Reservoir(s)	Transmission	Prevention
Rubella virus	Infected humans	Secretion contact Airborne	1. Immunization prior to pregnancy
Syphilis	Infected humans	Secretion contact	1. Serologic screening 2. Early therapy
Toxoplasmosis	Cat feces Rare meat	Ingestion ? Airborne	1. Avoidance of reservoir
Cytomegalovirus	Infected humans Blood products	Transfusion Secretions Contact	1. Avoidance of reservoir
Varicella	Infected humans	Airborne Secretion contact Lesion contact	1. Avoidance of reservoir 2. Zoster immune globulin to infant if onset of maternal infection is within 4 days before or after delivery
Bacterial infection	Multiple	Multiple	1. Early aggressive therapy to prevent secondary bloodstream infection

infected offspring than women not working in areas of high endemic disease. Three studies (51–53) have shown increased seroconversion of nurses working on pediatric wards, while two (54, 55) other studies document no increased seroconversion. Ahlfors et al looked more specifically at the incidence of actual infection in the children born to pediatric nurses and found no increased rate (54). Although the theoretic concern remains, there appears to be no increased risk to pregnant women working in settings of high endemic rates of CMV disease of their delivering congenitally infected infants.

Amniocentesis, internal fetal monitoring, and intrapartum fetal surgeries and transfusion require careful consideration as to benefit versus infection or other untoward complications. Scrupulous adherence to technique, including routine scrubs and the careful maintenance of equipment, coupled with careful observation and early diagnosis of the infectious complications may decrease the incidence or alter the otherwise devastating outcome.

NEONATAL INFECTION ACQUIRED DURING LABOR AND DELIVERY

The microorganisms colonizing the maternal birth canal are those that the baby will become colonized with at the time of rupture of the fetal membrane and/or during descent through the birth canal. Any microorganism may be present in the maternal birth canal, the usual and normal flora includes gram-negative Enterobacteriaciae, gram-positive anaerobic and aerobic cocci, specifically the streptococci, and fungi, specifically *Candida albicans. Listeria monocytogenes,* the group B streptococcus, *Neisseria gonorrhoeae, Neisseria meningitidis,* herpes simplex virus, cytomegalovirus, hepatitis virus, and *Chlamydia trachomatis* are all microorganisms which frequently colonize the birth canal and are associated with significant neonatal diease (Table 27.2).

The group B streptococcus (GBS) is found in 2 to 25% of normal mothers (56, 57). However, 42 to 72% (mean 58%) of babies delivered vaginally to women colonized with the organism will become colonized with the organism. To those who become colonized, only 1 to 2% will develop disease (56). The risk of GBS septicemia markedly increases to 10 to 15% (*a*) if the colonized baby is born at a gestational age less than 37 weeks, (*b*) if there is rupture of membranes greater than 24 hours prior to delivery, (*c*) if there is chorioamnionitis, or (*d*) if there is maternal GBS bacteremia.

Prevention of GBS septicemia in the newborn by administration of penicillin to the infant has been proposed. Boyer et al (58) and Yow et al (59) showed that one could significantly reduce vertical transmission if ampicillin is administered to the mother during labor. Siegal et al evaluated the study of intramuscular penicillin G administered to the neonate 1 hour after birth (60). There was a lower incidence of GBS disease, but a greater incidence of gram-negative septicemia

Table 27.2.   Etiology and Prevention of Vertically Acquired Neonatal Infection

Organism	Prevention
Group B streptococcus	1. Intrapartum ampicillin
Herpes simplex type	1. Intrapartum cultures 2. Cesarean section delivery for culture-positive or high risk mothers 3. Antiviral therapy
Hepatitis B	1. Hepatitis B immune globulin 2. Hepatitis B vaccine
Neisseria gonorrhoeae	1. Silver nitrate eyedrops 2. Erythromycin eyedrops 3. Chemoprophylaxis to infants born to culture-positive women
Chlamydia trachomatis	1. Erythromycin eyedrops
Listeria monocytogenes	
Candida albicans	
Staphylococcus aureus	1. Antiseptic bathing
Gram-negative Enterobacteriaciae	

and other penicillin-resistant organisms when compared to the control population. Pyati et al showed that in their study population from Chicago, 90% of infants were bacteremic prior to penicillin administration, and therefore such therapy was administered too late to prevent disease in their patients (61). Chemoprophylaxis should be considered in (a) the nonaffected sibling of a twin with GBS disease and (b) a woman with a previous history of delivering a child with GBS disease.

Hepatitis B is also vertically transmitted, and over 90% of infants born to mothers who are hepatitis B e antigen-positive will become infected with the virus. Although significant disease is unlikely in these infants, 85 to 90% of those who become infected will become chronic carriers of the virus (62). Vertical transmission has been effectively interrupted by the combined use of hepatitis B immune globulin and the hepatitis B vaccine in 94% of infants born to women who are hepatitis B e antigen-positive (63).

Herpes simplex virus is another microorganism that is most commonly acquired by colonization during parturition, and it can result in devastating neonatal disease. Approximately 1% of pregnant women have cytologically detectable primary or recurrent herpetic genital infections during pregnancy (64–66). If a vaginal delivery takes place or there is rupture of the fetal membranes for greater than 4 hours and if the infection is primary, there is a 40 to 60% risk of the baby's becoming clinically infected (64). Herpes simplex disease in the newborn is manifested as a cutaneous disease, as ocular or mucous membrane disease, as a disseminated disease, or as meningoencephalitis (67). The disease carries a 65% mortality risk, and the survivors have significant neurologic sequelae (68).

Cultures during pregnancy should be performed during the last trimester, and repeated negative cultures may be useful in allowing a mother to deliver vaginally. One positive culture during the third trimester should mandate scheduled abdominal delivery as this is an effective method of preventing vertical transmission.

Neonatal herpes simplex disease has been transmitted via fetal motor scalp electrodes (69, 70), from paternal sources (71, 72), from a maternal breast lesion (73), from hospital personnel with oral herpes virus infection (74), and from one baby to another in the nursery setting (75–79).

Treatment with antiviral therapy has altered the outcome of this otherwise devastating illness, but mortality figures even with therapy are approximately 40% (80). The most important therapeutic modality is preventive. Mothers with a significant past history for herpes simplex should be screened by cytology and culture during their pregnancies, and women in the third trimester of pregnancy with continued evidence of clinical, cytologic, or culture-proven disease should deliver by cesarean section prior to the onset of labor and rupture of the fetal membranes. Cesarean section is not indicated if amniotic fluid cultures reveal herpes simplex virus prior to delivery (81, 82). If fetal membranes have been ruptured for greater than 4 to 6 hours in a woman known to be culture-positive, vaginal delivery is indicated (83). If a woman has herpes simplex infection at another site, cesarean section delivery is not indicated (83).

Mothers with active disease at the time of delivery should have a private room. Personnel who have contact with the infected area should use gown and glove precautions, and contaminated articles should be double bagged (84, 85). The mother should be encouraged to see her infant in her room providing she employs scrupulous technique.

Infants born to mothers with suspected or proven genital herpes should be placed in contact isolation, with appropriate gown and glove use and double bagged disposal of contaminated articles.

POSTPARTUM INFECTION (NOSOCOMIAL AND FAMILY-ACQUIRED INFECTION)

Sources of infection for the newborn in the immediate neonatal period are multiple (Table 27.3). The sterile fetal environment is replaced by microorganisms from the inanimate environment, the mother, hospital personnel, and visitors. Organisms that normally colonize are potentially invasive in this host with immature immunity, and as a result aspects of infection control which are not required in other hospital settings are mandatory in the care of the neonate.

Colonization of the healthy term newborn usually can be documented on the second or third day of life. The nose and umbilicus generally become colonized with *Staphylococcus epidermidis* and α-hemolytic streptococci, and the gastrointestinal tract with *E. coli*, lactobaccilli, and anaerobes. In contrast, babies admitted to newborn intensive care units have a very different colonization pattern. A study by Goldmann et al showed that colonization is generally delayed be-

Table 27.3.   Route of Infection of the More Common Neonatal Infections

Congenital Infection	Vertically Acquired Infection	Postpartum Infection
Syphilis	Herpes simplex virus	Tuberculosis
Cytomegalovirus	Group B streptococcus	Hepatitis B
Rubella virus	Hepatitis B	Cytomegalovirus
Varicella	Gram-negative Entero-	Herpes simplex virus
Toxoplasmosis gondii	bacteriaciae	*Staphylococcus aureus*
	Staphylococcus aureus	*Staphylococcus epider-*
	Candida albicans	*midis*
	Listeria monocyto-	Enterovirus
	genes	Rhinovirus
	Neisseria gonorrhoeae	Group B streptococ-
	Chlamydia trachoma-	cus
	tis	Enterobacteriaciae

yond 8 days (86). When it does occur, *Klebsiella, Enterobacter,* or *Citrobacter* species replace *E. coli* as the most common stool flora and often colonize the nose, throat, and umbilicus. Virtually all infants remaining in the intensive care unit for a month or longer were heavily colonized with the more unusual flora.

Studies looking at the antibiotic resistance patterns of gram-negative rods found in newly colonized neonates in intensive care units that aminoglycoside usage is directly correlated with the appearance of microbial resistance to that specific aminoglycoside (87). However, infection rates do not correlate with the changing resistance patterns, and White et al showed that surveillance cultures of resistant enteric bacilli and antibiotic usage in a neonatal intensive care unit did not effect control of neonatal sepsis due to these enteric bacilli (88). Mayhall et al, in a series of sequential outbreaks of *Klebsiella pneumoniae* septicemia, showed that the gastrointestinal tract of the neonates was the infectious reservoir, and the epidemic strain was spread on the hands of hospital personnel (89). Poor aseptic technique with bag resuscitation, oropharyngeal suctioning, and the use of nasogastric tubes facilitated the inoculation of organisms carried on the hands of personnel.

Nosocomial infection of neonates in newborn intensive care populations ranges from 5 to 25%. Hemming et al, in a study of 904 infants, showed a 15.3% overall infection rate with 14% of the infections being bacteremias, 29.3% pneumonias, 8.1% postoperative wound infections, 4.5% urinary tract infections, and 4.0% meningitis (90). Nosocomial infection rates were significantly greater in infants with birth weights less than 1500 g. Townsend and Wenzel looked at 49 newborns with nosocomial bacteremia and matched cases

with 49 control subjects without bloodstream infection (91). There was a strong association between nosocomial infections at sites other than the bloodstream and the development of subsequent bacteremia. Goldmann et al (92) studied nosocomial infections in a neonatal intensive care unit and showed that there was an increased risk of infection associated with low birth weight, patent ductus arteriosus, surgery and multiple invasive support procedures. Their study also showed a significant decrease in the overall infection rates when a new facility was opened with a marked increase in patient space, more convenient sinks, better isolation facilities, and a staffing increase of 50%.

Epidemics

The nursery is a common site of nosocomial epidemics. Historically, major epidemics in nurseries prior to 1960 were caused by *Staphylococcus aureus* and group A streptococcus. In the 1960s and 1970s the major epidemic pathogens were the gram-negative bacilli. Although the major cause of neonatal bacteremia has shifted back to the gram-positive cocci, specifically *S. aureus* and the coagulase-negative staphylococci (93–95), these infections are not a result of a specific pathogenic strain transmitted from a common reservoir. Instead, they represent multiple strains from the skin flora of patients and staff contaminating and infecting invasive intravascular monitoring and access devices.

Nosocomial viral infection is probably a problem of underestimated magnitude. Viruses have been documented in multiple nursery outbreaks (96–100), and the reservoirs of infection are staff members, parents, siblings, and other infected patients. The major mode of transmission is direct inoculation by hospital personnel or family.

In 1960 Wolinsky et al, using babies and nurses colonized with specific phage types of *S. aureus*, showed that transmission of the organism was by direct contact and not the previously thought airborne route (101). Hand inoculation of organisms has been the most common route of transmission documented in epidemics. *S. aureus* (101–106), *Klebsiella* (107–112), *Proteus mirabilis* (113), *E. coli* (114, 115), and *Salmonella* (116–121) have all been spread from a common reservoir to the cases by direct hand inoculation of the pathogen.

Contaminated solutions are a potential source of nosocomial infection throughout the hospital. Epidemics in nuseries have been documented from the saline solution used to irrigate the eyes of infants at birth (122), from contaminated hexachlorophene solutions (123, 124), hand lotions (125–127), disinfectants (123, 124, 128, 129), and intravenous solutions (130–132).

Monitoring, supportive, and therapeutic equipment has been the source of sporadic and epidemic infection in newborn nurseries and, most specifically, critical care nurseries. Ventilatory equipment, pressure transducers for monitoring intra-arterial pressure, umbilical catheters, central venous catheters (long or short term), hyperalimentation, nasotracheal, and endotracheal tubes are only some of the types of equipment which are discussed in other chapters but carry the same if not greater risks to immune-immature newborns as to adults. Optimal maintenance and routine scrutiny of the equipment and procedures for potential breaks in technique and subsequent contamination are required. Patients with invasive equipment need to be assessed daily as to whether the device is absolutely necessary, because early removal is probably the most effective method of reducing the infection risks. If a patient does become infected with equipment in place, careful cultures of the devices as well as the patient should be carried out.

Environmental Cultures

Routine environmental culturing for bacterial contamination is indicated but only in the setting of investigation for a particular reservoir. Verification of sterile procedure in formula preparation and equipment maintenance may mandate specific routine surveillance culturing.

Hand Washing

Hand washing by nursery personnel remains the hallmark of effective interruption of the spread of potentially pathogenic bacteria between patients and between staff and patients (133, 134). With the understanding of the immunocompromised nature of the small infant, it is imperative that initial and subsequent colonization of the newborn be protected. Adequate and convenient hand washing facilities should be available (90), and strict hand washing policies should be established and enforced for all personnel entering the units. Hands are colonized with both a permanent and a transient flora (135). The permanent flora is generally not removed with routine hand washing methods, but these organisms can be reduced in number and inactivated by some antiseptics. By definition, transient flora is more easily removed by routine soap and water wash. In an attempt to reduce the resident flora and remove the transient flora, an iodophor or antiseptic soap sould be used (136, 137). Personnel with hand dermatitis usually have an increased number of bacteria with a potential for more pathogenic organisms on their hand. They should be treated, required to use gloves, and possibly removed from clinical patient care until their dermatitis is improved.

Isolation

Cohort isolation may be required during epidemic periods where infected or colonized staff can care for infected or colonized infants. Sporadic cases of specific infections should be isolated according to the routine guidelines. A closed Isolette system is one method of isolation and is sufficient for most newborn infections if a special area is not available.

Gowns

Gown use is traditional but of unproven advantage in interrupting transmission of microorganisms in the nursery setting. Studies to date that address this issue have shown that there is delay in the colonization of the umbilical cord when gowns are used (138), but multiple other studies (102, 139–144) show no difference in the incidence of staphylococcal colonization or in the incidence of infections in settings of gown use compared to no gown use. A recent study in a pediatric intensive care unit showed no change in hand washing rates, infection, or intravascular catheter colonization rates when gowns were employed (145). Gowns should be worn for specific isolation or for actual contact with or handling of infants.

Linens

The American Academy of Pediatrics in the *Standards and Recommendations for Hospital Care of Newborn Infants* recommends that linen in newborn intensive care, intermediate care, continuing care, and admission observation areas be autoclaved (146). Meyer et al showed that the bacterial contamination of nonautoclaved linens delivered to a newborn intensive care unit was limited to skin flora in very low numbers (147). Their study also showed that 75% of nurseries did not routinely autoclave linens. Linens and infant clothing have not been shown to be of particular importance as sources for nosocomial infection and therefore do not warrant special sterilization for this setting.

Employee Health

Employee health services should be very much involved with the staff providing care to neonates. Screening programs for serologic evidence of immunity to rubella and varicella should be effected and enforced. Susceptible individuals should be successfully immunized or prevented from patient contact if exposed. Employees working in intensive care nurseries who have patient and blood contact should receive the hepatitis B vaccine. Employees should be screened on a yearly basis for tuberculosis and should be alerted to report exposures and unusual respiratory illnesses. Personnel with streptococcal, staphylococcal, upper respiratory infections, gastroenteritis, dermatitis, open skin lesions, or active herpes simplex infections should avoid patient contact for the duration of their illness or per established guidelines (83–85).

During periods of epidemic infections in the nursery, employee health should effect clinical and laboratory screening for dermatitis, skin infections, respiratory illness, or other potential sources of the epidemic pathogen.

Active teaching and in-service programs on the specific immune deficiencies of the newborn and the high susceptibility of this patient population to infection, the need for scrupulous technique and device maintenance, and the requirement for hand washing are required for continuing education and motivate staff to maintain optimal standards of care.

Therapy

The most common bacterial etiologies of bloodstream infection in neonates are the Group B streptococcus and the Enterobacteriaciae, specifically *E. coli* and *Klebsiella* species. If the patient has been hospitalized for more than 72 hours, particularly if invasive monitoring and therapeutic equipment have been used, there is a much greater incidence of gram-positive infection, specifically *S. aureus* and the coagulase-negative staphylococci (93–95).

In the neonate with signs and symptoms of septicemia, initial empiric therapy should include antibiotics effective against the group B streptococcus and the Enterobacteriaciae. If the patient has been hospitalized for more than 72 hours and particularly if vascular access devices have been used, initial therapy for bacteremia should include antibiotics effective against *S. aureus* and the coagulase-negative staphylococcus. Nosocomial bacteremia and antibiotic resistance patterns within the specific unit should be used to guide initial therapy.

White blood cell transfusions should be considered as adjunctive therapy in the bacteremic infant with depleted bone marrow white blood cell stores. White blood cell transfusions have been shown in preliminary studies (148–150) to be effective in decreasing morbidity and reducing mortality in bacteremic infants.

SUMMARY

It is not the treatment but rather the prevention that is the goal of infection control for the newborn. This goal is effected through good prenatal screening, immunization, and early therapy of the mother prior to and during her pregnancy. Cautious care of the neonate with his known immature host defenses requires scrupulous hand washing, adequate staffing, space and isolation facilities, and a conscious attempt to minimize invasive support and monitoring equipment. An active employee health program is required to insure that this highly susceptible population is not exposed and subsequently infected with common viruses (e.g., herpes simplex, enteroviruses, respiratory syncytial viruses) and bacteria (e.g., staphylococcus, streptococcus).

"It may seem a strange principle to enunciate as the very first requirement in a hospital that it should do the sick no harm."

Florence Nightingale

References

1. Plotkin SA, Starr SE: Symposium on perinatal infections. *Clin Perinatol* 8:617–637, 1981.
2. Alford CA, Pass RF: Epidemiology of chronic congenital and perinatal infections of man. *Clin Perinatol* 8:397–414, 1981.

3. Harpin VA, Rutter N: Barrier properties of the newborn infant's skin. *J Pediatr* 102:419–425, 1983.

4. Miller ME: Chemotactic function in the human neonate: humoral and cellular aspects. *Pediatr Res* 5:487–492, 1971.

5. Pahwa S, Pahwa R, Grines E, Smithwick EM: Cellular and humoral components of monocyte and neutrophil chemotaxis in cord blood. *Pediatr Res* 11:677–680, 1977.

6. Klein RB, Fischer TJ, Gard SE, Biberstein M, Rich KC, Stiehm ER: Decreased mononuclear and polymorphonuclear chemotaxis in human newborns, infants, and young children. *Pediatrics* 60:467–472, 1977.

7. Mease AD, Fischer GW, Hunter KW, Ruyman FB: Decreased phytohemagglutinin-induced aggregation and C5a-induced chemotaxis of human neutrophils. *Pediatr Res* 14:142–146, 1980.

8. Kimura GM, Miller ME, Leake RD, Raghunathan R, Cheung ATW: Reduced concanavalin A capping of neonatal polymorphonuclear leucocytes. *Pediatr Res* 15:1271–1273, 1981.

9. McCracken GH, Eichenwald HF: Leucocyte function and the development of opsonic and complement activity in the neonate. *Am J Dis Child* 121:120–126, 1971.

10. Coen R, Grush O, Kauder E: Studies of bactericidal activity and metabolism of the leukocyte in full term neonates. *J Pediatr* 75:400–406, 1969.

11. Dassett JH, Williams RC Jr, Quie PG: Studies on interaction of bacteria, serum factors and polymorphonuclear leucocytes in mothers and newborns. *Pediatrics* 44:49–57, 1969.

12. Miller ME: Phagocytosis in the newborn infant: humoral and cellular factors. *J Pediatr* 74: 255–259, 1969.

13. Park BH, Holmes B, Good RA: Metabolic activities in leucocytes of newborn infants. *J Pediatr* 76:237–241, 1970.

14. Cocchi P, Marianelli L: Phagocytosis and intracellular killing of *Pseudomonas aeruginosa* in premature infants. *Helv Paediatr Acta* 22:110–118, 1967.

15. Mills EL, Thompson T, Bjorksten B, Filipovich D, Quie P: The chemoluminescence response and bactericidal activity of neutrophils from newborns and their mothers. *Pediatrics* 63:429–434, 1979.

16. Stiehm ER, Ammann AJ, Cherry JD: Elevated cord macroglobulins in the diagnosis of intrauterine infections. *N Engl J Med* 275:971–977, 1966.

17. Kohler PF, Farr RS: Elevation of cord over maternal IgG immunoglobulin—evidence for an active placental IgG transport. *Nature* 210:1070–1071, 1966.

18. Farman ML, Stiehm ER: Impaired opsonic activity but normal phagocytosis in low birth weight infants. *N Engl J Med* 281:926–931, 1969.

19. Gerdes JS, Yoder MC, Douglas SD, Polin RA: Decreased plasma fibronectin in neonatal sepsis. *Pediatrics* 72:877–881, 1983.

20. Holroyde CP, Oski FA, Gardner FH: The "pocked" erythrocyte: red-cell surface alterations in reticuloendothelial immaturity of the neonate. *N Engl J Med* 281:516–520, 1969.

21. Fray RE, Davis TP, Brown EA: *Clostridium welchii* infection after amniocentesis. *Br Med J* 288:901–902, 1984.

22. An assessment of the hazards of amniocentesis. Report to the Medical Research Council by their Working Party on Amniocentesis. *Br J Obstet Gynaecol* 85 (suppl 2):1–41, 1978.

23. United States National Institute of Child Health and Human Development Study Group. Midtrimester amniocentesis for prenatal diagnosis. Safety and accuracy. *JAMA* 236:1471–1476, 1976.

24. King-Lewis PA, Gardner SD: Congenital cytomegalic inclusion disease following intrauterine transfusion. *Br Med J* 2:603–605, 1969.

25. Scott JM, Henderson A: Acute villous inflammation in the placenta following intrauterine transfusion. *J Clin Pathol* 25:872–875, 1972.

26. Wagener MM, Rycheck RR, Yee RB, McVay JF, Buffenmyer CL, Harger JH: Septic dermatitis of the neonatal scalp and maternal endomyometritis with intrapartum internal fetal monitoring. *Pediatrics* 74:81–85, 1984.

27. Glaser JB, Engelberg M, Hammerschlag M: Scalp abscess associated with *Mycoplasma hominis* infection complicating intrapartum monitoring. *Pediatr Infect Dis* 2:468–470, 1983.

28. Cordero L, Anderson CW, Zuspan FP: Scalp abscess: a benign and infrequent complication of fetal monitoring. *Am J Obstet Gynecol* 146:126–130, 1983.

29. Koszalka MF Jr, Haverkamp AD, Orleans M, Murphy J: The effects of internal electronic fetal heart rate monitoring on maternal and infant infections in high-risk pregnancies. *J Reprod Med* 27:661–665, 1982.

30. Goldkrand JW: Intrapartum inoculation of herpes simplex virus by fetal scalp electrode. *Obstet Gynecol* 59:263–265, 1982.

31. Rehu M Haukkamaa M: Puerperal endometritis and intrauterine fetal heart rate monitoring. *Ann Clin Res* 12:133–135, 1980.

32. Fribourg S: Contamination of intrauterine pressure transducers. *Am J Obstet Gynecol* 135:551–552, 1979.

33. Baker DA, Mead PB, Gallant JM, Hayward RG, Hamel AJ: Water-borne contamination of intrauterine pressure transducers. *Am J Obstet Gynecol* 133:923–924, 1979.

34. Kaye EM, Dooling EC: Neonatal herpes simplex meningoencephalitis associated with fetal monitor scalp electrodes. *Neurology* 31:1045–1047, 1981.

35. Turbeville DF, Heath RE, Bowen FW, Killam AP: Complications of fetal scalp electrodes: a case report. *Am J Obstet Gynecol* 122:530–531, 1975.

36. Overturf GD, Balfour G: Osteomyelitis and sepsis: severe complications of fetal monitoring. *Pediatrics* 55:244–247, 1975.

37. Adams G, Purohit DM, Bada HS, Andres BF: Neonatal infection by herpes virus hominis type 2, a complication of intrapartum fetal monitoring. *Pediatr Res* 9:337, 1975.

38. Griffiths PD, Baboonian C: A prospective study of primary cytomegalovirus infection during pregnancy: final report. *Br J Obstet Gynaecol* 91:307–315, 1984.

39. Kaariainen L, Paloheimo J, Klemola E: Cytomegalovirus-mononucleosis: isolation of the virus and demonstration of subclinical infections after fresh blood transfusion in connection with open-heart

surgery. *Ann Med Exp Biol Fenn* 44:297–301, 1966.

40. Bayer WL: The effect of frozen blood on the relationship of cytomegalovirus and hepatitis virus to infection and disease. *In* Dawson RB, Barnes A Jr (eds): *Clinical and Practical Aspects of the Use of Frozen Blood.* Washington, DC, American Association of Blood Banks, 1977, pp 133–147.

41. Kumar A, Nankervis GA, Cooper AR, Gold E, Kumar ML: Acquisition of cytomegalovirus infection in infants following exchange transfusion: a prospective study. *Transfusion* 20:327–331, 1980.

42. Benson JW, Bodden SJ, Tobin JO: Cytomegalovirus and blood transfusion in neonates. *Arch Dis Child* 54:538–541, 1979.

43. Yeager AS, Grumet FC, Hafleigh EB, Arvin AM, Bradley JS, Prober CG: Prevention of transfusion-acquired cytomegalovirus infections in newborn infants. *J Pediatr* 98:281–287, 1981.

44. Sandler SG, Grumet FC: Posttransfusion cytomegalovirus infections. *Pediatrics* 69:650–653, 1982.

45. Welsh J, May JT: Breast milk and infant infection. *Med J Aust* 2:66–68, 1979.

46. Hayes K, Danks DM, Gibas H, Jack I: Cytomegalovirus in human milk. *N Engl J Med* 287:177–178, 1972.

47. Stagno S, Reynolds DW, Pass RF, Alford CA: Breast milk and the risk of cytomegalovirus infection. *N Engl J Med* 302:1073–1076, 1980.

48. Ballard RA, Drew WL, Hufnagle KC, Riedel PA: Acquired cytomegalovirus infection in preterm infants. *Am J Dis Child* 133:482–485, 1979.

49. Barness LA, Dallman PR, Anderson H, Collipp PJ, Nichols BL Jr, Walker WA, Woodruff CW: Human milk banking. *Pediatrics* 65:854–857, 1980.

50. Dworsky M, Stagno S, Pass RF, Cassady G, Alford C: Persistence of cytomegalovirus in human milk after storage. *J Pediatr* 101:440–443, 1982.

51. Yaeger AS: Longitudinal, serological study of cytomegalovirus infections in nurses and in personnel without patient contact. *J Clin Microbiol* 2:448–452, 1975.

52. Haneberg B, Bertnes E, Haukenes G: Antibodies to cytomegalovirus among personnel at a children's hospital. *Acta Paediatr Scand* 69:407–409, 1980.

53. Friedman HM, Lewis MR, Nemerofsky DM, Plotkin SA: Acquisition of cytomegalovirus infection among female employees at a pediatric hospital. *Pediatr Infect Dis* 3:233–235, 1984.

54. Ahlfors K, Ivarsson SA, Johnsson T: Risk of cytomegalovirus infection in nurses and congenital infection in their offspring. *Acta Paediatr Scand* 70:819–823, 1981.

55. Dworsky ME, Welch K, Cassady G, Stagno S: Occupational risk for primary cytomegalovirus infection among pediatric health-care workers. *N Engl J Med* 309:950–953, 1983.

56. Baker CJ, Barrett FF: Transmission of group B streptococci among parturient women and their neonates. *J Pediatr* 83:919–925, 1973.

57. Anthony BF, Okada DM, Hobel CJ: Epidemiology of the group B streptococcus: longitudinal observations during pregnancy. *J Infect Dis* 137:524–530, 1978.

58. Boyer KM, Gadzala CA, Burd LI, Fisher DE, Paton JB, Gotoff SP: Selective intrapartum chemoprophylaxis of neonatal group B streptococcal early-onset disease. I. Epidemiologic rationale. *J Infect Dis* 148:795–816, 1983.

59. Yow MD, Mason EO, Leeds LJ, Thompson PK, Clark DJ: Ampicillin prevents intrapartum transmission of group B streptococcus *JAMA* 241:1245–1247, 1979.

60. Siegal JD, McCracken GH, Rosenfeld CR: Penicillin prophylaxis of group B streptococcal infections in neonates. Status Program and Abstracts 21st Interscience Conference on Antimicrobial Agents and Chemotherapeutics, Chicago, 1981, no. 313.

61. Pyati SP, Pildes RS, Jacobs NM, Ramamurthy RS, Yeh TF, Devyani SR, Lilien LD, Amma P, Metzger WI: Penicillin in infants weighing two kilograms or less with early-onset group B streptococcal disease. *N Engl J Med* 308:1383–1389, 1983.

62. Stevens CE, Neuroth RA, Beasley RP, Szmuness W: HBeAg and anti-HBe detection by radioimmunoassay: correlation with vertical transmission of hepatitis B virus in Taiwan. *J Med Virol* 3:237–241, 1979.

63. Beasley RP, Hwang LY, Lee GC, Lan CC, Roan CH, Huang FY, Chen CL: Prevention of perinatally transmitted hepatitis B virus infections with hepatitis B immune globulin and hepatitis B vaccine. *Lancet* 2:1099–1102, 1983.

64. Nahmias AJ, Josey WE, Naib ZM, Freeman MG, Fernandez RS, Wheeler JH: Perinatal risk associated with maternal genital herpes simplex infection. *Am J Obstet Gynecol* 110:825–837, 1971.

65. Hanshaw JC: *Herpesvirus hominis* infections in the fetus and newborn. *Am J Dis Child* 126:546–555, 1973.

66. Nahmias AJ, Josey WE, Naib ZM: Significance of herpes simplex virus infection during pregnancy. *Clin Obstet Gynecol* 15:929–938, 1972.

67. Whitley RJ, Nahmias AJ, Visintine AM, Fleming CL, Alford CA: The natural history of herpes simplex virus infection of mother and newborn. *Pediatrics* 66:489–494, 1980.

68. Nahmias AJ, Visintine AM: Herpes simplex. In Remington JS, Klein JO (eds): *Infectious Diseases of the Fetus and Newborn Infant.* Philadelphia, WB Saunders, 1976, p 156.

69. Parvey LS, Chien LT: Neonatal herpes simplex virus infection introduced by fetal monitor scalp electrodes. *Pediatrics* 65:1150–1153, 1980.

70. Echeverria P, Miller G, Campbell AG, Tucker G: Scalp vesicles within the first week of life: a clue to early diagnosis of herpes neonatorum. *J Pediatr* 83:1062–1064, 1973.

71. Yeager AS, Ashley RL, Corey L: Transmission of herpes simplex virus from father to neonate. *J Pediatr* 103:905–907, 1983.

72. Douglas J, Schmidt O, Corey L: Acquisition of neonatal HSV-1 infection from a paternal source contact. *J Pediatr* 103:908–910, 1983.

73. Sullivan-Bolyai JZ, Fife KH, Jacobs RF, Miller Z, Corey L: Disseminated neonatal herpes simplex virus type 1 from a maternal breast lesion. *Pediatrics* 71:455–457, 1983.

74. Van Dyke RB, Spector SA: Transmission of her-

pes simplex virus type 1 to a newborn infant during endotracheal suctioning for meconium aspiration. *Pediatr Infect Dis* 3:153–156, 1984.

75. Linnemann CC, Light IJ, Buchman TG, Ballard JL, Roizman B: Transmission of herpes simplex virus type 1 in a nursery for the newborn. *Lancet* 1:964–966, 1978.

76. Hammerberg O, Watts J, Chernesky M, Luchsinger I, Rawls W: An outbreak of herpes simplex virus type 1 in an intensive care nursery. *Pediatr Infect Dis* 2:290–294, 1983.

77. Francis DP, Herrmann KL, MacMahon JR, Chavigny KH, Sanderlin KC: Nosocomial and maternally acquired *Herpesvirus hominis* infections: a report of four fatal cases in neonates. *Am J Dis Child* 129:889–893, 1975.

78. Halperin SA, Hendley JO, Nosal C, Roizman B: DNA fingerprinting in investigation of apparent nosocomial acquisition of neonatal herpes simplex. *J Pediatr* 97:91–93, 1980.

79. Buchman TG, Roizman B, Adams G, Stover BH: Restriction endonuclease fingerprinting of herpes simplex virus DNA: a novel epidemiological tool applied to a nosocomial outbreak. *J Infect Dis* 138:488–498, 1978.

80. Whitley RJ, Yeager A, Kartus P, Bryson Y, Connor JD, Alford CA, Nahmias A, Soong SJ: Neonatal herpes simplex virus infection: follow-up evaluation of vidarabine therapy. *Pediatrics* 72:778–785, 1983.

81. Amstey MS: Management of pregnancy complicated by genital herpes virus infections. *Obstet Gynecol* 37:515–520, 1971.

82. Visintine AM, Nahmias AJ, Josey WE: Relation of cytohistopathology of genital herpes simplex infection to cervical anaplasia. *Cancer* 33:1452–1458, 1973.

83. Kibrich S: Herpes simplex infection at term. What to do with mother, newborn and nursery personnel. *JAMA* 243:157–160, 1980.

84. Garner JS, Simmons B: CDC guidelines for isolation precautions in hospitals. *Infect Control* 4:281, 1983.

85. Valenti WM, Betts RF, Hall CB, Hruska JF, Douglas RG: Nosocomial viral infections: guidelines for prevention and control of respiratory viruses, herpesviruses, and hepatitis viruses. *Infect Control* 1:165–178, 1980.

86. Goldmann DA, Leclair J, Macone A: Bacterial colonization of neonates admitted to an intensive care environment. *J Pediatr* 93:288–293, 1978.

87. Franco JA, Eitzman DV, Baer H: Antibiotic usage and microbial resistance in an intensive care nursery. *Am J Dis Child* 126:318–321, 1973.

88. White RD, Townsend TR, Stephens MA, Moxon ER: Are surveillance of resistant enteric bacilli and antimicrobial usage among neonates in a newborn intensive care unit useful? *Pediatrics* 68:1–4, 1981.

89. Mayhall CG, Lamb VA, Bitar CM, Miller KB, Furse EY, Kirkpatrick BV, Markowitz SM, Veazey JM, Macrina FL: Nosocomial *Klebsiella* infection in a neonatal unit: identification of risk factors for gastrointestinal colonization. *Infect Control* 1:239–246, 1980.

90. Hemming VQ, Overall JC, Britt MR: Nosocomial infections in a newborn intensive care unit: results

of forty-one months of surveillance. *N Engl J Med* 294:1310–1316, 1976.

91. Townsend TR, Wenzel RP: Nosocomial bloodstream infections in a newborn intensive care unit: a case-matched control study of morbidity, mortality and risk. *Am J Epidemiol* 114:73–80, 1981.

92. Goldmann DA, Durbin WA, Freeman J: Nosocomial infections in a neonatal intensive care unit. *J Infect Dis* 144:449–459, 1981.

93. Fleer A, Sanders RC, Visser MR, Bijlmer RP, Gerards LJ, Kraaijeveld CA, Verhoff J: Septicemia due to coagulase negative staphylococci in a neonatal intensive care unit: clinical and bacteriologic features and contaminated parenteral fluids are a source of sepsis. *Pediatr Infect Dis* 2:426–431, 1983.

94. Munson DP, Thompson TR, Johnson DE, Rhame FS, VanDrunen N, Ferrieri P: Coagulase-negative staphylococci septicemia: experience in a newborn intensive care unit. *J Pediatr* 101:602–605, 1982.

95. Haley CE, Gregory WW, Donowitz LG, Wenzel RP: Neonatal intensive care unit bloodstream pathogens: emergence of gram positive bacteria as major pathogens. Abstracts of the Twenty-Second Interscience Conference on Antimicrobial Agents and Chemotherapeutics, 1982, abstract 691, p 187.

96. Brightman VJ, Scott TF, Westphal M, Boggs TR: An outbreak of coxsackie B-5 virus infection in a newborn nursery. *J Pediatr* 69:179–192, 1966.

97. McDonald LL, Geme JW Jr, Arnold BH: Nosocomial infection with echovirus type 31 in a neonatal intensive care unit. *Pediatrics* 47:995–999, 1971.

98. Modlin JF: Fatal echovirus 11 disease in premature neonates. *Pediatrics* 66:775–780, 1980.

99. Krajden S, Middleton PJ: Enterovirus infections in the neonate. *Clin Pediatr* 22:87–92, 1983.

100. Hall CB, Kopelman AE, Douglas RG, Geiman JM, Meagher MP: Neonatal respiratory syncytial virus infection. *N Engl J Med* 300:393–396, 1979.

101. Wolinsky E, Lipsitz PJ, Mortimer EA Jr, Rammelkamp CH Jr: Acquisition of staphylococci by newborns. Direct versus indirect transmission. *Lancet* 2:620–622, 1960.

102. Forfar JO, MacCabe AF: Masking and gowning in nurseries for the newborn infant; effect on staphylococcal carriage and infection. *Br Med J* 1:76–79, 1958.

103. Gezon HM, Thompson DJ, Rogers KD, Hatch TF, Rycheck RR, Yee RB: Control of staphylococcal infections and disease in the newborn through the use of hexachlorophene bathing. *Pediatrics* 51:331–344, 1973.

104. Nahmias AJ, Eickhoff TC: Staphylococcal infections in hospitals: recent developments in epidemiologic and laboratory investigation. *N Engl J Med* 265:74–81, 120–128, 177–182, 1961.

105. Williams JD, Waltho CA, Ayliffe GA, Lowbury EJ: Trials of five antibacterial creams in the control of nasal carriage of *Staphylococcus aureus*. *Lancet* 2:390–392, 1967.

106. Melish M, Glasgow LA: Staphylococcal scalded skin syndrome. The expanded clinical syndrome. *J Pediatr* 78:958–967, 1971.

107. Adler JL, Shulman JA, Terry PM, Feldman DB,

Skaliy P: Nosocomial colonization with kanamycin-resistant *Klebsiella pneumoniae*, types 2 and 11, in a premature nursery. *J Pediatr* 77:376–385, 1970.

108. Eisenach KD, Reber RM, Eitzman DV, Baer H: Nosocomial infections due to kanamycin-resistant, "R"-factor-carrying enteric organisms in an intensive care nursery. *Pediatrics* 50:395–402, 1972.

109. Hable KA, Matsen JM, Wheeler DJ, Hunt CE, Quie PG: *Klebsiella* type 33 septicemia in an infant in the intensive care unit. *J Pediatr* 80:920–924, 1972.

110. Kayyali MZ, Nicholson DP, Smith IM: A *Klebsiella* outbreak in a pediatric nursery: emergency action and preventive surveillance. *Clin Pediatr (Phila)* 11:422–426, 1972.

111. Donowitz LG, Marsik FJ, Fisher KA, Wenzel RP: Nosocomial *Klebsiella* bacteremia in a newborn intensive care unit caused by contaminated breast milk. *Rev Infect Dis* 3:716–720, 1981.

112. Hill HR, Hunt CE, Matsen JM: Nosocomial colonization with *Klebsiella*, type 26, in a neonatal intensive care unit associated with an outbreak of sepsis, meningitis, and necrotizing enterocolitis. *J Pediatr* 85:415–419, 1974.

113. Burke JP, Ingall D, Klein JO, Gezon HM, Finland M: *Proteus mirabilis* infections in a hospital nursery traced to a human carrier. *N Engl J Med* 284:115–121, 1971.

114. Boyer KM, Petersen NJ, Farzaneh I, Pattison CP, Hart MC, Maynard JE: An outbreak of gastroenteritis due to *E. coli* 0142 in a neonatal nursery. *J Pediatr* 86:919–927, 1975.

115. Kaslow RA, Taylor A Jr, Dweck HS, Bobo RA, Steele CD, Cassady G Jr: Enteropathogenic *Escherichia coli* infection in a newborn nursery. *Am J Dis Child* 128:797–801, 1974.

116. Abroms IF, Cochran WD, Holmes LB, Marsh EB, Moore JW: A *Salmonella newport* outbreak in a premature nursery with a 1-year followup. Effect of ampicillin following bacteriologic failure of response to kanamycin. *Pediatrics* 37:616–623, 1966.

117. Epstein HC, Hochwald A, Ashe R: *Salmonella* infection of the newborn infant. *J Pediatr* 38:723–731, 1951.

118. Leeder FS: An epidemic of *Salmonella panama* infections in infants. *Ann NY Acad Sci* 66:54–60, 1956.

119. Rubenstein AD, Fowler RN: Salmonellosis of the newborn with transmission by delivery room resuscitators. *Am J Public Health* 45:1109–1114, 1955.

120. Silverstolpe L, Plazikowski U, Kjellander J, Vahlne G: An epidemic among infants caused by *Salmonella muenchen*. *J Appl Bacteriol* 24:134–142, 1961.

121. Watt J, Wegman ME, Brown OW, Schliessmann DJ, Maupin E, Hemphill EC: Salmonellosis in a premature nursery unaccompanied by diarrheal disease. *Pediatrics* 22:689–705, 1958.

122. Plotkin SA, McKitrick JC: Nosocomial meningitis of the newborn caused by a *Flavobacterium*. *JAMA* 198:662–664, 1966.

123. Simmons NA: Contamination of disinfectants. *Br Med J* 1:842, 1969.

124. Ayliffe GA, Barrowcliff DF, Lowbury EJ: Contamination of disinfectants. *Br Med J* 1:505, 1969.

125. Morse LJ, Schonbeck LE: Hand lotions–a potential nosocomial hazard. *N Engl J Med* 278:376–378, 1968.

126. Morse LJ, Williams HL, Grenn FP Jr, Eldridge EE, Rotta JR: Septicemia due to *Klebsiella pneumoniae* originating from hand-cream dispenser. *N Engl J Med* 277:472–473, 1967.

127. Wargo EJ: Microbial contamination of topical ointments. *Am J Hosp Pharm* 30:332–335, 1973.

128. Simmons NA, Gardner DA: Bacterial contamination of a phenolic disinfectant. *Br Med J* 2:668–669, 1969.

129. Sanford JP: Disinfectants that don't (editorial). *Ann Intern Med* 72:282, 1970.

130. Felts SK, Schaffner W, Melley MA, Koenig MG: Sepsis caused by contaminated intravenous fluids. Epidemiologic, clinical and laboratory investigation of an outbreak in one hospital. *Ann Intern Med* 77:881–890, 1972.

131. Guynn JB Jr, Poretz DM, Duma RJ: Growth of various bacteria in a variety of intravenous fluids. *Am J Hosp Pharm* 30:321–325, 1973.

132. Lapage SP, Johnson R, Holmes B: Bacteria from intravenous fluids. *Lancet* 2:284–285, 1973.

133. Steere AC, Mallison GF: Handwashing practices for the prevention of nosocomial infections. *Ann Intern Med* 83:683–690, 1975.

134. Mortimer EA Jr, Lipsitz PJ, Wolinsky E, Gonzaga AJ, Rammelkamp CH Jr: Transmission of staphylococci between newborns. Importance of the hands to personnel. *Am J Dis Child* 104:289–295, 1962.

135. Price PB: The bacteriology of normal skin; new quantitative test applied to study of bacterial flora and disinfectant action of mechanical cleansing. *J Infect Dis* 63:301–318, 1938.

136. Brawley RL, Cabezudo I, Guenthner SH, Hendley JO, Wenzel RP: Evaluation of handwash agents using brief contact time. Program and Abstracts of the Twenty-Fourth Interscience Conference on Antimicrobial Agents and Chemotherapy, 1984, no. 520, p 184.

137. Maki D, McCormick R, Alvarado C, Hassemer C: Clinical evaluation of the degerming efficacy of seven agents for handwashing in hospitals. Program and Abstracts of the Twenty-Fourth Interscience Conference on Antimicrobial Agents and Chemotherapy, 1984, no. 522, p 184.

138. Renaud MT: Effects of discontinuing cover gowns on a postpartal ward on cord colonization of the newborn. *JOGN Nurs* 12:399–401, 1983.

139. Nauseef WM, Maki DG: A study of the value of simple protective isolation in patients with granulocytopenia. *N Engl J Med* 304:440–453, 1981.

140. Moylan JA, Kennedy BV: The importance of gown and drape barriers in the prevention of wound infection. *Surg Gynecol Obstet* 151:465–470, 1980.

141. Murphey D, Todd JK, Chao RK: The use of gowns and masks to control respiratory illness in pediatric hospital personnel. *J Pediatr* 99:746–750, 1981.

142. Agbayani M, Rosenfeld W, Evans H: Evaluation

of modified gowning procedures in a neonatal intensive care unit. *Am J Dis Child* 135:650–652, 1981.

143. Evans HE, Akpata SO, Baki A, Behrman RE: Bacteriologic and clinical evaluation of gowning in a premature nursery. *J Pediatr* 78:883–886, 1971.

144. Williams CP, Oliver TK Jr: Nursery routines and staphylococcal colonization of the newborn. *Pediatrics* 44:640–646, 1969.

145. Donowitz LG: Efficacy of the overgown in preventing nosocomial infection in a pediatric intensive care unit. *Pediatr Res* 18:182A, 1984.

146. *Standards and Recommendations for Hospital Care of Newborn Infants.* Evanston, IL, American Academy of Pediatrics, 1977, pp 118–199.

147. Meyer CL, Eitzen HE, Schreiner RL, Gfell MA, Moye L, Kleiman MB: Should linen in newborn intensive care units be autoclaved? *Pediatrics* 67:362–364, 1981.

148. Cairo MS, Rucker R, Bennetts GA, Hicks D, Worcester C, Amlie R, Johnson S, Katz J: Improved survival of newborns receiving leukocyte transfusions for sepsis. *Pediatrics* 74:887–892, 1984.

149. Laurenti F, Ferro R, Isacchi G, Panero A, Savignoni PG, Malagnino F, Palermo D, Mandelli F, Bucci G: Polymorphonuclear leucocyte transfusion for the treatment of sepsis in the newborn infant. *J Pediatr* 98:118–123, 1981.

150. Christensen RD, Rothstein G, Anstall H, Bybee B: Granulocyte transfusions in neonates with bacterial infection, neutropenia and depletion of mature marrow neutrophils. *Pediatrics* 70:1–6, 1982.

Chapter 28

The Special Problems of Nosocomial Infection in the Pediatric Patient

E. Lee Ford-Jones, M.D.

THE MAGNITUDE OF THE PROBLEM

At the Sixth Northern Pediatric Congress Meeting in Stockholm, Sweden in 1934, data were presented indicating that as many as 50% hospitalized patients acquired cross-infections, with small infants and patients with tuberculosis and diabetes being especially susceptible (1). A review of records of the Infants' and Children's Hospitals, Boston, in 1935 and 1936 indicated that 12.6% of 1455 infants admitted to hospital had febrile disturbances appearing sufficiently long after hospitalization to justify the assumption that they had been acquired in the hospital (1). With measles, chickenpox, German measles, polio, diphtheria and pertussis present in only 2.6% of patients being admitted, nosocomial contagious disease occurred only rarely, and the appearance of such contagious diseases led to such radical temporary improvement in the technique used in the ward that cross-infection was reduced. No nosocomial gastroenteritis occurred, but admissions for diarrhea were unusual (0.6%). Of all children remaining in the wards longer than 2 weeks, 26.6% acquired infections, accounting for 90% of all hospital infections. Others at the time identified the need for closed cubicles with outside exhaust for measles and varicella cases (1). Masks, confinement of each infant to a separate cubicle, exclusion of visitors, control of nurses' health, administration of cold vaccine to nurses, and employment of older nurses who would not be predisposed to catarrhal infection were recommended (1, 2). While the risk attributable to hospitalization was not known, it was hoped that control measures found effective in hospital would be of use in public health control. In a prospective review of 26 pediatric wards in 14 British hospitals in 1949, cross-infection was documented in 7.1% of patients during the hospital stay. Most common were acute respiratory infections (38%) and gastroenteritis (21%) (3).

Recent data on the problem of nosocomial infections in pediatric patients indicate that the problem is still with us. In general, the magnitude of the problem in pediatric hospitals remains poorly defined. There are few systematic reviews, and much information is based on reports of outbreaks of disease. Nosocomial infection rates between 2.3 and 12.6/100 admissions or discharges have been reported (1, 4–15) and are listed in Table 28.1. Lower rates of nosocomial infection were found in the National Nosocomial Infection Surveillance study (16) and varied depending on the type of hospital surveyed, as shown in Table 28.2. In general, surveillance methods varied widely, as did diagnostic criteria. For example, intravenous catheter-related infections were not always clearly defined (4), colonization was included in some studies (11, 13), positive wound cultures were required for a diagnosis of wound infection (11), and incubation periods for presumptive diagnoses of infectious respiratory and gastrointestinal infections have varied (4, 6). Noninfectious complications of hospitalization were included in one report (1).

Table 28.3 includes infection rates by service reported in the literature (4, 10, 13–15). The major problem areas have included the intensive care nursery and pediatric intensive care unit, neurosurgery, cardiovascular surgery, and oncology services (4, 10). These are all areas with severely compromised patients with prolonged stays undergoing many diagnostic and therapeutic interventions.

Infection rates in different anatomic sites vary widely (Table 28.4) (1, 4, 5, 10, 12, 13). The most comprehensive report to date (4) and the only

Table 28.1. Overall Nosocomial Infection Rates Reported in the Literature

Hospital	Year Reported	No. of Pediatric Beds	Infection Rate/100 Patients	Primary Method of Surveillance	Duration of Surveillance
Children's Hospital of Buffalo	1984	181	4.1	Review of nursing Kardex. All lab reports. Medical record discharges.	12 months
University of Virginia Hospital (5)	1981	Unknown	4.7	Review of nursing Kardex weekly to select high risk patients for chart survery	70 months
Strong Memorial Hospital (6–9)	1980	Unknown	2.3	Ward visits twice weekly. Viral lab reports.	17 months
Children's Hospital Medical Center (10)	1972	343	4.6	Ward visits to head nurses twice weekly. Bacteriology lab reports.	12 months
Adelaide Children's Hospital (11)	1970	Unknown	2.8	Ward visits to ward nurses thrice weekly. All lab reports.	33 months
Universityof Kentucky Hospital (12)	1967	Unknown	5.3	Review of mycology and bacteriology lab reports.	57 days
The Hospital for Sick Children, Toronto (13–15)	1962	609	6.5	Daily ward visits.	12 months
Infants' and Children's Hospitals, Boston (1)	1938	Unknown	12.6	Chart review.	24 months

Table 28.2. Infection Rates/100 Discharges by Site on Pediatric Services NNIS 1980 to 1982 (16)

Type of Hospital	Nosocomial Infection Rate at Different Sites of Infection*						
	UTI	SWI	LRI	CUT	BACT	Other	All Sites
Nonteaching	0.04	0.06	0.04	0.06	0.01	0.07	0.27
Small teaching	0.22	0.08	0.21	0.15	0.19	0.45	1.3
Large teaching	0.24	0.16	0.23	0.20	0.18	0.44	1.45

* UTI, urinary tract infection; SWI, surgical wound infection; LRI, lower respiratory infection; CUT, cutaneous; BACT, bacteremia.

one to include viral disease found that respiratory tract infections accounted for 23.9%, gastrointestinal infections 16.8%, blood 10.0%, and urinary tract, surgical wound, skin, and eye, each for about 8% of all nosocomial infections. Unlike adults, gastrointestinal infections are a major problem in children and urinary tract infections are not.

Risk Factors

Age. The attack rates were highest on infant wards (6.7%), lowest among adolescents (1.6%) and intermediate on wards housing toddlers and school-aged children (3.4% and 4.1%) (4). Others have found the infection rate during the first year of life to be twice that of subsequent age groups

Table 28.3. Overall Nosocomial Infection Rate by Service Reported in the Literature

Hospital	Nosocomial Infection Rate per 100 Admissions or Discharges												
	Intensive Care Nursery	Nursery	Pediatric ICU	Medical	Surgical	General Surgery	Neuro-surgery	Cardio-vascular	Ortho-paedic	Neurol-ogy	Tumor Therapy	Ear-Nose-Throat	Dental
Children's Hospital of Buffalo (4)	22.2	1.7	11.0	4.9	2.0	3.7	17.7	11.2					
Children's Hospital Medical Center (10)				4.2		4.2	18.6	4.7	3.9	1.0	21.4	0	0
The Hospital for Sick Children (13–15)				4.4	10.3								

(10), and a decrease in infection rates after the first 10 years of life has been reported by others (13–15). At a teaching hospital in Lagos, the 0 to 4 age group had the highest number of infections (17). A very low risk of 10 infections/1000 discharges during the first decade has been reported, but this study did not provide details of the population and surveillance methods (18).

Other host risk factors and length of stay have generally not been addressed (19), except for some viral respiratory disease in which the risk appears to be most related to the duration of hospitalization, with 45% of the infants hospitalized for 1 week or more becoming infected and the proportion continuing to increase with the length of hospitalization (20).

The Special Problem of Viral Disease

Viral pathogens are a major cause of nosocomial disease in pediatric patients. In a report comparing the relative importance of bacterial and viral pathogens, *Staphylococcus aureus* was identified as the most common pathogen, followed by rotavirus (4). Viruses—including rotavirus, respiratory syncytial virus, parainfluenza, adenovirus, echoviruses, coronavirus, calicivirus, and astrovirus—caused more infections than gram-negative bacilli. Respiratory infections of known etiology were more commonly caused by viruses than bacteria. All enteric infections were caused by viruses. In summary, viral agents caused 14.3% of all nosocomial infections and probably many more of the respiratory and enteric infections from which no infectious agent was recovered.

During 17 months of surveillance for viral infections at the Strong Memorial Hospital, the pediatric service had the highest rate of nosocomial viral infection, approximately 5-fold higher than that on the adult medical service (6). Viral infections occurred at a rate of 72.4/10,000 pediatric admissions, accounting for 35.4% of all nosocomial infections. Unlike adults in whom exogenous and endogenous viral infections (i.e., herpes simplex virus, cytomegalovirus varicella-zoster) were equally common, the pediatric infections were caused almost exclusively by RSV, adenovirus, and parainfluenza virus. In a review of new episodes of fever occurring in hospitalized children, one-third were associated with the recovery of respiratory viruses (21). Other presumptive cases of viral disease were reported during hospital-wide surveys and included 75 cases of measles, 25 cases of varicella, 5 cases of rubella,

Table 28.4. Proportional Distribution of Nosocomial Infections by Site of Infection

Hospital	Respiratory Tract (%)	Gastro-intestinal Tract (%)	Blood (%)	Urinary Tract (%)	Surgical Wound (%)	Skin (%)	Eye (%)	Miscellaneous (%)
Children's Hospital of Buffalo (4)*	23.9	16.8	10.0	8.9	8.4	8.0	7.9	16.0
Univerity of Virginia Hospital (5)	8.4		22.7	14.1	0.36			54.5
Children's Hospital Medical Center, Boston (10)	17.0	3.2	13.6	17.2	26.0	10.6		9.1
University of Kentucky Hospital (12)	35			5	30			30
The Hospital for Sick Children, Toronto (13)	41.8	20.0			13.5			24.7
Infants' and Children's Hospital, Boston (1)	59.8	0				15.6		

* Only center to include viral infections systematically.

2 cases of mumps, and 1 coxsackie B encephalitis (10, 11, 13).

Most reports of nosocomial viral infectious diseases have been investigations of recognized outbreaks. Rates of infection in hospitalized patients have not been compared to those in children at home or in day care facilities, but severe or fatal disease from a relatively uncommon community virus such as adenovirus 7 (22) has been attributed to hospitalization; and for several reasons, it would seem prudent to minimize the risk of occurrence of these infections and endeavor to defer them to an older age:

1. the severity of RSV is inversely related to age (23) with symptomatic infections occurring on re-exposure to this and other respiratory viruses throughout life. Infectious are particularly severe until 3 years of age (23–25).
2. Wheezing in as many as 10% of children may be attributable to bronchiolitis (26–29).
3. Intestinal infections occurring frequently in a normal host or in a patient whose nutritional status is already marginal can be an important determinant of nutritional health (30) and can lead to chronic intractable diarrhea in the young infant who is poorly adapted to fasting (31).
4. Infants with otitis media in early infancy are at high risk for chronic otitis media with effusion (32).
5. Both epidemiologic data and experimental evidence support the hypothesis that pri-

mary viral infection increases host susceptibility to secondary bacterial, fungal, and protozoal infection (33).

Efforts should be made to protect hospitalized children, particularly those less than 2 years of age, from these extra infections which may have serious sequelae.

Hall has identified a number of principles of nosocomial viral infections which distinguish them from bacterial infections (34):

1. They reflect the pattern of activity in the community rather than hospital bacterial flora;
2. The incidence, age of person affected, type of illness, and seasonal occurrence are typical of infection with that virus in the community;
3. They are constantly being introduced into the hospital since some children may be silently or asymptomatically shedding virus;
4. They may occur in any patient rather than just in high risk patients.

The incidence of nosocomial viral infections has probably been grossly underestimated for the following reasons: viral diagnostic services are not readily available; patients have not been followed after discharge (most cases of nosocomial varicella have been identified only after discharge (35, 36); asymptomatic infection is common; multiple or sequential infections may occur, and the necessary repeat cultures are not obtained; and infections are so common as to be considered "the norm." Additional studies are needed using

Table 28.5. Criteria for Nosocomial Viral Infection*

Virus	No. of Days from Onset of Illness
Respiratory	
Influenza	3
Respiratory syncytial	5
Parainfluenza	5
Adenovirus	7
Rhinovirus	3
Gastrointestinal	
Norwalk-like	2
Rotavirus	3
Exanthematous	
Measles	10
Mumps	18
Rubella	18
Roseola	10
Chickenpox	13
Picornavirus	
Echovirus	5
Coxsackievirus	5
Poliovirus	4–30
Hepatitis	
A	15–45
B	60–180
Non-A, non-B	18–89
Herpesvirus	
Herpes simplex	3
Herpes zoster	3
Cytomegalovirus	3
Viral respiratory illness (not cultured)	3

* From Valenti WM, Hall CB, Douglas RG, Menegus MA, Pincus PH: Nosocomial viral infections. 1. Epidemiology and significance. *Infect Control* 1:33–37, 1980.

standard diagnostic criteria such as those set forth by the Centers for Disease Control (CDC) with the appropriate modifications for viruses such as those seen in Table 28.5. Laboratory-based surveillance, including a review of all patients with positive viral cultures, a 4-fold rise in viral antibody titer between acute and convalescent sera, or a positive test for rotavirus by counterimmunoelectrophoresis, may be the most sensitive method of surveillance. This method detected 75% of infections as compared to 25% detection using ward visits by the infection control nurse (6).

Postoperative Wound Infections

Postoperative wound infections account for between 0.36 and 30% of nosocomial infections in pediatric patients (4, 5, 10, 12, 13) (Table 28.4). The highest proportion of wound infections is found in centers which have not included viral causes of nosocomial infections. One center has noted that wound infections constitute less than one-half of the infections acquired by surgical patients with the exception of the orthopaedic service, although infections following cutdown and procedures other than classical surgery were included in this report (10).

The frequency of postoperative wound infection at the Milwaukee Children's Hospital varied slightly by service, with an overall clean wound infection rate of 3.1% (37). Patients were followed for 1 month by questionnaire at the physician's office. Between 21% and 53% of wound infections in adults may go unrecorded because they appear after discharge (38). Children requiring simple day surgery procedures, which are generally clean, low risk surgery, were excluded from analysis, leaving perhaps a higher risk group to account for higher infection rates than those seen in adults. Twenty-five years ago, The Hospital for Sick Children in Toronto reported wound infection in 2.1% of patients undergoing clean surgery and 3.1% of patients following any surgical procedure (14). Higher rates have been reported by others (39), as shown in Table 28.6.

The subject of prophylactic antibiotics in children has recently been reviewed (40–43). There are virtually no studies documenting the efficacy of perioperative antibiotic prophylaxis of wound infection in children, although the principles should be the same in children as in adults (44), and the evidence of inappropriate use appears similar (37, 45, 46). Prophylactic antibiotics were given to 50% of patients undergoing clean surgery and continued for 4 days or more in about half of cases (37). Of antimicrobial agents used on surgical services at a large pediatric teaching hospital, 66% were considered inappropriate with respect to drug, dose, timing, duration, or indication (45). In another study, antibiotics were prescribed for 62% of children who had surgery, and prophylaxis, largely inappropriate, was the sole reason for antibiotic use in 73% of the patients (46). Retrospective case-control studies (47–52) on the value of shunt prophylaxis have demonstrated efficacy, but randomized controlled trials (53–56) to date, all with inadequate sample size, have not agreed as to the benefit of such prophylaxis. Infection following ventriculoperitoneal shunt surgery may ultimately have a negative effect on the child's intellectual function (57).

Two epidemics related to streptococcal carriage

Table 28.6. Number of Postoperative Wound Infections (%) by Classification of the Surgical Wounds

Reference	Wound Class				
	Clean	Clean-Contaminated	Contaminated	Dirty	Total
37	26 (3.1)	11 (7.8)	4 (17)	3 (10)	44 (4.2)
39	7 (3.5)	8 (16)	30 (37)		45 (13.6)

in pediatric surgeons have been described (58, 59). Anal carriage of group A streptococci was found in one orthopaedic surgeon who operated on three of four patients who developed wound infections following orthopaedic procedures (58). *Streptococcus equismilis* (Lancefield group C) was isolated from two postoperative orthopaedic wound infections performed by another surgeon within a 3-day period. He had perianal dermatitis from which *S. equismilis* was isolated, as well as colonization of the nose and rectum (59).

Bloodstream Infections

This subject is extensively reviewed in Chapter 19, and the problem in pediatric patients appears to differ very little from that in adults, although the amount of blood collected is often small, and there may therefore be some concern about the sensitivity of the test (60).

Endemic Infections

The etiology of bacteremias has been poorly defined to date. Bloodstream infections account for between 10 and 23% (4, 5, 10) of all nosocomial infections. In a report of nosocomial bacteremia from the Johns Hopkins Hospital, 1968 to 1974, the attack rate was 1.90/1000 patients for infants under 1 year of age excluding newborns (61). In 1984, Buffalo Children's Hospital (4) reported that 42% were caused by *Staphylococcus epidermidis*, reflecting trends observed in other populations and new information on its ability to cause serious infections (62–71). Twenty-four percent were caused by *S. aureus*. During the 12-month study, *Escherichia coli*, *Klebsiella*, streptococci, *Pseudomonas* and *Candida sp.* accounted for the remainder of infections, 13 of which were polymicrobial. Sixty percent of all cases of nosocomial bacteremia occurred in patients in intensive care areas (4) with attack rates 10-fold higher in these areas (2.8 and 2.1) than those in nonintensive care areas (0.2). An association with hyperalimentation was noted in 37% of patients, and in total 83% of all cases of nosocomial bloodstream infections were associated with the use of indwelling intravascular catheters, although the strength of this association is

not clear because the population from which the infected patients came was not described. At Children's Hospital, Boston in 1972, *E. coli* and *Klebsiella-Enterobacter* were the most common isolates; *S. epidermidis* was dismissed as a contaminant at that time except when associated with intravenous polyethylene catheters (10).

Device-Related and Epidemic Infections

There are few data on colonization of pediatric catheters (72, 73). The definition of an episode of bacteremia in the patient with an intravascular device which is not removed is controversial. If it is unclear whether a patient's Broviac catheter is the source of sepsis, quantitative bacteriologic techniques may be more sensitive and specific (74). In all nine positive catheter samples in one study of pediatric patients, the concentration of pathogens in cultures obtained through the catheter was 10 times as great as that observed in the peripheral venous sample. In two patients with septicemia not attributable to the catheter, quantitative cultures yielded low colony counts in the catheter sample. This method detected pathogens within 16 hours and identified infections with multiple organisms. Surveillance cultures taken through a Broviac catheter were not helpful in detecting impending septicemia.

In a report of patients with polymicrobial bacteremia, an intravascular device could be implicated in seven patients with polymicrobial bacteremia and in two patients with combined monomicrobial pseudobacteremia (75). Septic thrombophlebitis has been described following Teflon catheter insertion (*Klebsiella pneumoniae*, *S. epidermidis*) and venous cutdown (*Pseudomonas aeruginosa*) (76, 77). Subperiosteal abscess has also been described (77). Heparin locks have been used safely in cystic fibrosis patients (78). Prolonged use of lines for patients receiving total parenteral nutrition and chemotherapy has been associated with an infection rate of 2.68/1000 catheter use days (79). In some cases of central line infection, the infection may be adequately treated with antibiotics and without removal of the line (79, 80). Results of urokinase therapy have been variable (81,82).

Epidemic bacteremia in pediatric patients has been associated with contaminated infusion fluids including 5% dextrose in 0.2% sodium chloride to which potassium chloride had been added in the hospital's central pharmacy (*Enterobacter*) (83), heavily contaminated tops of intravenous bottles (*Enterobacter cloacae* and *Enterobacter agglomerans*) (84, 85), stored nonbacteriostatic saline used in a diagnostic tracer procedure (*Achromobacter xylosoxidans*) (86), and arterial pressure monitoring devices (*Pseudomonas maltophilia*) (87).

General host risk factors for nosocomial bacteremia include malnutrition (88) and age (89, 90), with the attack rate being highest in infants. Immunosupression is discussed in a subsequent section of this chapter. Nosocomial bacteremia with either one or more organisms may also be the result of Munchausen syndrome (91) or a child abuse variant, Munchausen syndrome by Proxy or Polle Syndrome (92, 93). One infant developed two episodes of bacteremia in hospital: one due to *P. aeruginosa* and the other due to *P. aeruginosa*, *Citrobacter freundii*, and *Klebsiella oxytoca* acquired when the mother used her husband's insulin syringes to inject contaminated water into the child's intravenous tubing (92). Another 4 ½-year-old child presented with "immunodeficiency disease" before the diagnosis of Polle syndrome was made (93, 94).

Respiratory Therapy

While this subject is dealt with in detail in Chapter 20, two points are worthy of emphasis. Aerosol therapy via croupettes is probably of little if any benefit in conditions characterized by pathology in the smaller airways, such as pneumonia and bronchiolitis. Of the mass of droplets produced by either the jet or ultrasonic nebulizer, (80 to 90%) are removed by the nose or oropharynx with nasal or normal mouth breathing (95). The possible benefits of a few milliliters of water in the lower respiratory tract should be weighed against the well known hazards of infection (96–98), uneven thermal environment, and the probable adverse psychological impact of therapy in most patients, and unnecessary use should be avoided.

Because of the minimal temperature decrease over the length of the Bain circuit in pediatric patients, humidifier temperatures must be kept significantly lower (i.e., 36.9 ± 1.9°C) than the recommended 50°C to avoid excessive airway temperature and thermal injury (99, 100). In a study of 14 pediatric patients ventilated for 99 days, 21.9% of cascade humidifier cultures and 46% of inspiratory tubing cultures were culture-positive (99), an incidence of colonization much lower than that found in Craven et al in an adult population (101). None of the patients exposed to this contaminated respiratory equipment developed respiratory disease as a result of therapy, although two became colonized with the same organism. *Acinetobacter calcoaceticus* was recovered from the cascade water in quantities of 10 to 20 organisms/ml (99).

Urinary Tract Infections

Although nosocomial urinary tract infections may account for between 5 and 17.2% of nosocomial infections in pediatric hospitals (4, 5, 10, 12), their true importance is difficult to assess because of the frequency of asymptomatic infections in nonhospitalized patients (1 to 2% of healthy school-age girls (102)) and the need for sterile urethral catheterization or bladder aspiration to obtain an uncontaminated urine in infants and young children. In healthy adolescent females undergoing spinal fusion, a statistically significant relationship between the number of straight catheterizations, the number of hours of urinary retention/stasis, and the subsequent development of urinary tract infections has been identified (103). Clean intermittent catheterization appears to be a safer and more effective means of regular bladder emptying than ileal loop diversion in the pediatric patient (104, 105).

Eye Infections

A recent cluster of 10 nosocomial eye infections in pediatric and adult patients resulting in blindness in three patients was traced to bacterial dispersion during tracheal suctioning (106). Only the left eye was infected in 9 cases; colony counts on settle plates were higher on the side opposite to the hand the nurse used to withdraw the catheter than on the same side, and the catheters tended to be withdrawn diagonally across the patient's face past uncovered and open eyes (106). Similarly, use of nasogastric tubes may be expected to cause eye infections, although this association has not been demonstrated.

Pediatric Intensive Care Unit

Endemic nosocomial infection rates in pediatric intensive care unit (ICU) patients have been reported as 11.0% in an 18-bed unit in a pediatric hospital (4) and 3% in a 16-bed unit which admits some children (107). Sixty percent of all nosocomial bloodstream infections occur there (4). As in the adult patient, multiple factors—including a depressed immune system due to underlying illness, invasive devices, exposure to antibiotic-resistant bacteria, emergency procedures performed without proper aseptic techniques, and the close proximity of patients to each other—may account for the high incidence.

Epidemic disease has been described. In three outbreaks due to *P. aeruginosa* and *E. cloacae* no source was identified, although some environmental contamination was documented (89, 90). Two outbreaks appeared to originate with a patient transferred from another hospital (89). The highest attack rates have been in neonates (89, 90). Intrinsic contamination of tracheal irrigant with *Pseudomonas pickettii* was documented in one outbreak (108). Control measures have been directed at removal of the source and improved infection control practices. In the outbreak of a gentamicin-resistant organism, gentamicin was withdrawn before the outbreak was controlled (90). The importance of viral infections in the ICU is now being recognized (109). Two clusters of nosocomial herpes simplex infections with two separate genetic strains were described in a pediatric ICU (110). Three nurses developed herpetic whitlow and a fourth acquired gingivostomatitis. The index case in the first cluster was a child with encephalitis and oral herpes. A 2-year-old girl acquired severe gingivostomatitis from one of three infected nurses (110). Additional information about risk factors is required (111–113).

Burn Units

There are few data on infections in children in burn units, although the susceptibility to bacterial wound infection and sepsis is well recognized. The care of the burned child does not differ from adults except for a greater probability of group A streptococcal sepsis. Nosocomial herpes simplex and varicella infections have been described (114).

Immunosuppressed Patients

Immunosuppressed patients are at high risk of nosocomial infections because of (a) impaired host defenses, (b) the need to perform invasive diagnostic or therapeutic procedures, and (c) alterations in normal flora. *S. aureus* bacteremias were preceded by a primary site of infection in

58% of 45 episodes. Primary sites of infection included an infected finger secondary to finger puncture for blood sampling, infected hyperalimentation lines, an intravenous catheter, a pierced ear lobe, a biopsy site, and a paracentesis site (115). In another series of *S. aureus* sepsis, primary sites similarly preceded 57% of episodes and included finger punctures for blood sampling (5) and intravenous catheter sites (10, 116).

Others have noted the emergence of *S. epidermidis* as an organism responsible for 12.7% of all septicemic episodes in a 30-month period (117). Unlike other groups who have associated the increased incidence of this pathogen with the use of long term indwelling catheters (79), they report two fatal episodes of *S. epidermidis* septicemia occurring in patients who did not have indwelling intravascular catheters. The incidence of sepsis was similar in patients with both peripheral and central lines, and antecedent throat and rectal colonization did not precede sepsis. They postulate two groups of patients who are undergoing intensive chemotherapy and prolonged hospitalization who are at risk for *S. epidermidis* septicemia. The first group have had significant prolonged breaks in the integument often with indwelling catheters, while the others have neoplastic disease in relapse with absolute granulocyte counts of less than $100/mm^3$/for 3 weeks or more.

Children with congenital immunodeficiency syndromes experience an increased severity of infection with parainfluenza virus (118, 119), respiratory syncytial virus (120), adenovirus (121), and rotavirus (122). Bacteria including *Clostridium difficile*, protozoa including *Cryptosporidium*, and other diarrheal agents may also be associated with overwhelming diarrhea, chronic infection, and death, particularly in bone marrow transplant recipients (123–125).

Alterations in Normal Flora

The three factors which seem to alter normal flora are (a) severity of illness, (b) duration of hospitalization, and (c) antibiotics (126). Antibiotic therapy was the main risk factor in determining the colonization rate of the external ear canal with potentially pathogenic flora in one study in which gram-negative bacilli or yeast were found in 58% of patients receiving antibiotic therapy, compared with 17% of patients hospitalized for 10 days or longer and only 3% of patients hospitalized for short periods (127). Thirty percent of children studied on admission to hospital had positive yeast isolates, with the percentage increasing with each week of hospitalization. By the fourth week, 80% of those still in hospital were colonized (128). The relative importance of confounding factors, such as antibiotics, corticosteroid therapy, intravenous therapy, parenteral alimentation, surgery, intravenous or urinary catheters, was not assessed. Asymptomatic nasopharyngeal colonization with *H. influenzae* type b of 11% of staff performing respiratory therapy in a pediatric chronic disease hospital has been documented (129).

MODES OF TRANSMISSION OF INFECTION IN THE PEDIATRIC HOSPITAL

The routes for acquisition of new organisms are multiple (Fig. 28.1) and include contact (both direct from one patient to another and indirect via contaminated fomites or droplets produced through coughing and sneezing), vehicles (for example, leafy vegetables contaminated with gram-negative organisms, water, food, drugs, blood products), and airborne (either droplet nuclei or dust particles or small particle aerosols < 10 μ mass median diameter which are contaminated with bacteria fungi or virus). Hospital construction and building materials can disseminate fungal spores which cause disease in immunocompromised patients. Insect transmission does not appear to be a major problem in North American hospitals.

The problem of infections in children is aggra-

vated by the normal behavior of the children themselves (130–134).

1. Toddlers between the ages of 2 and 4 years have been clocked at putting a hand or object in the mouth every 3 minutes.
2. Close contact of young children is almost constant unless children are specifically segregated.
3. Younger children are incontinent of feces before toilet training.
4. Younger children lack proper personal hygiene because of their age.

Of special concern in the pediatric facility are the role of visitors, contaminated fomites, and asymptomtic carriers of potential pathogens.

Visitors

The number of visitors may exceed the number of patients, and the parent-visitor may spend up to 24 hours a day and 7 days a week in the hospital. They may move freely in and out of waiting rooms, lobbies, cafeterias, washrooms, hallways, elevators, and may have contact with other children at home and in day care facilities, before returning to the patient's room. Parent-visitors often freely handle other children in a multibed room. The nurse, on the other hand, often spends less than 3 hours a day and the doctor less than 1 hour a day in the patient's room. Additional information is needed on the role of the parent-visitor in transmission (135, 136).

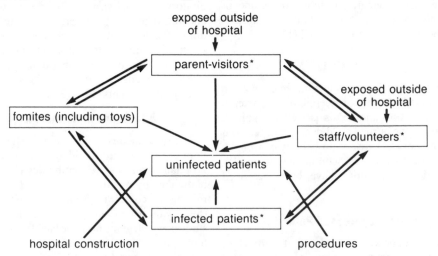

* symptomatic, asymptomatic, transient hand carriage

Figure 28.1.   Routes for acquisition of communicable diseases in the pediatric hospital. (Modified from Hall CB, Geiman JM, Douglas RG, Meagher MP: Control of nosocomial respiratory syncytial viral infections. *Pediatrics* 62:728–732, 1978.)

Fomites

Removal of respiratory and enteric viruses from contaminated surfaces may be important in control of nosocomial infection and is covered in detail in Chapter 18 and under respiratory and gastrointestinal infection control later in this chapter. Tremendous numbers of virus are excreted in respiratory secretions (137–139) and stool (140–142), and persistence of virus on surfaces for hours and even days may be common (143–146). Rotavirus, as well as hepatitis B, may be resistant to killing by routinely used disinfectants (147–152). Increased environmental contamination has been described during epidemic diarrheal disease in day care settings (145, 153, 154). Toys may be particularly important vectors (153, 154).

Asymptomatic Carriers

In Providence, in 1912, Chapin noted "Studies in hospitals and elsewhere have confirmed the belief that air is of minor importance in the spread of disease . . . the carrier is very important, if not the most important factor in the spread of the disease . . ." (155). This may be equally true today as incubationary and convalescent carriage are documented in children, parent-visitors, and staff as well as asymptomatic infection with many viral and bacterial pathogens.

PRIMARY PREVENTION AND PRE-EXPOSURE MANAGEMENT

Transmission of infection may be interrupted through efforts directed at the patient and parent-visitor, environment, and hospital personnel. Hand washing is of particular importance.

The Patient and Parent-Visitor

In considering this aspect of nosocomial infection prevention, the three traditional approaches to the control of infectious diseases in the host must be examined: immunization, chemoprophylaxis, and general infection control practice.

Immunization of Infants and Children

The best means of reducing the incidence of the vaccine-preventable diseases of childhood (diphtheria, pertussis, tetanus, polio, measles, mumps, and rubella) is by having a highly immune population (156). Particular attention must be paid to the immunization of premature infants, long stay patients, patients with nonpro-gressive and chronic diseases, neurologic disorders, and immigrants from nonimmune populations (157, 158). Enforcement of day care and school immunization requirements should be undertaken, and a comprehensive and accurate immunization record should be established for each newborn infant, maintained by the parent (156), and included in the hospital records.

Chemoprophylaxis

While this is more appropriately considered under treatment, prompt initiation of appropriate therapy may be successful in decreasing the reservoir of infectious agent in hospital even in situations where such therapy would not necessarily be recommended in outpatients, e.g., trimethoprim-sulfamethoxazole in enteropathogenic *E. coli* diarrhea, so that the risk of transmission to others is minimized.

General Infection Control Practices for Outpatients

Wherever possible, patients with an infectious disease, transmitted by the airborne route should be escorted through a separate entrance, avoiding waiting areas, into a single room in a separate area of the clinic for prompt assessment. While airborne disease transmission has not been documented in hospital clinics, measles has been contracted in a physician's office (159, 160). Patients at high risk of life-threatening disease from respiratory infection (e.g., the young infant (161), patients with congenital heart disease (162), and immunosuppressed patients (120)) should be similarly sent directly to a single room rather than remain in a common waiting area. Such patients who make repeated visits to the hospital may be identified by a card. Patients in observation areas should be managed according to general isolation guidelines, and high risk patients should be excluded from these areas. The hazards of immunosuppressed patient clinics have not been elucidated (135). A report of recovery of *P. aeruginosa* in dried sputum for more than 1 week and from sinks, soap, baths, toys, tables, brushes, cloths, and air in a cystic fibrosis clinic as compared to isolation cubicles where patients were treated suggested that it may be appropriate to segregate colonized and noncolonized patients and arrange for visits on separate days in the outpatient clinics (163). Pulmonary function laboratories in which these patients are tested should follow good infection control technique (164).

General Infection Control Practices for All Inpatients

Contagion Check. A communicable disease survey or "contagion check" is required for every pediatric patient. This survey should be completed prior to admission so that elective patients with infections may be excluded and appropriate ward placement and isolation implemented as indicated. This is particularly important during peak virus activity in the community. Essential components include the immunization history for measles, mumps, rubella, polio, diphtheria, pertussis, and tetanus; a history of exposure to varicella; any smptoms of infection, including cold, cough, vomiting, diarrhea, skin rash, or fever; and recent previous hospitalization requiring isolation (9). Infection control personnel must be available to review histories and physical findings at the request of admitting staff. It may be prudent to isolate patients transferred from other hospitals if the risk of colonization with resistant organisms acquired in that hospital is likely. This applies in particular to patients transferred from other hospitals in parts of the world with a high prevalence of methicillin-resistant *S. aureus* (e.g., Western Europe). Infants at high risk for severe or complicated RSV infection should not be electively admitted to the pediatric wards during an RSV outbreak (20).

Playroom. Restriction of children from the playrooms for the 48 hours after admission may be appropriate while the presence of infectious diseases previously overlooked or still in the incubationary phase on admission is ruled out. The use of nonporous toys which can withstand rigorous mechanical cleaning with running water

for at least 10 second, high level disinfection, or alternatively sterilization after use by infected patients and those with high rates of hand-mouth contact is desirable. Stuffed toys should be suspended out of reach or provided for personal use by selected patients. Floors should be kept clean since younger patients may use the floor as a playground (165).

General Infection Control Practices for Infected Inpatients

Isolation Precautions. Authoritative sources for isolation procedures are available (157, 166–169). With additional studies, it will be necessary to revise some recommendations (166). The importance of prompt isolation of all infected patients and those with presumed or possible infections, including those with colds or chronic diarrhea, until an infectious etiology has definitely been ruled out cannot be overemphasized. Isolation requirements should be routinely recorded in the admitting orders. The new CDC guidelines (166) have eliminated "reverse/protective isolation" for immunocompromised patients for reasons discussed in Chapter 29. Contact or "mini-strict" isolation—that is, masks for contact within 3 feet, gowns and gloves for physical contact—has been introduced as an alternative for uncertain isolation situations where small particle aerosol transmission is not likely (166, 167). Contact isolation is recommended for infants and young children with viral respiratory symptoms. Respiratory isolation is recommended for infants and children but not for adults with *H. influenzae* pneumonia. Cohorting as described in Table 28.7 may be appropriate if all patients are infected with the

Table 28.7. General Guidelines for Use of Cohort Isolation*

1. Patients should be separated into cohorts of infected ("dirty") and noninfected ("clean") patients.
2. Only persons with proven or suspected infection should be admitted to the infected cohort.
3. All exposed (potentially infected) individuals should be included with the cohort of infected patients. In some instances, the potentially infected cohort may be separated into a third cohort.
4. The infected cohort should be closed to new, uninfected admissions, and all new, uninfected admissions should be placed with the uninfected cohort.
5. Personnel working with the infected cohort should be immune to the illness in question by either previous history of illness or vaccination whenever possible.
6. Personnel should be assigned so that separate groups work with the infected and uninfected cohorts whenever possible. Crossover between cohorts should be discouraged to minimize the risk of cross-infection of the uninfected cohort.
7. When personnel must work in both areas, they should work in the "clean" area first, then work in the "dirty" area.
8. The infected cohort area will be closed as patients are discharged from the hospital and may be used for new, uninfected admissions after thorough cleaning of the area and its equipment.

* From Valenti WM, Menegus MA: Nosocomial viral infections. IV. Guidelines for cohort isolation, the communicable disease survey, collection and transport of specimens for virus isolation and consideration for the future. *Infec Control* 2:236–245, 1981.

same pathogen. Cohorting by clinical syndrome rather than by etiologic agent is generally unacceptable, but is often all that is possible in patients infected with viruses or enteric bacterial pathogens because of delays in specific diagnosis.

Gowns should be worn if patient contact is likely to lead to direct soiling of garments (166, 167) or if the organism is particularly contagious or virulent, e.g., methicillin-resistent *S. aureus*. Masks have not been shown to be of value in the prevention of nosocomial spread of RSV infection in either patients (170) or staff (171). Because coughs and sneezes result in the production of large particles which fall to the floor within about 3 feet of their origin, any exposure at this distance may be minimized by masks (167). In the case of smaller particles in which aerosol transmission can occur from highly contagious illnesses such as varicella, masks are thought to be of use (167). Gloves have been recommended when personnel have contact with the infected area of babies with diarrhea for aesthetic reasons (166) and as a reminder to wash hands (167).

Effects of Isolation. Little is known of the psychologic effects of isolation on the hospitalized child. Children in isolation may feel that they are being punished and rejected and may therefore be at risk of withdrawal and regression (172). Swedish workers have reported no negative effects of isolation provided that the child can observe the staff (165). Children raised in reverse isolation may experience difficulty with attachment behavior, although difficulties with emotional development may be modified (173, 174).

Diagnostic Investigations of Isolated Patients. These should be deferred if possible or scheduled at the end of the day in hospital areas where management of such cases has been clearly delineated (175).

Discharge. The charts of patients colonized with multiply resistant organisms which may persist for months should be identified on discharge so that the patients are isolated on subsequent admissions. Alternatively, parent letters or Medical-Alert bracelets may be provided. Ideally, convalescing infected patients should be discharged and readmitted for elective investigation to minimize problems associated with convalescent carriage of infective agents.

Visitors

It is advisable that visitors under 12 years of age be permitted only under special circumstances and after special arrangements have been made with the charge nurse or responsible phy-

sician. A "contagion check" as for an inpatient must be completed and the need for strict parental supervision of these sibling-visitors stressed. Parents should be instructed on hand washing before and after contact with their own child and the necessity of handling only their own child. Nosocomial pertussis (176), herpes (177), and RSV (20, 178) infections have been traced to parent-visitors, and their role in introduction of other respiratory and enteric pathogens is strongly suspected.

The Environment

Design of Facilities. The ideal design is not known. The pattern of transmission of RSV on the wards during outbreaks suggests that large open wards allow greater transmission than wards composed of smaller rooms (Table 28.8) (20, 179–182). Placement of each patient in a single room will almost certainly minimize the risk of nosocomial infection through facilitation of hand washing and disinfection but will not eliminate the risk (181, 183). It has been said that the sick child should be able to see adults (165). Some guidelines are available, and it appears that at least in the nursery population, increasing bed space per patient may result in a lower rate of infection (184), although others have not found this to be essential in adult populations (185). The importance of disinfection of the environment and toys has been discussed under "Methods of Transmission."

Hospital Personnel

The subject of employee health (169, 186–189) including the pregnant employee (190) is discussed in Chapters 12 and 13. The patterns of illness occurring in adult contacts are noted in Table 28.9. All staff should have completed a primary series of tetanus and diphtheria immunizations with boosters every 10 years, and all born after 1956 should have proof of immunity to measles. Rubella vaccination and annual tuberculosis skin testing should be conditions of employment. Mumps and polio protection is also advisable; pertussis immunization is not routinely required. Annual influenza immunization is recommended. The need for hepatitis B immunization of staff in pediatric facilities is unclear. One pediatric center has documented no increase in risk in a supposedly high risk population over a control population using hepatitis B surface antibody as a marker (191).

The need for careful education and screening

Table 28.8. Nosocomial Respiratory Virus Infection on Pediatric Wards with Differing Design and Infection Control Procedures Reported in the Literature

Reference	Agent	Time Course (Months)	No. (%) of Patient Contacts with Nosocomial Respiratory Infection
183	RSV	2	13
	Rhinovirus		2
	Parainfluenza virus Type 1		1
246	Parainfluenza 3	15	36 (18)
179	RSV	4	15
	Influenza A		16
	Parainfluenza		19
251	Influenza A	1	12 (70)
181	Rhinovirus	4	4 ⎫
	RSV		3 ⎬
	Parainfluenza type 3		2 ⎬ 15 (17)
	Influenza A and B		2 ⎬
	Symptomatic		4 ⎭
182	RSV	2	8 (19)
180	RSV	24	25 ⎫
	Influenza		18 ⎬
	Parainfluenza		12 ⎬ 169 (1.6)
	Adenovius		10 ⎬
	Rhinovirus		9 ⎬
	Symptomatic		95 ⎭
170	RSV	2	19 (37)
256	Influenza type C	12	17 (85)
22	Adenovirus type 7b	1	5 (1.0)

of all employees and students during a prework health evaluation, assessment at the time of acute illnesses, and meticulous follow-up of all exposures 24 hours of the day, 7 days of the week cannot be overemphasized in the pediatric hospital (188). An information sheet dealing with diseases and exposures such as that in Table 28.10 may be reviewed with all employees and students before employment to advise them of what they may acquire from and transmit to patients. This necessarily includes medical and surgical attending and research staff, house officers, nurses, support staff, ancillary personnel, and their students.

Disease in pediatric hospitals due to rubella,

herpes simplex, (110), influenza A, respiratory syncytial viruses (170, 192), pertussis (193, 194), varicella (35, 36, 195), scabies (196), mumps (197), respiratory and diarrheal pathogens has been traced to and from personnel. Infants on a pediatric ward have been exposed to a nurse with diphtheria but no disease occurred in contact infants (198).

Precautions for Special Patients

Pediatric Intensive Care Unit Patients

The pediatric ICU should be given high priority in an infection control program. Adherence to basic practices, such as hand washing and good device management, should be stressed and monitored through a surveillance program and appropriate epidemiologic studies as in the adult ICU.

Immunosuppressed Patients

Infections in immunosuppressed pediatric patients resemble those in adults (199). Efforts to minimize pathogenic endogenous flora include prophylactic antibiotics and antifungals, colonization and suppression therapy, isolation and surveillance cultures, as well as cytomegalovirus prophylaxis with immunoglobulins as described in Chapter 29 (200–205).

Immunization must be kept up to date because of the increased risk of exposure in hospitals and clinics and the increased severity of measles (206, 207) and polio (208). It is common practice to

Table 28.9. Patterns of Occurrence of Diseases in a Pediatric Hospital*

Pattern of Occurrence	Example
Manifestations of infection primarily in children	Herpes simplex
Infection affects children and hospital staff	Respiratory syncytial virus
Infection is inapparent in children, but is likely to be apparent in hospital staff	Hepatitis A virus
Infection is inapparent or mild in children and in adult contacts, but may have serious consequences for the fetus of a pregnant contact	Cytomegalovirus, rubella

* Modified from Goodman RA, Osterholm MT, Granoff DM, Pickering LK: Infectious diseases and child day care. *Pediatrics* 74:134–139, 1984.

Table 28.10. Occupational Health Infectious Diseases Information Sheet

If you have *diarrhea*—wash hands very carefully after using the bathroom and before touching patients or their equipment. Try to avoid working with children less than 2 years old and with those with metabolic defects.

If you have a *cold*—wash hands very carefully before touching patients or their equipment. Wear masks and gowns for any direct contact with patients less than 2 years of age. Minimize contact with infants, immunodeficient or congenital heart patients.

If you have a *cold sore*, cover it with a mask or Band-Aid and wash hands thoroughly before touching any patient. Avoid contct with burns, immunodeficient patient, patients with skin disease, and newborn infants.

If you have a constant *pain* in one area, watch carefully to be sure that shingles are not developing.

If you are exposed to chickenpox at work or home and have never had chickenpox, lived in the same house with or cared for someone with chickenpox, please check with occupational health or infectious diseases to determine if and when you should go on a leave of absence.

If you are exposed to measles and have never had measles or immunization against measles, please notify occupational health or infectious diseases before working.

If you are exposed to blood through contact with mucosa, eye, skin, please contact occupational health or infectious diseases to assess the need for hepatitis B prophylaxis.

If you are exposed to whooping cough and develop a cough, inform your doctor that you have had this contact so that he may take further tests and notify occupational health or infectious diseases before working.

If you have or are exposed to any other infections, please check with occupational health (daytime) or infectious diseases (nights and weekends) before working.

---

defer administration of all live virus vaccines until no less than 3 months after all immunosuppressed therapy has been discountinued (157), while administration of killed vaccines may continue since the majority will respond (209). Revaccination with DT-polio of previously adequately immunized children is recommended soon after cessation of therapy (210). Exposure of susceptibles to children excreting vaccine strains of poliovirus should be avoided. Although children receiving immunosuppressive therapy from leukemia make antibody less effectively than normal children, the majority will develop sufficient antibodies after immunization to modify natural infection favorably. Response to influenza vaccine appears adequate (211–213), although diminished responses may be noted in patients receiving long term chemotherapy for neoplastic diseases (212, 213).

Avoidance of urinary catheters, indwelling venous catheters, and frequent changes of steel needles is advisable (79). Meticulous skin preparation must antecede any break in the skin (115–117). Unusual presentations of highly communicable disease may pose problems. Measles pneumonia, for example, may be unaccompanied by rash (207). Sequelae from respiratory (118–121, 214–216) and enteric (122–125, 217, 218)

pathogens may be life-threatening or fatal. Patients likely to receive multiple blood transfusions should receive hepatitis B vaccine (157) because screening of donors for hepatitis B surface antigen is not 100% effective. There appears to be an increased incidence of chronic persistent and chronic active hepatitis in leukemic children (219, 220). Patients exposed to varicella or presenting with a rash should be instructed to seek immediate immunoglobulin prophylaxis and avoid the hematology/oncology clinics. Regular screening for varicella antibody using a sensitive and specific test, such as the fluorescent antibody membrane antigen test, is advisable in order to reduce unnecessary use of varicella-zoster immune globulin, although immunosuppressed history-negative, seropositive patients can occasionally develop mild disease (221). Patients should be moved from wards adjacent to or undergoing demolition or construction to minimize the risk of aspergillosis (222–224). Immunosuppressed patients exposed to active tuberculosis should receive rifampin and a second drug, e.g., ethambutol, for 6 months (157). Because *H. influenzae* infections have been described in an older age group (4 to 12 years) of immunosuppressed patients and infections may present without a focus, household and close contacts of those with *H. influenzae* disease should receive prophylaxis if there is an immunosuppressed child of any age in the household (225).

The National Institutes of Health in Bethesda have carried out a major and innovative campaign directed at patients to emphasize hand washing and to teach patients to protect themselves, so it is not uncommon for a child to inform a forgetful physician that his hands should be washed before examination (167).

Precautions for Specific Diseases

Prompt recognition of children with infectious diseases in need of isolation is essential.

Viral Respiratory Diseases

General guidelines may be found in Table 28.11. Influenza vaccine is recommended for high risk groups, including patients with congenital heart disease, cystic fibrosis, severe asthma and other chronic lung diseases (158, 226–232) as well as the immunosuppressed patient.

Diarrheal Diseases

General guidelines may be found in Table 28.12. Patients with acute vomiting or chronic diarrhea should be viewed as potentially infected and should be isolated until infection, particularly with *Salmonella* sp. and *E. coli*, has been ruled

Table 28.11.   Summary of Options for Control and Prevention of Nosocomial Respiratory Virus Infections

1. Prompt contact isolation of all patients ≤ 2 years old with any respiratory symptom including the common cold or cohorting of infected infants preferably by etiologic agent where individual isolation is not possible.
2. Hand washing.
3. Use of gowns if soiling is likely.
4. Cohorting to staff to infants infected by the same etiologic agent.
5. Isolation of high risk contact infants, i.e., infants with congenital heart disease, immunosuppressed patients, and premature infants with pulmonary problems, at distances greater than 6 feet from infected infants. Assign asymptomatic staff, preferably with long term pediatric experience, to their care.
6. Limitation of visitors.
7. Shorter hospital stay.
8. Avoidance of elective admissions and elective surgery.
9. During influenza A outbreaks, chemoprophylaxis with amantadine for unimmunized personnel and high risk patients. The use of influenza vaccine has been discussed under "Primary Prevention and Pre-exposure Management."

Table 28.12.   Control and Management of Nosocomial Gastroenteritis

1. Define the causative epidemic strain through studies for bacteria, viruses, and parasites. Strains should be typed if possible and antibiotic sensitivity patterns determined if appropriate. Failure to detect a pathogen is not a reason to stop enteric precautions in a child with acute diarrhea because unidentified, presumably contagious agents are common. Serologic tests are of no practical value.
2. Obtain a stool specimen (in consultation with laboratory staff) from all infants because asymptomatic carriage of organisms may perpetuate the outbreak. Ideally the stools of all staff (or at least ill staff) are also examined.
3. Remind staff of hand contamination with enteric pathogens following defecation.
4. Isolate the index case in a single room and isolate the roommate in the original room. This contact room should be closed to admissions for the duration of the incubation period (157). Since some of these patients will already be incubating the contagious diarrheal agent, they should not be transferred into a room with unexposed children.
5. Close the ward to all new admissions and reduce the ward census as rapidly as possible depending on the agent involved and the number of symptomatic children. Close the playroom. Counsel the family carefully on symptoms of disease, fluid management, and antibiotic therapy (if required) prior to discharge. Parents and other household contacts of infants should be instructed in the use of enteric precautions appropriate to the home. Disposal of stools and diapers and the need for careful hand washing after contact with the infant must be emphasized.

out. During community outbreaks, it may be appropriate to reduce enviromental contamination through weekly cleaning of infant and toddler rooms with concurrent bathing of each child and placement into a clean crib. Immunosuppressed patients, particularly those having undergone bone marrow transplant who are at risk of fatal disease in association with infection with enteric pathogens, infants and children in the first year of life who are at a higher risk of overwhelming sepsis and death with bacterial pathogens (233), and patients unable to adjust to fluid loss such as some metabolic patients, should not share personnel or be placed in rooms with staff caring for infected patients (233).

Multiply Resistant Organisms

The risk of transmission may be minimized by isolation of patients coming from other hospitals or other countries where multiply resistant organisms are endemic until nasal, rectal, and wound swabs are reported as negative. Patients once colonized may remain so for months and should be identified as such in the hospital chart for future admissions.

Aspergillus

Some cases of aspergillosis may be prevented by adherence to precautions taken at the time of construction as discussed under "Cutaneous and Other Fungal Infections Originating in Hospital" (222, 223, 234).

Hepatitis A

Prevention depends on the routine use of basic infection control practices including prompt isolation of patients with diarrhea regardless of whether or not an infectious process is suspected (235, 236).

Hepatitis B

Recommendations for the use of vaccine in pediatric patients are under review. Unvaccinated children born to infected patients and the institutionalized retarded probably provide the greatest risk (157).

Skin Infections

Patients with eczema who have secondary infections shed massive numbers of organisms, usually *S. aureus* and group A streptococcus. Care must be taken to avoid transmission from and to (e.g., herpes simplex) these patients.

Pediculosis

Although pediculosis is a widespread problem among school-age children, lice are unlikely to be transmitted to other patients except in ambulatory chronic care patients such as are on a psychiatric ward where visual screening of all residents at the time of admission is appropriate.

Scabies

Prevention of outbreaks requires screening of patients for skin problems and appropriate diagnostic tests. Color pictures in the ward procedure book may be of assistance.

SECONDARY PREVENTION CONTROL AND POSTEXPOSURE MANAGEMENT

This review of pediatric nosocomial infections by clinical syndrome includes the prevalence of agents in hospitalized children, nature and frequency of nosocomial outbreaks, information about mode of transmission, susceptibility and reinfection, and an approach to control and management.

Viral Respiratory Infections

Prevalence. A tremendous multiplicity of agents has been associated with viral respiratory illnesses in children. They generally vary in ability to cause specific syndromes, depending on the agent and the age of the patient. For example, the most common cause of wheezing associated with respiratory infection in children under 3 years of age is RSV, whereas *Mycoplasma pneumoniae* may be the most frequent isolate for school age children with wheezing illness (237). In a study of patients less than 5 years of age hospitalized with acute lower respiratory tract infection in which an exhaustive search for infectious agents was made, a viral pathogen, most commonly RSV, was identified in 63% of cases (238). Infection with multiple agents occurred in 5% of cases. Rhinovirus was associated with disease indistinguishable from RSV, parainfluenza, and adenovirus. *M. pneumoniae* is probably also important but was not diagnosed. In a study of patients with croup, 74.2% of all isolates were parainfluenza viruses, although RSV, influenza, and *M. pneumoniae* may also cause this clinical syndrome (239). Other countries including Sweden have similarly reported a high incidence of RSV (240), and indeed acute respiratory infections in children are a major global public health problem (241). In other parts of the world such as New Guinea, bacterial pneumonia may be more common than pneumonias caused by viruses (242).

Community epidemics of RSV occur regularly from midwinter to early spring, and during this period many children admitted to the hospital with respiratory symptoms are infected with RSV (243). During peak epidemic influenza virus activity, influenza virus may interfere with the spread of other major respiratory viruses (244). Repeated infections, often of severity equal to the primary infection in children, are the rule before 3 years of age on exposure to RSV (24), and indeed repeated infections with parainfluenza (25) and influenza (230) may occur throughout life.

Outbreaks. A review of nosocomial outbreaks can be found in Table 28.8. The spread within the hospital of RSV, parainfluenza, and influenza A viruses during the period of their respective community epidemics is probably the rule rather than the exception. In contrast, nosocomial adenoviral epidemics may occur during a time of minimal community activity (22). Cross-infection is commonly traced to infected infants on the same or adjacent wards. In one report of 11 nosocomial infections, only 2 were acquired from infected roommates, the remainder presumably being introduced by staff and visitors (181). Most infected staff are symptomatic (20, 245).

Mode of Transmission. There are two major routes of transmission of respiratory viruses. The first is by *small particle aerosols* (< 10 μm mass median diameter). Aerosols produced by coughing, sneezing, or talking can transmit infection from one person to another over a considerable distance. Influenza, varicella, and measles viruses exhibit patterns of spread compatible with this mechanism. Other viral agents, such as RSV and rhinovirus, can be transmitted by mechanisms requiring *close person-to-person contact*, usually defined as a distance less than 3 feet separating the two persons. Large droplets produced by coughing or sneezing may spread the infectious virus directly to the skin or mucous membranes of a susceptible host or may contaminate the donor's hands and spread via *hand-to-hand contact or indirectly, via contaminated fomites*. In either of the latter cases, infection of the susceptible host is the result of autoinoculation from transfer of virus from the hands to the mucous membranes of the eye, nose, or mouth. Contagiousness, therefore, depends on the quantity of virus in nasal secretions, the effectiveness with which infected secretions are propelled into the environment through coughing, sneezing, or carried on hands, and how long the infectious virus can survive in the environment.

Parainfluenza type 3, RSV, and influenza A virus may be recovered from the nasopharynx for up to 6 days before the onset of symptoms, although they are most common in the antecedent 24 to 48 hours (137). The duration and degree of shedding of RSV are related to the age of the host and severity of illness (138, 139), with young infants and those with lung consolidation shedding virus for longer periods of time (139). Viral excretion persists in high titers until considerable clinical improvement has occurred. Parainfluenza type 3 virus may be recovered for prolonged periods of time, from 12 (246) to 30 or 40 days (137). Shedding for 1 week following onset of influenza A and RSV disease caused by influenza A and RSV is common, while 37% of cultures for influenza B are still positive during week 2 (137).

RSV (143) and influenza A and B (144) viruses may persist on environmental surfaces, as shown in Table 28.13, providing an opportunity for

Table 28.13. Fomite Contamination by Virus

Agent	Source	Countertops (Hard, Nonporous)	Rubber Gloves	Paper Tissue	Cloth	Skin
RSV (143)	Freshly obtained infant secretions and	8 hr	1 1/2 hr	30–45 min	1–2 hr	20 min
	by hands touching these contaminated surfaces for up to 25 min					
Influenza A Influenza B (144)	Throat swab isolates passed once in tissue cultures and	24–48 hr 24–48 hr		8–12 hr 8–12 hr	8–12 hr 8–12 hr	5 min 5 min
	by hands touching these contaminated surfaces for up to 5 min					

hand contamination and subsequent autoinoculation. Inoculation of RSV into the eye or nose (247) and of parainfluenza into the nose or throat (the eye has not been studies) (25) results in infection in the susceptible. Hand-eye or hand-nose contact is a normal part of human behavior, occurring once every 2 to 3 person hours of observation, during Grand Rounds, and several times during a 20-minute infant feed (248, 249). Influenza infection is most efficiently induced in volunteers by fine particle aerosols, although the role in natural transmission is not known (250).

Respiratory Syncytial Virus

Outbreaks (170, 179–183, 192). Children who are infected on admission are sources of RSV and may cause symptomatic infections in 40 to 60% of contact infants and 50% of hospital staff (20). Case-control studies have shown that risk of infection with RSV is affected by duration of hospitalization and by ward design. Open wards have the highest rates of cross-infection (20, 179–182).

Mode of Transmission. Risk correlates with the closeness of person-to-person contact. Only those staff members who cuddle infected infants or touch possibly contaminated environmental surfaces immediately surrounding the infant become infected, suggesting that airborne spread is not important (20, 251).

Control and Management (Table 28.11) Complete control will be difficult until antiviral agents or vaccine is available to patients and staff. While ribavirin looks promising, delivery is cumbersome and often impractical. Teratogenicity will preclude widespread use in female hospital staff of childbearing age (252–254). Long term pediatric experience and exposure to patients for less than 30 hours/week have been associated with lower rates of infection in hospital staff (171). The use of gowns and masks when studied prospectively did not decrease the acquisition of symptomatic respiratory infections in patients (170) or medical personnel (171) caring for infants. Masks continue to be recommended for close contact of 3 feet or less by some authorities (166).

Parainfluenza Type 3

Outbreaks (179–181, 183, 246). Twenty percent of 197 hospitalized infants and children less than 18 months old who were in contact with parainfluenza 3 virus acquired infection, usually during a cluster of index community-acquired cases and between the fourth and fifteenth day of

hospitalization. Acquisition generally occurred after infants and children were removed from coupettes into low humidity environments (246).

Control and Management. See Table 28.11.

Influenza

Outbreaks (179–181, 255, 256). High fever was the major presenting finding occurring in a ward outbreak involving 12 or 29 (71%) children hospitalized more than 1 week. Although the presence of clinical illness can be used to identify patients infected with influenza, the proportion of asymptomatic influenza infection may be high (257). Influenza C was removed from one employee, and two others had serologic evidence of acute influenza C virus infection during an outbreak of influenza-like illness in employees in the pediatric clinic at the University of California, Los Angeles Hospital. Forty-six percent of children under 5 years of age lack antibody. In a survey of children's residence, fever, nasal discharge, and sneezing developed in 85% of 20 children and 22% of 9 staff with confirmation of influenza C infection in 65% of children and 13% of staff (256).

Control and Management (Table 28.11). The prophylactic efficacy of daily amantadine in reducing the incidence of influenza virus infection in children has been demonstrated (258–260). It prevented disease in 50% of recipients in a hospital for the mentally retarded (260). Staff and patients at risk for severe disease should be immunized (157, 158, 226–232).

Adenovirus

Outbreaks. In a 1-month outbreak of adenovirus type 7b disease in a children's hospital in San Diego, four patients who acquired the disease died (22). Extensive cross-coverage of nurses from different units, the use of nurses per diem and cross-coverage by respiratory therapists, house officers, phlebotomy teams, and dietary workers may also have been responsible for spread. Over a period of 2 months, 18 adenovirus type 3 infections occurred in patients aged 4 to 12 years on a ward to which an infected 7-year-old girl was admitted (261). Symptoms of fever and conjunctivitis were present. High titer adenovirus immune serum globulin, if available, may be of use in controlling the disease (262). Restriction enzyme analysis may provide a more rapid means of discriminating between patient isolates during a nosocomial outbreak (263, 264).

Control and Management (Table 28.11).

Vaccination of institutionalized infants during adenovirus outbreaks may be considered (264).

Morbidity Mortality and Cost

Prolongation of hospital stay by 5.8 to 11 days for children with pneumonia and upper respiratory infections has been reported (161). Over a 6-year period, 37% of infants hospitalized with congenital heart disease and RSV infection died. Most infections were nosocomially acquired. Pulmonary hypertension was present in 72% of cases (162). Similarly infected children immunosuppressed through malignancy or primary disease were at risk of more severe disease (120). In children in a transplant until at the time of a parainfluenza 3 outbreak, the frequency of rejection was generally increased, although outcome in terms of patient survival at 6 months was not affected (265). Occasional deaths may occur and hospitalization may be prolonged. The morbidity of influenza in children in general (257, 267, 268) and particulary in children with cancer (269) or chronic asthma (229) and the occurrence of repeated infections (230) with exposure to agents reaffirm the importance of reducing nosocomial disease. As well as lower respiratory disease, influenza may cause a nonspecific febrile illness and a variety of neurologic syndromes, including encephalitis, encephalopathy, meningitis, and Reye's syndrome. Types of underlying disease putting children at greatest risk, such as pre-existing heart disease, immunosuppressive disorders, chronic pulmonary disease, diabetes mellitus, chronic renal disease, neuromuscular disorders, and neoplasms (231), are generally extrapolated from adults. Adenovirus type 7 has a propensity to cause fatal disease in the immunocompromised host (22).

General Recommendations for Control and Management of Viral Respiratory Infections

Control measures are listed in Table 28.11. Hand washing with 3 to 10 seconds of rapidly running water before and after all patient contacts remains the single most effective method of reducing the incidence of nosocomial infection. Rapid viral diagnosis will allow identification of infectious patients to facilitate segregated patients at high risk of severe disease. A number of techniques are under investigation, including detection of viral antigens in respiratory secretions by fluorescent antibody (FA) and enzyme-linked immunosorbent assay (ELISA) and early detection of viral antigens in tissue culture (270, 271).

Diarrheal Diseases

Prevalence. Through population-based prospective studies in North America, annual rates of diarrhea during the first year of life have been estimated at 0.82 to 1.05/child (272–274). Rates in other parts of the world may be 5 times as high. In the day care situation the rate appears to be somewhat higher at 1.24 cases/year in the first 2 years with high attack rates in staff and family members (275). Seroepidemiologic data in developed and developing countries suggest that most children acquire antibody to rotavirus before 3 years of age (276–278). Among children admitted to hospital with gastroenteritis, viruses are recovered from 25 to 55% of patients, generally in the winter months and especially in those patients between 7 and 24 months of age (111, 279–286). Rotavirus diarrhea increases slightly in cool dry months (151, 287). Bacterial causes are identified in 5% or less of hospitalized patients with some exceptions (288). Agents such as *Salmonella edinburg* or *Vibrio cholerae* may circulate in hospital when there is little or no community activity (289, 290).

Complete epidemiologic data linking agents detected only by electron microscopy to disease are lacking, although fairly convincing evidence is available to show that noncultivatable adenovirus and calicivirus are indeed pathogens (287). A poor association of rotavirus with entities other than the classic fever-vomiting-diarrhea syndrome (284–286) indicates the need for serologic studies in determining the etiology of diarrhea (272). While susceptibility of infants and children to bacterial pathogens is virtually universal, susceptibility of staff to bacterial pathogens is variable. Repeated infections with the same or other subgroups of rotavirus are known to occur in all age groups, although repeated infections may be milder (291–295).

Outbreaks. Tables 28.14 and 28.15 summarize the outbreaks reported on pediatric wards. Diagnostic methods, incubation periods, assiduousness of case finding, and definition of the population at risk vary considerably. Rotavirus and adenovirus infections are probably grossly underestimated because of the lack of readily available diagnostic methods. Of 1173 patients with nosocomial gastroenteritis listed in Tables 28.12 and 28.13, viruses were implicated as the cause in 400 patients, *Salmonella* sp. in 489 patients, and other bacterial agents in the remainder. Multiple putative pathogens may circulate independently (296, 297, 299, 300, 303). An outbreak with a heterologous rotavirus population

Table 28.14. Nosocomial Viral and Mixed Diarrhea on Pediatric Wards Reported in the Literature

Reference	Agent (No.)	No. (%) of Patients with Nosocomial Infection*	Time Course
296	Rotavirus (6)	6 (23)	39 days
	Adenovirus (6)	6 (32)	3 days
297	Rotavirus (75)	213	1 year
	Minireovirus (58)		
	Adenovirus (31)		
	Picorna/parvovirus (38)		
	Astrovirus (11)		
298	Reovirus-like agent (10)	12 (20)	24 days
299	Astrovirus (14)	22 (5)	4 months
	Astrovirus + rotavirus (5)		
	Rotavirus (3)		
300	Rotavirus (1)	26 (16)	53 days
	Minirotavirus (10)		
	Calicivirus (7)		
	Picorna-paravirus (1)		
301	Calicivirus (7)	26 (77)	31 days
302	Calicivirus (4)	5 (83)	2 months
303	Rota (14)	77	1 year
	Salmonella (8)		
	Shigella (1)		
	E. coli (30)		
	Parasites (3)		
	E. histolytica (1)		
304	Adenovirus (5)	5	3 months
305	Rotavirus (22)	37	11 months
306	Rotavirus (8)	8	3 months
284	Rotavirus (6)	6 (.03)	11 months

* Includes patients with one or more of the following: clinical disease, pathogen in stool, or serologic evidence of infection.

Table 28.15. Nosocomial Bacterial Diarrhea on Pediatric Wards Reported in the Literature

Reference	Agent	No. (%) of Patients with Nosocomial Infection	Time Course (Months)
289	*Salmonella edinburg*	299	32
307	*Salmonella indiana* (MDR)*	46	13
308	*Salmonella heidelburg*	55	4
309	*Salmonella wandsworth*	7	4
310	*Salmonella muenchen*	28 (7)	1
311	*Salmonella havana* (MDR)	44	6
312	*Salmonella typhimurium* (MDR)	26 (44)	3
290	*Vibrio cholerae* (MDR)	216	7
313	*Shigella sonnei*	13	1

* MDR, multiple drug-resistant.

with mixed patterns has been described (314). In only 10 of 25 cases of nosocomial gastroenteritis was concordance with a presumed index case roommate demonstrated (300). With the availa- bility of tissue culture methods to recover rota- virus, asymptomatic shedding of rotavirus has been found in 15 to 60% of infants 7 to 24 months of age, much higher than in outbreaks using only less sensitive electron microscopic or counterimmunoelectrophoresis techniques (272). The prevalence of asymptomatic rotavirus carriage in outbreaks has been lower than this (Table 28.16). Asymptomatic and symptomatic staff have been identified during outbreaks, and incidental pathogens such as *Camphylobacter* sp. or *Salmonella* sp. have been uncovered during screening. Their role in transmission is unknown, although asymptomatic carriers may be important in the maintenance of neonatal rotaviral outbreaks (315).

The following issues have been identified as factors contributing to outbreaks: multibed rooms; overcrowding; roommate with diarrhea; temporal relationship to infected patient (either sharing ward or moving to the room following discharge of an infected patient); sharing a cot; eating with fingers from a communal plate; transport of diapers outside the patient's room for diagnostic tests; handling of infants by parents of other children; common playroom, scale, bathing, and feeding facilities; multiuse lubricants; failure to transfer long stay patients to an isolation ward; contamination of sodium hypochlorite; and inadequate kitchen procedures. Nosocomial gastroenteritis appears to be most prevalent in children under 2 years, although age-specific attack rates for nosocomial disease are not available.

Mode of Transmission. Because rotaviruses and fastidious adenoviruses have not been cultivatable in tissue culture until recently, there have been no systematic studies of the mechanism of transmission of these aspects which cause most cases of infantile diarrhea. Rotavirus and other agents causing diarrhea are excreted in very large numbers in the feces of patients, with 100×10^9 viral particles/g of stool being visible by electron microscopy and as many as 2000 infectious virions/ml detectable by tissue culture (140,141).

Table 28.16. Asymptomatic Carriage of Enteric Pathogens in Children during Nosocomial Outbreaks

Reference	Agent	No. Recovered/ No. of Children Examined
296, 298, 300, 303	Rotavirus	2/82
296, 304	Adenovirus	1/85
300	Minirotavirus	8/25
300, 301	Calicivirus	5/38
299	Astrovirus	0/10

Extrapolating from data on rotavirus antigen there may be 1 mg of virus/ml of infected stool (142). Even larger amounts of infectious organisms are shed in bacterial diarrheas. The infecting dose in children is unknown (316, 317).

Rotavirus has been recovered from a variety of hospital surfaces, and in studies of suspension of fecal matter survival for up to 10 days on nonporous surfaces has been demonstrated (140, 145, 151, 154). Solutions containing organic iodine, hypochlorite, or quaternary ammonium salts as the principal active ingredient(s) are ineffective in inactivating rotavirus. Phenol-based products give variable results. Products containing 60% ethanol or inorganic acid(s) are able to inactivate the virus (147, 148, 150). Products appearing effective in the suspension have not always been effective in the disinfection of rotavirus-contaminated surfaces (149).

Hand carriage of enteric pathogens is probably very important (318). The hands of all attendants working with 147 children under 5 years of age admitted to the International Center for Diarrheal Disease Research, Bangladesh, were washed thoroughly in a sterilized bowl with 100 ml of tap water within 4 hours of admission of the first four children each day (319). A total of 78.6% of the attendants of 70 patients with rotavirus diarrhea and 19.5% of the attendants of 77 patients without were positive for rotavirus antigen. The hand washings of attendants of younger children with rotavirus diarrhea contained more rotavirus antigen than the hand washings of attendants of older children. Hand contamination following defecation in convalescent carriers of *Salmonella* sp. has been described (320).

Environmental contamination has been demonstrated in elegant studies involving piglets in a nursery (321–323). Contamination of the facility with porcine rotavirus increased with continuous use, causing a progressive increase in the incidence of infection and death. One-day-old piglets were introduced to a nursery every 10 days for a 2-week period so that there was an overlap of younger and older piglets with no opportunity to clean and disinfect the facility. A repeatable pattern emerged; the first few litters were asymptomatic and showed a satisfactory weight gain. However, by the time the eighth litter was introduced (after 5 weeks of continuous operation), a mild diarrhea was noticed in older piglets. With subsequent litters more severe illness, including vomiting, occurred; and after 9 weeks of operations, 50% died of gastroenteritis. At this time all piglets were removed so that the nursery could be cleaned and the first litter of piglets entered 1 week later. The same pattern of illness emerged but was subsequently prevented by a thorough cleaning of the facility before the introduction of a new litter.

During outbreaks of diarrhea in day care centers, fecal coliforms are recovered significantly more frequently from classroom objects, including water taps, than during nonepidemic periods, but the role in transmission is unknown (153, 154). Persistence of *Salmonella* sp. in the inanimate environment for more than 1 week has been documented (324).

The spread of rotavirus among hospitalized patients and to children admitted to rooms previously occupied by infected patients suggests that a contaminated environment may be a factor in viral dissemination (296, 298, 306). The massive number of rotavirus particles commonly seen in feces of infected children could easily cause environmental contamination. Persistence of excretion to the ninth day of illness and beyond would provide ample opportunity for such contamination. In most young infants, there is either no demonstrable rotavirus at the time of cessation of diarrhea, or significantly less; older children, on the other hand, have higher titers persisting after diarrhea ceases (285). This refers to virus detectable by electron microscopy, a method which is probably much less sensitive than culture (142).

The respiratory route may be important in transmission of viral enteric pathogens, and recent work has shown that rotavirus can survive in the airborne state for several days (325). In a study of children hospitalized with pneumonia, the rotavirus was recovered from respiratory tract secretions from four patients, and in two patients for whom paired sera were available, the presence of antibody rises suggests that it may on occasion be associated with pneumonia (326). The potential for respiratory transmission requires further clarification but has been suspected in outbreaks (327, 328). Alternatively massive environmental contamination with virus and a low infecting dose could explain the transmission which mimics airborne transmission. The role of contamination of the environment in the spread of bacterial pathogens is less clearly understood.

Morbidity and Mortality. Patients with metabolic diseases are less able to handle problems in fluid balance associated with the tremendous fluid losses which may accompany any diarrhea, but particularly rotavirus. Bone marrow transplant recipients who acquired diarrhea had a higher mortality rate (56%) than those who did not (13%) (123).

Control and Management. A strictly monitored hand washing program after toilet activities and before eating/feeding resulted in a 50% decrease in the entire 35-week study period in two day care centers compared to two nonintervention centers (329). A similarly dramatic impact of a hand washing program on intrafamily transmission of diarrhea was demonstrated in Bangladesh (330). Current methods of control are included in Table 28.12 (280,331). Other methods of control have been described (332). An effective vaccine is ultimately required (333). Additional therapy for bacterial diarrhea is described below.

Bacterial Diarrhea

Clostridium sp. C. difficile is commonly found in the stools of normal children, being present in 33% of children less than 1 year of age, 10% of children between 1 and 2 years of age, and very rarely between 3 and 10 years of age (334–336). It has been found more frequently in children with diarrhea during day care center outbreaks (57%) compared to those without diarrhea (9%) (337). Nosocomial pediatric disease has not yet been described. *C. perfringens* from an unidentified food source has been implicated in a large nosocomial outbreak involving 61 patients including children (338).

Cryptosporidium sp. Person-to-person transmission has been suggested in 4 cases involving pediatric patients and hospital staff, although a common earlier source and other exposure was not been ruled out (339, 340). The identification of *Cryptosporidium* in 65% of symptomatic children in a day care center compared to 10% of controls suggests that epidemic disease in immunocompetent children can occur (341). Additional day care outbreaks continue to be described (342) and with improved diagnostic efforts may well be identified in hospitals around the world (343).

Salmonella sp. and E. coli. Outbreaks are listed in Table 28.13. The association of antibiotic therapy with colonization by multiresistant *Salmonella* and the proneness of young children to develop systemic disease have been noted (307, 308, 312). While common source outbreaks have been described (309), transmission has generally been related to hand carriage, serious patient overcrowding, suboptimal nursery facilities, poor architectural design, and contamination of the environment as in the adult. Children in the first year of life have increased attack rates of bacteremia and death with *Salmonella* and chronic diarrhea and death with enteropathogenic *E. coli* (233, 344, 345).

Antibiotic therapy to reduce stool carriage and thereby minimize the reservoir is controversial (307, 346). Stool cultures for *Salmonella* sp. have continued to be positive, and there is probably no indication for suppressive therapy. On the other hand, suppressive therapy for enteropathogenic *E. coli* may be worthwhile in the hospitalized child.

Shigella sp. An outbreak of shigellosis in pediatric staff has followed contamination of tuna salad in a hospital salad bar. Fifty-one percent of staff were colonized but no patient illness occurred, although the hospital was closed to new admissions for 3 days (347). Appropriate antibiotic treatment rapidly eliminates shigella from the stool. Therefore treatment of all infected children regardless of severity of disease is recommended be3cause of the high degree of contagiousness of shigellosis (344).

V. cholerae. Prophylactic antibiotic therapy may be of value (290).

Other. There have been no reports of nosocomial giardiasis or *Campylobacter* sp. to date.

Morbidity, Mortality, and Cost

Deaths directly attributable to nosocomial gastroenteritis infection have generally been caused by *Salmonella* infection (3, 233, 310, 312, 346). One estimate found the cost of reovirus diarrhea to be a prolongation of stay of 2.8 days at a cost of $836/infection (296). The indirect costs to the health care system (e.g., refusal of emergency admissions and curtailing of elective admissions) and to the family are unknown (310). Reduction of cholera spread through cross-infection in the children's infectious disease ward was said to reduce the number of cases in the hospital and the whole city drastically (290).

Previously Common Childhood Diseases

Pertussis

Following the introduction of pertussis vaccine, there has been a steady decline in the incidence of the disease. There are now 5 to 20 people dying of pertussis each year in the U.S., and the disease has been reduced to 1000 to 2000 cases a year. There is now an increasing incidence in many areas of the U.S. (348); the agent is exquisitely contagious with 100% of unvaccinated and 46%

of vaccinated household contacts acquiring infection. Nearly half of the cases may be asymptomatic, and their role in transmission is unknown (349). Age does offer protection with 81% of contacts less than 1 year of age developing pertussis compared to 8% of contacts older than 20 years. Similarly, a history of immunization offers some protection, with pertussis developing in 30% of those immunized compared with 82% of those not immunized. The vaccine efficacy rate was estimated at 63%. In one series, 9 of 10 asymptomatically infected children had received three or more DTP immunizations (350). Serologic response in asymptomatic infections suggests that this exposure may be important in maintaining immunity. Pertussis occurs in adults, even in those with a history of previous infection or immunization. Illness in adults is generally less severe and may be misdiagnosed as bronchitis or an upper respiratory tract infection unless paroxysmal symptoms develop. The relationship of symptoms to increasing age, immunization, or previous infection has not been carefully studied (351, 352).

Hospital staff have transmitted this disease in three outbreaks (193, 194)—one in 1969 involving 11 adults (staff and their contacts) in Denver (193), another in 1974 involving 135 staff members and spouses and 6 patients in Cincinnati (194). Disease appears to have been spread to another patient after his exposure to the index patient from day 8 to day 10 of erythromycin therapy, although transmission by asymptomatic staff cannot be ruled out (353). Failure to recognize the disease in a mother and hospital staff with paroxysmal coughing with subsequent removal from duty has resulted in nosocomial disease (176).

Some data suggest that prophylactic erythromycin is effective in preventing colonization and disease in immunized and unimmunized contacts (176, 353–355). In a pertussis outbreak at Cincinnati Children's Hospital, clinical disease developed in five of five colonized contacts before prophylaxis was initiated. After beginning erythromycin prophylaxis, clinical pertussis developed in only one of eight colonized contacts (194). Erythromycin administered 5 days after exposure failed to prevent disease in a 5-month-old patient (353). Additional studies of the value of prophylactic erythromycin are needed but difficult to design because of the variable exposures before prophylaxis is initiated. Erythromycin is useful in eradication of the organism from cases; there are no reports of bacteriologic relapse in patients treated for 14 days, and most patients appear to be rendered noninfectious after 10 days (355, 356). Vaccination has been used in outbreak control in room and ward contacts less than 7 years of age and in older children and staff (194).

The protocol for management is found in Table 28.17 (see also Tables 28.18–28.21). Intervention includes the following:

Contacts less than 7 years old who were previously immunized against pertussis should receive a booster dose of vaccine, preferably as DTP, unless a booster dose was given within the past 6

Table 28.17.   Protocol for Common Childhood Disease Exposure in Hospitalized Patients*

1. Isolate the contagious patient as defined in Table 28.18 and discharge if condition permits, especially if the patient has measles or chickenpox. If patient cannot be discharged, transfer to nearest isolation area, avoiding patient care areas during transport.
2. Delay admission to the exposed ward for an hour or so until the charts can be reviewed to determine who is susceptible.
3. Decide which patients were exposed to the disease. If the contagious patient used the play area, consider all other children using the play area to have been exposed. All other potential exposures in diagnostic facilities and operating room should be considered. Make a list of exposed patients. Determine their susceptibility as defined in Table 28.19. Private physicians should be notified if they have patients on the list, but the responsibility to isolate exposed susceptible patients who cannot be discharged should be clearly assigned to the pediatric representative on the hospital infection committee, nurse, or pediatric ward resident.
4. Identify high risk patients as defined in Table 28.20 who were exposed and require immediate prophylaxis as discussed in the text.
5. Discharge as many exposed susceptible patients as possible, before minimum of range of incubation period has elapsed since onset of exposure as defined in Table 28.21.
6. Move exposed susceptible who cannot be discharged before the time when a secondary case would be expected on the basis of the minimum of the incubation period. Put this exposed cohort under the proper isolation technique until after the maximum of range of incubation period as defined in Table 28.21.
7. Admit immune patients to floor without restrictions. Susceptible patients can be admitted provided the above precautions are followed carefully.
8. Decide which staff were exposed to the disease, including doctors, nurses, physiotherapists, radiology technicians, volunteers, students. Advise them of the need for prophylaxis or withdrawal from patient contact.

* Modified from Moffeth HL: Pediatric nosocomial infections in the community hospital. *Pediatr Infect Dis* 1:430–442, 1982.

Table 28.18.   Contagious Period of Common Childhood Diseases*

Disease	Earliest	Latest
Measles	4 days prior to onset of rash	4 days after onset of rash
Mumps	1–2 days before parotid swelling	5 days after onset of parotid swelling
Rubella	Few days before rash	Few days after rash
Pertussis	Catarrhal stage	Rarely after fourth week of disease; 7–10 days after initiation of 10–14-day course of erythromycin
Varicella	48 hours before rash	5–7 days after onset of last vesicle
Diphtheria	Onset of illness	2–4 weeks; 1–2 days after initiation of penicillin therapy

* Modified from Moffet HL: Pediatric nosocomial infections in the community hospital. *Pediatr Infect Dis* 1:430–442, 1982.

months. Because immunity conferred by vaccine is not absolute, all immunized and unimmunized contacts should also receive erythromycin prophylactically (40 mg/kg/day for 10 days). Con-

Table 28.19. Definitions of Susceptibility to Common Childhood Disease*

Measles	Those unable to provide documentation of (*a*) measles diagnosed by a physician (*b*) serologic confirmation of immunity, or (*c*) live measles vaccine on or after their first birthday.
Mumps	No practicable way of testing for susceptibility at the present time.
Rubella	Those unable to provide documentation of (*a*) serologic confirmation of immunity or (*b*) immunization.
Pertussis	No practicable way of testing for susceptibility at the present time.
Varicella	Those unable to provide documentation of (*a*) varicella diagnosed by a physician, (*b*) household exposure to varicella, or (*c*) serologic confirmation of immunity.

* Modified from Moffet HL: Pediatric nosocomial infections in the community hospital. *Pediatr Infect Dis* 1:430–442, 1982.

Table 28.20. Definitions of Patients at High Risk of Severe Disease from Common Childhood Diseases Who Require Special Intervention

Measles	All susceptibles
Mumps	None
Rubella	Suspect or confirmed pregnancy
Pertussis	Practically, all exposed
Diphtheria	Practically, all exposed
Varicella	Immunospressed patients (leukemia, lymphoma, congenital or acquired immunodeficiency, and recipients of 2 mg/kg/day of prednisone and other immunosuppressive treatment) Patients in plaster casts

Table 28.21. Incubation Period of Common Childhood Diseases*

Disease	Minimum (days)	Maximum (days)	Usual (days)
Measles	9	12	Same
Mumps	12	25	16–18
Rubella	14	21	16–18
Pertussis	7	14	7–10
Diphtheria	2	5 or longer	2–5
Varicella	10	21, 28 if VZIG given	10–14

* Modified from Moffet HL: Pediatric nosocomial infections in the community hospital. *Pediatr Infect Dis* 1:430–442, 1982.

tacts not previously immunized should receive erythromycin for 10 days after the contact is broken; if it is not possible to break the contact, they should be treated for the duration of the cough in the index patient, or until the patient has received 7 days of treatment with erythromycin. Pertussis immune globulin (human) has shown no prophylactic effect in controlled trials (157). Ultimately, elimination of this disease, which has plagued patients and physicians for years (357), will depend on improved vaccine (358–360).

Measles

Control of measles worldwide has met with variable success. Through a nationwide initiative to eliminate indigenous measles from the United States by October 1, 1982 through high immunization levels, aggressive surveillance, and vigorous response to cases, measles morbidity reached a new low of 3124 reported cases in 1981 (361). Young infants, susceptible adolescents, immigrants, and patients excluded from immunization for religious reasons continue to represent a potential risk to hospitalized patients. In 1980–1981, 205 cases were reported for an average of two importations/week with more than one-third of all importations from Mexico. Canada, and England and nearly one-quarter of cases associated with secondary transmission (160, 36!). Nosocomial measles was reported more commonly than varicella, rubella, and mumps in hospital-wide surveillance berfore 1972 (10, 11, 13). Airborne transmission in doctors' offices has been documented (159, 160). In one report, a 7-month-old Korean orphan infected four other children. One had arrived 5 minutes before the patient left the office but had no face-to-face contact with her. The other three patients arrived 65 to 75 minues after the index patient had left.

Only one used the same examining room, but all four shared the waiting room. Survival of measles virus in droplet nuclei for over 2 hours has been documented in the laboratory (362).

The protocol for management is found in Table 28.17.

Intervention for susceptible children ≥ 1 year of age exposed for < 5 days includes immunization. Children during the first year of life should receive 0.25 ml/kg of immune serum globin (IG) and active immunization at 15 months. Susceptible older children exposed for more than 5 days should receive IG, then be actively immunized 3 months afterward. Immunocompromised children should receive 0.5 ml/kg of IG even if they were immune prior to the onset of immunosuppression. The maximal dose should not exceed 15 ml of IG (157, 363, 364).

Mumps

Investigation of patients on a children' tuberculosis ward exposed to mumps indicated that all susceptibles, as identified by neutralizing antibody test, acquired disease (over 25% asymptomatically) despite isolation at the first sign of parotid swelling. Mumps virus was recovered as early as 2 days before and as late as 6 days after the onset of parotitis (365). An epidemic of mumps occurred in patients in the children's orthopaedic division of an Alaskan hospital. The index case was believed to be a new staff nurse who had been visiting her nephew with mumps (197), suggesting a possible role for the asymptomatic carrier in transmission. ELISA screening may be of use in determining susceptibility, although vaccination of immune individuals is not associated with complications (366). The protocol for management is found in Table 28.17. Exposed susceptible children ≥ 12 months of age should be immunized (367, 368).

Rubella

The special problem of rubella is discussed in Chapters 12 and 13. Shedding of rubella in a 4½-year-old boy with congenital rubella has been documented (369). The protocol for management is found in Table 28.17. Susceptibles ≥ 12 months of age should be immunized unless they are of childbearing age. These patients require serologic testing and, if they are seronegative, appropriate follow-up (157).

Diphtheria

Outbreaks of diphtheria occurred at two centers for the mentally retarded. Eight children between 3 and 10 years of age developed nasal diphtheria and a ninth individual, a 21-year-old nursing aide, presented with the pharyngeal form of disease (198). The potential for an increased incidence of clinical diphtheria exists as carriage and disease continue to be reported in indigenous and immigrant populations (370). A protocol for management of exposed patients is shown in Table 28.17. The need for additional management, including diphtheria toxoid, antitoxin, and penicillin, must be determined by individual circumstances. All hospital contacts should be kept under surveillance for 7 days (157, 371).

Polio

Immunization programs have reduced the number of cases of paralytic poliomyelitis to 7 in 1981, although certain unimmunized religious groups continue to be at risk (372–376). No nosocomial disease has been described, although a nursery school outbreak has been reported (377).

Varicella-Zoster Virus Infection

Prevalence. Varicella presents a major problem in pediatric hospitals because of the possibility of airborne spread (35, 36, 378–381) without direct contact and the severity of illness that may occur in immunosuppressed patients (221, 382–387). In the U.S. 82% of varicella cases occur in the first 9 years of life, although in tropical areas varicella occurs at a later age, as is reflected in susceptibility of 4.5% of pregnant women from New York versus 16% of those from tropical areas (388–391) and severe nosocomial outbreaks in the tropics (378, 392).

Outbreaks. Outbreaks are listed in Table 28.22 (35, 36, 39, 195, 393). Twenty-eight cases of nosocomial varicella have occurred on wards despite the use of full isolation precautions for patients with varicella, including single rooms, closed doors, and prohibition of physical contact (35, 36, 39, 195). One outbreak was related in time to the vacuuming of the index patient's room, although varicella virus has not been successfully recovered from skin scales or fomites (195). Brief operating room exposure on the day before the onset of rash in an 8-year-old boy in the tropics resulted in disease in 12 medical and surgical staff (392). Three cases have occurred in leukemic toddlers confined to cribs 50 to 100 feet from the index case with leukemia and extensive varicella skin lesions (36). Disease has occurred in a patient on isolation precautions during the entire exposure and who was confined to a room on the same ward as an index case with varicella

Table 28.22.   Outbreaks of Nosocomial Varicella Infection on Pediatric Wards Reported in the Literature

Reference	Disease in Index Case	No. (%) of Cases in Susceptible Patient Contact	Susceptibility Test Used	Time Course
195	Varicella	8 (22%)	History, age	21 days
36	Varicella	3 (13%)	History	21 days
	Varicella	4 (24%)	History	21 days
35	Varicella	13 (54%)	History, FAMA	23 days
393	Zoster	3	History	31 days

pneumonia who was being ventilated (35). Furthermore, three isolated wardmates of a patient with zoster also acquired varicella (393). Disease has also occurred in a susceptible physiotherapist in Boston who did not have direct patient care with infected children (35). Seventeen presumed nosocomial cases have been identified only after discharge (35, 36).

In a period of 34 months, more than 500 hospital employees and 209 patients were exposed to varicella-zoster virus (VZV) following 22 uncontrolled hospital introductions. Five introductions by employees followed acquisition of varicella outside the hospital (394). Additional outbreaks have been investigated by the CDC, and many earlier reports can be found (10, 11, 13, 379, 380).

Mode of Transmission. Varicella can occur in a susceptible person exposed to either varicella or zoster. Because zoster is not associated with respiratory shedding of viral particles, except potentially when lesions involve the nose or oropharynx, infection is more likely to occur after exposure to varicella than zoster (395). The path of entry into the susceptible host is assumed to be the upper respiratory tract. The infecting dose has not been established. There are different strains of VZV identifiable by DNA fingerprinting, but it is not clear whether there is more than one serotype (221, 388). VZV chickenpox is transmissible at the time of the exanthem, although it cannot be isolated from the respiratory tract after the exanthem appears or immediately before the eruption even in the presence of vesicular lesions in the mouth possibly because the virus is inactivated by local factors or because the culture systems are insensitive (388, 389, 395). One of three children studied did transmit infection to a classmate the day before the appearance of the first skin lesion, similar to the previously mentioned tropical operating room exposure (392, 395). It is not known whether asymptomatic

individuals carry the virus, although immune individuals can be asymptomatically infected as inferred by increases in antibody titers.

In spite of the relatively low infectivity of the virus on casual contact, transmission in an institutional environment occurs fairly readily. The thesis that airborne transmission of droplet nuclei, as well as contact infection, helps to spread the virus is supported by investigation of a hospital outbreak in which air-tracer studies of the movement of sulfur hexafluoride released in the room occupied by the index case clearly documented the preferential flow of air to adjacent rooms (35) with high occupant attack rates. A confirmatory report linked transmission of virus with the airflow from the isolation room to the corridor (195).

Susceptibility and Reinfection. If an assessment of susceptibility is being made solely on historical information to assess immune status, the interview should be conducted by experienced personnel (394, 396). Susceptibility obtained through history may be unreliable. Eight percent of adults who said they had not had chickenpox developed infection after household exposure; 2% of those who were unsure of their history and 0.2% of those who said they had had the disease developed chickenpox under similar circumstances. The attack rate among children with a negative history in the same household was 95% (388). An attempt should be made to elicit a past history of exposure to siblings or children with varicella; persons with previous household exposure to active cases are likely to be immune. Individuals who have attended an urban school or had previous occupational exposure, e.g., in nursery school, kindergarten, or a pediatric health care setting, also are likely to be immune (396).

Susceptibility may be reliably determined by such sensitive and specific test as the fluorescent antibody membrane antigen test, immune adherence hemagglutination assay (IAHA), and

ELISA, but these tests are not yet widely available (397, 398). A skin test developed in Japan to detect susceptibility to varicella has also proven very sensitive (400) but currently lacks a commercial manufacturer and may not be sensitive in the elderly (389).

Increases in both humoral and cell-mediated immunity to VZV that occur in the majority of VZV-immune adults exposed to varicella suggest that subclinical reinfection does occur (401). Clinical reinfection can occur, both in immunocompetent and immunosuppressed individuals but appears to be unusual and mild (401, 402). An immunosuppressed patient with repeatedly positive VZV immunofluorescent antibody titers but no history of chickenpox developed varicella pneumonia (383). Twenty-eight percent of patients with preimmunization antibody to VZV experience a mild clinical illness, suggesting that these history-negative, seropositive patients remain at risk for VZV infection (401–405).

High Risk Patients. In immunosuppressed patients, such as those with Hodgkin's disease, non-Hodgkin's lymphoma, or lymphocytic leukemia, particularly those with absolute leukopenia, visceral involvement (pneumonia, hepatitis, encephalitis) may occur in 32% and death in 7% (382). In bone marrow transplant recipients after high dosage radiochemotherapy, infections are particularly severe. They are to be considered at risk regardless of their varicella history or the immune status of the donor. Cell-mediated immunity may be depressed for 100 days after transplant, and the level of depression correlates with increased susceptibility (405). Less drastic immunosuppression, such as that following organ transplant, also increases the risk (384). Defects in cell-mediated immunity appear to be associated with greatest risk. Patients on high dose steroid therapy, such as for rheumatic fever or the nephrotic syndrome, have more severe disease, whereas patients on low dose schedules are not at increased risk (385). Recipients of low doses of steroids, e.g., 5 to 10 mg of prednisone/day, do not exhibit increased morbidity when they develop varicella. A dose of prednisone equivalent to 2 mg/kg of body weight/day is arbitrarily considered to confer increased risk even in those with otherwise normal immune function (385). The effect of inhaled steroids or steroids applied topically to large areas of the skin is unknown (396). Patients receiving cytotoxic drugs are at increased risk in direct proportion to the degree of aggressiveness of the therapy (396).

Exposure. It is well recognized that continu-

ing household exposure to chickenpox will result in infection in virtually 100% of susceptibles, but results of other types of exposure such as in hospitals are not predictable. In general, there is far less risk of transmission in these situations than following continuing household exposure, but in view of the high communicability, a liberal definition of exposure should be employed. A patient who has shared a hospital room containing four or fewer beds, or played for at least 1 hour with contagious children is said to have been exposed. Exposures may also occur in playrooms, X-ray department, and other locations in hospital (396).

Prevention: Varicella-Zoster Immune Globulin (VZIG)

VZIG can prevent chickenpox in exposed susceptible normal children. In a collaborative study in which 15 susceptible immunosuppressed children received zoster immune globulin (ZIG) within 3 days following exposure, there were no deaths and only one child developed progressive varicella, although a mortality rate of 7% and progressive disease in 30% were expected on the basis of previous studies at that time (386). Administration of zoster immune plasma 7 days after exposure did not prevent severe varicella from developing (383). Patients who develop 4-fold antibody rise from high titer ZIG have a significantly lower risk of death and complications (387). VZIG appears to offer protection for 3 to 4 weeks after administration. Patients receiving intravenous immune serum globulin every 4 weeks do maintain titers comparable to those patients receiving VZIG every 3 weeks. Because higher titers are achieved sooner after administration of intravenous immune serum globulin, it might be especially useful in patients receiving prophylaxis more than 4 days after exposure (407). VZIG can prolong the incubation period for up to 28 days, so exposed recipients who remain in hospital must be isolated for 10 to 28 days postexposure (396).

Vaccine. The vaccine, first available in Japan, is a live virus vaccine attenuated by multiple passage in cell culture capable of inducing immunity to varicella-zoster virus in a high percentage of normal (404) and immunocompromised (408–411) children. In a study by Gershon et al (409), over 90% of 191 study participants with leukemia showed an immune response after receiving two doses of vaccine. Eighty percent of leukemia vaccinees with subsequent household exposure have remained free of illness; the other 20% had a mild disease with about 50 vesicular lesions. The 4 of 22 patients exposed who did develop chickenpox acquired milder disease than might be expected in healthy children exposed to varicella. The attack rate of 18% was significantly lower than the 80 to 90% usually seen in healthy children with household exposure. Similar success has been documented in other patients with lymphoreticular malignancies, although 2 patients who had failed to develop significant lymphocyte stimulation to VZV antigen after immunization developed a blastogenic response on re-exposure. One household contact seroconverted, presumably due to the vaccine strain (412). This vaccine is unlikely to be recommended for normal children in the near future, since extensive studies will be needed to evaluate the potential risk of delaying natural infection (410, 411). Reinfection and latent infection appear to follow vaccination of immunosuppressed children just as they may follow natural infection. Normal children appear to acquire complete protection. Vaccine has been administered to 11 children before or immediately after exposure to a child with zoster who infected three cases of the ward contacts (393). Although all showed an antibody response, additional studies are needed to determine the safety of this procedure.

Control and Management

Management is summarized in Table 28.23 (396, 406, 413–415). Isolation of patients who have received vaccine, who may develop mild disease, is recommended because of the theoretical risk to ward patients based on secondary attack rates in households. Casual management on the wards is costly (416).

Pre-employment serologic or skin testing and varicella immunization would reduce the cost and turmoil of occupational exposure (394) but may not be necessary. To protect a semiclosed community against varicella adequately, all infants less than 6 months old may require immunization. The incidence of varicella has not been decreased in an institution using the vaccine since 1975, although the average rate of immune individuals in the population was maintained at more than 70%. Varicella outbreaks continued to occur, including children less than 6 months of age (417).

Invasive Bacterial Disease

H. influenzae

H. influenzae is transmitted by person-to-person contact via infected droplets of respiratory tract secretions. The respiratory tract is the portal of entry in cases of meningitis, and the upper respiratory tract remains colonized until effective antibiotic therapy has been instituted. Only one case of nosocomial disease has been described (418). A 4-month-old boy undergoing repeated subdural taps was hospitalized in the same room as a 4-month-old girl with *H. influenzae* osteomyelitis and septic arthritis who had received four doses of ampicillin, four doses of chloramphenicol, and three doses of oxacillin intravenously 24 hours and 50 minutes prior to his admission to that room. At day 11 of hospitalization, he developed meningitis with the strain of *H. influenzae* which had the same outer membrane protein profile as the index case (419). Lipopolysaccharide subtype may be used to distinguish some strains not differentiated by outer membrane protein (420). Two nosocomial cases occurred in a chronic care facility for the retarded in which 11% of the staff and 18% of the patients were

Table 28.23. Management of Nosocomial Varicella

1. Patients with varicella should be discharged if possible.
2. Patients with varicella who cannot be discharged should be placed under strict isolation or cohorted with other patients who have varicella in the same room.
3. Exposed susceptibles should be discharged as soon as possible.
4. Exposed susceptibles who cannot be discharged should be placed on strict isolation for 10 days after the first possible exposure to 21 days after the last possible exposure.
5. Exposed susceptibles at high risk should receive zoster immune globlin or varicella-zoster immune globulin and isolated for 10 to 28 days after the first and last exposures, respectively. It appears beneficial to discontinue chemotherapy or radiotherapy, if possible.
6. Exclude susceptible immunocompromised patients from admission to that ward.
7. Susceptible staff should not be allowed to work with patients with varicella-zoster infections, and a sign stating this may be placed on the door.
8. Susceptible staff, once exposed, should not be allowed to work with high risk patients from 10 days after the first possible exposure to 21 days after the last possible exposure.

colonized (129). Respiratory isolation is recommended until patients have completed 24 hours of treatment with ampicillin or chloramphenicol and theoretically until nasopharyngeal eradication of the organism has been achieved. The infected patient should receive rifampin prophylaxis, 20 mg/kg (600 mg maximum dose), given once daily for 4 days and usually initiated just prior to discharge from the hospital (421). Recently simultaneous administration of chloramphenicol and rifampin has been associated with subtherapeutic chloramphenicol levels, and this administration requires critical evaluation before a recommendation can be made. Rifampin can induce hepatic microsomal enzymes, and possibly its administration should be deferred until chloramphenicol administration is complete (422). Day care contacts should be managed according to local public health policy (423). If there are additional family members < 4 years of age or immunosuppressed children of any age in the family (157, 225), the entire family should be counseled. Vaccine is close to licensure and may be recommended for use in exposed 18- to 47-month-old children (424).

N. meningitidis

No nosocomial cases have been reported in the pediatric population (425, 426), although six cases occurred in children situated 100 cm nose-to-nose from the index case during a 6-day classroom epidemic (427, 428). The exposed patient should receive rifampin prophylaxis, 20 mg/kg (divided every 12 hours for 2 days), or sulfonamides if the strain is sensitive (157). Vaccine may be of use in outbreaks involving types a or c meningococcus (428).

S. pneumoniae

S. pneumoniae is presumably transmitted by person-to-person contact via infected droplets of respiratory tract secretions, but the low pathogenicity in the normal child precludes the need for prophylaxis.

Group A Streptococcus

Transmission of group A streptococcus on pediatric wards appears to be rare now, although children with the early phase of pharyngitis are effective disseminators of the agent. Outbreaks regularly occurred in rheumatic fever units prior to the availability of penicillin (429, 430). A 6-month-old infant with an infection of the skin superimposed on infantile eczema contaminated the ward environment (air, dust, and bed clothes). Twenty-five infants and 18 adults, including attending staff and visitors, developed infections (431). Therapeutic and prophylactic penicillin was recommended for control. When secondary cases are occurring, the environment is probably heavily contaminated (429–431). In detention centers and jails outbreaks have been controlled through identification and treatment of all cases plus environmental cleaning (432). A 10 day course of penicillin therapy for all entrants to an institution may be necessary (429–432). Food-borne outbreaks are more likely to be self-limiting (430).

S. aureus

An outbreak in a pediatric residental facility was controlled with the introduction of a relatively benign strain of S. aureus 502A following the failure of routine infection control measures (434).

Multiply Resistant Organisms

S. pneumoniae has been associated with nosocomial disease and death in pediatric patients in South Africa (88). In the day care center attended by an infected child, 27% of children, particularly those with a history of antibiotic use, were colonized (435).

Methicillin-resistant S. aureus and other multiply resistant organisms are very difficult to control once introduced (436) and may colonize patients for months following discharge. The CDC guidelines should be followed (166).

Fever

Device-related infections, influenza A and other intercurrent viral infections including echovirus, rhinovirus, coxsackie B, parainfluenza 3 and herpes simplex (255, 437–439), and endotoxemia (44) may present with fever. Presumed endotoxemia developed in two pediatric patients receiving total parenteral nutrition contaminated with endotoxin. A combination of equipment inadequacies, including failure to disassemble and sterilize a bypass valve and pressure gauge after bulk preparation of solution, and faulty laboratory testing in which the standard USP rabbit test for endotoxin was being performed with only one-tenth of the required solution, resulted in a slowly increasing level of pyrogen contamination which remained undetected until clinically significant pyrogen reactions occurred.

Cutaneous and Other Fungal Infections Originating in Hospital

Rhizopus sp.

Contaminated elastic bandages (Elastoplast) applied to a buttock abcess in a 7-year-old boy and the biopsy site of a 6-year-old girl both with lymphoblastic leukemia led to deep abscesses caused by *Rhizopus oryzae* which were successfully treated with topical and parenteral amphotericin B and surgical debridement (441, 442).

Aspergillosis sp.

Hospital renovations, particularly those resulting in a disturbance of dust in the false ceilings and problems with air handling systems, can lead to nosocomial aspergillosis of the skin and subcutaneous tissue, paranasal sinuses, and lungs in immunocompromised children, including those who have had bone marrow transplant (224). Disease occasionally occurs in immunocompetent children (443). Three children with hematologic disorders developed *A. flavus* infections at the point of contact with a paper-covered board or adhesive tape used to immobilize the extremity during intravenous therapy for 5, 7, and 14 days, respectively (234). The initial lesion was an erythematous papule which progressed to an ulcer with a central black necrotic eschar. All died, and in two the cause of death was overwhelming fungal infection. Cross-circulation as a result of air backflow through a common duct during an exhaust for shutdown was temporally related to pulmonary, sinus, and periorbital infections in five patients with acute leukemia (222). The introduction of routine cleaning procedures for air conditioning equipment and rooms was followed by only two cases in the next 12 months. A 2-year-old patient died of disseminated *A. fumigatus* following repair of a tetralogy of Fallot. Although the source was not proven, the event was associated with hospital construction and a pigeon roost on an air conditioner outside of the operating room (444). Environmental review is recommended at the time of a case of *Aspergillus* endocarditis because of the likelihood of airborne inoculation of the heart during operation (444). In other cases, no environmental source has been recognized. Early diagnosis requires prompt biopsy of any new lesion. Serology while specific is not sensitive, and the value of surveillance, cultures, and prophylactic antifungal therapy is unclear (445, 446). Prevention and control measures have included the following: establishing impervious barriers between patients and construction areas to prevent dissemination of dust, cleaning renovated areas well before occupancy, moving high risk immunosuppressed patients from adjacent and lower floors to an area of the hospital not under construction, installing dampers to isolate airflow to each unit, vacuuming false ceilings and ventilation ducts; disinfecting air ducts and removing and replacing high efficiency, particulate air filters. Intensive air filtration in the rooms of high risk patients may be of value.

Miscellaneous Infections

Legionnaire's Disease

L. pneumophilia infection appears to be fairly common subclinical or minor infection in early life with detectable antibody titers in many school-aged children (447–449). Very rarely it is associated with pneumonia in children (450–453). Almost all pediatric cases have occurred in severely immunodeficient children (450–454). Fatal nosocomial disease is extremely rare but did develop in a 13-year-old girl following bone marrow transplantation. Prevention and control of the infection have recently been reviewed and are discussed in Chapter 20 (455, 456).

Hepatitis A

Hepatitis A infections in hospitals are generally the result of transmission from clinically anicteric patients with fecal incontinence who are in the prodromal phase of illness when the diagnosis is not suspected (236, 457–462). These are summarized in Table 28.24. Most cases occur in staff; nosocomial disease in children is rarely documented (236). Levels of virus in stool are usually at their highest at or before elevated levels of liver enzymes occur (235), although fecal shedding can continue until at least 2 weeks after the onset of dark urine (463). The virus may survive drying for more than 1 month. Failure to isolate a patient with explosive diarrhea in whom hepatitis A (235, 236, 457) was ultimately diagnosed has resulted in additional cases in staff and patients (236, 457). Staff in contact with two patients on enteric precautions (457, 458) acquired the infection. Hematologic transmission has been postulated following the occurrence of hepatitis A in a baby who received blood from a man who developed hepatitis A 28 days after donating blood (460).

Although attack rates are generally higher in nurses who presumably have prolonged patient contact (25% of susceptibles) (459), disease has

Table 28.24. Outbreaks of Hepatitis A among Pediatric Hospital Personnel and Patients Reported in the Literature*

Reference	Index Patient	Total No. of Secondary Cases	Attack Rate
457	18-month-old boy with shigellosis	14	20
458	21-month-old child with Down's syndrome, amebic liver abscess, and dysentry	4	3
461	23-month-old child with Down's syndrome and congenital heart disease	4	Unknown
460	1-month-old girl with osteomyelitis	10	Unknown
459	34-month-old girl with Down's syndrome and colostomy for imperforate anus	8	10 (12% of susceptibles)
236	1-year-old girl with congenital heart disease	19	18.5 (12% of susceptibles)

* From Krober MS, Bass JW, Brown JD, Lemon SM, Rupert KJ: Hospital outbreak of hepatits A: risk factors for spread. Pediatr Infect Dis 3:296–299, 1984.

Table 28.25. Attack Rate for Exposed Susceptible Hospital Personnel Reported in the Literature*

Position	No. Exposed	Blood Samples Obtained	Susceptible (IgG Antibody-Negative)	No. of Cases of Hepatitis	Attack Rate (% of Susceptibles)
Physicians	11	11	10	1	10
Nurses	11	16	16	4	25
Nursing assistants	29	28	20	3	15
Medical students	4	4	4	0	0
Other exposed personnel†	25	22	18	0	0
Total	80	81	68	8	12

* From Krober MS, Bass JW, Brown JD, Lemon SM, Rupert KJ: Hospital outbreak of hepatitis A: risk factors for spread. Pediatr Infect Dis 3:296–299, 1984.
† Includes intensive care unit, operating room, catheterization laboratory, and pulmonary service personnel.

been reported in an infectious disease consultant, "a scrupulous hand washer" who stayed 1 hour at the bedside (458). Transmission among adults may be less common in view of the failure of 21 susceptibles to hepatitis A virus to acquire the infection from continent adults (462, 464). Attack rates are given in Table 28.25.

When hepatitis A is diagnosed in a child who is found retrospectively to have had diarrhea during hospitalization before the diagnosis of hepatitis is made, immune serum globulin, 0.02 ml/ kg, might be of use in hospital personnel exposed during the period of diarrhea provided that less than 2 weeks have elapsed (157, 235, 458). The risk of transmission appears to be greater if the index case is young, mentally retarded, or fecally incontinent.

Hepatitis B

Although high rates of infection are found among homosexuals, patients on chronic hemo- dialysis, intravenous drug abusers, those of Asian descent, and those receiving frequent blood trans- fusion (157), there is a paucity of data on the incidence of hepatitis B in pediatric institutions. In one pediatric hemodialysis unit, 58% of the patients had at least one positive hepatitis B sur- face antigen (HBsAg) determination (465). Vac- cine administration was effective in preventing hepatitis in 10 children with chronic renal failure who were immunized and followed for 16 to 33 months (466). The prevalence in pediatric oncol- ogy units has varied from 20% of patients by radioimmunoassay (RIA) (HBsAg) and 8% of DNA (anti-HBs) (467) in one center to 1% by RIA (HBsAg), 10% RIA (anti-HBs), and 7% (anti-HBc) (468) in another center. This may be explained by "third generation" testing through RIA and reversed passive hemagglutination tech- niques and the exclusive use of blood and blood products from volunteer blood donors in the second study. In the second study the prevalence was higher among those receiving chemotherapy (19%) than among those not receiving chemo- therapy (7%).

Horizontal, non-parenteral transmission of hepatitis B virus via the exchange among children of objects contaminated with oral secretions such as chewing gum was the explanation given for 15 cases among 21 people in two families (470). Human biting was recognized as a probable mode of transmission in an outbreak in a residential institution for the mentally retarded (471). Both of these methods in addition to the traditional parenteral route may be important in a pediatric hospital. Classroom transmission to students sharing a room with mentally retarded chronic hepatitis B carriers appears to be low (1.8%) in a facility with a strong continuing health education program. These results should not be extrapolated to the residential setting (472). Infants born to carrier mothers who do not receive currently recommended prophylaxis (473) will continue to provide a reservoir of the virus if basic infection control measures are not followed.

In one Canadian pediatric hospital 28.3% of foreign-born, high risk staff but only 2.7% of north American-born, high risk personnel were anti-HBs-positive (191). This may be an under- estimation of the problem because the nature of the screening was not stated and only one marker was included. The recommendations for the use of hepatitis B vaccine are currently under review. Adequate environmental disinfection is impor- tant (152). The risk to pediatric health care per- sonnel may not be as high as that reflected in adult studies (474, 475) and is discussed in Chap- ters 12 and 13.

Non-A, Non-B Hepatitis

During two nosocomial outbreaks of non-A, and non-B hepatitis in a cardiovascular surgical unit in Japan, the incidence of 21.8% in the population between 1 and 19 years of age was lower than the 43% incidence observed in adults (476).

Cytomegalovirus Infections

The hazard of transfusion-related CMV infec- tion and employee health-related issues are de- scribed elsewhere. Studies of CMV have found infection rates for preschool-aged children in the U.S. to range from 5 to 30% with early acquisition more common among children of lower socio- economic status (477). Childrearing practices can greatly influence the incidence of infection so that in populations from New Guinea, the Hebrides, and kibbutzim in Israel, the rates are very high. Fifty-seven percent of children enrolled in group day care have been found to shed CMV in the urine, significantly more than either the rate of viruria or seropositivity among children in home care (478). Children less than 12 months of age at enrollment to this study had an increase in saliva excretion or viruria from 10% at entry to more than 80% 1 year later. While the inci- dence of nosocomial acquisition in pediatric fa- cilities outside of the nursery is unknown, the potential for transmission through routes other than blood may be great depending on the pop- ulation hospitalized, and ultimately immuniza- tion is desirable (479, 480).

The value of gown and mask isolation proce- dures in children with leukemia was studied dur- ing a 22-month period. The infection rate in the 13 months following the introduction of isolation was not associated with a decreased incidence of infection in the immunocompromised host (481, 482), supporting the importance of other modes of transmission now known to include blood (483, 484).

Acquired Immunodeficiency Syndrome (AIDS)

Of 35 children with AIDS there have now been six reported whose sole risk factor for AIDS was receipt of blood transfusions (485, 486). Two boys, aged 7 and 10 years, with severe hemophilia A have developed immunodeficiency, presumably secondary to treatment with factor VIII concentrate (487). The prevalence of AIDS among hemophiliacs is currently under study (488). Although secondary cases have not been observed among medical personnel caring for patients with AIDS, current precautions are recommended for all patients with newly recognized severe cellular immunodeficiency and opportunistic infection, pending exclusion of AIDS (489).

Scabies

The prevalence of scabies varies among preschool and young school-age children. Sexually active adolescents are at risk of acquiring scabies. The failure to observe the mite (*Sarcoptes scabiei* var. *hominis*) without magnification contributes to the increased risk of secondary transmission to staff and tertiary transmission to other patients or residents. Primary intimate contact with an infected person is probably required, although fomite transmission may be significant, particularly for Norwegian scabies which can survive for 2 to 3 days off the skin surface (490). Patients with persistent pruritus with or without extensive crusting or scaling of skin require confirmatory skin scraping (196). If scrapings from two or more patients are positive and if one or more staff members exhibit pruritus or show positive scrapings, it is necessary to administer simultaneous mass treatment or prophylaxis. However, personnel with little direct patient contact (e.g., housekeepers) may be omitted. Sensitivity to the emotional needs of personnel is essential. If scabies is identified in patients or staff, post-treatment surveillance is essential because active infestations may occur 1 to 3 months after apparently successful treatment (196, 490–492). Treatment protocols should be readily available on all wards for use 24 hours a day.

Parvovirus

A report of nosocomial parvovirus infection follows reports of an association between serum parvovirus-like virus and bone marrow aplasia. A 12-year-old patient with sickle cell anemia who became severely anemic with absent reticulocytes seroconverted to parvovirus between 9 and 11 days after contact in hospital with a 4-year-old girl who had serologic evidence of a recent parvovirus infection (493). The mode of transmission of this agent and the true incidence of infection are unknown (494).

References

1. McKhann CF, Steeger A, Long AP: Hospital infections. A survey of the problem. *Am J Dis Child* 55:579–599, 1938.
2. Harries EHR: Infection and its control in children's wards. *Lancet* 2:173–178, 1935.
3. Watkins AG, Lewis-Fanning E: Incidence of cross-infection in children's wards. *Br Med J* 2:616–619, 1949.
4. Welliver RC, McLaughlin, S: Unique epidemiology of nosocomial infections in a children's hospital. *Am J Dis Child* 138:131–135, 1984.
5. Wenzel RP: Surveillance and reporting of hospital-acquired infections. In Wenzel RP (ed): *Handbook of Hospital Acquired Infections.* Boca Raton, FL, CRC Press, 1981, p 44.
6. Valenti WM, Hall CB, Douglas RG, Menegus MA, Pincus PH: Nosocomial viral infections. 1. Epidemiology and significance. *Infect Control* 1:33–37, 1980.
7. Valenti WM, Betts RF, Hall CB, Hruska JF, Douglas RG: Nosocomial viral infections. II. Guidelines for prevention and control of respiratory viruses, herpesviruses and hepatitis viruses. *Infect Control* 1:165–177, 1980.
8. Valenti WM, Hruska JF, Menegus MA, Freeburn MJ: Nosocomial viral infections. III. Guidelines for prevention and control of exanthematous viruses, gastroenteritis viruses, picornoviruses, and uncommonly seen viruses. *Infect Control* 2:38–49, 1981.
9. Valenti WM, Menegus MA: Nosocomial viral infections. IV. Guidelines for cohort isolation, the communicable disease survey, collection and transport of specimens for virus isolation and considerations for the future. *Infect Control* 2:236–245, 1981.
10. Gardner P, Carles DG: Infections acquired in a pediatric hospital. *J Pediatr* 81:1205–1210, 1972.
11. Cooper RG, Sumner C: Hospital infection data from a children's hospital. *Med J Aust* 2:1110–1113, 1970.
12. McNamara MJ, Hill MC, Balows A, Tucker EB: A study of the bacteriologic patterns of hospital infections. *Ann Intern Med* 66:480–488, 1967.
13. Roy TE, McDonald S, Patrick ML, Keddy JA: A survey of hospital infection in a pediatric hospital. *Can Med Assoc J* 87:531–538, 1962.
14. Roy TE, McDonald S, Patrick ML, Keddy JA: A survey of hospital infection in a pediatric hospital. *Can Med Assoc J* 87:592–599, 1962.
15. Roy TE, McDonald S, Patrick ML, Keddy JA: A survey of hospital infection in a pediatric hospital. *Can Med Assoc J* 87:656–660, 1962.
16. Hughes JM, Culver DH, White JW, Jarvis WR, Morgan WM, Munn VP, Mosser JL, Emori TG: Nosocomial infection surveillance, 1980–1982. *CDC Surveillance Summaries* 32(no. 455):1–17, 1983.

17. Daniel SO: An epidemiological study of nosocomial infections at the Lagos University Teaching Hospital. *Public Health Lond* 91:13–18, 1977.
18. Gross P, Rapuano C, Adrignolo A, Shaw B: Nosocomial infections: decade-specific risk. *Infect Control* 4:145–147, 1983.
19. Freeman J, McGowan JE: Risk factors for nosocomial infection. *J Infect Dis* 138:811–819, 1978.
20. Hall CB: The nosocomial spread of respiratory syncytial viral infection. *Annu Rev Med* 34:311–19, 1983.
21. Konerding K, Moffet, HL: New episodes of fever in hospitalized children. *Am J Dis Child* 120:515–519, 1970.
22. Straube RC, Thompson MA, Van Dyke RB, Wadell G, Connor JD, Wingard D, Spector SD: Adenovirus type 7b in children's hospital. *J Infect Dis* 147:814–819, 1983.
23. Hall CB: Respiratory syncytial virus infections. In Feigin RD, Cherry JD (eds): *Textbook of Pediatric Infectious Diseases.* Philadelphia, WB Saunders, 1981, vol 2, p 1250.
24. Henderson TW, Collier AM, Clyde WA, Denny FW: Respiratory-syncytial virus infections, reinfections and immunity. *N Engl J Med* 300:530–534, 1979.
25. Hall CB: Parainfluenza viruses. In Feigin RD, Cherry JD (eds): *Textbook of Pediatric Infectious Diseases.* Philadelphia, WB Saunders, 1981, p 1239.
26. McConnochie DM, Roghmann KJ: Bronchiolitis as a possible cause of wheezing in childhood: new evidence. *J Pediatr* 74:1–10, 1984.
27. Stokes GM, Milner AD, Hodges GC, Groggins R: Lung function abnormalities after acute bronchiolitis. *J Pediatr* 98:871–874, 1981.
28. Gurwitz D, Mindorff C, Levison H: Increased incidence of bronchial reactivity in children with a history of bronchiolitis. *J Pediatr* 98:551–555, 1981.
29. Hall CB, Hall WJ, Gala CL, MaGill FB, Leddy JP: Long-term prospective study in children after respiratory syncytial virus infection. *J Pediatr* 105:358–364, 1984.
30. Heird WC, Winters RW: Total parenteral nutrition. *J Pediatr* 86:2–16, 1975.
31. Hamilton JR: Gastrointestinal disease: an important cause of malnutrition in childhood. In Suskin RM (ed): *Textbook of Pediatric Nutrition.* New York, Raven Press, 1981, pp 465–474.
32. Marchant CD, Shurin PA, Turczyk VA, Wasikowski DE, Tutihasi MA, Kinney SE: Course and outcome of otitis media in early infancy: a prospective study. *J Pediatr* 104:826–831, 1984.
33. Mills EL: Viral infections predisposing to bacterial infections. *Annu Rev Med* 35:469–479, 1984.
34. Hall CB: Nosocomial viral respiratory infections: perennial weeds on pediatric wards. *Am J Med* 70:670–676, 1981.
35. LeClair JM, Zaia JA, Levine MJ, Congdon RG, Goldmann DA: Airborne transmission of chickenpox in a hospital. *N Engl J Med* 302:450–453, 1980.
36. Scheifele D, Bonner M: Airborne transmission of chickenpox. *N Engl J Med* 303:281–282, 1980.
37. Davis, SD, Sobocinski K, Hoffman RG, Mohr B, Nelson DB: Postoperative wound infections in a children's hospital. *Pediatr Infect Dis* 3:114–116, 1984.
38. Rosendorf LL, Octavio J, Estes JP: Effect of methods of postdischarge wound infection surveillance on reported infection rates. *Am J Infect Control* 11:226–229, 1983.
39. Doig CM, Wilkinson AW: Wound infections in a children's hospital. *Br J Surg* 63:647–650, 1976.
40. Brunell PA, Chairman, Committee on Infectious Disease, American Academy of *Pediatrics*, 1983–1984: Antimicrobial prophylaxis in pediatric surgical patients. *Pediatrics* 74:437–439, 1984.
41. Feder HM: Chemoprophylaxis in ambulatory pediatrics. *Pediatr Infect Dis* 2:251–256, 1983.
42. Scheifele DW: Prophylactic antibiotics in children. *Pediatr Infect Dis* 1:420–424, 1982.
43. Chang JHT: The use of antibiotics in pediatric abdominal surgery. *Pediatr Infect Dis* 3:195–198, 1984.
44. Simmons BP: Guideline for prevention of surgical wound infections. *Infect Control* 3:189–196, 1982.
45. Naqui SH, Dunkle LM, Timmerman KJ, Feichley RM, Stanley DL, O'Connor D: Antibiotic usage in a pediatric medical center. *JAMA* 242:1981–1984, 1979.
46. Kesler RW, Guhlow LJ, Saulsbury FT: Prophylactic antibiotics in pediatric surgery. *Pediatrics* 69:1–3, 1982.
47. Ajir F, Levin AB, Duff TA: Effect of prophylactic methicillin on cerebrospinal fluid shunt infections in children. *Neurosurgery* 9:6–8, 1981.
48. Klein DM: Comparison of antibiotic methods in the prophylaxis of operative shunt infections. *Concepts Pediatr Neurosurg* 4:131–141, 1983.
49. McCullough DC, Kane JG, Presper JH, Wells M: Antibiotic prophylaxis in ventricular shunt surgery. *Child's Brain* 7:182–189, 1980.
50. Savitz MH, Katz SS: Rationale for prophylactic antibiotics in shunt surgery. *Neurosurgery* 9:142–144, 1981.
51. Venes JL: Control of shunt infection. Report of 150 consecutive cases. *J Neurosurg* 45:311–314, 1979.
52. Welch K: Residual shunt infection in a program aimed at its prevention. *Z Kinderchir* 28:374–377, 1979.
53. Bayston R. Antibiotic prophylaxis in shunt surgery. *Dev Med Child Neurol* 17 (suppl 35):99–103, 1975.
54. Haines SJ, Taylor F: Prophylactic methicillin for shunt operations: effects on incidence of shunt malfunction and infection. *Child's Brain* 9:10–22, 1982.
55. Schmidt K, Gjerris R, Osgaard O: Antibiotic prophylaxis in cerebrospinal fluid shunting. A prospective randomized trial in 152 hydrocephalic patients. Presented at the Seventh European Congress of Neurosurgery, Brussels, Belgium, 1983.
56. Wang EEL, Prober CG, Hendrick BE, Hoffman HJ, Humphreys RR: Prophylactic sulfamethoxazole and trimethoprim in ventriculoperitoneal shunt surgery. *JAMA* 251:1174–1177, 1984.
57. McLone DG, Czyzewski D, Raimondi AJ, Sommers RC: Central nervous system infections as a limiting factor in the intelligence of children with

myelomeningocele. *Pediatrics* 70:338–342, 1982.

58. Richman DD, Breton SJ, Goldmann DA: Scarlet fever and group A streptococcal surgical wound infection traced to an anal carrier. *J Pediatr* 90:387–390, 1977.

59. Goldmann DA, Breton SJ: Group C streptococcal surgical wound infection transmitted by an anorectal and nasal carrier. *Pediatrics* 61:235–237.

60. Kennaugh JK, Gregory WW, Powell KR, Hendley JO: The effect of dilution during culture on detection of low concentrations of bacteria in blood. *Pediatr Infect Dis* 3:317–318, 1984.

61. Spengler RF, Greenough WB, III, Stolley PD: A descriptive study of nosocomial bacteremias at the Johns Hopkins Hospital, 1968–1974. *Johns Hopkins Med J* 142:77–84, 1978.

62. Fulginiti VA: *Staphylococcus epidermidis* septicemia in children: an emerging and difficult problem. *JAMA* 252:1054, 1984.

63. Feigin RD, Schackelford PG, Campbell J, Lyles TO, Schechter M, Lins RD: Assessment of the role of *Staphylococcus epidermidis* as a cause of otitis media. *Pediatrics* 52:569–576, 1973.

64. Crowe MJ, Ward OC: *Staphylococcus epidermidis* as a cause of meningitis. *Irish J Med Sci* 146:113–115, 1977.

65. Stratton CW: Endemic staphylococcal pseudobacteremia. *Infect Control* 2:251–252, 1981.

66. Christensen GD, Parisi JT, Bisno AL, Simpson WA, Beachey EH: Characterization of clinically significant strains of coagulase negative staphylococci. *J Clin Microbiol* 18:258–269, 1983.

67. Lowy FD, Hammer SM: *Staphylococcus epidermidis* infections. *Ann Intern Med* 99:834–39, 1983.

68. Gray ED, Peters G, Verstegen M, Regelman WE: Effect of extracellular slime substance from *Staphylococcus epidermidis* on the human cellular immune reponse. *Lancet* 1:365–367, 1984.

69. Peters G, Locci R, Pulverer G: Adherence and growth of coagulas-negative staphylococci on surfaces of intravenous catheters. *J Infect Dis* 146:479–482, 1982.

70. Archer GL, Karchmer AW, Vishniavsky N, Johnston JL: Plasmid-pattern analysis for the differentiation of infecting from non-infecting *Staphylococcus epidermidis. J Infect Dis* 149:913–920, 1984.

71. Franson TR, Sheth NK, Rose HD, Sohnle PG: Scanning electron microscopy of bacteria adherent to intravascular catheters. *J Clin Microbiol* 20:500–505, 1984.

72. Peter G, Lloyd-Still JD, Lovejoy FH: Local infection and bacteremia from scalp vein needles and polyethylene catheters in children. *J Pediatr* 80:78–83, 1972.

73. Ashkenazi S, Mirelman D: Adherence of bacteria to pediatric intravenous catheters and needles and its relation to phlebitis in animals. *Pediatr Res* 18:1361–1366, 1984.

74. Raucher HS, Hyatt AC, Barzilai A, Harris MB, Weiner MA, LeLeiko NS, Hodes DS: Quantitative blood cultures in the evaluation of septicemia in children with Broviac catheters. *J Pediatr* 104:29–33, 1984.

75. Frommell GT, Todd JK: Polymicrobial bacter-

76. Sears N, Grosfield JL, Weber TR, Kleiman, MB: Suppurative thrombophlebitis in childhood. *Pediatrics* 68:630–632, 1981.

77. Jupiter JB, Ehrlich MG, Novelline RA, Leeds HC, Keim D: The association of septic thrombophlebitis with subperiosteal abscesses in children. *J Pediatr* 101:690–693, 1982.

78. Hodder SL, Stern RC: Safety of long duration needles for administration of antibiotics to cystic fibrosis patients. *J Pediatr* 90:312–314, 1981.

79. Shapiro ED, Wald ER, Nelson KA, Spiegelman KN: Broviac catheter-related bacteremia in oncology patients. *Am J Dis Child* 136:679–681, 1982.

80. Wang EEL, Prober CG, Ford-Jones L, Gold R: The management of central intravenous catheter infections. *Pediatr Infect Dis* 3:110–113, 1984.

81. Haffer AAM, Rench MA, Ferry GD, Seavy DE, Edwards MS: Failure of urokinase to resolve Broviac catheter-related bacteremia in children. *J Pediatr* 104:256–258, 1984.

82. Delaplane D, Scott JP, Riggs TW, Silverman BL, Hunt CE: Urokinase therapy for a catheter-related right atrial thrombus. *J Pediatr* 100:149–152, 1982.

83. Edwards KE, Allen JR, Miller MJ, Yogev R, Hoffman PC, Klotz R, Marubio S, Burkholder E, Williams T, Davis AT: *Enterobacter aerogenes* primary bacteremia in pediatric patients. *Pediatrics* 62:304–306, 1978.

84. Matsaniotis NS, Syriopoulou VP, Theodoridou MC, Tzanetou KG, Mostrou GI: *Enterobacter* sepsis in infants and children due to contaminated intravenous fluids. *Infect Control* 5:471–477, 1984.

85. Goldmann DA: Intravenous fluid contamination, Aegean-style. *Infect Control* 5:469–470, 1984.

86. McGuckin MB, Thorpe RJ, Koch KM, Alavi A, Staum M, Abrutyn E: An outbreak of *Achromobacter xylosoxidans* related to diagnostic tracer procedures. *Am J Epidemiol* 115:785–793, 1982.

87. Fisher MC, Long SS, Roberts EM, Dunn JM, Balsara RK: *Pseudomonas maltophilia* bacteremia in children undergoing open heart surgery. *JAMA* 246:1571–1574, 1981.

88. Berkowitz FE: Bacteremia in hospitalized Black South African Children: a one-year study emphasizing nosocomial bacteremia and bacteremia in severely malnourished children. *Am J Dis Child* 138:551–556, 1984.

89. Morehead CD, Houck PW: Epidemiology of *Pseudomonas* infections in a pediatric intensive care unit. *Am J Dis Child* 124:564–570, 1972.

90. Anderson EL, Hieber JP: An outbreak of gentamicin-resistant *Enterobacter cloacae* infections in a pediatric intensive care unit. *Infect Control* 4:148–152, 1983.

91. Scully RE, Mark EJ, McNeely BU: Munchausen's syndrome. *N Engl J Med* 311:108–115, 1984.

92. Liston TE, Levine PL, Anderson C: Polymicrobial bacteremia due to Polle syndrome: the child abuse variant of Munchausen by proxy. *Pediatrics* 72:211–213, 1983.

93. Pickering LK, Kohl S: Munchausen syndrome by

proxy. *Am J Dis Child* 135:288, 1981.

94. Kohl S, Pickering LK, Dupree E: Child abuse presenting as immunodeficiency disease. *J Pediatr* 93:466–468, 1978.

95. Wolfsdorf J, Swift DL, Avery ME: Mist therapy reconsidered: an evaluation of the respiratory deposition of labelled water aerosols produced by jet and ultrasonic nebulizers. *Pediatrics* 43:799–808, 1969.

96. Moffet HL, Williams T: Bacteria recovered from distilled water and inhalation therapy equipment. *Am J Dis Child* 114:7–12, 1967.

97. Moffet HL, Allan D, Williams T: Survival and dissemination of bacteria in nebulizers and incubators. *Am J Dis Child* 114:13–20, 1967.

98. Moffet HL, Allan D: Colonization of infants exposed to bacterially contaminated mists. *Am J Dis Child* 114:21–25, 1967.

99. Trapana Y, MacIntyre DS, Holzman BH, Cleary T, Mora J: Surveillance study of pediatric patients receiving respiratory therapy, using the Bain circuit system. *Am J Infect Control* 10:128–132, 1982.

100. Holzman BH, Trapana Y, Mora J, Macintyre S: A modified Mapleson D system for long term mechanical ventilation of infants and children. *Crit Care Med* 9:481–486, 1981.

101. Craven DE, Connolly MG, Lichtenberg DA, Primeau PJ, McCabe WR: Contamination of mechanical ventilators with tubing changes every 24 to 48 hours. *N Engl J Med* 306:1506–1509, 1982.

102. Drummond KN: Infection of the urinary tract. In Behrman RE, Vaughan VC (eds): *Nelson Textbook of Pediatrics*, ed 12. Philadelphia, WB Saunders, 1983, pp 1367–1372.

103. Wade GH: The relationship between urinary retention, multiple straight catheterizations, and the incidence of urinary tract infection in the female adolescent following a posterior spinal fusion. *Orthop Nurs* 1:23–27, 1982.

104. Crooks KK, Enrile BG: Comparison of the ileal conduit and clean intermittent catheterization for myelomeningocele. *Pediatrics* 72:203–206, 1983.

105. Ehrlich O, Brem AS: A prospective comparison of urinary tract infections in patients treated with either clean intermittent catheterization or urinary diversion. *Pediatrics* 70:665–669, 1982

106. Hilton E, Uliss A, Samuels S, Adams AA, Lesser ML, Lowy FD: Nosocomial bacterial eye infections in intensive care units. *Lancet* 1:1318–1320, 1983.

107. Donowitz LG, Wenzel RP, Hoyt J: High risk of hospital-acquired infection in the ICU patient. *Crit Care Med* 6:355–357, 1982.

108. Gardner S, Shulman ST: A nosocomial common source outbreak caused by *Pseudomonas pickettii*. *Pediatr Infect Dis* 3:420–422, 1984.

109. Jeffries DJ: Viruses and intensive care. *Intensive Care Med* 9:105–107, 1983.

110. Adams G, Stover BH, Keenlyside RA, Hooton TM, Buchman TG, Roizman B, Stewart JA: Nosocomial herpetic infections in a pediatric intensive care unit. *Am J Epidemiol* 113:126–132, 1981.

111. Holzman BH, Scott GB: Control of infection and techniques of isolation in the pediatric intensive care unit. *Pediatr Clin North Am* 28:703–721, 1981.

112. Moodie PS, Feldt RH, Kaye MP: Measurement of postoperative output by thermodilution at flows applicable to the pediatric patient. *Crit Care Med* 7:130, 1979.

113. Pollack MM, Reed TD, Holbrook PR: Bedside pulmonary artery catheterization in pediatrics. *Crit Care Med* 7:141, 1979.

114. Foley FD, Greenawald KA, Nash G, Pruitt BA: Herpes virus infection in burned patients. *N Engl J Med* 181:652–656, 1970.

115. Miser JS, Miser AW: *Staphylococcus aureus* sepsis in childhood malignancy. *Am J Dis Child* 134:831–833, 1980.

116. Ladisch S, Pizzo PA: *Staphylococcus aureus* sepsis in children with cancer. *Pediatrics* 61:231–234, 1978.

117. Friedman LE, Brown AE, Miller DR, Armstrong D: *Staphyloccoccus epidermidis* septicemia in children with leukemia and lymphoma. *Am J Dis Child* 138:715–719, 1984.

118. Delage G, Brochu P, Pelletier M, Jasmin G, Lapointe N: Giant cell pneumonia caused by parainfluenza virus. *J Pediatr* 94:426–429, 1979.

119. Jarvis WR, Middleton PJ, Gelfand EW: Parainfluenza pneumonia in severe combined immunodeficiency. *J Pediatr* 94:423–429, 1979.

120. Hall CB, MacDonald NE, Klemperev MK, Ettinger LJ: Respiratory syncytical virus infection in immunocompromised children. *Pediatr Res* 15:613, 1981.

121. Zahradnik, JM, Spencer MJ, Porter DD: Adenovirus infection in the immunocompromised patient. *Am J Med* 68:725–732, 1980.

122. Saulsbury FT, Winkelstein JA, Yolken RH: Chronic rotavirus infection in immunodeficiency. *Pediatrics* 97:61–65, 1980.

123. Yolken RH, Bishop CA, Townsend TR, Bolyard EA, Bartlett J, Santos GW, Saral R: Infectious gastroenteritis in bone marrow-transplant recipients. *N Engl J Med* 306:1009–1012, 1982.

124. Townsend TR, Bolyard EA, Yolken RH, Beschorner WE, Bishop CA, Burns WH, Santos GW, Saral R: Outbreak of coxsackie Al gastroenteritis: a complication of bone-marrow transplantation. *Lancet* 1:820–823, 1982.

125. Miller RA, Holmberg RE, Clausen CR: Life-threatening diarrhoea caused by *Cryptosporidium* in a child undergoing therapy for acute lymphocytic leukemia. *J Pediatr* 103:256–259, 1983.

126. Mackowiak PA: The normal microbial flora. *N Engl J Med* 307:83–92, 1982.

127. Ostfeld E, Rubinstein E, Gazit E, Smetana Z: Effect of systemic antibiotics on the microbial flora of the external ear canal in hospitalized children. *Pediatrics* 60:364–366, 1977.

128. Marks MI, Mark S, Brazeau M: Yeast colonization in hospitalized and nonhospitalized children. *J Pediatr* 87:524–527, 1975.

129. Shapiro EP, Wald ER: Efficacy of rifampin in eliminating pharyngeal carriage of *Haemophilus influenza* type b. *Pediatrics* 66:5–8, 1980.

130. Schuman SH: Day-care associated infection: more than meets the eye. *JAMA* 249:76, 1983.

131. Kim K, Du Pont HL, Pickering LK: Outbreaks of diarrhea associated with *Clostridium difficile* and its toxin in day-care centers: evidence of person-to-person spread. *J Pediatr* 102:376–382, 1983.

132. Marwick C, Simmons K: Changing childhood

disease pattern linked with day care boom. *JAMA* 251:1245–1251, 1984.

133. Goodman RA, Osterholm MT, Granoff DM, Pickering LK: Infectious diseases and child day care. *Pediatrics* 74:134–139, 1984.

134. Bartlett AV (Chairman, Child Day Care Infectious Disease Study Group): Public health considerations of infectious diseases in child day care centers. *Pediatrics* 105:683–701, 1984.

135. Hughes WT, Townsend TR: Nosocomial infections in immunocompromised children. *Am J Med* 70:412–416, 1981.

136. Editorial: Why not child visitors? *Br Med J* 3:510–511, 1968.

137. Frank AL, Taber LH, Wells CR, Wells JM, Glezen WP, Paredes A: Patterns of shedding of myxoviruses and paramyxoviruses in children. *J Infect Dis* 144:433–441, 1981.

138. Hall CB: The shedding and spreading of respiratory syncytial virus. *Pediatr Res* 11:236–239, 1977.

139. Hall CB, Douglas RG, Geiman JM: Respiratory syncytial virus infections in infants: quantitation and duration of shedding. *J Pediatr* 89:11–15, 1976.

140. Flewett TH: Rotavirus in the home and hospital nursery. *Br Med J* 287:568–569, 1983.

141. Vesikari T, Sarkkinen HK, Maki M: Quantitative aspects of rotavirus excretion in childhood diarrhoea. *Acta Paediatr Scand* 70:717–721, 1981.

142. Ward RL, Knowlton DR, Pierce MJ: Efficiency of human rotavirus propagation in cell culture. *J Clin Microbiol* 19:748–753, 1984.

143. Hall CB, Douglas RG, Geiman JM: Possible transmission by fomites of respiratory syncytial virus. *J Infect Dis* 147:98–102, 1980.

144. Bean B, Moore BM, Steiner B, Peterson LR, Gerding DN, Balfour HH: Survival of influenza viruses on environmental surfaces. *J Infect Dis* 146:47–51, 1982.

145. Keswick BH, Pickering LK, DuPont HL, Woodward WE: Survival and detection of rotaviruses on environmental surfaces in day care centers. *Appl Environ Microbiol* 46:813–816, 1983.

146. Kilbrick S: The persistence of virus in the environment of patients with Kaposi's varicelliform eruption. *Am J Dis Child* 98:609–611, 1959.

147. Sattar SA, Raphael RA, Lochnan H, Springthorpe VS: Rotavirus inactivation by chemical disinfectants and antiseptics used in hospitals. *Can J Microbiol* 29:1464–1469, 1983.

148. Tan JA, Schnagl RD: Inactivation of a rotavirus by disinfectants. *Med J Aust* 1:19–23, 1981.

149. Sattar SA: Proceedings of the 4th International Symposium on Neonatal Diarrhoea, 1984, pp 90–99.

150. Sattar SA, Raphael RA, Springthorpe VS: Rotavirus survivial in conventionally treated drinking water. *Can J Microbiol* 30:653–656, 1984.

151. Moe K, Shirley JA: The effects of relative humidity and temperature on the survivial of human rotavirus in faeces. *Arch Virol* 72:179–186, 1982.

152. Kobayashi H, Tsuzuki M, Koshimizu K, Toyama H, Yoshihara N, Shikata T, Abe K, Mizuno K, Otomo N, Oda T: Susceptibility of hepatitis B virus to disinfectants or heat. *J Clin Microbiol* 20:214–216, 1984.

153. Ekanem EE, Dupont HL, Pickering LK, Selwyn BJ, Hawkins CM: Transmission dynamics of enteric bacteria in day-care centers. *Am J Epidemiol* 118:562–572, 1983.

154. Weniger BA, Futtenbur AJ, Goodman RA, Juranek DD, Wahlquist SD, Smith JD: Fecal coliforms on environmental surfaces in two daycare centers. *Appl Environ Microbiol* 45:733–735, 1983.

155. Chapin CV: Preface. In Chapin CV (ed): *The Sources and Modes of Infection.* Boston, FH Gilson, 1912, p vii.

156. Recommendations of the Immunization Practices Advisory Committee, Centers for Disease Control, Department of Health and Human Services, Atlanta, Georgia: General recommendations on immunization. *Ann Intern Med* 98:615–622, 1983.

157. Report of the Committee on Infectious Diseases: *The 1982 Red Book,* ed 19. Evanston, IL, American Academy of Pediatrics, 1982.

158. Fulginiti VA: Immunizations: current controversies. *J Pediatr* 101:487–494, 1982.

159. Imported measles with subsequent transmission in a pediatrician's office—Michigan. *Clin Paediatr (Phila)* 23:291, 1984.

160. Foulon G, Klein-Zabban ML, Gnansou-Nezzi L, Martin-Bouyer G: Preventing the spread of measles in children's clinics. *Lancet* 2:1498–1499, 1983.

161. Hall CB, Kopelman AE, Douglas RG Jr, Geiman JM, Meagher MP: Neonatal respiratory syncytial virus infection. *N Engl J Med* 300:393–396, 1979.

162. MacDonald NE, Hall CB, Suffin SC, Alexson C, Harris PJ, Manning JA: Respiratory syncytial viral infection in infants with congenital heart disease. *N Engl J Med* 307:397–399, 1982.

163. Zimakoff J, Noiby N, Rosendal K, Guilbert JP: Epidemiology of *Pseudomonas aeruginosa* infection and the role of contamination of the environment in a cystic fibrosis clinic. *J Hosp Infect* 4:31–40, 1983.

164. Isles A, Maclusky I, Corey M, Gold R, Prober C, Fleming P, Levison H: *Pseudomonas cepacia* infection in cystic fibrosis: an emerging problem. *J Pediatr* 104:206–210, 1984.

165. Putsep E: Pediatric patients. In Putsep E (ed): *Modern Hospital.* London, Lloyd-Luke, 1981, pp 86–88.

166. Garner JS, Simmons BP: CDC guideline for isolation in hospital. *Infect Control* 4:245–328, 1983.

167. Pizzo P: Isolation techniques in hospitals. *Pediatr Infect Dis* 2:94–98, 1983.

168. Moffet HL: Pediatric nosocomial infections in the community hospital. *Pediatr Infect Dis* 1:430–442, 1982.

169. Gardner P, Oxman MN, Breton S: Hospital management of patients and personnel exposed to communicable diseases. *Pediatrics* 56:700–709, 1975.

170. Hall CB, Douglas RG: Nosocomial respiratory syncytial virus infections. Should gowns and masks be used? *Am J Dis Child* 135:512–515, 1981.

171. Murphy D, Todd JK, Chao RK, Orr I, McIntosh K: The use of gowns and masks to control respiratory illness in pediatric hospital personnel. *J Pediatr* 99:746–750, 1981.

172. Robertson BA: The child in hospital. *SA Med J* 51:749–752, 1977.

173. Dalton R: The assessment and enhancement of

development of a child being raised in reverse isolation. *J Am Acad Child Psychol* 20:611–622, 1981.

174. Freedman DA, Montegomery JR, Wilson R, Bealmean PM, South MA: Further observations on the effect of reverse isolation from birth on cognitive and affective development. *J Am Acad Child Psychol* 15:593–603, 1976.

175. Riley HD Jr: Hospital-associated infections. *Pediatr Clin North Am* 16:701–734, 1969.

176. Valenti WM, Pincus PH, Messner MK: Nosocomial pertussis. Possible spread by a hospital visitor. *Am J Dis Child* 134:520–521, 1980.

177. Light IJ: Postnatal acquisition of herpes simplex virus by the newborn infant: a review of the literature. *Pediatrics* 63:480–482, 1979.

178. Crane LR, Kish HA, Ratanatharathorn V, Merline JR, Raval MF: Fatal syncytial virus pneumonia in a laminar airflow room. *JAMA* 246:366–368, 1981.

179. Gardner PS, Court SDM, Brockelbank JT, Downham MAPS, Weightman D: Virus cross-infection in paediatric wards. *Br Med J* 2:571–575, 1973.

180. Sims DG: A two-year prospective study of hospital-acquired respiratory virus infection on paediatric wards. *J Hyg (Lond)* 86:335–342, 1981.

181. Wenzel RP, Deal EC, Hendley JO: Hospital-acquired viral respiratory illness on a pediatric ward. *Pediatrics* 60:367–371, 1977.

182. Hall CB, Geiman JM, Douglas RG, Meagher MP: Control of nosocomial respiratory syncytial viral infections. *Pediatrics* 62:728–732, 1978.

183. Ditchburn K, McQuillin J, Gardner PS, Court SDM: Respiratory syncytial virus in hospital cross-infection. *Br Med J* 3:671–673, 1971.

184. Goldmann DA, Durbin WA, Freeman J: Nosocomial infections in a neonatal intensive care unit. *J Infect Dis* 144:449–459, 1981.

185. Maki DG, Alvarado CJ, Hassemer CA, Zilz MA: Relation of the inanimate hospital environment to endemic nosocomial infection. *N Engl J Med* 307:1562–1566, 1982.

186. Williams W: Guideline for infection control in hospital personnel. *Infect Control* 4:326–348, 1983.

187. Brown TC, Kreider SD, Lange WR: Guidelines for employee health services in hospitals, clinics, and medical research institutions. *J Occup Med* 25:771–773, 1983.

188. Klein JO: Management of infections in hospital employees. *Am J Med* 70:919–923, 1981.

189. Geddes AM: Immunization of hospital staff against infectious diseases. *J Hosp Infect* 2:205–206, 1981.

190. Gurevich I, Tafuro P: Caring for the infectious patient: risk factors during pregnancy. *Infect Control* 5:482–488, 1984.

191. Hamel L, Spika J: Prevalence of one hepatitis B marker among personnel in a pediatric hospital—Quebec. *Can Dis Weekly Rep* 9:197–198, 1983.

192. Hall CB, Douglas RG Jr, Geiman JM, Messner MK: Nosocomial respiratory syncytial virus infection. *N Engl J Med* 293:1343–1346, 1975.

193. Kurt TL, Yeager AS, Guenette S, Dunlop S: Spread of pertussis by hospital staff. *JAMA* 221:264–267, 1972.

194. Linnemann CC, Ramundo N, Perlstein PH, Minton SD, Englender GS, McCormick, JB, Hayes PS: Use of pertussis vaccine in an epidemic involving hospital staff. *Lancet* 2:540–543, 1975.

195. Gustafson TL, Lavely GB, Brawner ER, Hutcheson RH, Wright PF, Schaffner W: An outbreak of airborne nosocomial varicella. *Pediatrics* 70:550–556, 1982.

196. Bernstein B, Mihan R: Hospital epidemic of scabies. *J Pediatr* 83:1086–1087, 1973.

197. Sparling D: Transmission of mumps. *N Engl J Med* 280:276, 1976.

198. Breton JP, Martineau G: Outbreak of diphtheria—Quebec. *Can Dis Weekly Rep* 4:1–2, 1977.

199. Schaffner W: Infections in compromised hosts: an overview. *Infect Control* 4:452–453, 1983.

200. Frazier JP, Kramer WG, Pickering LK, Culbert S, Brandt K, Frankel LS: Antimicrobial therapy of febrile children with malignancies and possible sepsis. *Pediatr Infect Dis* 3:40–45, 1984.

201. Commers JR, Pizzo PA: Empiric antifungal therapy in the management of the febrile granulocytopenic cancer patient. *Pediatr Infect Dis* 2:56–60, 1983.

202. Pizzo PA, Robichaud KJ, Edwards BK, Schumaker C, Kramer BS, Johnson A: Oral antibiotic prophylaxis in patients with cancer: a double-blind randomized placebo-controlled trial. *J Pediatr* 102:125–133, 1983.

203. Kramer BS, Pizzo PA, Robichaud KJ, Witebsky F, Wesley R: Role of serial microbiologic surveillance and clinical evaluation in the management of cancer patients with fever and granulocytopenia. *Am J Med* 72:561–568, 1982.

204. Pizzo PA, Robichaud KJ, Gill FA, Witebsky FG: Empiric antibiotic and antifungal therapy for cancer patients with prolonged fever and granulocytopenia. *Am J Med* 72:101–111, 1982.

205. Pizzo PA: Infectious complications in the child with cancer. *J Pediatr* 98:341–354, 1981.

206. Ninane J, Chessells JM: Serious infections during continuing treatment of acute lymphoblastic leukemia. *Arch Dis Child* 56:841–844, 1981.

207. Enders JF, McCarthy K, Mitus A, Cheatham WJ: Isolation of measles virus at autopsy in cases of giant-cell pneumonia without rash. *N Engl J Med* 201:875–881, 1959.

208. Davis LE, Bodian D, Price IJ, Butler D, Vickers JH: Chronic progressive poliomyelitis secondary to vaccination of an immunodeficient child. *N Engl J Med* 297:241–245, 1977.

209. van der Does-van den Berg A, Hermans J, Nagel J, van Steenis G: Immunity of diphtheria, tetanus and poliomyelitis in children with acute lymphocytic leukemia after cessation of chemotherapy. *Pediatrics* 67:222–229, 1981.

210. Kung FH, Orgel HA, Wallace WW, Hamburger RN: Antibody production following immunization with diphtheria and tetanus toxoids in children receiving chemotherapy during remission of malignant disease. *Pediatrics* 74:86–89, 1984.

211. Smithson WA, Siem RA, Ritts RE, Gilchrist GS, Burgert ED Jr, Ilstrup DM, Smith TF: Response to influenza virus vaccine in children receiving chemotherapy for malignancy. *J Pediatr* 93:633–634, 1978.

212. Brown AE, Steinherz PG, Miller DR, Armstrong D, Kellick MG: Immunization against influenza in children with cancer: results of a three dose trial. *J Infect Dis* 145:124–126, 1982.

213. Sumaya CV, Williams TE: Persistence of antibody after the administration of influenza vaccine to children with cancer. *Pediatrics* 69:226–229, 1982.

214. Rubin RH, Wolfson JS, Cosimi AB: Infection in the renal transplant recipient. *Am J Med* 70:405–411, 1981.

215. Craft AW, Reid MM, Gardner PS, Jackson E, Kernahan J, McQuillin J, Noble TC, Walker W: Virus infections in children with acute lymphoblastic leukemia. *Arch Dis Child* 54:755–759, 1979.

216. Iacuone JJ, Wong KY, Bove KE, Lampkin BC: Acute respiratory illness in children with acute lymphoblastic leukemia. *J Pediatr* 90:915–919, 1977.

217. Hoecker JL, Pickering LIC, Groschel D: Current concepts of bacteremia in children with malignancies. *Cancer* 44:1939–1944, 1979.

218. Johnson JR, Yolken RH, Goodman D, Winkelstein JA: Prolonged excretion of group A coxsackievirus in an infant with agammaglobulinemia. *J Infect Dis* 146:713, 1982.

219. Malone W, Novak R: Outcome of hepatitis in children with acute leukemia. *Am J Dis Child* 134:584–587, 1980.

220. Masera G, Locasciulli A, Jankovic JG, Rossi MR, Recchia M, Uderzo C: Hepatitis B and childhood acute lymphoblastic leukemia. *J Pediatr* 99:98, 1981.

221. Zaia JA, Levin MJ, Preblud SR, Leszczynski J, Wright GG, Ellis RJ, Curtis AC, Valerio MA, LeGore J: Evaluation of varicella-zoster immune globulin: protection of immunosuppressed children after household exposure to varicella. *J Infect Dis* 147:737–743, 1983.

22. Mahoney DH, Steuber CP, Starling KA, Barrett FF, Goldberg J, Fernback DJ: An outbreak of aspergillosis in children with acute leukemia. *J Pediatr* 95:70–72, 1979.

223. Berkow RL, Weisman SJ, Provisor AJ, Weetman RM, Baehner RL: Invasive aspergillosis of paranasal tissues in children with malignancies. *J Pediatr* 103:49–53, 1983.

224. Peterson PK, McGlave P, Ramsay NKC, Rhame F, Cohen E, Perry GS III, Goldman AI, Kersey J: A prospective study of infectious diseases following bone marrow transplantation: emergence of *Aspergillus* and cytomegalovirus as the major causes of mortality. *Infect Control* 4:81–84, 1983.

225. Bartlett AV, Zusman J, Daum RS: Unusual presentations of *Haemophilus influenzae* infections in immunocompromised patients. *J Pediatr* 102:55–58, 1983.

226. Wright PI, Okabe N, McKee KT, Maassab HF, Karzon DT: Cold-adapted recombinant influenza A virus vaccine in seronegative young children. *J Infect Dis* 146:71–79, 1982.

227. Recommendations of the Immunization Practices Advisory Committee, CDC: Prevention and control of influenza. *Ann Intern Med* 101:218–222, 1984.

228. Hoffman P, Dixon RE: Control of influenza in hospital. *Ann Intern Med* 87:725–728, 1977.

229. Bell TD, Chai H, Berlow N, Daniels G: Immunization with killed influenza virus in children with chronic asthma. *Chest* 73:14–145, 1978.

230. Frank AL, Taber LH, Glezen WP, Paredes A, Couch RB: Reinfection with influenza A (H3N2) virus in young children and their families. *J Infect Dis* 140:829–836, 1979.

231. Eickhoff TC, Sherman IL, Serfling RE: Observations on excess mortality associated with epidemic influenza. *JAMA* 176:776–782, 1961.

232. Glezen WP, Payne AA, Snyder DN, Downs TD: Mortality and influenza. *J Infect Dis* 146:313–321, 1982.

233. Schroeder SA, Asergoff B, Brachman PS: Epidemic salmonellosis in hospitals and institutions: a-five year review. *N Engl J Med* 279:674–678, 1968.

234. Prystowsky SD, Vogelstein B, Ettinger DS, Merz WG, Kaizer H, Sulica VI, Zinkham WH: Invasive aspergillosis. *N Engl J Med* 295:655–658, 1976.

235. Alter MJ: Nosocomial hepatitis A infection: can we wash our hands of it? *Pediatr Infect Dis* 3:294–295, 1984.

236. Reed CM, Gustafson TL, Siegel J, Duer P: Nosocomial transmission of hepatitis A from a hospital-acquired case. *Pediatr Infect Dis* 3:300–303, 1984.

237. Henderson FW, Clyde WA, Collier AM, Denny FW: The etiologic and epidemiologic spectrum of bronchiolitis in pediatric practice. *J Pediatr* 95:183–190, 1979.

238. Paisley JW, Lauer BA, McIntosh K, Glode MP, Schachter J, Rumak C: Pathogens associated with acute lower respiratory tract infection in young children. *Pediatr Infect Dis* 3:14–19, 1984.

239. Denny FW, Murphy TF, Clyde WA, Collier AM, Henderson FW: Croup: an 11-year study in a pediatric practice. *Pediatrics* 71:871–876, 1983.

240. Eriksson M, Forsgren M, Sjoberg S, von Sydow M, Wolontis S: Respiratory syncytial virus infection in young hospitalized children. *Acta Paediatr Scand* 72:47–51, 1983.

241. Chretien J, Holland W, Macklem P, Murray J, Woolcock A: Acute respiratory infections in children. *N Engl J Med* 310:982–984, 1984.

242. Shann F, Gratten M, Germer S, Linnemann V, Hazlett D, Payne R: Aetiology of pneumonia in children in Goroka hospital, Papua New Guinea. *Lancet* 2:537–541, 1984.

243. Tyeryar FJ: National Institute of Allergy and Infectious Diseases: report of a workshop on respiratory syncytial virus and parainfluenza viruses. *J Infect Dis* 148:588–598, 1983.

244. Hall CB, Douglas RG Jr: Respiratory syncytial virus and influenza: practical community surveillance. *Am J Dis Child* 130:615–620, 1976.

245. Glezen WP: Viral pneumonia as a cause and result of hospitalization. *J Infect Dis* 147:765–770, 1983.

246. Mufson MA, Mocega HE, Krause HE: Acquisition of parainfluenza 3 virus infection by hospitalized children. 1. Frequencies, rates and temporal data. *J Infect Dis* 128:141–147, 1973.

247. Hall CB, Douglas RG, Schnabel KC, Geiman JM: Infectivity of respiratory syncytial virus by various

routes of inoculation. *Infect Immun* 33:779–783, 1981.

248. Gwaltney JM, Hendley JO: Rhinovirus transmission. *Am J Epidemiol* 107:357–361, 1978.

249. Gwaltney JM, Moskalski PB, Hendley JO: Hand-to-hand transmission of rhinovirus colds. *Ann Intern Med* 88:463–467, 1978.

250. Boyer KM, Cherry JD: Influenza viruses. In Feigin RD, Cherry JD (eds): *Textbook of Pediatric Infectious Diseases.* Philadelphia, WB Saunders, 1981, p 1302.

251. Hall CB, Douglas RG Jr: Modes of transmission of respiratory syncytial virus. *J Pediatr* 99:100–103, 1981.

252. Taber LH, Knight V, Gilbert BE, McLung HW, Wilson SZ, Norton J, Thurson JM, Gordon WH, Atmar RL, Schlaudt WR: Ribavirin aerosol treatment of bronchiolitis associated with respiratory syncytial virus infection. *Pediatrics* 72:613–618, 1983.

253. Hall CB, McBride JT, Walsh EE, Bell DM, Gala CL, Hildreth S, Ten Eyck LG, Hall WJ: Aerosolized ribavirin treatment of infants with respiratory syncytial viral infection. *N Engl J Med* 308:1443–1447, 1983.

254. Nicholson KG: Properties of antiviral agents. *Lancet* 2:562–564, 1984.

255. Hall CB, Douglas RG: Nosocomial influenza infection as a cause of intercurrent fevers in infants. *Pediatrics* 55:673–677, 1975.

256. Katagiri S, Ohizumi A, Homma M: Outbreak of type C influenza in a children's home. *J Infect Dis* 148:51–56, 1983.

257. Paisley JW, Bruhn FW, Lauer BA, McIntosh K: Type A2 influenza viral infections in children. *Am J Dis Child* 132:34–36, 1978.

258. Payler DK, Purdham PA: Influenza A prophylaxis with amantadine in a boarding school. *Lancet* 1:502–504, 1984.

259. Nicholson KG: Antiviral therapy. *Lancet* 2:617–621, 1984.

260. Quilligan JJ, Hirayama M, Baernstein HD: The suppression of A₂ influenza in children by the chemoprophylactic use of amantadine. *J Pediatr* 69:572–575, 1966.

261. Barr J, Kjellen L, Svedmyr A: Hospital outbreak of adenovirus type 3 infections. *Acta Paediatr* 47:365–382, 1958.

262. Dagan R, Schwartz RH, Insel RA, Menegus MA: Severe diffuse adenovirus 7a pneumonia in a child with combined immunodeficiency: possible therapeutic effect of human immune serum globulin containing specific neutralizing antibody. *Pediatr Infect Dis* 3:246–251, 1984.

263. Brown M, Petric M, Middleton PJ: Silver staining of DNA restriction fragments for the rapid identification of adenovirus isolates: application during nosocomial outbreaks. *J Virol Meth* 9:87–98, 1984.

264. Wadell G, Varsanyi TM, Lord A, Sutton RNP: Epidemic outbreaks of adenovirus 7 with special reference to the pathogenicity of adenovirus genome type 7b. *Am J Epidemiol* 112:619–627, 1980.

265. De Fabritus AM, Riggio RR, David DS, Senterfit LB, Cheigh JS, Stenzel KH: Parainfluenza type 3 in a transplant unit. *JAMA* 241:384–386, 1979.

266. Dykes AC, Cherry JD, Nolan CE: A clinical, epidemiologic, serologic and virologic study of influenza C virus infection. *Arch Intern Med* 140:1295–1298, 1980.

267. Glezen WP: Consideration of the risk of influenza in children and indications for prophylaxis. *Rev Infect Dis* 2:408–420, 1980.

268. Laraya-Cuasay LR, DeForest A, Huff D, Lischne H, Huang NN: Chronic pulmonary complications of early influenza virus infection in children. *Am Rev Respir Dis* 116:617–624, 1977.

269. Feldman S, Webster RG, Sugg M: Influenza in children and young adults with cancer. *Cancer* 39:350–353, 1977.

270. Hendry RM, McIntosh K: Enzyme-linked immunosorbent assay for detection of respiratory syncytial virus infection: development and description. *J Clin Microbiol* 16:324–328, 1982.

271. Eriksson M, Forsgren M, Sjöberg S, von Sydow M, Wolontis S: Respiratory syncytial virus infections in young hospitalized children. *Acta Paediatr Scand* 72:47–51, 1983.

272. DuPont HL: Rotaviral gastroenteritis—some recent developments. *J Infect Dis* 149:663–666, 1984.

273. Gurwith M, Wenman W, Hinde D, Feltham S, Greenberg H: A proscpetive study of rotavirus infection in infants and young children. *J Infect Dis* 144:218–224, 1981.

274. Koopman JS, Turkish VJ, Monto AS, Gouvea V, Srivastava S, Isaacson RE: Patterns and etiology of diarrhea in three clinical settings. *Am J Epidemiol* 119:114–123, 1984.

275. Sullivan P, Woodward WE, Pickering LK, DuPont HL: Longitudinal study of occurrence of diarrheal disease in day care center. *Am J Public Health* 74:987–991, 1984.

276. Brandt CD, Kim HW, Rodriguez WJ, Arrobio JO, Jeffries BC, Stallings EP, Lewis C, Miles AJ, Chanock RM, Kapikian AZ, Parrott RH: Pediatric viral gastroenteritis during eight years of study. *J Clin Microbiol* 18:71–78, 1983.

277. Appleton H, Buckley M, Robertson MH, Thom BT: A search for fecal viruses in new-born and other infants. *J Hyg (Camb)* 81:279–283, 1978.

278. Black RE, Greenberg HB, Kapikian AZ, Brown KH, Becker S: Acquisition of serum antibody to Norwalk virus and rotavirus and relation to diarrhoea in a longitudinal study in young children in rural Bangladesh. *J Infect Dis* 145:483–489, 1982.

279. Kapikian AZ, Kim HW, Wyatt RG, Cline WL, Arrobio JO, Brandt CD, Rodriguez WJ, Sack DA, Chanock RM, Parrott RH: Human reovirus-like agent as the major pathogen associated with "winter" gastroenteritis in hospitalized infants and young children. *N Engl J Med* 294:965–972, 1976.

280. Holzel HS, Cubitt WD: Enteric viruses in hospital-acquired infection. *J Hosp Infect* 3:101–104, 1982.

281. Sebodo T, Soenarto Y, Rohde JE, Ryan NJ, Taylor BJ, Luke RJK, Bishop RF, Barnes GL, Holmes IH, Ruck BJ: Aetiology of diarrhoea in children aged less than two years in central Java. *Lancet* 1:490–491, 1977.

282. Truant AL, Chonmaitree T: Incidence of rotavirus infection in different age groups of pediatric patients with gastroenteritis. *J Clin Microbiol* 16:568–569, 1982.

283. Espejo RT, Calderon E, Gonzalez N, Salomon A, Maruscelli A, Romero P: Presence of two distinct types of rotavirus in infants and young children hospitalized wth acute gastroenteritis in Mexico City, 1977. *J Infect Dis* 139:474–477, 1979.

284. Champsaur H, Henry-Amar M, Goldszmidt D, Prevot J, Bourjouane M, Questiaux E, Bach C: Rotavirus carriage; asymptomatic infection and disease in the first two years of life. II. Serological response. *J Infect Dis* 149:675–682, 1984.

285. Champsaur H, Questiaux E, Prevot J, Henry-Amar M, Goldszmidt D. Bourjouane M, Bach C: Rotavirus carriage; asymptomatic infection and disease in the first two years of Life. I. Virus shedding. *J Infect Dis* 149:667–674, 1984.

286. Walther FJ, Bruggeman C, Daniels-Bosman SM, Pourier S, Grauls G, Stals F, Bogaard AVD: Symptomatic and asymptomatic rotavirus infections in hospitalized children. *Acta Paediatr Scand* 72:659–663, 1983.

287. Blacklow NR, Cukor G: Viral gastroenteritis. *N Engl J Med* 304:397–406, 1981.

288. Persson BL, Thoren A, Tufvesson B, Walder M: Diarrhoea in Swedish infants. *Acta Paediatr Scand* 71:909–913, 1982.

289. Hirsch W, Sapiro-Hirsch R, Berger A, Winter ST, Mayer G, Merzbach D: *Salmonella edinburg* infection in children. *Lancet* 1:828–829, 1965.

290. Mhalu FS, Mtango FDE, Msengi AE: Hospital outbreaks of cholera transmitted through close person-tc-person contact. *Lancet* 2:82–84, 1984.

291. Kapikian AZ, Wyatt RG, Levine MM, Yolken RH, Vankirk DH, Dolin R, Greenberg HB, Chanock RM: Oral administration of human rotavirus to volunteers. *J Infect Dis* 147:95–106, 1983.

292. Kim HW, Brandt CD, Kapikian AZ, Wyatt RG, Arrobio JO, Rodriguez WJ, Chanock RM, Parrott RH: Human reovirus-like agent infection: occurrence in adult contacts of pediatric patients with gastroenteritis. *JAMA* 238:404–407, 1977.

293. Rodriguez WJ, Kim HW, Brandt CD, Yolken RH, Richard M, Arrobio JO, Schwartz RH, Kapikian AZ, Chanock RM, Parrott RH: Common exposure outbreak of gastroenteritis due to type 2 rotavirus with high secondary attack rate within families. *J Infect Dis* 140:353–357, 1979.

294. Wenman WM, Hinde D, Feltham S, Gurwith M: Rotavirus infection in adults: results of a prospective family study. *N Engl J Med* 301:303–306, 1979.

295. Elmwood AF, Abbott GD, Fergusson DM, Jennings LC, Allan JM: Spread of rotavirus within families: a community based study. *Br Med J* 287:575–577, 1983.

296. Flewett TH, Bryden AS, Davies H, Morris CA: Epidemic viral enteritis in a long-stay children's ward. *Lancet* 1:4–5, 1975.

297. Middleton PJ, Szymanski MT, Petric M: Viruses associated with acute gastroenteritis in young children. *Am J Dis Child* 131:733–737, 1977.

298. Ryder RW, McGowan JE, Hatch MH, Palmer EL: Reovirus-like agent as a cause of nosocomial diarrhoea in infants. *J Pediatr* 90:698–702, 1977.

299. Kurtz JB, Lee TW, Pickering D: Astrovirus associated gastroenteritis in a children's ward. *J Clin Pathol* 30:948–952, 1977.

300. Spratt HC, Marks MI, Gomersall M, Gill P, Pai CH: Nosocomial infantile gastroenteritis associated with minirotavirus and calicivirus. *J Pediatr* 93:922–926, 1978.

301. Chiba S, Sakuma Y, Kogasaka R, Akihara M, Horino K, Nakao T, Fukui S: An outbreak of gastroenteritis associated with calicivirus in an infant home. *J Med Virol* 4:249–254, 1979.

302. Cubitt WD, McSwiggan DA, Artstall S: An outbreak of calicivirus infection in a mother and baby unit. *J Clin Pathol* 33:1095–1098, 1980.

303. Ruiz-Gomez J, Espinosa-Larios EL, Becerril P, Munoz-Hernandez O, Chacon-Garcia A, Vargas-de la Rosa R, Gutierrez G: Etiology of hospital-acquired infectious diarrhoea. *Arch Invest Med (Mex)* 13:213–218, 1982.

304. Yolken RH, Lawrence F, Leister F, Takiff HE, Strauss SE: Gastroenteritis associated with enteric adenovirus in hospitalized infants. *J Pediatr* 101:21–26, 1982.

305. Noone C, Banatvala JE: Hospital acquired rotaviral gastroenteritis in a general pediatric hospital. *J Hosp Infect* 4:297–299, 1983.

306. Chapin M, Yatabe J, Cherry JD: An outbreak of rotavirus gastroenteritis on a pediatric unit. *Am J Infect Control* 11:88–91, 1983.

307. Adler JL, Anderson RL, Boring JR, Nahmias AJ: A protracted hospital-associated outbreak of *Salmonella* is due to a multiple-antibiotic-resistant strain of *Salmonella indiana. J Pediatr* 77:970–975, 1970.

308. Rice PA, Craven PC, Wells JG: *Salmonella heidelberg* enteritis and bacteremia. An epidemic on two pediatric wards. *Am J Med* 60:509–516, 1976.

309. Im SWK, Chow K, Chau PY: Rectal thermometer mediated cross-infection with *Salmonella wandsworth* in a paediatric ward. *J Hosp Infect* 2:171–174, 1981.

310. Kumarasinghe G, Hamilton WJ, Gould JDM, Palmer SR, Dudgeon JA, Marshall WC: An outbreak of *Salmonella muenchen* infection in a specialist paediatric hospital. *J Hosp Infect* 3:341–344, 1982.

311. Makarem EH: Outbreak of multiple drug-resistant *Salmonella havanna* originating in pediatric wards of two hospitals in Shiraz, Iran—in vitro susceptibility patterns. *J Trop Pediatr* 28:14–19, 1982.

312. Robins-Browne RM, Rowe B, Ramsaroop R, Naran AD, Threlfall EJ, Ward LR, Lloyd DA, Mickel RE: A hospital outbreak of multiresistant *Salmonella typhimurium* belonging to phage type 193. *J Infect Dis* 147:210–216, 1983.

313. Pickering LK, Evans DJ, Munoz O: Prospective study of enteropathogens in children with diarrhoea in Houston and Mexico. *J Pediatr* 93:383–388, 1978.

314. Konno T, Sato T, Kitaoka S, Katsushima N, Sakamoto M, Yazaki N, Ishida N: Changing RNA patterns in rotaviruses of human origin: demonstration of a single dominant pattern at the start of an epidemic and various patterns thereafter. *J Infect Dis* 149:683–687, 1984.

315. Totterdell BM, Chrystie IL, Banatvala JE: Rotavirus infections in a maternity unit. *Arch Dis Child* 51:924–928, 1976.

316. Lemp GJ, Woodward WE, Pickering LK, Sullivan PS, DuPont HL: The relationships of staff to the

incidence of diarrhoea in day-care centers. *Am J Epidemiol* 120:750–758, 1984.

317. Pickering LK, Woodward WE: Diarrhoea in day-care centers. *Pediatr Infect Dis* 1:47–52, 1982.

318. World Health Organization Sub-group of the Scientific Working Group on Epidemiology and Etiology: *Rotavirus and Other Viral Diarrhoeas.* Geneva, World Health Organization, 1979 (WHO/DDC/EPE/79.2).

319. Samadi AR, Huq MI, Ahmed QS: Detection of rotavirus in handwashings of attendants of children with diarrhoea. *Br Med J* 286:188, 1983.

320. Pether JVS, Scott RJD: *Salmonella* carriers: are they dangerous? A study to identify finger contamination with *Salmonella* by convalescent carriers. *J Infect* 5:81–88, 1982.

321. Middleton PJ: Role of viruses in pediatric gastrointestinal disease and epidemiologic factors. In Tyrrell PAJ, Kapikian AZ (eds): *Virus Infections of the Gastrointestinal Tract.* New York, Marcel Dekker, 1982, pp 211–225.

322. Lecce JG, King MW, Dorsey WB: Rearing regimen producing piglet diarrhea (rotavirus) and its relevance to acute infantile diarrhea. *Science* 199:776–778, 1978.

323. Lecce JG, King MW, Mock R: Reovirus-like agent associated with fatal diarrhoea in neonatal pigs. *Infect Immun* 14:816–825, 1976.

324. Watt J, Wegman M, Brown W, Schiliessman M, Maupin E, Hemphill E: Salmonellosis in a premature nursery unaccompanied by diarrheal disease. *Pediatrics* 22:689–705, 1958.

325. Sattar SA: Rotavirus survival in air. *Appl Environ Microbiol* 47:879–889, 1984.

326. Santosham M, Yolken RH, Quiroz E, Dillman L, Oro G, Reeves WC, Sack RB: Detection of rotavirus in respiratory secretions of children with pneumonia. *J Pediatr* 103:583–585, 1983.

327. Foster SO, Palmer EL, Gary GW, Martin ML, Heriman KL, Beasley P, Sampson J: Gastroenteritis due to rotavirus in an isolated Pacific Island group: an epidemic of 3,439 cases. *J Infect Dis* 141:32–39, 1980.

328. Gordon AG: Rotavirus infections and the sompe syndrome. *J Infect Dis* 146:117–118, 1982.

329. Black RE, Dykes AC, Anderson KE, Wells JG, Sinclair SP, Gary GW, Hatch MD, Gangarosa EJ: Handwashing to prevent diarrhea in day-care centers. *Am J Epidemiol* 113:446–451, 1981.

330. Khan MU: Interruption of shigellosis by handwashing. International Center for diarrhoeal disease research. *Trans R Soc Trop Med Hyg* 76:no. 2, 1982.

331. Taylor MRH, Keane CT, Kerrison IM, Stronge JL: Simple and effective measures for control of enteric cross infection in a children's hospital. *Lancet* 1:863–867, 1979.

332. Berger R, Hadziselimovic F, Just M, Reigel P: Effect of feeding human milk on nosocomial rotavirus infection in an infant ward. *Dev Biol Standard* 53:219–228, 1983.

333. Vesikari T, Isolauri E, D'Hondt E, Delem A, Andre FE, Zissis E: Protection of infants against rotavirus diarrhoea by Rit 4237 attenuated bovine rotavirus strain vaccine. *Lancet* 1:977–981, 1984.

334. Jarvis WR, Feldman RA: *Clostridium difficile* and

gastroenteritis—how strong is the association in children? *Pediatr Infect Dis* 3:4–6, 1984.

335. Holzel HS, Cubitt WD: Enteric viruses in hospital-acquired infection. *J Hosp Infect* 3:101–104, 1982.

336. Larson HE, Barclay FE, Honour P, Hill ID: Epidemiology of *Clostridium difficile* in infants. *J Infect Dis* 146:727–733, 1982.

337. Kim K, DuPont HL, Pickering LK: Outbreaks of diarrhoea associated with *Clostridium difficile* and its toxin in day-care centers: evidence of person-to-person transmission. *J Pediatr* 102:376–382, 1983.

338. Yamagishi T, Sakamoto K, Sakurai S, Konishi K, Daimon Y, Matsuda M, Gyobu Y, Kubo Y, Kodama H: A nosocomial outbreak of food poisioning caused by enterotoxigenic *Clostridium perfringens. Microbiol Immunol* 27:291–296, 1983.

339. Collier AC, Miller RA, Meyers JD: Cryptosporidiosis after marrow transplantation: person-to-person transmission and treatment with spiramycin. *Ann Intern Med* 101:205–206, 1984.

340. Baxby D, Hart A, Taylor A: Human cryptosporidiosis: a possible cause of hospital cross infection. *Br Med J* 287:1760–1761, 1983.

341. Alpert G, Bell LM, Kirkpatrick CE, Budnick LD, Campos JM, Friedman HM, Plotkin SA: Cryptosporidiosis in a day-care center. *N Engl J Med* 311:860–861, 1984.

342. Bohan G, et al: Crtyptosporidiosis among children attending day-care centers—Georgia, Pennsylvania, Michigan, California, New Mexico. *MMWR* 33:599–601, 1984.

343. Bogaerts J, Lepage P, Rouvroy D, Vandepitte J: *Crytosporidium* spp, a frequent cause of diarrhea in central Africa. *J Clin Microbiol* 20:874–876, 1984.

344. Fekety R: Recent advances in management of bacterial diarrhoea. *Rev Infect Dis* 5:246–257, 1983.

345. Behera SK, Mohapatra SS, Kar S, Das D, Panda C: Clinical profile of *E. coli* diarrhoea in hospitalized children (Part II). *Indian Pediatr* 16:249–254, 1979.

346. Palmer SR, Rowe B: Investigation of outbreaks of *Salmonella* in hospitals. *Br Med J* 287:891–893, 1983.

347. Lampert J, Plotkin S, Campos J, Trendler M, Schlagel D: Shigellosis in a children's hospital—Pennsylvania. *MMWR* 32:498–499, 1979.

348. Geller RJ: The pertussis syndrome: a persistent problem. *Pediatr Infect Dis* 3:182–196, 1984.

349. Mertsola J, Ruuskanen O, Eerola E, Vilijanen MK: Intrafamilial spread of pertussis. *J Pediatr* 103:359–363, 1983.

350. Broome CV, Preblud SR, Bruner B, McGowan JE, Hayes PS, Harris PP, Elsea W, Fraser DW: Epidemiology of pertussis, Atlanta, 1977. *J Pediatr* 98:362–367, 1981.

351. Linnemann CC, Nasenbeny J: Pertussis in the adult. *Annu Rev Med* 28:179–185, 1977.

352. Trollfors B, Rabo E: Whooping cough in adults. *Br Med J* 283:696–697, 1981.

353. Halsey NA, Welling MA, Lehman RM: Nosocomial pertussis: a failure of erythromycin treatment and prophylaxis. *Am J Dis Child* 134:521–522, 1980.

354. Altemeier WA, Ayoub EM: Erythromycin prophylaxis for pertussis. *Pediatrics* 59:623–625, 1977.
355. Bass JW: Use of erythromycin in pertussis outbreaks. *Pediatrics* 72:748–749, 1983.
356. Bass JW, Harden LB: Treatment and prophylaxis failure of erythromycin in pertussis. *Am J Dis Child* 134:1178–1179, 1980.
357. Gordon JE, Hood RI: Whooping cough and its epidemiological anomalies. *Am J Med Sci* 222:333–361, 1951.
358. Brunell PA, Chairman, Committee on Infectious Diseases, 1983–1984, American Academy of Pediatrics: Committee on Infectious Diseases: pertussis vaccine. *Pediatrics* 74:303–305, 1984.
359. Fulginiti VA: A new pertussis vaccine: hope for the future? *J Infect Dis* 148:146–147, 1983.
360. Sato Y, Kimura M, Fukumi H: Development of a pertussis component vaccine in Japan. *Lancet* 1:122–126, 1984.
361. Doglo J: Measles. *MMWR* 33:349–351, 1984.
362. DeJong JG, Winkler KC: Survival of measles virus in air. *Nature* 201:1054–1055, 1964.
363. Murphy MD, Brunell PA, Lievens AW, Shehab, ZM: Effect of early immunization on antibody response to reimmunization with measles vaccine as demonstrated by enzyme-linked immunosorbent assay (ELISA). *Pediatrics* 74:90–93, 1984.
364. Walsh JA: Selective primary health care: strategies for control of diseases in the developing world. IV. Measles. *J Infect Dis* 5:330–340, 1983.
365. Brunell PA, Brickman A, O'Hare D, Steinberg S: Ineffectiveness of isolation of patients as a method of preventing the spread of mumps. *N Engl J Med* 279:1357–1361, 1968.
366. Shehab ZM, Brunell PA, Cobb E: Epidemiological standardization of a test for susceptibility to mumps. *J Infect Dis* 149:810–812, 1984.
367. Recommendation of the Immunization Practices Advisory Committee, Centers for Disease Control, Department of Health and Human Services; Atlanta, Georgia; Mumps vaccine. *Ann Intern Med* 98:192–194, 1983.
368. Lewis E, Chernesky MA, Rawls ML, Rawls WE: Epidemic of mumps in a partially immune population. *Can Med Assoc J* 121:751–754, 1979.
369. Shewmon DA, Cherry JD, Kirby SE: Shedding of rubella virus in a 4½-year-old boy with congenital rubella. *Pediatr Infect Dis* 1:342–343, 1982.
370. Nelson LA, Peri BA, Reiger CHL, Newcomb RW, Rothberg RM: Immunity to diphtheria in an urban population. *Pediatrics* 61:703–710, 1978.
371. Palmer SR, Balfour AH, Jephcott AE: Immunization of adults during an outbreak of diphtheria. *Br Med J* 1:624–626, 1983.
372. Robbins FC: (Poliomyelitis) Summary and recommendations. *Rev Infect Dis* 6:596–600, 1984.
373. Weller TH: Poliomyelitis: its global demise? *Pediatrics* 74:442, 1984.
374. Horstmann DM: Control of poliomyelitis: a continuing paradox. *J Infect Dis* 146:540–549, 1982.
375. Immunization Practices Advisory Committee, Centers for Disease Control; Atlanta, Georgia: Poliomyelitis prevention. *Ann Intern Med* 96:630–634, 1982.
376. Alexander E: Inactivated poliomyelitis vaccination. Issues reconsidered. *JAMA* 251:2710–2712, 1984.
377. Patterson WJ, Bell EJ: Poliomyelitis in a nursery school in Glasgow. *Br Med J* 2:1574–1576, 1963.
378. Venkitaraman, John TJ: Chickenpox outbreak in staff and students of a hospital in the tropics. *Lancet* 2:165, 1982.
379. Judelsohn RG: Varicella-outbreak. Atlanta, Public Health Service, Centers for Disease Control, 1971, EPI-71-98-2.
380. Meyers JD, MacQuarrie MB, Witte JJ: Varicella outbreak. Atlanta, Public Health Service, Centers for Disease Control, 1974, EPI-74-93-2.
381. Thomson FH: The aerial conveyance of infection. *Lancet* 1:341–344, 1916.
382. Feldman S, Hughes WT, Daniel CB: Varicella in children with cancer: seventy-seven cases. *Pediatrics* 56:388–397, 1975.
383. Balfour HH, Groth KE: Zoster immune plasma prophylaxis of varicella: a follow-up report. *J Pediatr* 94:743–748, 1979.
384. Feldhoff CM, Balfour HH, Simmons RL, Najarian JS, Maner SM: Varicella in children with renal transplant. *J Pediatr* 98:25–31, 1981.
385. Falliers CJ, Ellis EF: Corticosteroids and varicella. *Arch Dis Child* 40:593–599, 1965.
386. Balfour HH, Groth KE, McCullough J, Kalis JM, Marker SC, Nesbit TS, Simmons RL, Najarian JS: Prevention or modification of varicella using zoster immune plasma. *Am J Dis Child* 131:693–696, 1977.
387. Orenstein WA, Heymann DL, Ellis RJ, Rosenberg RL, Nakano J, Halsey NA, Overturf GD, Hayden GF, Witte JJ: Prophylaxis of varicella in high-risk children: dose-response effect of zoster immune globulin. *J Pediatr* 98:368–373, 1981.
388. Weller T: Varicella and herpes zoster. *N Engl J Med* 309:1362–1368, 1983.
389. Weller T: Varicella and herpes zoster. *N Engl J Med* 309:1434–1440, 1983.
390. Gershon AA, Raker R, Steinberg S, Olstein BT, Drusin LM: Antibody to varicella zoster virus in parturient women and their offspring during the first year of life. *Pediatrics* 58:692–696, 1976.
391. Varicella-zoster virus affecting immigrant nurses. *Lancet* 2:154–155, 1980.
392. Venkitaraman AR, John TJ: Chickenpox outbreak in staff and students of a hospital in the tropics. *Lancet* 2:165, 1982.
393. Asano Y, Iwayama S, Miyata T, Yazaki T, Ozaki T, Tsuzuki K, Ito S, Takahashi M: Spread of varicella in hospitalized children having no direct contact with an indicator zoster case and at its prevention by a live vaccine. *Biken J* 23:157–161, 1980.
394. Myers MG, Rasley DA, Hierholzer WJ: Hospital infection control for varicella zoster virus infection. *Pediatrics* 70:199–202, 1982.
395. Brunell PA: Contagion and varicella-zoster virus. *Pediatr Infect Dis* 1:304–307, 1982.
396. Brunnell PA (Chairman American Academy of *Pediatrics*, Committee on Infectious Diseases): Expanded guidelines for use of varicella zoster immune globulin. *Pediatrics* 72:886–889, 1983.
397. Shehab Z, Brunell PA: Enzyme-linked immunosorbent assay for susceptibility to varicella. *J Infect*

Dis 148:472–476, 1983.

398. Hutter JJ, Minnich LL, Ray G: Varicella-zoster antibody titers in children with leukemia and lymphoma: relationship of titer to varicella-zoster infection. *Am J Dis Child* 138:56–59, 1984.

399. Deleted in proof.

400. Steele RW, Coleman MA, Fiser M, Bradsher RW: Varicella zoster in hospital personnel: skin test reactivity to monitor susceptibility. *Pediatrics* 70:604–608, 1982.

401. Arvin AM, Koropchak CM, Wittek AE: Immunologic evidence of reinfection with varicella-zoster virus. *J Infect Dis* 148:200–205, 1983.

402. Gershon AA, Steinberg SP, Gelb L: Clinical reinfection with varicella-zoster virus. *J Infect Dis* 149:137–142, 1984.

403. Balfour HH Jr, Bean B, Laskin OL: Acyclovir halts progression of herpes zoster in immunocompromised patients. *N Engl J Med* 308:1448–1453, 1983.

404. Weibel RE, Neff BJ, Kuter BJ, Guess HA, Rothenberger CA, Fitzgerald AJ, Connor KA, McLean AA, Hilleman MR, Buynak EB, Scolnick EM: Live attenuated varicella virus vaccine: efficacy trial in healthy children. *N Engl J Med* 310:1409–1415, 1984.

405. Bogger-Goren S, Bernstein JM, Gerson AA, Ogra PL: Mucosal cell-mediated immunity to varicella zoster virus: role in protection against disease. *J Pediatr* 105:195–199, 1984.

406. Recommendations of the Immunization Practices Advisory Committee, Centers for Disease Control, Atlanta, Georgia: Varicella-zoster immune globulin for the prevention of chickenpox. *Ann Intern Med* 100:859–865, 1984.

407. Paryani SG, Arvin AM, Koropchak CM, Dobkin MB, Wittek AE, Amylon MD, Budinger MD: Comparisons of varicella zoster antibody titers in patients given intravenous immune serum globulin or varicella zoster immune globulin. *J Pediatr* 105:200–205, 1984.

408. Gershon AA, Steinberg SP, Gelb L, Galasso G, Borkowsky W, LaRussa P, Ferrara A: Live attenuated varicella vaccine. Efficacy for children with leukemia in remission. *JAMA* 252:355–362, 1984.

409. Gershon A, Steinberg S, Gelb L: Efficacy of live attenuated varicella vaccine in children with acute leukemia remission. *JAMA* 252:355–362, 1984.

410. Gershon AS: The success of varicella vaccine. *Pediatr Infect Dis* 3:500–502, 1984.

411. McIntosh K: Varicella vaccine: decisions a little nearer. *N Engl J Med* 310:1456–1457, 1984.

412. Brunell PA, Shehab Z, Geiser C, Waugh JE: Administration of live varicella vaccine to children with leukemia. *Lancet* 2:1069–1073, 1982.

413. Brawley RL, Wenzel RP: An algorithm for chickenpox exposure. *Pediatr Infect Dis* 3:502–504, 1984.

414. Hayden GF, Meyers JD, Dixon RE: Nosocomial varicella. Part II. Suggested guidelines for management. *West J Med* 130:300–303, 1979.

415. Meyers JD, MacQuarrie MB, Merigan TC: Nosocomial varicella. Part I. Outbreak in oncology patients at a children's hospital. *West J Med* 130:196–199, 1979.

416. Hyams PJ, Stuewe MCS, Heitzer V: Herpes zoster causing varicella (chickenpox) in hospital employ-

ees: cost of a casual attitude. *Am J Infect Control* 12:2–5, 1984.

417. Baba K, Yabuuchi H, Takahashi M, Gershon AA, Ogra PL: Seroepidemiologic behaviour of varicella zoster virus infection in a semiclosed environment after introduction of V2V vaccine. *J Pediatr* 105:712–716, 1984.

418. Bryson YJ: The use of acyclovir in children. *Pediatr Infect Dis* 3:345–348, 1984.

419. Barton LL, Granoff DM, Barenkamp SJ: Nosocomial spread of *Haemophilus influenzae* type b infection documented by outer membrane protein subtype analysis. *J Pediatr* 102:820–824, 1983.

420. Inzana TJ, Pichichero ME: Lipopolysaccharide subtypes of *Haemophilus influenzae* type b from an outbreak of invasive disease. *J Clin Microbiol* 20:145–150, 1984.

421. Brunell PA. (Chairman Committee on Infectious Diseases 1983–1984): Revision of recommendation for use of rifampin prophylaxis of contacts of patients with *Haemophilus influenzae* infections. *Pediatrics* 74:301–302, 1984.

422. Prober CG: Pharmacologic interaction of rifampin and chloramphenicol. *N Engl J Med* 312:788–789, 1985.

423. Daum R, Gilsdorf J, Granoff D, Murphy T, Osterholm M: Guidelines for dealing with the guidelines: rifampin prophylaxis for day care contacts of patients with serious *Haemophilus influenzae* type b infections. *J Pediatr* 105:761–763, 1984.

424. Peltola H, Kayhty H, Virtanen M, Makela H: Prevention of *Haemophilus influenzae* type b bacteremic infections with the capsular polysaccharide vaccine. *N Engl J Med* 310:1561–1566, 1984.

425. Cohen MS, Steere AC, Baltimore R, von Graevenitz A, Pantelick E, Camp B, Root RK: Possible nosocomial transmission of group y *Neisseria meningitidis* among oncology patients. *Ann Intern Med* 91:7–12, 1979.

426. Rose HD, Lonz IE, Sheth NK: Meningococcal pneumonia. A source of nosocomial infection. *Arch Intern Med* 141:575–577, 1981.

427. Feigin RD, Baker CJ, Herwaldt LA, Lampe RM, Mason EO, Whitney SE: Epidemic meningococcal disease in an elementary-school classroom. *N Engl J Med* 307:1255–1257, 1982.

428. Nelson JD: How preventable is bacterial meningitis? *N Engl J Med* 307:1265–1267, 1982.

429. Ayton M: An outbreak of streptococcal infection in a children's ward. *Nursing Times*, May 7, 1981, pp 4–7.

430. Editorial: Streptococci in institutions. *Lancet* 1:311–312, 1981.

431. Loosli CG, Smith MHD, Cline J, Nelson L: The transmission of hemolytic streptococcal infections in infant wards with special reference to "skin dispersers." *Am J Dis Child*, pp 342–359.

432. Colling, A, Kerr F, Maxted WR, Widdowson JP: Streptococcal infection in a junior detention center: a five year study. *J Hyg* 85:331–341, 1980.

433. Ryder RW, Lawrence DN, Nitzkin JL, Feeley JC, Merson MH: An evaluation of penicillin prophylaxis during an outbreak of food-borne streptococcal pharyngitis. *Am J Epidemiol* 106:139–144, 1977.

434. Steele RW, Ashcraft EW, Payton TS, Eisenach KD: Recurrent staphylococcal infection in a pe-

diatric residential care facility. *Am J Infect Control* 11:217–220, 1983.

435. Radetsky MS, Istre GR, Johansen TL, Parmelee SW, Lauer BA, Wiesenthal AM, Glode MP: Multiple resistant pneumococcus causing meningitis: its epidemiology within a day-care centre. *Lancet* 2:771–773, 1981.

436. Bartzokas CA, Paton JH, Gibson MF, Graham R, McLoughlin GA, Croton RS: Control and eradication of methicillin-resistant *Staphylococcus aureus* on a surgical unit. *N Engl J Med* 311:1422–1425, 1981.

437. Artenstein MS, Weinstein L: Hospital-acquired enterovirus infections. *N Engl J Med* 267:1005–1010, 1962.

438. Suzuki N, Ishikawa K, Horiuchi T, Shibazaki M, Soda K: Age-related symptomatology of ECHO 11 virus infection in children. *Pediatrics* 65:284–286, 1980.

439. Parrott RH, Huebner RJ, McCullough NB, Wolf SI, Naiden E: The hospital as a factor in the occurrence of coxsackie viruses in various illness groups. *Pediatrics* 15:255–262, 1955.

440. Stansfield SA, Ford-Jones EL: Pyrogen contamination of total parenteral nutrition solutions: a case report. *Can J Hosp Pharm* 1:21–28, 1983.

441. Keys TF, Haldorson AM, Rhodes KH, Roberts GD, Fifer EZ: Nosocomial outbreak of rhizopus infections associated with Elastoplast® wound dressings—Minnesota. *MMWR* 27:33–34, 1978.

442. Dennis JE, Rhodes KH, Cooney DR, Roberts GD: Nosocomial rhizopus infection (zygomycosis) in children. *J Pediatr* 96:824–828, 1980.

443. Corrall CJ, Merz WA, Rekedal K, Hughes WT: *Aspergillus* osteomyelitis in an immunocompetent adolescent: a case report and review of the literature. *Pediatrics* 70:455–460, 1982.

444. Barst RJ, Prince AS, Neu HC: *Aspergillus* endocarditis in children. *Pediatrics* 68:73–78, 1981.

445. Rinaldi MG: Invasive aspergillosis. *Rev Infect Dis* 5:1061–1077, 1983.

446. Gerson SL, Talbot GH, Hurwitz S, Strom BL, Lusk EJ, Cassileth PA: Prolonged granulocytopenia: the major risk factor for invasive pulmonary aspergillosis in patients with acute leukemia. *Ann Intern Med* 100:345–351, 1984.

447. Orenstein WA, Overturf GD, Leedom JM, Alvarado R, Geffner M, Fryer A, Chan L, Haynes V, Starc T, Portnoy B: The frequency of *Legionella* infection prospectively determined in children hospitalized with pneumonia. *J Pediatr* 403–405, 1981.

448. Andersen RD, Lauer BA, Fraser DW, Hayes PS, McIntosh K: Infections with *Legionella pneumophila* in children. *J Infect Dis* 143:386–390, 1981.

449. Muldoon RL, Jaecker DL, Kiefer HK: Legionnaires' disease in children. *Pediatrics* 67:329–332, 1981.

450. Ryan ME, Feldman S, Pruitt B, Fraser DW: Legionnaires' disease in a child with cancer. *Pediatrics* 64:951–953, 1979.

451. Cutz E, Thorner PS, Rao P, Toma S, Gold R, Gelfand EW: Disseminated *Legionella pneumophila* infection in an infant with severe combined immunodeficiency. *J Pediatr* 100:760–762, 1982.

452. Kovatch AL, Jardine DS, Dowling JN, Yee RB, Pasculle AW: Legionellosis in children with leukemia in relapse. *Pediatrics* 73:811–815, 1984.

453. Sturm R, Staneck JL, Myers JP, Wilkinson HW, Cottrill CM, Towbin RB: Pediatric Legionnaires' disease: diagnosis by direct immunofluorescent staining of sputum. *Pediatrics* 68:539–543, 1981.

454. Helms CM, Massanari M, Zeitler R, Streed S, Gilchrist MJR, Hall N, Hausler WJ Jr, Sywassink J, Johnson W, Wintermeyer L, Hierholzer WJ Jr: Legionnaires' diseases associated with a hospital water system: a cluster of 24 nosocomial cases. *Ann Intern Med* 99:172–178, 1983.

455. Best M, Goetz A, Yu VL: Heat eradication measures for control of nosocomial Legionnaires' disease: implementation, education, cost analysis. *Am J Infect Control* 12:26–30, 1984.

456. Myerowitz RL: Nosocomial Legionnaires' disease and other nosocomial *Legionella* pneumonias. *Infect Control* 4:107–110, 1983.

457. Ellsbury E, Owosekun O, Mackey K, Ten Eyck O, Mahoney LE: Outbreak of viral hepatitis in the staff of a pediatric ward—California. *MMWR* 26:77–78, 1977.

458. Orenstein WA, Wu E, Wilkins J, Robinson K, Francis DP, Timko N, Wayne R: Hospital-acquired hepatitis A: report of an outbreak. *Pediatrics* 67:494–497, 1981.

459. Krober MS, Bass JW, Brown JD, Lemon SM, Rupert KJ: Hospital outbreak of hepatitis A: risk factors for spread. *Pediatr Infect Dis* 3:296–299, 1984.

460. Seeberg S, Brandberg A, Hermodsson S, Larsson P, Lundgren S: Hospital outbreak of hepatitis A secondary to blood exchange in a baby. *Lancet* 1:1155–1156, 1981.

461. Rhame FS, VanDrunen N, Cameron S: An outbreak of nosocomial hepatitis A. Abstracts of the Eighth Annual Conference of the Association of Practioners in Infection Control. Atlanta, 1981.

462. Goodman RA, Carder CC, Allen JR, Orenstein WA, Finton RJ: Nosocomial hepatitis A transmission by an adult patient with diarrhea. *Am J Med* 73:220–226, 1982.

463. Coulepis AG, Locarnini SA, Lehmann NI, Gust ID: Detection of hepatitis A virus in the faeces of patients with naturally acquired infections. *J Infect Dis* 141:151–156, 1980.

464. Papaevangelou GJ, Roumeliotou-Karayannis AJ, Contoyannis PC: The risk of nosocomial hepatitis A and B virus infections for patients under care without isolation precautions. *J Med Virol* 7:143–148, 1981.

465. Fine RN, Malekzadeh MH, Wright HT: Hepatitis B in a pediatric hemodialysis unit. *J Pediatr* 86:349–355, 1975.

466. Nivet H, Drucker J, Dubois F, Goudreau A, Coursaget P, Rolland JC, Grenier P, Maupas P: Vaccine against hepatitis B in children: prevention of hepatitis in a pediatric hemodialysis unit. *Int J Pediatr Nephrol* 3:25–28, 1982.

467. Steinberg SC, Alter HJ, Leventhal BG: The risk of hepatitis transmission to family contacts of leukemia patients. *J Pediatr* 87:753–756, 1975.

468. Tabor E, Gerety RJ, Mott M, Wilbur J: Prevalence of hepatitis B in a high-risk setting: a serologic study of patients and staff in a pediatric oncology unit. *Pediatrics* 61:711–715, 1978.

469. Deleted in proof.

470. Leichtner AM, Leclair J, Goldmann DA, Schumacher RT, Gewolb IH, Katz AJ: Horizontal nonparenteral spread of hepatitis B among children. *Ann Intern MEd* 94:346–349, 1981.
471. Cancio-Bello TP, de Medina M, Shorey J, Valledor MD, Schiff ER: An institutional outbreak of hepatitis B related to a human biting carrier. *J Infect Dis* 146:652–656, 1982.
472. Williams C, Weber T, Cullen J, Kane M: Hepatitis B transmission in school contacts of retarded HB$_s$A$_g$ carrier students. *J Pediatr* 103:192–196, 1983.
473. Chin J: Prevention of chronic hepatitis B virus infection from mothers to infants in the United States. *Pediatrics* 71:289–292, 1983.
474. Dienstag JL, Ryan DM: Occupational exposure to hepatitis B virus in hospital personnel: infection or immunization? *Am J Epidemiol* 115:26–39, 1982.
475. Mulley AG, Silverstein MD, Dienstag JL: Indications for use of hepatitis B vaccine, based on cost-effectiveness analysis. *N Engl J Med* 307:644–651, 1983.
476. Ohori N, Nagatsuka Y, Kanno A, Abe Y, Ishaida N: Two distinct types of non-A non-B hepatitis in a cardiovascular survey unit. *J Med Virol* 11:105–113, 1983.
477. Plotkin SA, Michelson S, M de R, Alford CA, Starr SE, Parkman PD, Pagano JS, Rapp F: The pathogenesis and prevention of human cytomegalovirus infection. *Pediatr Infect Dis* 3:67–74, 1984.
478. Pass RF, Hutto C, Reynolds, DW, Polhill RB: Increased frequency of cytomegalovirus infection in children in group day-care. *Pediatrics* 74:121–126, 1984.
479. Hanshaw JB: The launching of a cytomegalovirus vaccine. *Am J Dis Child* 136:291–292, 1982.
480. Plotkin SA: Prevention of cytomegalovirus disease. *Pediatr Infect Dis* 3:1–4, 1984.
481. Henson D, Siegel SE, Fuccillo DA, Matthew E, Levine AS: Cytomegalovirus infections during acute leukemia. *J Infect Dis* 126:469–481, 1972.
482. Cox F, Hughes WT: The value of isolation procedures for cytomegalovirus infections in children with leukemia. *Cancer* 36:1158–1161, 1975.
483. Stagno S: Isolation precautions for patients with cytomeyalovirus infection. *Pediatr Infect Dis* 1:145–147, 1982.
383. Adler S: Transfusion-associated cytomegalovirus infections. *Rev Infect Dis* 5:977–993, 1983.
485. Thomas PA, Jaffe HW, Spira TJ, Reiss R, Guerrero IC, Auerbach D: Unexplained immunodeficiency in children. *JAMA* 252:639–644, 1984.
486. Ammann AJ, Cowan MJ, Wara DW, Weintrub P, Dritz S, Goldman H, Perkins HA: Acquired immunodeficiency in an infant: possible transmission by means of blood products. *Lancet* 1:956–958, 1983.
487. Gill JC, Menitove JE, Wheeler D, Aster RH, Montgomery RR: Generalized lymphadenopathy and T-cell abnormalities in hemophilia A. *J Pediatr* 103:18–22, 1983.
488. Meyer PR, Modlin RW, Powars D, Ewing D, Parker JW, Taylor CR: Altered distribution of T-lymphocyte subpopulations in lymph nodes from patients with acquired immunodeficiency-like syndrome and hemophilia. *J Pediatr* 103:407–410, 1983.
489. Eickhoff TC, Chairman, Axnick KJ, Brimhall D, Cole WR, Dixon RE, Garner JS, Gibbs RS, Hall CB, Schaffner W, Washington JH II, Brocks L: (A hospital wide approach to AIDS): Recommendations of the Advisory Committee on Infections within Hospitals. *Am Hosp Assoc* 5:242–248, 1984.
490. Burkhart CG: Scabies: an epidemiologic reassessment. *Ann Intern Med* 98:498–503, 1983.
491. Ginsburg CM: Scabies. *Pediatr Infect Dis* 3:133–134, 1984.
492. Belle EA, D'Souza TJ, Zarzour JY, Lemieux M, Wong CC: Hospital epidemic of scabies: diagnosis and control. *Can J Public Health* 70:133–135, 1979.
493. Evans JPM, Rossiter MA, Kumaran TO, Marsh GW, Mortimer PP: Human parvovirus aplasia: case due to cross-infection in a ward. *Br Med J* 288:681, 1984.
494. Editorial: Bone marrow aplasia and parvovirus. *Lancet* 2:21–22, 1983.

Chapter 29

Infections in the Elderly

Peter A. Gross, M.D., and Jerome F. Levine, M.D.

INTRODUCTION

It has been assumed that infections, both community-acquired as well as nosocomial, are more common in the elderly. This assumption is gradually being placed on a firmer scientific foundation. The interaction between immune senescence, age-associated diseases, concomitant use of diagnostic and therapeutic modalities, and normal physiologic and anatomic changes of aging is being carefully examined (1).

A precise *definition* of the elderly finds no consensus. The years 60, 65, and 70 have all been selected as the dividing point; yet, there are no consistent markers of senescence. Therefore, we will simply specify the year or period defined by individual authors. The purpose of this chapter is to review infections in the elderly. Although nosocomial infections will be highlighted, information on community-acquired infections will also be included.

Incidence

The elderly hospitalized patient is more likely to develop a nosocomial infection than is the younger adult patient (2–4). The decade-specific risk is approximately 10/1000 discharged patients from birth to the fifth decade (40 to 49 years). Thereafter, the rate rises sharply to peak at 100/1000 discharges after 70 years of age (3).

While length of stay is approximately 2 days longer in the elderly patient, it does not account for the higher risk. The daily rate of infection is 0.43% in patients under 60 years compared to 0.63% in older patients (4).

Urinary tract infections account for the majority of nosocomial infections in the elderly. The daily rate in one study rose from a low of 0.03% in younger patients to 0.28% in the ninth decade.

Respiratory tract infections are the next most common nosocomial infection in both of the above studies. The daily rate of infection rose from a stable level of 0.6% in younger patients to 15% in the elderly (4).

When all types of nosocomial infection are considered together, the elderly have a dispropor-tionate percentage. Twenty-three to 24% of the hospital discharges occur in those over 60 years of age, yet 37 to 64% of all nosocomial infections appear in this age group (3, 4). The elderly clearly are not only more likely to develop a nosocomial infection, but as a group they contribute a majority of nosocomial infections despite having a minority of the total admissions. The observations require that one develop a better understanding of the unique risk factors that predispose the elderly to an increased risk of nosocomial infection acquisition.

Mortality

Mortality from nosocomial infections is difficult to delineate since the patients who die have diseases of multiple organ systems. Nosocomial infections were present in 32% of patients who died in a study done at Hackensack Medical Center and Columbia Presbyterian Medical Center (5). In those who died with a nosocomial infection, it was assessed to directly contribute to death in 60% of the patients. In this group, patients were terminal on admission and were typically in their sixties with metastatic carcinoma. The fatal infections in this setting were usually lower respiratory tract infections. In the other patients with nosocomial infections, the infections were assessed not to have contributed to death. In this group, the patients typically were in their late seventies and had complications of arteriosclerotic cardiovascular disease. The most common infection was of the urinary tract.

In a separate study of *Klebsiella* bacteremia, the source of infection was also shown to influence mortality. Pulmonary and abdominal infections were associated with mortality in patients with a nonfatal underlying disease, while urinary tract and intravenous site infections were not (6).

Prevention

That prevention of nosocomial infections will decrease hospital costs is clear as pointed out earlier (see Chapter 3 on costs of nosocomial infections). Whether prevention of nosocomial infections will decrease mortality is not clear. In a study at Hackensack Medical Center, nosocomial infections were thought to be related to death only in patients who were classified as not being terminal at the time of hospital admission (7).

HOST DEFENSES

Consideration of normal defenses should include not only the immune defenses of the host but also the physiologic and anatomic barriers. All are significantly altered as the human host ages. In addition, age-associated disorders, such as cancer and diabetes, further impair the aging host's ability to defend itself against infection. Although not usually thought of as a host defense, the common infection control barrier techniques, such as those used to prevent transmission by the airborne route and by hands, should be considered a defense for the host.

Immune System

It is generally agreed that the function of *T lymphocytes* is adversely affected in the elderly (8–10). Despite the decrease in function, the absolute numbers of circulating T lymphocytes are usually unchanged. Clinically, anergy to common skin test antigens is seen. In the laboratory, a decrease in mitogen responsiveness and clonal proliferation and a reduction in thymopoietin and various lymphokines are observed. Furthermore, suppressor T cell activity is increased. Whether reconstitution of T cell function with thymic hormones is possible is a topic of current investigation.

The humoral immune response is also affected, particularly T cell-dependent *B lymphocyte* responsiveness. The elderly seem less likely to respond to new antigens, such as those found in vaccines. The levels of certain immunoglobulin classes—IgG and IgA—increase with age, and autoantibodies are known to increase with age. The interaction of these autoantibodies with surface immunoglobulin on the B lymphocyte may be one of the factors responsible for inhibiting the formation of new antibodies. In addition, autoantibodies may inhibit fixation of complement onto the cell surface and may alter phagocytosis.

The effect of aging on the *secretory antibody* system in the respiratory and gastrointestinal tract is unknown. *Polymorphonuclear leukocyte* function and count appear to be normal in the elderly, although studies in the hospitalized patient are few. While some *complement* components may

be reduced, assays for the classic and alternative pathways are normal.

Physiologic and Anatomic Barriers

There are numerous normal physiologic and anatomic changes associated with aging (11).

In the *respiratory tract*, the cough reflex is impaired, ciliary function is diminished, and oral flora may be altered. Emphysema and chronic bronchitis become common in the aged even in the absence of a history of cigarette smoking. The impaired host defenses conspire to affect adherence and clearance of the mucosal surfaces and thereby predispose to the development of pneumonia.

In the *nervous system*, recent memory decreases and several significant perceptual changes occur. An increase in pain tolerance, a decrease in hearing and visual acuity, a diminution in the sense of balance, and a diminished sense of thirst all occur. These changes subject the patient to physical trauma to the skin and bones, failure to take medication properly, and the development of dehydration.

The *skin* of the elderly patient becomes thinner and drier. It loses elasticity and fat and receives less circulation. The clinical outcome is an increased susceptibility to injury and the development of decubitus ulcers, the most common infection in nursing homes.

The *skeletal system* begins to undergo significant changes in the third decade of life. Calcium intake is usually inadequate, especially in women, and contributes to the development of osteoporosis. Osteomalacia and disk degeneration also occur. Clinically, fractures are common.

Transit time through the *colon* decreases. Awareness to call is less, and diverticulosis develops. These all contribute to the appearance of constipation, diverticulitis, and intestinal obstruction.

In the *urinary tract*, renal function decreases, prostatic hypertrophy develops in males, pelvic floor relaxation occurs in females along with the development of cystoceles, and incontinence is common and is aggravated by sedative abuse. Clinically, a normal serum creatinine gives the physician the impression that normal doses of drugs can be used. Foley catheters are used for incontinence and increase the chance of a urinary tract infection. Urinary tract obstruction may result from an enlarged prostate.

Finally, changes occur in the *endocrine system*. Hyperthyroidism is more common and occasionally presents as the apathetic type. Changes in sexuality may be likened to General Douglas MacArthur's "old soldier" who faded away.

Age-Associated Disorders

The noninfectious diseases associated with aging may directly or indirectly affect host defenses. Cancer of the lung, urinary tract, or gastrointestinal tract may obstruct the lung, ureters, or colon, respectively. A secondary infection behind the tumor may then develop. Pernicious anemia is associated with achlorhydria, and tuberculosis is more common in this setting. Diabetes mellitus adversely affects polymorphonuclear function. Sclerosis of the cardiac valves predisposes to endocarditis, and endothelial aortic plaques to *Salmonella* aortitis. Chronic pulmonary disease is aggravated by the emphysema and chronic bronchitis of the aged. Furthermore, alcohol abuse affects oropharyngeal colonization, the risk of aspiration, mucociliary clearance and pulmonary macrophage function.

Malnutrition

Protein-calorie malnutrition is more common in the hospitalized elderly patient. Death rates and the incidence of infection are higher in the malnourished elderly, just as they are higher in the malnourished younger patient (12). Normal physiologic changes in the sense of taste and smell tend to decrease appetite, thereby favoring a tendency toward malnutrition (13). The occurrence of specific vitamin and mineral deficiencies is currently being evaluated.

Infection Control Barriers

The recognition of the role of hand and airborne transmission of nosocomial pathogens in the elderly should be included as one of the host defenses (14, 15). This topic is discussed in Chapter 30.

BACTEREMIA
Incidence and Case-Fatality Ratio

As with many other infections in the elderly, the incidence of bacteremia increases with age. The incidence above 70 years is 3 times that below 30 years. The proportion of elderly hospitalized patients who have nosocomial versus community-acquired infections varies depending on the study population. At Boston City Hospital and Grady Memorial Hospital, McGowan and colleagues found community-acquired bacter-

emia was more common, whereas in Denver, Weinstein and associates found nosocomial bacteremia was twice as frequent (16–18).

The case-fatality ratio again is correlated with age: above age 70, the ratio rises to over 50%. In the hospital and in the long-term care facility, mortality from bacteremia depends on the type of microorganism. Gram positive bacteremia is two to three times more frequently fatal than gram negative bacteremia, particularly in those patients with an underlying illness that by itself has a relatively good prognosis (19, 20). Other investigators have also pointed out the high mortality from nosocomial *Staphylococcus aureus* bacteremia in the elderly (21).

In a controlled study that matched patients for age and primary diagnosis, bacteremia was associated with not only a significantly higher mortality, but also an increased morbidity and cost of hospitalization (22).

Source and Microbial Etiology

The most common source in the long term care facility is the urinary tract, followed by skin and soft tissue sites and the respiratory tract (20). The most common microorganisms in the long term care facility are the gram-negative rods (67%), followed by gram-positive cocci (24%), and a mixture of the two groups (9%). The most frequent gram-negative rods are *Escherichia coli*, *Proteus* species, and *Klebsiella* species. Among gram-positive cocci, *Staphylococcus aureus* predominates.

Clinical Manifestation and Therapeutic Approach

Clinical manifestations of bacteremia in the elderly are different than in younger adults. Vascular collapse, vomiting, oliguria, and leukocytosis are not the rule. More often, the elderly present with confusion, agitation, or stupor. The lack of fever in many bacteremic patients confounds the diagnosis further (23). The physician caring for the elderly is in a position similar to the neonatologist who has to diagnose a potentially lethal infection based on a paucity of clinical clues.

The recommended number of blood cultures required to detect bacteremia has decreased with the growing appreciation that the initial ones drawn are positive in 80 to 90% of cases. A minimum of two and a maximum of four sets of blood cultures should be drawn. Each set must be drawn at a different time, and the presence or absence of fever at the time of drawing is irrelevant. Two should be drawn to permit assessment of a possible contaminant in one. For example, *Staphylococcus epidermidis*, once thought to be a common contaminant of blood cultures, is now known to be a not infrequent cause of significant and occasionally fatal bacteremia (24).

Therapy should be instituted rapidly. Antibiotic therapy should be appropriate for the suspected organisms at the site of infection and should be based on the predicted sensitivity of those organisms for the particular hospital. Dosage selection and monitoring for side effects of therapy are critical because of the altered pharmacokinetics of antibiotics in the elderly.

PNEUMONIA
Epidemiology and Etiology

Among the many infections to which the aged are susceptible, pneumonia and influenza combined cause the greatest mortality (25). In a study of patient deaths from nosocomial infections in the acute care hospital, Gross and associates reported that the lower respiratory tract was the most common site causally related to or contributory to death (5). Additionally, a comprehensive review of 1700 autopsies at the Jewish Home and Hospital for the Aged in New York City noted that 41% of these patients had anatomic evidence of pneumonia either alone or associated with other diseases (26). A depressed state of consciousness due to sedative administration, and cerebral vascular disease are major predisposing factors and are more common in the elderly (27). Colonization of the oropharynx followed by aspiration associated with poor bronchial clearance mechanisms results in pneumonia (28). Valenti and associates demonstrated that colonization of the oropharynx with gram-negative bacilli increased with age and with decreasing ability for self-care (29). However, this study was only a single-culture survey. A prospective analysis in a skilled nursing facility by Irwin and co-investigators revealed that 14% of their elderly patients showed only transient colonization and did not demonstrate a direct association with an increased risk of gram-negative bacillary pneumonia (30). Moreover, the colonization was continually changing over an extended period of time. Further data are necessary to clarify the conflicting results.

In the analysis of the data for the Study on the Efficacy of Nosocomial Infection Control

(SENIC Project), age was shown to be a significant risk factor for nosocomial pneumonia (2). Other factors that may have an important etiologic role in the increased incidence of pneumonia in this population included depressed mucociliary clearance mechanisms (31), pressure of prior antimicrobial therapy (32), respiratory tract instrumentation, and increased salivary protease activity with loss of the fibronectin coating of epithelial cells in acutely ill patients (33).

Most studies on the etiology of nosocomial pneumonia in the elderly have reported on bacterial pneumonia. The enteric gram-negative bacilli and *Pseudomonas* species account for the majority of bacterial pneumonias, although *S. aureus* is still a prominent pathogen (34). The role of viruses and anerobes is porly understood due to the absence of well controlled studies. However, several outbreaks of respiratory syncytial virus in the elderly have been published (35, 36). Also, the mortality of hospital-acquired influenza A virus infection in the elderly has been high (37). Certainly, long term prospective studies to clarify and extend these reports in the elderly are needed.

Clinical Approach

Clinically, nosocomial pneumonia in the geriatric patient ranges from typical symptoms of fevers, chills, and productive cough to a more subtle and indolent presentation of malaise and confusion (38). Sputum production and fevers can be absent or minimal. Likewise, physical examination may be unrevealing. Chest roentgenograms can be atypical and resolution delayed (39). Differential diagnosis includes noninfectious illnesses such as pulmonary emboli, tumor, and lipoid pneumonia. The diagnosis could also be difficult since adequate sputum may not be available. Blood cultures, urine and blood for counterimmunoelectrophoresis, or latex agglutination can be helpful. Furthermore, bronchoscopy, transtracheal aspiration, and open lung biopsy are also indicated in selected patient populations, such as immunocompromised individuals with pulmonary infiltrates.

Control

Precautions and control of nosocomial pneumonias as outlined by the CDC guidelines are important (40). Prophylactic antibiotics have not been shown to be efficacious to reduce the incidence of nosocomial pneumonia in high risk patients. Additionally, endotracheal antibiotic administration or aerolization may transiently reduce colonization, but deaths from pneumonia are not prevented and resistant bacteria may emerge (41). Bacterial interference to prevent colonization by gram-negative bacilli has been reported, but conclusive data are still lacking (42).

URINARY TRACT INFECTIONS
Epidemiology

Urinary tract infections account for approximately 40% of all nosocomial infections in the acute care hospital (43). The prevalence of urinary tract infections increases with age; it is approximately 1% in ambulatory young women and increases to approximately 20% among women over the age of 70. Infections are rarely seen in men under the age of 50 and occur in approximately 4% of men over the age of 70 (20). Among institutionalized patients of both sexes, the incidence of bacteriuria is between 25 and 50% (44, 45). In institutions where men and women have been simultaneously investigated, the incidence tends to be greater in females than males, though the difference is less marked than in younger patients (46, 47). In a study of bacteriuria in elderly ambulatory patients over a 10-year period in Greece, Dontas and investigators reported that bacteriuric patients had a significantly reduced survival of 30 to 50% compared to nonbacteriuric patients (47). However, this study demonstrated only an association and not a causal relationship between asymptomatic bacteriuria and increased mortality. Nevertheless, Platt and co-workers reported that the onset of bacteriuria in a hospitalized catheterized patient was associated with a 3-fold increase in mortality (48). The reasons for this association could not be delineated from this study.

The risk factors for the increased incidence of urinary tract infections in the elderly include bladder dysfunction, increased prostate size, relaxation of pelvic musculature, and concomitant illness. Seventy percent of elderly patients in one long term care facility were found to have urinary dysfunction, with 38% of the patients incontinent and 20% having an indwelling Foley catheter in place (49). The role of long term catheterization in the pathogenesis of urinary tract infections is discussed in Chapter 21. Condom catheters in the elderly have been shown by some investigators to contribute to urinary tract infections in that population (50, 51).

Microbial Etiology

Etiologically, E. coli is the most prevalent organism isolated in patients with urinary tract infections in the acute care hospital (52). However, in a prospective study of bacteriuric patients with chronic indwelling Foley catheters, Proteus and Providencia species were the most frequently isolated bacteria (53). Interestingly, once Providencia gained access to the urinary tract, it had a tendency to persist for longer periods of time as compared to the duration of episodes of bacteriuria due to the Enterobacteriace and Pseudomonas species (53).

Therapy

Therapeutically, all symptomatic infections need to be treated, but the signs and symptoms of infections in elderly patients are variable, as noted previously. Controversy exists as to the appropriate treatment of asymptomatic infections in this population. Nicolle and co-workers reported that antibiotic therapy was ineffective in curing bacteriuria and preventing relapse among noncatheterized institutionalized men (44). Their study tended to support the concept that the kidney and prostate are common sites of infection among elderly men. In addition, antibiotics could result in superinfection, emergence of resistant organisms, and drug-related adverse reactions (44, 54). However, further studies are needed before extrapolating the data to other geriatric groups, such as women and ambulatory men.

ENDOCARDITIS

Endocarditis in the aged has been assumed to differ in several aspects from the same disease presenting in young adults. Precise conclusions, however, cannot be drawn from the literature because of numerous differences in study group composition. In addition, most studies in the elderly do not include younger patients from the same institutions (55–58). The numbers of elderly patients studied in the largest series are still small and range from 29 to 57. In the studies conducted in the general population, the number studied range from 60 to 408 (59–62). With these limitations in mind, the unique aspects of endocarditis in the elderly will be reviewed.

Age Distribution

Endocarditis appears to be *more common in the elderly* in recent years. The average age of patients in published studies has risen from 31 years in the 1920s to 57 in the 1970s (59).

Predisposing Factors

This increase in mean age may be a result of the increased numbers of hospitalized elderly exposed to invasive procedures. Nosocomial bacteremia and the subsequent development of endocarditis have been related to intravascular devices, prosthetic heart valves and hips, joints, decubitus ulcers, postoperative wound infections following gastrointestinal surgery, and genitourinary tract manipulation (55, 56, 63). These predisposing factors are present more frequently in the elderly patient with endocarditis. Nevertheless, no apparent predisposing factor is found in approximately half of the elderly, unlike the situation in younger adults.

Underlying Heart Diseases

The distribution of underlying heart disease differs in the elderly: calcific aortic stenosis, atherosclerotic heart disease, and prosthetic heart valves are all more common in the elderly. While rheumatic heart disease is less common, the valve most frequently involved in the elderly is the aortic valve, while in the young adult, the mitral valve is the more common site of infection. The most common finding, however, is no predisposing heart disease in the elderly patient; this finding is unusual in the younger patient.

Infecting Microorganism

The frequency of the various organisms is similar in young and old adults. Streptococci are the most commonly encountered and are found in approximately 45% of cases (59). *Streptococcus viridans* is the most common of the streptococci followed by enterococcus. Staphylococci, particularly *S. aureus*, account for approximately 21%. Gram-negative bacilli and fungi are relatively uncommon.

Culture-negative cases make up a variable percentage in the reported series (0 to 20%). In up to 60% of these cases, the diagnosis was not suspected before the patient died. When the elderly patient complains of weight loss, neoplasm is often considered. When the patient presents with hemiplegia, a cerebrovascular accident is diagnosed. Back pain is considered a sign of degenerative disk disease, and heart failure is usually considered a natural consequence of arteriosclerotic cardiovascular disease. Confusion is considered a sign of senility. Slight azotemia or anemia may be ignored. Yet any of these signs and symptoms may be a manifestation of endocarditis in the elderly.

Table 29.1. Endocarditis: Clinical Presentation*

Feature	Range of Occurrence (%)	
	In Elderly	In All Ages
Fever	87	99
Heart murmurs	80	91
Congestive heart failure	43	19
Neurologic manifestations	25	23
Cutaneous manifestations	33	40
Splenomegaly	21	43

* Adapted from reference 59.

Clinical Manifestations

A comparison of the occurrence of the clinical signs and symptoms in the young and the old is shown in Table 29.1. Fever is less common in the elderly because of alteration in thermoregulatory control and the presence of azotemia or congestive heart failure. Reported series vary: some report fever in 50%, others in 100%. A heart murmur is heard less often and is often considered insignificant in the elderly. Neurologic complications have been thought to be more common in the elderly. In Gantz's review, the incidence was approximately equal in both age groups. The cutaneous manifestations and splenomegaly, however, were less common in the elderly (59).

In the only study where young and old adults came from the same institution, many of these differences disappeared (64). Whether the experience of Tan and associates is atypical cannot be stated now.

Laboratory Signs

Virtually all elderly patients had an elevated sedimentation rate, two-thirds were anemic, and less than one-third have had leukocytosis. In young adults, two-thirds typically had leukocytosis. The presence of a positive rheumatoid factor depended more on the duration of the infection. The association of a false positive rheumatoid test with age, however, could be misleading.

Mortality

In most series, mortality in the aged patient with endocarditis was clearly higher than in younger patients (44 to 72% versus 14 to 33%). The one exception is Tan et al's study where mortality was 0% (64). They reported, however, only patients infected with *S. viridans*. In another publication from the same laboratory, the mortality was 90% in a series of patients with *S. aureus* endocarditis (65). These differences emphasize the need for additional studies to compare endocarditis in the young and the old at the same institution.

MENINGITIS
Mortality

Since the introduction of penicillin, most deaths from bacterial meningitis have occurred in the elderly. Prior to 1946, the median age of patients who died from meningitis was 11.5 years (66). In recent years the median age is 64 years. The higher mortality in the elderly may be due to other associated chronic debilitating illnesses, delay in diagnosis, and infection with gram-negative bacilli and *S. aureus*.

Incidence

The incidence of bacterial meningitis in the aged has tripled to 15 cases/100,000 (66). The cause for the observed increased incidence is not clear, but increased case reporting, diminished host defenses, corticosteroid use, and earlier recognition in confused patients are all cited.

Organisms

Streptococcus pneumoniae is the single most common pathogen. It is responsible for more than 50% cases (67). *Neisseria meningitidis* accounts for 16% and *Haemophilus influenzae* for 2%, in contrast to significantly higher proportions in young adults and children. Gram-negative bacilli as a group account for 8% and *Listeria monocytogenes* for 7%, figures significantly higher than those in younger age groups. A small percentage of cases remain undiagnosed despite cerebrospinal fluid (CSF) findings consistent with purulent meningitis.

The vast majority of cases are community-acquired. Hodges and Perkins found only 5% (18 of 349 cases) of meningitis to be hospital-acquired (68). The etiologic agents in order of likelihood were gram-negative bacilli, unknown agents, staphylococci, and streptococci. *Pseudomonas* species were encountered most often among the gram-negative bacilli.

Among neurosurgical patients, the usual hospital pathogens cause nosocomial meningitis. Gram-negative bacilli and *S. epidermidis* are most frequently found (68–71). Infection is acquired by bacteremia from a distant pneumonia, urinary tract infection, or decubitus ulcer; from direct inoculation during neurosurgery or head trauma; or from a contiguous sinusitis or otitis.

Clinical Findings

In community-acquired cases, the clinical findings that distinguish the old from the younger adults at the time of diagnosis are an increased incidence of mental status changes (89% versus 53%), presence of paresis (22% versus 9%), and other neurologic abnormalities. Fever and nuchal rigidity are not less common in the older adults (72). The clinical conditions that more frequently complicate the clinical course in the old compared to the younger adults are pneumonia (41% versus 6%), neurologic deficits (28% versus 19%), motor seizures (30% versus 0%), hydrocephalus (9% versus 0%), and urinary tract infection (17% versus 0%).

In nosocomial cases with gram-negative bacillary meningitis, a 1- to 2-week history of mild fever and lethargy is typical (67) even without antibiotic therapy. Other causes for delay in diagnosis occur when symptoms of meningitis are attributed to stroke, psychosis, or prolonged postoperative course. A stiff neck may be attributed to cervical osteoarthritis.

Clues to Diagnosis

Evaluation of the CSF requires special attention to the gram stain. *H. influenzae* and other gram-negative bacilli may not be readily distinguished. *Acinetobacter* species may resemble the more common gram-negative diplococcus, *N. meningitidis*. *L. monocytogenes* may occasionally resemble the gram-positive diplococcus, *S. pneumoniae*. Furthermore, *L. monocytogenes* infection may initially present with a predominance of lymphocytes.

Gram-negative meningitis presents with two different types of illness. When Foley catheters, vertebral osteomyelitis, decubitus ulcers, and urinary tract instrumentation are the predisposing factors, the onset is abrupt and the diagnosis is obvious. Enteric bacteria and *Pseudomonas aeruginosa* are commonly found. The other clinical presentation follows craniotomy or myelography, and the onset is both insidious and difficult to distinguish from the postoperative course. The diagnoses in one series were not made for 2 to 19 days (6.6 days mean).

L. monocytogenes should be considered in the patient with a lymphoproliferative disorder or in one being treated with corticosteroids. Even an otherwise normal elderly adult may acquire this organism. *H. influenzae* not uncommonly causes pneumonia in the elderly but rarely is the cause of meningitis (73).

While *N. meningitidis* is unusual in the elderly, an epidemic was reported from a mental institution where an influenza outbreak occurred simultaneously (74). *S. aureus* is responsible for 15% of cases of nosocomial meningitis (69). It should be considered in infections following a craniotomy, myelography, sinusitis, and osteomyelitis. *S. epidermidis* meningitis may occur following craniotomy or placement of a ventricular shunt or reservoir.

Anaerobic meningitis has been reported after laminectomy and in association with head and neck malignancies. *Bacteroides fragilis* and anaerobic streptococci are usually responsible (75, 76). Enterococcus arising from a urinary tract infection or infected heart valves can seed the meninges (77), and *Pasturella multocida* has been reported once to cause meningitis following hemodialysis (75).

Initial treatment of nosocomial meningitis requires one or more antibiotics that will include gram-negative rods, streptococci, and staphylococci. *Listeria* may also have to be considered. In the past, chloramphenicol plus gentamicin was the usual therapeutic combination. Gentamicin now is considered a poor choice for several reasons: renal function is normally diminished in the elderly and renal toxicity is more likely to occur in the elderly; cerebrospinal fluid levels of gentamicin are neither predictable nor reliable; and in the presence of ventriculitis this dilemma is compounded. In addition, use of a potentially ototoxic drug in someone whose sense of balance may already be compromised is a poor idea.

A third generation cephalosporin—such as cefotaxime, cefoperazone, or moxalactam—or one of the second generation drugs—cefuroxime— should be considered. Piperacillin could be added to cefotaxime to improve coverage of *Pseudomonas*. Penicillin has to be added to moxalactam to cover streptococci. However, the methyltetrazolethiol side chain is present in cefoperazone and moxalactam. It is responsible for adenosine 5'-diphosphate-induced platelet aggregation and disulfiram-like reactions. Reduction of vitamin K-producing gut organisms is also more likely with these third generation cephalosporins. In the presence of a neurosurgical procedure, vancomycin should be added to cover for resistant staphylococci, and in the immunosuppressed host, ampicillin or penicillin should be considered for *Listeria*. When a specific organism is isolated, therapy should be changed to the most appropriate antibiotic.

The goal of prevention of nosocomial meningitis can best be met by meticulous attention to neurosurgical technique and wound care. Prophylactic antibiotics are recommended for neurosurgical procedures although its efficacy is unclear. In one series 27 of 35 patients with meningitis had been given prophylactic antibiotics (70). Pneumococcal vaccine probably can prevent pneumococci associated with pneumococcal pneumonia and should be given to the elderly. Whether monovalent type A and C meningococcal vaccines should be used in the nursing home is unclear.

TUBERCULOSIS
Incidence

Tuberculosis is still a prevalent disease in the elderly and is the result primarily of recrudescence of dormant infection (78). Though Powell and Farer reported in 1980 that among persons over the age of 65 there was an increase in the incidence of tuberculosis, they did not think that this population of patients was at an increased risk for the disease (79). However, data presented by Stead and Lofgren from Arkansas disputed the report (80). They reviewed the incidence of tuberculosis in Arkansas and demonstrated that not only does the incidence increase among the elderly, but that this group was indeed at a higher risk for this disease.

Tuberculin Reactivity

The rate of reversion of a previous positive tuberculin skin reactor to negative is about 5%/ year (81). Loss of reactivity could be the result of true anergy or loss of sensitivity of the T cells over time due to the disappearance of the tubercle bacilli and lack of re-exposure to the organism (80). If the latter were true, then it may be hypothesized that an elderly patient with negative tuberculin reactivity could be susceptible to infection if exposed. Furthermore, a positive skin reaction may correlate with persistant tubercle bacilli and hence risk of recrudescence of old infection. Supporting this concept was an outbreak of tuberculosis in a nursing home recently reported by Stead (82). Among these patients, there was a low level of tuberculin reactivity, and it was interesting to note that there were several cases of primary tuberculosis in that subpopulation. This epidemic was also associated with significant morbidity and mortality. Thus, elderly individuals with a negative tuberculin skin test may indeed be more susceptible to infection and hence the likelihood of nosocomial outbreaks. Since early detection and appropriate treatment of both new cases of active tuberculosis and recent converters can stop the spread of the disease, enhanced surveillance among nursing home residents is indicated.

Clinical Features

Several features of the clinical presentation of pulmonary tuberculosis in the elderly need to be stressed. Though weight loss, cough, and weakness are noted frequently, the mildness and chronicity of these symptoms are often attributed to other problems, such as the aging process alone (83, 84). Night sweats, hemoptysis, and chest pain are less frequent than in younger patients. As noted by Rubin, a prominent feature of tuberculosis in the elderly as compared to younger patients is the frequent ocurrence of other morbid conditions, such as chronic obstructive pulmonary disease, diabetes mellitus, and malignancy (84). On physical examination, fever is infrequent, and there are few clues to a specific diagnosis (85, 86). Radiographically, though most elderly persons with pulmonary tuberculosis have classic postprimary disease (apical scarring, cavitary formation), recent studies have reported almost one-third of adults to have atypical patterns with lower lung field infiltrates and mass lesions (87). Thus, the diagnosis of tuberculosis must be considered in all elderly patients with abnormal chest X-ray findings.

As with pulmonary tuberculosis, the highest case rates of extrapulmonary tuberculosis occur in the elderly (88). These sites include kidneys, meninges, and bone. Miliary tuberculosis in the older patient may be associated with nonspecific signs and symptoms of fever, weight loss, and weakness (89, 90). Concomitant illness can also obscure the clinical presentation.

Therapy

Current drug therapy for active tuberculosis has been reviewed in detail elsewhere and is beyond the scope of this chapter (91, 92). Isoniazid (INH) chemoprophylaxis may be important to prevent nosocomial outbreaks in chronic care facilities. However, the age-related incidence of INH hepatitis and adverse reactions need to be defined more clearly. For example, though approximately 20% of patients over the age of 55 will experience some adverse effect to INH, the incidence of hepatitis in a recent U.S. Public Health Service study decreased from 2,300/100,000 patients for the 50 to 64 age group to 800/100,000 in those over 64 (93). However, since a smaller sample size may have attributed to this decline, more data are needed to elucidate the true risk of hepatitis in the elderly.

INFECTIONS IN THE CHRONIC CARE FACILITY

Scope of Problem

Approximately 5% of the elderly over the age of 65 are nursing home (NH) residents at any given time (94). However, 25 to 28% of the elderly spend 3 weeks or more in a long term care facility at some period after the age of 65 years. However, as noted by several investigators, epidemiologic data, infection surveillance, and control measures have received little attention (95, 96). Previously, nosocomial infections have referred to infections acquired in the acute hospital setting, but the term clearly needs to be expanded to the long term facility.

Nursing home patients are at an increased risk for infection for a variety of reasons: underlying diseases that may predispose them to infection, clustering of patients in closed quarters, and frequent use of invasive devices such as the Foley catheter (96–98). Also, immobility, fecal incontinence, and the frequent prescribing of sedatives and tranquilizers are other important risk factors (96). The increased incidence of oropharyngeal colonization with gram-negative bacilli, a potential predisposing factor for pneumonia in this population, has been previously reported (29).

These issues were addressed by Garibaldi and co-workers in a prevalence study of several skilled care nursing homes in Salt Lake City, Utah (99). Among 532 patients surveyed (193 men and 339 women), 97 infections were noted, a prevalance of 16.2%. Infected decubitus ulcers, conjunctivitis, urinary tract infections, and pneumonia were the most frequent types of infection recorded. They reported a high incidence of bacteriuria in catheterized patients. Disturbing was the frequent colonization in the urinary tract of these patients with multiple antibiotic-resistant organisms. The frequent and spontaneous variations in the bacteria isolated from the urinary tract of catheterized geriatric patients reported by Alling and co-workers underscore the need for appropriate cultures and antimicrobial susceptibility testing of symptomatic patients (100).

Impact of Staff

Another area of great importance identified by Garibaldi et al's study was the potential impact of the nursing home staff on infection control policies. They noted the following: relatively higher percentage of nonprofessional to professional staff; high ratio of patients to staff, particularly during the evening shifts; lack of compensation for sick leave, discouraging the staff from remaining home when ill; inadequate immunization requirements for the staff; and frequent turnover of nonprofessional employees, disrupting infection control in-service educational programs. These issues must be carefully studied in order to implement corrective actions. Furthermore, prospective, baseline, epidemiologic data are needed to elucidate clearly the impact of the nursing home staff, types of infection, organisms, and patterns of transmission to establish guidelines for infection control.

FEVER OF UNKNOWN ORIGIN

Finding the cause of a fever of unknown origin in the elderly patient may be even more perplexing than in the younger adult. This difference occurs because the history of the symptoms may be more difficult to elicit, and the physical signs of the disease process may be more occult in the elderly patient.

The study of this disease entity in the elderly is further obfuscated by the knowledge that the thermoregulatory mechanisms are altered with age (101). The body core temperature is typically at least 1°C lower in the elderly. This observation may lead physicians to underdiagnose fever of unknown origin and other diseases commonly associated with fever.

Definition

The current definition for the specific entity of fever of unknown origin was described by Petersdorf and Beeson in 1961 (102). They defined it as an illness that was associated with a fever of 38.3°C (101°F) on several occasions and was present for at least 3 weeks; during one of those weeks, the patient should have been in the hospital and have had the "standard" tests done, such as a chest film, blood count, blood culture, and other

tests appropriate to the patient's complaints and physical findings.

Although elderly patients may tend to have no fever and less elevation of their body temperature with illness, the above definition is the one still used in the elderly. With that caveat in mind, one can examine what is know of fever of unknown origin in the elderly.

Distribution of Diseases

No investigator has reviewed a series of cases accumulated in the same institution. The only published study of this entity in the elderly is by Esposito and Gleckman (103, 104). They gathered from the literature 111 cases of patients 65 years and older with fever of unknown origin. Their cases were usually community-acquired and not nosocomial. As there is no series of nosocomial cases, the entity as described in the community will be reviewed.

In Esposito and Gleckman's series, common diseases again presented in subtle and atypical ways. However, the distribution of cases among the major categories of disease differed from that observed in younger adults (Table 29.2). Connective tissue disorders appeared to be more common in the elderly while miscellaneous diseases were less common. Additional series should be accumulated in the elderly to confirm their observations.

Infections

Infections remain the most common disease category in all ages. In the aged, however, intraabdominal infections are more common than endocarditis. Often a history of abdominal surgery, diverticulitis, or inflammatory bowel disease is not available. In some instances, abdominal abscesses may occur in the absence of a history

Table 29.2. Fever of Unknown Origin in Adults*

Category	For Adults 65 Years and Above (%)	For Adults of All Ages (%)
Infection	36	36
Neoplasm	24	19
Connective tissue disorder	26	15
Miscellaneous	9	23
Undiagnosed	5	7

* Adapted from references 102 and 103.

of prior surgery or bowel disease. Hepatic abscesses, in particular, are more common in the elderly. The classical signs and symptoms of peritoneal tenderness may be missing when the patient has a perforated viscus associated with diverticulitis or empyema of the gallbladder.

Endocarditis may go unsuspected because antimicrobials prescribed for a fever rendered the blood cultures negative. Peripheral manifestations of endocarditis may be less common in the elderly. The distribution of organisms, however, is similar. The valvular disease most commonly found is calcific disease of the aortic or mitral annulus.

Extrapulmonary tuberculosis, especially the disseminated form, should be sought. A search for retroperitoneal nodes, urine culture for acid-fast bacilli, and a bone marrow, liver, or epididymis biopsy may be helpful. Negative skin tests with purified protein derivative should not dissuade the clinician.

Neoplasms

In the neoplasm group, lymphoma is the most common disorder as it is in younger adults. Loss of appetite, weakness, and weight loss may be confused with the "normal process of aging." A search for localized disease in the abdomen should be pursued.

Connective Tissue Disorders

Giant cell arteritis is the most common entity in the connective tissue disease group. Most patients with this disorder are women and they present initially with fever, malaise, and myalgias. Later, they may develop headache, jaw claudication, or visual changes. A temporal artery biopsy should be considered. Polyarteritis is the next most commonly encountered disorder. Systemic lupus erythematosus and the rheumatic disorders are unusual in the aged.

Miscellaneous Disorders

The miscellaneous category is smaller in the elderly than in younger adults. Factitious fever is unusual, but pulmonary emboli and drug fever are more likely.

Undiagnosed Diseases

As in most series on fever of unknown origin, a small percentage never fall into any of the diagnostic categories. The patient who continues to have progressive weight loss probably has a serious disorder. The others are more likely to have a self-limited, benign disorder.

Outcome

The mortality of elderly patients with fever of unknown origin is higher than in younger adults just as it is with most other diseases in the elderly. While most of the disease entities are serious, most of them are also potentially treatable, and the evaluation should be vigorously pursued.

Evaluation

Antipyretics and antibiotics should be discontinued. A careful history of pre-existing medical problems and surgical procedures, medication use, domestic and foreign travel, and animal exposure should be sought. Family members may be helpful in gathering this information. Laboratory tests that often direct attention to the problem are complete blood count and differential, sedimentation rate, liver ezymes, antinuclear antibodies, rheumatoid factor, stool and blood cultures, and certain specific serologic studies. Febrile agglutinins are invariably worthless. Radiographic procedures include a careful assessment of the chest film and combined use of the gallium scan, ultrasonogram, and computed tomography for intra-abdominal pathology. Ventilation-perfusion scans for pulmonary emboli and combined liver-lung scans for subphrenic abscesses are also useful. A biopsy of the liver, bone marrow, lymph node, or temporal artery is often helpful.

IMMUNIZATION*

Just as prevention of measles, mumps, and rubella is the aim of preventive public health programs in the young, so should the prevention of influenza and pneumococcal disease be the target of public health efforts in the old. The impact of respiratory tract infections with influenza virus and *S. pneumoniae* is relatively small in the young compared to the impact of these infections in the elderly. Immune senescence, age-associated diseases, concomitant use of diagnostic and therapeutic modalities, and normal physiologic and anatomic changes of aging all conspire to make the morbidity and mortality from influenza and pneumococcal infections significant in the elderly.

---

* See also Chapter 12 on immunizations.

Influenza Vaccine

Influenza virus is the only major human virus that is genetically unstable. This characteristic is the prime factor that makes control of the disease difficult. As a result of the genetic instability, the virus changes in minor ways ("antigenic drift") frequently and in major ways infrequently ("antigenic shift").

Antigenic drift occurs every 2 to 3 years for influenza A viruses and less frequently for influenza B. Antigenic shift occurs at intervals of 10 or more years for influenza A and does not occur with influenza B. Antigenic drift is associated with local or regional epidemics while antigenic shift is characterized by world-wide pandemics.

The influenza vaccine is updated annually to take into account the changes in prevalent influenza strains. Given the vagaries in predicting the prevalent strains, the vaccine contains the epidemic strains most of the time. Because of the frequent changes in vaccine composition, annual immunization is necessary to protect against new strains. The vaccines in recent years have had two influenza A viruses (an H3N2 strain and an H1N1 strain) and one influenza B strain.

Epidemics of influenza virus infection have been associated with 10,000 or more deaths 15 times in the years between 1957 and 1982. Antigenic drift of an influenza A or B strain has been followed by an epidemic in all but one instance. Only one epidemic was due to a major antigenic shift in the influenza A virus, and that was in 1968. Ten thousand excess deaths occurred as recently as the winter of 1982–1983, and this epidemic was due to antigenic drift, that is, a relatively minor change in the influenza A strain (105).

When excess deaths due to influenza and pneumonia are studied it is apparent that the mortality in those above 65 years is far in excess of that seen in younger persons (106–108). Whether age is the key factor or more likely the underlying disease is not clear. But it is likely that the chronic disorders associated with age, such as chronic respiratory diseases, cardiovascular diseases, and diabetes, are significant risk factors.

Transmission of influenza virus in the hospital is a frequent finding during community outbreaks of influenza. Introduction by hospital personnel and visitors permits easy access of the virus to hospitalized patients where the elderly are particularly susceptible (109).

The significant and frequent impact of influenza on the population, therefore, is readily apparent. What is also readily apparent but not widely appreciated is that influenza vaccine is clearly effective in reducing the morbidity and mortality from influenza virus infection. Several studies have documented a reduction in respiratory illness rates, hospitalization rates, and mortality in the elderly (110–112). However, these studies were not randomized, prospective, placebo-controlled clinical trials. Conducting such idealized studies in the elderly, however, probably will never be possible given the ethical dictates of our society.

The side effects of influenza immunization are typically benign and short lived. Local reactions, such as pain and redness at the injection site, occur in about one-third of vaccinees and last for 1 to 2 days. Systemic reactions, such as fever and myalgias, occur in a few percent of vaccines and last for 1 to 2 days.

Allergic reactions are extremely rare and are usually due to egg proteins. Therefore, anyone who has had an anaphylactic reaction on eating eggs should not receive influenza vaccine.

Guillain-Barré syndrome was associated with the swine influenza vaccine given in 1976. The reasons for this association remain unclear. Subsequent influenza vaccines, however, have not been associated with an increased frequency of Guillain-Barré syndrome (105).

The current vaccines are inactivated vaccines, not live attenuated virus vaccines. The vaccine is composed of either whole virus inactivated by formalin or detergent-treated whole virus vaccine (so-called split product or subunit vaccine) which is also formalin-inactivated (113). The route of administration for the vaccine is subcutaneous. Smaller doses given intradermally may be immunogenic, but this route has not been tested in vaccine efficacy studies and is therefore not recommended for routine use.

The target groups for immunization since 1963 have been persons who are at high risk of lower respiratory tract complications and death following influenza virus infection. Currently, the elderly with chronic disorders of the cardiovascular or pulmonary systems, diabetes, renal disease, severe anemia, or compromised immune function are considered at greatest risk when their medical condition has required regular medical follow-up or hospitalization in the preceding year. Residents of nursing homes and other chronic care facilities are also in this high risk group.

Medical personnel can transmit influenza to high risk persons. So physicians, nurses, and other personnel who have close contact with high risk elderly patients should also be immunized.

After the immunization needs of these two groups have been met, vaccine should be made available to otherwise healthy individuals over the age of 65 years because they are at moderately increased risk of serious illness compared to the general population (105).

After influenza appears in the community, vaccination can still be given. For optimal protection, amantadine should be given for 2 weeks after vaccination until immunity develops (114). Giving amantadine for the entire influenza season, however, is not a cost-effective alternative to vaccination and may be associated with significant side effects.

Pneumococcal Vaccine

Pneumococcal pneumonia is still the most common community-acquired pneumonia. The incidence of pneumococcal pneumonia increases with age beginning at 40 years; and over 60 years, the incidence doubles. As a cause of hospital-acquired pneumonia, it is rare. Despite the widespread use of effective antibiotics, the mortality from pneumococcal bacteremia is as high as 40% in high risk patients. The mortality associated with pneumococcal meningitis is even higher (105).

The conditions likely to place a person at high risk of serious complications from pneumococcal pneumonia are sickle cell anemia, Hodgkin's disease, multiple myeloma, cirrhosis, alcoholism, nephrotic syndrome, renal failure, chronic pulmonary diseases, other causes of splenic dysfunction, and a history of splenectomy or organ transplant.

Other patient groups may also be at greater risk of acquiring pneumococcal infection or of developing severe complications of infection. The groups include those with diabetes mellitus, congestive heart failure, and immunosuppressive conditions. Patients with a cerebrospinal fluid leak from a skull fracture or neurosurgical procedure may develop recurrent meningitis due to the pneumococcus.

Pneumococcal vaccine has been a subject of investigation for many decades. Polysaccharide vaccines were tested as early as the 1930s. The current multivalent polysaccharide vaccines were licensed within the past 10 years. In 1977 a 14-valent vaccine was approved for use, and in 1983 a 23-valent vaccine was licensed. The 23 bacterial types in the latest vaccine include 87% of the strains responsibe for bacteremic pneumococcal disease in the United States (115). The 14-valent vaccine covered 71% of the strains (116).

While patients with the above conditions are considered at high risk, the precise degree of risk has not been clearly defined. A large scale study was done in the elderly by Kaufman in the 1940s (117). There were more than 5000 persons each in the vaccinated and unvaccinated groups. He demonstrated a 79% protective efficacy against types 1, 2, and 3. However, the incidence of the other types increased in the vaccinated group compared to the control group. Importantly, the vaccine was more effective in the first year following vaccination than it was in subsequent years.

Multivalent vaccines have been recently tested in South African miners and in New Guinea, where the incidence of pneumococcal disease is high (118, 119). While vaccine efficacy was high, the relevance of these studies to vaccine efficacy in the elderly is unclear. In two studies recently conducted in the elderly, a low incidence of pneumococcal disease prevented an adequate test of vaccine efficacy (120). In another study, vaccine efficacy was estimated to be 70% for all patients over 55 years of age (121).

Vaccination is indicated in all those considered at high risk as described previously. In addition, it is now recommended in all adults over 65 years of age. Caution should be taken to administer vaccine to patients scheduled for splenectomy 2 weeks before the procedure. In addition, when vaccinating immunosuppressed patients, vaccine should be given so as to provide the longest interval possible between vaccination and initiation of immunosuppressive therapy.

Pneumococcal vaccine can be given at the same time as influenza vaccine without any adverse effect on immunogenicity of either vaccine (122).

Consideration should be given to providing vaccine at the end of hospitalization for high risk patients. Two-thirds of persons who will develop serious pneumococcal disease are likely to be hospitalized within 5 years of that illness (123). Consequently, a concerted effort to immunize patients at the time of discharge will reach most of the target population. Third-party payers will reimburse for pneumococcal vaccine.

Administration of pneumococcal vaccine is associated with local pain and redness at the injection site in about half of the vaccine recipients. Less than 1% of vaccinees will develop systemic symptoms of fever and myalgias. Allergic reactions are rare.

Revaccination is not currently recommended because arthus reactions and systemic reactions are common following a second dose (124). Persons who have received the 14-valent vaccine should not be revaccinated with the newer 23-valent vaccine.

The duration of immunity is thought to be at least 5 years, and reactions to revaccination may be less as immunity wanes. This phenomenon is currently being investigated.

Other Vaccines

Immunity to tetanus toxoid may wane in many elderly persons either because booster immunizations were not maintained or because a complete primary series was never received. These reasons account in part for the above average susceptibility to tetanus in the elderly (125).

Immunization with adult Td (tetanus and diphtheria toxoids) should be assured every 10 years in the primary care setting and at the time of penetrating trauma. At the time of trauma, if the history of prior immunization is questionable, human tetanus immune globulin should be administered in conjunction with tetanus toxoid (126).

Many elderly persons are likely to spend time traveling in foreign countries. In most developing countries and many developed countries the childhood diseases (measles, rubella, mumps, diphtheria, and polio) are still common. Adequate protection against these diseases should be assured if exposure is likely.

For polio, the killed inactivated vaccine (IPV—Salk vaccine) given subcutaneously is preferred to the live attenuated oral vaccine (OPV—Sabin vaccine). The incidence of vaccine-associated polio, while small, is, nevertheless, increased in adults following OPV administration (127).

The indications for vaccines against yellow fever, cholera, hepatitis B, meningococcal meningitis, typhoid, plague, Japanese encephalitis, and rabies should be reviewed for each person and for each travel itinerary. Smallpox vaccine should no longer be administered (128).

SKIN INFECTIONS

Prevalence

Skin infections are common problems in the elderly and include pressure sores or decubitus ulcers (99), streptococcal infections (129), herpes zoster (130, 131), and occasionally parasitic and fungal infections (132, 133). Garibaldi et al, in a study of infections in the nursing home, noted that infected pressure sores were the leading sites of infection, with a prevalence rate of 6% (99). Bliss and co-workers reported that 35% of patients in geriatric institutions have decubitus ulcers (134).

Predisposing Factors

Geriatric patients are particularly predisposed to pressure sores due to a number of factors, including reduced physical activity, malnutrition, dehydration, and underlying sytemic illness. The primary factor in the development of a decubitus ulcer is unrelieved pressure. Studies have shown that the greatest tissue damage is deep at a bony interface, not at a more superficial skin surface (135). The sacrum, ischial tuberosities, dorsal spine, and heels are particularly susceptible to pressure sores. As blood and lymphatics become compromised, localized tissue ischemia results. In general, the greater the pressure the less time neeeded to produce necrosis. Other important local factors in the pathogenesis of pressure sores are shearing forces (136), friction, and moisture (135). Complications of infected pressure ulcers include sepsis (137, 138), osteomyelitis (139), gangrenous crepitant cellulitis (140), and tetanus (141).

Microbial Etiology

Microbiologically, these infections tend to be polymicrobial with an average of four isolates per patient (three aerobes + one anerobe) (142). The aerobes include *Proteus* species, *E. coli*, enterococcus, *Staphylococcus*, and *Pseudomonas* species. The anerobes include *Bacteroides fragilus*, *Peptostreptococcus*, and *Clostridium perfringens*.

Therapy

The most important method of therapy is prevention, with quality nursing care of prime importance. A scoring system to identify high risk patients has been successfully utilized to reduce the incidence of decubitus ulcers in several institutions (143). Other modalities to reduce pressure sores include rotation of patient at a minimum of 2-hour intervals and the use of special beds or mattresses. Once a decubitus ulcer occurs, wound care includes control of any active infection, debridement of tissue, nutritional support, and relief of the pressure. The actual number of aerobic bacteria needed to cause local skin infection is 10^5 organisms/g of tissue (144). The infective dose of anerobes has not been determined yet. However, antibiotics alone, either topical or systemic, have not been shown to lower bacterial counts effectively in chronically contaminated wounds or to promote healing. If there is an area of surrounding cellulitis or if sepsis is suspected, appropriate parenteral antibiotics are necessary. Though a number of enzymatic agents which attack undenatured collagen and necrotic debris without damaging granulation tissue are available as adjuncts to debridement, their precise role has not been fully evaluated in carefully controlled studies.

Herpes Zoster

As cellular immunity wanes with increasing age, reactivation of varicella-zoster virus leading to clinical herpes zoster has been well documented (145). The attack rate is approximately 9/1000 in those over the age of 60. The most frequent sites of involvement are the spinal nerves T3 to L2 and the fifth cranial nerve. Outbreaks of zoster in geriatric centers has been described, suggesting that exogenous transmission following exposure to another infected person with either chickenpox or zoster is possible (146). Thus, appropriate isolation precautions for patients with herpes zoster in the nursing home setting should be instituted if an outbreak has occurred.

INFECTIOUS DIARRHEA

Incidence

There appears to be a higher mortality in the elderly with infectious diarrhea than for other age groups, though comprehensive epidemiologic data on the morbidity and mortality are lacking (147). For example, the incidence of *Salmonella* bacteremia is more common in patients over the age of 60 than in younger persons (148). Interestingly, one published survey has suggested that traveler's diarrhea may occur less frequently in the elderly, though the reasons were not clear (149). In a survey of diarrhea in the elderly in a chronic care setting, Pentland and Pennington reported that fecal impaction causing diarrhea occurred in 16% of patients, laxative abuse in 6%, antibiotic use in 11%, and inflammatory bowel disease in 4%. Viral agents were associated with 34% of cases of diarrhea and bacterial agents with 14% of cases in the study (150).

Etiology

Age-related changes in the gastrointestinal tract that may predispose the elderly to infectious diarrhea include gastric atrophy and achlorhydria (151), prolongation of gut transient time due to impaired motility (152), and vascular insufficiency. The role of local intestinal immunity in the elderly is still controversial.

A large number of agents have been implicated in producing diarrhea, including bacterial (*Salmonella, Shigella, Campylobacter*), viral (Norwark agent, rotavirus), and parasitic (*Entamoeba histolytica*). The clinical features of these infec-

tions are reviewed in Chapter 24. Of interest are the well documented outbreaks of both Norwark virus and rotavirus in a chronic care institution (153, 154). The latter agent is usually considered a serious illness in infancy and not in the elderly. However, viral agents may, in fact, be the leading cause of infectious diarrhea in the elderly. These organisms are transmitted via the fecal-oral route, and enteric precautions are an effective infection control method during an outbreak in an institutional setting.

References

1. Schneider EL: Infectious diseases in the elderly. *Ann Intern Med* 98:395–400, 1983.
2. Haley RW, Hooton TM, Culver DH, Stanley RC, Emori TG, Hardison CD, Quade D, Shachtman RH, Schaberg DR, Shah BV, Schatz GD: Nosocomial infections in U.S. hospitals, 1975–1976: estimated frequency by selected characteristics of patients. *Am J Med* 70:947–959, 1981.
3. Gross PA, Rapuano C, Adrignolo A, Shaw B: Nosocomial infections: decade-specific risk. *Infect Control* 4:145–147, 1983.
4. Saviteer SM, Samsa GP, Rutala WA: Nosocomial infection in the elderly: decade-specific rates per hospital day. Program and Abstracts of the Twenty-Fourth Interscience Conference on Antimicrobial Agents and Chemotherapy, American Society for Microbiology, 1984, no. 515, p 183.
5. Gross PA, Neu HC, Van Antwerpen C, Aswapokee N: Deaths from nosocomial infections: experience in a university hospital and a community hospital. *Am J Med* 68:219–223, 1980.
6. Montgomerie JZ, Ota JK: *Klebsiella* bacteremia. *Arch Intern Med* 140:525–527, 1980.
7. Gross PA, Van Antwerpen C: Nosocomial infections and hospital deaths. A case-control study. *Am J Med* 75:658–661, 1983.
8. Phair JD: Aging and infection: a review. *J Chronic Dis* 32:535–540, 1979.
9. Gardner I: The effect of aging on susceptibility to infection. *Rev Infect Dis* 2:801–810, 1980.
10. Weksler ME: Senescence of the immune system. *Med Clin North Am* 67:263–272, 1983.
11. American College of Physicians: *Medical Knowledge Self-Assessment Program VI. Syllabus, Part 2. Geriatrics.* Philadelphia, American College of Physicians, 1982, pp 298–301.
12. Bienia R, Ratcliff S, Barbour GL, Kummer M: Malnutrition in the hospitalized geriatric patient. *J Am Geriatri Soc* 30:433–436, 1982.
13. Rivlin RS: Nutrition and aging: some unanswered questions. *Am J Med* 71:337–340, 1981.
14. Harris AA, Levin S, Trenholme GM: Selected aspects of nosocomial infections in the 1980s. *Am J Med* 77:3–10, 1984.
15. Nicolle LE, McIntyre M, Zacharias H, MacDonell JA: Twelve-month surveillance of infections in institutionalized elderly men. *J Am Geriatric Soc* 32:513–519, 1984.
16. McGowan JE Jr, Barnes MW, Finland M: Bacteremia at Boston City Hospital: occurrence and mortality during 12 selected years (1935–1972), with special reference to hospital-acquired cases.

J Infect Dis 132:316–335, 1975.

17. McGowan JE Jr, Parrott PL, Duty VP: Nosocomial bacteremia—potential for prevention of procedure-related cases. *JAMA* 237:2727–2729, 1977.
18. Weinstein MP, Reller LB, Murphy JR, Lichtenstein KA: The clinical significance of positive blood cultures: a comprehensive analysis of 500 episodes of bacteremia and fungemia in adults. I. Laboratory and epidemiologic observations. *Rev Infect Dis* 5:35–53, 1983.
19. Setia U, Gross PA: Bacteremia in a community hospital. *Arch Intern Med* 137:1698–1701, 1977.
20. Setia U, Serventi I, Lorenz P: Bacteremia in a long-term care facility. Spectrum and mortality. *Arch Intern Med* 144:1633–1635, 1984.
21. Rosendal K, Jessen O, Faber V, Bentzon MW: Frequency, phage types and antibiotic resistance of *Staphylococcus aureus* isolated from blood cultures in Denmark 1975–1981. *Scand J Infect Dis* (Suppl) 41:19–29, 1983.
22. Rose R, Hunting KJ, Townsend TR, Wenzel RP: Morbidity/mortality and economics of hospital-acquired blood stream infections: a controlled study. *South Med J* 70:1267–1269, 1977.
23. Gleckman R, Hibert D: Afebrile bacteremia. A phenomenon in geriatric patients. *JAMA* 248:1478–1481, 1982.
24. Ponce De Leon S, Wenzel RP: Hospital-acquired bloodstream infections with *Staphylococcus epidermidis*. Review of 100 cases. *Am J Med* 77:639–644, 1984.
25. Ebright JR, Ryter MW: Bacterial pneumonia in the elderly. *J Am Geriatric Soc* 28:220–223, 1980.
26. Gerber IE: Terminal pneumonia in the aged. *Mt Sinai J Med* 47:166, 1980.
27. Huxley EJ, Viroslav J, Gram WR, Pierle AK: Pharyngeal aspiration in normal adults and patients with depressed consciousness. *Am J Med* 64:564, 1978.
28. Johanson WG, Pierce AK, Sanford JP, Thomas GD: Nosocomial respiratory infections with gram-negative bacilli: the significance of colonization of the respiratory tract. *Ann Intern Med* 77:701, 1972.
29. Valenti WM, Trudell RG, Bentley DW: Factors predisposing to oropharyngeal colonization with gram-negative bacilli in the aged. *N Engl J Med* 298:1108, 1978.
30. Irwin RS, Whitaker S, Pratter MR, Millard CE, Tarpey JT, Corwin RW: The transiency of oropharyngeal colonization with gram-negative bacilli in residents of a skilled nursing facility. *Chest* 81:31, 1982.
31. Campbell EJ, Lefrek SS: How aging affects the structure and function of the respiratory system. *Geriatrics* 33:68, 1974.
32. La Force FM: Hospital-acquired gram-negative rod pneumonia—an overview. *Am J Med* 70:664, 1981.
33. Woods DE, Straus DC, Johanson WG: Role of salivary protease activity in gram-negative bacilli to adherence mammalian buccal epithelial cells in vivo. *J Clin Invest* 68:1435, 1981.
34. Espersen F, Gabrielsen J: Pneumonia due to *Staphylococcus aureus* during mechanical ventilation. *J Infect Dis* 144:19, 1981.

35. Garvie DG, Gray J: Outbreak of respiratory syncytial viruses infection in the elderly. *Br Med J* 281:1253, 1980.
36. Mathur U, Bentley DW, Hall CB: Concurrent respiratory syncytial virus and influenza A infections in the institutionalized elderly and chronically ill. *Ann Intern Med* 93:44, 1980.
37. Kapila R, Lintz DI, Tecson FT, Ziskia L, Louria DB: A nosocomial outbreak of influenza A. *Chest* 71:576, 1977.
38. Dhar S, Shastri SR, Lenora RA: Aging and the respiratory system. *Med Clin North Am* 60:1121, 1976.
39. Oswald NC, Simon G, Shooterra: Pneumonia in hospital practice. *Br J Dis Chest* 55:109, 1961.
40. Simmons BP, Wong ES: CDC guidelines for the prevention and control of nosocomial infections. Guidelines for prevention of nosocomial pneumonia. *Am J Infect Control* 11:230, 1983.
41. Feeley TW, du Moulin GC, Hedley-Whyte J, Bushnell LS, Gilbert JP, Feingold DS: Aerosol polymyxin and pneumonia in seriously ill patients. *N Engl J Med* 293:471, 1975.
42. Sprunt K, Redman W: Evidence suggesting importance of role of interbacterial inhibition in maintaining balance of normal flora. *Ann Intern Med* 68:579, 1968.
43. Turck M, Stamm W: Nosocomial infection of the urinary tract. *Am J Med* 70:651, 1981.
44. Nicolle LE, Bjornson J, Harding GKM, MacDonell JA: Bacteriuria in elderly institutionalized men. *N Engl J Med* 309:1420, 1983.
45. Freedman LR: Interstitial renal inflammation, including pyelonephritis and urinary tract infection. In Ealley LE, Gottschall CW (eds): *Strauss and Welt's Diseases of the Kidney*, ed 3. Boston, Little, Brown, and Co, 1979, p 817.
46. Bentzen A, Vejlsgaaro R: Asymptomatic bacteriuria in elderly subjects. *Dan Med Bull* 27:101, 1980.
47. Dontas AS, Kasviki-Charvati P, Papanayiotou PC, Marketos SG: Bacteriuria and survival in old age. *N Engl J Med* 304:939, 1981.
48. Platt R, Polk BF, Murdock B, Rosner B: Mortality associated with nosocomial urinary tract infection. *N Engl J Med* 307:637, 1982.
49. Jewett MAS, Fernie GR, Holliday PJ, Dim ME: Urinary dysfunction in a geriatric long-term care population: prevalence and patterns. *J Am Geriatr Soc* 29:211, 1981.
50. Fierer J, Ekstrom M: An outbreak of *Providencia stuartii* urinary tract infections: patients with condom catheters are a reservoir of the bacteria. *JAMA* 245:1553, 1981.
51. Hirsh DD, Fainstein V, Musher DM: Do condom catheter collecting systems cause urinary tract infection? *JAMA* 242:340, 1979.
52. Sherman FT, Tucci V, Libow LS, Isenberg HD: Nosocomial urinary tract infection in a skilled nursing facility. *J Am Geriat Soc* 28:456, 1980.
53. Warren JW, Tenney JH, Hoopes JM, Muncie HL, Anthony WC: A prospective microbiologic study of bacteriuria in patients with chronic indwelling urethral catheters. *J Infect Dis* 146:719, 1982.
54. Breitenbucher RB: Bacterial changes in the urine samples of patients with long-term indwelling catheters. *Arch Intern Med* 144:1585–1588, 1984.

55. Robbins N, Demaria A, Miller MH: Infective endocarditis in the elderly. *South Med J* 73:1335–1338, 1980.

56. Applefeld MM, Hornick RB: Infective endocarditis in patients over age 60. *Am Heart J* 88:90, 1974.

57. Thell R, Martin FH, Edwards JE: Bacterial endocarditis in subjects 60 years of age and older. *Circulation* 51:174, 1975.

58. Habte-Gabr E, January LE, Smith IM: Bacterial endocarditis: the need for early diagnosis. *Geriatrics* 28:164, 1973.

59. Gantz NM: Infective endocarditis. In Gleckman RA, Gantz NM (eds): *Infections in the Elderly.* Boston, Little, Brown, and Co, 1983, p 217.

60. Rabinovich S, Evans J, Smith IM, January LE: A long-term view of bacterial endocarditis: 337 cases 1924 to 1963. *Ann Intern Med* 63:185, 1965.

61. Friedberg CK, Goldman HM, Field LE: Study of bacterial endocarditis. Comparisons in ninety-five cases. *Arch Intern Med* 107:74, 1961.

62. Lerner PI, Weinstein L: Infective endocarditis in the antibiotic era. *N Engl J Med* 274:199, 1966.

63. Guze LB, Pearce ML: Hospital acquired bacterial endocarditis. *Arch Intern Med* 112:56, 1963.

64. Tan JS, Watanakunakorn C, Terhune CA Jr: *Streptococcus viridans* endocarditis: favorable prognosis in geriatric patients. *Geriatrics* 28:68, 1973.

65. Watanakunakorn C, Tan JS: Diagnostic difficulties of staphylococcal endocarditis in geriatric patients. *Geriatrics* 28:168, 1973.

66. Fraser DW, Henke CE, Feldman RA: Changing patterns of bacterial meningitis in Olmstead County, Minnesota, 1935–1970. *J Infect Dis* 128:300, 1973.

67. Berk SL: Bacterial meningitis. In Gleckman RA, Gantz NM (eds): *Infections in the Elderly.* Boston, Little, Brown, and Co, 1983, p 235.

68. Hodges GR, Perkins RL: Hospital-associated bacterial meningitis. *Am J Med Sci* 271:335, 1976.

69. Buckwold FJ, Hand R, Hansebout RR: Hospital-acquired bacterial meningitis in neurosurgical patients. *J Neurosurg* 46:494, 1977.

70. Mangi RJ, Quintiliani R, Andriole VT: Gram-negative bacillary meningitis. *Am J Med* 93:253, 1980.

71. Berk SL, McCabe WR: Meningitis caused by gram-negative bacilli. *Ann Intern Med* 93:253–260, 1980.

72. Gorse GJ, Thrupp LD, Nudleman KL, Wyle FA, Hawkins B, Cesario TC: Bacterial meningitis in the elderly. *Arch Intern Med* 144:1603–1607, 1984.

73. Stein JA, DeRossi R, Neu HC: Adult *Haemophilus influenzae* meningitis. *NY State J Med* 69:1760–1766, 1969.

74. Young LS, LaForce FM, Head JJ, Feeley BS, Bennett JV: A simultaneous outbreak of meningococcal and influenza infections. *N Engl J Med* 287:5–9, 1972.

75. Cherubin CE, Marr JS, Sierra MF, Becker S: *Listeria* and gram-negative bacillary meningitis in New York City 1972–1979. *Am J Med* 71:199–209, 1981.

76. Chernik NL, Armstrong D, Posner JB: Central nervous system infections in patients with cancer. *Medicine* 52:563–581, 1973.

77. Ryan JL, Pachner A, Andriole VT, Root RK: Enterococcal meningitis: combined vancomycin and rifampin therapy. *Am J Med* 68:449–451, 1980.

78. Stead WW: Pathogenesis of pulmonary tuberculosis among older persons. *Am Rev Respir Dis* 91:811–822, 1965.

79. Powell KE, Farer LS: The rising age of the tuberculosis patient: a sign of success and failure. *J Infect Dis* 142:946–948, 1980.

80. Stead WW, Lofgren JP: Does the risk of tuberculosis increase in old age? *J Infect Dis* 147:951–955, 1983.

81. Grzybowski S, Allen EA: The challenge of tuberculosis in decline: a study based on the epidemiology of tuberculosis in Ontario, Canada. *Am Rev Respir Dis* 90:707–720, 1964.

82. Stead WW: Tuberculosis among elderly patients: an outbreak in a nursing home. *Ann Intern Med* 94:606–610, 1981.

83. Wilkens EG: Incidence and onset of pulmonary tuberculosis in old men. *Br Med J* 1:883–886, 1956.

84. Rubin EH: Pulmonary tuberculosis in the aged. *Am Rev Tuberculosis* 26:516–519, 1936.

85. Myers JA, Anderson HR: The significance of tuberculosis among the aged. *Am Rev Respir Dis* 21:541–545, 1930.

86. Freeman JT, Heiken CA: The geriatric aspect of pulmonary tuberculosis. *Am J Med Sci* 202:29–38, 1941.

87. Hadlock FP, Park SK, Awe RJ, Miuera M: Unusual radiographic findings in adult pulmonary tuberculosis. *AJR* 134:1015–1018, 1980.

88. Centers for Disease Control: *Tuberculosis in the United States, 178.* HHS Publication no. (CDC) 80-8322. Atlanta, Centers for Disease Control, 1980, 57 pp.

89. Sahn SA, Neff TA: Miliary tuberculosis. *Am J Med* 56:495–505, 1974.

90. Slavin RE, Walsh TJ, Pollack AD: Late generalized tuberculosis: a clinical pathologic analysis and comparison of 100 cases in the preantibiotic and antibiotic eras. *Medicine* 59:352–366, 1980.

91. Fox W: The chemotherapy of pulmonary tuberculosis: a review. *Chest* 76 (suppl):785–796, 1979.

92. Dutt AK, Stead WW: Short-course treatment regimen for patients with tuberculosis. *Arch Intern Med* 140:827–829, 1980.

93. Kopanoff DI, Snider DE Jr, Caras GJ: Isoniazid-related hepatitis. A U.S. Public Health Service cooperative surveillance study. *Am Rev Respir Dis* 117:991–1001, 1978.

94. United States Bureau of the Census: Demographic aspects of aging and the older population in the United States. *Current Population Reports Series* 23, no. 59 (revised). Washington, DC, US Government Printing Office, 1978, 68 pp.

95. Sherman FT, Libow LS: Infection in long-term care facilities. *Ann Intern Med* 90:855–856, 1979.

96. Magnussen MH, Robb SS: Nosocomial infections in a long-term care facility. *Am J Infect Control* 8:12–17, 1980.

97. Cohen ED, Hierholzer WJ, Schilling CR, Snydman DR: Nosocomial infections in skilled nursing facilities: a preliminary survey. *Public Health Rep*

94:162–165, 1979.

98. Standfast SJ, Michelsen PB, Baltch AL, Smith RP, Latham EK, Spellacy AB, Venezia RA, Andritz MH: A prevalence survey of infection in a combined acute and long-term care hospital. *Infect Control* 5:177–184, 1984.

99. Garibaldi RA, Brodine S, Matsumiya S: Infections among patients in nursing homes: policies, prevalence and problems. *N Engl J Med* 305:731–735, 1981.

100. Alling B, Brandberg A, Seeberg S, Svanborg A: Aerobic and anaerobic microbial flora in the urinary tract of geriatric patients during long care. *J Infect Dis* 127:34–38, 1973.

101. Fox RH, MacGibbon R, Davies L, Woodward PM: Problem of the old and the cold. *Br Med J* 1:21–24, 1973.

102. Petersdorf RG, Beeson PB: Fever of unexplained origin: report on 100 cases. *Medicine* 40:1–30, 1961.

103. Esposito AL, Gleckman RA: Fever of unknown origin in the elderly. *J Am Geriatr Soc* 26:498–505, 1978.

104. Esposito AL: Fever of unknown origin. In Gleckman RA, Gantz NM (eds): *Infections in the Elderly*. Boston, Little, Brown, and Co, 1983, pp 137–157.

105. Prevention and control of influenza: recommendations of the Immunization Practices Advisory Committee, Centers for Disease Control. *Ann Intern Med* 101:218–222, 1984.

106. Eickhoff TC, Sherman IL, Serfling RE: Observations on excess mortality associated with epidemic influenza. *JAMA* 176:776–782, 1961.

107. Barker WH, Mullooly JP: Impact of epidemic type A influenza in a defined adult population. *Am J Epidemiol* 112:798–811, 1980.

108. Barker WH, Mullooly JP: Pneumonia and influenza deaths during epidemics: implications for prevention. *Arch Intern Med* 142:85–89, 1982.

109. Van Voris LP, Belshe RB, Shaffer JL: Nosocomial influenza B virus infection in the elderly. *Ann Intern Med* 96:153–158, 1982.

110. Fedson DS, Kessler HA: A hospital-based influenza immunization program, 1977–78. *Am J Public Health* 73:442–445, 1983.

111. Galasso GJ, Tyeryar FJ Jr, Cate TR, Couch RB, Glezen WP, Gross PA, Kasel JA, Webster RG, Wright PF: Clinical studies of influenza vaccines—1976. *J Infect Dis* 136 (suppl):S341–S742, 1977.

112. Glezen WP: Serious morbidity and mortality associated with influenza epidemics. *Epidemiol Rev* 4:25–44, 1982.

113. Gross PA, Ennis FA: Influenza vaccine: split product versus whole virus types—how do they differ? (Editorial) *N Engl J Med* 296:567–568, 1977.

114. Horadam VW, Sharp JG, Smilack JD, Schonberger LB: Pharmacokinetics of amantadine hydrochloride in subjects with normal and impaired renal function. *Ann Intern Med* 94:454–458, 1981.

115. Update: pneumococcal polysaccharide vaccine usage—United States. Recommendations of the Immunization Practices Advisory Committee, Centers for Disease Control. *Ann Intern Med* 101:348–350, 1984.

116. Broome CV, Facklam RR: Epidemiology of clinically significant isolates of *Streptococcus pneumoniae* in the United States. *Rev Infect Dis* 3:277–281, 1981.

117. Kaufman P: Pneumonia in old age: active immunization against pneumonia with pneumococcus polysaccharide; results of a six year study. *Arch Intern Med* 79:518–531, 1947.

118. Austrian R, Douglas RM, Schiffman G, Coetzee AM, Koornhof HJ, Hayden-Smith S, Reid RDW: Prevention of pneumococcal pneumonia by vaccination. *Trans Assoc Am Physicians* 89:184–194, 1976.

119. Riley ID, Tarr PI, Andrews M, Pfeiffer M, Howard R, Challands P, Jennison G, Douglas RM: Immunization with a polyvalent pneumococcal vaccine. Reduction of adult respiratory mortality in a New Guinea Highlands community. *Lancet* 1:1338–1341, 1975.

120. Austrian R: Surveillance of pneumococcal infection for field trials of polyvalent pneumococcal vaccines. Report DAB-VDP-12-84. Bethesda, MD, *National Institutes of Health*, 1980, pp 1–82.

121. Shapiro ED, Clemens JD: A controlled evaluation of the protective efficacy of pneumococcal vaccine for patients at high risk for serious pneumococcal infections. *Ann Intern Med* 101:325–330, 1984.

122. DeStefano F, Goodman RA, Noble GR, McClary GD, Smith SJ, Broome CV: Simultaneous administration of influenza and pneumococcal vaccines. *JAMA* 247:2551–2554, 1982.

123. Fedson DS, Chiarello LA: Previous hospital care and pneumococcal bacteremia: importance for pneumococcal immunization. *Arch Intern Med* 143:885–889, 1983.

124. Borgono JM, McLean AA, Vella PP, Woodhour AF, Canepa I, Davidson WL, Hilleman MR: Vaccination and revaccination with polyvalent pneumococcal polysaccharide vaccines in adults and infants (40010). *Proc Soc Exp Biol Med* 157:148–154, 1978.

125. Levine L, Wyman L: Survey of immunity by serologic methods: results of three successive surveys of samples of the Massachusetts population for diphtheria and tetanus antitoxin. *N Engl J Med* 272:23–26, 1965.

126. Toxoids: adult immunization: recommendations of the Immunization Practices Advisory Committee, Centers for Disease Control. *MMWR* 33:10S–12S, 1984.

127. Both live-virus and inactivated-virus vaccines: poliomyelitis: recommendations of the Immunization Practices Advisory Committee, Centers for Disease Control. *MMWR* 33:20S–21S, 1984.

128. Committee on Immunization, Council of Medical Societies, American College of Physicians: *Guide for Adult Immunization*. Philadelphia, American College of Physicians, 1985, p 132.

129. Ruben FL, Norden CW, Heisler B, Korica Y: An outbreak of *Streptococcus pyogenes* infections in a nursing home. *Ann Intern Med* 101:494–496, 1984.

130. Rahman M: Outbreak of *Streptococcus pyogenes* infections in a geriatric hospital and control by mass treatment. *J Hosp Infect* 2:63–69, 1981.

131. Burgoon CT, Burgoon JS, Baldridge GD: The natural history of herpes-zoster. *JAMA* 164:265–270, 1957.

132. Jacobson JA, Kolts RL, Conti M, Burke JP: Hospital-acquired myiasis. *Infect Control* 1:319–320, 1980.

133. Peachey RDG, English MP: An outbreak of *Trichophyton rubrum* infection in a geriatric hospital. *Br J Dermatol* 91:389–397, 1974.

134. Bliss MR, McLaren R, Exton-Smith AN: Preventing pressure sores in hospitals: controlled trial of large-celled ripple mattresses. *Br Med J* 1:394–397, 1967.

135. Reuler JB, Cooney TG: The pressure sore: pathophysiology and principles of management. *Ann Intern Med* 94:661–666, 1981.

136. Reichel SM: Shearing force as a factor in decubitus ulcers in paraplegics. *JAMA* 166:762–763, 1958.

137. Galpin JE, Chow AW, Bayer AS, Guzo LC: Sepsis associated with decubitus ulcers. *Am J Med* 61:346–350, 1976.

138. Bryan CS, Dew CE, Reynolds KL: Bacteremia associated with decubitus ulcers. *Arch Intern Med* 143:2093–2095, 1983.

139. Waldvogel FA, Vasey H: Osteomyelitis: the past decade. *N Engl J Med* 303:360–369, 1980.

140. Feingold DS: The diagnosis and treatment of gangrenous and crepitant cellulitis. In Remington JS, Swartz MN (eds): *Current Clinical Topics in Infectious Diseases.* New York, McGraw-Hill, 1981, pp 259–277.

141. La Force FM, Young LS, Bennett JV: Tetanus in the United States (1965–1966). Epidemiologic and clinical features. *N Engl J Med* 280:571–574, 1969.

142. Chow AW, Galpin JE, Guze LB: Clindamycin for treatment of sepsis caused by decubitus ulcers. *J Infect Dis* 135 (suppl):65–68, 1971.

143. Norton D, McLaren R, Exton-Smith AN: *An Investigation of Geriatric Nursing Problems in Hospital.* Edinburgh, Churchill Livingstone, 1975, 238 pp.

144. Constantian MB, Jackson HS: Biology and care of the pressure ulcer wound. In Constantian MB (ed): *Pressure Ulcers, Principles and Technique of Management.* Boston, Little, Brown, and Co, 1980, pp 69–100.

145. Bergen R, Florent G, Just M: Decrease of the lymphoproliferative response to varicella-zoster antigen in the aged. *Infect Immunol* 32:24–27, 1981.

146. Rahman M: Outbreak of chickenpox and herpes zoster in a geriatric hospital. *Br J Clin Pract* 33:291–293, 1979.

147. Blacklow NR: Infectious diarrhea. In Gleckman RA, Gantz N (eds): *Infections in the Elderly.* Boston, Little, Brown, and Co, 1983, pp 153–175.

148. Blaser MJ, Feldman RA: *Salmonella* bacteremia reports to the Centers for Disease Control, 1968–1979. *J Infect Dis* 143:743–746, 1981.

149. Kendrick MA: Summary of study on illness among Americans visiting Europe, March 31, 1969–March 30, 1970. *J Infect Dis* 126:684–685, 1972.

150. Pentland R, Pennington CR: Acute diarrhea in the elderly. *Age Ageing* 9:90–92, 1980.

151. Giannella RA, Broitman SA, Zamcheck N: Influence of gastric acidity on bacterial and parasitic enteric infections. *Ann Intern Med* 78:271–276, 1973.

152. Sprintz H: Pathogenesis of intestinal infections. *Arch Pathol* 87:556–562, 1969.

153. Gustafson TL, Kobylik B, Hutcheson RH, Schaffner W: Protective effect of anticholinergic drugs and psyllium in a nosocomial outbreak of Norwalk gastroenteritis. *J Hosp Infect* 4:367–374, 1983.

154. Marrie TJ, Lee SH, Faulkner RS, Ethier J, Young CH: Rotavirus infection in a geriatric population. *Arch Intern Med* 142:313–316, 1982.

Chapter 30

Infection Prevention in the Compromised Host

Gerald R. Donowitz, M.D.

INTRODUCTION

The immune-compromised host represents a subpopulation of patients in whom hospital-acquired infection remains a major source of morbidity and mortality. Numbers of patients with immune defects continue to grow as advances are made in therapeutic strategies in hematology-oncology, rheumatolgy, and organ transplantation. Before examining the issues involved in prophylaxis of infection, one needs a brief review of the pathogenesis of infection in this group of patients. Specifically, risk factors for infection, sites of infections, and origin of infection need to be discussed.

PATHOGENESIS OF INFECTION IN THE COMPROMISED HOST

Normal host defenses can be undermined in one of three ways: (*a*) by underlying disease, (*b*) by therapy for disease, or (*c*) by iatrogenic manipulation of the patient within the hospital setting. While genetic defects in cellular and humoral host defense have been well characterized, our emphasis will be on acquired host defense defects. Certain acquired disease states are associated with specific defects in host defense. Patients with Hodgkin's disease have defects in T cell function as measured by both in vitro and in vivo techniques (1–3). The severity of the defects usually progresses as the underlying disease worsens (4). Patients with multiple myeloma have abnormal humoral immunity with low levels of normal immunoglobulin due to increased turnover, decreased synthesis, or both (5–9). Patients with chronic lymphocytic leukemia may have defects in both T cell and humoral immunity (8). Most recently, patients with acquired immune deficiency syndrome (AIDS) have been shown to have a profound depression of cell-mediated immunity associated with depression of lymphocyte numbers and an array of in vitro and in vivo defects in T cell activity (9–13). Nevertheless, the association of a given underlying disease state with a specific host defense defect or series of defects must be viewed as only a "first approximation" of the state of the patients' immune defense status. As disease progresses, and as patients become debilitated, a variety of host defense defects can be acquired because of inanition, independent of the defects first noted (14).

In some cases, it is the therapy for disease rather than the disease itself that brings about an immune suppressed state. Neutropenia associated with the marrow suppressive chemotherapy used for leukemia, lymphoma, and bone marrow and organ transplantation has been clearly identified as one of the most important risk factors for the development of infection (15). The association of neutrophil counts of less than 500 to 1000 cells/mm^3 and the number of days spent with severe infection, fever, or on antibiotics have been clearly established by Bodey and substantiated by others for an array of bacterial and fungal infections (16–19). The use of steroids as part of therapeutic regimens and transplantation protocols has been associated with host defense defects including depression of neutrophil chemotaxis (20–22), decreased leukocyte adherence (23), depressed monocyte bactericidal activity (24), and decreased endocytosis and clearing of particles by the reticuloendothelial system (25). Lymphocyte functions—including antigen processing, lymphocyte proliferation, response to cell mediators, and cell-mediated cytotoxicity—have all been shown to be affected adversely by steroids (26–31). Such cytotoxic agents as cyclophosphamide, 5-fluorouracil, and methotrexate have been shown to depress various aspects of immune function, including humoral and cellular immunity (32).

The hospital in which most immune-compromised patients find themselves for prolonged periods of time must be viewed as a hostile environment and yet another important risk factor for infection. Routine hospital procedures represent important infection risks: peripheral, central, and right atrial catheters, as well as urinary catheters breach the physical barriers normally established by the skin and mucous membranes and allow for colonization and subsequent infection. The use of broad spectrum antibiotics (33), nebulizers, and inhalational equipment (34, 35) has been associated with colonization of the respiratory tract with hospital pathogens which can and do go on to cause subsequent pneumonias. Exposure to potential pathogens may occur within the hospital via hand-to-hand transmission, food sources, hospital equipment, and contaminated air or water supplies (36, 37).

The means by which an immune-compromised host actually develops on infection are central to the issue of prevention. Schimpff and colleagues (37) in a classic series published in 1972 established the importance of endogenous flora in causing infection in the immune-suppressed host. They showed that in patients with acute nonlymphocytic leukemia, organisms that caused infections colonized the patient prior to the infectious episode. Eighty-six percent of the organisms were shown to be part of the patients' endogenous flora and could be isolated from the gingiva, nose, axilla, urine, or rectum. Of importance was that 47% of infections were caused by organisms that were acquired by patients and became part of their endogenous microbiologic flora only *after* hospitalization.

Based on these considerations, infection prevention in the immune-compromised host must deal with three basic issues: (*a*) prevention of acquisition of hospital-associated pathogens, (*b*) suppression or elimination of endogenous pathogens, and (*c*) reversal of host defense defects. As a fourth issue, efforts at prevention should address infections caused by specific pathogens which have been identified with well defined subpopulations of immune-suppressed patients.

MINIMIZING ACQUISITION OF HOSPITAL FLORA—THE PROTECTED ENVIRONMENT

Isolation of patients as a means of preventing acquisition of nosocomial pathogens remains one of the most basic, yet one of the most controversial, aspects of infection prevention in the compromised host.

Simple Reverse Isolation

Simple reverse isolation (use of gowns, gloves, and masks for those having contact with the patient) has not proven to be an efficacious means of reducing infection. In a controlled, prospective study, Nauseef and Maki compared simple reverse isolation with standard hospital care in 43 episodes of severe neutropenia (38). No statistically significant differences were noted in the overall incidence of infection, time of onset of initial infection, or number of days of fever.

Protective Isolation

More sophisticated means of creating a protected environment have been of interest since at least the 1950s. It was during this time that techniques were developed to maintain germ-free animal colonies (39). As subsequent observations showed that germ-free mice and rats with leukemia could tolerate higher doses of radio- and chemotherapy with less infection, these isolation techniques were applied to humans (40–42). Early isolation systems, the "life islands," consisted of a plastic bag or bubble supported over a bed through which filtered air was passed (43, 44). More refined air filtering systems were employed in the 1960s using techniques developed by the National Aeronautics and Space Administration (NASA). High efficiency particulate air (HEPA) filters were developed which filtered particles greater than 0.3 μm in diameter with 99.97% efficiency (45). As a subsequent development in air handling, unidirectional flow of air or laminar air flow, was shown to reduce air turbulence and decrease air contamination (46, 47). Laminar air flow (LAF) rooms were developed where air was circulated through HEPA filters at 90 to 140 feet/minute with approximately 100 air exchanges within the room/hour. As long as personnel and equipment were kept "down wind" of the patient, direct person-to-person or equipment-to-person transmission of organisms could be minimized.

The effect of these facilities on patients' environmental exposure to potential pathogens has been clearly documented. In a microbiologic assessment of protected environments, Bodey and Johnston (46) sampled air from life islands, LAF rooms, and regular hospital rooms. Five organisms/1000 feet^3 were isolated in the LAF rooms compared to 31 organisms/1000 feet^3 in the life island rooms and 3064 organisms/1000 feet^3 in the regular hospital rooms. While nearly 60% of air samples from hospital rooms contained potential pathogens, only 1.0% of LAF room samples did versus 21.4% of life island air samples, a statistically significant difference ($p < 0.01$). Similar results have been noted by others (48, 49).

Although the microbiologic effects of the protected environments appear clear, their overall clinical impact on changing the course of disease remains a question. One of the problems in evaluating the efficacy of protected environments is the paucity of data concerning their use alone without other infection prevention measures.

In the study of Yates and Holland (50), patients with acute myelocytic leukemia were randomized to receive protective isolation alone, protective isolation with oral and topical antibiotics for gut and skin sterilization, oral and topical antibiotics with reverse isolation procedures in a conventional room, or routine ward care. For the first 3 weeks of the study, no protection from severe infections was afforded by any of the isolation procedures. However, after day 23, no further infections occurred in the patients in protective isolation while infections occurred at the same rate in patients treated without protective isolation. Statistically fewer pneumonias and fewer infections with *Pseudomonas aeruginosa* were noted in the isolated patients. No significant differences in incidence of infection or in mortality were noted in isolated patients receiving oral and topical antibiotics and isolated patients who did not. While infectious deaths were less common in the groups receiving oral and topical antibiotics, death from hemorrhage was more frequent. In a study of similar design, Dietrich et al studied patients with acute leukemia who were assigned to protective isolation, protective isolation with oral and topical antibiotics, or treatment under standard ward conditions (51). While use of protective isolation significantly lowered rates of bacterial colonization, no statistically significant differences were noted in overall numbers of infections. However, fewer documented pneumonias were noted in patients in isolation. Patients in isolation using antibiotic decontamination tended to have less severe infections than patients in isolation not receiving antibiotics, though the differences were not statistically significant.

Total Protected Environment

Many more studies have been carried out examining the role of a "total protected environment"—that is, protective isolation and antibiotic decontamination of the gut, skin, and mucosal surfaces. An excellent review of the literature has been provided by Pizzo and Levine (52). It should be emphasized that half of the more than one dozen studies carried out at the time of this review were nonrandomized, relying on historical controls for comparison. While all the studies quoted showed fewer infections developing in patients in total protected environments, more weight must be given to those studies in which prospective randomized controls were utilized.

The studies of Yates and Holland (50) and Dietrich et al (51) showed that oral and topical antibiotic regimens used in conjunction with protective isolation led to more frequent sterility of body sites than did protective isolation alone. However, as previously noted, this approach did not lead to significant differences in overall infection rates.

In the studies of Schimpff et al (53) and Levine et al (54) the total protected environment was compared either to oral antibiotic prophylaxis alone or to routine ward care. In each case, use of the total protected environment was associated with a more sterile environment for the patient as judged by lower numbers of organisms in air samples, fewer stool cultures positive for potential pathogens, and fewer organisms acquired after hospitalization. Infectious complications were reduced by over 50% in Levine et al's study by use of the total protected environment compared to routine care. Severe infections, septicemia, pneumonia, and disseminated fungal disease were reduced by over 70%. In the presence of severe neutropenia, patients in a total protective environment spent less time with infections. No differences were noted between ward care and oral antibiotic prophylaxis used alone. Schimpff et al's study also clearly documented the utility of the total protected environment in reducing total infections, severe infections, and bacteremias compared to patients on a routine ward. However, unlike Levine et al's study, use of oral antibiotics alone was also associated with a significant decrease in risk of infections.

Rodriquez et al (55) examined protective isolation with either intravenous or oral antibiotic prophylaxis compared to antibiotic prophylaxis given without protective isolation. Overall infection rates for patients in protective isolation were less than those outside the protective isolation, though the difference was not statistically significant. At neutrophil counts below 100 neutrophils/mm^3 and between 101 and 500 neutrophils/mm^3, the number of days with infection was less in patients in protective isolation. Fewer septicemias and pneumonias were noted and statistically fewer infectious deaths occurred in patients within the protected environment.

While the majority of patients studied have been those with acute leukemia and chemotherapy-related neutropenia, protected environments have been studied with other patient groups as well. Navari et al (56) assigned patients with aplastic anemia receiving allogeneic marrow transplants to receive a total protected environment versus a conventional, nonprotected environment versus prophylactic white cell transfusions. Approximately one-third of patients were placed into each category by availability rather than random assignment. Infections and septicemia were significantly less in the group of patients in a total protected environment. Compared to patients receiving prophylactic white cell transfusions, a significantly decreased incidence of infection was noted for patients within the protected environment from the day of engraftment to day 100 only. Buckner et al randomized bone marrow transplant recipients to a total protected environment versus routine care (57). Again fewer infections were noted in patients within the protected environment.

With the exception of the series by Dietrich et al (51), all studies quoted have shown a reduction in infection due to use of the total protected environment. However, the general utility of this technique still needs to be defined. Several series have demonstrated that several weeks are needed before the effect of protective isolation can be seen. Since profound neutropenia has been the most important host defense defect associated with infection in the patient groups studied, patients without prolonged, profound neutropenia would not seem to be reasonable candidates for protective isolation or the total protected environment. Furthermore, although reduction of infection rates has been demonstrated by use of protected environments, a recent review suggests that some of the differences noted in the most widely cited studies could be attributed to differences in patient population and intensity of supporting care (58).

Various problems have been associated with protective isolation. The cost of purchasing and installing a single LAF unit is approximately $35,000. Increased nursing and supportive staff is usually necessary for caring for patients in protective isolation. Maintaining a sterile environment and acceptable diet requires close and constant interaction between housekeeping, dietary, and sterile supplies personnel. While psychologic response to isolation is usually good (59), most centers screen their patients carefully for suitability for isolation, and up to 20% of patients reviewed may be deemed unsuitable (50). As discussed below, the oral nonabsorbable antibiotic protocols used in the total protected environment are associated with a variety of problems, including gastrointestinal (GI) symptoms, colonization with drug-resistant organisms, and superinfection.

The final and most important question to be raised concerning the usefulness of protective isolation procedures is whether their use makes any significant long term difference to the patient as far as overall survival or development of significant complications. In the review of protected environments by Pizzo and Levine (52), a dozen randomized and nonrandomized studies were examined. If one considers only randomized studies, the majority, which deal with patients with acute leukemia, indicate no significant differences in remission rates or in survival. Because of relatively small numbers and lack of homogeneity of patient groups, it is difficult to assess the differences between these studies and those few which did show a difference in patient survival. Lack of improved survival has been noted for patients with solid tumors, sarcomas, and lymphomas (60, 61).

The results of studies with patients undergoing bone marrow transplantation may be more hopeful. In patients with aplastic anemia or leukemia who received bone marrow transplantation, use of LAF has been associated with a delay in onset of significant graft versus host disease (57). In a decrease in the incidence of graft versus host disease as well as a delay in onset was noted in patients treated within LAF compared to controls. While these differences were not statistically significant, survival by day 100 was significantly greater in the patients treated in LAF rooms versus those treated conventionally. In a larger series, use of LAF was associated with both a significant decrease in the incidence of clinically significant graft versus host disease and an increased probability of survival (62).

In summary, the utility of protective isolation and the total protected environment remains unproven. The high cost of establishing and maintaining protective isolation units, the increased demand for nursing and supporting personnel, and the problems with use of gut sterilization regimens are out of proportion to the benefits that have thus far been demonstrated. The lack of beneficial effects may be in part due to the patient population studied most frequently, that is, the neutropenic leukemic. Overall prognosis for this group of patients, despite advances in chemotherapeutic regimens and supportive services, remains guarded at best. As experience is gained with other populations and with other treatment modalities, such as bone marrow transplantation, patient subpopulations may be defined in which use of protected environments will allow for increased overall survival. Until this occurs, use of protective isolation and the total protected environment should be reserved for clearly monitored, select, clinical trials.

MINIMIZING ACQUISITION OF HOSPITAL FLORA—FOOD HANDLING

Means of reducing acquisition of hospital-associated pathogens aside from protective isolation have been developed as specific risks have been identified. The importance of food as a means of acquiring potential pathogens has only recently been fully appreciated. In 1971, Shooter et al showed that *E. coli*, *P. aeruginosa* and *Klebsiella* species could be cultured from 30 to 50% of food samples from hospitals, canteens, and school kitchens with many samples containing more than 1000 colonies/g (63). Only hot food appeared free of this degree of contamination. Similar observations were made by Kominos et al who found that over 80% of samples of tomatoes, 27% of samples of salads, as well as numbers of other raw vegetables contained *Pseudomonas* sp. (64). Subsequent studies showed that *Serratia* and *Enterobacter* species were also frequently present in vegetables, often in high titer (greater than 1000 colonies/g) (65). Casewell and Phillips found that isolates of *Klebsiella* species found in food were more prevalent in clinical specimens (66). As with the work of Shooter et al (63), only hot food was relatively free of contamination.

How bacteria in food affect the immune-suppressed host is not clear. The number of organisms required to create a high risk situation for infection is undefined. Ingestion of up to 10^6 organisms has not been associated with GI tract colonization (67). However in the presence of antibiotics which change the natural flora of the gut, foodborne bacteria have been shown to colonize the gut with as few as 10 to 100 organisms (68, 69). Since many impaired hosts, especially

those with neutropenia, spend a significant portion of their hospitalization on antibiotics, and since an average portion of salad may harbor as many as 5000 organisms (63), the potential danger of foodborne bacteria as a source of GI tract colonization becomes quite real.

While sterility of food was the initial aim of many programs (70), foods with *low* bacterial counts have been shown to be acceptable as far as safety and are more palatable than sterile diets (71, 72). As a practical matter, examination of a variety of processed and prepackaged foods has shown that over two-thirds have low bacterial counts and can be used safely (73).

For patients who are not in a total protected environment, food handling practices can be less rigid and should rely on common sense (69). Use of low microbial cooked or processed foods, and avoidance of relatively contaminated foods (raw vegetables, cold meats, etc) allow for a wide range of food choices while minimizing exposure to potential pathogens.

REDUCTION OF ENDOGENOUS FLORA
Oral and Systemic Antibiotic Prophylaxis
Oral Nonabsorbable Antibiotics

As pointed out above, development of infection in the compromised host occurs as a result of colonization with potential pathogens, over half of which are part of the patients' endogenous flora prior to hospitalization (37). Suppression of this endogenous flora represents the second major component of infection prevention in the immune-suppressed patient.

Since the GI tract is the major site of colonization, gastrointestinal decontamination with antibiotics received early and ongoing attention. Oral, nonabsorbable antibiotics have been most widely used. While various agents have been used on rotating as well as on fixed schedules, the combination of gentamicin, vancomycin, and nystatin (GVN) has emerged as one of the most consistently utilized regimens (50, 53, 54, 60). Liquid preparations rather than capsules or tablets have been used to provide more prolonged contact with mucous membranes, a practice which may enhance effectiveness (74).

Ample microbiologic data exist documenting the effect of oral antibiotic regimens on gut flora. Priesler et al studied 21 patients with acute leukemia receiving induction chemotherapy (72). The use of GVN led to no growth in 85% of aerobic stool cultures and in 75% of anaerobic stool cultures. However, fungal cultures of stool were sterile in only 20% of samples. In the study of Bodey and Rosenbaum (75), virtually all bacterial pathogens were eliminated within 2 weeks by the regimen of vancomycin, gentamicin and either amphotericin B, candicidin, or nystatin. As with Priesler et al's study, only 44% of fungal isolates initially noted were eliminated. The findings of significant suppression of anaerobic and anerobic gut flora and only partial suppression of fungal species have been substantiated by others using GVN as well as a variety of other oral antibiotic regimens (50, 54, 76, 77). Significant reductions in gut flora have been demonstrated in routine ward settings, as well as in protected environments (52, 54).

The kinetics of gut suppression by oral non-absorbable antibiotics has been studied by King (78). Using a regimen of kamanycin, vancomycin, and nystatin, King noted effects on fecal flora as early as 24 hours, with maximal effects on both aerobic and anaerobic flora occurring between 3 and 5 days. After 5 days, isolates of fungal and aminoglycoside-resistant aerobic bacilli began to emerge. While oral antibiotic regimens reduce bacterial counts in the stool, it is important to note that suppression rather than sterilization occurs (75–77). Forty to 70% of organisms originally isolated can be cultured again once antibiotics are discontinued, usually within the first week and as early as the first 3 days (76, 79). Furthermore, new organisms may be acquired even in the presence of antibiotic prophylaxis. In the study of Bodey and Rosenbaum (75), 73 new organisms were cultured only after prophylactic antibiotics were begun, with fungi and anaerobes predominating. In the series of Hahn et al (77) a total of 274 potential pathogens were acquired during 87 patient trials; on the average, one new potential pathogen was acquired every 30 days. In this series *Candida* species and aerobic gram-negative bacilli were most commonly isolated. Newly acquired stool isolates have been thought to come either from the environment or other body sites, or they occur as mutations of previously cultured strains (76). Development of gentamicin resistance has been noted in 12 to 30% of the organisms (72, 77).

The effect of the vancomycin component of the GVN regimen has been examined. Bodey showed that without vancomycin, suppression of anerobes in the gut was markedly decreased (76). Bender et al examined 38 patients, most of whom had acute leukemia and were randomized to receive GVN or GN (80). Use of vancomycin was associated with more complete suppression of gut aerobes, especially group D streptococcal species. The effect of vancomycin on anaerobes was indeterminate. The degree of colonization with yeasts and gentamicin-resistant organisms was noted equally in both groups. Of note was that vancomycin was identified as the most unpalatable component in the GVN regimen and was the most likely agent to cause nausea and vomiting. Consequently, the GN regimen was more tolerable and was associated with greater compliance than the GVN regimen.

Despite the reduction of potentially pathogenic flora in the gut, studies examining the effect of nonabsorbable antibiotics in reducing infections in the immune-suppressed patient when used alone distinct from their use in protected environments have been inconclusive. Only a small number of prospective, randomized trials exist.

Schimpff et al (53) studied the effect of GVN used in a ward setting versus GVN used in a protected environment versus no antibiotics on a ward setting alone. Compared to the ward setting alone, nonabsorbable antibiotics led to almost half the number of infections. Results were comparable to those when the antibiotics were used within a protected environment. Severe infections and bacteremias were significantly reduced. However, only when antibiotics were used in a protected environment were there noted statistically significant numbers of patients without infections, without severe infection, or without bacteremias. Utilizing a regimen of framycetin, colistin sulphate, and nystatin (FRACON), Storring et al studied 113 patients treated for acute non-lymphoblastic leukemia (81). Fifty-eight patients received no antibiotics, and 55 patients received the FRACON regimen. Both groups were housed in single rooms, with simple reverse isolation. Patients receiving FRACON therapy had fewer febrile episodes and required less antibiotics. The greatest differences were noted at neutrophil counts of less than $100/\mu l$. Statistically significant differences in microbiologically documented infections and bacteremias were also noted in the FRACON-treated group.

Despite the positive results from these two studies, others have not demonstrated a significant effect of prophylactic antibiotics on the incidence of infections. Levine et al (54) studied the effect of GVN with or without a protected environment, compared to routine ward care. While GVN suppression of gut flora was similar with or without the protected environment, GVN in a nonprotected environment did not reduce the incidence of infection, sepsis, or pneumonia. Of the 18 severe infections in which a site and an organism were identified, one-half were due to organisms' colonizing the orophanynx, a site relatively unaffected by prophylactic antibiotics. In the study of Yates and Holland, GVN utilized with conventional reverse isolation was unsuccessful in preventing the acquisition of severe infection compared to routine ward care and was only effective in infection reduction when used in a protected environment (50). Similar results were noted by Lohner et al, who compared the use of vancomycin, polymicin, kanamycin, and nystatin with or without a protected environment (82). While similar degrees of gut suppression were achieved, patients in a protected environment had significantly fewer microbiologically proven infections, had fewer days with infection, and received fewer days of antibiotics than patients receiving antibiotics in a nonprotected environment.

Given the lack of consistent results regarding the efficacy of oral nonabsorbable antibiotics on infection in the compromised host, it is not surprising that their effect on patients' overall clinical course is unimpressive. Examining the two series in which antibiotics significantly decreased infections, only the study by Schimpff et al (53) showed a significant increase in remission rates in those patients receiving antibiotics alone. No such findings were noted by Storring et al (81).

Various problems associated with oral nonabsorbable antibiotics make their widespread use even less appealing than do their inconsistent effects. GVN is not well tolerated by most patients. Odor, taste, and aftertaste of the regimen, especially the vancomycin component, are unpleasant as judged by patients as well as impartial nursing and support staff (74). Nausea, vomiting, and diarrhea are frequently observed. Since the drugs are given on every 4- to 6-hour schedules, and since longer intervals between doses are associated with less effective microbial suppression, 85% of the doses must be taken for maximum effectiveness by patients who may already be feeling ill from chemotherapy-related mucositis or colitis (74, 83). Abnormal serum levels of carotene and folate, and abnormal gastrointestinal absorption of D-xylose have been documented as indications of malabsorption caused by nonabsorbable antibiotics (84). Embarking on a prophylactic antibiotic regimen and then discontinuing it while patients are still neutropenic has been associated with higher than predicted incidences of serious bacterial infections, especially with aerobic gram-negative bacilli (53). A rebound phenomenon by the suppressed but not eradicated organisms is thought to be the cause. Development of aminoglycoside resistance of organisms persisting in the stool has been noted in 12 to 30% of isolates (76, 77) during up to 54% of antibiotic courses (78). Finally, the cost of oral nonabsorbable regimens is approximately $100/day.

Systemic Antibiotics

In a small number of studies, systemic antibiotics have been used instead of or with oral antibiotics. In an early series by Rodriquez et al (55), patients with acute leukemia were randomized to receive either parenteral or oral antibiotics both with and without a protected environment. No significant differences in infection rates were noted. However, in a similar study involving patients with extensive small cell bronchogenic carcinoma, parenteral antibiotics were more effective than oral antibiotics in reducing the incidence of overall infection and of documented infections (85). Prophylactic intravenous antibiotics were compared to combined intravenous-oral regimens in patients with acute leukemia who were being treated in a protected environment (86). While an increased incidence of fevers of unknown etiology and of major infections occurred in patients receiving parenteral antibiotic prophylaxis, no significant differences were noted in either duration of complete remissions or overall success of therapy.

Selective Suppression of Gut Flora

Because of the various problems encountered, attempts have been made to modify selectively rather than totally suppress gut flora. These efforts have been based on colonization resistance, a concept developed by van der Waaij who, using a germ-free animal model, observed that an intact population of gut anaerobes prevented gut colonization with exogenous aerobic organisms (68, 87). Since studies by Naff (88), Knothe (89), and Hargadon et al (90) demonstrated that Enterobacteriaceae were reduced in the gut of patients taking trimethoprim-sulfamethoxazole (T-SMX) while anaerobic organisms were left intact, this drug as well as nalidixic acid, an agent with a similar effect, became the objects of extensive investigation. Preliminary support for the use of T-SMX as gut prophylaxis in the compromised host came from Hughes et al (91). In a randomized, double-blind, placebo-controlled study, T-SMX was studied as prophylaxis against *Pneumocystis carinii* infections in pediatric patients with malignancy. Not only was the incidence of *Pneumocystis* infection significantly reduced, but the incidences of bacterial sepsis, pneumonias other than those caused by *Pneumocystis*, and localized infections were also reduced. The only adverse effect was a statistically significant increase in oral candidiasis. Since Hughes et al's work in 1977, nearly 20 series involving approximately 1000 patients have been published examining the utility of selective gut prophylaxis as a means of preventing infections in a variety of immune-suppressed hosts. Despite extensive investigation, however, findings remain inconsistent.

Gurwith et al (92) examined the affect of prophylactic T-SMX on patients with malignancy and granulocytopenia. Compared to untreated controls, fewer febrile episodes were noted in the T-SMX-treated group during all degrees of granulocytopenia except in those in whom neutrophil counts fell below $10/mm^3$. Fewer bacteremias, urinary tract infections, and soft tissue infections were noted. When infections did occur, the time of onset was delayed. No significant increase in fungal infections or infections with T-SMX-resistant organisms were noted. In similar studies comparing T-SMX prophylaxis to placebo or untreated controls, a decreased incidence of infections in patients receiving T-SMX has been noted (93–97). However, the lower numbers of febrile days and diminished episodes of bacteremias noted by Gurwith et al have not been confirmed by others (94, 96, 98, 99).

Compared to trimethoprim alone, T-SMX in one comparative study was associated with more complete gut suppression. Although infection rates were lower in patients receiving T-SMX, the difference was not statistically significant (100).

In a limited number of studies, T-SMX was compared to or used in association with oral, nonabsorbable antibiotics. T-SMX plus nystatin was shown to be equivalent to gentamicin and nystatin in preventing infections in patients who were neutropenic (101). The T-SMX regimen was better tolerated, a factor which led to better patient compliance. Furthermore, while the daily cost of the T-SMX/nystatin regimen was $4.90, that of gentamicin/nystatin was $66.00. In a se-

ries of patients either with acute leukemia or undergoing bone marrow transplantation, T-SMX was shown to be superior to neomycin and colistin in preventing infections (102). T-SMX used in association with a nonabsorbable antibiotic regimen including framycetin sulphate, colistin sulphate, and nystatin (FRACON) proved more effective in decreasing infections, reducing days of fever, and delaying the onset of infections than the nonabsorbable antibiotic regimen used alone (103).

Compared to nalidixic acid, T-SMX appeared more effective in delaying onset of first infection, reducing the number of total infections, and reducing the number of episodes of bacteremia in patients undergoing initial induction chemotherapy for acute leukemia (104).

Despite the ease of twice a day scheduling, decreased cost, and increased compliance, major problems have been recognized with use of T-SMX. Some series have reported no significant differences in overall infection rate, febrile episodes, or incidence of bacteremias with T-SMX compared to untreated controls (97, 105). While differences in patient population, and duration and severity of granulocytopenia have been offered as possible explanations for these findings, no significant differences in these parameters between the studies showing a positive response and those showing an equivocal response are discernible. Hackbarth et al have suggested that the suppressive effect of T-SMX in blood cultures may have diminished the efficiency of laboratory recovery of organisms, making results appear more favorable in the T-SMX-treated groups (106). An increased incidence of fungal colonization, fungal infection, and death due to fungal infection has been reported, even when oral antifungal prophylaxis has been administered (93, 97, 103, 107). Furthermore, an increased incidence of T-SMX-resistant organisms has been detected in patients receiving T-SMX. Since T-SMX resistance results from a transmissible plasmid that also codes for resistance to carbenicillin, this phenomenon could have important epidemiologic and therapeutic ramifications (108). In some series, prolongation of profound neutropenia was noted in patients receiving T-SMX (98, 99, 103, 104). Finally, the overall impact of T-SMX on the clinical course of underlying disease has been unimpressive. Although decreased mortality from gram-negative sepsis has been reported (109), overall deaths as well as remission rates have remained unaffected (99, 109).

More involved means of preserving colonization resistance have been attempted using a regimen of neomycin, polymyxin B, amphotericin, and nalidixic acid (110, 111). As with use of T-SMX or nalidixic acid alone, the goal has been to suppress aerobic bacteria in the gut, while allowing the anaerobic flora to persist. Compared to untreated, nonrandomized controls, this regimen has been associated with a decrease in the number of acquired major infections after the first week of prophylaxis, although the number of febrile days and minor infections remained unchanged. Results were similar with or without use of protected environment, topical decontamination procedures, or specially prepared food.

As with the use of protective isolation and total protected environments, the use of oral nonabsorbable antibiotics as a means of reducing infection in the compromised host should be viewed as useful in a limited group of patients in a well defined clinical setting. Profound prolonged neutropenia (<100 neutrophils/μl for 2 weeks or more) has been suggested as a prerequisite for use of oral nonabsorbable antibiotic regimens (112). Lesser degrees of neutropenia are associated with lower infection rates and less significant impact of prophylactic antibiotics. A strong nursing staff must be present to provide for regular administration of drugs and for close vigilance to insure that most drug doses are taken. Facilities and personnel to obtain and process surveillance cultures are needed to determine the emergence of significant antibiotic resistance patterns. Most importantly, a group of patients needs to be defined in whom prolonging infection-free periods or reducing the incidence of infection via oral nonabsorbable antibiotics improves response rates and long term survival.

Topical Antibiotic Prophylaxis

Topical antibiotic regimens have been used widely in total protected environments. Skin decontamination usually involves daily showers and shampoos with povidone-iodine, chlorhexidene, or other antibacterial solutions, as well as routine cleaning of the axilla, groin, and perineum. Mucosal surfaces (nose and mouth) have been treated with sprays and ointments composed of a variety of antibacterial and antifungal agents, including polymyxin B, vancomycin, neomycin, bacitracin, and nystatin (50, 54, 75). Unfortunately, specific studies have not been conducted examining the role of these regimens in reducing colonization and subsequent infection apart from the other components of the total protected environment.

The effect of topical agents, both in decreasing colonization as well as infection, therefore, can only be estimated. Studies by Levine et al (54) and Bodey and Rosenbaum (75) demonstrated that bacterial and fungal flora in the oral cavity were rarely eliminated and that organisms persist at levels of 10^5 to 10^6. Skin decontamination is often incomplete, with the groin and perirectal area representing the sites of highest bacterial persistence. While the use of povidone-iodine-impregnated swabs has been shown to reduce the incidence of axillary infection in patients with acute nonlymphocytic leukemia, the effect of topical regimens in reducing infectious risks in the compromised host remains unclear (113).

PROPHYLAXIS OF SPECIAL PATHOGENS
Viruses

Patients undergoing bone marrow or organ transplantation, as well as those with chemotherapy-induced bone marrow failure, are at high risk of developing herpes simplex virus infections due to reactivation of latent virus (114–116). Incidences of up to 40% have been reported, especially in patients with positive herpes simplex serologies prior to therapy (117–119). Acyclovir, a guanine derivative, is preferentially incorporated into cells infected with herpes viruses where it is transformed by a viral thymidine kinase and phosphorylated. It then inhibits viral DNA synthesis. Used prophylactically, acylovir, both orally and intravenously, has been shown in double-blind, placebo-controlled studies to prevent herpes simplex disease in patients with leukemia and in patients receiving bone marrow transplantation (117–121). Once prophylaxis is stopped, recurrence of infection is common, indicating that the drug affects reactivation of the virus rather than its latency.

Varicella-zoster infection is a severe infection in children who are immune-suppressed (122). Use of zoster immune globulin (ZIG) obtained from patients recovering from herpes zoster infection, varicella-zoster immune globulin (VZIG) obtained from plasma of volunteer donors screened for high titers of varicella-zoster antibiotics, or zoster immune plasma (ZIP) has been shown to be effective in ameliorating disease (123–125). The clinical attack rate of varicella in immune-compromised patients, exposed to viruses but receiving passive immunization, ranges from 20 to 68% (123, 124, 126). This is lower than the usual 80 to 90% attack rate noted in household exposures (127). Complication rates of about 7% have been reported in immunized patients compared to the 30% complication rate in high risk children not receiving immune prophylaxis (122, 123, 128). While the natural subclinical attack rate is about 5%, the subclinical attack rate in immunized, immune-suppressed children has been reported to be as high as 33% (123). The only major drawback of passive immunization is that exposure to varicella-zoster virus must be recognized so that prophylaxis can be given.

Although human interferon and transfer factor have been suggested as means of preventing varicella-zoster infection, they remain experimental (128). Similarly, a live attenuated varicella vaccine has been available for over 10 years (129). However, only small numbers of compromised patients have been evaluated (130).

Cytomegalovirus (CMV) infection is a common infectious problem in various compromised hosts. In renal transplant recipients, it has been associated with superinfection or co-infection with fungi, bacteria, and protozoa (131, 132), renal allograft rejection (133–135), glomerulopathy (136), and an array of clinical syndromes ranging from fever to disseminated disease (134–140). The majority of cases of interstitial pneumonia in bone marow transplant recipients, and up to 26% of pneumonias of any kind, will be due to CMV (141–143). A variety of agents have proven ineffective against CMV infections (144–146). However, in bone marrow transplant recipients not receiving leukocyte transfusions (a recognized risk factor for CMV infection) passive immunization with CMV immune globulin has been associated with a significant reduction not only in infection rate (147) but also in the incidence of symptomatic infection and of interstitial pneumonia (148, 149). Complete protection against CMV in patients receiving CMV hyperimmune globulin has been reported (150).

Since blood products are a source of CMV exposure, screening programs have been developed to ensure that only CMV-seronegative donors are used for immune-suppressed hosts. In a preliminary report, use of prescreened, seronegative blood products was more effective than CMV immune globulin in preventing infection in marrow recipients from seronegative donors (151). Interferon has been used in renal transplant recipients and has been shown to delay the onset of CMV excretion and decrease the incidence of viremia (152). A live attenuated CMV vaccine has been developed (153) and used in renal transplant recipients (154). The overall utilization and safety of these latter means of CMV prophylaxis remain unproven.

Protozoa

Trimethoprim-sulfamethoxazole (T-SMX) was first shown in the early 1970s to prevent the development of *P. carinii* infection in an animal model (155). Using this as the basis for human investigation, Hughes et al demonstrated that T-SMX (5 mg/kg of trimethoprim, 20 mg/kg of sulfamethoxazole/day) could prevent disease in a highly susceptible population of children and young adults with malignancy (91). Widespread use of T-SMX has not developed because of concerns that T-SMX may be associated with development of resistance in *Pneumocystis* (156) and because T-SMX is not well tolerated by all patient populations (157–159). T-SMX prophylaxis against *P. carinii* is therefore recommended only for patients in geographic areas where a high incidence of disease can be documented.

Immunoprophylaxis of Bacterial Infections

Core glycolipid, a component of bacterial cell walls, is common to a wide variety of gram-negative rods. Human antibody to core glycolipid from a mutant *E. coli* has been shown to be effective in reducing morbidity from gram-negative bacteremia and shock (160). A trial of prophylactic antibody in severely neutropenic patients has failed to demonstrate an effect on the incidence of gram-negative infection, mortality due to gram-negative infection, or even number of febrile days (161).

Pneumococcal vaccine, containing polysaccharide from the pneumococcal strains responsible for the majority of infections, has been used in a variety of immune-compromised hosts. Patients with Hodgkin's disease undergoing therapy have demonstrated low and inconsistent responses (162, 163). Subnormal responses have also been noted in patients with chronic lymphocytic leukemia, myeloma (164–166) and in certain patients with solid tumors (167). Normal antibody responses have been noted in patients with lymphoma and chronic myelocytic leukemia if vaccine was given before chemotherapy, irradiation, or splenectomy (168, 169). Whether even low rises in antibody offer protection remains unclear. However, no definitive evidence has been produced showing that use of vaccine prevents pneumococcal disease in immune-suppressed patients (168, 170, 171).

Prophylaxis in the Splenectomized Patient

Patients who undergo splenectomy are at an increased risk of infection. In an extensive review of over 2000 cases, Singer noted a sepsis rate of

4.25% and a death rate from sepsis of 2.25% (172). This represents an increased risk of death from sepsis over the general population of 225-fold (173). The risk of postsplenectomy sepsis is related to the age of the patient, the cause for splenectomy, and the interval of time since splenectomy. Younger patients have greater risks for life-threatening infections. Children under 1 year of age have a 50% chance of developing sepsis (172); the risk of sepsis in adults has been estimated at between 1 and 2% (174, 175). Patients undergoing splenectomy for thalassemia or those receiving chemotherapy, irradiation, or immune-suppressive therapy are at higher risk for infection than patients splenectomized because of trauma. The risk of sepsis is greatest during the first year after splenectomy. Twenty percent of episodes occur within the first 6 months, 30% occur within the first year, and 66% occur within the first 2 years (172, 177, 178). However, episodes of fatal sepsis have occurred as long as 40 years postsplenectomy (179).

Encapsulated organisms most commonly cause infection in splenectomized patients. *Streptococcus pneumoniae* causes about 50% of cases, with *Haemophilus influenzae, Neisseria* species, and a variety of other gram-negative organisms also playing important roles (172, 177, 178). Because of the predominance of the pneumococcus in causing disease, penicillin prophylaxis for several years after splenectomy has been recommended (177, 178). No prospective, randomized trial with adequate numbers of patients has been carried out to document the efficacy of this practice. Although pneumococcal vaccine has been recommended, it is most effective if it can be given at least 2 weeks before the splenectomy is performed (180).

REVERSAL OF HOST DEFENSE DEFECTS—GRANULOCYTE TRANSFUSIONS

Since granulocytopenia is one of the most important risk factors for the development of infection, granulocyte transfusion as a means of prophylaxis has received a great deal of interest. The major conceptual and technologic problem involved is that of trying to provide adequate numbers of cells for transfusion. In a normal 70-kg patient, the usual daily turnover of granulocytes is approximately 10^{11}, which can be increased up to 10 times during active infection. Since the half-life of a circulating granulocyte is about 6 hours, an ongoing supply of large numbers of granulocytes is necessary to approximate a normal physiologic response. Available techniques provide only about 10^{10} neutrophils under optimal conditions, but often not even this amount can be obtained (181).

The majority of studies of prophylactic granulocyte transfusions have been carried out in neutropenic leukemics or in patients undergoing bone marrow transplantation. Alternate day transfusions of 1.2^{10} to 1.5^{10} neutrophils were attempted by Ford and Cullen (182) and Schiffer et al (183) in small numbers of patients with acute nonlymphocytic leukemia. A decrease in serious infections was noted only in the latter series, although statistical significance was not achieved. Neither study demonstrated significant differences in the number of days spent on antibiotics, number of febrile days, or, most importantly, remission rates.

Daily granulocyte transfusions have been utilized by a number of investigators. Clift et al evaluated the effect of granulocyte transfusion in 29 patients with aplastic anemia or acute leukemia undergoing bone marrow transplantation compared to 40 transplanted but nontransfused controls (184). Although the incidence of infection and sepsis was significantly reduced in the patients receiving transfusion, the incidence of fever was greater. No differences in outcome or long term survival were noted. Winston et al evaluated the efficacy of daily granulocyte transfusions used with oral nonabsorbable antibiotics compared to nonabsorbable antibiotics used alone (185). The incidence of sepsis was decreased in the group of patients receiving transfusions, but the difference was not statistically significant. There were no significant differences in the number of total infections, number of localized infections, days of fever, or days spent on antibiotics. The incidence of leukemic relapse and graft versus host disease as well as the mortality rates were comparable.

The largest series has been that of Strauss et al, who examined the effect of daily granulocyte transfusions in 54 patients with leukemia (186). The incidence of bacterial sepsis was decreased in the transfused group compared to the nontransfused controls (9% versus 27%, respectively; $p < 0.01$). As with previous studies, however, there were no differences in overall infection rates, recovery rates, or duration of survival.

Given the high cost of granulocyte harvest and transfusion (187), the lack of effect on overall infection rates and outcome, and the fact that various adverse reactions have been associated with granulocyte transfusions (183, 185, 186, 188,

189), little enthusiasm exists in recent reviews for this technique as a means of prophylaxis (190–192).

References

1. Aisenberg AC: Quantitative estimation of the reactivity of normal and Hodgkin's disease lymphocytes with thymidine-2^{14}C. *Nature* 205:1233–1235, 1965.
2. Gatti RA, Good RA: The immunological deficiency diseases. *Med Clin North Am* 54:281–307, 1970.
3. Graze PR, Perlin E, Royston I: In vitro lymphocyte dysfunction in Hodgkin's disease. *J Natl Cancer Inst* 56:239–243, 1976.
4. Aisenberg AC: Studies on delayed sensitivity in Hodgkin's disease. *J Clin Invest* 41:1964–1970, 1962.
5. Fahey JL, Scoggins R, Ute JP, Szwed CF: Infection, antibody response and gamma globulin components in multiple myeloma and macroglobulinemia. *Am J Med* 35:698–707, 1963.
6. Lippincott SW, Korman S, Forg C, Stickley E, Wolins W, Hughs WL: Turnover of labeled normal gamma globulin in multiple myeloma. *J Clin Invest* 39:565–572, 1960.
7. Marks J: Antibody formation in myelomatosis. *J Clin Pathol* 6:62–63, 1953.
8. Sweet DL Jr, Golomb HM, Ultmann JE: The clinical features of chronic lymphocytic leukaemia. *Clin Hematol* 61:185–207, 1977.
9. Masur H, Michelis MA, Greene JB, Onorato I, Vande Stouwe RA, Holzman RS, Wormser G, Brettman L, Lange M, Murray HW, Cunningham-Rundles S: An outbreak of community-acquired *Pneumocystis carinii* pneumonia: initial manifestation of cellular immune dysfunction. *N Engl J Med* 305:1431–1438, 1981.
10. Siegal FP, Lopez C, Hammer GS, Brown AE, Kornfeld SJ, Gold J, Hassett J, Hirschman SZ, Cunningham-Rundles C, Adelsberg BR, Parham DM, Siegal M, Cunningham-Rundles S, Armstrong D: Severe acquired immunodeficiency in male homosexuals, manifested by chronic perianal ulcerative herpex simplex lesions. *N Engl J Med* 305:1439–1444, 1981.
11. Gottlieb MS, Schroff R, Schanker HM, Weisman JD, Peng Thim Fan DO, Wolf RA, Saxon A: *Pneumocystis carinii* pneumonia and mucosal candidiasis in previously healthy homosexual men. *N Engl J Med* 305:1425–1431, 1981.
12. Small CB, Klein RS, Friedland GH, Moll B, Emeson EE, Spigland I: Community acquired opportunistic infections and defective cellular immunity in heterosexual drug abusing and homosexual men. *Am J Med* 74:433–441, 1983.
13. Stahl RE, Friedman-Kien A, Dubin R, Marmor M, Zolla-Pazner S: Immunologic abnormalities in homosexual men: relationship to Kaposi's sarcoma. *Am J Med* 73:171–178, 1982.
14. Keusch GT: The effects of malnutrition on host defenses and the metabolic sequence of infections. In Grieco MH (ed): *Infections in the Abnormal Host.* New York, Yorke Medical Books, 1980, pp 210–223.
15. Bodey GP, Buckley M, Sathe YS, Freireich EJ: Quantitative relationships between circulating leukocytes and infections in patients with acute leukemia. *Ann Intern Med* 64:328–340, 1966.
16. Kurrle E, Bhaduri S, Krieger D, Gaus W, Heimpel H, Pflieger H, Arnold R, Vanek E: Risk factors for infections of the oropharynx and the respiratory tract in patients with acute leukemia. *J Infect Dis* 144:128–136, 1981.
17. Chang HY, Rodriquez V, Narboni G, Bodey GP, Luna MA, Freireich EJ: Causes of death in adults with acute leukemia. *Medicine* 55:259–268, 1976.
18. Degregorio MW, Lee WMF, Linler CA, Jacobs RA, Ries CA: Fungal infections in patients with acute leukemia. *Am J Med* 73:543–548, 1982.
19. Young RC, Bennett JE, Vogel CL, Carbone PP, DeVita VT: Aspergillosis: the spectrum of disease in 98 patients. *Medicine* 49:147–173, 1970.
20. Boggs DR, Athens JW, Cartwright GE, Wintrobe MM: The effect of adrenal glucocorticosteroids upon the cellular composition of inflammatory exudates. *Am J Pathol* 44:763–773, 1964.
21. Peters WP, Holland JF, Hansjoerg S, Senn H, Rhomberg W, Banerjee T: Corticosteroid administration and localized leukocyte mobilization in man. *N Engl J Med* 286:342–345, 1972.
22. Perper RJ, Sanda M, Chinea G, Oronsky AL: Leukocyte chemotaxis in vivo. II. Analysis of the selective inhibition of neutrophil or mononuclear cell accumulation. *J Lab Clin Med* 84:394–406, 1974.
23. MacGreger RR, Spagnulo PJ, Lentnek AL: Inhibition of granulocyte adherence by ethanol, prednisone, and aspirin, measured with an assay system. *N Engl J Med* 291:642–646, 1974.
24. Rinehart JJ, Sagore AL, Balcerzak SO, Ackerman GA, LoBuglio AF: Effects of corticosteroid therapy on human monocyte function. *N Engl J Med* 292:236–241, 1975.
25. Atkinson JP, Schreiber AD, Frank MM: Effects of corticosteroids and splenectomy on the immune clearance and destruction of erythrocytes. *J Clin Invest* 52:1509–1517, 1973.
26. Weston WL, Mandell JM, Yeckley JA, Krueger GG, Clamen HN: Mechanism of cortisol inhibition of adoptive transfer of tuberculin sensitivity. *J Lab Clin Med* 82:366–371, 1973.
27. Fauci AS, Dale DC: The effect of in vitro hydrocortisone on subpopulations of human lymphocytes. *J Clin Invest* 53:240–246, 1974.
28. Clamen HN: Corticosteroids and lymphoid cells. *N Engl J Med* 287:388–397, 1972.
29. Weston WL, Clamon HN, Krueger CG: Site of action of cortisol in cellular immunity. *J Immunol* 110:880–883, 1973.
30. Stavy L, Cophen IR, Feldman M: The effect of hydrocortisone on lymphocyte-mediated cytolysis. *Cell Immunol* 7:302–312, 1973.
31. Fauci AS (moderator), NIH Conference: Glucorticosteroid therapy: mechanisms of action and clinical considerations. *Ann Intern Med* 84:305–315, 1976.
32. Santos GW, Owens AH Jr, Sensenbrenner LL: Effects of selected cytotoxic agents on antibody production in man; a preliminary report. *Ann NY Acad Sci* 114:404–423, 1964.
33. Feingold DS: Hospital-acquired infections. *N Engl J Med* 283:1384–1391, 1970.

34. Reinarz JA, Pierce AK, Mays BB, Anford JP: The potential role of inhalation therapy equipment in nosocomial pulmonary infection. *J Clin Invest* 44:831–839, 1965.

35. Ringrose RE, McKown B, Felton FG, Barclay BO, Muchmore HG, Rhoades ER: A hospital outbreak of *Serratia marcescens* associated with ultrasonic nebulizers. *Ann Intern Med* 69:719–729, 1968.

36. Schimpff SC, Young VM: Epidemiology and prevention of infection in the compromised host. In Rubin RH, Young LS (eds): *Clinical Approach to Infection in the Compromised Host.* New York, Plenum, 1981, p 12.

37. Schimpff SC, Young VM, Greene WH, Vermeulen GD, Moody MR, Wiernik PA: Origin of infection in acute nonlymphocytic leukemia: significance of hospital acquisition of potential pathogens. *Ann Intern Med* 77:707–714, 1972.

38. Nauseef WM, Maki DG: A study of the value of simple protective isolation in patients with granulocytopenia. *N Engl J Med* 304:448–453, 1981.

39. Reyniers JA, Trexler PC: The germfree technique and its application to rearing animals free from contamination. In Reyniers JA (ed): *Micrurgical and Germ-Free Methods.* Springfield, IL, Charles C Thomas, 1943, p 114.

40. Pollard M, Sharon N: Chemotherapy of spontaneous leukemia in germ-free AKR mice. *J Natl Cancer Inst* 45:677–680, 1970.

41. Reyniers JA, Trexler PC, Scruggs W, Wagner M, Gordon HA: Observation on germ-free and conventional albino rats after total body X-radiation (abstract). *Radiat Res* 5:591, 1956.

42. White LP, Claflin EF: Nitrogen mustard: diminution of toxicity in axenic mice. *Science* 140:1400–1401, 1963.

43. Levenson SM: Application of the technology of the germ-free laboratory to special problems of patient care. *Am J Surg* 107:710–722, 1964.

44. Haynes BW Jr, Hench ME: Hospital isolation system for preventing cross contamination by staphylococci and *Pseudomonas* organisms in burn wounds. *Ann Surg* 162:641–649, 1965.

45. Hall LB: NASA requirements for the sterilization of spacecraft. *Proc Natl Conf Spacecraft Steril Technol (NASA Suppl)* 108:25–36, 1966.

46. Bodey GP, Johnston D: Microbiological evaluation of protected environment during patient occupancy. *Appl Microbiol* 22:828–835, 1971.

47. Michaelsen GS, Vesley D, Halbert MM: Laminar air flow studied as and in care of low resistance patient. *Hospitals* 41:91–106, 1967.

48. Shadomy S, Ginsberg M, Laconte M, Zieger E: Evaluation of a patient isolator system. *Arch Environ Health* 11:191–200, 1985.

49. Young VM, Moody MR, Clinical gnotobiotics. *Am J Clin Nutr* 30:1911–1920, 1977.

50. Yates JW, Holland JF: A controlled study of isolation and endogenous microbial suppression in acute myelocytic leukemia patients. *Cancer* 32:1490–1498, 1972.

51. Dietrich M, Gaus W, Vossen J, van der Waaij D, Wendt F: Protective isolation and antimicrobial decontamination in patients with high susceptibility to infection. *Infection* 5:107–114, 1977.

52. Pizzo PA, Levine AS: The utility of protected environment regimens for the compromised host: a clinical assessment. *Prog Hematol* 10:311–332, 1977.

53. Schimpff SC, Greene WH, Young VM, Fortner CL, Hauser J, Priesler H, Goldstein IM, Seidler F, Simon R, Perry S, Bennett JE, Henderson ES: Infection prevention in acute nonlymphocytic leukemia: laminar air flow room reverse isolation with oral nonabsorbable antibiotic prophylaxis. *Ann Intern Med* 82:351–358, 1975.

54. Levine AS, Siegel SE, Schriber AD, Hauser J, Preisler H, Goldstein IM, Seidler F, Simon R, Seymour P, Bennett JE, Henderson ES: Protected environment and prophylactic antibiotics: a prospective controlled study of their utility in the therapy of acute leukemia. *N Engl J Med* 288:477–484, 1973.

55. Rodriquez V, Bodey GP, Freireich EG, McCredie KB, Gutterman JU, Keating MJ, Smith TL, Gehan EA: Randomized trial of protected environment-prophylactic antibiotics in 145 adults with acute leukemia. *Medicine* 57:253–266, 1978.

56. Navari RM, Buckner CD, Cleft RA, Storb R, Sanders JE, Stewart P, Sullivan KM, Williams B, Counts GW, Meyers JD, Thomas ED: Prophylaxis of infection in patients with aplastic anemia receiving allogeneic marrow transplants. *Am J Med* 76:564–572, 1984.

57. Buckner DC, Cleft RA, Sanders JE: Protective environment for marrow transplant recipients: a prophylactic study. *Ann Intern Med* 89:893–910, 1978.

58. Armstrong D: Protected environments are discomforting and expensive and do not offer meaningful protection. *Am J Med* 76:685–689, 1984.

59. Holland J, Plumb M, Yates J, Harris S, Tuttolvmondo A, Holmes J, Holland JF: Psychological response of patients with acute leukemia to germ-free environments. *Cancer* 40:871–879, 1977.

60. Bodey GP, Rodriquez V, Cabanillas F, Freireich EJ; Protected environment-prophylactic antibiotic program for malignant lymphoma: randomized trial during remission induction chemotherapy. *Am J Med* 66:74–81, 1979.

61. Bodey GP, Rodriquez V, Murphy WK, Burgess MA, Benjamin RS: Protected environment-prophylactic antibiotic program for malignant sarcomas: randomized trial during remission induction chemotherapy. *Cancer* 47:2422–2429, 1981.

62. Strob R, Prentice RL, Buckner DC, Clift RA, Appelbaum F, Deeg J, Doney K, Hansen JA, Mason M, Sanders JE, Singer J, Sullivan KM, Witherspoon RP, Thomas ED: Graft versus host disease and survival in patients with aplastic anemia treated by marrow grafts from HLA-identical siblings: beneficial effect of a protective environment. *N Engl J Med* 308:302–307, 1983.

63. Shooter RA, Cooke EM, Faiers MC, Breaden AL, O'Farrell SM: Isolation of *Escherichia coli, Pseudomonas aeruginosa* and *Klebsiella* from food in hospitals, canteens and schools. *Lancet* 2:390–392, 1971.

64. Kominos SD, Copeland CE, Grosiak B, Postic B: Introduction of *Pseudomonas aeruginosa* into a

hospital via vegetables. *Appl Microbiol* 24:567–570, 1972.

65. Wright C, Kominos SD, Yee RB: Enterobacteriaceae and *Pseudomonas aeruginosa* recovered from vegetable salads. *Appl Environ Microbiol* 31:453–454, 1976.

66. Casewell M, Phillips I: Food as a source of *Klebsiella* species for colonization and infection of intensive care patients. *J Clin Pathol* 31:845–849, 1978.

67. Buck AC, Cooke EM: The fate of ingested *Pseudomonas aeruginosa* in normal persons. *J Med Microbiol* 2:521–525, 1969.

68. Van der Waaij D, Berghuis JM, Lekkerkerk JEC: Colonization resistance of the digestive tract of mice during systemic antibiotic treatment. *J Hyg* 70:605–610, 1972.

69. Remington JS, Schimpff SC: Please don't eat the salads. *N Engl J Med* 304:433–435, 1981.

70. Reimer AO, Tillotson JL: Food service procedures for reverse isolation. *J Am Diet Assoc* 48:381–384, 1966.

71. Watson P, Bodey GP: Sterile food service for patients in protected environments. *J Am Diet Assoc* 56:515–520, 1970.

72. Preisler HJ, Goldstein IM, Henderson ES: Gastrointestinal sterilization in the treatment of patients with acute leukemia. *Cancer* 26:1076–1081, 1970.

73. Pizzo PA, Purvis DS, Waters C: Microbiological evaluation of food items for patients undergoing gastrointestinal decontamination and protected isolation. *J Am Diet Assoc* 81:272–279, 1982.

74. Newman KA, Schimpff SC, Wade JC: Antibiotic prophylaxis for infection for patients with granulocytopenia. In Verhoef J, Peterson PK, Quie PG (eds):*Infections in the Immunocompromised Host—Pathogenesis, Prevention, and Therapy.* New York, Elsevier/North-Holland, 1980, p 187.

75. Bodey GP, Rosenbaum B: Effect of prophylactic measures in the microbial flora of patients in protected environment units. *Medicine* 53:209–228, 1974.

76. Bodey GP; Antibiotic prophylaxis in cancer patients: regimens of oral nonabsorbable antibiotics for prevention of infection during induction of remission. *Rev Infect Dis* 3 (suppl):S259–S268, 1981.

77. Hahn DM, Schimpff SC, Fortner CL, Smyth AC, Young VM, Wiernik PH: Infection in acute leukemia patients receiving oral nonabsorbable antibiotics. *Antimicrob Agents Chemother* 13:958–964, 1978.

78. King K: Prophylactic nonabsorbable antibiotics in leukemic patients. *J Hyg (Camb)* 85:141–151, 1980.

79. Bodey GP: Oral antibiotic prophylaxis in protected environment units: effect of nonabsorbable and absorbable antibiotics on the fecal flora. *Antimicrob Agents Chemother* 1:343–347, 1972.

80. Bender JF, Schimpff SC, Young VM, Fortner CL, Brouillet MD, Love LJ, Wiernik PH: Role of vancomycin as a component of oral nonabsorbable antibiotics for microbial suppression in leukemic patients. *Antimicrob Agents Chemother* 15:455–460, 1979.

81. Storring RH, McElwain TJ, Jameson B, Wiltshaw E: Oral non-absorbable antibiotics prevent acute infection in acute non-lymphoblastic leukemia. *Lancet* 1:837–841, 1977.

82. Lohner D, Debusscher L, Prevost JM, Klastersky J: Comparative randomized study of protected environment plus oral antibiotics versus oral antibiotics alone in neutropenic patients' cancer treatment. *Cancer Treat Rep* 63:363–368, 1979.

83. Bodey GP, Hart J, Freireich EJ, Frei E III: Studies of a patient isolation unit and prophylactic antibiotics in cancer chemotherapy: general techniques and preliminary results. *Cancer* 22:1018–1026, 1968.

84. Cohen MH, Crearen PF, Fossieck BE, Johnston AV, Williams CL: Effect of oal prophylactic broad spectrum nonabsorbable antibiotics on the gastrointestinal absorption of nutrients and methotrexate in small cell bronchogenic carcinoma patients. *Cancer* 38:1556–1559, 1976.

85. Valdivieso M, Cabanillos F, Keating M, Borkley HT, Murphy WK, Frazier H, Chen T, Bodey GP: Effect of intensive induction chemotherapy for extensive disease small cell bronchogenic carcinoma in protected environment-prophylactic antibiotic units. *Am J Med* 76:405–412, 1984.

86. Bodey GP, Keating MJ, McCredie KB, Elting L, Rosenbaum B, Freireich EJ; Prospective randomized trial of antibiotic prophylaxis in acute leukemia. *Am J Med* 78:407–416, 1985.

87. van der Waaij D, Berghuis-De Vries JM: Selective elimination of Enterobacteriaceae species from the digestive tract in mice and monkeys. *J Hyg (Camb)* 72:205–211, 1974.

88. Naff H: On the changes in the intestinal flora induced in man by Bactrim. *Pathol Microbiol* 37:1–22, 1971.

89. Knothe H: The effect of a combined preparation of trimethoprim and sulfamethoxazole following short term and long term administration on the flora of the human gut. *Chemotherapy* 18:285–296, 1973.

90. Hargadon MT, Young VM, Schimpff SC, Wade JC, Minah GE: Selective suppression of alimentary tract microbial flora as prophylaxis during granulocytopenia. *Antimicrob Agents Chemother* 1:343–347, 1972.

91. Hughes WT, Kuhn S, Chaudhany S, Feldman S, Verzosa M, Aur RJA, Pratt C, George SL: Successful chemoprophylaxis for *Pneumocystis carinii* pneumonia. *N Engl J Med* 297:1419–1426, 1977.

92. Gurwith MJ, Brunton JL, Lank BA, Harding GKM, Ronald AR: A prospective controlled investigation of prophylactic trimethoprim/sulfamethoxazole in hospitalized granulocytopenic patients. *Am J Med* 66:248–256, 1979.

93. Estey E, Maksymiuk A, Smith T, Fainstein V, Keating M, McCredie KB, Freireich EJ, Bodey GP: Infection prophylaxis in acute leukemia: comparative effectiveness of sulfamethoxazole and trimethoprim, ketoconazole, and a combination of the two. *Arch Intern Med* 144:1562–1568, 1984.

94. Henry SA: Chemoprophylaxis of bacterial infections in granulocytopenic patients. *Am J Med* 67:645–652, 1984.

95. Kauffman CA, Leipman MK, Bergman AG, Mioduszewski J; Trimethoprim/sulfamethoxazole prophylaxis in neutropenic patients. *Am J Med* 74:599–607, 1983.

96. EORTC International Antimicrobial Therapy Project Group: Trimethoprim-sulfamethoxazole in the prevention of infection in neutropenic patients. *J Infect Dis* 150:372–379, 1984.

97. Henry SA, Armstrong D, Kempin S, Gee T, Arlen Z, Clarkson B: Oral trimethoprim/sulfamethoxazole in attempt to prevent infection after induction chemotherapy for acute leukemia. *Am J Med* 77:663–666, 1984.

98. Gualtieri RJ, Donowitz GR, Kaiser DL, Hess CE, Sande MA: Double blind randomized study of prophylactic trimethoprim/sulfamethoxazole in granulocytopenic patients with hematologic malignancies. *Am J Med* 74:934–940, 1983.

99. Dekker AW, Rozenberg-Arska M, Sixma JJ, Verhoef J: Prevention of infection by trimethoprim-sulfamethoxazole plus amphotericin B in patients with acute non-lymphocytic leukemia. *Ann Intern Med* 95:558–559, 1981.

100. Bow EJ, Louie TJ, Riben PD, McNaughton RD, Harding GKM, Ronald AR: Randomized controlled trial comparing trimethoprim/sulfamethoxazole and trimethoprim for infection prophylaxis in hospitalized granulocytopenic patients. *Am J Med* 76:223–233, 1984.

101. Wade JC, Schimpff SC, Hargadon MT, Fortner CL, Young VM, Wiernik PH: A comparison of trimethoprim-sulfamethoxazole plus nystatin with gentamicin plus nystatin in the prevention of infections in acute leukemia. *N Engl J Med* 304:1057–1062, 1981.

102. Watson JG, Powles RL, Lason DN, Morgenstean GR, Jameson B, McElwain TJ, Judson I, Lumley H, Kay HEM: Co-trimoxazole versus nonabsorbable antibiotics in acute leukemia. *Lancet* 1:6–9, 1982.

103. Enno A, Darrell J, Hows J, Catovsky D, Goldman JM, Galton DAG: Co-trimoxazole for prevention of infection in acute leukemia. *Lancet* 2:395–397, 1978.

104. Wade JC, deJongh CA, Newman KA, Crowley J, Wiernik PH, Schimpff SC: Selective antimicrobiol modulation as prophylaxis against infection during granulocytopenia: trimethoprim-sulfamethoxazole vs nalidixic acid. *J Infect Dis* 147:624–634, 1983.

105. Weiser B, Longe M, Fialk MA, Singer C, Szatrowski TH, Armstrong D: Prophylactic trimethoprim-sulfamethoxazole during consolidation chemotherapy for acute leukemia. *Ann Intern Med* 95:436–438, 1981.

106. Hackbarth CJ, Ernst JD, Sande MA: Inhibition of isolation of *Escherichia coli* in blood cultures by trimethoprim-sulfamethoxazole. *J Infect Dis* 147:964–965, 1983.

107. Bavisotto L, Maki DG: Does TMP-SMX prophylaxis in acute non-lymphocytic leukemia (ANLL) predispose to fungal infection? *Clin Res* 29:726A, 1981.

108. Wilson JM, Guiney DG: Failure of oral trimethoprim-sulfamethoxazole prophylaxis in acute leukemia—isolation of resistant plasmids from strains of Enterobacteriaceae causing bacteremia. *N Engl J Med* 306:16–20, 1982.

109. Riben PD, Louie TJ, Lank BA, Kornachuk E, Gurwith MJ, Harding GKM, Ronald AR: Reduction in mortality from gram-negative sepsis in neutropenic patients receiving trimethoprim/sulfamethoxazole therapy. *Cancer* 51:1587–1592, 1983.

110. Guiot HFL, van der Meer JWM, van Furth R: Selective antimicrobial modulation of human microbial flora: infection prevention in patients with decreased host defense mechanisms by selective elimination of potentially pathogenic bacteria. *J Infect Dis* 143:644–654, 1981.

111. Guiot HFL, van den Broek, van der Meer JWM, van Furth R: Selective antimicrobial modulation of the intestinal flora of patients with acute non-lymphocytic leukemia: a double blind placebo control study. *J Infect Dis* 147:615–623, 1983.

112. Schimpff SC: Infection prevention during profound granulocytopenia: new approaches to alimentary canal microbial suppression. *Ann Intern Med* 93:358–361, 1980.

113. Murillo J, Schimpff SC, Brouillet MD: Axillary lesions in patients with acute leukemia. *Cancer* 49:1493–1496, 1979.

114. Elfenbein GJ, Saral R: Infectious disease during immune recovery after bone marrow transplantation. In Allen JC (ed): *Infection and the Compromised Host.* Baltimore, Williams & Wilkins, 1971, p 157.

115. Meyers JD, Fluornoy N, Thomass ED: Infection with herpes simplex virus and cell mediated immunity after marrow transplant. *J Infect Dis* 142:338–346, 1980.

116. Pass RF, Whitley RJ, Whelchel JD, Diethelm AG, Reynolds DW, Alford CA: Identification of patients with increased risk of infection with herpes simplex virus after renal transplantation. *J Infect Dis* 140:487–492, 1979.

117. Gluckman E, Devergee A, Melo R: Prophylaxis of herpes infection after bone marrow transplantation by oral acyclovir. *Lancet* 2:706–708, 1983.

118. Saral R, Ambinder RF, Burns WH; Acyclovir prophylaxis against herpes simplex virus infections in patients with leukemia. *Ann Intern Med* 99:773–776, 1983.

119. Hann IM, Prentice HG, Blacklock HA: Acyclovir prophylaxis against herpes virus infection in severely immunocompromised patients: randomized double blind trial. *Br Med J* 287:384–388, 1983.

120. Wade JC, Newton B, Flouring N, Meyers JD: Oral acyclovir for prevention of herpes simplex virus reactivation after marrow transplantation. *Ann Intern Med* 100:823–828, 1984.

121. Saral R, Burns WH, Laskn OL, Santos GW, Lietman PS; Acyclovir prophylaxis of herpes simplex virus infections: a randomized double-blind controlled trial in bone marrow transplant recipient. *N Engl J Med* 305:63–67, 1981.

122. Feldman S, Hughes W, Daniel C: Varicella in children with cancer. Seventy-seven cases. *Pediatrics* 56:388–397, 1975.

123. Gershon AA, Steinberg S, Brunell PA: Zoster immune globulin: a further assessment. *N Engl J*

Med 290:243–245, 1974.

124. Zaia JA, Levin MJ, Preblud SR, Leszczynski J, Wright GG, Ellis RJ, Curtis AC, Valiero MA, LeGore J: Evaluation of varicella zoster immune globulin: protection of immune-suppressed children after household exposure to varicella. *J Infect Dis* 147:737–743, 1983.

125. Balfocin HH, Groth KE, McCullough J, Kalis JM, Marker SC, Nesbit ME, Simmons RL, Najarian JS: Prevention or modification of varicella using zoster immune plasma. *Am J Dis Child* 131:693–696, 1977.

126. Judelsohn RG, Meyers JD, Ellis RJ, Thomas EK: Efficacy of zoster immune globulin. *Pediatrics* 53:476–480, 1974.

127. Ross AH, Leuchner E, Reitman G: Modification of chickenpox in family contacts by administration of gamma globulin. *N Engl J Med* 267:369–376, 1962.

128. Gershon AA: Immunoprophylaxis of varicella-zoster infections. *Am J Med* 76:672–677, 1984.

129. Takahashi M, Otsuka T, Okuno Y, Asano Y, Yazaki T: Live vaccine used to prevent the spread of varicella in children in hospital. *Lancet* 2:1288–1290, 1974.

130. Brunnell P, Geiser C, Shehab Z, Waugh JE: Administration of live varicella vaccine to children with leukemia. *Lancet* 2:1069–1072, 1982.

131. Chatterjee SN, Fiala M, Weiner J, Stewart JA, Stacey B, Warner N: Primary cytomegalovirus and opportunistic infections: incidence in renal transplant patients. *JAMA* 240:2446–2449, 1978.

132. Rand KH, Polland RB, Merigan TC: Increased pulmonary superinfections in cardiac transplant patients undergoing primary cytomegalovirus infection. *N Engl J Med* 298:951–953, 1978.

133. Peterson PK, Balfour HH, Marker SC, Fryd DS, Howard RJ, Simmons RL: Cytomegalovirus disease in renal allograft recipients: a prospective study of the clinical features, risk factors and impact on renal transplantation. *Medicine* 59:283–300, 1980.

134. Betts RF, Freeman RB, Douglas RG, Talley TE: Clinical manifestation of renal allograft derived primary cytomegalovirus infection. *Am J Dis Child* 131:759–763, 1977.

135. Rubin RH, Cosimi AB, Tolkoff-Rubin NE, Russell PS, Hirsch MS: Infectious disease syndromes attributable to cytomegalovirus and their significance among renal transplant recipients. *Transplantation* 24:458–464, 1977.

136. Richardson WP, Colvin RB, Cheeseman SH, Tolkoff-Rubin NE, Herrin JT, Cosimi AB, Collins AB, Hirsch MS, McCluskey RT, Russell PS, Rubin RH; Glomerulopathy associated with cytomegalovirus viremia in renal allografts. *N Engl J Med* 305:57–63, 1981.

137. Simmons RL, Lopez C, Balfour H Jr, Kalis J, Rattazzi LC, Najarian JS: Cytomegalovirus: clinical, virological correlation in renal transplant recipients. *Ann Surg* 180:623–631, 1974.

138. Fryd DS, Peterson PK, Ferguson RM, Simmons RL, Balfour HH Jr, Najarian JS: Cytomegalovirus as a risk factor in renal transplantation. *Transplantation* 30:436–449, 1980.

139. Kanich RE, Craighead JE: Cytomegalovirus infec-

tion and cytomegalic inclusion disease in renal homotransplant recipients. *Am J Med* 40:874–882, 1966.

140. Anderson Hk, Spencer ES: Cytomegalovirus infection among renal allograftrecipients. *Acta Med Scand* 186:7–19, 1969.

141. Winston DJ, Gale RP, Meyer DV, Young LS: Infectious complications of human bone marrow transplantation. *Medicine* 58:1–31, 1979.

142. Meyers JP, Spencer HC, Watts JC, Gregg MB, Stewart JA, Troupin RH, Thomas ED: Cytomegalovirus pneumonia after human marrow transplantation. *Ann Intern Med* 82:181–188, 1975.

143. Neiman PE, Reeves W, Ray G, Flournoy N, Lerner KG, Stale GE, Thomas ED: A prospective analysis of interstitial pneumonia and opportunistic viral infection among recipients of bone marrow grafts. *J Infect Dis* 136:754–767, 1977.

144. Meyers JD, McGuffin RW, Bryson YJ, Cantell K, Thomas ED: Treatment of cytomegalovirus pneumonia after marrow transplantation with combined vidarabine and human leukocyte interferon. *J Infect Dis* 146:80–84, 1982.

145. Jones JF, Minnich LL, Jeter WS, Fulginitc VA, Wedgewood RJ: Treatment of childhood combined Epstein-Barr virus/cytomegalovirus infection with oral bovine transfer factor. *Lancet* 2:122–124, 1981.

146. Ch'ien LT, Cannon NJ, Whitly RJ, Diethelm AG, Dismukes WE, Scott CW, Buchanan RA, Alford CA: Effect of adenine arabinoside on cytomegalovirus infections. *J Infect Dis* 130:32–39, 1974.

147. Meyers JD, Leszczynski J, Zaia JA, Flournoy N, Newton B, Snydman DR, Wright GG, Levin MJ, Thomas ED: Prevention of cytomegalovirus infection by cytomegalovirus immune globulin after marrow transplantation. *Ann Intern Med* 98:442–446, 1983.

148. Winston DJ, Pollard RB, Ho WG, Gallagher JG, Rosmussen LE, Huang SNY, Lin CH, Gossett TG, Merigan TC, Gale RP: Cytomegalovirus immune plasma in bone marrow transplant recipients. *Ann Intern Med* 97:11–18, 1982.

149. Winston DJ, Ho WG, Lin CH, Budinger MD, Champlin RE, Gale RP: Intravenous immunoglobulin for modification of cytomegalovirus infections associated with bone marrow transplantation: preliminary results of a controlled trial. *Am J Med* 76:128–133, 1984.

150. Condie RM, O'Reilly RJ: Prevention of cytomegalovirus infection by prophylaxis with an intravenous, hyperimmune, native, unmodified cytomegalovirus globulin; randomized trial in bone marrow transplant recipients. *Am J Med* 76:134–141, 1984.

151. Bowden RA, Sagers M, McIver J, Leszczywnski J, Flournoy N, Thomas ED, Meyers JA: Comparative trial of intravenous cytomegalovirus globulin and sero negative blood products for the prevention of primary cytomegalovirus infection following marrow transplant (abstract). *Clin Res* 33:395A, 1985.

152. Cheeseman SH, Rubin RH, Stewart JA, Tolkoff-Rubin NE, Cosmi AB, Cantell K, Gilbert J, Winkle S, Herrin JT, Black PH, Russell PS, Hirschi MS: Controlled clinical trial of prophylactic hu-

man-leukocyte interferon in renal transplantation: effects on cytomegalovirus and herpes simplex virus infections. *N Engl J Med* 300:1345–1349, 1979.

153. Plotkin SA, Farguhar J, Hornberger E: Clinical trials of immunization with the towne 125 strain of human cytomegalovirus. *J Infect Dis* 134:470–475, 1976.

154. Glazer JP, Friedman HM, Grossman RA, Starr SE, Barker CF, Perloff LJ, Huang ES, Plotkin SA: Live cytomegalovirus vaccination of renal transplant candidates: a preliminary trial. *Ann Intern Med* 91:676–683, 1979.

155. Hughes WT, McNabb PC, Markres TD: Efficacy of trimethoprim and sulfamethoxazole in the prevention and treatment of *Pneumocystiis carinii* pneumonitis. *Antimicrob Agents Chemother* 5:289–293, 1974.

156. Hugh WT, Feldman S, Chaudhary SC, Ossi MJ, Cox F, Sanyal SK: Comparison of pentamidine isethionate and trimethoprim-sulfamethoxazole in treatment of *Pneumocystis carinii* pneumonia. *J Pediatr* 92:285–291, 1978.

157. Kouals JA, Hiemenz JW, Macher AM, Stover D, Murray HW, Shelhamer J, Lane HC, Urmacher C, Honig C, Longo DL, Parker MM, Natanson L, Parrillo JE, Fauci AS, Pizzo PA, Masur H: *Pneumocystis carinii* pneumonia: a comparison between patients with the acquired immune deficiency syndrome and patients with other immuno-deficiencies. *Ann Intern Med* 100:663–671, 1984.

158. Gordin FM, Simon GL, Wofsy CB, Mills J: Adverse reactions to trimethoprim-sulfamethoxazole in patients with the acquired immunodeficiency syndrome. *Ann Intern Med* 100:495–499, 1984.

159. Bradley PD, Warden GD, Maxwell JG, Rothstein G: Neutropenia and thrombocytopenia in renal allograft recipients treated with trimethoprim-sulfamethoxazole. *Ann Intern Med* 93:560–562, 1980.

160. Ziegler EJ, McCuthan JA, Fierer J, Glauser MP, Asodd JC, Douglas H, Braude AI: Treatment of gram negative bacteremia and shock with human antiserum to a mutant *Escherichia coli. N Engl J Med* 307:1225–1230, 1982.

161. McCutchan JA, Wolf JL, Ziegler EJ, Braude AL; Ineffectiveness of single dose human antiserum to core glycolipid (*E. coli* J5) for prophylaxis of bacteremic gram negative infections in patients with prolonged neutropenia. *Schweiz Med Wochenschr* S14:40–45, 1983.

162. Siber G, Witzman SA, Aisenberg AC, Weinstein HJ, Schiffman G: Impaired antibody response to pneumococcal vaccine after treatment for Hodgkin's disease. *N Engl J Med* 299:442–448, 1978.

163. Minor DR, Schiffman G, McIntosh LS: Response of patients with Hodgkin's disease to pneumococcal vaccine. *Ann Intern Med* 90:887–892, 1979.

164. Lazarus HM, Lederman M, Lubin A, Herzig RH: Pneumococcal vaccination: the response of patients with multiple myeloma. *Am J Med* 69:419–424, 1980.

165. Predeim L, Schiffman G, Mailland J, Schlueter W: Pneumococcal vaccine response in chronic lymphocytic leukemia and multiple myeloma (abstract). *Clin Res* 27:753A, 1979.

166. Schmid GP, Smith RP, Baltch AL, Hall CA: Antibody response to pneumococcal vaccine in patients with multiple myeloma. *J Infect Dis* 143:590–597, 1981.

167. Ammann AJ, Schiffman G, Addiego JE, Wora WM, Wora DW: Immunization of immunosuppressed patients with pneumococcal polysaccharide vaccine. *Rev Infect Dis* 3 (suppl):S160–S167, 1981.

168. Young LS: Immunoprophylaxis and serotherapy of bacterial infection. *Am J Med* 76:664–671, 1984.

169. Siber GR, Weitzman SA, Aisenberg AC: Antibody response of patients with Hodgkin's disease to protein and polysaccharide antigens. *Rev Infect Dis* 3:S144–S159, 1981.

170. Broome CV, Facklam RR, Fraser DW: Pneumococcal disease after pneumococcal vaccination: an alternative method to estimate the efficacy of pneumococcal vaccine. *N Engl J Med* 303:549–552, 1980.

171. Shapiro ED, Clemens JD: A controlled evaluation of the protective efficacy of pneumococcal vaccine for patients at high risk of serious pneumococcal infections. *Ann Intern Med* 101:325–330, 1984.

172. Singer DB: Postsplenectomy sepsis. In Rosenberg HS, Bolande RP (eds): *Perspectives in Pediatric Pathology.* Chicago, Yearbook, 1973, vol 1, p 285.

173. Dancer CC, Korns RF, Schuman LM: *Infectious Diseases.* Cambridge, Harvard University Press, 1968, p 134.

174. Zarrabl MH, Rosner F: Serious infections in adults following splenectomy for trauma. *Arch Intern Med* 144:1421–1424, 1984.

175. Schwortz PE, Sterioff S, Mucha P, Melton LJ, Offord KP: Postsplenectomy sepsis and mortality in adults. *JAMA* 248:2279–2283, 1982.

176. Desser RK, Ultmann JE: Risk of severe infection in patients with Hodgkin's disease or lymphoma after diagnostic laparotomy and splenectomy. *Ann Intern Med* 77:143–146, 1972.

177. Ellison EC, Fabri PJ: Complications of splenectomy. *Surg Clin North Am* 63:1313–1330, 1983.

178. Francke EL, Neu HC: Postsplenectomy infection. *Surg Clin North Am* 61:135–155, 1981.

179. Gopal V, Bisno AL: Fulminant, pneumococcal infections in "normal" asplenic hosts. *Arch Intern Med* 137:1526–1530, 1977.

180. Centers for Disease Control: Update: pneumococcal polysaccharide vaccine usage—United States. *Ann Intern Med* 101:348–350, 1984.

181. French JE, Solomon JM, Fratantoni JC: Survey on the current use of leukapheresis and collection of granulocyte concentrates. *Transfusion* 22:220–225, 1982.

182. Ford JM, Cullen MH; Prophylactic granulocyte transfusions. *Exp Hematol* 5 (suppl):65–72, 1977.

183. Schiffer CA, Aisner J, Daly PA, Schimpff SC, Wiernik PH: Alloimmunization following prophylactic granulocyte transfusion. *Blood* 54:766–774, 1979.

184. Clift RA, Sanders JE, Thomas ED, Williams B, Buckner CA: Granulocyte transfusions for the prevention of infection in patients receiving bone-marrow transplants. *N Engl J Med* 298:1052–1057, 1978.

185. Winston DJ, Ho WG, Young LS, Gale RP: Pro-

phylactic granulocyte transfusions during human bone marrow transplantation. *Am J Med* 68:893–897, 1980.

186. Strauss RG, Connett JE, Gale RP, Bloomfield CD, Herzig GP, McCullough J, Maguire LC, Winston DJ, Ho WG, Strmp DC, Miller WV, Koepke JA: A controlled trial of prophylactic granulocyte transfusions during initial induction chemotherapy for acute myelogenous leukemia. *N Engl J Med* 305:597–603, 1981.

187. Rosenshein MS, Farewell VT, Price TH, Larson EB, Dale AC: The cost effectiveness of therapeutic and prophylactic leukocyte transfusion. *N Engl J Med* 302:1058–1062, 1980.

188. Hersman J, Meyers JD, Thomas ED, Buckner CD, Cleft R: The effect of granulocyte transfusions on the incidence of cytomegalovirus infection after allogeneic marrow transplantation. *Ann Intern Med* 96:149–152, 1982.

189. Wright DG, Robichand KJ, Pizzo P, Deisseroth AB: Lethal pulmonary reactions associated with combined use of amphotericin B and leukocyte transfusion. *N Engl J Med* 304:1185–1189, 1981.

190. Young LS: Prophylactic granulocytes in the neutropenic host. *Ann Intern Med* 96:240–242, 1982.

191. Wright DG: Leukocyte transfusions: thinking twice. *Am J Med* 76:637–644, 1984.

192. Clift RA, Buckner CD: Granulocyte transfusions. *Am J Med* 76:631–636, 1984.

Chapter 31

New Aspects of Case-Control Studies and Clinical Trials

Timothy R. Townsend, M.D.

INTRODUCTION

Methods for the design and analysis of epidemiologic studies have become increasingly sophisticated over the past few decades. Among the many reasons for this, two seem to stand out as highly significant. First, as causes of morbidity and mortality have shifted in developed nations from acute infectious diseases, where cause and effect are closely related in time and space, to more "chronic" diseases, such as cancer and heart disease, where exposure to the often multiple causal factors may have occurred years prior to the observed effect, simple methods of assessing causality have become inadequate. Second, computers have permitted the manipulation of data in ways that were too cumbersome by hand and the development of mathematical models to analyze large data sets. Over the past decade, as the understanding of infectious diseases has become more sophisticated, the methods of design and analysis, originally used to study heart disease and cancer, increasingly are being applied to studies relating to infectious diseases. A natural extension of this trend is the use of the same methods in studies involving nosocomial infections, one of the most important infectious causes of morbidity and mortality in the U.S. today. The study of nosocomial infections lends itself well to the use of these methods because, as discussed below, nosocomial infections (the outcome variable) usually do not have a single causal risk factor but are due to a complex interaction between factors related to the host, the infectious parasite, and the environment.

A single chapter in a book cannot cover in detail all elements of design and analysis of epidemiologic studies. However, many of these methods are being used in studies of nosocomial infections, and the results of these studies are appearing in the scientific literature. Therefore, this chapter can serve the 2-fold purpose of, first,

acquainting the reader with the basic concepts involved in the study methods so that interpretation of the scientific literature is possible and, second, providing the investigator with basic tools for the design and analysis of the most commonly used study methods, the clinical trial and the case-control study. For the investigator this chapter provides only an overview, and prior to initiating a study one needs to review many of the books and articles cited here and to consult a good statistician.

STUDY DESIGNS

A disease may be studied from two perspectives: an experimental or an observational approach. An observational approach is one where "nature takes its course" in that the investigator does not intervene or manipulate factors in the disease process. In experimental studies, on the other hand, the investigator controls chosen factors that may be of importance in the disease process. Both the observational and experimental approaches are used to examine cause and effect relationships between a disease and various factors thought to be important for that disease. Clinical trials are a particular type of experimental approach which are limited to studies of human disease, confined for ethical reasons to certain manipulations of risk factors, and performed in an organized clinical setting. Case-control studies are a particular type of observational approach whereby selected individuals, some with and some without the disease, are compared rather than simply enumerated (e.g., surveillance). Case-control studies are not limited by common usage to human disease, but for the purposes of this chapter will be.

Clinical Trials

The design characteristics, conduct, and basic methods of analysis of clinical trials have been well described (1–3). Only selected aspects of clinical trials will be included here.

The cause and effect relationship between one or more factors and a disease may be examined from a cause-to-effect approach. Stated in its simplest form, an investigator can study two groups of people: one group containing people that possess a particular factor thought to be important in causing the disease of interest and the other group containing people similar to the first group except that they lack the factor. The investigator observes both groups over time for the development of the disease. If the occurrence of the disease is much higher in the group possessing the factor of interest, the investigator might conclude that the factor is causally related to the disease. In a clinical trial, the same cause-to-effect approach is used except that rather than finding people with and without the factor of interest, the investigator manipulates the conditions of the experiment by assigning the factor to some of the people and withholding it from others. The investigator then follows both groups for the occurrence of disease, which should be more common in the group assigned to receive the factor if the factor causes the disease. If the group of people prior to the initiation of the clinical trial were homogeneous with respect to other factors, such as age, sex, race, etc., if the method of assigning the risk factor was unbiased, and if the groups of people were large enough to determine if the occurrence of disease was different in the two groups, then the investigator's claim of a cause and effect relationship would be strengthened.

An investigator must be careful to balance the need for a homogeneous study population with the need that it not be too homogeneous. If the population is not homogeneous enough, then factors that are also important in causing the disease may be present and by chance alone may occur more commonly in the study group exposed to the assigned risk factor, which would enhance the apparent importance of the assigned risk factor, or in the group from which the assigned risk factor was withheld, which would lessen, negate, or reverse the influence of the assigned risk factor. On the other hand, if the study population is too homogeneous, the applicability of the results of the study to the general population may be limited. For example, if a particular antibiotic was compared to a placebo to prevent postoperative wound infections and the study population was a highly homogeneous population with heart-lung transplants, the results

of the study could not be easily applied to general surgical patients in community hospitals. In a later section, there will be a more extensive discussion of comparability of study groups since the issue of confounding is often more of a problem in case-control studies. In addition, the size of study groups needed to determine whether the occurrence of disease (clinical trials) or risk exposure (case-control studies) is different will be discussed later.

Randomization

In a clinical trial, the method of assignment of the factor of interest must be unbiased. This is necessary to avoid any systematic selection of one type of patient into one or the other of the study groups, thereby obscuring or enhancing the effect of the assigned factor. For example, if an investigator truly thinks that antibiotic X is better than antibiotic Y in preventing postoperative wound infections, there would be a temptation to use X in the highest risk patients. Of course, at the end of the study with a greater number of high risk patients treated with antibiotic X, that drug may actually appear to prevent fewer wound infections than treatment Y, not because it is a less effective drug but because it was used in patients who were more likely to develop the outcome variable, postoperative wound infection. To avoid the bias in the method of assignment, the method of assignment must assure the following: The treatment (factor of interest) must be unknown ("masked" or "blinded") to the investigator, the study subject, and all study personnel who could influence patient or treatment selection or evaluation; future assignments cannot be predicted from past assignments; the order of assignments is reproducible; the methods for generation and administration of the assignments must be documented; the process of making assignments must have known mathematical properties (to permit the use of statistical analyses); and there must be sufficient documentation so deviations from the assignment can be detected (3). Commonly used methods of assignment, such as birth dates, Social Security numbers, hospital numbers, coin flips (nonreproducible), sequential odd-even, etc, fail to satisfy the above requirements. Such methods are haphazard and not random. Randomization is a process in which the probability of a given outcome (e.g., a coin toss) is known but in which the occurrence of a particular outcome for a specific repetition of the process is not known in advance of that particular repetition. Furthermore, it cannot be predicted with any greater certainty than for any other repetition of the process, and it is the only method which satisfies the above requirements.

Summarized in its simplest form, when study patients are to be randomized to two groups, A and B, a randomization scheme can be devised using a table of random numbers which can be found in the appendix of most biostatistics textbooks. Table 31.1 gives a typical example. Notice that each row of numbers is separated by a space at every fifth digit. This is only for ease of reading and has no mathematical meaning. To use a table of random numbers to allocate patients to the two treatment groups A and B, arbitrarily select either a row or column and decide whether you will read left to right or right to left. If one had chosen the third column of numbers in Table 31.1 (9,0,4,3,7) and decided to read left to right (columns beginning with 9, then 4, then 8, then 2, then 0, then 0, etc), the random sequence would begin 9,0,4,3,7,4,1,6,2,5,8, etc. To assign patients to group A or B, use an odd-even designation for A and B in which, for example, A is even and B is odd. The first patient allocated is allocated to groups B because the first random number 9 is odd; the second patient is allocated to group A because the second random number 0 is even; the third patient to group A because the third random number 4 is even, etc.

If one had chosen instead row 1 in Table 31.1 (5,0,9,4,8,2,0,0,0,2), of the first 10 patients allocated 8 would have been in group A (even numbers). Even in a table of random numbers there can be long strings of numbers with similar characteristics due to chance alone. If an investigator's study was small or was performed over a long time period in which patient characteristics might change, a process called blocking might be used to avoid imbalances in the study groups. Blocking is a method by which after a predetermined number of patients have been entered, the allocations into study groups are equal. For example, if the blocking was set up for every tenth patient with five in group A and five in group B, then after the tenth, twentieth, thirtieth, etc patient entered, the groups would be of equal size (5, 10, 15, respectively). The Moses-Oakford Assignment

Algorithm is quite useful in devising block randomization, and for more sophisticated allocation methods using three or four groups the reader is referred to a more detailed text (3).

A final word concerns a common misconception concerning randomization. The objective of randomization is to remove bias from the method of allocating patients into treatment groups, not to assure that the treatment groups are "equal" with respect to underlying characteristics. In fact, if enough patient characteristics are tabulated once patients are randomized to their respective groups, there is a high probability that one or more characteristics will be "significantly different" (at the 0.05 level) between the groups, assuming a normal distribution of characteristics in the study population.

Case-Control Studies

As with clinical trials, many excellent descriptions of case-control study methodologies have been written (1, 2). Only selected aspects will be included here.

In contradistinction to a clinical trial, the cause and effect relationship between one or more factors and a disease is examined from an effect-to-cause approach in a case-control study. The effect, the disease of interest, has already occurred in the cases, and the investigator looks back in time to the past history of the cases to examine the presence or absence of certain factors that may be important for the development of disease. The investigator also selects another group of people, hopefully similar in most respects to the cases, and looks back in time to the past history of the controls to determine the presence or absence of the same factors sought in the past history of the cases. If exposure to one or more factors has occurred more commonly among cases as compared to controls, the investigator might conclude that the factor (or factors) is causally related to the disease. It should be pointed out that in the strictest sense an observational study such as a case-control study cannot prove causality; an experimental study is usually necessary. This is not to say that a case-control study cannot come close to proving a cause and effect relationship. For example, to date no clinical trials (for ethical reasons) have proven on a biochemical basis the exact cause of lung cancer to be cigarette smoking, but most if not all well designed case-control studies have "proved" the cause and effect relationship.

The selection of a control group is of prime importance in case-control studies. Ideally, the

Table 31.1.   Table of Random Numbers

50948	20002	30976
75019	05217	76305
36466	62481	75779
70326	62660	90279
41757	96488	37231

controls should be identical in every respect to the cases except for the single factor which causes the disease in the cases. In reality, this is not possible. Even identical twins have different environmental exposures. As a practical matter, the method of selecting controls is first to characterize the cases as best as possible so that the "population universe" from which the cases came can be determined. The controls should then come from that "universe." For example, if an investigator was studying risk factors for Foley catheter-related urinary tract infections in patients following bladder cancer surgery, then both cases and controls must come from catheterized postoperative patients with bladder cancer. Controls should not be orthopaedic surgery patients.

Since in reality controls cannot be identical to cases except for the causal disease factor, two methods are used to minimize differences in characteristics in cases and controls which may confound the relationship between the causal factor and the disease: matching and adjustment. Adjustment will be discussed later.

Matching

Matching is pairing two or more persons on the basis of a similar or identical characteristic. Matching is rarely used in clinical trials because it is too cumbersome to identify two persons with similar characteristics within a short time during the recruitment phase of the study. On the other hand, matching is commonly used in case-control studies. Controls may be matched to cases on nearly any characteristic: age, sex, weight, race, hospital service, type of operation, etc. When a case and a control are matched on a particular characteristic, the effect of that characteristic is eliminated as a cause of the disease and the influence of other causal factors that are different between the cases and controls can then be examined. As a general rule, an investigator should match only on characteristics that are risk factors for the disease independently of the risk factor of interest. For example, birth weight in newborn infants is a risk factor for nosocomial infection (4). If one wanted to examine other risk factors, such as exposure to invasive procedures, one might match on birth weight to remove its influence on infection risk.

If matching is used, an analysis using statistical methods designed specifically for matched-pair analysis must be used. If matching occurs during control selection and unmatched analysis of the data is used, the differences between cases and controls will be lessened (odds ratio biased toward unity).

With the increasing availability of computerized databases in hospitals today and the apparent ease of searching these databases for controls that can be matched to cases, there is a strong temptation to use a matched study design. However, many authorities now caution against using the matched study design, and before deciding on a matched or unmatched design the reader should consider Schlesselman's discussion of the advantages and disadvantages of each (5). The two most compelling arguments against matched designs are: first, in the analysis one cannot fully investigate the interaction between the matching variable(s) and the exposure of interest, and, second, if multiple exposures are being examined the matching variable(s) may be confounders (vide infra) for some of the exposures and not for others, thereby leading to a loss of efficiency in the analysis of the nonconfounders. With better methods of analysis available for unmatched designs (stratified analysis, logistic regression) matched-pair designs should be used only when there is a specific good reason to do so and with a full understanding of the limitations of matching.

RISK MEASUREMENT

Risk may be defined as the chance or probability of a particular event, such as the "risk" of a postoperative wound infection following surgery. One can avoid exposure to that risk by not having the surgery. Therefore, having surgery can be considered exposure to a risk factor for postoperative wound infection. A risk factor can, of course, be a personal characteristic, such as age, or having a disease, cancer. The measurement of risk forms the basis of epidemiologic study, and the most important methods of risk measurement, incidence and prevalence, relative risk, and odds ratios will be discussed.

Incidence and Prevalence

Incidence is the number of new cases of a disease occurring in a specified time period among a population at risk for the disease. Incidence may be expressed mathematically as a conditional probability statement:

$$I = C/N \qquad 1$$

where I is the incidence rate, C the number of new cases in a specified time period, and N the population free of disease at the start of the time period. The incidence is conditional on all cases at risk being disease free at the beginning of the time period and is the average risk or chance that disease will occur during the time period. If 100 persons are hospitalized for 7 days and two of them develop nosocomial bacteremia during their hospitalization, the incidence per week is 2/100 (2%). Likewise, the risk or chance of bacteremia is 2/100 (2%). Incidence, therefore, is a direct measure of risk of a disease.

Prevalence, on the other hand, is the number of cases of a disease present in a population at risk for that disease at a point in time, irrespective of when the cases had their onset of disease. If on a particular day 100 hospitalized patients were evaluated for nosocomial bacteremia and three were found, one whose bacteremia first started on the day of evaluation and two whose bacteremia started 1 day and 2 days, respectively, before the evaluation, the prevalence of bacteremia would be 3/100 (3%). Prevalence, therefore, depends on the duration of the disease. If incidence, based on the time period of 1 day, were calculated for the above example, it would be 1/98 because the "old" cases that started 1 and 2 days before would not be included in either the numerator or the denominator (they are not disease-free at the beginning of the interval). Incidence and prevalence can be related in a steady state where neither incidence nor disease duration depends on time (6):

$$P = dI \qquad\qquad 2$$

where P is prevalence, d is average duration of the disease, and I is incidence. From equation 2 it is apparent that a higher prevalence can occur if either the duration of the disease is longer (e.g., better supportive care) or the incidence is higher. For this reason, in case-control studies where disease causation is of prime interest, only incident or new cases should be used in order to remove the influence of factors relating to disease duration.

Relative Risk

Assume a study of two populations that are equal in all characteristics except that one population is exposed to a factor thought to be important in causing a particular disease. If, after a period of time, a number of cases of the disease occur, the relationship between exposure to the factor and the occurrence of the disease can be shown in a 2×2 table as in Table 31.2.

Table 31.2. Relationship between an Exposure to a Factor and a Disease Occurrence

Exposure	Disease		Total
	Yes	No	
Yes	a	b	$a + b$
No	c	d	$c + d$
Total	$a + c$	$b + d$	$N(a + b + c + d)$

The incidence, from equation 1, among those exposed is $I_e = a/a + b$, and the incidence among those not exposed is $I_u = c/c + d$. Since incidence is a measure of risk of a disease, one can compare the risk among those exposed to those not exposed:

$$\text{let } P_1 = I_e \text{ (proportion exposed)}$$
$$P_2 = I_u \text{ (proportion unexposed)} \qquad 3$$
$$R = \frac{P_1}{P_2} = \frac{a/a + b}{c/c + d}$$

The comparison of the incidence (risk) among exposed to the incidence (risk) among the unexposed is called relative risk. In clinical trials (or other effect-to-cause cohort studies) the relative risk may be calculated directly. If the relative risk deviates from unity (1.0, implying the risk in the exposed is the same as the risk in the unexposed) the factor can be said to either cause (> unity or a positive association) the disease or be protective (< unity or negatively associated) against the disease.

The concept of relative risk is quite useful in expressing the relationship between an exposure and a disease. For example, assume that during a 3-month period all of the surgeons at a hospital who performed a particular operation had a 2% incidence of postoperative wound infection. However, surgeon A had an incidence of 5% and surgeon B had an incidence of 10%. The relative risk of infection of patients of surgeon A would be 5%/2% = 2.5 and of surgeon B 10%/2% = 5 compared to patients of all the other surgeons. The strength of the association between postoperative wound infection and being a patient of surgeon B ($R = 5$) is stronger than that for being a patient of surgeon A ($R = 2.5$).

In a hospital setting, relative risk can be used to analyze surveillance data, as in the example above, or to analyze more formally planned studies. Relative risk can only be used with incidence data. If a case-control study method is used, relative risk usually cannot be calculated.

Odds Ratio

The probability of an event is expressed by a number from 0 to 1 indicating how likely an event is to occur, where 0 represents an event that is impossible and 1 represents an event certain to occur. Odds are the ratio of the probability of an event's occurring (p) and the probability of the event's not occurring ($q = 1-p$). For example, if the probability of developing a nosocomial infection following exposure to some risk factor is 5%, the probability of not developing one is $1-0.05 = 95\%$, so the odds are $0.05/0.95 = 0.053$. Notice that for rather uncommon diseases the probability (0.05) is nearly equal to the odds (0.053).

The calculation of the odds ratio employs the same principles used to calculate relative risk except that odds instead of incidence are used. For example, in Table 31.2, if 100 ($a + b$) patients were exposed and $a = 5$ and $b = 95$ and 100 ($c + d$) patients were not exposed and $c = 1$ and $d = 99$, the odds of disease following exposure would be a/b (5/95) and the odds of disease following no exposure would be c/d (1/99). The ratio of the odds of disease in the exposed and unexposed is called the odds ratio,

$$OR = \frac{a/b}{c/d} = \frac{ad}{bc}. \qquad 4$$

In the example,

$$OR = \frac{5/95}{1/99} = \frac{5 \times 99}{95 \times 1} = 5.21.$$

In case-control studies the odds ratio only approximates the relative risk, because relative risk is derived from incidence data, and incidence usually cannot be determined from a case-control study unless all or a sample of all possible cases and all possible controls in a population are studied. The odds ratio is a close approximation of relative risk as shown for both large and small studies in Table 31.3.

Since many recently published studies of nosocomial infections have used the case-control design, the reader should be familiar with odds ratios. Odds ratios have the same use and interpretation as relative risk except odds ratios only approximate the strength of the association between an exposure and a disease. For example, assume that Table 31.3 depicts a hypothetical case-control study of eight cases of nosocomial urinary tract infection following cytoscopy. The exposure of interest is the cystoscope used in room 2. Eleven of 25 uninfected controls were cytoscoped in room 2 and six of the eight infected patients were also cystoscoped in room 2. The odds ratio of 3.82 means that patients cystoscoped in room 2 were 3.82 times as likely to develop an infection compared to patients not cystoscoped in room 2.

Confounding

An association between two or more variables is said to exist when there is an interdependence between them. The entire basis for statistical testing is the null hypothesis indicating no association between two variables. Relative risk and odds ratios are measures of the strength of association: the farther the deviation from unity, the stronger the association. However, an association does not imply a cause and effect relationship. For example, duration of Foley bladder catheterization is

Table 31.3. Hypothetical Large and Small Study Comparing Relative Risk and Odds Ratio

A.	Exposure	Disease Yes	Disease No	Total	
	Yes	36	983	1019	$R = \dfrac{36/1019}{16/1006} = 2.22$
	No	16	990	1006	
	Total	52	1973	2025	
					$OR = \dfrac{36 \times 990}{16 \times 983} = 2.27$

B.	Exposure	Disease Yes	Disease No	Total	
	Yes	6	11	17	$R = \dfrac{6/17}{2/16} = 2.82$
	No	2	14	16	
	Total	8	25	33	
					$OR = \dfrac{6 \times 14}{2 \times 11} = 3.82$

associated with an increased risk of nosocomial urinary tract infection (7). Although there may be a statistically significant association between duration of catheterization and infection, it is obvious that time per se does not cause infections; microorganisms do.

Confounding is the effect of a variable that partially or totally accounts for the apparent association (or lack of association—a masking effect) between a study variable and the disease of interest. A confounding variable must itself be a risk factor for the disease of interest, and it must be associated with the study variable of interest (it, however, cannot be a variable that is a result of the study exposure). A hypothetical example of a case-control study of 160 neonates with bacteremia and 180 neonates without bacteremia is shown in Table 31.4. An odds ratio of 3.47 shows a strong association between umbilical artery catheterization and bacteremia. However, it is apparent that gestational age is a risk factor for bacteremia (10 of 160 full terms versus 150 of 180 prematures had bacteremia, $OR = 0.013$) and gestational age is associated with the study variable (catheterization) of interest (150 of 180 prematures had catheters versus 80 of 160 full

terms, $OR = 0.2$). In this example the apparent association, bacteremia and catheterization, is largely explained by the confounding of gestational age because when the influence of gestational age is removed (e.g., adjusted for) by examining the relationship between catheterization and bacteremia among infants of similar gestational ages, the association disappears ($OR = 1$) or becomes less strong ($OR = 1.68$).

From an operational point of view, particularly in case-control studies where confounding variables may be unknown at the time the study starts, it is wise to regard all variables as potential confounders. During the analysis phase of the study one can then define the true confounding variables as those that are risk factors (not as a consequence of the study exposure) which, when controlled for through stratification, adjustment, etc., appreciably alter the effect of the variable of interest on the disease of interest.

SAMPLE SIZE AND POWER

In planning a study or in evaluating a published study in which the relationship between a risk factor and a disease is examined, one must know

Table 31.4. Gestational Age Confounding the Association between Umbilical Artery Catheterization and Nosocomial Bacteremia (Hypothetical Data)

A.	Catheterization	Bacteremia		
		Yes	No	
	Yes	130	100	$OR = \dfrac{130 \times 80}{30 \times 100} = 3.47$
	No	30	80	

B.	Gestational Age	Bacteremia		
		Yes	No	
	Full term	10	150	$OR = \dfrac{10 \times 30}{150 \times 150} = 0.013$
	Premature	150	30	

C.	Gestational Age	Catheterization		
		Yes	No	
	Full term	80	80	$OR = \dfrac{80 \times 30}{150 \times 80} = 0.20$
	Premature	150	30	

D.	Full term: Catheterization	Bacteremia		Total	
		Yes	No		
	Yes	5	75	80	$OR = \dfrac{5 \times 75}{5 \times 75} = 1.0$
	No	5	75	80	
	Total	10	150	160	
	Premature: Catheterization				
	Yes	127	23	150	$OR = \dfrac{127 \times 7}{23 \times 23} = 1.68$
	No	23	7	30	
	Total	150	30	180	

if a sufficiently large number of study subjects were included to avoid two types of error: (a) concluding that the exposure is associated with the disease when in fact it is not; or (b) concluding that the exposure is not associated with the disease when in reality it is.

The first error is called a Type I error and the probability of its occurrence is α or the level of statistical significance. The second error is called a Type II error and its probability of occurrence is β. The probability of *not* making a Type II error, $1-\beta$, is called the power of the study. It also indicates the probability that the odds ratio differs from unity.

These probabilities can be mathematically expressed in terms of the normal distribution curve with a mean of zero and a variance of one (8). $Z\alpha$ is the point on the abscissa axis to the right of which is $100(\alpha)\%$ (or $\frac{\alpha}{2}$ for two sided) of the area under the curve and Z_β is the point on the abscissa axis to the right of which is $100(\beta)\%$ of the area under the curve. Table 31.5 shows several unit normal deviates for $Z\alpha$ and $Z\beta$ for commonly used values of α and β.

To calculate the number of study subjects needed to avoid Type I and II errors, several estimates must be made. In a clinical trial one must estimate the incidence rate (P_c) of the outcome in the control group. In a case-control study one must estimate the frequency of the exposure of interest (P_o) in the control group. Both of these estimates will usually come from previous studies or surveys but in some cases will only be a best guess. The second estimate needed to calculate a sample size is the estimated relative risk (R) that has clinical importance. Sometimes small changes in risk are important. For example, a 5% reduction in bacteremia associated with a new intravascular catheter would be important if that catheter was used nationwide. Finally, the desired level of significance (α) and study power $(1-\beta)$ are chosen: traditionally $\alpha = 0.05$ and β either 0.10 or 0.20.

Table 31.5. z_α and z_β for Commonly Used Values of α and β

α or β	Z_α or Z_β (One-Sided Test)	Z_α (Two-Sided Test)
0.01	2.33	2.58
0.025	1.96	2.24
0.05	1.64	1.96
0.10	1.28	1.64
0.20	0.84	1.28
0.30	0.52	1.04

The sample size formula for unmatched case-control studies as shown by Schlesselman is as follows (5):

$$n = \frac{[Z_\alpha \sqrt{2\bar{p}\bar{q}} + Z_\beta \sqrt{p_1 q_1 + p_0 q_0}]^2}{(p_1 - p_0)^2} \quad 5$$

where

$$p_1 = \frac{p_0 R}{[1 + p_0 (R - 1)]}$$

$$\bar{p} = 1/2 \, (p_1 + p_0)$$

$$\bar{q} = 1 - \bar{p}$$

$$q_1 = 1 - p_1$$

$$q_0 = 1 - p_0$$

n = the number of subjects in either the case or control group ($2n$ is the total study population).

Suppose one wanted to do a case-control study of Foley catheter-related urinary tract infection. One type of catheter had been in use for a number of years (old) in the hospital and about 2 years ago a new one was introduced and was used with about equal frequency as the old one. There were suspicions that the old one was associated with more infections. How many catheterized patients would be needed to study the relationship between infection and use of the two catheters? If one assumes that use (exposure) of the new catheter among catheterized patients is 30% $(p_o = 0.30)$, the suspected increase in risk of infection associated with the old catheter is 50% $(R = 1.5)$, and one wants only a 5% (α) chance of falsely concluding that the old catheter is associated with infection and a 20% (β) chance of falsely concluding that the old catheter is not associated with infection, then the calculation of the number of subjects needed for study would be as follows: $p_o = 0.30$, $p_1 = (0.30)(1.5)/[1 + (0.3)(1.5) - 1)] = 0.39$, $\bar{p} = 0.30 + 0.39/2 = 0.345$, $\bar{q} = 1 - 0.345 = 0.655$, $q_1 = 1 - 0.39 = 0.61$, $q_0 = 1 - 0.30 = 0.70$, $Z_\alpha = 1.64$ (one-sided, one is interested in only the old catheter being worse, not either better or worse), $Z_\beta = 0.84$,

$$n = \frac{[1.64\sqrt{(2)(0.345)(0.655)} + 0.84 \sqrt{(0.39)(0.61) + (0.30)(0.70)}]^2}{(0.39 - 0.30)^2}$$

$$n = 342.$$

Therefore, 342 catheterized infected patients would be selected and 342 catheterized uninfected patients would be selected. This number would be needed if the assumed risk of infection with the old catheter was 50% greater than the new catheter. The number needed would increase if any of the following assumptions changed: a lower frequency of use of the new catheter (p_o), less difference in risk (R approaching unity), or more stringent error (α or β) criteria.

Suppose that the above hypothetical study was performed but due to lack of funds or unavailability of numbers of patients only 260 catheterized infected patients and 260 catheterized uninfected patients could be included in the study. The results of the study showed the odds ratio (estimated relative risk) for infection associated with the old catheter to be 1.5. Since there are fewer patients in the study, the investigator may not be as confident that the old catheter is associated with 50% more infections. Maybe there really is no difference ($R = 1$). To find out, the investigator would calculate the power ($1 - \beta$) of the study by using the sample size formula rearranged to solve for Z_β

$$Z_\beta = \frac{[\sqrt{n(p_1 - p_o)^2} - Z_\alpha \sqrt{2\,p\,q}]}{\sqrt{p_1\,q_1 + p_o\,q_o}} \qquad 6$$

Using the study example

$$Z_\beta = \frac{[\sqrt{(260)(0.39 - 0.30)^2} - 1.64\,\sqrt{(2)(0.345)(0.655)}]}{\sqrt{(0/39)(0.61 + (0.3)(0.7)}}$$

$$Z_\beta = 0.52.$$

From Table 31.5 (or any table of area under the unit deviate curve) a Z_β of 0.52 corresponds to β of 0.30 so power $= 1 - 0.3 = 0.7$.

The investigator's conclusion then is that the study has a 70% probability that the odds ratio differs from unity (the catheters are the same in terms of risk of infection).

For sample size and power calculations for case-control studies where there are unequal numbers of cases and controls and for sample size and power calculations for clinical trials where discrete and continuous data are used the reader should consult other texts (3, 5). Of particular note in clinical trials involving nosocomial infections where the possibility that the rate of occurrence of the outcome may be low (5 to 20%), the chi-square approximation may be inappropriate and the following formula for sample

size and power using the inverse sine transformation approximation might be used (3):

$$n_c = \frac{(Z_\alpha + Z_\beta)^2\,(\lambda + 1)/\lambda}{4\,[\sin^{-1}\sqrt{p_c} - \sin^{-1}\sqrt{p_t}]^2} \qquad 7$$

where

n_c = number in control group;

n_t = number in each treatment group;

$\lambda = n_t/n_c$ (allocation ratio);

p_c = expected event rate (proportion) in control group;

p_t = expected event rate (proportion) in treated group.

Power $= 1 - \beta = 1 - \phi\,(A)$ A = proportion of area under unit deviate curve to left of A

$$A = \frac{Z_\alpha - 2\,|\sin^{-1} P_c - \sin^{-1} P_t\,|}{\sqrt{1/n_c + 1/n_t}}. \qquad 8$$

It must be stressed that sample size calculations are to be used as estimates for planning a study. They are based on assumptions (P_o and R for case-control studies) over which the investigator has no control, and the assumptions cannot be predicted as to whether they are correct or not prior to the study. Sample size estimates only answer the investigator's question "am I in the ball park." Power calculations, based on the study's data are more useful.

DATA ANALYSIS
Point Estimate and Confidence Interval of the Odds Ratio

In virtually every study of nosocomial infection (or other biologic phenomenon, for that matter) it is nearly impossible to study the entire universe of patients relevant to the study. Platt et al reported on the relationship between mortality and nosocomial urinary tract infection (adjusted OR = 2.8; 95% confidence intervals, 1.5–5.1) among 1458 patients at the New England Deaconess Hospital (9). Platt did not study all patients in the world who had ever died to see if they had had a nosocomial urinary tract infection: he took a sample of that universe.

If repeated samples of a universe are taken, the numerical results of these samples, if plotted on a graph, will describe a normal or Gaussian curve.

For example, if the study described above were repeated in hospitals, A, B, C, D, etc, and the adjusted odds ratios were found to be 2.8, 1.7, 3.2, 2.4, etc, and the results were plotted, they would distribute themselves normally around a mean value. Ninety-five percent of odds ratios would be within 2 standard deviations of the mean of all the odds ratios and 2½% would be greater and 2½% would be less than the odds ratios, exactly 2 standard deviations greater and less, respectively, than the mean value. Since Platt et al performed only one sample of the universe, they can only estimate whether the odds ratio they found was within 2 standard deviations of the mean of the universe. They can make an estimate from their data as to the range of values where the mean of the odds ratio of the universe can be found on the normal curve. By calculating 95% confidence limits based on their data, they can be 95% confident (probability of 0.95) that the mean odds ratio of the universe lies within 2 standard deviations of the odds ratio described from their study. (The reader is referred to several excellent sources for the mathematical derivation and explanation of the central limit theorem (10, 11).)

The point estimate of the odds ratio $(\widehat{OR})$ is calculated from a 2×2 contingency table as shown previously in equation 4. For convenience in mathematical computation so that an $\widehat{OR} = $ one becomes zero, the natural log (ln) of the odds ratio is used:

$$w = \ln \widehat{OR}. \qquad 9$$

Approximate confidence limits can be calculated using $Z_\alpha = 1.96$ (two sided) and the notation found in Table 31.2 from the following formulas:

$$\text{var } (\ln \widehat{OR}) \simeq \left(\frac{1}{a} + \frac{1}{b} + \frac{1}{c} + \frac{1}{d}\right) \qquad 10$$

$$\ln \widehat{OR} \pm Z_\alpha \sqrt{\frac{1}{a} + \frac{1}{b} + \frac{1}{c} + \frac{1}{d}} \qquad 11$$

$$\widehat{OR}_L = \widehat{OR} \exp \left[-Z_\alpha \sqrt{\text{var } (\ln OR)}\right] \qquad 12$$
$$\widehat{OR}_U = \widehat{OR} \exp \left[+Z_\alpha \sqrt{\text{var } (\ln OR)}\right]$$

Using the hypothetical data in Table 31.3A, an example of the calculation of $\widehat{OR} \pm 95\%$ confidence limits (CL) would be as follows:

$$w = \ln 2.27 = 0.82, \text{ var } (\ln \widehat{OR})$$

$$\simeq \left(\frac{1}{36} + \frac{1}{983} + \frac{1}{16} + \frac{1}{990}\right)$$

$$= 0.0923, \ 0.82 \pm (1.96)\ (\sqrt{0.0923})$$

$$= 0.82 \pm 1.96 \times 0.3038, \ \widehat{OR}_L$$

$$= 2.27 \exp [-0.595] = 1.25, \ \widehat{OR}_U$$

$$= 2.27 \exp [+0.595] = 4.11.$$

A simpler operational approach rather than using equation 12 would be to calculate the natural log confidence intervals $(0.82 - 0.595 = 0.225)$ $(0.82 + 0.595 = 1.415)$ from equation 11 then take the antilogs of 0.225 and 1.415.

The interpretation of the hypothetical study in Table 31.3A, therefore, is the point estimate of the odds ratio is 2.27 and from the data of that study it is estimated that there is a 95% chance that the mean of the odds ratios, if the entire universe were studied, would be somewhere between 1.25 and 4.11. The confidence interval does not include unity $(\widehat{OR} = 1)$, so one can state with 95% confidence that sampling variation is an unlikely explanation for the association between the exposure and the disease seen in the hypothetical study.

Adjustment for Confounding

In the previous section on confounding it was apparent from Table 31.4 that the variable gestational age was a risk factor for the disease, bacteremia, and associated with the study variable of interest, umbilical artery catheterization. Gestational age was therefore a confounding variable. By arranging the data into strata containing infants of similar gestational age and examining the relationship between bacteremia and catheterization, one could hold the influence of gestational age constant. This stratification is a method, therefore, of removing bias from a comparison which was confounded. Since the influence of gestational age is removed, the odds ratios expressing the relationship between bacteremia and catheterization may be thought of as "adjusted" for the effects of gestational age. The "unadjusted" OR of 3.47 is confounded by gestational age; however, it is not clear which of the "adjusted" odds ratios, the one for prematures $(OR = 1.68)$ or the one for full terms $(OR = 1.0)$, is the correct overall expression of the relationship between bacteremia and catheterization in this hypothetical study. A number of techniques have been devised to give an adjusted summary odds ratio for stratified data (5). One of the more commonly used is the Mantel-Haenszel method (12).

The Mantel-Haenszel method is a weighted average of odds ratios from a series of 2×2 contingency tables. The formulas needed to calculate the weighed summary odds ratio and confidence limits (intervals) are as follows (2×2 table notation from Table 31.2).

$$\widehat{OR} = \frac{\sum\limits_{i=1}^{k} \left(\frac{a_i d_i}{N_i}\right)}{\sum\limits_{i=1}^{k} \left(\frac{b_i c_i}{N_i}\right)} \qquad 13$$

$$\text{var (ln } \widehat{OR}) \simeq \frac{\sum w_i^2 v_i}{(\sum w_i)^2} \qquad 14$$

where

$$w_i = b_i c_i / N_i$$

$$v_i = \frac{(a_i + c_i)}{a_i c_i} + \frac{(b_i + d_i)}{b_i d_i}$$

Using the data from the hypothetical study in Table 31.4, the Mantel-Haenszel odds ratio adjusted for gestational age (summary odds ratio for the two 2×2 tables stratified for gestational age):

$$\widehat{OR_1} = \frac{5 \times 75}{5 \times 75} = 1.0 \qquad \widehat{OR_2} = \frac{125 \times 7}{23 \times 23} = 1.68$$

$$\frac{a_1 d_1}{N_1} = \frac{5 \times 75}{160} = 2.34 \qquad \frac{a_2 d_2}{N_2} = \frac{127 \times 7}{180} = 4.94$$

$$\frac{b_1 c_1}{N_1} = \frac{5 \times 75}{160} = 2.34 \qquad \frac{b_2 c_2}{N_2} = \frac{23 \times 23}{180} = 2.94$$

from equation 13,

$$\text{adjusted } \widehat{OR} = \frac{2.34 + 4.94}{2.34 + 2.94} = 1.38$$

$$w_1 = \frac{75 \times 5}{160} = 2.34$$

$$w_2 = \frac{23 \times 23}{180} = 2.94$$

$$v_1 = \frac{10}{5 \times 5} + \frac{150}{75 \times 75} = 0.43$$

$$v_2 = \frac{150}{127 \times 23} + \frac{30}{23 \times 7} = 0.24$$

from equation 14,

$$\text{var (ln } \widehat{OR}) \simeq \frac{(2.34)(0.43) + (2.94)(0.24)}{(2.34 + 2.94)^2}$$

$$= 0.159$$

from equations 9 and 11,

$$w = \ln \widehat{OR} = \ln 1.38 = 0.32$$

$$0.32 \pm 1.96 \sqrt{0.159} \text{ or } 0.32 \pm 0.7815$$

taking antilogs

$$1.38, (0.63)(3.20).$$

Whereas the unadjusted $\widehat{OR}$ of 3.47 (confidence intervals of 2.12 and 5.64) appeared to show a strong association between bacteremia and catheterization by virtue of the confidence interval excluding unity, the adjusted odds ratio of 1.38 indicates no association because the confidence interval (0.63)(3.02) includes unity.

A word of caution regarding the use of the Mantel-Haenszel method. In the example given the adjusted $\widehat{OR}$ for full term infants (1.0) is similar to the $\widehat{OR}$ for premature infants (1.68). Had there been considerable difference, such as 1.0 and 2.85, for example, the Mantel-Haenszel method should not have been used. Such wide disparity would suggest an interaction, either additive or multiplicative, between the variables, and a different analytic method would be more appropriate. In such a situation expert biostatistical consultation should be sought.

Logistic Regression

Suppose in the hypothetical study shown in Table 31.4 that other confounding factors—such as exposure to antibiotics, mechanical ventilation, surgical procedures, underlying illness, and parenteral fluids other than the umbilical artery catheter—were suspected as being important. To stratify on each of these variables and to calculate a Mantel-Haenszel adjusted odds ratio would be difficult. Many of the resulting 2×2 tables would contain very small numbers. To deal with this problem, a method called multiple logistic regression has been devised.

The logistic model states that the probability of a disease depends on a set of variables and that the variables relate to the disease and to each other as described in the following mathematical model (5):

$$Px = \left(d = \frac{1}{x}\right)$$

$$= \frac{1}{\{1 + \exp[-(\beta_o + \beta_1 x_1 + \beta_2 x_2 \cdots \cdot \beta_p x_p)]\}}. \qquad 15$$

Variables which are risk factors or confounders are represented as $x_1, x_2, x_3 \cdots x_p$. The term d

equals 1 when the disease or outcome of interest is present and equals 0 when it is absent. The terms β are coefficients that indicate how each corresponding x influences the risk of the disease or outcome of interest and are calculated directly from the study data. These coefficients usually are calculated by the maximum likelihood method, which requires a computer to perform the iterative calculations.

Table 31.6 shows coefficients calculated for four variables which were part of a study of postoperative wound infections (B Koblin, TR Townsend, S Self, M Stephens, R Lawson, V Gott, BF Polk, unpublished data). If one chose to examine the risk of infection in a white female, whose surgery lasted 1 hour and who had been operated on within the previous month, from equation 15,

$$P_x = \frac{1}{\{1 + \exp[-(-3.6519 - 0.2593 + 0.4284 + 0.3790 + 1.0230)]\}}$$

$$= \frac{1}{1 + \exp(2.0808)} = 0.11.$$

Therefore, the risk of infection (P_x) would be 11/100 (11%) for a person with the characteristics (variables) listed. Odds ratios and confidence limits can be calculated, interactions between variables can be examined, and formulas are available for use with matched case-control study designs (5).

Logistic regression is a useful analytic tool because it permits the analysis of the influence of multiple exposures on the disease of interest, and small numbers resulting from infrequent exposures are less of a problem compared to the Mantel-Haenszel method. Logistic regression can be applied to most studies where the disease of interest is present in some patients ($d = 1$) and absent in others ($d = 0$) and exposure variables ($X_1 \ldots X_p$) are measured. A major criticism,

Table 31.6. Coefficients Calculated from Multiple Logistic Regression Analysis of Postoperative Wound Infection Study Data

Variable	Parameter	Coefficient
X_0 intercept	β_0	−3.6519
X_1 sex (f/m)	β_1	−0.2593
X_2 race (w/b)	β_2	0.4284
X_3 operating room time (1-hour increments)	β_3	0.3790
X_4 surgery within 1 month (y/n)	β_4	1.0230

however, of using logistic regression, particularly the stepwise logistic models, is the reliance on an arbitrarily chosen level of significance in evaluating the importance of different variables. The level of statistical significance may not be indicative of the level of clinical or biologic significance. Expert biostatistical consultation can be a valuable asset to any investigator planning to use logistic regression analysis.

SUMMARY

This chapter was designed to assist the reader in understanding some of the underlying concepts in the design and analysis of clinical trials and case-control studies. Such understanding should help in the interpretation of published studies which use modern methods of design and analysis, and such understanding should help investigators to design and analyze studies. It is important that studies be analyzed in a logical fashion from the simple to the complex. Errors are often made by simply jumping to a computer and plugging data into a logistic regression formula. Statistical significance does not imply biologic significance; and in any given study, factors that are found not to be statistically significant (possibly due to small sample size or bias in study design or execution) may be biologically important. As computers and statistical packages proliferate, investigators run the risk of losing touch with their data and failing to present them completely to the scientific reading public. There is still a need for simple and thorough examination of study data, and through this process the biologic relevance of the study can be determined.

References

1. Townsend TR: Designing a study to answer infection-control questions. In Wenzel RP (ed.): *Handbook of Hospital Acquired Infections*. Boca Raton, FL, CRC Press, 1981, p 581.
2. Lilienfeld AM, Lilienfeld DE: *Foundations of Epidemiology*, ed 2. New York, Oxford University Press, 1980, p 3.
3. Meinert CL: *Clinical Trials: Design, Conduct, and Analysis*. New York, Oxford University Press, in press.
4. Hemming VG, Overall JC, Britt MR: Nosocomial infections in a newborn intensive-care unit. *N Engl J Med* 294:1310–1316, 1976.
5. Schlesselman JJ: *Case-Control Studies: Design, Conduct, Analysis*. New York, Oxford University Press, 1982, p 6.
6. Freeman J, Hutchinson GB: Prevalence, incidence and duration. *Am J Epidemiol* 112:707–723, 1980.
7. Kunin CM, McCormack RC: Prevention of catheter-induced urinary-tract infections by sterile

closed drainage. *N Engl J Med* 274:1155–1161, 1966.

8. Armitage P: *Statistical Methods in Medical Research*. Oxford, Blackwell Scientific Publications, 1971, p 72.

9. Platt R, Polk BF, Murdock B, Rosner B: Mortality associated with nosocomial urinary tract infection. *N Engl J Med* 307:637–642, 1982.

10. Leaverton PE: Statistical inference. In Leaverton PE (ed): *A Review of Biostatistics*, ed 2. Boston, Little, Brown, and Co, 1978, p 36.

11. O'Brien PC, Shampo MA: Estimation from samples. *Mayo Clin Proc* 56:274–276, 1981.

12. Mantel N, Haenszel W: Statistical aspects of the analysis of data from retrospective studies of disease. *J Natl Cancer Inst* 22:719–748, 1959.

Chapter 32

Statistical Concepts in Infection Control

Donald L. Kaiser, Dr.P.H.

INTRODUCTION

Statistics, or more precisely, probabilities, should play an important role in the conduct of effective hospital infection control programs. Statistical applications derived from the realities of probability distributions will substantially influence program and study design, determine sampling techniques, establish sensitivity criteria for determining the importance of events, and provide a foundation for the analysis of virtually all results.

The increasing availability of computers and statistical analysis programs means that powerful statistical techniques can be available to any researcher. The professionals involved in infection control programs will have been exposed to these techniques to some extent, as most medical and nursing school programs will include at least some instruction in beginning statistics. Finally, there are presently several dozen comprehensive statistical textbooks in print which are oriented toward clinical data and problems.

Despite plentiful resources, the researcher or practitioner in infection control still faces the major challenge of understanding *how* and *why* specific statistical methods are applied to their problems. Thus, this chapter will concentrate on the *conceptual* aspects of statistics, leaving the simpler matter of the discovery of formulas and algorithms (from books and computer programs) to the individual reader.

The chapter will examine considerations in research design, the statistics of description (and their alternatives), the basics of statistical analysis for populations, groups, and relationships (or etiologies), nonparametric alternatives to the more commonly known parametric tests, and the more complex methods associated with identifying outcomes which may arise from multiple causes.

For the reader who desires greater depth and detail, there are ample sources available (1–8). Commonly available statistical packages are SPSS (9), SAS (10), BMDP (11), Minitab (12), INDAS (13), and COSAP (14). Time spent on the following pages will provide the reader with a foundation from which to approach these sources and others.

DESIGNING STUDIES

The most important design issue to be considered in the planning of a study is that of sampling. Classically, one regards any set of subjects as a sample drawn from some larger population. Even an exhaustive sample (all known subjects) from a hospital should still be regarded as only a sample of all possible patients with a given condition and provided a certain treatment. When the characteristics of a sample are understood, inferences can be made and findings extended to larger populations. Three sample characteristics are particularly important:

1. *Representation*, which considers the source and nature of the population sample (e.g., did every population member have an equal chance of being selected for the sample?);
2. *Precision*, which describes how exactly experimental conditions can be defined;
3. *Consistency*, which indicates whether each sample member is treated in the same manner, thus giving the overall sample an acceptable degree of internal homogeneity.

As it is intended that inference be drawn from observed results in samples, these characteristics are useful criteria in the assessment of potential study designs.

Retrospective Studies

Retrospective studies gather samples and information by going back to past events and measurements. Such studies can, under the proper circumstances, be extremely useful. Retrospective data have already been gathered. The investigator does not have to wait for the occurrence of events; those events wait patiently to be collected and quantified. As a result, retrospective studies usually are less expensive to conduct and can proceed rapidly (if the data have been effectively organized).

There are usually some drawbacks to retrospective studies. These become more obvious if one thinks in terms of the criteria established above. Because the studies are retrospective, the investigator has rarely controlled subject selection, and the exact nature of the *representation* of the sample may be unknown. Changes in referral patterns, individual physician practices (predisposition for types of treatment), and shifts in populations are major external forces which can alter the representation of retrospective samples. Further, even in the most thorough data systems (automated or otherwise), there are usually compromises or gaps in the *precision* with which treatment information has been recorded. Finally, it is likely that the *consistency* of subject treatment has been compromised by inevitable changes in method or technique; this is especially true for infrequent events that require extensive historical research.

Confronted with these realities, the investigator has two major strategies available. First, one may study retrospectively only those cases where sufficient information is available to make representation clear, where one can make certain the precise definition of the circumstances of the case, and where salient aspects of the cases appear to be consistent with other cases chosen for the sample. Alternatively, one may choose less strict definitions, while retaining the requirement of relatively complete information, and hope that any differences among cases which do appear can be rationalized as irrelevant to the major points of the study.

Complete information concerning retrospective cases will, moreover, permit a more precise definition of the population from which the cases were drawn. Any study from which an investigator hopes to draw inference for some larger reality (and most studies do make such an attempt, either implicit or explicit) must characterize the underlying population as clearly as possible. The problem in retrospective studies is that clarity in case selection and definition is frequently poor and almost always irremediable. The past is history; thus we must rely on historians to understand it. If our clinical and experimental historians were imperfect, we may have no alternatives.

One potential alternative identified above is to focus the population of inference by choosing only those cases which may be precisely characterized. While this places a bias on the sample, it may not be a fatal bias if the population of inference is sufficiently numerous in the larger population and sufficiently interesting to potential users of the research results.

Finally, it is useful to identify subjects who may be used as controls for the study. In so doing, it is important to understand the *exact* nature of the available control subjects. That is, in *precisely* what ways do they differ from the cases which are the subject of the study. If, for example, one identified controls which were identical to cases in every measurable way, except for the presence of a nosocomial infection, most analyses would be relatively uninteresting. That is, whatever contributed to the occurrence of the infection was not measured (had such factor or factors been measured then, of course, the controls would *not* be identical). Commonly, one is concerned with the nature of the risk of acquiring an infection. Thus, one must be certain that similarity is achieved in characteristics which lie outside the realm of relevant risk (age, race, sex, and underlying disease are common choices), but which leave risk areas to be represented in their naturally occurring variety.

This approach is by no means as easy as it has been made to sound. Given the complexities of the medical care environment, there are frequently hidden operators (referral patterns, patient selection, diagnostic and treatment choices, etc) which produce bias in subpopulations. Thus, for example, patients provided a particular course of treatment may be intrinsically different from those experiencing a different treatment, in ways other than simply what treatment was provided. The choice may have been made on the basis of the perception of their disease, individual physician preference, prior treatment at another institution, and so on. Simply put, in retrospective studies observations commonly are not what they appear to be; unmeasured contributing factors strongly influence behavior and events within the medical care system.

Prospective Studies

A prospective study plans future data collection according to (*a*) a predefined plan of subject definition and identification, (*b*) a clearly established treatment and assignment protocol, and (*c*) consistent criteria both for the data to be collected and for the standards of measurement. Prospective studies are generally more expensive and time consuming than their retrospective counterparts (though some would argue that there are no true counterparts in the retrospective mode). Furthermore, many problems cannot practically be examined prospectively (except perhaps in multicenter trials) because the ocurrence of the events required to define a case is too infrequent.

However, prospective studies do provide a precision and control which can never be paralleled with retrospective data collection. If one has a problem which occurs with sufficient frequency and an ability to identify and effect patient care activities uniformly, then a prospective study is the only reasonable approach. The patient population is described and assembled, subjects are randomly (perhaps with some stratification) assigned to treatment groups, rigorously defined treatments are applied, and measurements are made. Inference can be made from the results to a well understood population.

Even the best study environment can be compromised by poor practices. For example, the design of the study is intimately linked to the underlying hypothesis of the study. A clear-cut hypothesis leads to clean study, e.g., "administering drug A will change the outcome of *X*." Two groups (or perhaps two measurements on the same group, if physiologically feasible) are implied by such an idea, with a relatively simple statistical approach to identifying the probable outcome. Even such a simple amendment as an additional treatment (drug B perhaps) adds substantially to the complexity of the experiment. For example, is the action of A antagonistic (or inhibitory, or identical) to B? Is the reverse true? What about the combined effects of A and B? Does the order of administration make a difference? And so it goes.

The reality is that *simple questions make the best experiments.* If one cannot state the hypothesis in a simple sentence, then the eventual design will probably be too complex to be successful. This is true not only because of intrinsic design complexities, but also because experiments almost never go as planned. For instance, subjects may not be identified as rapidly as planned, or materials will be late, or the answer will be desired earlier than planned. In short, some set of circumstances will intrude on even the most carefully made plans, requiring adjustment that will almost certainly compromise the experiment. Therefore, in the interest of both efficiency and sanity, one

should keep the questions as simple as possible. Remember that totally successful, simple experiments have probably secured more recognition (and funding) than partially successful, complex ones.

With simple designs, patients can be identified and placed in a pool for random assignment to study groups. In some designs, patients may be crossed over from one treatment to another. Carryover of treatment effect and the potential for spontaneous temporal changes should be very carefully considered when planning crossover studies (with crossover designs not used if either phenomenon is likely to be present), and treatment sequence should be randomly assigned to avoid temporal bias. Crossover studies have the advantage of providing very good control subjects (the treated subjects themselves), thus eliminating a major source of random variability.

When subjects are placed in single treatment groups, assignment is often carried out with separate randomization patterns for individual strata of the eligible subjects. That is, males are randomized separately from females, or older patients separately from younger. Obviously, the number of strata one might use could get quite large. The advantage is an assurance that control and treatment groups are individually composed from representative populations using relatively small numbers of subjects (randomization itself would have this outcome with sufficiently large groups, but the approach is risky and expensive). The disadvantage is an added element of complexity to the study, and it is especially bothersome when complex strata are used.

Summary

The above concepts suggest that one should use prospective techniques wherever possible in hospital infection control programs. In fact, most effective nosocomial infection control information systems are actually one form of prospective design. Case identification, measurement principles, and monitoring procedures are established prospectively, with cases allowed to follow a natural course within this framework. Certainly, in the absence of such a finite program, and in the case of infrequently occurring events, some retrospective data collection must be utilized. In either case, the key elements are simplicity and precision. The principle of simplicity should be compromised only under the most dire circumstances. Compromises of precision are much less under investigator control and have consequences which usually are less troublesome.

DATA EXAMINATION

Before one can begin mathematical calculations on data, it is prudent to examine those data to make certain (*a*) that the data are as we expected them to be and (*b*) that the realities of the data are consistent with the intrinsic assumptions of the mathematical methods.

Point *a* deals with the issue of variability. Variability can arise from many sources, but the two which are most important for this discussion are variability due to inaccuracy or inconsistency of method and variability due to innate differences in subjects.

Considering the first source, measurement methods clearly do change over time, both in the short run (from assay to assay or day to day) and over longer periods (with variation in manufacturer's lots of materials, technician changes, etc). This type of variability is usually much greater than simple errors of measurement, which generally arise from human error or the inadequacies of specific measurement techniques. Controls or standards for measurement help to identify the magnitude of this type of variability, relative to the magnitude of a measurement's actual value, or the change in the value of a measurement. Depending on the amount of the variability, alternative mathematical techniques may need to be used in analysis.

Variability in a set of subjects can also arise from the fact that subjects actually belong in two or more relatively homogeneous groups, rather than in one large, heterogeneous set. Thus to evaluate, for example, hemoglobin values for a set of men and women would introduce variability because such values are intrinsically different for men and women. A more appropriate strategy would be to consider hemoglobin values (and such analyses as we might conduct on those values) separately for men and women.

Once one has explored the variability of data and its sources, one should plan the mathematical and statistical analysis and compare the methods selected with the realities of the data. For example, calculating the mean value for a set of data carries an assumption about the underlying distribution of variability in the data (see discussion under "Descriptive Statistics," below). If empirical examination of the data suggests that these assumptions have been grossly violated, then one must re-examine the justification for their use and consider alternatives.

Knowing what one should look for, what approach to data examination should be used? Descriptive statistics can be calculated for examining data, as shall be presented in the next section. However, at this preliminary stage, one should employ graphic techniques to gain the fullest insight. The most useful graphic is the histogram. A histogram is a bar chart (either horizontal or vertical) in which the position of the bar along an axis indicates the range of values being represented, and the length (or height) indicates the number of observations (subjects) with values in the range.

A histogram (Fig. 32.1) is really just a way of looking at a distribution curve. Instead of the smooth, continuous curve of a density distribution, the histogram is broken down into ranges. Examining data in this manner permits decisions about the presence of subpopulations, the appropriateness of planned mathematical techniques, and the nature of variability in an experiment.

DATA ANALYSIS

Once it has been assured that the proper data have been collected in the proper way and that

	1-4	5-9	10-14	15-19	20-24	25-29	30-34	35-39	40-44
14			XXX	XXX		XXX			
13			XXX	XXX		XXX	XXX		
12			XXX	XXX		XXX	XXX		
11		XXX	XXX	XXX		XXX	XXX		
10		XXX	XXX	XXX		XXX	XXX		
9		XXX	XXX	XXX	XXX	XXX	XXX		
8		XXX	XXX	XXX	XXX	XXX	XXX	XXX	
7		XXX	XXX	XXX	XXX	XXX	XXX	XXX	XXX
6		XXX	XXX	XXX	XXX	XXX	XXX	XXX	XXX
5	XXX	XXX	XXX	XXX	XXX	XXX	XXX	XXX	XXX
4	XXX	XXX	XXX	XXX	XXX	XXX	XXX	XXX	XXX
3	XXX	XXX	XXX	XXX	XXX	XXX	XXX	XXX	XXX
2	XXX	XXX	XXX	XXX	XXX	XXX	XXX	XXX	XXX
1	XXX	XXX	XXX	XXX	XXX	XXX	XXX	XXX	XXX

Figure 32.1.   A histogram.

anomalies of variability have been recognized, it is possible to begin data analysis. The most frequent choice for data analysis is the use of some sort of *statistic*. A statistic is nothing more than a number, calculated according to an established formula, which represents an aspect of a set of data or relationships among multiple aspects. There are statistics which describe and statistics which test. Both types provide powerful tools for understanding data because, *for most types of data distributions*, the behavior of statistics has been investigated both theoretically and empirically and is well understood. Thus a certain type of outcome can be related to a known probability distribution and used to test a hypothesis.

Descriptive Statistics

A common use of statistics is to describe. The most prevalent descriptive statistics are those which describe the average (or middle) value for a set and those which describe the dispersion (or variability). The usual purpose of descriptive statistics is to provide some estimate of the characteristics of the underlying population from which the sample was drawn. Thus, these statistics are also referred to as inferential.

The middle or average value of a set of sample observations (such as height) can be represented with several different types of statistics, each suited to different circumstances. The most commonly used is the mean (more correctly, the *arithmetic mean*), which is simply the average of a set of data, calculated as the sum of the set of data values, divided by the quantity of values which have been summed. While commonly used, it is also commonly *mis*used by being applied to (*a*) data with outlying data points (which pull the result toward the outlying points and away from the real middle), (*b*) data with distributions which are truncated by natural barriers (such as physiologic maxima and minima), and (*c*) data containing more than one inherent distribution (i.e., a set of data with *more than one* true average). The arithmetic mean is *properly* applied to data which have a *more or less* normal (Gaussian) distribution (most statistics books will provide a decent discussion of this idea).

The advantage of the arithmetic mean is that it is possible, using the mean, to calculate a statistic of variability (see discussion of standard deviation, below) which has properties that have been exploited by statisticians over the years. Their work has led to test statistics (see "Testing Hypotheses," below) which have proven effectiveness and a vast body of supporting literature.

While there are ways of dealing statistically with other types of averages, the techniques generally are not as elegant or familiar as those associated with the arithmetic mean.

The representation of the average which is most like the arithmetic mean is the *geometric mean*, calculated as the antilog of the arithmetic mean of the log of the values. The geometric mean is more cumbersome to employ than the arithmetic mean for subsequent analyses (it is usually better to transform the measurements to a log scale and then do more elaborate calculations). This type of mean is the most apropriate way of examining such things as bacterial growth and dilution data.

Other useful measures of the average (see a statistics text for a more detailed discussion) are the *median* or middle value (50th percentile), which is useful for damping out the effect of outlier values, and the *mode*, which is an expression of the middle using the most prevalent value.

Once the middle has been described by a statistic, it still remains to provide a measure of the deviation or variability around that middle. While several measures of variability exist, those used more often are based directly on *variance*. Variance is the sum of the squared deviations of all data values from the arithmetic mean. The deviations are squared to accommodate the reality that half the variance is on one side of the mean and half on the other. Squaring prevents these values from cancelling each other. Derived from variance are (*a*) the *mean variance* (the average deviation; variance divided by number of data points minus 1), (*b*) the *standard deviation* (the square root of the mean variance; extracting the square root returns the measure to the original measurement scale), (*c*) the *coefficient of variation* (the standard deviation divided by the mean; calculated to adjust for the reality that even with a comparable variable, standard deviations increase as the mean increases), and (*d*) the *standard error of the mean* (the standard deviation divided by the square root of the number of data points).

All of these measures of variability, except the standard error of the mean, are simply different ways of representing the variability of *individual points* around the sample mean. In this respect, these measures are, like the mean, *estimators* of the characteristics of the large population from which the sample was drawn. A slightly different concept applies for the standard error of the mean. This parameter is an expression of the accuracy of the mean as an estimator of the population mean. In other words, the standard

This mathematical model provides an ideal null hypothesis. If X has no effect, then Y will always equal A, and B will equal 0. Thus, if a way can be devised for estimating B (in the same sense as we estimate a mean) for a sample, and if an expression for the variability of B as an estimate of the larger population can be calculated (in the same sense as an SEM), then one can test the null hypothesis $B = 0$ and accept or reject, thereby rejecting or supporting (respectively) an experimental hypothesis of linear effect of increasing X.

The least squares algorithm provides a method of estimating B, and a standard error for B, using a technique which fits a line to the experimental data. The method will find a line for any data in which there are measures of variable Y associated with corresponding values of X. The extent or closeness of fit of the line is evaluated largely in terms of the value of the standard error of B. The nature of the fit will depend on a combination of (a) the magnitude of the changes in Y produced by changes in X (the steepness of the line), (b) the consistency of those changes (distribution of individual points around the line), and (c) the range of X values over which the relationship was tested (the length of the line). The likelihood that the null hypothesis is true is decreased by (a) increased strength (size of B) of the relationship between X and Y, (b) more consistency in those changes (tighter fit of individual points to the line), and (c) increased range of X values over which the relationship was tested. As characteristic a increases, the value of B moves away from 0, and as characteristics b and c improve, the standard error of B decreases. Such changes, in some combination, make it increasingly less likely that the null hypothesis is true and, by inference, more likely that the experimental hypothesis (X effects Y in a linear fashion) is true.

Two cautions are necessary in using linear regression. First, the mathematics of regression will produce a line for *every* set of data, regardless of the appropriateness of a linear function. Thus, one may have remarkably consistent responses in one's data but fail to show a significant linear relationship because the response simply *is not linear*. This points back to the principle developed earlier, that one ought to examine one's data graphically before plunging into mathematical techniques which can obscure the true nature of an effect. Second, linear functions are among the more fastidious types of relationships which one can propose (as well as being anathema to many physiologic pathways, which almost always

have intrinsic limits and controls, making simple linear increase or decrease unlikely). A failure to develop a significant linear function should not necessarily be regarded as a failure for the experiment. There are less elegant models. For example, high doses can be hypothesized to produce a larger effect than low doses will return the hypothesis to a test of means as discussed above.

Regression is a very flexible technique when applied to circumstances where effect is linear (or within a restricted range of linearity from some overall relationship that has high and/or low limits). Multiple regression considers the simultaneous effects of multiple causal factors. Linear functions of individual Xs (separate causal factors considered either singly or in combination) can be compared to see whether the effect of one factor is larger than the effect of another. Finally, special types of regression have been devised for special circumstances (killing curves; dose curves; outcomes which are categorical in nature, lived versus died; and systems where causal variables are themselves related). While regression is a powerful tool, it also has much more complexity, making the potential for misuse greater than with the simpler techniques.

Testing Hypotheses without Parameters

Tests of means and slopes share the common characteristic of being *parametric* tests. That is, a statistic (the mean or the slope) is calculated which describes the effect, and that statistic is examined to evaluate a hypothesis. There are circumstances (probably more numerous than one might imagine) where examination of data will show that a statistic does not provide an appropriate representation of results. It has already been shown that certain types of distributions cannot be properly represented using a mean. These types of distributions are relatively common in medicine, where fundamental physiology imposes limits on how a characteristic may vary (while leaving the subject organism still alive). Thus, one will also commonly have a need for tests of effect under conditions where a parameter should not be calculated.

Fortunately, there are a group of tests called *nonparametric*, which use other methods of examining effects. While these tests have been around for a long time, they are generally not as well known or understood as parametric tests. The tests can be thought of as being in two categories.

Category one contains tests that are the approximate equivalent of tests of means. Instead of using a mean, these tests consider the *relative* magnitude of results through the use of the ranking of data points. That is, in a set of data the highest value is ranked 1, the second highest is ranked 2, and so on. While this represents a certain lack of precision, it is a technique which can deal with unusual distributions in a mathematically acceptable manner.

It is beyond the scope of the present discussion to deal with these methods in any great detail. However, there are equivalents to the paired test (sign test, signed rank test), the unpaired test (rank sum test), and the multiple group test (Kruskal-Wallis test).

Category two consists of tests involving tables, where the phenomena under consideration are measured in categorical terms. These tests use the chi-square statistic to evaluate whether the rate of occurrence of phenomena is consistent or shows some deviation that might be the result of causation (i.e., being in a particular category for one measurement, such as sex, predisposes a subject to being in a particular category when measured in some other way, such as morbidity). To continue with the above example, this provides a method for evaluating the incidence of infection in males versus the incidence in females. If the rates are comparable, then the rates for each group should be about the same as the rates of incidence for both groups combined. The chi-square statistic provides a mechanism for assessing deviation in discrete events from hypothetical quantities (the number of cases we would expect from a sample of a certain size, given some underlying rate of occurrence). Tables of results can thus be evaluated with this statistic for many different kinds of discrete phenomena.

The statistics of nonparametric tests are frequently very different from their parametric counterparts (this is especially true for the chi-square statistic). For this reason, nonparametric statistics shoud be examined carefully by the reader, using a statistics text which pays particular attention to this area of mathematics (see Fleiss (17) and Conover (18) for especially good treatments).

SUMMARY

The above discussion deals in a conceptual way with the fundamental techniques of statistics which are applied to infection control programs

and research activities. No attempt has been made to provide an exhaustive reference for the practitioner who wishes to use these methods. Rather, it is the goal to provide some understanding of the directions in which to head when confronted with specific problems or ideas. There is no substitute for the statistics textbook, data analysis computer program, or statistician in generating hypotheses and analysis for a specific problem.

Some general principles do bear repeating.

1. One should be very explicit with oneself and others about the design of the experiment. On the facts of the design will rest both an understanding of the idea underlying the experiment and the appropriateness of extending the results to other sets of subjects.
2. Keep the purpose of the experiment (the relationships to be examined) as simple as possible. Two simple experiments are probably worth five complex ones, both in terms of the certainty of the meaning of the results, and in terms of the dollars-to-decimal-points ratio (the experimental cost of specific pieces of new information).
3. Examine data carefully with graphic techniques before submerging results in a vat of statistical analysis. Not only will a better understanding of the experiment itself be gained, but also one will be able to be more certain about the correctness of the analysis.
4. Remember that hypotheses can only be disproven. A forced recognition of the null hypothesis will keep experimental ideas cleaner and more interpretable.
5. Always run your ideas past a trained biostatistician, even when you are dead certain that your techniques are correct. Far from being a ploy to keep biostatisticians working, this point is a recognition that even the simplest of problems can have hidden characteristics to trap the unwary or partially educated.

With these ideas firmly in mind, one is suitably armed to pursue research. It is impractical to learn everything ahead of time. Science is certainly as much an experiential craft as it is a rigid discipline, and one must be aware that experience holds as much education as formal training.

References

1. Daniel WW: *Biostatistics: A Foundation for Analysis in the Health Sciences.* New York, John Wiley & Sons, 1983.

2. Feinstein AR: *Clinical Biostatistics.* St Louis, CV Mosby, 1977.
3. Lewis AE: *Biostatistics,* ed 2., New York, Van Nostrand Reinhold, 1984.
4. Armitage P: *Statistical Methods in Medical Research.* Oxford, Blackwell Scientific Pubications, 1971.
5. Murphy EA: *Biostatistics in Medicine.* Baltimore, Johns Hopkins University Press, 1982.
6. Ingelfinger JA, Mosteller F, Thibodeau LA, Ware JH: *Biostatics in Clinical Medicine.* New York, Macmillan, 1983.
7. Rosner B: *Fundamentals of Biostatistics.* Boston, Duxbury, 1982.
8. Brown BW Jr, Hollander M: *Statistics: A Biomedical Introduction.* New York, John Wiley and Sons, 1977.
9. *SPSS, Statistical Package for the Social Sciences.* New York, McGraw-Hill, 1975.
10. *SAS, Statistical Analysis System.* Cary, NC, SAS Institute, 1984.
11. *BMDP, BMDP Statistical Software.* Berkeley, University of California Press, 1981.
12. *Minitab.* University Park, PA, Pennsylvania State University, 1982.
13. *INDAS.* Nashville TN, S & H Computer Systems, 1985.
14. *COSAP.* Appleton, WI, Lawrence University, 1983.
15. Dunn OJ, Clark VA: *Applied Statistics: Analysis of Variance and Regression.* New York, John Wiley & Sons, 1974.
16. Searle SR: *Linear Models.* New York, John Wiley & Sons, 1971.
17. Fleiss JL: *Statistical Methods for Rates and Proportions.* New York, John Wiley & Sons, 1981.
18. Conover WJ: *Practical Nonparametric Statistics,* ed 2. New York, John Wiley & Sons, 1980.

Chapter 33

Using the Literature

Richard A. Peterson, M.S.L.S.

The purpose of this chapter is to summarize the major books and journals on hospital-acquired infections, to describe the most important indexes and data bases used to access the literature of nosocomial infections, and, finally, to give an overview of the options for document delivery of materials identified. For additional information both Chen (1) and Morton (2) provide comprehensive guides to the medical literature.

MONOGRAPHS

Several "core" lists of the medical literature are available (3–5), the most notable being the Brandon list, now in its eleventh revision. These lists are useful for identifying the major books and journals in the general specialties such as internal medicine, infectious diseases, and laboratory methods. However, only one title directly concerned with hospital-acquired infections appears in these lists: the American Hospital Association's *Infection Control in the Hospital*. Useful sources to consult for current titles on nosocomial infections include *Books in Print*, *National Library of Medicine Current Catalog*, book reviews found in the various journals, and publishers' flyers and catalogs.

Produced annually by Bowker, *Books in Print* lists all in print and forthcoming titles from more than 16,300 publishers. An alternative subset of *Books in Print* is *Medical Books and Serials in Print*, a biannual Bowker publication. Updates are provided by *Forthcoming Books in Print*, a bimonthly cumulative publication, also from Bowker. In addition to author and title entries, subject access to these sources is provided by the separate subject guides that utilize Library of Congress subject headings. *Books in Print* is also available online through Bibliographic Retrieval Services and Dialog Information Service.

The *National Library of Medicine Current Catalog* is a bibliographic listing of citations to publications cataloged by the National Library of Medicine. It is issued quarterly with an annual cumulation. Subject access is by NLM Medical Subject Headings. The *Current Catalog* is also available online as CATLINE through the National Library of Medicine.

Book reviews in the medical journals provide qualitative descriptions of new books, but often lag well behind the publication date compared to the more current, but nonqualitative, *Current Catalog* and *Books in Print*. Publishers' flyers and catalogs provide another means of current awareness, but obviously list only a portion of all available titles.

The following subject headings, depending on a particular library's classification scheme, should be consulted to determine the library's holdings on cross-infection. The corresponding call numbers are also included if browsing the shelves is preferred.

1. Dewey Decimal Classification (6) and Library of Congress Subject Headings (listed below): 614 and 616
2. Library of Congress Subject Headings (7) and Classification (8, 9):
   Cross Infection RA969
   Nosocomial Infections RA969
   Surgical Wound Infections RD98.3
   Communicable Diseases—hospitals RA969
   Communicable Diseases—nursing RT95
   Isolation (Hospital Care) RA975.5
   Hospitals-Disinfection RA969
   Hospitals-Hygiene RA969
   Laminar Flow Clean Rooms RA969.43
3. National Library of Medicine Medical Subject Headings (10) and Classification (11):
   Cross Infection WC195, WX167
   Communicable Diseases—nursing WY153
   Patient Isolation WX167
   Patient Isolators WX147
   Surgical Wound Infection WO185
   Environment, Controlled WX165, WX218

Below is an annotated bibliography of selected recent titles on infection control in hospitals.

The APIC Curriculum for Infection Control Practice. Barbara M Soule, ed. Dubuque, Kendall/ Hunt Publishing Company, 1983. Contains a detailed overview of infection control for daily use or as an aid when preparing for certification examination (12).

Clinial Microbiology and Infection Control. Elaine Larson. Boston, Blackwell Scientific Publications, 1984. Designed for the health care practitioner as a basic source with clinical applications from the field of microbiology.

Departmental Procedures for Infection Control Programs. Charles P Craig and David N Reifsnyder, eds. Oradell, NJ, Medical Economics, 1977. Offers recommended guidelines for establishing infection control procedures, broken down by 24 hospital departments.

Epidemiology for the Infection Control Nurse. Elizabeth Barrett-Conner et al, eds. St Louis, CV Mosby, 1978. Provides examples, guides, specific details, and general approaches to infection control programs (13).

Epidemiology of Hospital-Associated Infections. Peter C Fuchs. Chicago, American Society of Clinical Pathologists, 1979. Gives an overview of nosocomial infections, describes the epidemiology of hospital infections, and provides a guide for conducting a hospital epidemiology program (14).

Fundamentals of Infection Control: An In-Service Orientation Program. Charles P Craig, ed. Oradell, NJ, Medical Economics, 1983. Useful teaching resource for in-service programs and self-review reference for students (15).

Fungal Infection in the Compromised Patient. DW Warnock and MD Richardson, eds. New York, John Wiley & Sons, 1982. For the experienced infection control practitioner. Describes the relation between the deficient or absent immunologic defenses of the compromised patient and fungal diseases. Diagnosis, manifestations, and treatment of frequent fungal diseases are discussed in detail (16).

Guidelines for Prevention and Control of Nosocomial Infections. Atlanta, Centers for Disease Control, 1983. Consolidates CDC recommendations and updates into single source. Recommendations are ranked according to scientific studies and practical experience.

Handbook of Hospital Acquired Infections. Richard P Wenzel ed. Boca Raton, FL, CRC Press, 1981. Highly referenced textbook for the experienced infection control practitioner and physician epidemiologist.

Hospital-Acquired Infections: Guidelines to Laboratory Methods. MT Parker, ed. Copenhagen, World Health Organization, 1978. Covers the more important laboratory tests and demonstrates how the work of the laboratory can be integrated with the rest of the hospital infection control activities.

Hospital-Associated Infections in the Compromised Host. Gerald P Bodey and Victorio Rodriquez, eds. (*Handbook on Hospital Associated Infections,* vol 2) New York, Dekker, 1979. Discusses hospital-acquired infections in relation to the compromised host's weakened immune system, including diagnosis and treatment.

Hospital-Associated Infections in the General Hospital Population and Specific Measures of Control. Dieter Groschel, ed. (*Handbook on Hospital Associated Infections,* vol 3) New York, Dekker, 1979. Discusses types of infections and methods of control by body system, for the new infection control practitioner (ICP) or student (17, 18).

Hospital Infection Control: Principles and Practice. Mary Castle. New York, John Wiley, 1980. Provides excellent practical instruction and advice for the beginning ICP (19).

Hospital Infection Control Policy and Procedure Manual. Gary Lee Stanley. Herrin, IL, Hospital and Physician Consulting Service, 1977. Detailed 2-volume loose-leaf set to be used as a guide for establishing individual policies and procedures.

Hospital Infections. John V Bennet and Phillip S Brachman, eds. Boston, Little, Brown, and Co, 1979. Well written reference on the epidemiology and control of hospital infections. Written for the hospital epidemiologist, ICP, microbiologist, and architect (20).

Infection and the Perioperative Period. Alix Mathieu and John F. Burke. New York, Grune & Stratton, 1982. Covers the relation of surgical procedures and development of infection and also includes practical guidelines for prevention and treatment of infections.

Infection Control. Lucille M Arking and Barbara J McArthur, eds. (*Nursing Clinics of North America.* 15: no. 4). Philadelphia, WB Saunders, 1980. Targeted for a nursing audience, this symposium gives a good overview on the nursing process as it relates to infection control (21, 22).

Infection Control: A Policy and Procedure Manual. Monica B Palmer. Philadelphia, WB Saunders, 1984. Useful handbook of practical information for use by the beginning ICP, as a teaching tool, and as a guide for establishing and maintaining an infection control program.

Infection Control: An Integrated Approach. Mary Yarbrough. St Louis, CV Mosby, 1983. Excellent work on the role of the ICP in the hospital, skills required of the ICP, and infections of specific body systems (23).

Infection Control in Critical Care. Marilyn A Roderick, ed. Rockville, MD, Aspen Systems, 1983. Offers a guide for developing or improving infection control programs in critical care units. Covers identification, control, and prevention of nosocomial infections (24, 25).

Infection Control in Long-Term Care Facilities. Philip W Smith. New York, John Wiley & Sons, 1984. A good reference on the effects of aging on the immunological system and infectious diseases in the elderly (26).

Infection Control in the Hospital, ed 4. Chicago, American Hospital Association, 1979. A standard reference in the field of infection control, contains useful information for both the novice and the experienced practitioner (27).

Infection Control Manual, ed 2. C Meshelany. Oradell, NJ, Medical Economics, 1979. Looseleaf guide for infection control programs in hospitals, clinics, and nursing homes.

Infection: Prevention and Control, ed 2. Elaine C Dubay and Reba D Grubb. St Louis, CV Mosby, 1978. Provides an overview of infection control and offers a suggested policy and procedure manual.

Infections in Surgery, Basic and Clinical Aspects. J Mck Watts, et al, eds. New York, Churchill Livingstone, 1981. Well organized compilation of papers presented at Symposium on Infection in Surgery by experts in the field, for the hospital epidemiologist, ICP, and researcher (28).

Manual for Review and Update of Hospital Department Safety, Environmental, and Infection Control Policies. Frank D Murphy. Fond du Lac, WI, Health Tech Services, 1980. Suggested guidelines for updating infection control policies and procedures.

Manual of Infection Control in Respiratory Care. Arthur J McLaughlin. Boston, Little, Brown, and Co, 1983. Written for respiratory care personnel as a convenient and concise source on infection control.

Manual on Control of Infection in Surgical Patients, ed 2. The Committee on Control of Surgical Infections of the Committee on Pre- and Postoperative Care of the American College of Surgeons, William A Altemeier, et al, eds. Phil-

adelphia, JB Lippincott, 1983. Provides authoritative and current information on the cause, prevention, and treatment of surgical infections.

Model Department Safety, Environmental, and Infection Control Policies for Hospitals. Frank D Murphy. Boston, GK Hall, 1981. Provides a model for the construction of an infection control policy and procedure manual.

Nosocomial Infections. Richard E Dixon. New York, Yorke Medical, 1981. A compilation of papers presented at the Second International Conference on Nosocomial Infections sponsored by the CDC. Discusses current concepts of nosocomial infections by site and offers challenges for the future (29).

Occurrence, Diagnosis, and Sources of Hospital-Associated Infections. Willson J Fahlberg and Dieter Groschel, eds. (*Handbook on Hospital Associated Infections,* vol 1). New York, Dekker, 1978. An introduction to a planned 10-volume handbook series, this work presents an overview of infection control principles for the student or beginning ICP (30, 31).

Surgical Infections. J Wesley Alexander, ed. (*Surgical Clinics of North America* 60: no. 1). Philadelphia, WB Saunders, 1980. Excellent reference for the ICP on epidemiology, pathogenesis, and prevention of postoperative infections (32).

PERIODICALS

Only a handful of journals exist that are specifically devoted to hospital-acquired infections; not one of these journals is included in the "core" lists mentioned in the previous section. A survey of the 1984 *Index Medicus* identified over 130 other non-nosocomial disease specialty journal titles containing articles indexed under the term "cross-infection." The number of articles published in the literature of other specialties and multidisciplinary journals necessitates the use of indexes, abstracts, and online data bases to provide effective access to the journal literature; the following section is devoted to these alternative information sources.

Useful sources for identifying journal titles by broad subject category include *Ulrich's International Periodicals Directory* (RR Bowker), *Ulrich's Irregular Serials and Annuals* (RR Bowker), and *The Standard Periodical Directory* (Oxbridge Communications). Subscription rates and publishers' addresses are also included. Several of the index/abstract and data base producers also publish their own lists of journals covered;

these include *List of Journals Abstracted* (Excerpta Medica), *List of Journals Indexed in Index Medicus* (National Library of Medicine), *Serial Sources for the BIOSIS Data Base* (BioSciences Information Service), and *Science Citation Index Guide and List of Source Publications* (Institute for Scientific Information). These sources are useful for translating the journal abbreviations used in the corresponding indexes/abstracts and online data bases to the full title. Below are the journal titles identified in the above sources devoted exclusively to hospital-acquired infections.

American Journal of Infection Control. St Louis, CV Mosby, 1980–, bimonthly. Previously published as *APIC Journal* (1978–1979) and *APIC Newsletter* (1973–1977). Official publication of the Association for Practitioners in Infection Control. Contains original articles pertaining to the prevention, surveillance, and control of infections in health care institutions, and their relationship to the community. Also contains reviews of books and literature from other journals. Indexed in *Biological Abstracts, Current Contents, Cumulative Index to Nursing and Allied Health Literature, Excerpta Medica, Hospital Literature Index, Index Medicus,* and *Nursing Abstracts.*

Hospital Infection Control. Atlanta, American Health Consultants, 1974–, monthly. Covers the subject of infections acquired by patients in hospitals and how to prevent acquisition of such infections. Indexes in *Index Medicus* and *Hospital Literature Index.*

Infection Control. Thorofare, NJ, Charles B Slack, 1980–, monthly. Includes articles on all aspects of infection control. Indexed in *Current Contents, Cumulative Index to Nursing and Allied Health Literature, Hospital Literature Index,* and *Index Medicus.*

Journal of Hospital Infection. London, Academic Press, 1980–, quarterly. Published for the Hospital Infection Society. Includes book reviews. Indexed in *Index Medicus.*

Infection Control Digest. Chicago, American Hospital Association, 1980–, monthly. For ICPs in hospitals.

ABSTRACTS AND INDEXES

The secondary journals, or abstracts and indexes, offer the ICP an efficient means to access the literature. To perform even the simplest subject search effectively requires the use of one or more of the sources listed below or their online counter-parts described in the following section. The information query determines which

source(s) to consult. While there are varying degrees of overlap between the abstracts and indexes, all serve to complement each other (33–36).

Biological Abstracts. Philadelphia, Biosciences Information, 1926–, semimonthly. Abstracts to the life sciences research literature. Covers over 8000 serials and includes many indexes: author, biosystematic, generic, concept, and subject. Cumulative indexes are produced semiannually. Useful source for information on drugs and infectious disease causative agents. Should be used for comprehensive searches.

Biological Abstracts RRM. Philadelphia, Biosciences Information, 1980, monthly. Abstracts to the life sciences research literature. Covers books, book chapters, reports, reviews, and meetings. Includes the same indexes as listed above with a semiannual cumulative index. Also to be used for the most comprehensive searches.

Chemical Abstracts. Columbus, OH, Chemical Abstracts Service, 1907–, weekly. Abstracts to the chemical literature, including pharmacology. As with the above two titles, should only be used to perform comprehensive literature searches.

Current Contents: Life Sciences. Philadelphia, Institute for Scientific Information, 1958–, weekly. Includes table of contents for over 1130 journals and 600 new multiauthor books/year. Title word and author indexes with triannual cumulative index. Unsurpassed as a current awareness tool, this title offers the most rapid manual retrieval of the literature.

Current Contents: Clinical Practice. Philadelphia, Institute for Scientific Information, 1973–, weekly. Includes table of contents of over 790 journals and 400 new multiauthor books/year. Title word and author indexes with triannual cumulative index. Useful when utilized for the most current clinical literature.

Excerpta Medica. Amersterdam, The Netherlands, Princeton, NJ, Excerpta Medica, 1946–, 10 to 30 issues/year depending on section. Includes abstracts to over 3500 journals, divided into 52 sections, and is the largest and most expensive biomedical abstracting service in existence. Useful sections include Drug Literature Index (Section 37), Health Economics and Hospital Management (Section 36), Internal Medicine (Section 6), Microbiology (Section 4), Pharmacology (Section 30), and Virology (Section 47). The continued "title splitting" into additional sections requires using more than one section to perform most searches (37). The average 12-month turnaround time between article publication and appearance in the abstract (38) results in a tool that is best used primarily for retrospective searching of the medical literature.

Hospital Literature Index. Washington, DC, US Government Printing Office, 1945–, quarterly with annual cumulation. Produced by the American Hospital Association with the assistance of the National Library of Medicine. Selectively indexes approximately 670 journals for articles on hospital and health facility administration. Useful for comprehensive searching on topics such as the economics of infection control or administration of hospital policies and procedures.

Index Medicus. Washington, DC, US Government Printing Office, 1879–, monthly with annual cumulation. Produced by the National Library of Medicine; covers all aspects of the biomedical literature; indexes 2695 journals. Includes a separate section indexing review articles: Bibliography of Medical Reviews. Its relatively inexpensive price and broad coverage of the biomedical literature have made this an essential tool for medical libraries. Criticisms (39, 40) include the time lag between article publication and appearance in the index (3 to 12 months), and the inconvenience of having to go through each monthly issue before the annual cumulation is available. To be used as a primary tool for retrospective searches of the biomedical literature.

Abridged Index Medicus. Washington, DC, US Government Printing Office, 1970–, monthly with annual cumulation. Produced by the National Library of Medicine; indexes 100 English-language clinical journals. Designed for the individual practitioner and small hospital libraries. Useful when exhaustive research is unnecessary and offers a means to deal with the massive amounts of medical literature by indexing only the "core" clinical journals (41).

International Pharmaceutical Abstracts. Washington, DC, American Society of Hospital Pharmacists, 1964–, semimonthly. Abstracts to the pharmacy literature, covers over 700 journals, each issue contains only a subject index that cumulates twice a year, author index appears only in semiannual index. Useful for comprehensive searching of the drug literature.

Science Citation Index. Philadelphia, Institute for Scientific Information, 1961–, bimonthly with annual and 5-year cumulations. Indexes over 2500 journals. Includes author, title word, and citation indexes. Most useful for retrieving information on topics not adequately defined by other indexes that use controlled vocabulary and most importantly for citation searching. The citation searching is particularly useful for comprehensive searching. The citation index is used to progress from older, known publications to more recent, related articles which cite them. The unique advantages of citation searching are further described in detail by Garfield (42).

ONLINE VERSUS MANUAL SEARCHING

The advent of computerized literature searching in the 1960s provided researchers an optional approach to searching the literature to supplement traditional manual searching. When both online services and indexes are available, manual searching is effective for single term searches, for browsing the literature, or when only a few references are needed. Online searching should be the choice for multiterm searches or when there does not exist a suitable subject heading for a particular topic. The pros and cons of manual versus online searching (43, 44) are summarized below.

Advantages to Online Searching

Speed. The time required to search a topic and print out the citations online is considerably less than a manual search, especially when several concepts are combined.

Coordinate Searching. Multiple concepts can be combined using Boolean logic to retrieve the most relevant articles.

More Access Points. Several fields such as age groups, words in the abstract, date of publication, author affiliation, and language are only searchable online.

Currency. The data online is usually more current than the particular data base's print counterpart.

Multiple Data Bases. Access to many data bases allows for more comprehensive searching.

Cost Effectiveness. Less person-hours are required to perform and print out the results online than manually.

Disadvantages to Online Searching

Coverage. Online data bases only cover a limited time frame—generally from 1970 to the present. Indexes offer the only access to earlier literature.

Finances. Although online searching is more cost-effective, the requester is usually charged for online time, whereas use of a library's indexes incurs no charges.

Availability. Occasional computer for telecommunications problems can make the system unaccessible when needed.

ONLINE DATA BASES VENDORS

The indexes and abstracts described in the previous section all have computerized counterparts which can be accessed by medical libraries with online search services. Prices for searching the data bases are determined by several factors, including online connect time, data base royalties, telecommunications charges (UNINET $8.00/hour, TYMENET $14.00/hour, or TELENET $8.00/hour), citation charges, and offline page charges. The various systems that make the various data bases available for searching charge different connect charges, offer varying contract options based on projected use, and operate during different schedules. In addition to price variations, other factors determine which system to select (45, 46) such as system software and hours on online availability. The systems include the following:

Bibliographic Retrieval Services (BRS), 1200 Rt 7, Latham, NY 12100. (800) 833-4707; (800) 553-5566 in New York. Hours (EST): Monday to Saturday 6:00 a.m. to 4:00 a.m., Sunday 6:00 a.m. to 2:00 p.m. and 7:00 p.m. to 4:00 a.m., total = 149 hours/week. Offers volume discounts.

BRS/Saunders Colleague, jointly produced by Bibliographic Retrieval Services and WB Saunders Publishing Company, 1290 Avenue of the Americas, New York, NY 10019. (800) 833-4707; (800) 553-5566 in New York. Hours (EST): Monday to Saturday 6:00 a.m. to 4:00 a.m., Sunday 6:00 a.m. to 2:00 p.m. and 7:00 p.m. to 4:00 a.m., total = 149 hours/week. A user-friendly, menu-driven system for end user searching of the BRS medical data bases at rates less than the command-driven BRS system above (47). Other BRS data bases are also searchable at the regular rates. Offers discounts for volume use and also searching during nonprime time.

DIALOG Information Services, 3460 Hillview Avenue, Palo Alto, CA 94304. (800) 227-1960; (800) 982-5838 in California. Hours (EST): Monday to Thursday 12:00 midnight to 10:00 p.m., Friday 12:00 midnight to 8:00 p.m., Saturday 8:00 a.m. to 8:00 p.m., down on Sunday, total = 120 hours/week. Offers volume discounts.

DIALOG Knowledge Index. Available through DIALOG Information Services, provides user-friendly access to 16 of the DIALOG data bases during evening hours at reduced rates (48). Hours (EST): Monday to Thursday 6:00 p.m. to 5:00

a.m., Friday 6:00 p.m. to 12:00 midnight, Saturday 8:00 a.m. to 12:00 midnight, Sunday 3:00 p.m. to 5:00 a.m., total = 80 hours/week.

MEDLARS Management Section, National Library of Medicine, 8600 Rockville Pike, Bethesda, MD 20209. (301) 496-6193; (800) 638-8480. Hours (EST): Monday to Friday 3:00 a.m. to 9:00 p.m., Saturday 8:30 a.m. to 5:00 p.m., down on Sunday, total = 98.5 hours/week. Offers discounts for nonprime time usage.

System Development Corporation (SDC), 2500 Colorado Avenue, Santa Monica, CA 90406. (800) 421-7229; (800) 352-6689 in California. Hours (EST): Monday to Thursday all day except 9:45 p.m. to 10:15 p.m., Friday 3:00 a.m. to 8:00 p.m., Saturday 8:00 a.m. to 7:00 p.m., Sunday 7:00 p.m. to 3:00 a.m., total 130 = hours/week.

SPECIFIC ONLINE DATA BASES

BIOSIS, the online version of *Biological Abstracts* and *Biological Abstracts RRM*, available through BRS and BRS Colleague ($51 to $70/hour plus $0.08 to $0.17/citation), DIALOG ($60 to $75/hour plus $0.057 to $0.19/citation), and DIALOG Knowledge Index ($24/hour). Covers 1969 to the present. Produced by Biosciences Information Service, 2100 Arch Street, Philadelphia, Pennsylvania 19103, (800) 523-4806, (215) 568-4016 in Pennsylvania.

CA Search, corresponds to print editions of *Chemical Abstracts*, available through BRS and BRS Colleague ($54 to $73/hour plus $0.08 to $0.23/citation), DIALOG ($61 to $76/hour plus $0.056 to $0.18/citation), and SDC ($48 to $68/hour plus $0.20/citation). Covers 1967 to the present on DIALOG and SDC, 1970 to the present on BRS. Produced by Chemical Abstracts Service, PO Box 3012, Columbus, OH 43210. (800) 848-6533; (614) 421-3698 in Ohio.

Comprehensive Core Medical Library, provides full text searching and retrieval of over 20 medical books and several journals including *Annals of Internal Medicine, British Medical Journal, The Lancet, Medical Letter,* and *The New England Journal of Medicine.* Produced and available only through BRS ($36 to $55/hour plus $0.05/citation) and BRS Colleague ($17 to $32/hour).

EMBASE, corresponds to print volumes of *Excerpta Medica* in addition to an additional 1000 journals or 40% more not covered in print version, available through BRS and BRS Colleague

($55 to $74/hour plus $0.30/citation), and DIALOG ($69 to $84/hour plus $0.19 to $0.38/citation). Covers 1974 to the present on DIALOG and 1980 to the present on BRS. Produced by Elsevier Science Publishers BV/Excerpta Medica, PO Box 1527, 1000 BM Amsterdam, The Netherlands. (020) 5803-911. North American office at 52 Vanderbilt Avenue, New York, NY 10017. (212) 867-9040. Although more expensive to search than MEDLINE, an advantage (49) is the extensive foreign literature coverage. The data base is also limited to medical sciences with minimal coverage of allied health sources.

HEALTHLINE, online version of *Hospital Literature Index*, available through BRS ($15 to $35/hour plus $0.05/citation), BRS Colleague ($17 to $32/hour), NLM ($4.50 to $7.25/hour plus the following: $0.01/search statement, $0.01/citation, $0.01/carriage return, $0.06 to $0.12/100 disk accesses, and $0.08 to $0.12/1000 character charges), and DIALOG ($20 to $35/hour). Covers 1975 to the present. Produced by the National Library of Medicine, address is listed above.

International Pharmaceutical Abstracts, provides online coverage to its print counterpart under the same name, available through BRS ($26.50 to $45.50/hour plus $0.05/citation), BRS Colleague ($17 to $32/hour), DIALOG ($40 to $55/hour), and DIALOG Knowledge Index ($24/hour). Covers 1970 to the present. Produced by American Society of Hospital Pharmacists, 4630 Montgomery Avenue, Bethesda, MD 20814. (301) 657-3000.

MEDLINE, online edition of *Index Medicus*, *Index to Dental Literature*, and *International Nursing Index*, in addition to 600 journals not covered in the print indexes, available through BRS ($19 to $39/hour plus $0.05/citation), BRS Colleague ($17 to 32/hour), DIALOG ($20 to $35/hour), DIALOG Knowledge Index ($24/hour), and NLM (same price for HEALTHLINE listed above). Covers 1966 to the present. Produced by the National Library of medicine; the address is listed above. As a price comparison of the other data bases described in this section reveals, MEDLINE is the most economical data base for retrospective searching. Other advantages (49, p 70) include the depth of indexing and the broad coverage of subjects; allied health and basic life sciences are well covered in addition to medicine. MEDLINE is also noted for its high degree of indexing consistency (50). A disadvantage is the limited foreign coverage when compared to EMBASE.

PREMED, provides rapid access to the most recent 3 to 4 months of 108 clinical journals prior to being entered in the MEDLINE file, both produced and available only through BRS ($16 to $35/hour plus $0.10/citation) and BRS Colleague ($17 to $32/hour). Address is listed above.

SCISEARCH, a multidisciplinary science and technology and data base, online equivalent to *Science Citation Index*, available through DIALOG ($50 to $165/hour—the higher price is for nonsubscribers of the print counterpart). Covers 1974 to the present. The advantages (51) are as follows: the most extensive data base coverage for the pure and applied science, the citation indexing that allows for searching of papers that have cited a particular earlier paper, and currency. Comparisons of other data bases (52) have confirmed that SCISEARCH provides the most up-to-date online retrieval. The drawback is that subject searching is limited to title words only; there are no abstracts to search and also no controlled vocabulary of subject headings.

Data Base	No. of Citations/Publication Year					
	1985	1984	1983	1982	1981	1980
BIOSIS	0	129	162	206	312	168
CA Search	0	6	5	11	7	14
Comprehensive Core	1	48	35	3	12	0
EMBASE	0	166	426	455	470	474
HEALTHLINE	0	207	397	395	366	336
International Pharmaceutical Abstracts	0	3	3	15	5	2
MEDLINE	0	377	632	629	577	488
PREMED	0	9	0	0	0	0
SCISEARCH	0	96	138	130	175	132

At the bottom of the previous page are the results of a search performed on the above data bases on January 7, 1985 to give an indication of the amount of information available directly related to hospital-acquired infections. The following phrases were entered with the Boolean operator "or": nosocomial, cross-infection, hospital infection(s), hospital-acquired infection(s), and infection control.

DOCUMENT DELIVERY

After identifying relevant literature, there are two basic options to select for obtaining the materials. The first is to utilize the Regional Medical Library (RML) Network defined by the National Library of Medicine, and the second is to use the various commercial document delivery suppliers, such as Information on Demand, University Microfilms International, and the Institute for Scientific Information's The Genuine Article.

During the period between the end of September, 1982 and January, 1983, the RML Network was reconfigured from 11 to seven regions, although the basic principles for routing interlibrary loan requests remained the same (53). Libraries remain categorized in a hierarchical arrangement starting with the basic units (hospital libraries), to resource libraries (medical school libraries), to a regional medical library designated for each region. Requests for materials not owned at the basic units within a region are routed to the resource libraries and, if necessary, to the RML. Materials may also be requested from other regions if unavailable in the requestor's region. The final source to be used ultimately is the National Library of Medicine. The basic goal of the RML program is to provide health professionals, wherever located, with improved access to biomedical information. Individual libraries participating in the RML program are free to establish their own loan policies, but a $6.00/item ceiling on any loan is the national standard. Medical libraries all have their individual procedures for accepting requests for materials and need to be contacted to obtain information on their document delivery services. For additional information on the nearest library, contact the appropriate RML from the list below.

Region 1 RML: New York Academy of Medicine, 2 E 103rd Street, New York, NY 10029. (212) 876-8200. States served: CT, DE, MA, ME, NH, NJ, NY, PA, RI, VT, and Puerto Rico.

Region 2 RML: University of Maryland Health Sciences Library, 111 S Greene Street, Baltimore, MD 21201. (301) 528-7546. States served: AL, FL, GA, MD, MS, NC, SC, TN, VA, WV, and the District of Columbia.

Region 3 RML: University of Illinois at Chicago, Library of the Health Sciences, 1750 W Polk Street, Chicago, IL 60612. (312) 996-8974. States served: IA, IL, IN, KY, MI, MN, ND, OH, SD, WI.

Region 4 RML: University of Nebraska, Leon S McGoogan Library of Medicine, University of Nebraska Medical Center, 42nd Street and Dewey Avenue, Omaha, NE 68105. (402) 541-4006. States served: CO, KS, MO, NE, UT, WY.

Region 5 RML: University of Texas, Health Science Center at Dallas, 5323 Harry Hines Blvd., Dallas, TX 75235. (214) 688-2626. States served: AR, LA, NM, OK, TX.

Region 6 RML: University of Washington, Health Sciences Library, Seattle, WA 98105. (206) 543-5530. States served: AK, ID, MT, OR, WA.

Region 7 RML: UCLA Biomedical Library, Los Angeles, CA 90024. (213) 825-5781. States served: AZ, CA, HI, NV.

The National Library of Medicine's National Biomedical Serials Holdings Database (SERHOLD) (54) was developed in January, 1982, to support automated routing of interlibrary loan requests and to produce a variety of union lists for use in the RML Network. There are presently holdings and location data for over 1000 biomedical libraries. The interlibrary routing system (DOCLINE) is presently under development and will serve as the automated interface between borrowers and lenders in the RML Network and the National Library of Medicine.

The second option for obtaining materials is through the various commercial document delivery suppliers. Descriptions of the major suppliers can be found in *Document Retrieval: Sources and Services* (San Francisco, the Information Store). The primary advantage of the commercial suppliers is quicker turnaround time for processing requests, but the charges may be substantially higher than will be found in the RML Network.

Examples of the commercial suppliers are listed below:

Information on Demand, PO Box 9550, Berkeley, CA 94709. (800) 227-0750 or (415) 841-1145. Advertised as the world's largest commercial document delivery service. Prices range from $7.00 to $14.00/item with additional charges for rush service.

The Genuine Article (formerly OATS), Institute for Scientific Information, 3501 Market Street, Philadelphia, PA 19104. (800) 532-1851. Provides all articles listed in *Current Contents*. Prices begin at $7.50/item plus $2.00 for every additional 10 pages.

University Microfilms International, 300 N Zeeb Road, Ann Arbor, MI 48106. (800) 732-0616 or (313) 761-4700 (collect) in Michigan, Alaska, and Hawaii. Provides copies from more than 7500 of the most frequently indexed and requested periodicals. Provides multidisciplinary coverage; consequently, only the major medical journals are available. One of the most economical suppliers with prices ranging from $4.00 to $8.00/item depending on volume of use. Articles are shipped within 48 hours of receipt with same-day shipment available for an additional charge.

References

1. Chen C: *Health Sciences Information Sources.* Cambridge, MIT Press, 1981.
2. Morton LT (ed): *Use of the Medical Literature,* ed 2. London, Butterworth, 1977.
3. Allyn R: A library for internists. *Ann Intern Med* 96:385–401, 1982.
4. Brandon AN, Hill DR, Gustave L, Levy JW: Selected list of books and journals for the small medical library. *Bull Med Libr Assoc* 73:176–205, 1985.
5. Wender RW, Parrish JW, Holman KG, Thompson CM, Callard JC: primary physician's book list. *Postgrad Med* 71:74–83, 1982.
6. Dewey M: *Dewey Decimal Classification and Relative Index.* Albany, Forest Press, 1979.
7. *Library of Congress Subject Headings,* ed 9. Washington, DC, Library of Congress, 1980.
8. *Library of Congress Classification: Medicine,* ed 4. Washington, DC, Library of Congress, 1980.
9. *Library of Congress Classification Schedule: A Cumulation of Additions and Changes through 1983.* Detroit, Gale, 1984.
10. *Medical Subject Headings: Annotated Alphabetic List, 1985.* Bethesda, MD, National Library of Medicine, 1984.
11. *National Library of Medicine Classification: A Scheme for the Shelf Arrangement of Books in the Field of Medicine and its Related Sciences,* ed 4. Bethesda, MD, National Library of Medicine, 1978.
12. Roepe D (reviewer), Soule BM (ed): *The APIC Curriculum for Infection Control Practice,* book review. *Infect Control* 5:407–408, 1984.
13. Wolf ZM, Topol EG, Pizzi ER, Creed J (reviewer), Barrett-Conner E: *Epidemiology for the Infection Control Nurse,* book review. *Top Clin Nurs* 1:85–87, 1979.
14. Troyer SR (reviewer), Fuchs PC: *Epidemiology of Hospital-Associated Infections,* book review. *Am J Infect Control* 9:56–57, 1981.
15. Crow S (reviewer), Craig CP: *Fundamentals of Infection Control: An In-service Orientation Program,* book review. *Infect Control* 5:455, 1984.
16. Valdon C (reviewer), Warnock DW: *Fungal Infection in the Compromised Patient,* book review. *Am J Infect Control* 12:66–67, 1984.
17. Conti MT (reviewer), Groschel D: *Hospital-Associated Infections in the General Hospital Population and Specific Measures of Control,* book review. *Am J Infect Control* 10:41–42, 1982.
18. Hadley K (reviewer), Groschel D: *Hospital-Associated Infections in the General Hospital Population and Specific Measures of Control,* book review. *Infect Control* 1:221, 1980.
19. Campbell A (reviewer), Castle M: *Hospital Infection Control: Principles and Practice,* book review. *Am J Infect Control* 9:130–131, 1981.
20. DeGroot-Kosolcharoen J (reviewer), Bennet JV, Brachman PS: *Hospital Infections,* book review. *Am J Infect Control* 9:22, 1981.
21. Bolyard E (reviewer), Arking LN, McArthur BJ: *Infection Control,* book review. *Infect Control* 2:447–448, 1981.
22. Krause SL (reviewer), Arking LN, McArthur BJ: *Infection Control,* book review. *Am J Infect Control* 9:98, 1981.
23. Crow S (reviewer), Yarbrough M: *Infection Control: An Integrated Approach,* book review. *Infect Control* 5:407, 1984.
24. Crow S (reviewer), Roderick MA: *Infection Control in Critical Care,* book review. *Infect Control* 4:237–238, 1983.
25. Marositz C (reviewer), Roderick MA: *Infection Control in Critical Care,* book review. *Am J Infect Control* 12:66–67, 1984.
26. Crow S (reviewer), Smith PW: *Infection Control in Long-Term Care Facilities,* book review. *Infect Control* 5:500, 1984.
27. Goldmann DA (reviewer): *Infection Control in the Hospital,* book review. *Infect Control* 2:114–116, 1980.
28. DeGroot-Kosolcharoen J (reviewer), McK Watts J: *Infections in Surgery, Basic and Clinical Aspects,* book review. *Am J Infect Control* 10:119, 1982.
29. Matsumiya S (reviewer), Dixon RE: *Nosocomial Infections,* book review. *Am J Infect Control* 9:131–132, 1981.
30. Blowers R (reviewer), Fahlberg WF, Groschel D (eds): *Occurrence, Diagnosis, and Sources of Hospital Associated Infections,* book review. *J Clin Pathol* 32:637, 1979.
31. Mattson KL (reviewer), Fahlberg WF, Groschel D (eds): *Occurrence, Diagnosis, and Sources of Hos-*

pital Associated Infections, book review. *Am J Infect Control* 9:132, 1981.

32. Olson M (reviewer), Alexander JW: *Surgical Infections,* book review. *Am J Infect Control* 9:56, 1981.

33. Dalcourt JL, Braude RM: Determination of overlap in coverage of *Excerpta Medica* and *Index Medicus* through SERLINE. *Bull Med Lib Assoc* 64:324–325.

34. Humphrey SM: *Index Medicus* and the *Science Citation Index. Br Med J* 286:892–893, 1983.

35. Poyer RJ: Journal article overlap among *Index Medicus, Science Citation Index, Biological Abstracts,* and *Chemical Abstracts. Bull Med Libr Assoc* 72:353–357.

36. Wilkinson D: A comparison of drug literature coverage by *Index Medicus* and *Drug Literature Index. Bull Med Libr Assoc* 61:431–2.

37. La Rocco A: *Excerpta Medica* abstracting journals: a case study of costs to medical school libraries. *Bull Med Libr Assoc* 65:255–262, 1977.

38. Sutherland FM: Indexes, abstracts, bibliographies and reviews. In Morton LT (ed): *Use of the Medical Literature.* London, Butterworth, 1977, p 55.

39. Jackson MF: The *Index Medicus:* why it works and when it doesn't. *Bull Med Libr Assoc* 54:325–328, 1966.

40. Welch J: Are you making the most of *Index Medicus. Br Med J* 285:1105–6, 1982.

41. Committed selection: *Abridged Index Medicus,* editorial. *N Engl J Med* 282:220–221, 1970.

42. Garfield E: *Citation Indexing: Its Theory and Application in Science, Technology, and Humanities.* New York, John Wiley & Sons, 1979.

43. Chen C: *Online Bibliographic Searching: A Learning Manual.* New York, Neal-Schuman, 1981, pp 5–6.

44. Egeland J, Foreman G: Reference services: searching and search techniques. In Darling L, Bishop D, Colaianni LA (eds): *Handbook of Medical Library Practice,* ed 4. Chicago, Medical Library Association, 1982, pp 189–190.

45. Burroughs S, Kyle S: Searching the MEDLARS files on NLM and BRS: a comparative study. *Bull Med Libr Assoc* 67:15–24, 1979.

46. Feinglos SJ: MEDLINE at BRS, DIALOG, and NLM: is there a choice? *Bull Med Libr Assoc* 71:6–12, 1983.

47. Baker CA: COLLEAGUE: a comprehensive online medical library for the end user. *Med Ref Serv Q* 3:13–26, 1984.

48. Ojala M: Knowledge index: a review. *Online* 7:31–34, 1983.

49. Boorkman JA: Online bibliographic databases. In Boorkman JA, Roper FW: *Introduction to Reference Sources in the Health Sciences.* Chicago, Medical Library Association, 1984, pp 77–78.

50. Funk ME: Indexing consistency in MEDLINE. *Bull Med Libr Assoc* 71:176–183.

51. Savage GS: SCISEARCH on DIALOG. *Database* 1:50–67, 1978.

52. Snow B: Online database coverage of pharmaceutical journals. *Database* 7:12–26.

53. Arenales D: New Regional Medical Library Configuration Announced. *NLM News* 38:1–3, 1983.

54. Fishel MR: National Biomedical Serials Holdings Database (SERHOLD). *NLM News* 39:1–4, 1984.

Index

Isopropyl alcohol, 258, 262
  cost, 263
  inactivation of
    HTLV-III, 265
    lymphadenopathy-associated virus, 265
  microbiocidal activity, 264
  properties, 263
  use of dilution, 263
  virucidal activity, 264
IV (*see* entries beginning with Intravenous)

Japanese encephalitis vaccine, 554
J-5 antisera, 328, 330
JK diphtheroids, 250
  colonization, 217
  environmental source, 206–207
  human reservoir, 207, 217
Joint Commission on Accreditation of Hospitals, 234, 243
Joint prostheses (*see also* Implantable joints)
  mechanical loosening, 388–389
  radiologic evaluation, 389
  types of, 385–386
Joint replacement
  incidence, 385
  morbidity, 385
Journal of Hospital Infection, 604
Justice, principle of, 49–50

Keratitis, 440, 441, 445, 447
  outcome, 450
Kirby-Bauer disk diffusion test, 208, 212
Klebsiella, 285
  antibiotic resistance patterns, 218–219
  bacteremia, 287, 288, 290, 302–303, 499, 543
  catheter-related sepsis, 311
  colonization, 217
    of newborn, 486
  environmental source, 207
  epidemics caused by, 95, 96
  in food, 564
  hemodialysis-associated infection, 398
  human reservoir, 207, 217
  in median sternotomy infections, 365
  as nosocomial pathogen, 290
  percentage distribution by site of infection, 73
  pneumonia, 322–323
    treating, 327
Klebsiella pneumoniae
  bacteremia, 288
  burn wound infection, 367
  contamination of arterial pressure fluids, 305
  gastroenteritis, 419
    in developing areas, 428
  necrotizing enterocolitis, 408
  prosthetic joint infections, 387
  pseudobacteremia, 223
  wound infections, 346
Knee prostheses, 386
Killetschka, Jacob, 4

Laboratory-acquired infection, 192
β-Lactamase, 238
  for pneumonia, 327–328
  susceptibility testing, 209
Lactobacilli, colonization of newborn, 485–486

Laminar air flow, 561–562
  for burn treatment, 373
  effectiveness in reducing infection, 563
  in joint replacement, 390, 392–393
  in operating room, 349
Lancefield precipitin procedure, 212
Lassa virus, 17, 103
Latex agglutination procedures, 212
Law
  civil, 26
  criminal, 26
  principles of, 27
  procedural issues, 27–28
Law suit, 26
Lazaretto(s), 3
Lectins, in adherence to airway mucosa, 325
Legal cases
  Anderson v. Lutheran Deaconess Hospital, 27
  Baines v. Baker, 29
  Barrella v. Richmond Memorial Hospital, 45
  *Baxter County Newspapers, Inc. v. Medical Staff of
    Baxter General Hospital*, 36
  Belle Bonfils Memorial Blood Bank v. Hansen, 45
  Best v. Stapp, 27
  Board v. Bisshopp, 29
  Booker v. Duke Medical Center, 45
  Brannan v. Lankenau Hospital, 30–31
  Broughton v. Cutter Laboratories, 45
  Carroll v. St. Luke's Hospital of Newburgh, 36
  City of Edmond v. Parr, 26
  Cocco v. Maryland Commission Medical Discipline, 38
  Cornfeldt v. Tongen, 45
  Crowe v. John W. Harton Memorial Hospital, 31
  Cummings v. Fondak, 46
  DeBattista v. Argonaut-Southwest Insurance Co., 45
  Derrick v. Ontario Community Hospital, 30
  Doss v. United States, 31
  Drexel v. Union Prescription Centers, Inc., 31
  Durden v. American Hospital Supply Corporation, 45
  Ellis v. International Platex, Inc., 47
  Farley v. County of Nassau, 36
  Feinstein v. Massachusetts General Hospital, 45
  Fisher v. Sibley Memorial Hospital, 45
  French Drug Company, Inc. v. Jones, 31
  Gadd v. News-Press Publishing Co., 36–38
  Gammill v. United States, 30, 45
  Garza v. Keillor, 31
  Gill v. Hartford Accident Indemnity Co., 30
  Gilmore v. St. Anthony Hospital, 45
  Good Samaritan Hospital Association v. Simon, 38
  Haas v. Tegtmeier, 30
  Kathleen K. v. Robert B., 47
  Kehm v. Proctor and Gamble Manufacturing, 47
  Kernall v. United States, 31
  Killeen, v. Reinhardt, 31
  King v. Retz, 31
  LaRocca v. Dalsheim, 45
  Leary v. Rupp, 31
  LeFever v. American Red Cross, 46
  Lennon v. United States, 31
  Lipari v. Sears, Roebuck & Co., 30
  Livingston v. Gribetz, 47
  Matter of DeMarco, 45
  McCormack v. Lindberg, 46
  McLean v. United States, 31–32